Core Radiology

A Visual Approach to Diagnostic Imaging

Core Radiology

A Visual Approach to Diagnostic Imaging

Jacob Mandell

Radiology Residency, Class of 2013,
Brigham and Women's Hospital, Boston, MA, USA

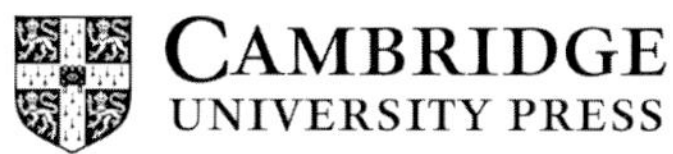

CAMBRIDGE
UNIVERSITY PRESS

University Printing House, Cambridge CB2 8BS, United Kingdom

One Liberty Plaza, 20th Floor, New York, NY 10006, USA

477 Williamstown Road, Port Melbourne, VIC 3207, Australia

314–321, 3rd Floor, Plot 3, Splendor Forum, Jasola District Centre, New Delhi – 110025, India

79 Anson Road, #06–04/06, Singapore 079906

Cambridge University Press is part of the University of Cambridge.

It furthers the University's mission by disseminating knowledge in he pursuit of education, learning and research at the highest international levels of excellence.

www.cambridge.org
Information on this title: www.cambridge.org/9781107679689

First published 2013
10th printing 2021

Printed in Singapore by Markono Print Media Pte Ltd

A catalogue record for this publication is available from the British Library

ISBN 978-1-107-67968-9 Paperback

Additional resources for this publication at www.cambridge.org/delan

For my wife Julie and our sons Baylor and Cameron.

You are the most amazing family I can ask for.

CONTENTS

ACKNOWLEDGEMENTS

A thousand thanks to my parents Karen and Fred, Julie's parents May and Henry, and my sisters Hinda and Becky. Your support and love is essential for everything we do.

This book would not have been possible without the unwavering support of Dr. Barbara Weissman, the Brigham and Women's Radiology Residency program director and my unofficial mentor. Thank you for actually saying "that's a great idea!" when I told you about the book a couple months after you met me, and for not acting too surprised when I actually finished it three years later.

This book would be a pale shadow of its current form without the invaluable contributions from each faculty and resident contributor, listed individually on the following pages. Thank you so much for investing so many hours in this project.

Thanks to Dr. Amir Zamani for kindly allowing me to use images from your teaching files and to Dr. Peter Doubilet and Dr. Steven Seltzer for your early and very helpful advice.

CONTRIBUTORS

Juan Carlos Baez, MD
Resident in Radiology,
Brigham and Women's Hospital

Beryl R. Benacerraf, MD
Clinical Professor of Radiology and
Obstetrics and Gynecology,
Harvard Medical School

Scott Britz-Cunningham, MD, PhD
Staff Radiologist, Department of Nuclear Medicine,
Brigham and Women's Hospital
Assistant Professor of Radiology,
Harvard Medical School

Paul M. Bunch, MD
Resident in Radiology,
Brigham and Women's Hospital

Michael J. Callahan, MD
Director, Computed Tomography
Division Chief, Abdominal Imaging
Department of Radiology,
Boston Children's Hospital
Assistant Professor of Radiology,
Harvard Medical School

Jeffrey Forris Beecham Chick, MD
Resident in Radiology,
Brigham and Women's Hospital

Sona A. Chikarmane, MD
Resident in Radiology,
Brigham and Women's Hospital

Mary Elizabeth Cunnane, MD
Staff Radiologist,
Massachusetts Eye and Ear Infirmary
Instructor of Radiology,
Harvard Medical School

Pamela Deaver Ketwaroo, MD
Resident in Radiology,
Brigham and Women's Hospital

Christine M. Denison, MD
Staff Radiologist, Division of Breast Imaging,
Brigham and Women's Hospital
Assistant Professor of Radiology,
Harvard Medical School

Naman S. Desai, MD
Resident in Radiology,
Brigham and Women's Hospital

Alexandra Fairchild, MD
Resident in Radiology,
Brigham and Women's Hospital

Ritu R. Gill, MD, MPH
Staff Radiologist, Division of Thoracic Imaging,
Brigham and Women's Hospital
Assistant Professor of Radiology,
Harvard Medical School

Alisa Suzuki Han, MD
Staff Radiologist, Division of Angiography and
Interventional Radiology,
Brigham and Women's Hospital
Instructor of Radiology,
Harvard Medical School

Michael Hanley, MD
Staff Radiologist,
Division of Thoraco-Abdominal Imaging,
University of Virginia Health System
Assistant Professor of Radiology,
University of Virginia School of Medicine

Timothy P. Killoran, MD
Staff Radiologist, Division of Angiography and
Interventional Radiology,
Brigham and Women's Hospital
Instructor of Radiology,
Harvard Medical School

Meaghan M. Mackesy, MD
Resident in Radiology,
Brigham and Women's Hospital

Jonathan Opraseuth, MD
Resident in Radiology,
Brigham and Women's Hospital

Sanjay Prabhu, MBBS, DCH, MRCPCH, FRCR
Director, Radiology Advanced Image Analysis Lab,
Staff Radiologist, Boston Children's Hospital
Instructor in Radiology,
Harvard Medical School

Sughra Raza, MD
Associate Director of Breast Imaging,
Brigham and Women's Hospital
Associate Professor of Radiology,
Harvard Medical School

Julie A. Ritner, MD
Staff Radiologist, Divisions of Ultrasound and Breast Imaging, Brigham and Women's Hospital
Instructor in Radiology,
Harvard Medical School

Justin R. Routhier, MD
Resident in Radiology,
Brigham and Women's Hospital

Ari Sacks, MD
Resident in Radiology,
Brigham and Women's Hospital

Cheryl A. Sadow, MD
Staff Radiologist, Division of Abdominal Imaging and Intervention, Brigham and Women's Hospital
Assistant Professor of Radiology,
Harvard Medical School

Asha Sarma, MD
Resident in Radiology,
Brigham and Women's Hospital

Nehal Shah, MD
Staff Radiologist, Division of Musculoskeletal Imaging and Intervention,
Brigham and Women's Hospital
Instructor in Radiology,
Harvard Medical School

Jeffrey Y. Shyu, MD
Resident in Radiology,
Brigham and Women's Hospital

Kirstin M. Small, MD
Staff Radiologist, Division of Musculoskeletal Imaging and Intervention,
Brigham and Women's Hospital
Instructor in Radiology,
Harvard Medical School

Stacy E. Smith, MD
Section Head and Barbara N. Weissman Distinguished Chair of Musculoskeletal Imaging and Intervention
Associate Director, Radiology Residency Program,
Brigham and Women's Hospital
Assistant Professor of Radiology,
Harvard Medical School

Darryl B. Sneag, MD
Resident in Radiology,
Brigham and Women's Hospital

Shreya Sood, MD
Resident in Radiology,
Brigham and Women's Hospital

Michael Steigner, MD
Staff Radiologist, Division of Non-invasive Cardiovascular Imaging,
Brigham and Women's Hospital
Instructor in Radiology,
Harvard Medical School

Barbara N. Weissman, MD
Vice Chair, Department of Radiology,
Section Head Emeritus, Musculoskeletal Imaging
Director, Radiology Residency Program
Brigham and Women's Hospital
Professor of Radiology,
Harvard Medical School

Ged Wieschhoff, MD
Resident in Radiology,
Brigham and Women's Hospital

Jeremy R. Wortman, MD
Resident in Radiology,
Brigham and Women's Hospital

Gregory L. Wrubel, MD
Clinical Fellow in Diagnostic Neuroradiology,
Brigham and Women's Hospital

1 Thoracic Imaging

Contents

ANATOMY

Lobar and segmental anatomy

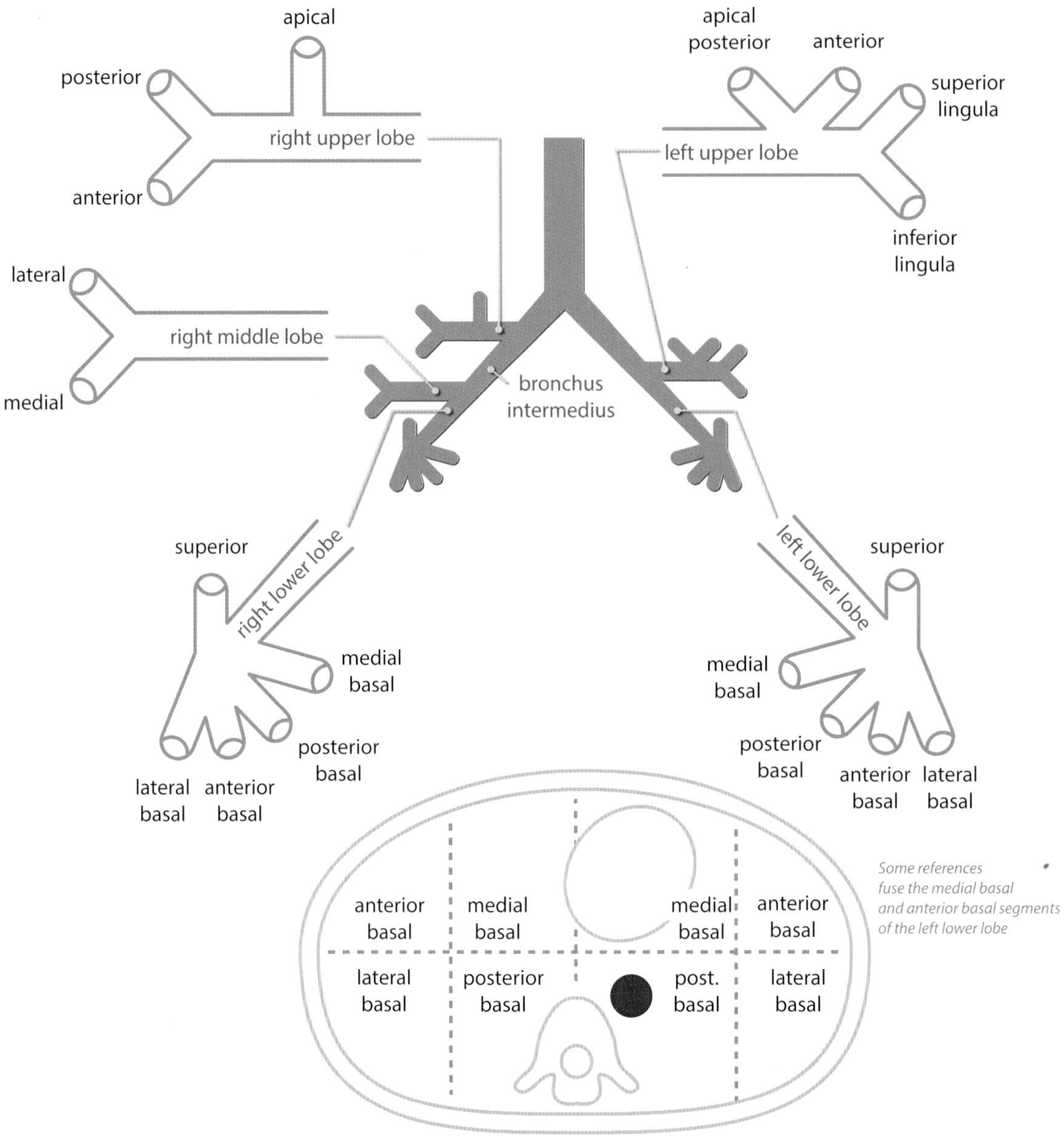

Interlobar fissures

- The minor fissure separates the right upper lobe (RUL) from the right middle lobe (RML) and is seen on both the frontal and lateral views as a fine horizontal line.
- The major (oblique) fissures are seen only on the lateral radiograph as oblique lines.
  On the right, the major fissure separates the RUL and RML from the right lower lobe.
  On the left, the major fissure separates the left upper lobe from the left lower lobe.
- The azygos fissure is an accessory fissure present in less than 1% of patients, seen in the presence of an azygos lobe. An azygos lobe is an anatomic variant where the right upper lobe apical or posterior segments are encased in their own parietal and visceral pleura.

Overview of atelectasis

- Atelectasis is loss of lung volume due to decreased aeration. Atelectasis is synonymous with collapse.
- Direct signs of atelectasis are from lobar volume loss and include:

Displacement of the fissures.	Vascular crowding.

- Indirect signs of atelectasis are due to the effect of volume loss on adjacent structures and include:

Elevation of the diaphragm.	Overinflation of adjacent or contralateral lobes.
Rib crowding on the side with volume loss.	Hilar displacement.
Mediastinal shift to the side with volume loss.	

- Air bronchograms are *not* seen in atelectasis when the cause of the atelectasis is central bronchial obstruction, but air bronchograms can be seen in subsegmental atelectasis. Subsegmental atelectasis is caused by obstruction of small peripheral bronchi, usually by secretions.
- Subsegmental atelectasis and mild fever are both commonly encountered in postsurgical patients, although it has been proposed that there is no causative relationship between atelectasis and postoperative fever.

Mechanisms of atelectasis

- **Obstructive** atelectasis occurs when alveolar gas is absorbed by blood circulating through alveolar capillaries but is not replaced by inspired air due to bronchial obstruction.

  Obstructive atelectasis can cause lobar atelectasis, which is complete collapse of a lobe, discussed on the following page.

  Obstructive atelectasis occurs more quickly when the patient is breathing supplemental oxygen since oxygen is absorbed from the alveoli more rapidly than nitrogen.

  In general, obstructive atelectasis is associated with volume loss. In critically ill ICU patients, however, there may be rapid transudation of fluid into the obstructed alveoli, causing superimposed consolidation.

  In children, airway obstruction is most often due to an aspirated foreign object. In contrast to adults, the affected side becomes hyperexpanded in children due to a ball-valve effect.

  Subsegmental atelectasis is a subtype of obstructive atelectasis commonly seen after surgery or general illness, due to mucus obstruction of the small airways.
- **Relaxation** (passive) atelectasis is caused by relaxation of lung adjacent to an intrathoracic lesion causing mass effect, such as a pleural effusion, pneumothorax, or pulmonary mass.
- **Adhesive** atelectasis is due to surfactant deficiency.

  Adhesive atelectasis is seen most commonly in neonatal respiratory distress syndrome, but can also be seen in acute respiratory distress syndrome (ARDS).
- **Cicatricial** atelectasis is volume loss from architectural distortion of lung parenchyma by fibrosis.

Lobar atelectasis

- Lobar atelectasis is usually caused by central bronchial obstruction (obstructive atelectasis), which may be secondary to mucus plugging or an obstructing neoplasm.

  If the lobar atelectasis occurs acutely, mucus plugging is the most likely cause.

  If lobar atelectasis is seen in an outpatient, an obstructing central tumor must be ruled out.
- Lobar atelectasis, or collapse of an entire lobe, has characteristic appearances depending on which of the five lobes is collapsed.

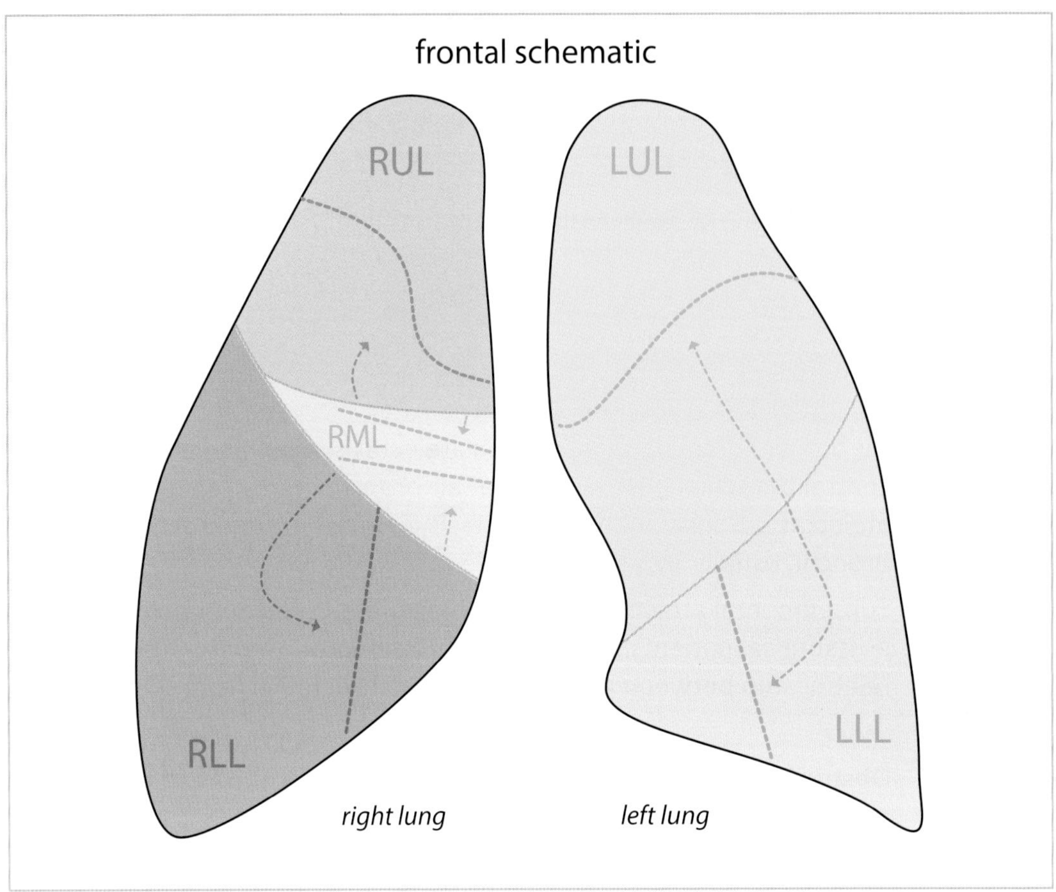

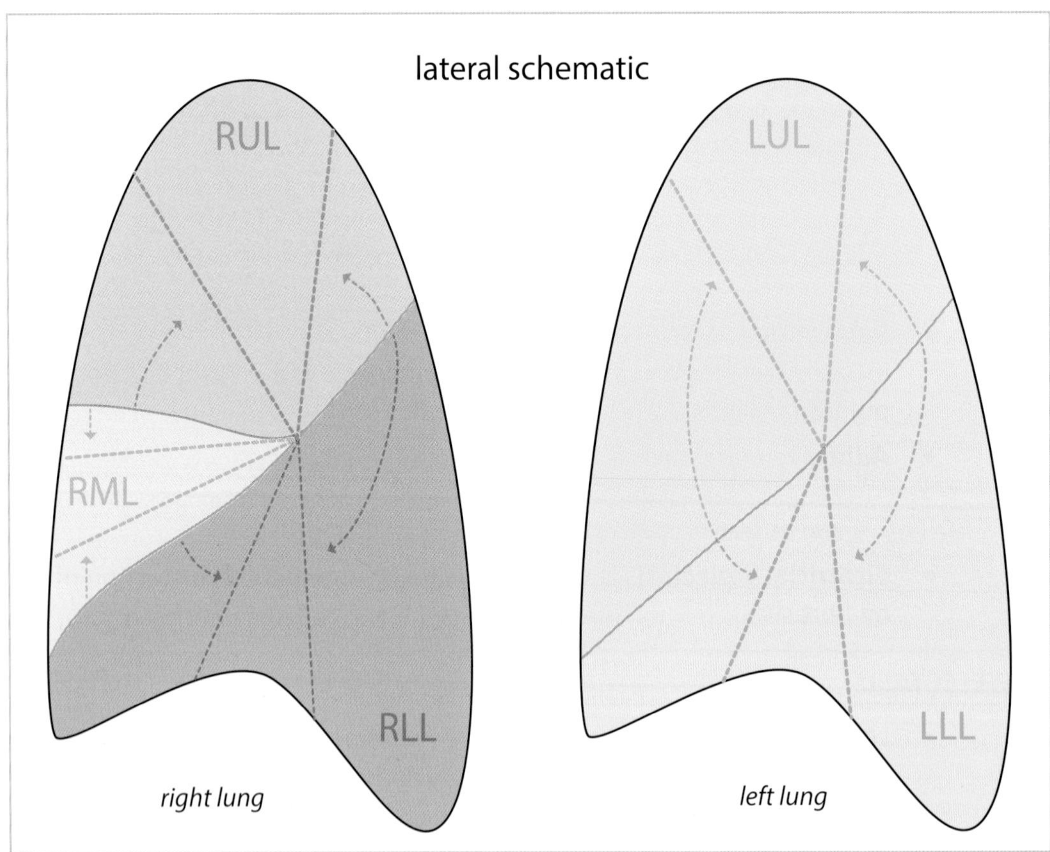

- Each of the five lobes tends to collapse in a predictable direction, as shown above.

Left upper lobe atelectasis

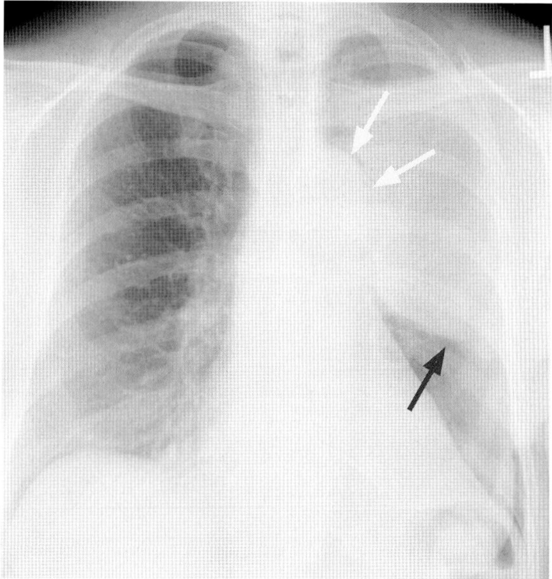

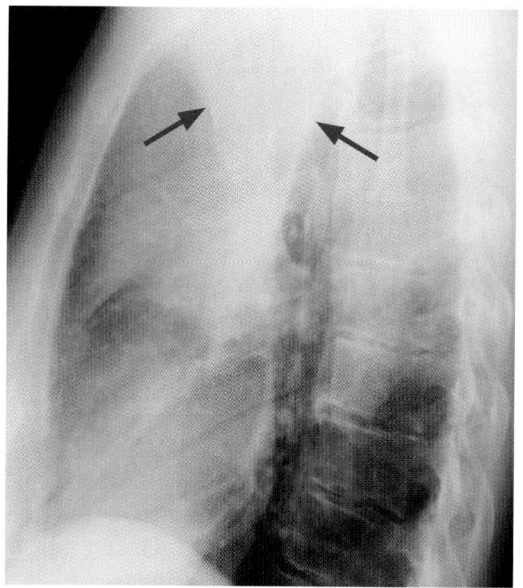

Left upper lobe collapse and *luftsichel* sign: Frontal radiograph (left image) shows a veil-like left upper lung opacity representing the collapsed left upper lobe (red arrow). A crescent of air lateral to the aortic arch is the *luftsichel* (yellow arrows). The lateral view (right image) shows the anterior wedge-shaped collapsed left upper lobe (red arrows). *Case courtesy Ritu R. Gill, MD, MPH, Brigham and Women's Hospital.*

- The *luftsichel* (*air-sickle* in German) sign of left upper lobe collapse is a crescent of air seen on the frontal radiograph, which represents the interface between the aorta and the hyperexpanded superior segment of the left lower lobe.
- It is important to recognize left upper lobe collapse and not mistake the left lung opacity for pneumonia, since a mass obstructing the airway may be the cause of the lobar atelectasis.

Right upper lobe atelectasis

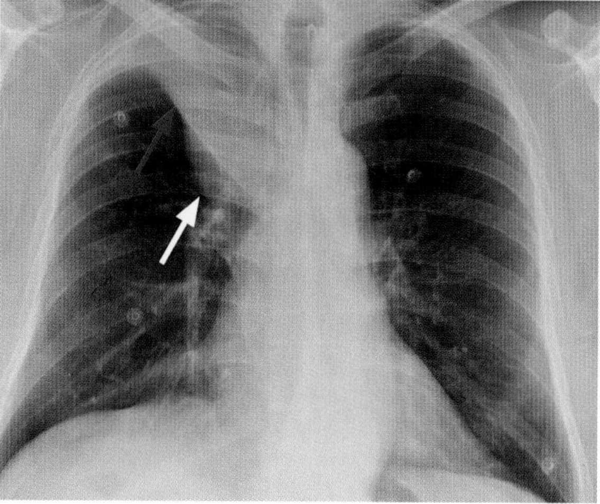

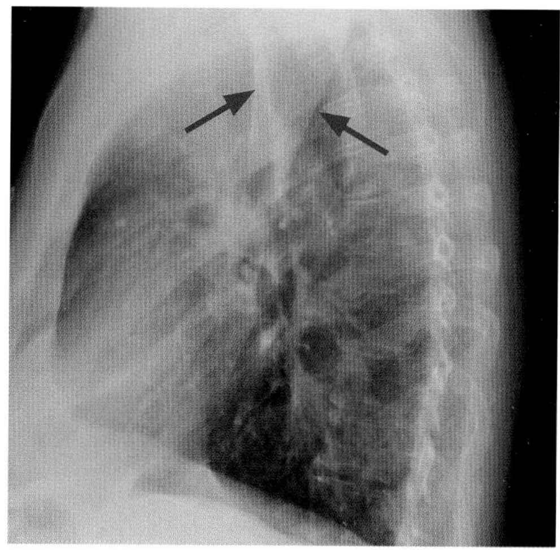

Right upper lobe collapse and *Golden's S* sign: Frontal radiograph (left image) shows a right upper lobe opacity with superior displacement of the minor fissure (red arrow) and a convex mass (yellow arrow). Lateral radiograph (right image) shows the wedge-shaped collapsed RUL projecting superiorly (red arrows).

- *The reverse S sign of Golden* is seen in right upper lobe collapse caused by an obstructing mass. The central convex margins of the mass form a reverse S. Although the sign describes a *reverse* S, it is also commonly known as *Golden's S* sign. Similar to left upper lobe collapse, a right upper lobe collapse should raise concern for an underlying malignancy, especially with a Golden's S sign present.
- The juxtaphrenic peak sign is a peridiaphragmatic triangular opacity caused by diaphragmatic traction from an inferior accessory fissure or an inferior pulmonary ligament.

Left lower lobe atelectasis

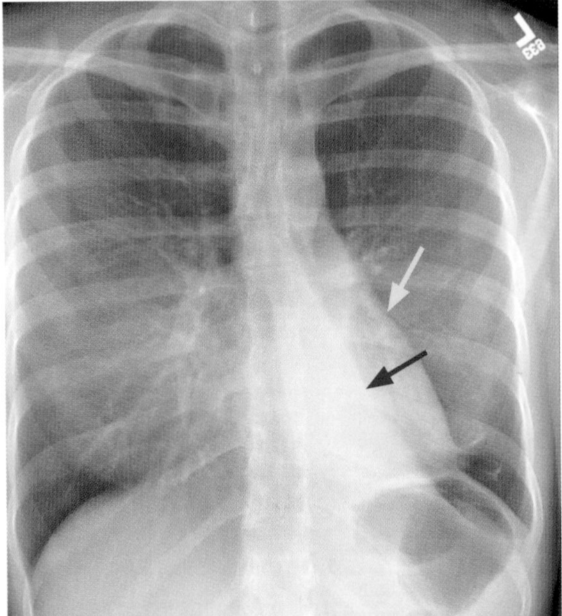

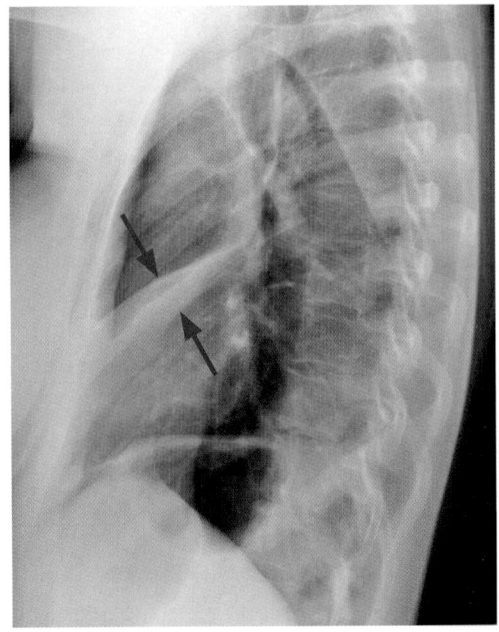

Left lower lobe collapse: Frontal and lateral radiographs demonstrate a triangular retrocardiac opacity representing the collapsed left lower lobe (red arrows). There is loss of concavity of the left heart border (the *flat waist* sign; yellow arrow).

Case courtesy Ritu R. Gill, MD, MPH, Brigham and Women's Hospital.

- In left lower lobe collapse, the heart slightly rotates and the left hilum is pulled down.
- The *flat waist* sign describes the flattening of the left heart border as a result of downward shift of hilar structures and resultant cardiac rotation.

Right lower lobe atelectasis

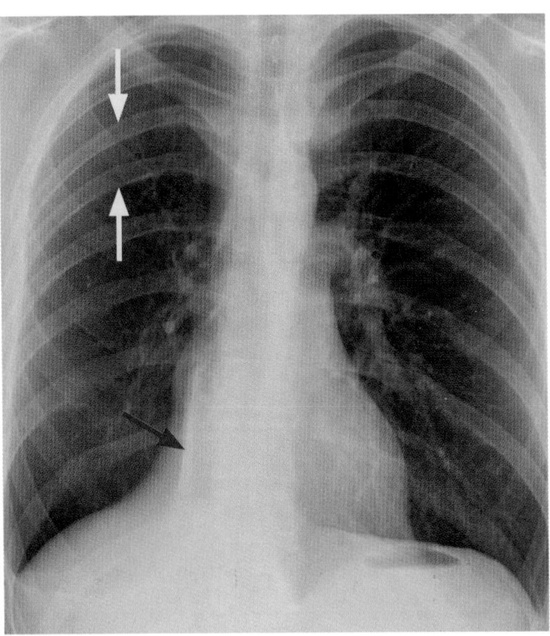

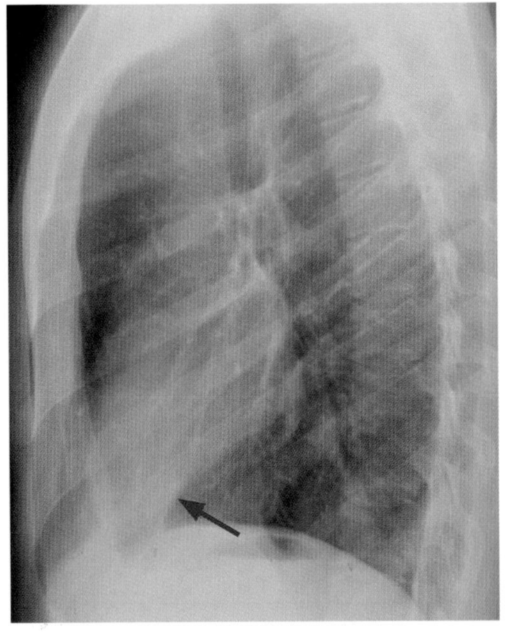

Right lower lobe collapse: Frontal radiograph shows an abnormal vertically oriented interface medial to the right heart border (red arrow), which corresponds to a wedge-shaped opacity projecting over the heart on the lateral view (red arrow) and represents the collapsed right lower lobe. On the frontal radiograph, there is subtle crowding of the ribs (yellow arrows) in the right hemithorax due to volume loss.

- Right lower lobe atelectasis is the mirror-image of left lower lobe atelectasis.
- The collapsed lower lobe appears as a wedge-shaped retrocardiac opacity.

Right middle lobe atelectasis

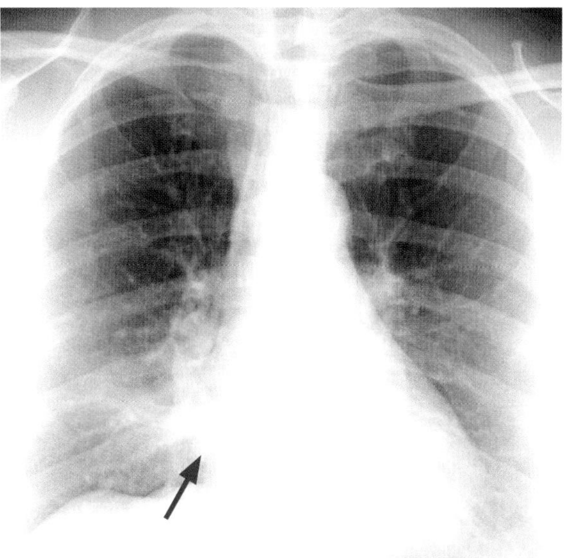

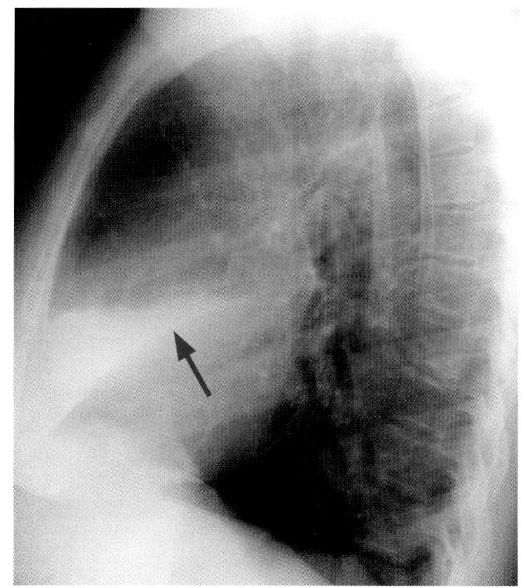

Right middle lobe atelectasis: Frontal chest radiograph shows an indistinct opacity in the right lung with focal silhouetting of the right heart border (arrow). There is elevation of the right hemidiaphragm due to volume loss. The lateral radiograph shows a wedge-shaped opacity (arrow) projecting over the mid-heart representing the collapsed right middle lobe.

Case courtesy Ritu R. Gill, MD, MPH, Brigham and Women's Hospital.

- The findings of right middle lobe atelectasis can be subtle on the frontal radiograph. Silhouetting of the right heart border by the collapsed medial segment of the middle lobe may be the only clue. The lateral radiograph shows a wedge-shaped opacity anteriorly.

ROUND ATELECTASIS

- Round atelectasis is focal atelectasis with a round morphology that is *always* associated with an adjacent pleural abnormality (e.g., pleural effusion, pleural thickening or plaque, pleural neoplasm, etc.).
- Round atelectasis is most common in the posterior lower lobes.
- All five of the following findings must be present to diagnose round atelectasis:

  1) Adjacent pleura must be abnormal.

  2) Opacity must be peripheral and in contact with the pleura.

  3) Opacity must be round or elliptical.

  4) Volume loss must be present in the affected lobe.

  5) Pulmonary vessels and bronchi leading into the opacity must be curved — this is the *comet tail* sign.

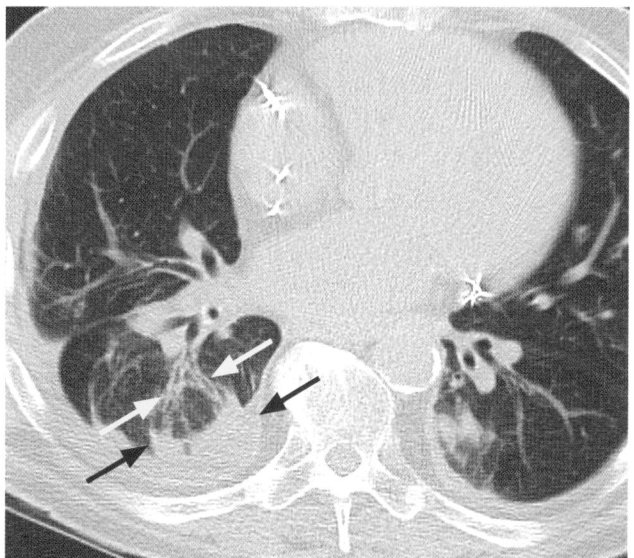

Round atelectasis: Noncontrast CT shows a rounded opacity in the medial right lower lobe (red arrows). This example meets all five criteria for round atelectasis including adjacent pleural abnormality (effusion), opacity in contact with the pleura, round shape, volume loss in the affected lobe, and the *comet tail* sign (yellow arrows) representing curved vessels and bronchi leading to the focus of round atelectasis.

ESSENTIAL ANATOMY

Secondary pulmonary lobule (SPL)

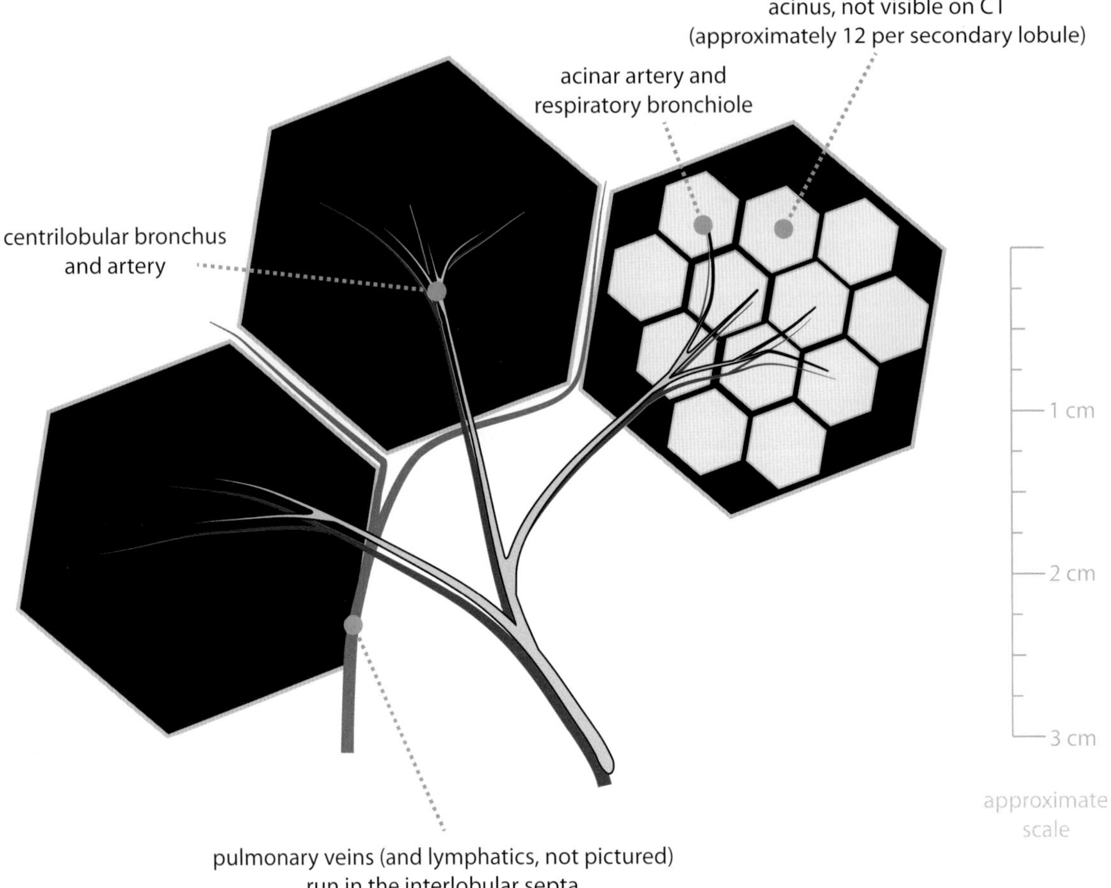

- The secondary pulmonary lobule (SPL) is the elemental unit of lung function.
- Each SPL contains a central artery (the aptly named centrilobular artery) and a central bronchus, each branching many times to ultimately produce acinar arteries and respiratory bronchioles.

  On CT, the centrilobular artery is often visible as a faint dot. The centrilobular bronchus is not normally visible.

  The acinus is the basic unit of gas exchange, containing several generations of branching respiratory bronchioles, alveolar ducts, and alveoli.

  There are generally 12 or fewer acini per secondary lobule.
- Pulmonary veins and lymphatics collect in the periphery of each SPL.
- Connective tissue, called interlobular septa, encases each SPL.

  Thickening of the interlobular septa can be seen on CT and suggests pathologic enlargement of either the venous or lymphatic spaces, as discussed on subsequent pages.
- Each SPL is between 1 and 2.5 cm in diameter.

Consolidation and ground glass

- Consolidation and ground glass opacification are two very commonly seen patterns of lung disease caused by abnormal alveoli. The alveolar abnormality may represent either filling of the alveoli with fluid or incomplete alveolar aeration.
- Consolidation can be described on either a chest radiograph or CT, while ground glass is generally reserved for CT.
- Although consolidation often implies pneumonia, both consolidation and ground glass are nonspecific findings with a broad differential depending on chronicity (acute versus chronic) and distribution (focal versus patchy or diffuse).

Consolidation

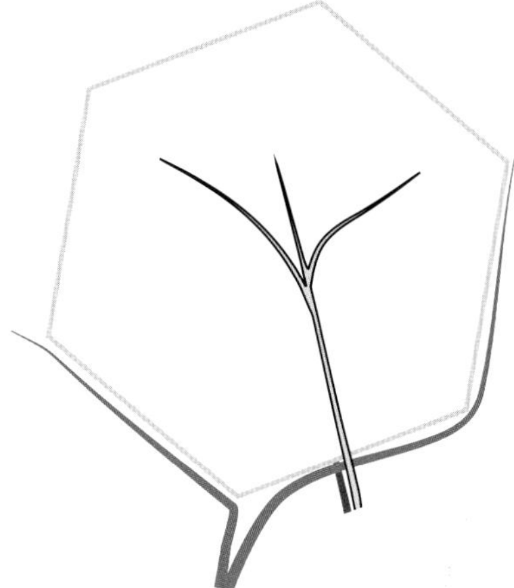

Schematic demonstrates complete filling of the alveolus with obscuration of the pulmonary vessels. The bronchus is visible as an air bronchogram.

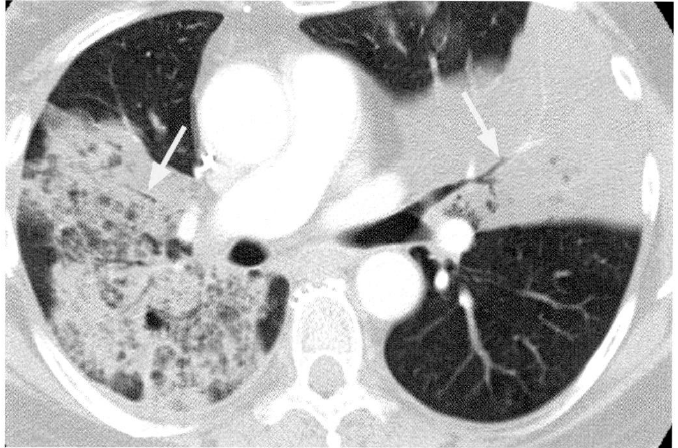

Consolidation: Contrast-enhanced CT shows bilateral consolidative opacities, more densely consolidated on the left. There are bilateral air bronchograms (arrows). Although these imaging findings are nonspecific, this was a case of multifocal bronchioloalveolar carcinoma.

- Consolidation is histologically due to complete filling of affected alveoli with a liquid-like substance (commonly remembered as *blood, pus, water,* or *cells*).
- Pulmonary vessels are **not** visible through the consolidation on an unenhanced CT.
- *Air bronchograms* are often present if the airway is patent. An air bronchogram represents a lucent air-filled bronchus (or bronchiole) seen within a consolidation.
- Consolidation causes silhouetting of adjacent structures on conventional radiography.
- **Acute consolidation** is most commonly due to pneumonia, but the differential includes:

> **Pneumonia** (by far the most common cause of acute consolidation).
>
> **Pulmonary hemorrhage** (primary pulmonary hemorrhage or aspiration of hemorrhage).
>
> **Acute respiratory distress syndrome (ARDS)**, which is noncardiogenic pulmonary edema seen in critically ill patients and thought to be due to increased capillary permeability.
>
> **Pulmonary edema** may cause consolidation, although this is an uncommon manifestation.

- The differential diagnosis of **chronic consolidation** includes:

> **Bronchioloalveolar carcinoma** mucinous subtype, a form of adenocarcinoma.
>
> **Organizing pneumonia**, which is a nonspecific response to injury characterized by granulation polyps which fill the distal airways, producing peripheral rounded and nodular consolidation.
>
> **Chronic eosinophilic pneumonia**, an inflammatory process characterized by eosinophils causing alveolar filling in an upper-lobe distribution.

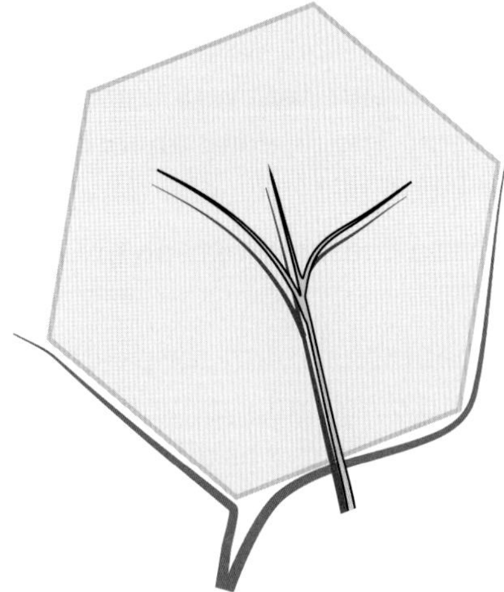

Schematic demonstrates complete hazy filling of the alveolus. The pulmonary vessels are still visible.

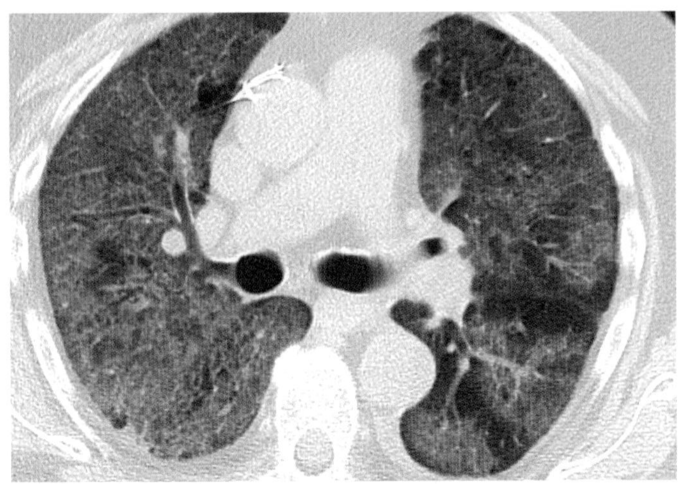

Ground glass opacification: Noncontrast CT shows diffuse ground glass opacification (GGO). The pulmonary architecture, including vasculature and bronchi, can be still seen, which is characteristic for GGO. Although these imaging findings are nonspecific, this was a case of acute respiratory distress syndrome (ARDS).

- Ground glass opacification is histologically due to either partial filling of the alveoli (by blood, pus, water, or cells), alveolar wall thickening, or reduced aeration of alveoli (atelectasis).
- Ground glass is usually a term reserved for CT. CT shows a hazy, gauze-like opacity, through which pulmonary vessels are still visible.

  The term ground glass was originally described for unenhanced CT as enhanced vessels are visible in consolidation as well; however, in common practice ground glass is used for any type of CT.
- As with consolidation, air bronchograms may be present.
- **Acute ground glass** opacification has a similar differential to acute consolidation, since many of the entities that initially cause partial airspace filling can progress to completely fill the airspaces later in the disease. The differential of acute ground glass includes:

  Pulmonary edema, which is usually dependent.

  Pneumonia. Unlike consolidation, ground glass is more commonly seen in atypical pneumonia such as viral or *Pneumocystis jiroveci* pneumonia.

  Pulmonary hemorrhage.

  Acute respiratory distress syndrome (ARDS).
- **Chronic ground glass** opacification has a similar but broader differential diagnosis compared to chronic consolidation. In addition to all of the entities which may cause chronic consolidation, the differential diagnosis of chronic ground glass also includes:

  Bronchioloalveolar carcinoma, which tends to be focal or multifocal.

  Organizing pneumonia, typically presenting as rounded, peripheral chronic consolidation.

  Chronic eosinophilic pneumonia, usually with an upper-lobe predominance.

  Idiopathic pneumonias, which are a diverse group of inflammatory responses to pulmonary injury.

  Hypersensitivity pneumonitis (HSP), especially the subacute phase. HSP is a type III hypersensitivity reaction to inhaled organic antigens. In the subacute phase there is ground glass, centrilobular nodules, and mosaic attenuation.

  Alveolar proteinosis, an idiopathic disease characterized by alveolar filling by a proteinaceous substance. The distribution is typically central, with sparing of the periphery.

Diffuse but central-predominant ground glass

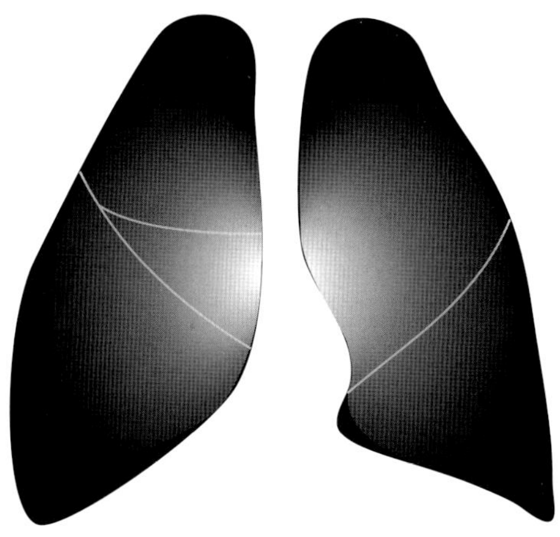

Coronal schematic shows central-predominant ground glass attenuation.

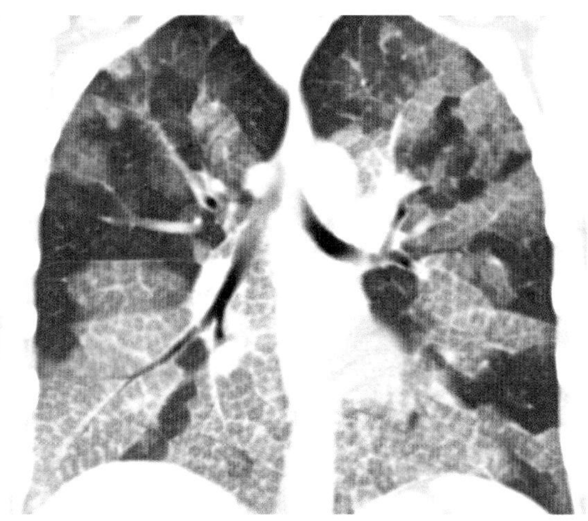

Coronal CT demonstrates central-predominant ground glass and associated septal thickening (the *crazy paving* pattern) in a case of alveolar proteinosis.

- The differential diagnosis for **ground glass in a central distribution** includes:

> **Pulmonary edema**.
>
> **Alveolar hemorrhage**.
>
> ***Pneumocystis jiroveci* pneumonia**.
>
> **Alveolar proteinosis**.

Peripheral ground glass or consolidation

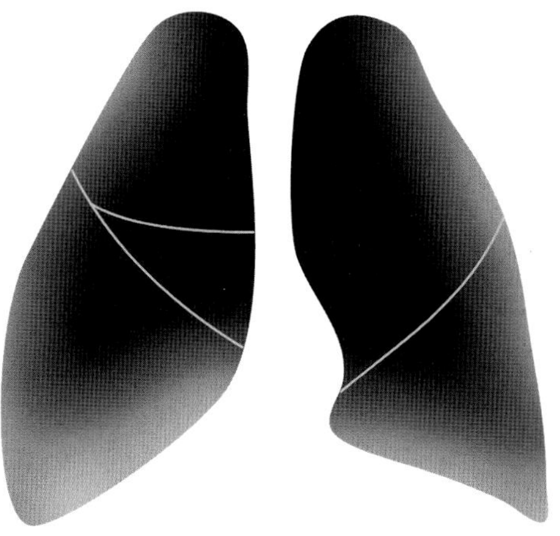

Coronal schematic demonstrates peripheral ground glass.

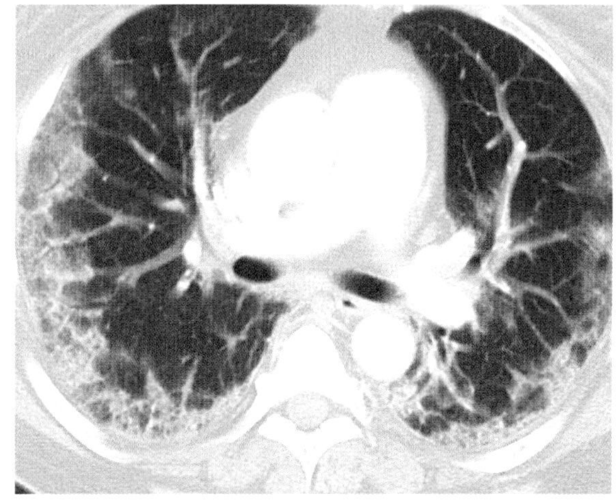

Axial CT shows peripheral and subpleural ground glass attenuation. This was a case of organizing pneumonia.

- The differential diagnosis for **peripheral consolidation or ground glass** includes:

> **Organizing pneumonia**.
>
> **Chronic eosinophilic pneumonia**, typically with an upper lobe predominance.
>
> **Atypical or viral pneumonia**.
>
> **Pulmonary edema.** Peripheral pulmonary edema tends to be noncardiogenic in etiology, such as edema triggered by drug reaction. Peripheral consolidation/ground glass is unusual for cardiogenic pulmonary edema.

Interlobular septal thickening – smooth

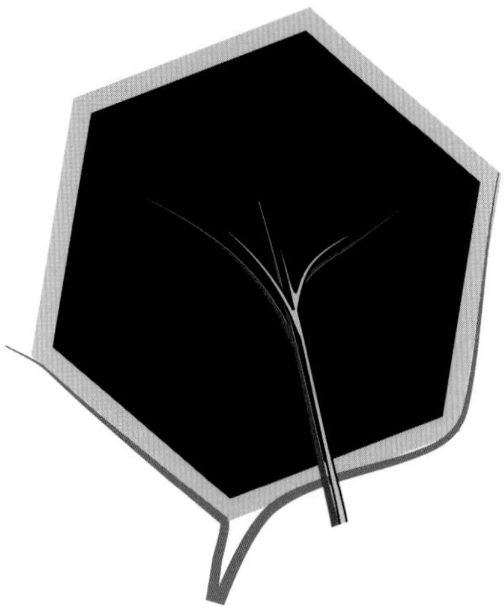

Schematic demonstrates smooth interlobular septal thickening.

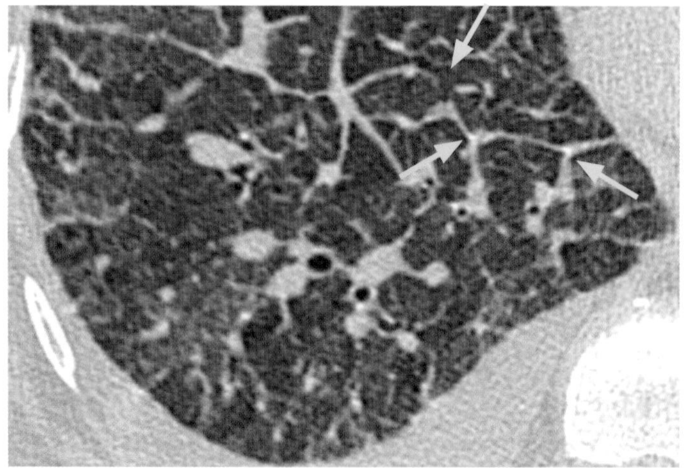

Smooth interlobular septal thickening: CT demonstrates smooth thickening of the interlobular septa (arrows) in pulmonary edema.

Courtesy Ritu R. Gill, MD, MPH, Brigham and Women's Hospital.

- Conditions that dilate the pulmonary veins cause smooth interlobular septal thickening.
- By far the most common cause of **smooth interlobular septal thickening** is pulmonary edema; however, the differential diagnosis for smooth interlobular septal thickening is identical to the differential for central ground glass:

> **Pulmonary edema** (by far the most common cause of smooth interlobular septal thickening).
>
> **Pulmonary alveolar proteinosis**.
>
> **Pulmonary hemorrhage**.
>
> **Atypical pneumonia**, especially *Pneumocystis jiroveci* pneumonia.

Interlobular septal thickening – nodular, irregular, or asymmetric

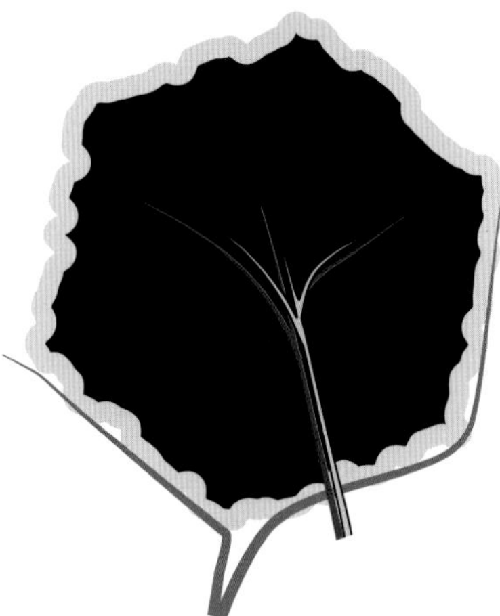

Schematic demonstrates irregular and nodular interlobular septal thickening.

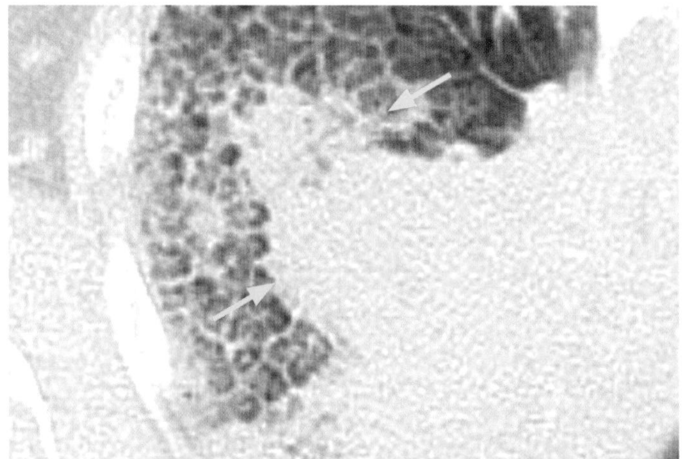

Nodular septal thickening: CT shows a dominant mass in the right lung (yellow arrows) with peripheral nodularity and septal thickening. This was a case of lymphangitic carcinomatosis.

- **Nodular, irregular, or asymmetric septal thickening** tends to be caused by processes that infiltrate the peripheral lymphatics, most commonly lymphangitic carcinomatosis and sarcoidosis:

> **Lymphangitic carcinomatosis** is tumor spread through the lymphatics.
>
> **Sarcoidosis** is an idiopathic, multi-organ disease characterized by noncaseating granulomas, which form nodules and masses primarily in a lymphatic distribution.

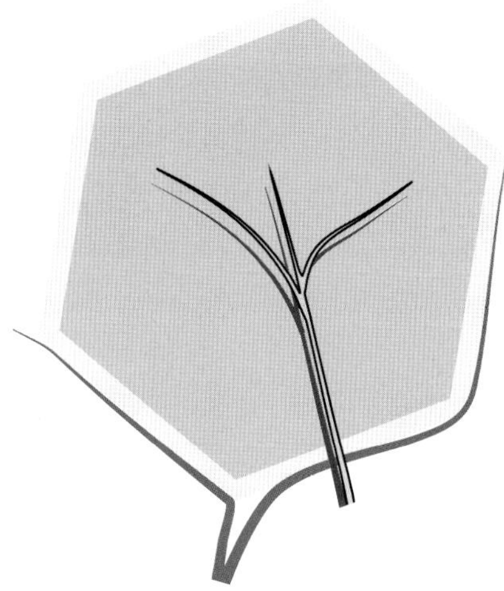

Schematic demonstrates interlobular septal thickening and ground glass opacification.

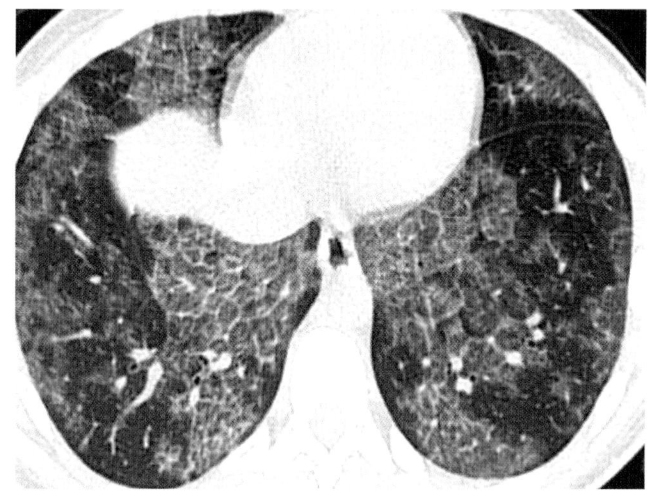

Axial CT shows interlobular septal thickening in regions of ground glass opacification, representing *crazy paving.* This was a case of alveolar proteinosis, the entity in which crazy paving was first described.

- *Crazy paving* describes interlobular septal thickening with superimposed ground glass opacification, which is thought to resemble the appearance of broken pieces of stone.
- Although nonspecific, this pattern was first described for alveolar proteinosis, where the ground glass opacification is caused by filling of alveoli by proteinaceous material and the interlobular septal thickening is caused by lymphatics taking up the same material.
- The differential diagnosis for **crazy paving** includes:

Alveolar proteinosis.

***Pneumocystis jiroveci* pneumonia**.

Organizing pneumonia.

Bronchioloalveolar carcinoma, mucinous subtype.

Lipoid pneumonia, an inflammatory pneumonia caused by a reaction to aspirated lipids.

Acute respiratory distress syndrome.

Pulmonary hemorrhage.

Centrilobular nodules

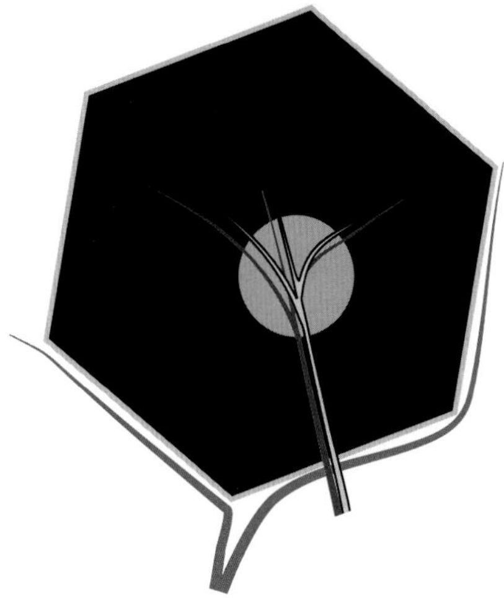

Schematic demonstrates a centrilobular nodule, located at the center of the pulmonary lobule.

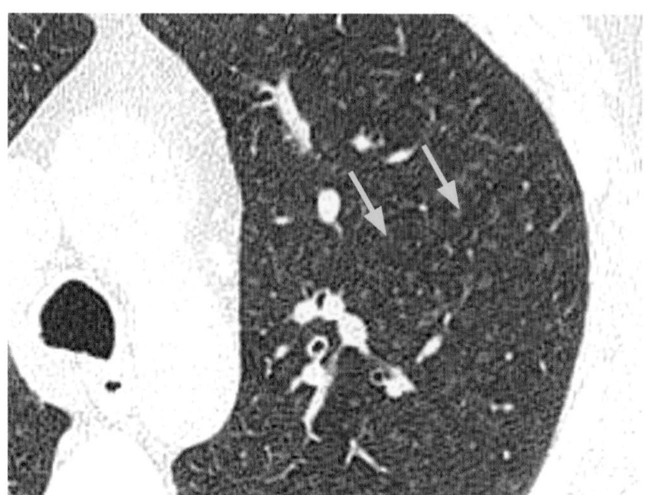

Axial CT demonstrates innumerable subcentimeter centrilobular nodules of ground glass attenuation (arrows). None of the nodules extends to the pleural surface, which is typical of a centrilobular distribution. This was a case of respiratory bronchiolitis interstitial lung disease (RB-ILD).

Courtesy Ritu R. Gill, MD, MPH, Brigham and Women's Hospital.

- Centrilobular nodules represent opacification of the centrilobular bronchiole (or less commonly the centrilobular artery) at the center of each secondary pulmonary lobule.
- On CT, multiple small nodules are seen in the centers of secondary pulmonary lobules. Centrilobular nodules never extend to the pleural surface. The nodules may be solid or of ground glass attenuation, and range in size from tiny up to a centimeter.
- Centrilobular nodules may be caused by infectious or inflammatory conditions.
- **Infectious** causes of **centrilobular nodules** include:

> **Endobronchial spread of tuberculosis** or atypical mycobacteria. Atypical mycobacteria are a diverse spectrum of acid-fast mycobacteria that do not cause tuberculosis. The typical pulmonary manifestation of atypical mycobacteria is a low-grade infection typically seen in elderly women, most commonly caused by *Mycobacterium avium-intracellulare*.
>
> **Bronchopneumonia**, which is spread of infectious pneumonia via the airways.
>
> **Atypical pneumonia,** especially **mycoplasma pneumonia**.

- The two most common **inflammatory** causes of **centrilobular nodules** include hypersensitivity pneumonitis (HSP) and respiratory bronchiolitis interstitial lung disease (RB-ILD), both exposure-related lung diseases. More prominent centrilobular nodules are suggestive of HSP.

> **HSP** is a type III hypersensitivity reaction to an inhaled organic antigen. The subacute phase of HSP is primarily characterized by centrilobular nodules.
>
> **Hot tub lung** is a hypersensitivity reaction to inhaled atypical mycobacteria, with similar imaging to HSP.
>
> **RB-ILD** is an inflammatory reaction to inhaled cigarette smoke mediated by pigmented macrophages.
>
> **Diffuse panbronchiolitis** is a chronic inflammatory disorder characterized by lymphoid hyperplasia in the walls of the respiratory bronchioles resulting in bronchiolectasis. It typically affects patients of Asian descent.
>
> **Silicosis**, an inhalation lung disease that develops in response to inhaled silica particles, is characterized by upper lobe predominant centrilobular and perilymphatic nodules.

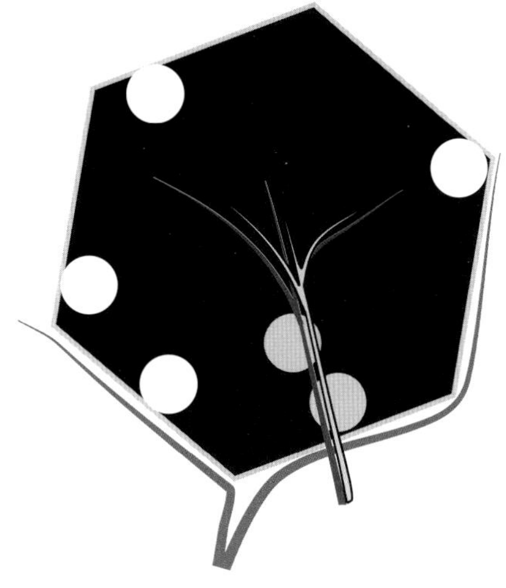

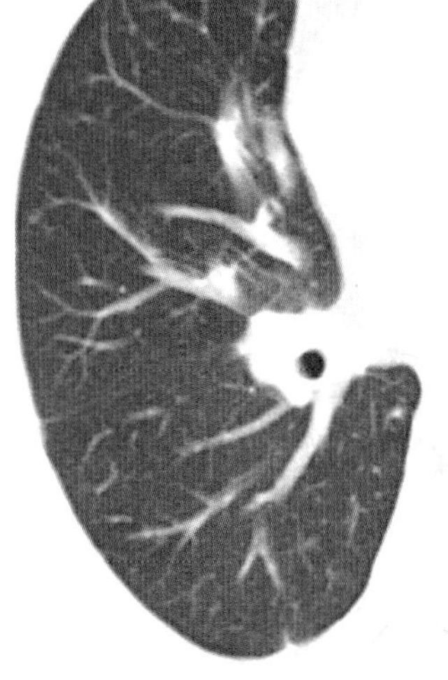

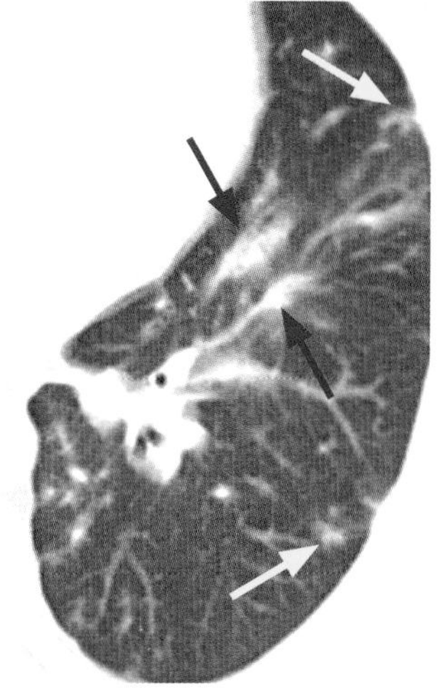

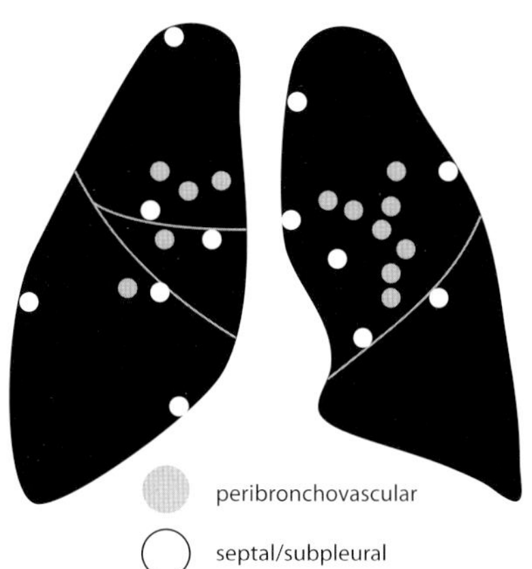

Perilymphatic nodules:

Schematic of the secondary pulmonary lobule (top left image) demonstrates two of the three distributions of perilymphatic nodules. The gray nodules are located along the bronchovascular bundle and the white nodules are located along the interlobular septa.

Schematic of the lungs (left image) demonstrates the peribronchovascular and subpleural/fissural distribution.

Axial CT (top right image) demonstrates multiple subpleural/fissural nodules (yellow arrows) and nodules along the bronchovascular bundles (red arrows). This was a case of sarcoidosis.

- Perilymphatic nodules follow the anatomic locations of pulmonary lymphatics, which can be seen in three locations in the lung:
  1) Subpleural.
  2) Peribronchovascular.
  3) Septal (within the interlobular septa separating the hexagonal secondary pulmonary lobules).
- Sarcoidosis is by far the most common cause of perilymphatic nodules, typically with an upper-lobe distribution. The nodules may become confluent creating the *galaxy* sign. The differential of **perilymphatic nodules** includes:

Sarcoidosis.

Pneumoconioses (silicosis and coal workers pneumoconiosis) are reactions to inorganic dust inhalation. The imaging may look identical to sarcoidosis with perilymphatic nodules, but there is usually a history of exposure (e.g. a sandblaster who develops silicosis).

Lymphangitic carcinomatosis.

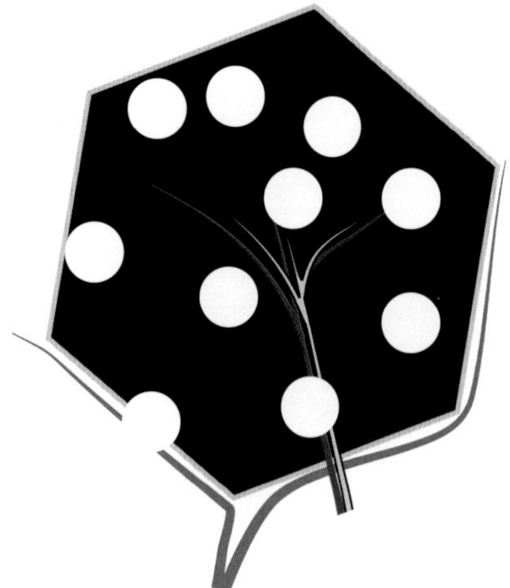

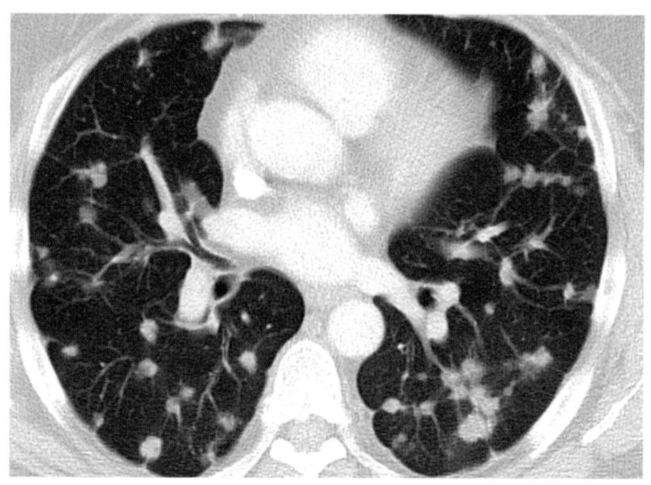

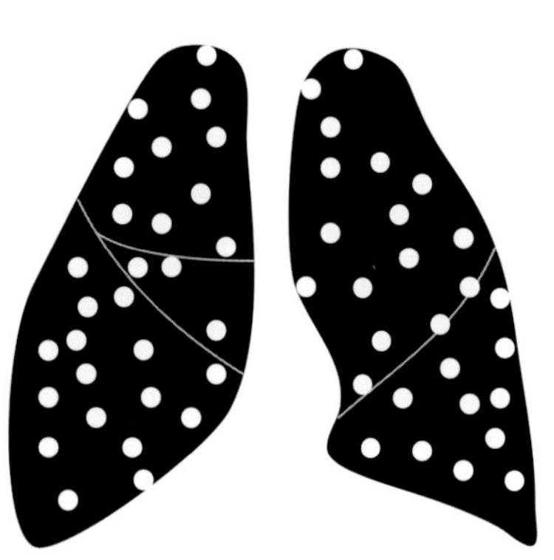

Random nodules:

Schematic of the secondary pulmonary lobule (top left image) demonstrates nodules distributed randomly throughout the SPL.

Schematic of the lungs (bottom left image) demonstrates nodules scattered randomly. Some of the nodules are in close contact with the pleural surface.

Axial CT (top right image) demonstrates multiple random nodules. Some of the nodules abut the pleural surface. This was a case of metastatic colon cancer.

- **Randomly distributed nodules** usually occur via hematogenous spread and have an angiocentric distribution. The differential of random nodules includes:

Hematogenous metastases.

Septic emboli. Embolic infection has a propensity to cavitate but early emboli may be irregular or solid.

Pulmonary Langerhans's cell histiocytosis (PLCH), a smoking-related lung disease that progresses from airway-associated and random nodules to irregular cysts. PLCH is usually distinguishable from other causes of random nodules due to the presence of cysts and non-angiocentric distribution.

- A ***miliary*** **pattern** is innumerable tiny random nodules disseminated hematogenously, suggestive of the appearance of millet seeds. The differential of miliary nodules includes:

Disseminated tuberculosis.	**Disseminated fungal infection.**	**Disseminated hematogenous metastases.**

Miliary nodules: Axial CT shows innumerable tiny nodules distributed randomly throughout both lungs in a miliary pattern. This was a case of miliary tuberculosis.

Case courtesy Ritu R. Gill, MD, MPH, Brigham and Women's Hospital.

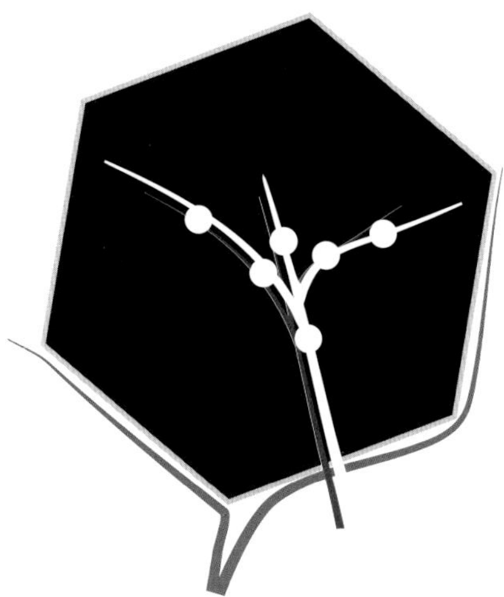

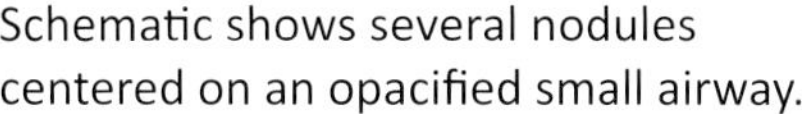

Schematic shows several nodules centered on an opacified small airway.

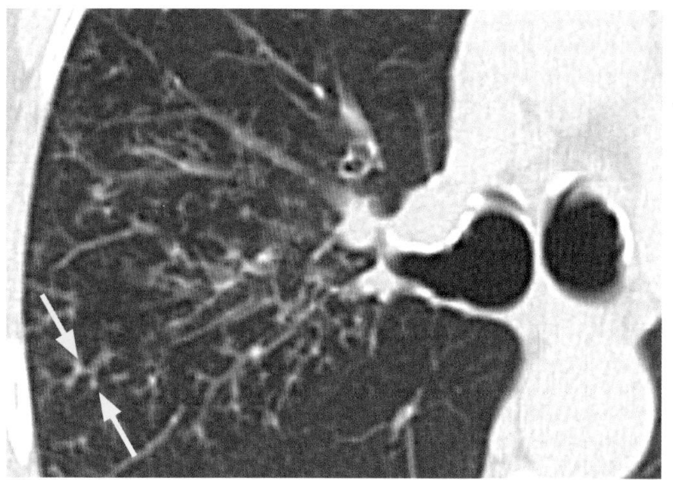

Tree-in-bud nodularity: Axial CT show numerous small nodules (arrows) "budding" off of linear branching structures in the right middle lobe. This case was secondary to atypical mycobacteria.

- Tree-in-bud nodules are multiple small nodules connected to linear branching structures, which resembles a budding tree branch in springtime as seen on CT. The linear branching structures represent the impacted bronchioles, which are normally invisible on CT, and the nodules represent impacted terminal bronchioles. Tree-in-bud nodules are due to mucus, pus, or fluid impacting bronchioles and terminal bronchioles.
- **Tree-in-bud nodules** are almost always associated with small airways infection, such as endobronchial spread of tuberculosis. The differential of tree-in-bud nodules includes:

Mycobacteria tuberculosis and **atypical mycobacteria**.

Bacterial pneumonia.

Aspiration pneumonia.

Airway-invasive aspergillus. Aspergillus is an opportunistic fungus with several patterns of disease. The airway-invasive pattern is seen in immunocompromised patients and may present either as bronchopneumonia or small airways infection.

Solitary cavitary nodule/mass

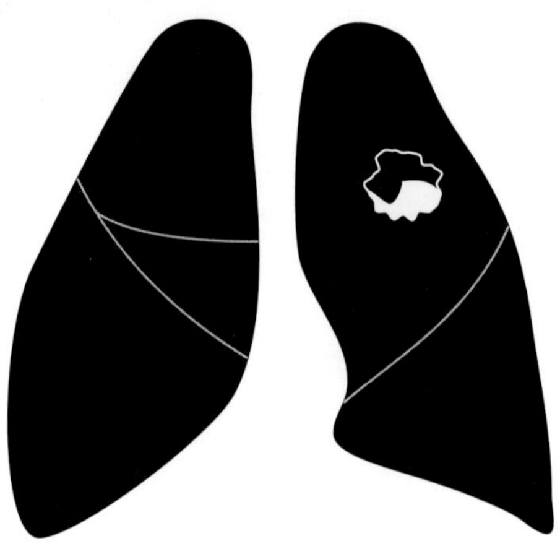

Coronal schematic demonstrates a single cavitary lesion.

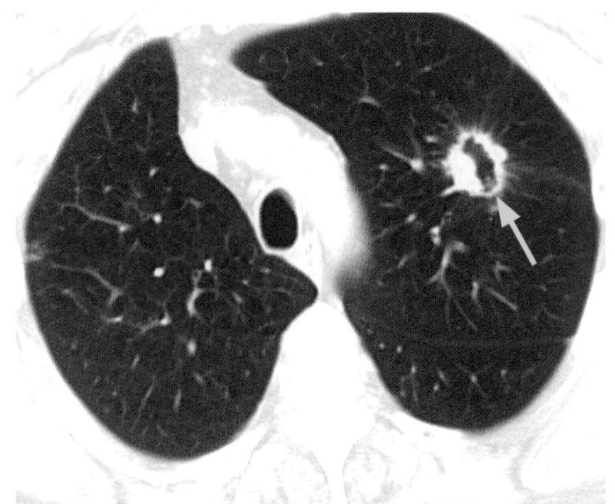

Axial CT shows a single spiculated cavitary lesion in the left upper lobe (arrow). This was a case of squamous cell carcinoma.

- A cavitary lesion has a thick, irregular wall, often with a solid mural component. Although the findings of benign and malignant cavitary nodules overlap, a maximum wall thickness of ≤4 mm is usually benign and a wall thickness >15 mm is usually malignant. Spiculated margins also suggest malignancy.
- A **solitary cavitary lesion** is most likely cancer or infection.

Primary bronchogenic carcinoma. While both squamous cell and adenocarcinoma can cavitate, squamous cell cavitates more frequently. Small cell carcinoma is never known to cavitate.

Tuberculosis classically produces an upper-lobe cavitation.

Multiple cavitary nodules

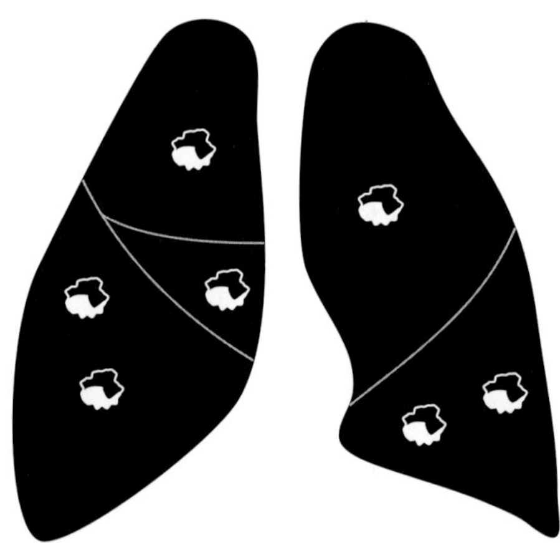

Coronal schematic shows numerous cavitary lesions bilaterally.

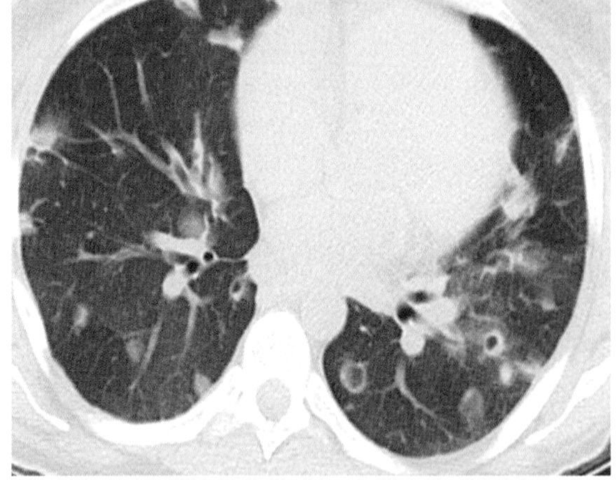

Axial CT shows numerous cavitary and noncavitary lesions bilaterally, in a random distribution. This was a case of tricuspid endocarditis and septic emboli.

Case courtesy Michael Hanley, MD, University of Virginia Health System.

- **Multiple cavitary lesions** are typically vascular or spread through the vascular system:

Septic emboli.

Vasculitis, including Wegener granulomatosis, which is especially prone to cavitate.

Metastases, of which squamous cell carcinoma and uterine carcinosarcoma are known to cavitate.

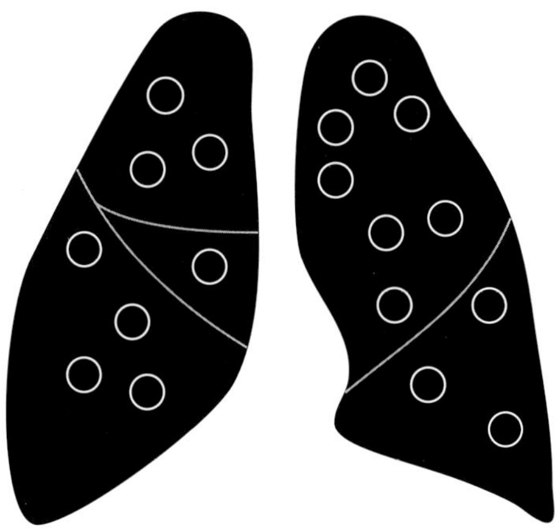

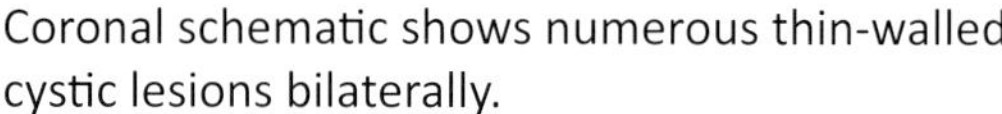

Coronal schematic shows numerous thin-walled cystic lesions bilaterally.

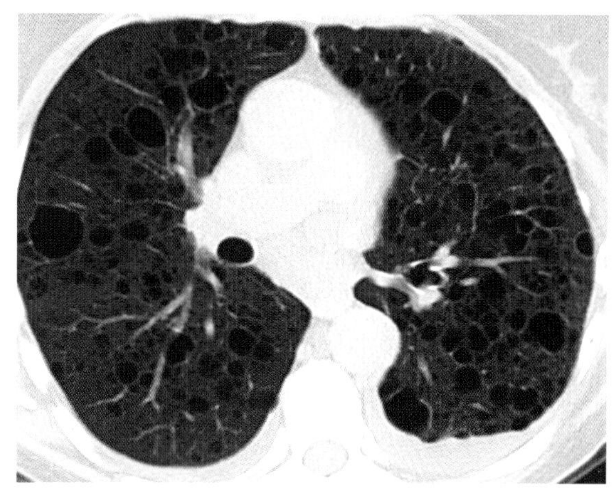

Axial CT shows bilateral thin-walled cysts that are of varying sizes but are predominantly regular in shape. There is a small left pleural effusion. This was a case of lymphangioleiomyomatosis.

- A cyst is an air-containing lucency with a thin, nearly imperceptible wall. In general, cystic lung disease is usually due to a primary airway abnormality.
- The differential diagnosis for multiple lung cysts includes:

Lymphangioleiomyomatosis (LAM), a diffuse cystic lung disease caused by smooth muscle proliferation of the distal airways. LAM causes uniformly distributed, thin-walled cysts in a diffuse distribution. It is classically associated with chylous effusion, as demonstrated in the above right case.

Emphysema, which tends to be upper-lobe predominant in a smoker.

Pulmonary Langerhans cell histiocytosis, which features irregular cysts and nodules predominantly in the upper lungs.

Diffuse cystic bronchiectasis. Bronchiectasis is dilation of the bronchioles. Although cystic fibrosis is the most common cause of bronchiectasis and has an upper-lobe predominance, congenital or post-infectious causes can have a diffuse or lower-lobe distribution.

***Pneumocystis jiroveci* pneumonia**, which features cysts in late-stage disease.

Lymphoid interstitial pneumonia (LIP), an exceptionally rare disease usually associated with Sjögren syndrome and characterized by alveolar distortion from lymphocytic infiltrate and multiple cysts.

- The differential for a single cyst includes:

Bulla. A bulla is an air-filled cyst measuring >1 cm. A giant bulla occupies at least 30% of the volume of the thorax.

Bleb. A bleb is a air-filled cystic structure contiguous with the pleura measuring <1 cm. Rupture of a bleb is the most common cause of spontaneous pneumothorax.

Pneumatocele, which is an air-filled space caused by prior lung trauma or infection.

Lower lobe fibrotic changes

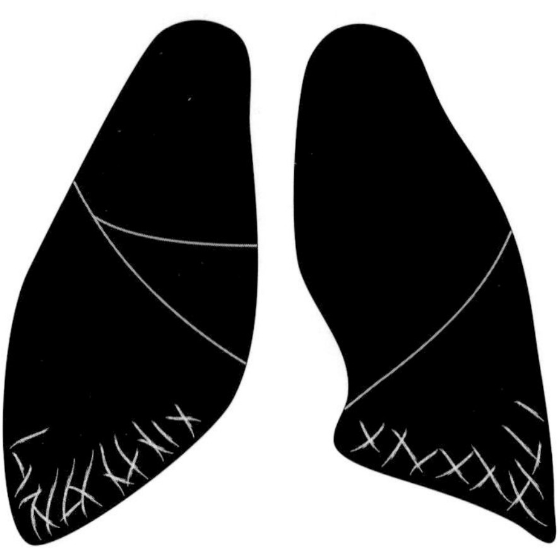

Coronal schematic shows basal-predominant fibrotic changes.

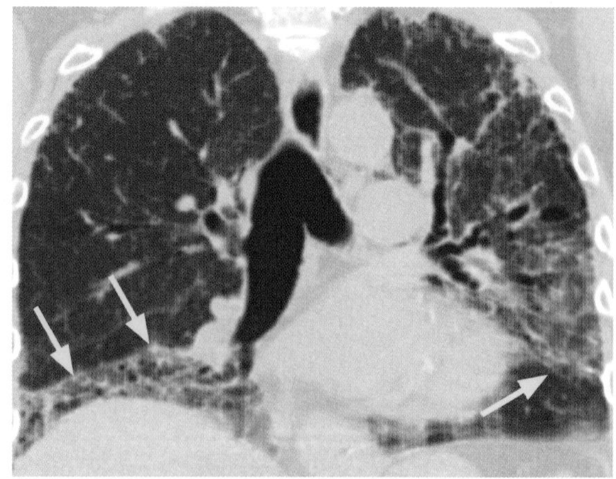

Coronal CT shows bibasilar fibrosis and honeycombing (arrows), with relative sparing of the upper lobes. This was a case of idiopathic pulmonary fibrosis.

- The differential diagnosis of basal-predominant fibrotic change includes:

Idiopathic pulmonary fibrosis (IPF), which is a clinical syndrome of progressive pulmonary fibrosis of unknown etiology and is most common cause of basilar fibrosis. It almost always features basilar honeycombing.

End-stage asbestosis. Asbestosis is an asbestos-induced inflammatory process ultimately producing pulmonary fibrosis. Usually other signs of asbestos exposure are present, such as pleural plaques.

Nonspecific interstitial pneumonia (NSIP), fibrotic form. NSIP is an idiopathic pneumonia. It is a lung response to injury commonly associated with collagen vascular disease and drug reaction. The two histologic subtypes are cellular and fibrotic forms, of which the latter may produce basal-predominant fibrosis. In contrast to IPF, honeycombing is usually absent.

Upper lobe fibrotic changes

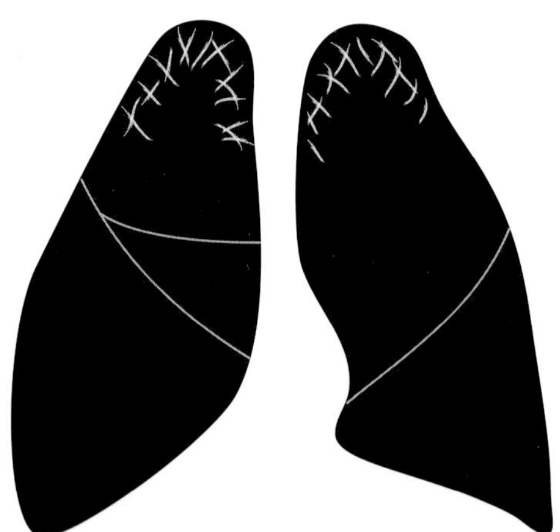

Coronal schematic shows fibrotic changes in the upper lobes.

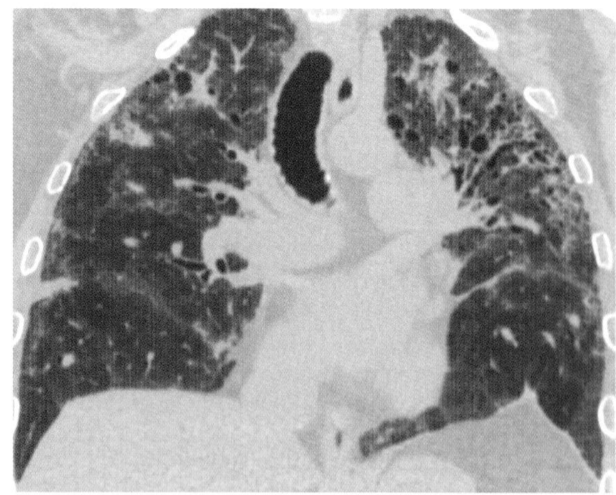

Coronal CT shows upper-lobe predominant subpleural fibrosis and traction bronchiectasis. A pathologic diagnosis was not established in this case.

- Although IPF is the most common cause of pulmonary fibrosis, fibrosis primarily affecting the upper lobes should raise concern for an alternative diagnoses, such as:

End-stage sarcoidosis. Sarcoidosis is a disease that primarily affects the upper lobes. The late stage of sarcoidosis leads to upper-lobe predominant fibrosis.

Chronic hypersensitivity pneumonitis may cause upper-lobe fibrosis in long-standing disease.

End-stage silicosis. The late stage of silicosis may lead to fibrosis with an upper lobe predominance.

Pulmonary infection

Clinical classification of pneumonia

Community-acquired pneumonia (CAP)

- *S. pneumoniae* is the most common cause of community-acquired pneumonia (CAP).
- Atypical pneumonia, including *Mycoplasma*, viral, and *Chlamydia*, typically infects young and otherwise healthy patients.

  Mycoplasma has a varied appearance and can produce consolidation, areas of ground glass attenuation, centrilobular nodules, and tree-in-bud nodules.
- *Legionella* most commonly occurs in elderly smokers. Infections tend to be severe.

  Peripheral consolidation often progresses to lobar and multifocal pneumonia.
- Infection by *Klebsiella* and other gram-negatives occurs in alcoholics and aspirators.

  Klebsiella classically leads to voluminous inflammatory exudates causing the *bulging fissure* sign.

Hospital acquired pneumonia (HAP)

- Hospital acquired pneumonia (HAP) occurs in hospitalized patients and is due to aspiration of colonized secretions. HAP is caused by a wide variety of organisms, but the most important pathogens include MRSA and resistant gram-negatives including *Pseudomonas*.

Health care associated pneumonia (HCAP)

- Health care associated pneumonia is defined as pneumonia in a nursing home resident or in a patient with a >2 day hospitalization over the past 90 days. Pathogens are similar to HAP.

Ventilator associated pneumonia (VAP)

- Ventilator associated pneumonia is caused by infectious agents not present at the time mechanical ventilation was started. Most infections are polymicrobial and primarily involve gram-negative rods such as *Pseudomonas* and *Acinetobacter*.

Pneumonia in the immunocompromised patient

- Any of the above pathogens, plus opportunistic infections including *Pneumocystis*, fungi such as *Aspergillus*, *Nocardia*, CMV, etc., can be seen in immunocompromised patients.

Radiographic patterns of infection

Lobar pneumonia

- Lobar pneumonia is consolidation of a single lobe. It is usually bacterial in origin and is the most common presentation of community acquired pneumonia.
- The larger bronchi remain patent, causing air bronchograms.

Lobular pneumonia (bronchopneumonia)

- Lobular pneumonia manifests as patchy consolidation with poorly defined airspace opacities, usually involving several lobes, and most commonly due to *S. aureus*.

Interstitial pneumonia

- Interstitial pneumonia is caused by inflammatory cells located predominantly in the interstitial tissue of the alveolar septa causing diffuse or patchy ground glass opacification. It can be caused by viral pneumonia, *Mycoplasma*, *Chlamydia*, or *Pneumocystis*.

Round pneumonia

- Round pneumonia is an infectious mass-like opacity seen only in children, most commonly due to *Streptococcus pneumoniae*.
- Infection remains somewhat confined due to incomplete formation of pores of Kohn.

Pulmonary abscess

- Pulmonary abscess is necrosis of the lung parenchyma typically due to *Staphylococcus aureus*, *Pseudomonas*, or anaerobic bacteria.
- An air–fluid level is almost always present.
- An abscess is usually spherical, with equal dimensions on frontal and lateral views.

Pulmonary gangrene

- Pulmonary gangrene is a very rare complication of pneumonia where there is extensive necrosis or sloughing of a pulmonary segment or lobe. Pulmonary gangrene is a severe manifestation of pulmonary abscess.

Empyema

- Empyema is infection within the pleural space.
- There are three stages in the development of an empyema:
    1) **Free-flowing exudative effusion**: Can be treated with needle aspiration or simple drain.
    2) **Development of fibrous strands**: Requires large-bore chest tube and fibrinolytic therapy.
    3) **Fluid becomes solid and jelly-like**: Usually requires surgery.
- Although pneumonia is often associated with a parapneumonic effusion, most pleural effusions associated with pneumonia are *not* empyema, but are instead a sterile effusion caused by increased capillary permeability.
- An empyema conforms to the shape of the pleural space, causing a longer air–fluid level on the lateral radiograph. This is in contrast to an abscess, discussed above, which typically is spherical and has the same dimensions on the frontal and lateral radiographs.
- The *split pleura* sign describes enhancing parietal and visceral pleura of an empyema seen on contrast-enhanced study.

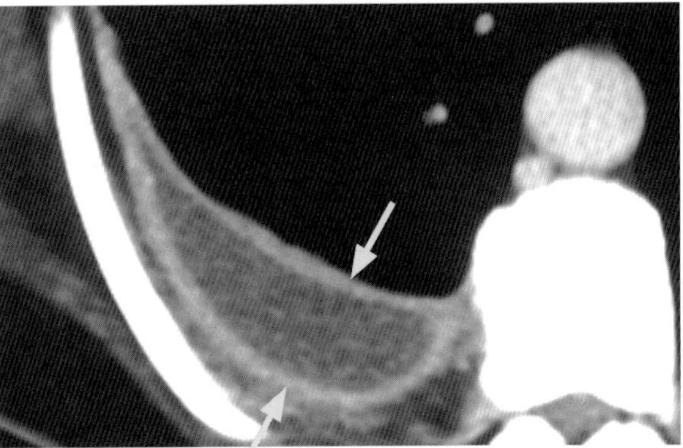

Split pleura sign: Contrast-enhanced CT shows enhancement of the thickened visceral and parietal pleural layers (arrows), which encase a pleural fluid collection.

The split pleura sign is seen in the majority of exudative effusions, although it is not specific. Similar findings can be seen in malignant effusion, mesothelioma, fibrothorax, and after talc pleurodesis.

Case courtesy Ritu R. Gill, MD, MPH, Brigham and Women's Hospital.

Pneumatocele

- A pneumatocele is a thin-walled, gas-filled cyst that may be post-traumatic or develop as a sequela of pneumonia, typically from *Staphylococcus aureus* or *Pneumocystis*.
- Pneumatoceles almost always resolve.

Bronchopleural fistula (BPF)

- Bronchopleural fistula (BPF) is an abnormal communication between the airway and the pleural space. It is caused by rupture of the visceral pleura. By far the most common cause of BPF is surgery; however, other etiologies include lung abscess, empyema, and trauma.
- On imaging, new or increasing gas is present in a pleural effusion. A connection between the bronchial tree and the pleura is not always apparent, but is helpful when seen.
- The treatment of BPF is controversial and highly individualized.

Empyema necessitans

- Empyema necessitans is extension of an empyema to the chest wall, most commonly secondary to tuberculosis. Other causative organisms include *Nocardia* and *Actinomyces*.

TUBERCULOSIS (TB)

- Tuberculosis (TB), caused by *Mycobacterium tuberculosis,* remains an important disease despite remarkable progress in public health and antituberculous therapy over the past century. Tuberculosis remains a significant problem in developing countries. In the United States, TB is seen primarily in the immigrant population and immunocompromised individuals.
- Initial exposure to TB can lead to two clinical outcomes:

  1) **Contained disease (90%)** results in calcified granulomas and/or calcified hilar lymph nodes. In a patient with normal immunity, the tuberculous bacilli are sequestered with a caseating granulomatous response.

  2) **Primary tuberculosis** results when the host cannot contain the organism. Primary tuberculosis is seen more commonly in children and immunocompromised patients.

- **Reactivation (post-primary)** TB is reactivation of a previously latent infection.

Primary tuberculosis

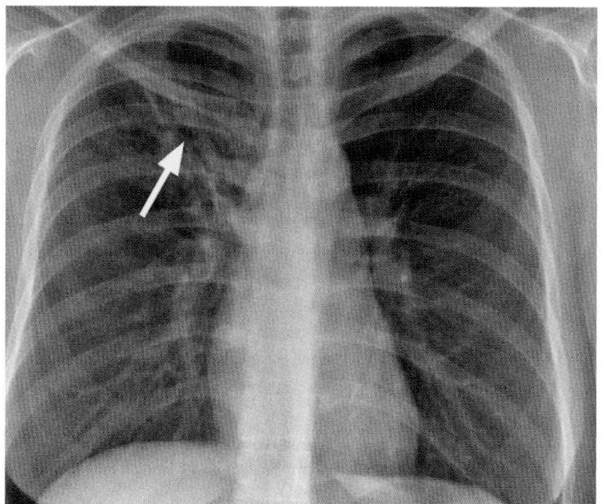
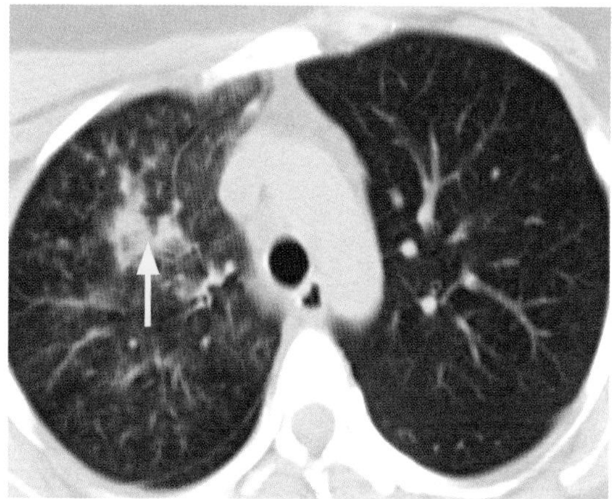

Primary tuberculosis: Chest radiograph (left image) shows a vague right upper lung opacity (arrow). CT shows a patchy opacification (arrow) in the lower portion of the right upper lobe with adjacent tree-in-bud nodularity. The patient's sputum grew *Mycobacterium tuberculosis.*

Case courtesy Ritu R. Gill, MD, MPH, Brigham and Women's Hospital.

- Primary tuberculosis represents infection from the first exposure to TB. Primary TB may involve the pulmonary parenchyma, the airways, and the pleura. Primary TB often causes adenopathy.
- As many as 15% of patients infected with primary TB have no radiographic changes and the imaging appearance of primary tuberculosis is nonspecific.
- The four imaging manifestations of primary TB (of which any, none, or all may be present) are ill-defined consolidation, pleural effusion, lymphadenopathy, and miliary disease. Primary TB may occur in any lobe, but the most typical locations are the lower lobes or right middle lobe. It can be difficult to distinguish between primary and post-primary TB, and in clinical practice, the treatment (antituberculous therapy) is the same.
- Classic imaging findings are not always seen, but include:

  Ghon focus: Initial focus of parenchymal infection, usually located in the upper part of the lower lobe or the lower part of the upper lobe.

  Ranke complex: *Ghon focus* and lymphadenopathy.

- Cavitation is rare in primary TB, in contrast to reactivation TB.

- Adenopathy is common in primary TB, typically featuring central low-attenuation and peripheral enhancement, especially in children. In contrast, post-primary TB does not feature prominent adenopathy.

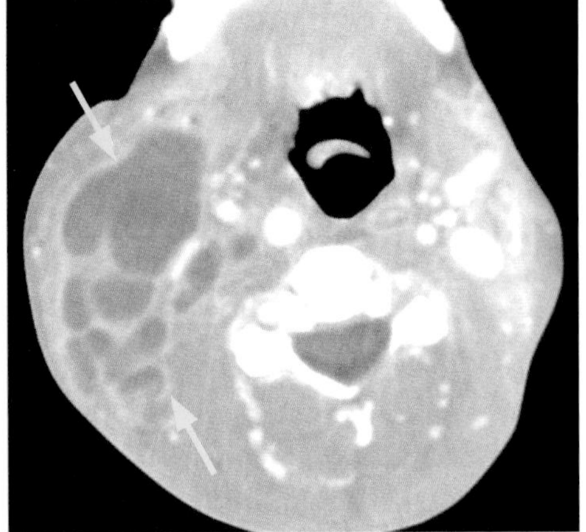

Tuberculous adenopathy: Contrast-enhanced neck CT shows marked right-sided adenopathy (arrows) with peripheral enhancement and central necrosis.

Case courtesy Ritu R. Gill, MD, MPH, Brigham and Women's Hospital.

Reactivation (post-primary) tuberculosis

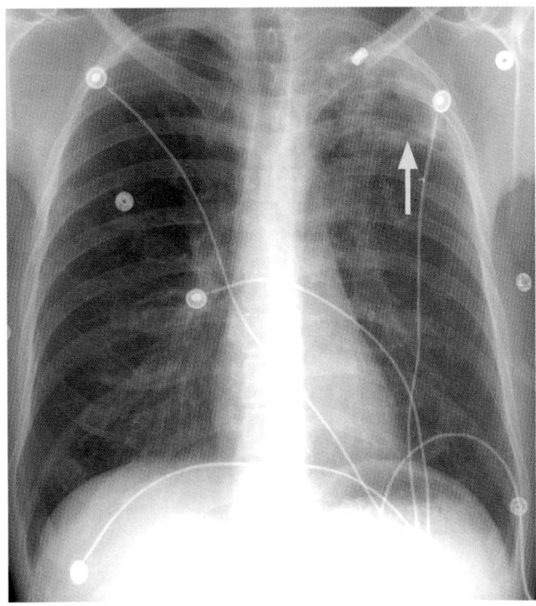

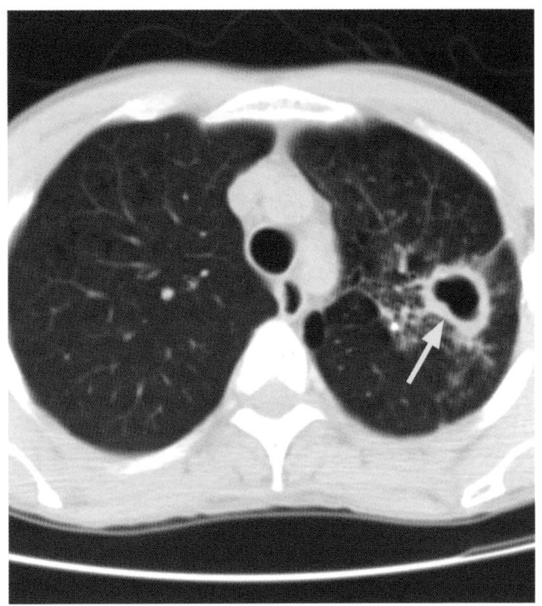

Reactivation TB: Frontal chest radiograph (left image) shows a cavitary lesion in the left upper lobe (arrow), confirmed by CT (arrow). There was no significant mediastinal adenopathy. The differential diagnosis of this appearance would include cavitary primary lung cancer, which would be expected to feature a thicker wall.

Case courtesy Michael Hanley, MD, University of Virginia Health System.

- Reactivation TB, also called post-primary TB, usually occurs in adolescents and adults and is caused by reactivation of a dormant infection acquired earlier in life. Clinical manifestations of reactivation TB include chronic cough, low-grade fever, hemoptysis, and night sweats.
- Reactivation TB most commonly occurs in the upper lobe apical and posterior segments.
- In an immunocompetent patient, the imaging hallmarks of reactivation TB are upper-lobe predominant disease with cavitation and lack of adenopathy. Focal upper lobe consolidation and endobronchial spread are common. Although not specific to TB, tree-in-bud nodules suggest active **endobronchial spread**.
- In an immunosuppressed patient (such as HIV), low-attenuation adenopathy is a typical additional finding, similar to the adenopathy seen in primary TB. Low density lymph nodes may mimic immune reconstitution syndrome in HIV patients.
- A tuberculoma is a well-defined rounded opacity usually in the upper lobes.

Healed tuberculosis

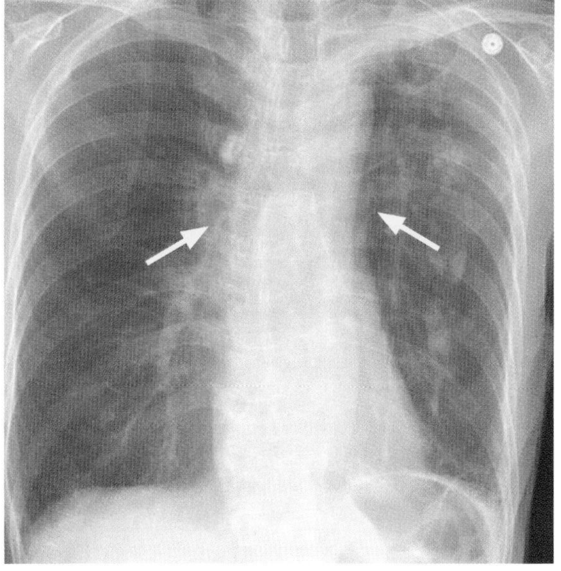

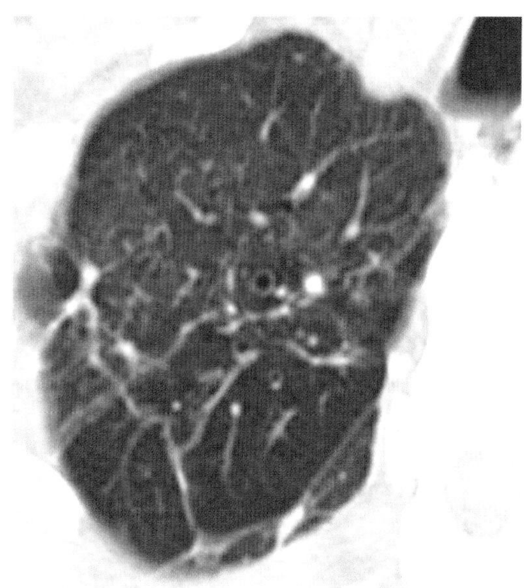

Healed tuberculosis: Radiograph shows scarring, volume loss, and superior hilar retraction (arrows). CT shows apical scarring.

Case courtesy Ritu R. Gill, MD, MPH, Brigham and Women's Hospital.

- Healed TB is evident on radiography as apical scarring, usually with upper lobe volume loss and superior hilar retraction.
- Calcified granulomas may be present as well, which indicate containment of the initial infection by a delayed hypersensitivity response.

Miliary tuberculosis

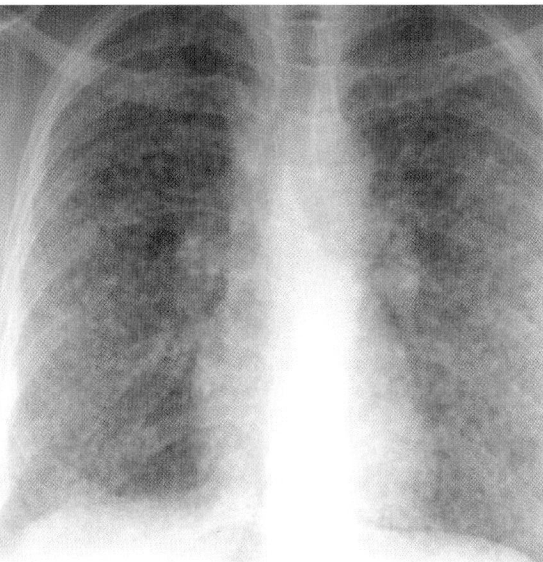

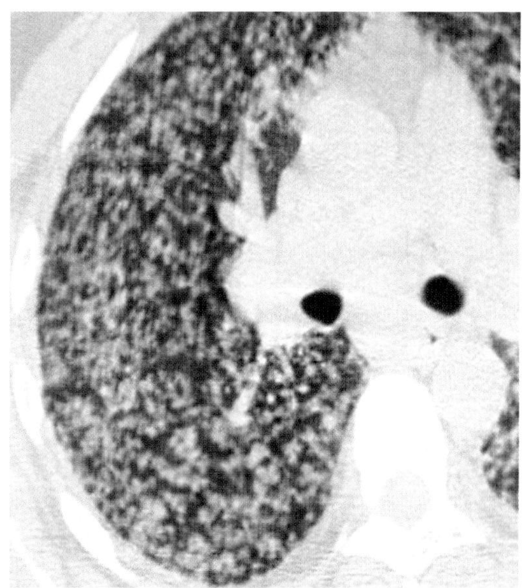

Miliary tuberculosis: Radiograph and CT show innumerable tiny nodules in a random pattern, reflecting hematogenous seeding of tuberculosis.

Case courtesy Ritu R. Gill, MD, MPH, Brigham and Women's Hospital.

- Miliary tuberculosis is a diffuse random distribution of tiny nodules seen in hematogenously disseminated TB.
- Miliary TB can occur in primary or reactivation TB.

ATYPICAL MYCOBACTERIA

Atypical mycobacteria infection

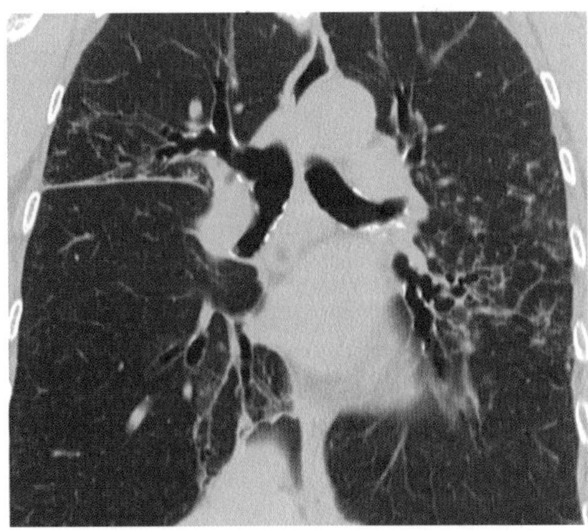
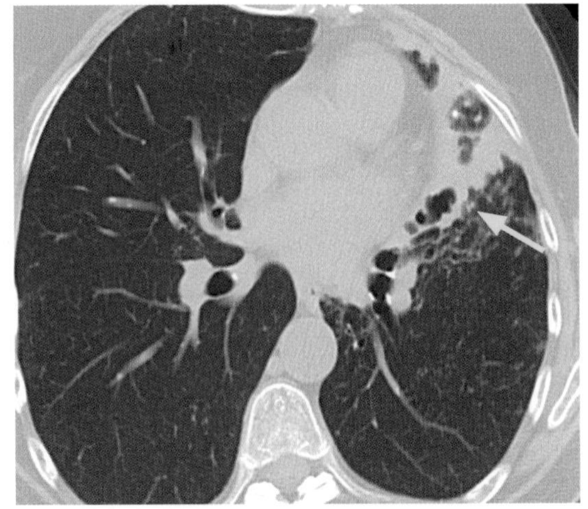

Mycobacterium avium intracellulare infection: Coronal (left) and axial CT show right upper lobe and lingular tree-in-bud opacities and bronchiectasis, with more focal consolidation in the lingula (arrow).

- The classic presentation of atypical mycobacteria is an elderly woman with cough, low-grade fever, and weight loss, called *Lady Windermere* syndrome. *Mycobacterium avium intracellulare* and *M. kansasii* are the two most common organisms.
- Classic radiographic findings are bronchiectasis and tree-in-bud nodules, most common in the right middle lobe or lingula.

"Hot-tub" lung

- "Hot-tub" lung is a hypersensitivity pneumonitis in response to atypical mycobacteria, which are often found in hot tubs. There is no active infection and the typical patient is otherwise healthy. Imaging is similar to other causes of hypersensitivity pneumonitis, featuring centrilobular nodules.

ENDEMIC FUNGI

- Endemic fungi can cause community acquired pneumonia in normal individuals, with each subtype having a specific geographic distribution. Most infected patients are asymptomatic.

Histoplasma capsulatum

- *Histoplasma capsulatum* is localized to the Ohio and Mississippi river valleys, in soil contaminated with bat or bird guano.
- The most common sequela of infection is a calcified granuloma. A less common radiologic manifestation is a pulmonary nodule (histoplasmoma), which can mimic a neoplasm.
- Chronic infection can mimic reactivation TB with upper lobe fibrocavitary consolidation.
- Fibrosing mediastinitis is a rare complication of *Histoplasma* infection of mediastinal lymph nodes leading to pulmonary venous obstruction, bronchial stenosis, and pulmonary artery stenosis. Affected lymph nodes tend to calcify.

Coccidioides immitis and *Blastomyces dermatitidis*

- *Coccidioides immitis* is found in the southwestern US and has a variety of radiologic appearances, including multifocal consolidation, multiple pulmonary nodules, and miliary nodules.
- *Blastomyces dermatitidis* is found in central and southeastern US. Infection is usually asymptomatic, but may present as flu-like illness that can progress to multifocal consolidation, ARDS, or miliary disease.

- Immunosuppressed patients are susceptible to the same organisms that infect immunocompetent patients; however, one must be aware of several additional opportunistic organisms that may present in the immunocompromised.
- An immunocompromised patient with a focal air space opacity is most likely to have a bacterial pneumonia (most commonly pneumococcus), but TB should also be considered if the CD4 count is low.
- In contrast, multifocal opacities have a wider differential diagnosis including *Pneumocystis* pneumonia and opportunistic fungal infection such as *Cryptococcus* or *Aspergillus*.

***Pneumocystis jiroveci* pneumonia**

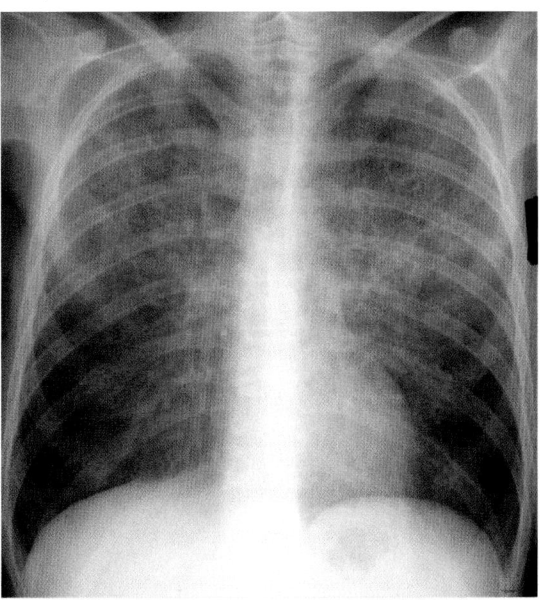

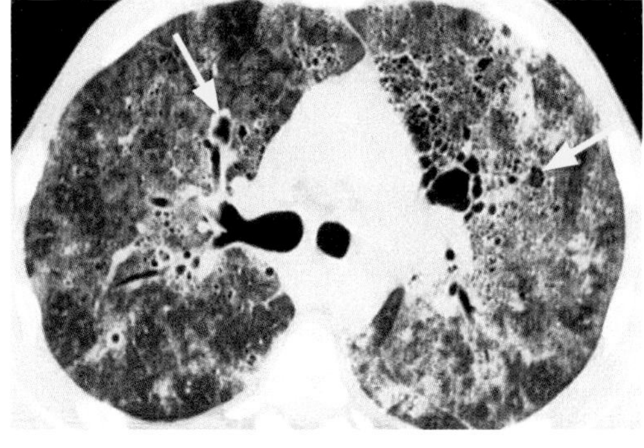

Pneumocystis pneumonia with cystic change: Radiograph (top left image) shows multiple upper-lobe predominant small nodular opacities. CT (top image) better defines the nodular opacities as being primarily centrilobular in distribution, with confluent ground glass attenuation and multiple small cysts/pneumatoceles (arrows).

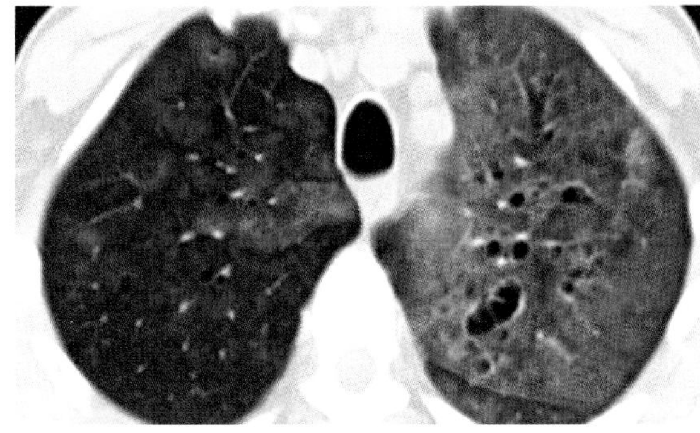

Axial CT in a different patient with *pneumocystis* pneumonia (bottom left image) shows asymmetric ground glass opacification in the left lung, with numerous thin-walled cysts. The right lung features centrilobular ground glass anteriorly.

Cases courtesy Ritu R. Gill, MD, MPH, Brigham and Women's Hospital.

- *Pneumocystis jiroveci* (previously called *Pneumocystis carinii*) is an opportunistic fungus that may cause pneumonia in individuals with CD4 counts <200 cells/cc. The incidence of *Pneumocystis* pneumonia is decreasing due to routine antibiotic prophylaxis.
- Chest radiograph findings can be normal but a classic finding of *Pneumocystis* pneumonia is **bilateral perihilar (central) airspace opacities** with peripheral sparing.
- The classic CT appearance is geometric **perihilar ground glass opacification**, sometimes with *crazy paving* (ground glass and thickening of the interlobular septa).
- A normal CT rules out *Pneumocystis* pneumonia; however, the disease can hide in a normal chest radiograph.
- *Pneumocystis* pneumonia has a propensity to cause upper lobe pneumatoceles, which may predispose to pneumothorax or pneumomediastinum.

Cryptococcus neoformans

- *Cryptococcus* is an opportunistic organism and is the most common fungal infection in AIDS patients. Pulmonary infection usually coexists with cryptococcal meningitis.

  Typically CD4 count is less than 100 cells/cc in affected individuals.

- In the immunosuppressed, *Cryptococcus* can have a wide range of appearances ranging from ground glass attenuation to focal consolidation to cavitating nodules. *Cryptococcus* can also present as miliary disease, often associated with lymphadenopathy or effusions.

Aspergillus

Overview of *Aspergillus*

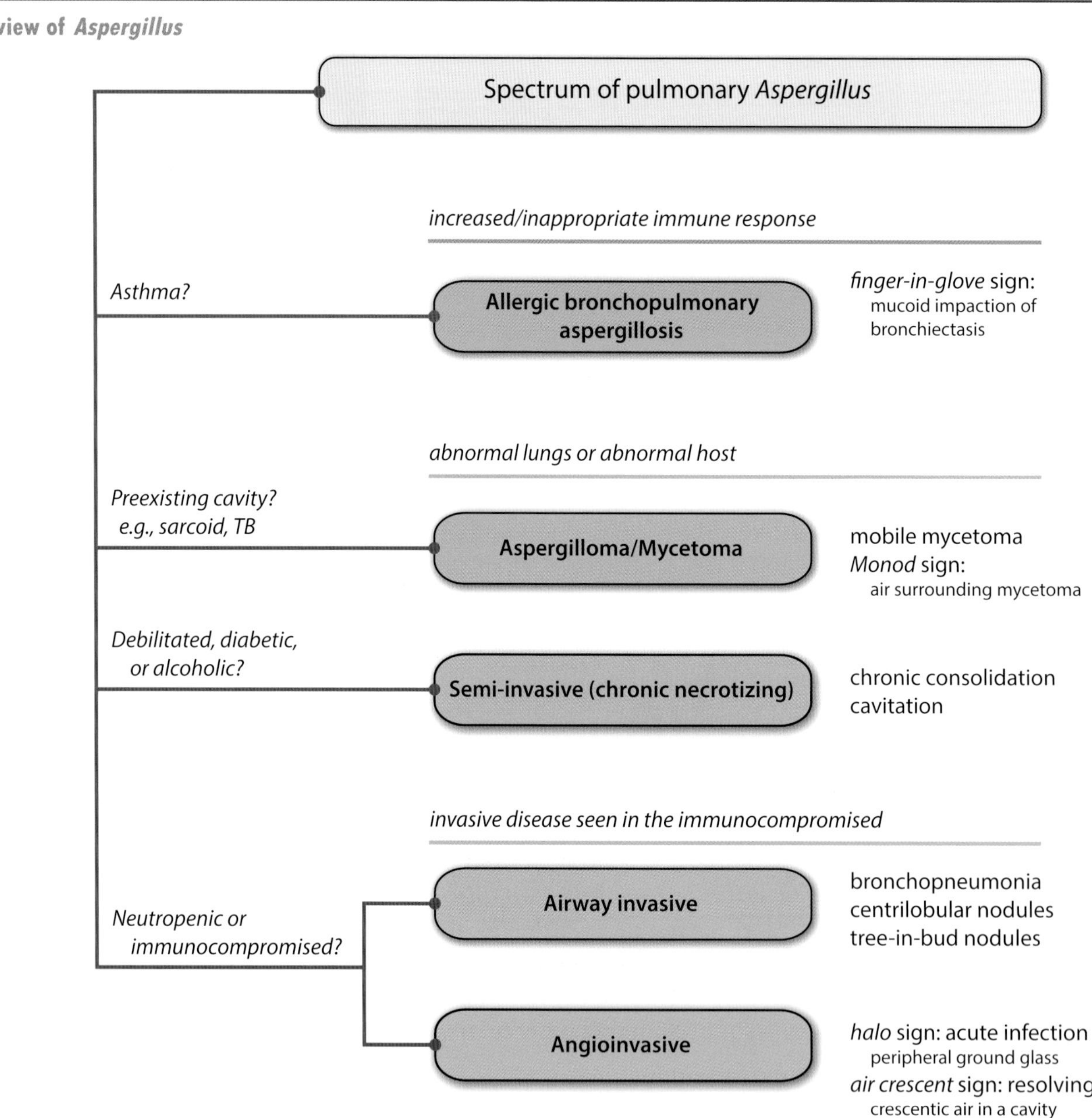

- *Aspergillus* is a ubiquitous soil fungus that manifests as five distinct categories of pulmonary disease. *Aspergillus* only affects individuals with abnormal immunity or preexisting pulmonary disease. Depending on the manifestation, the predisposing abnormality may include asthma, immunocompromised state, prior infection, or structural/congenital abnormality.

Allergic bronchopulmonary aspergillosis (ABPA)

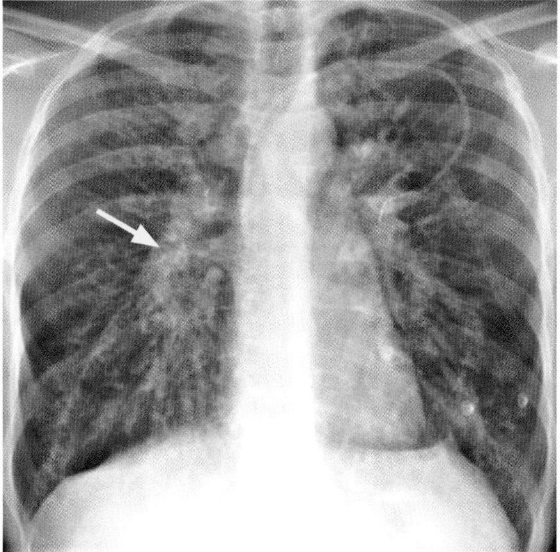
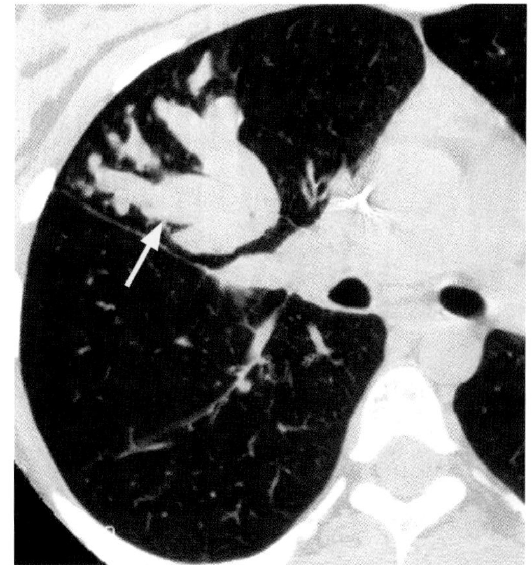

Finger-in-glove sign of ABPA: Chest radiograph shows upper-lobe predominant bronchiectasis with branching perihilar opacities most prominent on the right (arrow). CT shows dense bronchial mucoid impaction representing the *finger-in-glove* sign (arrow).

Case courtesy Ritu R. Gill, MD, MPH, Brigham and Women's Hospital.

- Allergic bronchopulmonary aspergillosis (ABPA) is a hypersensitivity reaction to aspergillus seen most commonly in patients with long-standing asthma.
- Patients present clinically with recurrent wheezing, low-grade fever, cough, and sputum production. The sputum contains fragments of aspergillus hyphae.
- The key finding on CT is upper lobe bronchiectasis and mucoid impaction, which can be high attenuation or even calcified. This combination of mucoid impaction within bronchiectatic airways represents the *finger-in-glove* sign.

  The *finger-in-glove* sign is not specific to ABPA and can also been seen in segmental bronchial atresia and many other diseases including cystic fibrosis (less commonly seen on a case-by-case basis).

Saprophytic aspergillosis (aspergilloma)

- An aspergilloma is a conglomeration of intertwined aspergillus fungal hyphae and cellular debris (a mycetoma or "fungus ball") in a *preexisting pulmonary cavity.*

  The aspergilloma is mobile and will change position when the patient is imaged in a different position.

- The most common causes of a preexisting cavity are prior tuberculosis and sarcoidosis.

  Less common causes include congenital anomalies such as bronchogenic cyst or sequestration, and post-infectious/post-traumatic pneumatocele.

- If an aspergilloma is symptomatic, hemoptysis is the most common symptom.
- When a crescent of air is seen outlining the mycetoma against the wall of the cavity, the correct term is *Monod* sign. The *air crescent* sign is reserved for angioinvasive aspergillus.

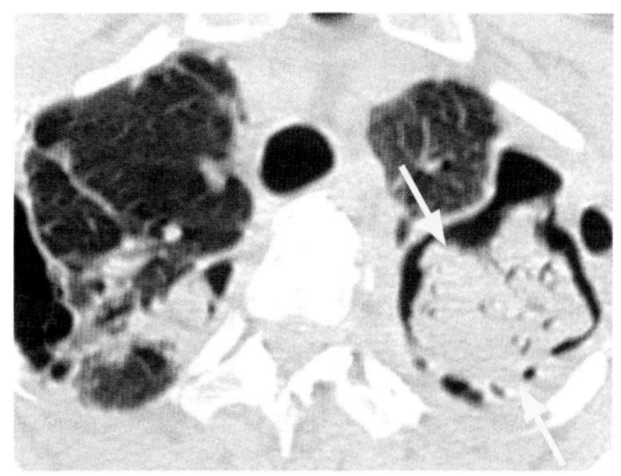

Aspergilloma and *Monod* sign: CT shows an irregular opacity (arrows) resting dependent within a left upper lobe cavity, representing an aspergilloma (arrows). The *Monod* sign is the curvilinear air surrounding the aspergilloma. This patient has prior TB with biapical scarring and prior left apical cavitation.

Case courtesy Ritu R. Gill, MD, MPH, Brigham and Women's Hospital.

Semi-invasive (chronic necrotizing) aspergillosis

- Semi-invasive aspergillosis is a necrotizing granulomatous inflammation (analogous in pathology to reactivation TB) in response to chronic aspergillus infection. Semi-invasive aspergillosis is seen in debilitated, diabetic, alcoholic, and COPD patients.
- Clinical symptoms include cough, chronic fever, and less commonly hemoptysis.
- On CT, there are segmental areas of consolidation, often with cavitation and pleural thickening, which progress slowly over months or years.

Airway-invasive aspergillosis

- Airway-invasive aspergillosis is aspergillus infection deep to the airway epithelial cells. It is seen only in the immunocompromised, including neutropenic and AIDS patients.
- The spectrum of clinical disease ranges from bronchiolitis to bronchopneumonia.
- The main CT findings of airway-invasive aspergillosis are centrilobular and tree-in-bud nodules. When bronchopneumonia is present, radiograph and CT findings are indistinguishable from other causes of bronchopneumonia, such as *Staph. aureus*.

Angioinvasive aspergillosis

- Angioinvasive aspergillosis is an aggressive infection characterized by invasion and occlusion of arterioles and smaller pulmonary arteries by fungal hyphae. Angioinvasive aspergillosis is seen almost exclusively in the severely immunocompromised, including patients on chemotherapy, stem cell or solid organ transplant recipients, and in AIDS.
- The CT *halo* sign represents a halo of ground glass attenuation surrounding a consolidation. The ground glass is thought to correspond to hemorrhagic infarction of the lung.

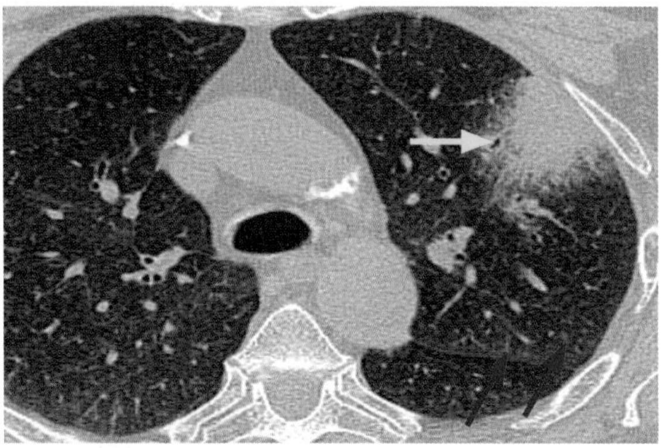

Halo sign: CT shows a left upper lobe mass with peripheral ground glass (yellow arrow), representing pulmonary hemorrhage.

There are also numerous ground glass centrilobular nodules (red arrows), likely representing bronchiolitis from superimposed airway-invasive aspergillosis.

Case courtesy Michael Hanley, MD, University of Virginia Health System.

The *halo* sign is not specific to angioinvasive aspergillosis, and can also be seen in viral infection, Wegener granulomatosis, Kaposi sarcoma, hemorrhagic metastasis, and others.

- The *air crescent* sign, visually similar to the Monod sign surrounding a mycetoma, represents a crescent of air from retraction of infarcted lung. It a good prognostic sign as it indicates that the patient is in the recovery phase.

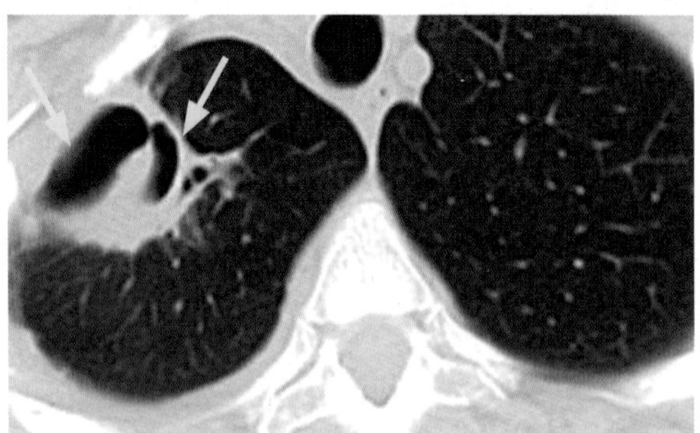

Air crescent sign: Noncontrast CT shows a cavitary lesion in the right upper lung with a crescent-shaped air collection anteriorly (arrows).

Case courtesy Ritu R. Gill, MD, MPH, Brigham and Women's Hospital.

PULMONARY EDEMA

Overview of pulmonary edema

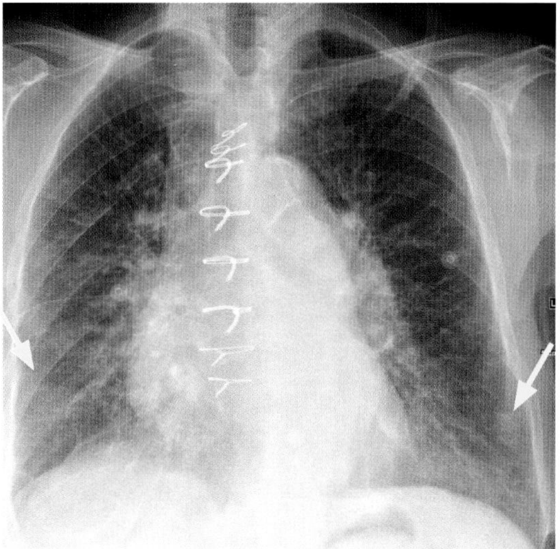

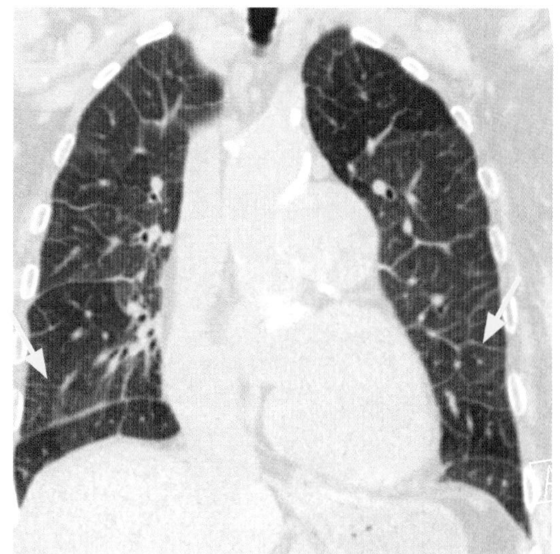

Mild pulmonary edema: Radiograph demonstrates moderate enlargement of the cardiac silhouette and sternotomy wires. There are increased interstitial markings with Kerley B lines (arrows). Chest CT shows smooth interlobular septal thickening (arrows), corresponding to the Kerley B lines seen on radiography. Mild geographic ground glass attenuation likely corresponds to early alveolar filling.

- The radiographic severity of pulmonary edema typically progresses through three stages, corresponding to progressively increased pulmonary venous pressures.
- **Vascular redistribution** is the first radiographic sign of increased pulmonary venous pressure. Imaging shows increased caliber of the upper lobe vessels compared to the lower lobe vessels.
- **Interstitial edema** is caused by increased fluid within the pulmonary veins, which surround the periphery of each hexagonal secondary pulmonary lobule. On radiography, there are increased interstitial markings, indistinctness of the pulmonary vasculature, peribronchial cuffing, and Kerley B and A lines.

  Kerley B lines are seen at the peripheral lung and represent thickened interlobular septa.

  Kerley A lines radiate outward from the hila and may represent dilation of lymphatic channels. They are not thought to be clinically relevant.
- **Alveolar edema** is caused by filling of the alveoli with fluid. On imaging, perihilar (central) opacifications are present. Pleural effusions and cardiomegaly are often present.
- CT findings of pulmonary edema include dependent ground glass opacification and interlobular septal thickening. Intrathoracic causes of pulmonary edema, such as heart failure, generally cause patchy ground glass, while systemic cause of pulmonary edema (e.g., sepsis or low protein states) often cause diffuse ground glass.
- Pulmonary edema is usually symmetric and dependent. A classic cause of asymmetric pulmonary edema is isolated right upper lobe pulmonary edema, caused by acute mitral regurgitation secondary to myocardial infarction and papillary muscle rupture.
- A complication of aggressive thoracentesis is **reexpansion pulmonary edema**, caused by rapid reexpansion of a lung in a state of collapse for more than three days.

Vascular pedicle

- The vascular pedicle is the transverse width of the upper mediastinum.

  The right border of the vascular pedicle is the interface of the superior vena cava (SVC) and the right mainstem bronchus.

  The left border of the vascular pedicle is the lateral border of the takeoff of the subclavian from the aorta.
- The vascular pedicle width is normally <58 mm.
- An interval increase in vascular pedicle width (both >63 and >70 mm have been proposed as cutoffs) on sequential supine AP ICU-type chest radiographs generally correlates with increased pulmonary capillary wedge pressure (>18 mm Hg) and fluid overload.

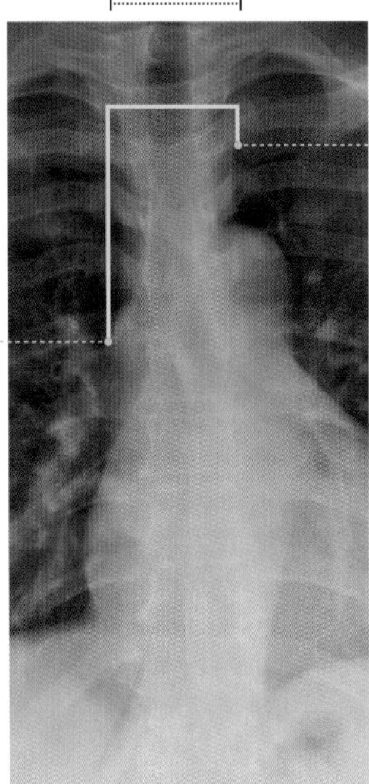

SUPPORT DEVICES

Endotracheal tube

- The endotracheal tube tip should be approximately 4–6 cm above the carina with the neck in neutral alignment. However, in situations with low pulmonary compliance (e.g., ARDS), a tip position closer to the carina may reduce barotrauma.
- Direct intubation of either the right or left mainstem bronchus (right mainstem bronchus far more common) is an emergent finding that can cause complete atelectasis of the un-intubated lung.

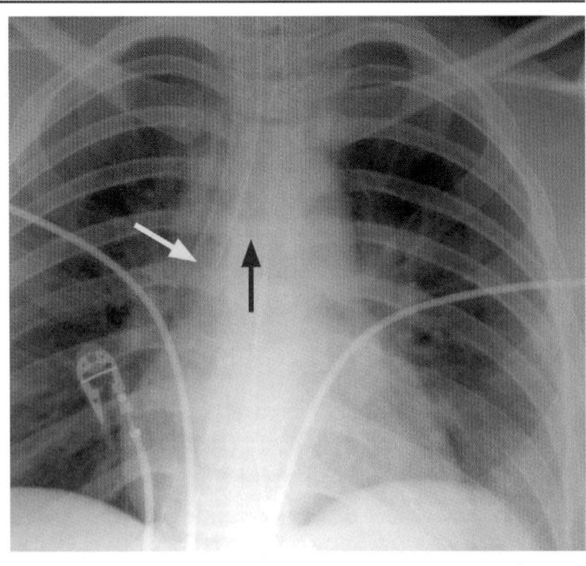

Right mainstem bronchus intubation: Chest radiograph shows the endotracheal tube terminating in the right mainstem bronchus (yellow arrow), a few centimeters distal to the carina (red arrow).

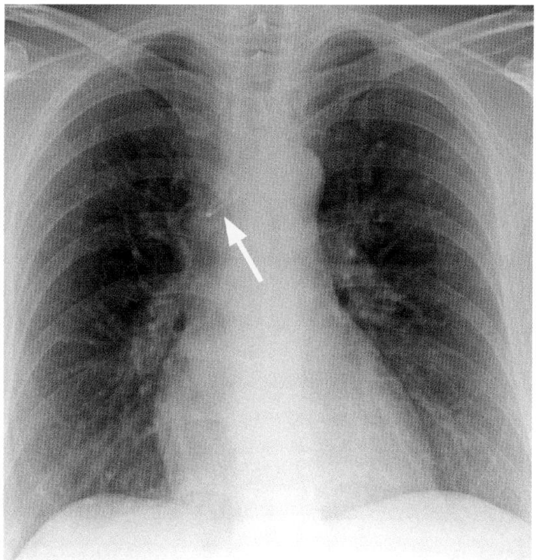

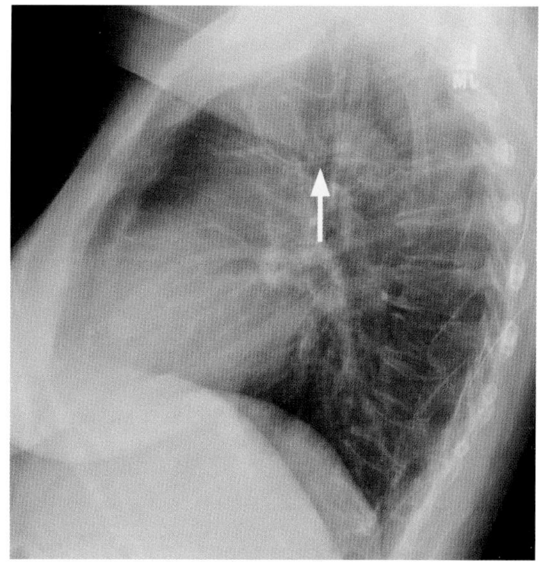

Peripherally inserted central catheter (PICC) in the azygos vein: Frontal radiograph shows a left-sided PICC coursing medially at the confluence of the brachiocephalic vein and the SVC (arrow). Lateral radiograph shows that the PICC curves anteriorly before heading inferiorly and posteriorly into the azygos vein (arrow).

Case courtesy Beatrice Trotman-Dickenson, MD, Brigham and Women's Hospital.

- The tip of a central venous catheter, including a PICC, should be in lower SVC or the cavoatrial junction. Azygos malposition is seen in approximately 1% of bedside-placed PICCs. Azygos malposition is associated with increased risk of venous perforation and catheter-associated thrombosis, and repositioning is recommended.
- A dialysis catheter should be located in the right atrium.

Pulmonary artery catheter

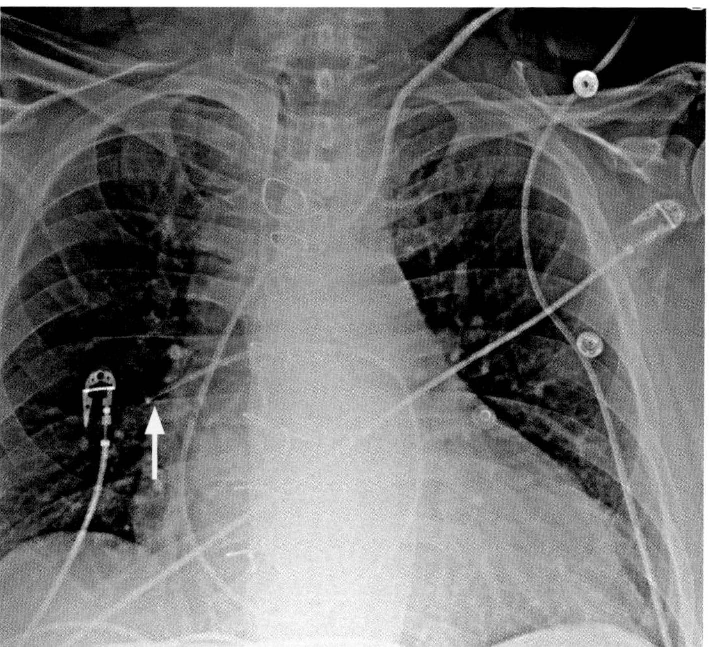

Normal position of a Swan–Ganz pulmonary artery catheter:

Chest radiograph with a sharpening filter applied shows a left internal jugular pulmonary artery catheter that takes a normal course through the SVC, right atrium, tricuspid valve, right ventricle, pulmonic valve, and finally the right pulmonary artery (arrow).

- The tip of a Swan–Ganz pulmonary artery catheter should be in either the main, right, or left pulmonary artery.
- If the tip is distal to the proximal interlobar pulmonary artery, there is a risk of pulmonary artery rupture or pseudoaneurysm. Other complications of pulmonary artery catheter placement include intracardiac catheter knot and arrhythmia.

LUNG CANCER

CLINICAL OVERVIEW OF LUNG CANCER

Epidemiology

- Lung cancer is the leading cause of cancer death in the USA.
- Including all stages and subtypes, the 5-year survival is 15%.

Risk factors for lung cancer

- Tobacco smoking is thought to cause 80–90% of lung cancers.

  Almost all cases of squamous cell and small cell carcinoma are seen in smokers.

  Adenocarcinoma is also associated with smoking, but primary bronchogenic carcinoma arising in a lifelong nonsmoker with no history of secondhand exposure is almost always adenocarcinoma.
- Occupational and environmental exposures, including beryllium, radon, arsenic, etc., remain an important risk factor for lung cancer. Asbestos exposure increases the risk of lung cancer by a factor of five, synergistic with smoking.
- Pulmonary fibrosis increases the risk of lung cancer by a factor of ten.
- Pulmonary scarring, such as from prior TB, also increases the risk of lung cancer.

SOLITARY PULMONARY NODULE

Overview of the solitary pulmonary nodule

- Pulmonary nodules are very common and the vast majority are benign; however, nodules are often followed with serial CT scans to screen for development of lung cancer.
- Calcified nodules are usually benign.
- Although less commonly seen, ground glass nodules (or mixed attenuation nodules containing both solid and ground glass) are more likely to be malignant than a solid nodule.

Nodule morphology essentially diagnostic for a benign etiology

- Central, laminar, and diffuse calcification are almost always benign.
- Popcorn calcification, suggestive of a pulmonary hamartoma, is benign.
- Intra-lesional fat, suggestive of hamartoma or lipoid granuloma, is benign.

Nodule morphology suggesting, but not diagnostic for, a benign etiology

- Small nodules are usually benign. A nodule <3 mm has a 0.2% chance of being cancer and a 4–7 mm nodule is malignant in 2.7% of cases.
- Any calcification in a small nodule is usually benign.
- Non-round shape, including oblong, polygonal, triangular, or geometric is probably benign.
- Subpleural location is often benign.
- Clustering of nodules suggests an infectious process.

Nodule morphology suggesting malignancy

- Large size is the single most important risk factor for malignancy, regardless of morphology: 0.8 to 3 cm nodules have 18% risk of being lung cancer and masses >3 cm have a very high chance of being malignant.
- Irregular edge or spiculated margin is concerning.
- Round shape (as opposed to oblong) is suggestive of malignancy.
- A cavitary nodule or nodule containing small cystic spaces is suspicious for malignancy.

Follow-up of pulmonary nodule

- Follow-up is not recommended for a solitary pulmonary nodule if the nodule is small (<4 mm) and the patient doesn't have a history of smoking or other risk factors.
- Any interval nodule growth is suspicious. A 26% increase in diameter (for instance, from 1.0 to 1.26 cm) is a doubling in volume.
  - Doubling time for lung cancers ranges from 42 days in very aggressive tumors to over 4 years in indolent lesions such as bronchioloalveolar carcinoma.
- A nodule that has not changed in size over 2 years is very likely, but not definitely, benign. Follow-up of ground glass nodules, which are often indolent bronchioloalveolar carcinoma, may be appropriate beyond 2 years.
- A decrease in size of a suspicious nodule on a single follow-up study is not sufficient to establish a benign etiology.
  - Transient decrease in size of a malignant lesion can occur with collapse of aerated alveoli or necrosis.
- The Fleischner Society (2005) suggests the following follow-up recommendations for noncalcified nodules in patients older than 35 without a history of malignancy. A high-risk patient is defined as a patient with a history of smoking or other risk factors for lung cancer.
  - Nodule ≤4 mm
    - Low-risk: No follow-up needed.
    - High-risk: At least one follow-up at 12 months. If unchanged, no further follow-up.
  - Nodule >4 and ≤6 mm
    - Low-risk: At least one follow-up at 12 months. If unchanged, no further follow-up.
    - High-risk: At least two follow-ups at 6–12 months and 18–24 months if no change.
  - Nodule >6 and ≤8 mm
    - Low-risk: At least two follow-ups at 6–12 months and 18–24 months if no change.
    - High-risk: At least three follow-ups at 3–6 months, 9–12, and 24 months if no change.
  - Nodule >8 mm
    - Regardless of risk, either PET, biopsy, or at least three follow-ups at 3, 9, and 24 months.

Histologic subtypes of lung cancer

- Lung cancer can be thought of as two types: "Small cell" and all other histologic types that are not small cell, such as adenocarcinoma, squamous cell carcinoma, etc. However, although previously small cell and non-small cell used separate staging systems, the 2009 staging revision unifies the staging of all types.
- Small cell is usually disseminated at diagnosis and has a much worse prognosis.

Adenocarcinoma

- Adenocarcinoma is the most common subtype of lung cancer. It is related to smoking, but less strongly than squamous cell.
- Adenocarcinoma tends to occur in the peripheral lung.
- The typical radiographic appearance of adenocarcinoma is of a pulmonary nodule, which often has a spiculated margin due to reactive fibrosis.
- Cavitation can occur but is less commonly seen compared to squamous cell.
- A useful pathologic marker is TTF-1 (thyroid transcription factor), which is positive in primary lung adenocarcinoma and negative in pulmonary metastases from an extrathoracic adenocarcinoma.

Squamous cell carcinoma (SCC)

- Squamous cell carcinoma (SCC) is slightly less common today than adenocarcinoma. Prior to filtered cigarettes, SCC was more common.
- The majority of SCC arise centrally from main, lobar, or segmental bronchi, where the tumor tends to cause symptoms early due to bronchial obstruction. SCC may also present as a hilar mass.
- Common radiographic findings are lobar atelectasis, mucoid impaction, consolidation, and bronchiectasis. SCC has a propensity to cavitate.

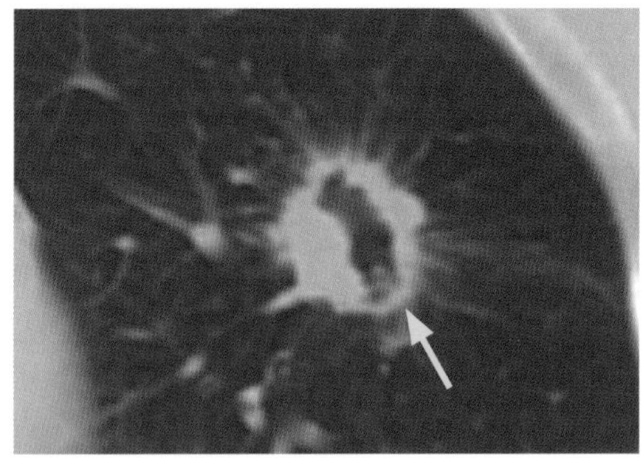

SCC: Axial CT shows a spiculated cavitary lesion (arrow) shown at pathology to be squamous cell carcinoma.

Bronchioloalveolar carcinoma (BAC)

- Bronchioloalveolar carcinoma (BAC) refers to a spectrum of well-differentiated adenocarcinoma that demonstrates *lepidic* growth. The hallmark of lepidic growth is a spreading of malignant cells using the alveolar walls as a scaffold.

  The opposite of *lepidic* growth is *hilic* growth, demonstrated by most other forms of lung cancer, which describes cancer growth by invasion and destruction of lung parenchyma.

- A spectrum of lesions have been called BAC ranging from small peripheral tumors with 100% survival to lesions causing widespread advanced disease. Despite this variability, BAC is most commonly indolent and is often negative on PET.
- To create more uniformity in the pathological, clinical, and research domains, a new classification for the spectrum of the adenocarcinoma subtypes formerly called BAC has recently been proposed. This classification is primarily based on the pathology of the lesion and differentiation of these entities on imaging is difficult. In clinical radiologic practice, this spectrum of lesions is routinely still referred to as BAC. This textbook will continue the common practice and refer to these lesions as BAC.

Adenomatous hyperplasia (AAH): A precursor lesion. **Adenocarcinoma in situ**: A preinvasive lesion. **Minimally invasive adenocarcinoma**.	**Adenocarcinoma, predominantly invasive with some nonmucinous lepidic component:** Formerly nonmucinous BAC. **Invasive mucinous adenocarcinoma:** Formerly mucinous BAC. Nonmucinous and mucinous subtypes of BAC occur with approximately equal prevalence.

- **Nonmucinous BAC** (*adenocarcinoma, predominantly invasive with some nonmucinous lepidic component*) classically presents as a ground glass or solid nodule with air bronchograms and has a better prognosis compared to the mucinous subtype.

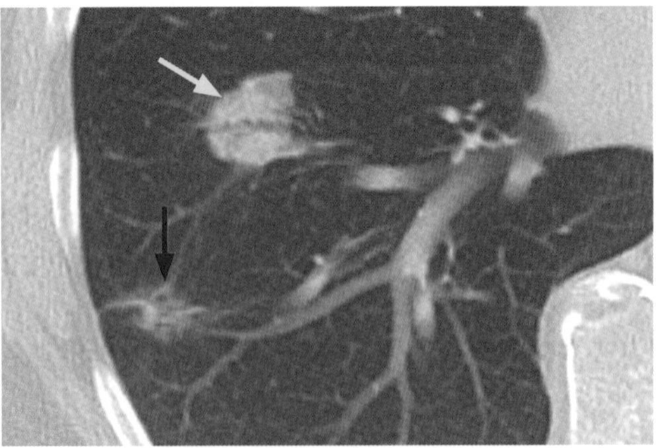

Nonmucinous BAC (multifocal): Axial CT shows a solid nodule with air bronchograms (yellow arrow) and a more peripheral ground glass nodule (red arrow).

- **Mucinous BAC** (*invasive mucinous adenocarcinoma)* tends to present with chronic consolidation. It has a worse prognosis compared with non-mucinous BAC.

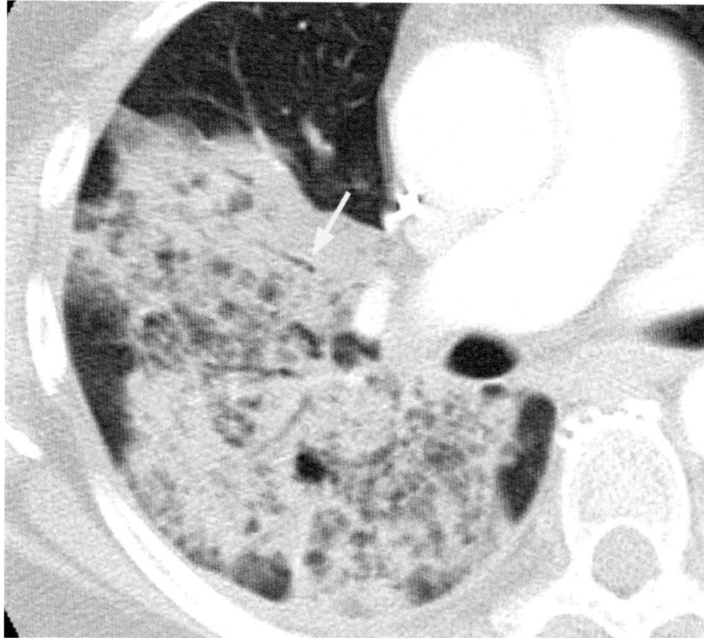

Mucinous BAC: Axial contrast-enhanced CT shows a right lower lobe consolidative opacity with air bronchograms (arrow).

Mucinous BAC is an important differential consideration for chronic ground glass or consolidation, often with air bronchograms.

The *CT angiogram* sign (not imaged above) describes the especially prominent appearance of enhancing pulmonary vessels seen in a low attenuation, mucin-rich consolidation of mucinous BAC.

Small cell carcinoma

- Small cell carcinoma is the third most common lung cancer cell type (after adenocarcinoma and squamous cell). Neoplastic cells are of neuroendocrine origin and are associated with various paraneoplastic syndromes.
- Small cell carcinoma is strongly associated with smoking.
- Small cell tends to occur in central bronchi with invasion through the bronchial wall, typically presenting as a large hilar or parahilar mass. Involvement of the SVC may cause SVC syndrome. Small cell rarely presents as a solitary pulmonary nodule.
- Small cell is considered a disseminated disease and is generally not amenable to surgery.

Large cell carcinoma

- Large cell carcinoma is a wastebasket pathologic diagnosis for tumors that are not squamous, adenocarcinoma, or small cell. Large cell carcinoma is strongly associated with smoking and has a poor prognosis.
- Large cell carcinoma often occurs in the lung periphery, where it presents as a large mass.

Carcinoid tumor

- Neoplastic carcinoid cells originate from neuroendocrine cells in the bronchial walls.
- A common presentation of carcinoid is an endobronchial mass distal to the carina, which may cause obstructive atelectasis. Up to 20% of cases present as a pulmonary nodule.
- Carcinoid may be typical (low-grade) or the more aggressive atypical variant. Typical carcinoids without nodal or distant metastases have an excellent prognosis (92% 5-year survival). Atypical carcinoids tend to arise peripherally and have a worse prognosis.
- Diffuse idiopathic pulmonary neuroendocrine cell hyperplasia (DIPNECH) is an extremely uncommon precursor lesion to typical carcinoid tumor, characterized by multiple foci of neuroendocrine hyperplasia or tumorlets (carcinoid foci <5 mm in size) and bronchiolitis obliterans.

Solitary pulmonary nodule or lung mass

- A nodule is defined as <3 cm and a mass is >3 cm.
- Adenocarcinoma, including subtypes formerly called BAC, comprises approximately 50% of cancers presenting as a solitary pulmonary nodule.

Segmental or lobar atelectasis

- Atelectasis due to bronchial obstruction is a common presentation of lung cancer.
- Despite the presence of atelectasis, volume loss is variable, secondary to the volume-displacing effects of desquamated cells, mucus, and fluid.
- Obstructive pneumonia is a common presentation of lung cancer, caused by bronchial obstruction and parenchymal consolidation by inflammatory cells and lipid-laden macrophages.
- If two foci of atelectasis are present simultaneously that cannot be explained by a single endobronchial lesion, a benign process is much more likely. However, CT and bronchoscopy are still needed for workup.

Consolidation

- Consolidation that is indistinguishable from pneumonia can be seen with BAC (mucinous subtype). Although BAC and pneumonia may appear similar, BAC is usually a non-resolving consolidation with (near) normal white blood cell count.

Hilar mass

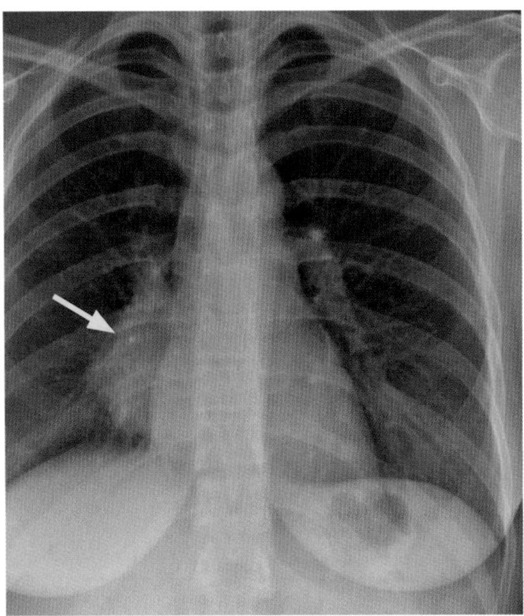

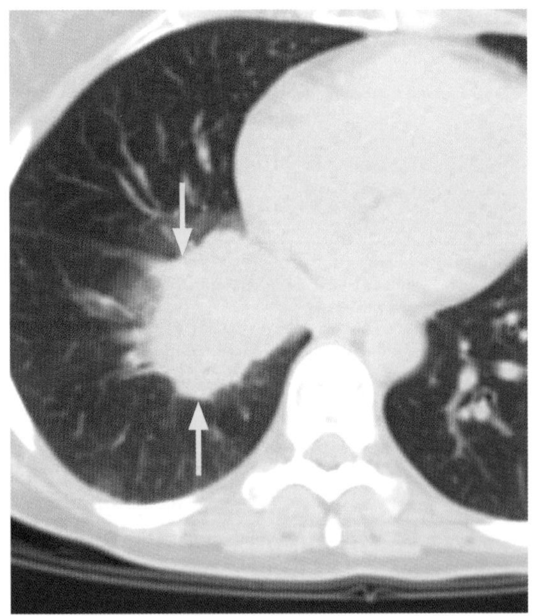

Lung cancer presenting as a hilar mass: Frontal radiograph (left image) shows a right paramediastinal opacity (arrow), which does not silhouette the right heart border. CT shows a large right infrahilar mass (arrows).

- A hilar mass is a common presentation of squamous cell and small cell carcinoma.
- Hilar enlargement may be due to a primary central tumor or nodal metastasis from a parenchymal neoplasm.
- Tumor may compress and narrow the bronchus. A tapered bronchus is highly specific for lung cancer.

Superior sulcus tumor

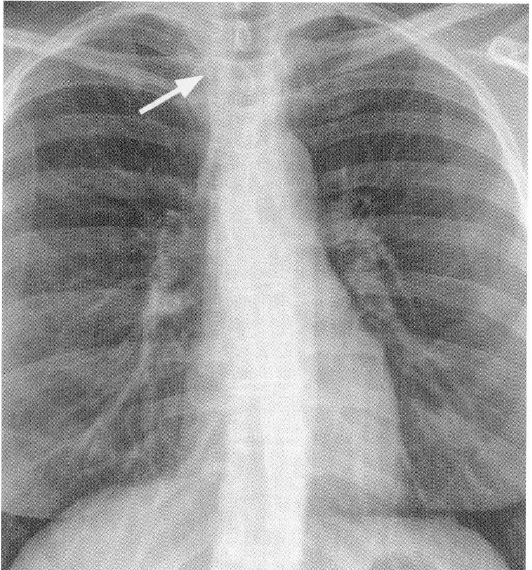

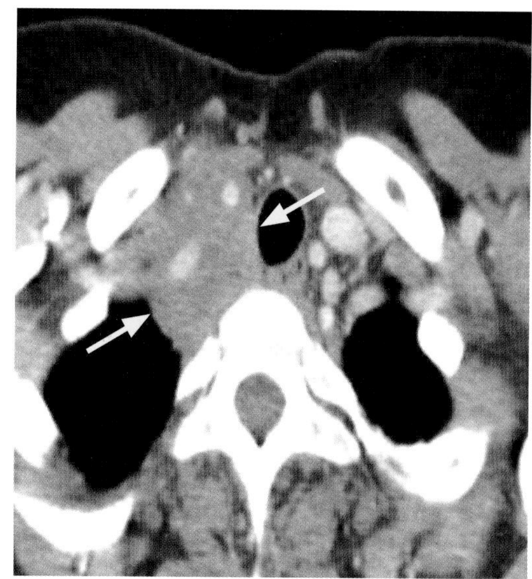

Superior sulcus tumor: Chest radiograph shows nearly imperceptible increased opacity in the right apex (arrow). A superior sulcus mass is clearly evident on CT (arrows), with encasement of the vasculature and effacement of the superior mediastinal fat.

Case courtesy Ritu R. Gill, MD, MPH, Brigham and Women's Hospital.

- A superior sulcus tumor is a lung cancer occurring in the lung apex.
- A Pancoast tumor is a type of superior sulcus tumor with involvement of the sympathetic ganglia causing a Horner syndrome, with ipsilateral ptosis, miosis, and anhidrosis.
- A superior sulcus tumor is a stage T3 tumor. The staging of lung cancer is subsequently discussed.

Lymphangitic carcinomatosis

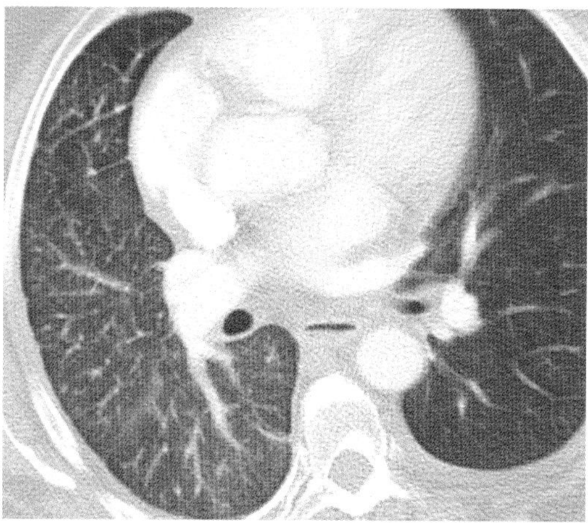

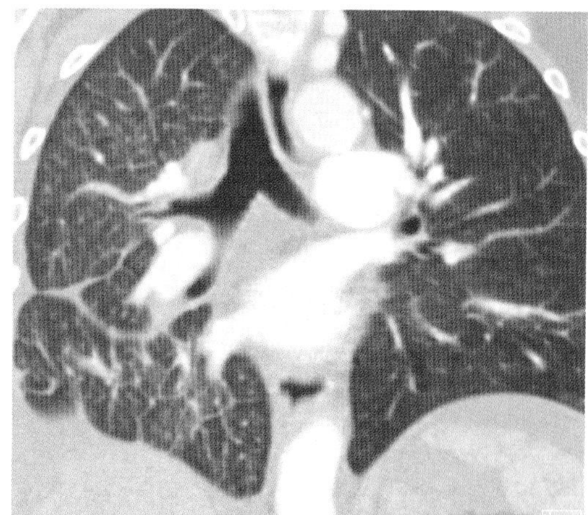

Lymphangitic carcinomatosis: Axial (left image) and coronal CT shows asymmetric, nodular septal thickening of the right lung in a patient with metastatic uterine sarcoma. Aside from a trace effusion, the left lung is clear.

Case courtesy Ritu R. Gill, MD, MPH, Brigham and Women's Hospital.

- Lymphangitic carcinomatosis represents diffuse spread of neoplasm through the pulmonary lymphatics, typically seen in late-stage disease.
- On imaging, carcinomatosis manifests as nodular interlobular septal thickening, which is usually asymmetric.

Pleural effusion

- Pleural effusions are relatively common in lung cancer, and may be due to lymphatic obstruction or pleural metastases.
- A *malignant* effusion is the presence of malignant cells within the effusion. A malignant effusion is an M1a lesion, which precludes curative resection. Not all effusions associated with lung cancer are malignant effusions, so cytologic evaluation is necessary.

Pneumothorax

- Pneumothorax is not a common presentation of lung cancer, but can be seen with peripheral tumors that cavitate or invade into the pleura.

STAGING OF LUNG CANCER

Overview of lung cancer staging

- The 7th edition of the TNM system, published in 2009, is based on data collected on over 100,000 patients with lung cancer from 1990 to 2000.
- Staging of small cell lung cancer was previously simplified to "limited-stage" or "extensive-stage." The new 7th TNM system, however, recommends that the same TNM staging system be used for both small cell and non-small cell lung cancer.

Stage	T	N	M
IA	Up to T1b	N0	M0
IB	T2a	N0	M0
IIA	Up to T2a (or T2b if N0)	N1	M0
IIB	T2b (or T3 if N0)	N1	M0
IIIA	Up to T3 (or T4 if N0–1)	N2	M0
IIIB	Any T (or T4 if N2)	N3	M0
IV	Any T	Any N	**M1a** or **M1b**

Treatment based on staging

- For early stages up to IIB and sometimes IIIA, surgery is usually performed. Neoadjuvant or adjuvant chemotherapy and radiotherapy can be used.
- Stage IIIB (N3 - contralateral or supraclavicular nodes; or T4/N2) is unresectable.
- Stage IV disease is generally not treated surgically unless there is a solitary adrenal or brain metastasis.

T (tumor)

- T1: Tumor ≤3 cm surrounded by lung or visceral pleura.

  T1a: Tumor ≤2 cm; 5-year survival rate 77%; T1b: >2 and ≤3 cm; 5-year survival rate 71%.
- T2: Tumor >3 cm and ≤7 cm, or local invasion of the visceral pleura, or endobronchial lesions >2 cm from the carina.

  T2a: >3 and ≤5 cm; 5-year survival rate 58%; T2b: >5 and ≤7 cm; 5-year survival rate 49%.
- T3: Tumor >7 cm, or local invasion of chest wall, diaphragm, pleura, or superior sulcus tumor, or endobronchial lesion <2 cm from carina.

  T3: 5-year survival rate 35%.

  T3: Separate tumor nodule in the same lobe; 5-year survival rate 28%.
- T4: Separate tumor nodule in a different lobe in the ipsilateral lung, or tumor of any size with invasion of mediastinal structures including carina, heart, great vessels, or vertebral bodies.

  T4: 5-year survival rate 22%.

N (nodes)

- The color coding of the lymph nodes on the diagram below represents the nodal staging of lung cancer for an example left-sided mass:

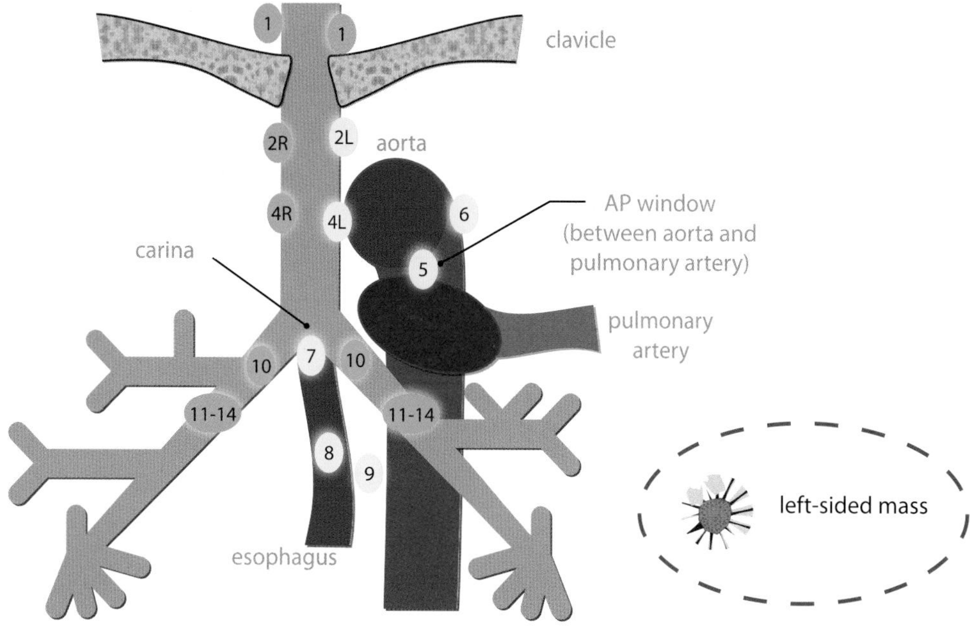

N1: ipsilateral hilar nodes and intrapulmonary nodes
10 - hilar
11 - interlobar (adjacent to interlobar bronchi)
12 - lobar (adjacent to lobar bronchi)
13 - segmental
14 - subsegmental

N2: ipsilateral mediastinal nodes
2 - upper paratracheal
3 - prevascular (anterior to aorta, not shown)
4 - paratracheal
5 - subaortic (AP window)
6 - paraaortic
7 - subcarinal
8 - paraesophageal
9 - pulmonary ligament

N3: 1 - supraclavicular nodes (any side)
any contralateral node

- the boundary between right and left for level 2 and 4 lymph nodes is set as the left lateral border of the trachea due to flow of lymphatic drainage
- in this example of a left-sided primary, the right-sided nodes are drawn in orange to demonstrate N3 due to contralaterality

- N0: No lymph node metastases.
- N1: Ipsilateral hilar or intrapulmonary lymph nodes.
- N2: Ipsilateral mediastinal nodes.
- N3: Contralateral lymph nodes or supraclavicular nodes on either side.

M (metastasis)

- M0: No metastatic disease.
- M1a: Local thoracic metastatic disease.

  Separate tumor nodule in contralateral lung; 5-year survival rate 3%.

  Malignant pleural or pericardial effusion; 5-year survival rate 2%.

- M1b: Distant or extrathoracic metastatic disease.

  Median survival 6 months. *1-year* survival rate 22%.

Example staging: Stage IIIA

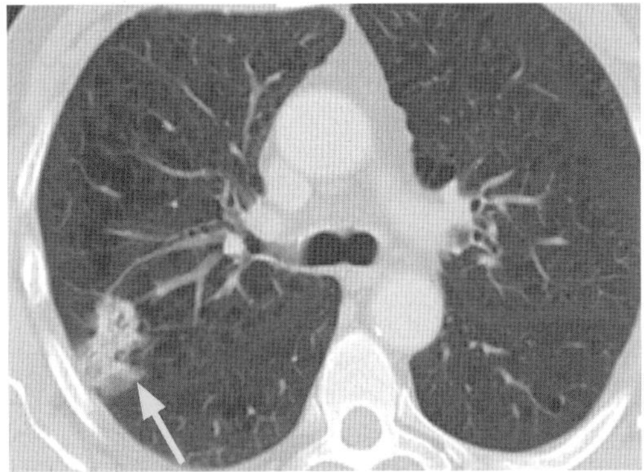

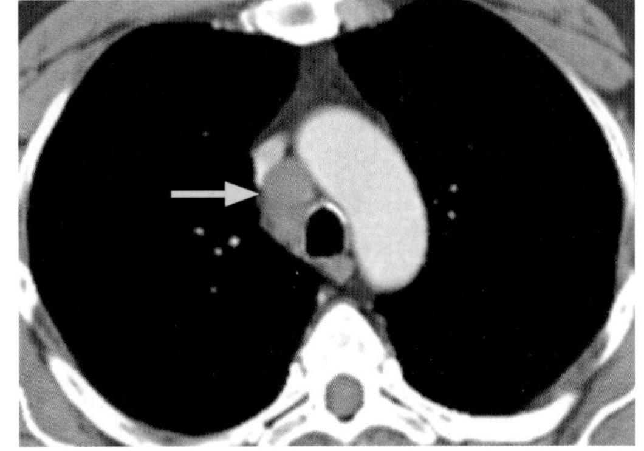

Stage IIIA lung cancer: Axial CT in lung windows (left image) shows a right upper lobe peripheral mass (arrow) that abuts the pleura. There is diffuse centrilobular emphysema. Soft-tissue window CT shows ipsilateral right paratracheal adenopathy (arrow). The T staging is T2 (both for size >3 cm and invasion of pleura) and the N staging is N2 for ipsilateral mediastinal nodes. The overall stage is therefore IIIA and this tumor is resectable.

Case courtesy Ritu R. Gill, MD, MPH, Brigham and Women's Hospital.

Example staging: Stage IV

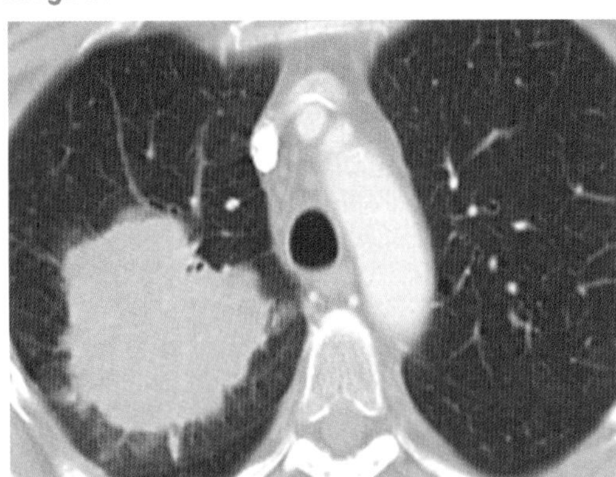

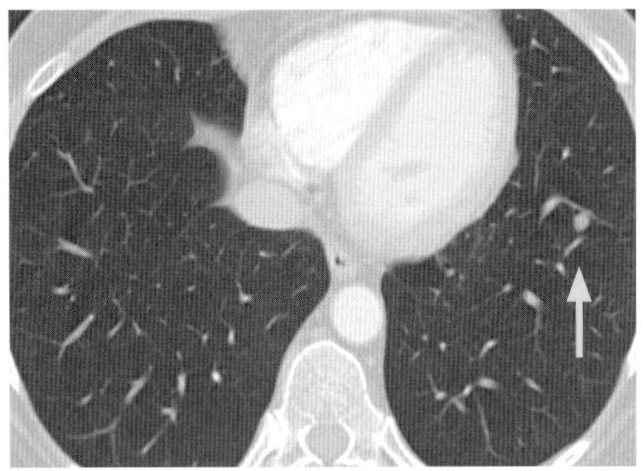

Stage IV lung cancer: Axial CT (left image) shows a dominant, spiculated right upper lobe T2 mass. More inferiorly (right image), a small contralateral nodule (arrow) is present. This nodule was determined to be malignant on follow-up, for an M staging of M1a and stage IV disease.

Case courtesy Ritu R. Gill, MD, MPH, Brigham and Women's Hospital.

Example staging: Stage IV

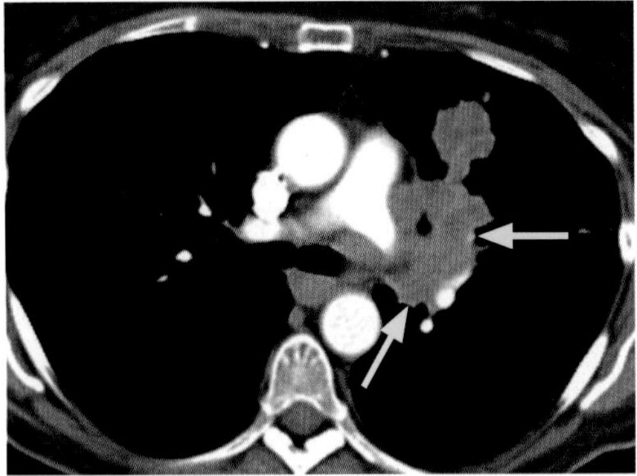

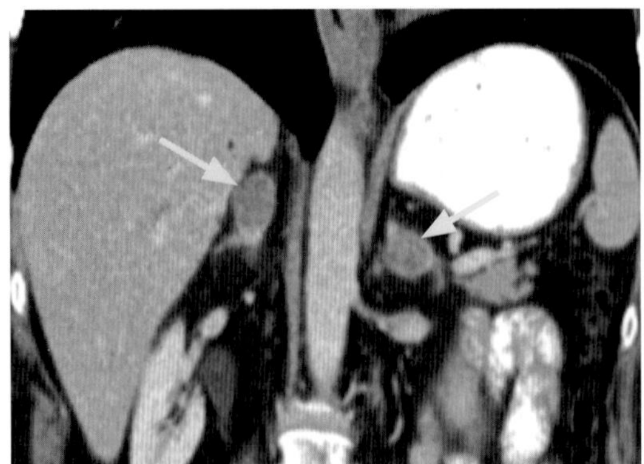

Stage IV lung cancer: Axial CT (left image) shows a left upper lobe mass with ipsilateral hilar adenopathy (arrows). Coronal CT through the upper abdomen shows bilateral adrenal masses (arrows), which were confirmed to be metastases (M1b), representing stage IV disease.

Case courtesy Ritu R. Gill, MD, MPH, Brigham and Women's Hospital.

PULMONARY VASCULAR DISEASE

PULMONARY HYPERTENSION

Definition of pulmonary hypertension

- Clinically, the term *pulmonary hypertension* is used to encompass both pulmonary arterial and pulmonary venous hypertension. The term *pulmonary arterial hypertension* (PAH) is generally reserved for the WHO class 1 entities, discussed below.
- It may be clinically difficult to distinguish pulmonary arterial from pulmonary venous hypertension. Further complicating the distinction, venous hypertension may be a cause of arterial hypertension.
- Pulmonary arterial hypertension is defined as pulmonary arterial systolic pressure ≥25 mm Hg at rest or ≥30 mm Hg during exercise.
- Elevated pulmonary venous pressures are present when pulmonary capillary wedge pressure (an approximation of pulmonary venous pressure) is ≥18 mm Hg.

Overview of pulmonary hypertension classification

- There are a number of causes of pulmonary hypertension including chronic thromboembolic disease, chronic respiratory disease, chronic heart disease, and idiopathic causes.
- The classification in widest use in the radiology literature is the hemodynamic division of precapillary and postcapillary etiologies.

> In **precapillary causes** of pulmonary hypertension, the primary abnormality is either the pulmonary arterial system or pulmonary arterial blood flow. Abnormalities of the pulmonary parenchyma leading to chronic alveolar hypoxia are also included in this category.
>
> In **postcapillary causes** of pulmonary hypertension, an abnormality of the pulmonary veins or elevation of pulmonary venous pressure leads to pulmonary arterial hypertension.

- In contrast, the World Health Organization (WHO) clinical classification, based on the 2003 World Symposium on Pulmonary Hypertension, describes five groups of pulmonary hypertension based on etiology. There is no correlation between the pre/postcapillary classification and the WHO classification, and in fact there can be both pre- and postcapillary etiologies within a single WHO group.

> Group 1: **Pulmonary arterial hypertension** (PAH).
>
> Primary pulmonary hypertension (PPH) may be idiopathic or familial.
>
> Congenital left-to-right shunts, such as atrial septal defect (ASD) and ventricular septal defect (VSD), may cause PAH and shunt reversal (Eisenmenger syndrome).
>
> PAH may be caused by pulmonary venous or capillary involvement, such as pulmonary veno-occlusive disease and pulmonary capillary hemangiomatosis.
>
> Group 2: **Pulmonary venous hypertension**.
>
> Left-sided heart disease (left atrial, left ventricular, or mitral/aortic valve disease) may cause elevated pulmonary venous pressure in chronic disease.
>
> Group 3: **Pulmonary hypertension associated with chronic hypoxemia**.
>
> COPD, interstitial lung disease, and sleep apnea can cause pulmonary hypertension in chronic disease.
>
> Group 4: **Pulmonary hypertension due to chronic thromboembolic disease**.
>
> Group 5: **Pulmonary hypertension due to miscellaneous disorders**.
>
> Sarcoidosis is a rare cause of pulmonary hypertension.
>
> Compression of pulmonary vessels, which can be due to neoplasm, fibrosing mediastinitis, etc., may cause pulmonary hypertension.

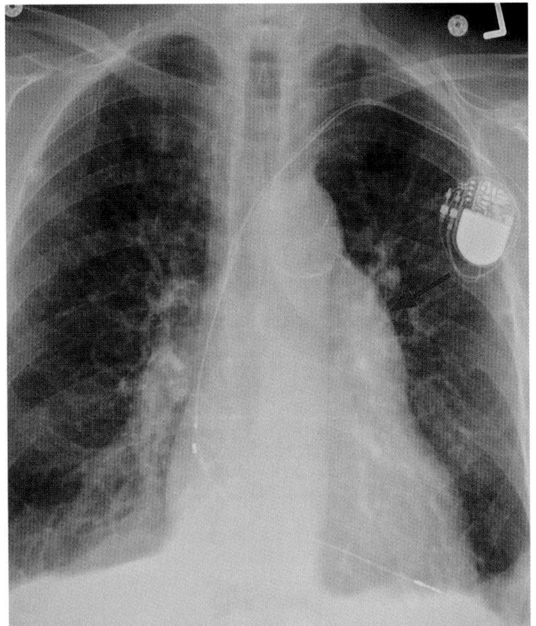

Pulmonary hypertension:

Chest radiograph shows an abnormal convex mediastinal bulge representing an enlarged main pulmonary artery (red arrow).

Noncontrast CT (bottom left image) and gated contrast-enhanced cardiac CT (bottom right image) show that the pulmonary arterial plaque has both calcified (arrow in noncontrast image) and noncalcified (arrow in contrast-enhanced image) components. The diameter of the main pulmonary artery (PA) is clearly larger than that of the aortic root, suggesting pulmonary hypertension.

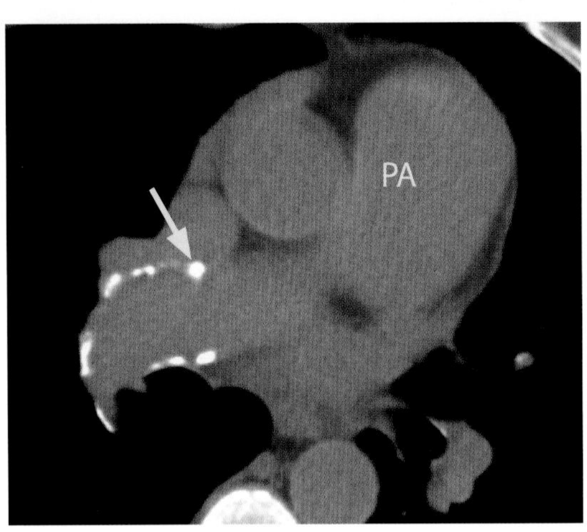

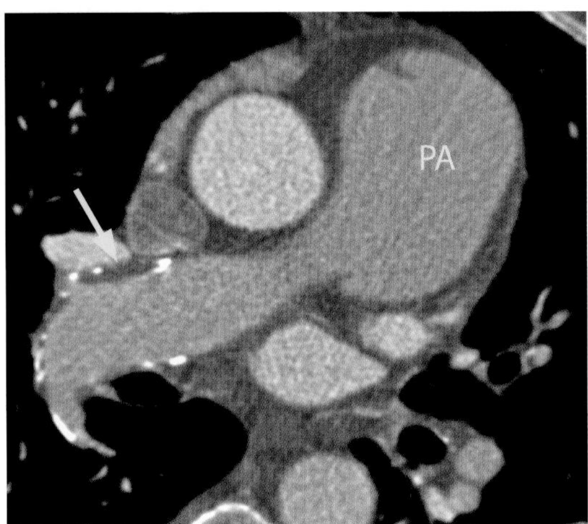

- A main pulmonary artery diameter ≥2.9 cm suggests the presence of pulmonary hypertension, although pulmonary hypertension may be present in a normal caliber pulmonary artery. A main pulmonary artery diameter larger than the aortic root diameter is also suggestive of pulmonary hypertension.
- Pulmonary artery calcifications are pathognomonic for chronic pulmonary artery hypertension.
- Pulmonary hypertension may cause mosaic attenuation due to perfusion abnormalities, most commonly seen in chronic thromboembolic pulmonary hypertension (CTEPH).
- Pulmonary hypertension may be associated with ground glass centrilobular nodules, especially in pulmonary veno-occlusive disease.
- An enlarged pulmonary artery can mimic a mediastinal mass. The *hilum convergence* sign is helpful to confirm that the apparent "mass" in fact represents the pulmonary artery. The *hilum convergence* sign describes the appearance of hilar pulmonary artery branches converging into an enlarged pulmonary artery.
- In contrast, the *hilum overlay* sign describes the visualization of hilar vessels through a mass. It indicates that a mediastinal mass is present, which cannot be in the middle mediastinum. Usually this means the mass is in the anterior mediastinum.

Primary pulmonary hypertension (PPH) – WHO group 1, precapillary

- The pathologic hallmark of primary pulmonary hypertension (PPH) is the *plexiform lesion* in the wall of the muscular arteries, which is a focal disruption of the elastic lamina by an obstructing plexus of endothelial channels. There is a relative paucity of prostacyclins and nitric oxide expressed by endothelial cells.
- PPH may be idiopathic (females > males) or familial (approximately 10% of cases).
- On imaging, there is typically enlargement of the main pulmonary arteries with rapidly tapering peripheral vessels.

Pulmonary hypertension due to left-to-right cardiac shunts – WHO group 1, precapillary

- Congenital left-to-right cardiac shunts, such as ventricular septal defect (VSD), atrial septal defect (ASD), and partial anomalous pulmonary venous return, cause increased flow through the pulmonary arterial bed. This chronically increased flow may eventually lead to irreversible vasculopathy characterized by pulmonary hypertension and reversal of the congenital shunt, known as Eisenmenger syndrome.
- Imaging of PAH secondary to a congenital shunt is similar to that of PPH. There is enlargement of the central and main pulmonary arteries, with peripheral tapering.

Pulmonary veno-occlusive disease – WHO group 1, postcapillary

- PAH secondary to pulmonary veno-occlusive disease is caused by fibrotic obliteration of the pulmonary veins and venules. Pulmonary veno-occlusive disease may be idiopathic but is associated with pregnancy, drugs (especially bleomycin), and bone marrow transplant.
- Imaging features pulmonary arterial enlargement. Pulmonary edema and ground glass centrilobular nodules are often present.

Pulmonary venous hypertension – WHO group 2, postcapillary

- Left-sided cardiovascular disease leads to elevated pulmonary venous pressure, which is a cause of pulmonary hypertension.
- Any left-sided lesion may cause pulmonary venous hypertension, including left ventricular outflow tract lesions, mitral stenosis, and obstructing intra-atrial tumor/thrombus.

Pulmonary hypertension associated with hypoxemic lung disease – WHO group 3, precapillary

- COPD, sleep apnea, and interstitial lung disease can all lead to pulmonary hypertension.
- Chronic hypoxic vasoconstriction is thought to invoke vascular remodeling leading to hypertrophy of pulmonary arterial vascular smooth muscle and intimal thickening.
- Chronic lung disease can further contribute to obliteration of pulmonary microvasculature through emphysema and the perivascular fibrotic changes of pulmonary fibrosis.

Chronic thromboembolic pulmonary hypertension (CTEPH) – WHO group 4, precapillary

- Chronic occlusion of the pulmonary arterial bed can lead to pulmonary arterial hypertension, which is a complication affecting 1–5% of patients who develope acute pulmonary embolism (PE). Due to the high prevalence of PE, a PE-protocol CT is typically the first step in workup of newly diagnosed pulmonary hypertension.
- Characteristic imaging features are peripheral, eccentric filling defects (in contrast to acute emboli which tend to be central) in the pulmonary arterial tree. Fibrous strands are sometimes visible on cross-sectional imaging. Mosaic perfusion may be present.
- CTEPH may cause secondary corkscrew bronchial arteries that are tortuous and dilated.
- Treatment of CTEPH is surgical thromboendarterectomy (similar to carotid endarterectomy).

Fibrosing mediastinitis – WHO group 5, postcapillary

- Progressive proliferation of fibrous tissue within the mediastinum may lead to encasement and compression of mediastinal structures. The most common causes of fibrosing mediastinitis are histoplasmosis and tuberculosis.
- Fibrous encasement of the pulmonary veins leads to permanent histological changes within the endothelial cells.
- Fibrosing mediastinitis may also encase the pulmonary arteries, creating a pre-capillary pulmonary hypertension.
- Imaging features of fibrosing mediastinitis include increased mediastinal soft tissue, often with calcified lymph nodes due to prior granulomatous infection.

Pulmonary embolism (PE)

Clinical diagnosis

- Diagnosis of pulmonary embolism (PE) can be challenging because the presenting symptoms are both common and nonspecific, including dyspnea, tachycardia, and pleuritic chest pain.
- Most pulmonary emboli originate in the deep veins of the thighs and pelvis. The risk factors for deep venous thrombosis are widely prevalent in a hospital environment, including:

  Immobilization, malignancy, catheter use, obesity, oral contraceptive use, and thrombophilia.

  Approximately 25% of patients with PE don't have any identifiable risk factor.
- The Wells score assigns point values to clinical suspicion and various symptoms suggestive of pulmonary embolism.
- D-dimer is sensitive for thromboembolic disease and has a high negative predictive value, but is of little value in the typical inpatient population as there are many false positives.

Imaging of pulmonary embolism

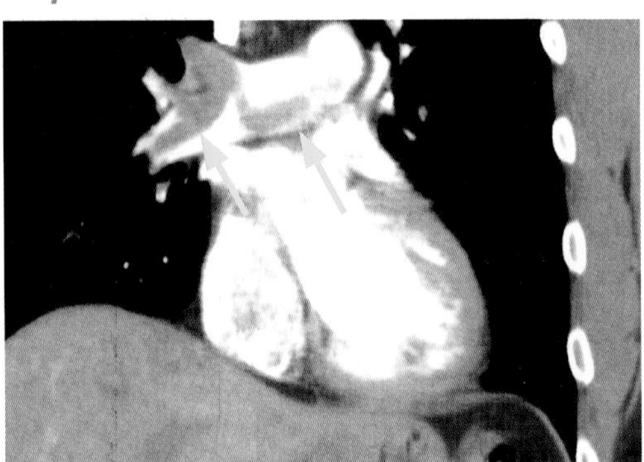

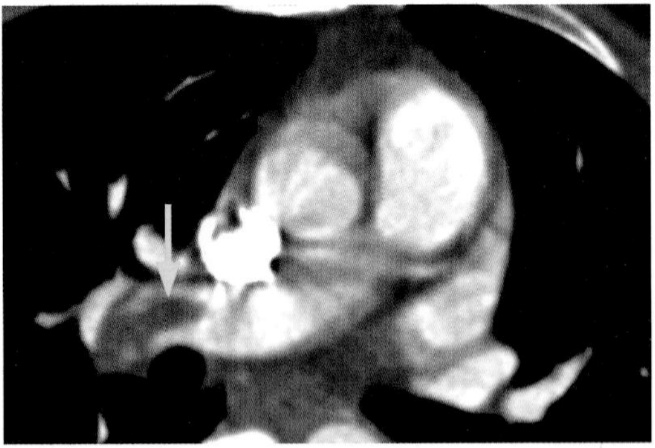

Massive pulmonary embolism: CT pulmonary angiogram shows a large, nearly-occlusive filling defect in the right main pulmonary artery (arrows) extending proximally to the bifurcation.

- CT pulmonary angiogram is the most common method to image for PE, where an embolism is typically seen as a central intraluminal pulmonary artery filling defect. Pulmonary emboli tend to lodge at vessel bifurcations.
- An eccentric, circumferential filling defect suggests chronic thromboembolic disease.
- Associated pulmonary abnormalities are commonly seen in patients with PE, including wedge-shaped consolidation, pleural effusion, and linear bands of subsegmental atelectasis. These findings, however, are nonspecific. In particular, pleural effusions and consolidation are seen approximately equally in patients with or without pulmonary embolism.

Plain film evaluation of pulmonary embolism

- While a CT pulmonary angiogram is the standard tool to evaluation for pulmonary embolism, it is important to be aware of plain film findings that could suggest pulmonary embolism in case the diagnosis is not clinically suspected.
- The *Fleischner* sign describes widening of the pulmonary arteries due to clot.

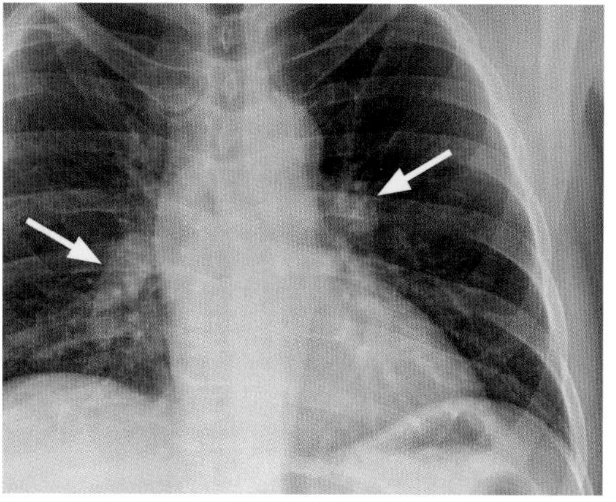

Current radiograph

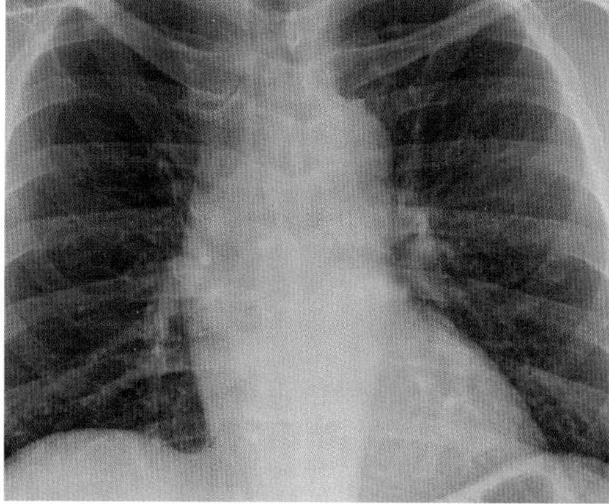

Prior radiograph

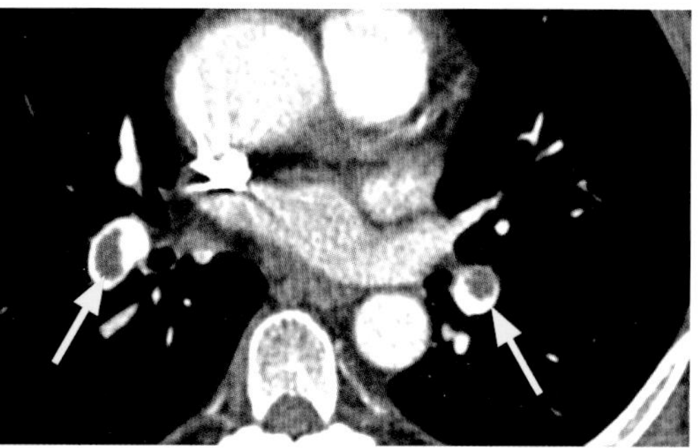

Fleischner sign: Current chest radiograph (top left image) shows relative enlargement of both pulmonary arteries (arrows), which is a new finding compared to the prior radiograph. Subsequently performed CT pulmonary angiogram (left image) shows bilateral pulmonary emboli (arrows).

Case courtesy Robert Gordon, MD, Brigham and Women's Hospital.

- *Hampton's hump* is a peripheral wedge-shaped opacity representing pulmonary infarct.
- *Westermark* sign is regional oligemia in the lung distal to the pulmonary artery thrombus.

Cardiac evaluation

- Pulmonary embolism may cause acute right heart strain. After evaluation of the pulmonary arterial tree, one should always examine the heart for imaging findings of right heart dysfunction.
- Massive PE may cause acute right ventricular dilation with bowing of the intraventricular septum to the left. An elevated RV:LV ratio (caused by RV enlargement) is linearly correlated with increased mortality.

Pitfalls of CT pulmonary angiogram

- Hilar lymph nodes may simulate large PE.
- Cardiac motion causes blurring of the left lower lobe pulmonary arteries, which may simulate small peripheral emboli.
- Respiratory motion overall decreases accuracy in evaluation of small pulmonary arteries.
- Mucus-impacted bronchi may simulate PE.
- Transient disruption of contrast bolus occurs when unopacified blood from the IVC enters the right atrium and is pumped into the lungs.
- Unopacified pulmonary veins may simulate PE on a single CT slice; however, one may distinguish between a pulmonary artery and vein by tracing the vessel back to the heart.

Idiopathic interstitial pneumonias

Overview of idiopathic interstitial pneumonias

- The lung has a limited repertoire of responses to injury. Common responses to injury range from recruiting lymphocytes or macrophages, increasing inflammatory debris, and instigating a fibrotic reaction.
- The idiopathic interstitial pneumonias (IIPs) are seven different patterns of injury response. These patterns can be associated with collagen vascular disease, drug reaction, occupational exposure, or they may be idiopathic.
- A disease can only be classified as an IIP if there is no other explanation for the pathologic changes.
- Each of the seven entities has both a clinical syndrome and a separate pathologic diagnosis. Sometimes the clinical syndrome and the pathologic terms have different names and sometimes they share the same name, but in every case there is an acronym!
- In order to understand the histopathological responses to injury, it is important to review the normal alveolar anatomy.

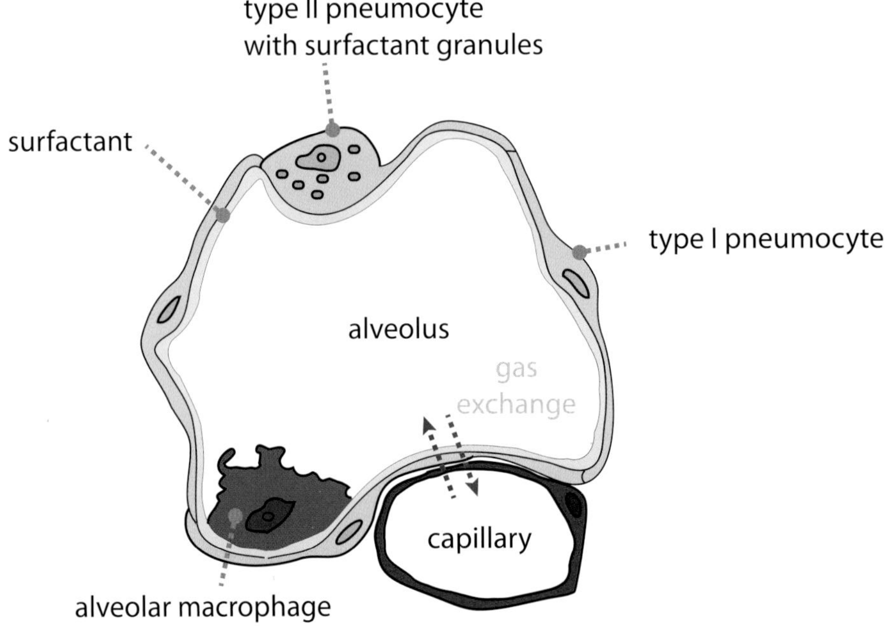

Normal alveolus:

Type I pneumocytes form alveolar wall and participate in gas exchange.

Type II pneumocytes produce surfactant, which prevents atelectasis.

Alveolar macrophages ingest and process inhaled particulate materials.

Idiopathic pulmonary fibrosis (IPF)

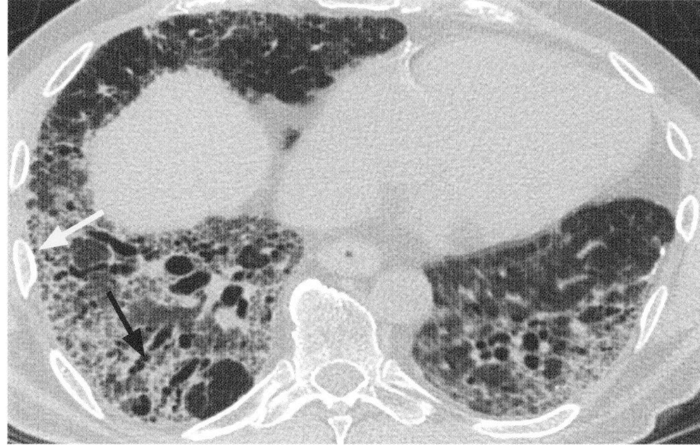

IPF: Noncontrast CT shows bibasilar subpleural honeycombing (yellow arrow) and traction bronchiectasis with cystic change (red arrow).

- Idiopathic pulmonary fibrosis (IPF) is the most common idiopathic interstitial pneumonia and has the second-worse prognosis of all, with a mean survival of 2–4 years. The mean survival of IPF is not much different compared to lung cancer. Of all the interstitial pneumonias, only acute interstitial pneumonitis (AIP) has a worse prognosis.
- Clinical symptoms of IPF include dry cough and dyspnea.
- IPF usually affects patients >50 years old.
- The pathologic diagnosis corresponding to the clinical syndrome of IPF is usual interstitial pneumonia (UIP), which features interstitial fibroblastic foci and chronic alveolar inflammation.

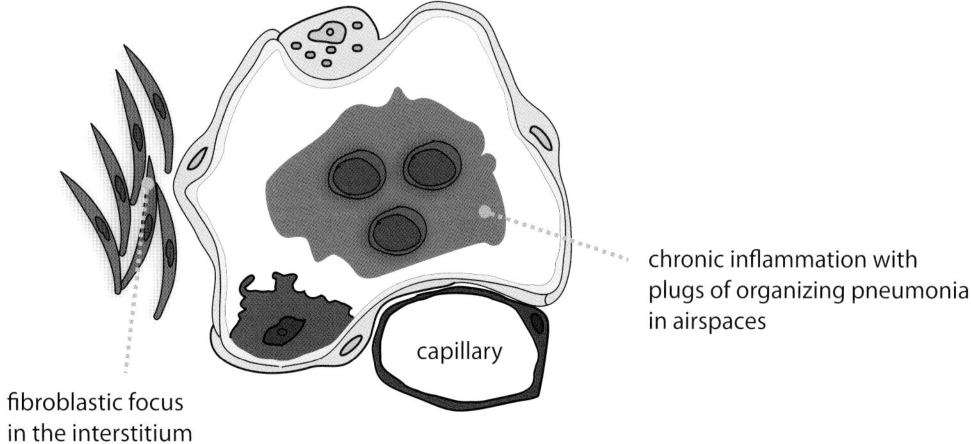

- IPF is the clinical syndrome of UIP with unknown cause and is the most common cause of UIP. IPF has a much worse clinical outcome compared to secondary causes of UIP.
- Other triggers of lung injury that may result in a UIP pattern include:
  - Collagen vascular disease (rheumatoid arthritis much more commonly than scleroderma).
  - Drug injury.
  - Asbestosis. An imaging clue to the presence of asbestosis is calcified plaques indicative of prior asbestos exposure.
- On imaging, early UIP features irregular reticulation in the posterior subpleural lung bases.
- In later stages of UIP, reticulation becomes fibrosis, traction bronchiectasis develops, and posterior subpleural honeycombing becomes prominent. The lung bases are most severely affected. The CT diagnosis of late UIP is very specific based on these findings, in particular the presence and posterior basal location of honeycombing. Surgical biopsy can often be avoided if these characteristic imaging features are present.

Nonspecific interstitial pneumonitis (NSIP)

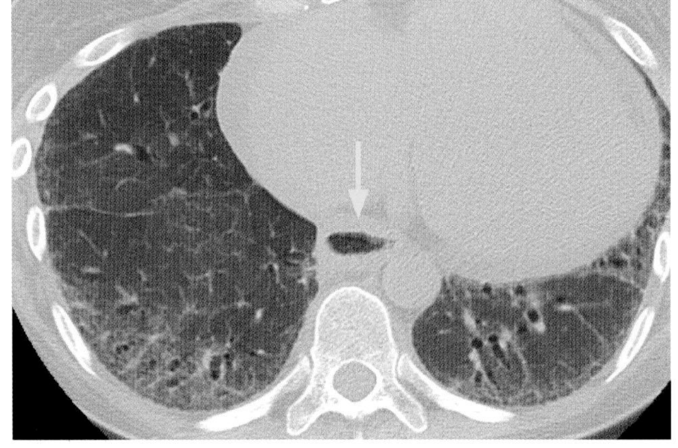

NSIP: Axial CT shows posterior basal predominant subpleural reticulation, mild ground glass attenuation, and mild traction bronchiectasis. This presentation likely represents the fibrotic subtype of NSIP.

Esophageal dilation (arrow) is a clue to the presence of scleroderma, which is often associated with NSIP.

Case courtesy Ritu R. Gill, MD, MPH, Brigham and Women's Hospital.

- Nonspecific interstitial pneumonitis (NSIP) is both the name of the clinical syndrome and the corresponding pathologic diagnosis. Affected patients are typically younger (40–50 years old) compared to IPF. Symptoms are similar to IPF with chronic dry cough and dyspnea.
- Histologically, NSIP features thickened alveolar septa from chronic inflammation. In contrast to IPF/UIP, there is less fibrotic change.

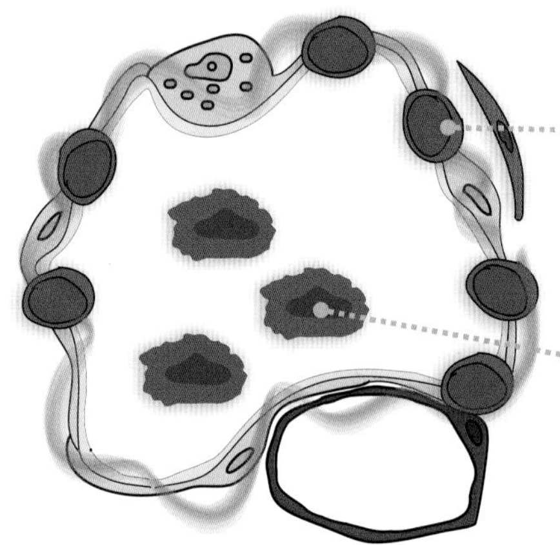

septal thickening (causing ground glass attenuation) due to chronic inflammation and collagen deposition

unlike IPF, there are no interstitial fibroblastic foci

nonpigmented macrophages in alveoli

- NSIP has a better 5-year survival compared to IPF. Unlike IPF, NSIP does respond to steroids.
- NSIP may be idiopathic or associated with other diseases. NSIP is the most common pulmonary manifestation in patients with collagen vascular disease.
  - NSIP may also be caused by drug reaction or occupational exposure.
  - NSIP may be associated with dermatomyositis.
- There are two forms of NSIP. An important imaging feature of NSIP, regardless of the form, is the presence of ground glass opacities (GGO), which are nearly always bilateral. A key feature differentiating NSIP from IPF is the presence of ground glass in NSIP.
- **Fibrotic NSIP** predominantly features GGO with fine reticulation and traction bronchiectasis.
  - Honeycombing is usually absent in NSIP. If honeycombing is present, consider UIP.
  - Fibrotic NSIP has a worse prognosis compared to cellular NSIP, but a better prognosis compared to UIP.
- **Cellular NSIP** also features GGO, but without significant fibrotic changes.
  - Cellular NSIP is much less common than fibrotic NSIP and has a better prognosis compared to fibrotic NSIP.
- A key imaging finding (not always seen but very specific) is sparing of immediate subpleural lung. This feature is NOT seen in UIP, and can be seen in both cellular and fibrotic NSIP.
- Like UIP, NSIP tends to affect the posterior peripheral lower lobes. Other diagnoses should be considered (e.g., chronic hypersensitivity pneumonitis or sarcoidosis) if there is primarily upper lobe disease.

Cryptogenic organizing pneumonia (COP)

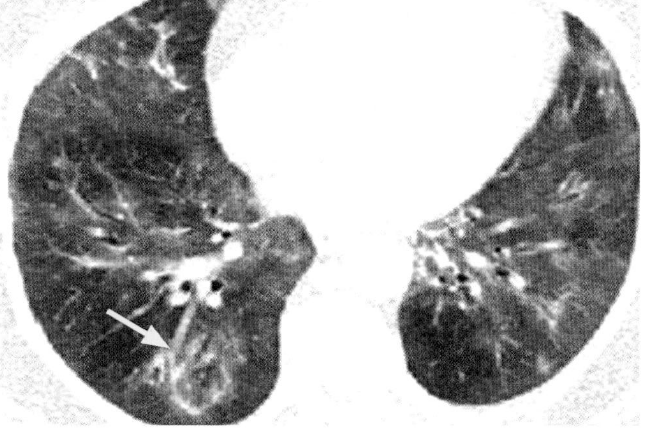

COP: Axial CT shows patchy consolidative and ground glass opacities in a peribronchovascular distribution. There is a *reverse halo* or *atoll* sign in the right lower lobe (arrow), where a central lucency is surrounded by a peripheral opacity.

Case courtesy Seth Kligerman, MD, University of Maryland.

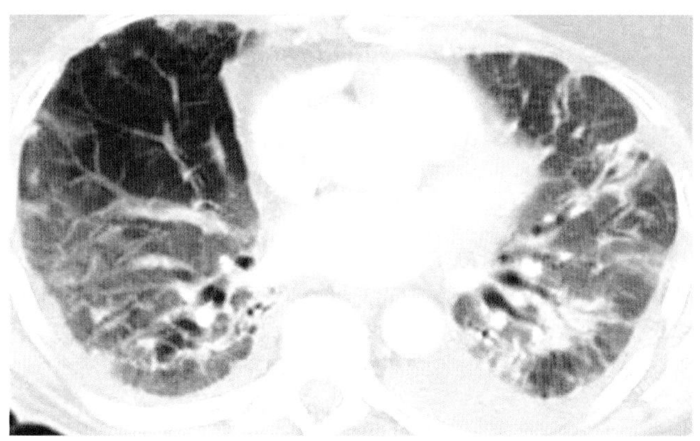

Contrast-enhanced CT in a different patient with COP shows patchy consolidation in a peribronchial and subpleural location.

Case courtesy Ritu R. Gill, MD, MPH, Brigham and Women's Hospital.

- Cryptogenic organizing pneumonia (COP) is the clinical syndrome of organizing pneumonia (OP) without known cause. The clinical syndrome of COP was previously called bronchiolitis obliterans organizing pneumonia (BOOP), which is a term still in general use.
- COP clinically responds to steroids with a good prognosis and may resolve completely, although recurrences are common.
- Organizing pneumonia (OP) is the pathologic pattern of granulation tissue polyps that fill the distal airways and alveoli. Organizing pneumonia may be a response to infection, drug reaction, or inhalation.

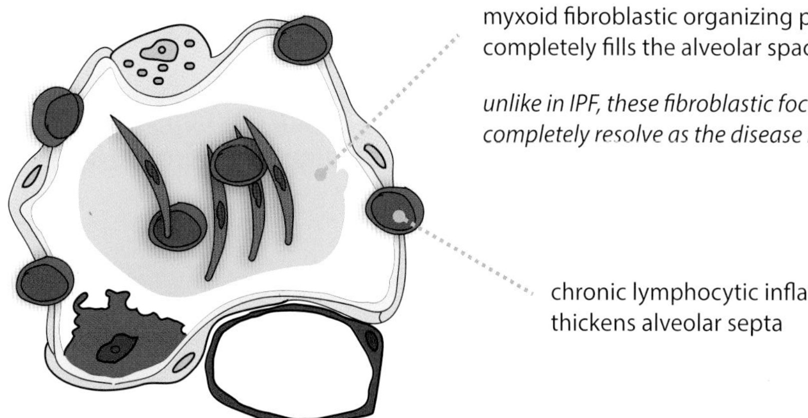
myxoid fibroblastic organizing pneumonia completely fills the alveolar spaces
unlike in IPF, these fibroblastic foci completely resolve as the disease regresses
chronic lymphocytic inflammation thickens alveolar septa

- CT of OP shows mixed consolidation and ground glass opacities in a peripheral and peribronchovascular distribution. The *reverse halo* sign (also known as the *atoll* sign) is relatively specific for OP and features a central lucency surrounded by a ground glass halo.

  The reverse halo sign should not be confused with the halo sign that is typical of invasive aspergillus, which shows a central opacity with peripheral ground glass.

Respiratory bronchiolitis–interstitial lung disease (RB-ILD)

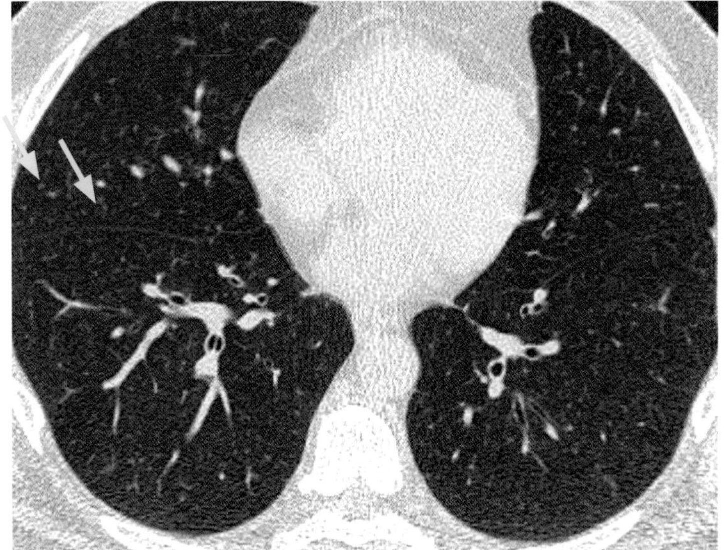

RB-ILD: Axial CT shows innumerable subtle ground glass centrilobular nodules (arrows). This case does not feature ground glass opacification. Centrilobular nodules are a nonspecific finding, and the other common disease featuring centrilobular nodules is hypersensitivity pneumonitis.

Case courtesy Ritu R. Gill, MD, MPH, Brigham and Women's Hospital.

- Respiratory bronchiolitis–interstitial lung disease (RB-ILD) is both the clinical syndrome and the pathologic diagnosis of this smoking-related interstitial lung disease.
- Respiratory bronchiolitis (RB, without the ILD) is very common in smokers, where pigmented macrophages are found in respiratory bronchioles. RB is usually asymptomatic, but if symptoms are present (usually cough and shortness of breath), the clinical syndrome is called RB-ILD.
- Histologically, RB-ILD is characterized by sheets of macrophages filling the terminal airways, with relative sparing of the alveoli.

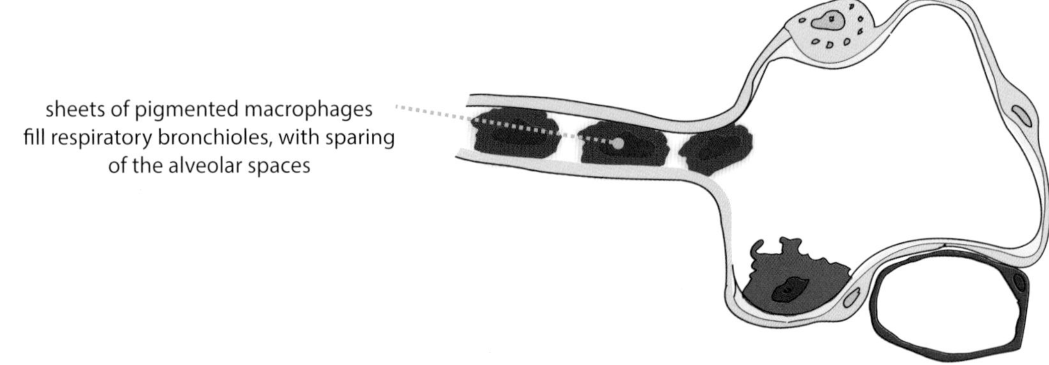
sheets of pigmented macrophages
fill respiratory bronchioles, with sparing
of the alveolar spaces

- The key imaging features of RB-ILD are centrilobular nodules and patchy ground glass opacities. In contrast to NSIP, the distribution of ground glass in RB-ILD is more random than the peripherally predominant pattern of NSIP.

Desquamative interstitial pneumonia (DIP)

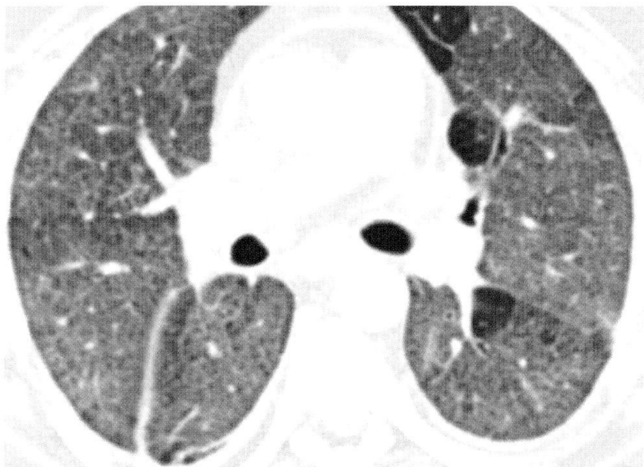

DIP: Axial CT shows extensive ground glass opacities. This is a nonspecific pattern.

Case courtesy Ritu R. Gill, MD, MPH, Brigham and Women's Hospital.

- Like RB-ILD, desquamative interstitial pneumonia (DIP) is both the clinical syndrome and the pathologic diagnosis. RB, RB-ILD, and DIP represent a continuous spectrum of smoking-related lung disease.
- Like RB, brown-pigmented macrophages are involved in DIP; however, sheets of these abnormal macrophages also extend into the alveoli in DIP.

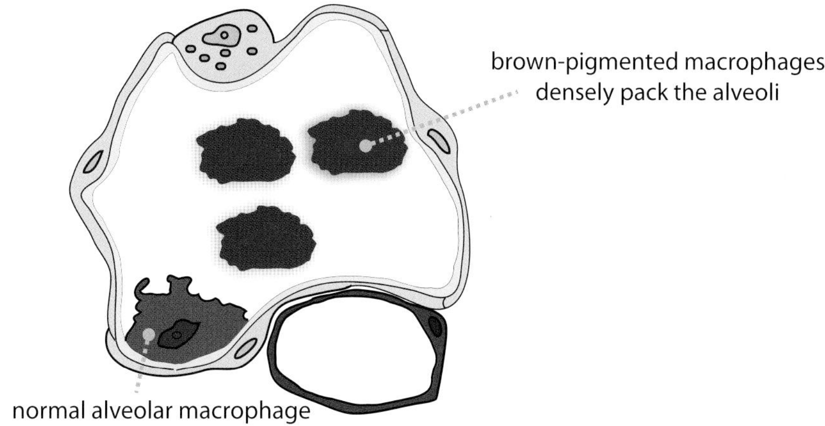
brown-pigmented macrophages
densely pack the alveoli
normal alveolar macrophage

- Imaging of DIP shows diffuse basal-predominant patchy or subpleural ground glass opacification, more extensive than RB-ILD. Although the predominant abnormality is ground glass, a few cysts may also be present.

Lymphoid interstitial pneumonia (LIP)

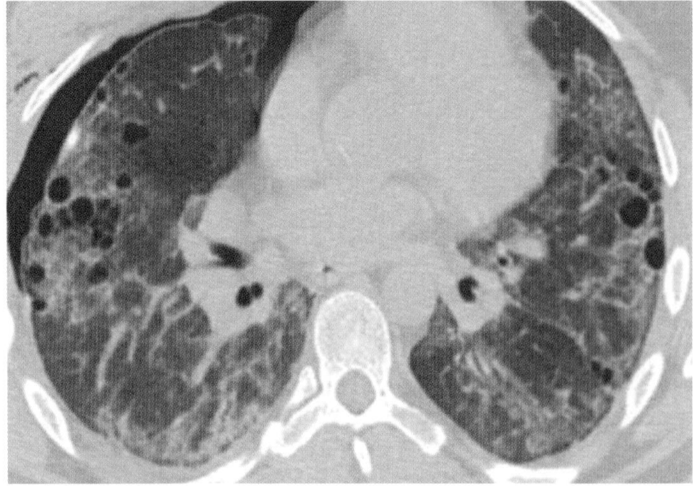

LIP: Unenhanced axial CT shows patchy ground glass opacities, scattered perivascular cysts, and a right-sided pneumothorax.

Case courtesy Ritu R. Gill, MD, MPH, Brigham and Women's Hospital.

- Lymphoid interstitial pneumonia (LIP) is both a clinical syndrome and the pathologic diagnosis. LIP is exceptionally rare as an isolated idiopathic disease and is more commonly associated with Sjögren syndrome or HIV.
- The histologic hallmark of LIP is diffuse infiltration of the interstitium by lymphocytes and other immune cells, with resultant distortion of the alveoli.

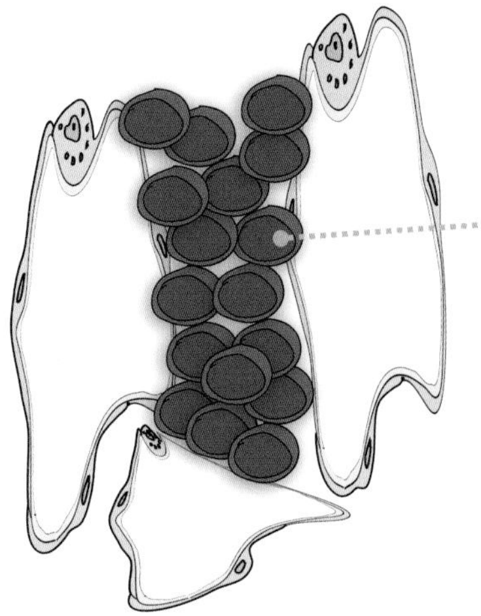

lymphocytes expand alveolar septa forming germinal centers, secondarily compressing alveoli

- Imaging findings of LIP include diffuse or lower-lobe predominant ground glass. Scattered thin-walled perivascular cysts are often present, which are thought to be due to air trapping from peribronchiolar cellular debris. LIP may be complicated by pneumothorax in advanced disease.

Acute interstitial pneumonia (AIP)

- Acute interstitial pneumonia (AIP), synonymous with diffuse alveolar damage (DAD), is the pathologic diagnosis seen in the clinical syndrome of acute respiratory distress syndrome (ARDS). Unlike the other IIPs, AIP is the only syndrome with an acute onset and has the worst prognosis.
- The primary cause of AIP is surfactant destruction.
- Two phases of AIP are recognized: Early (exudative) and chronic (organizing).
- **The early (exudative) phase** features hyaline membranes, diffuse alveolar infiltration by immune cells, and noncardiogenic pulmonary edema.

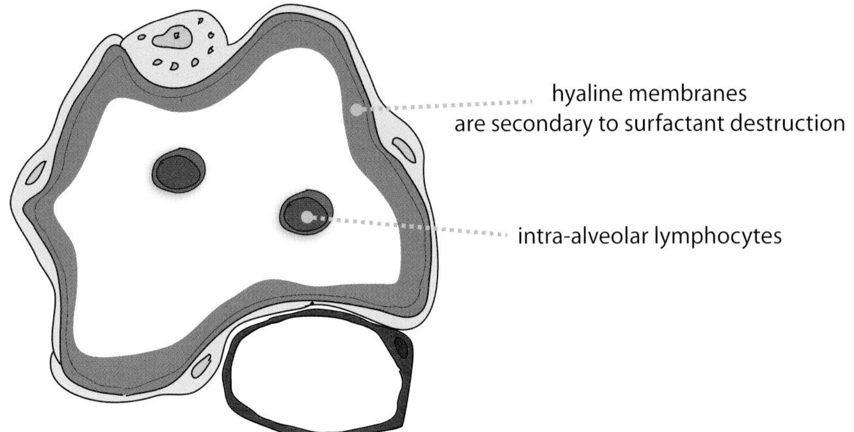
hyaline membranes
are secondary to surfactant destruction
intra-alveolar lymphocytes

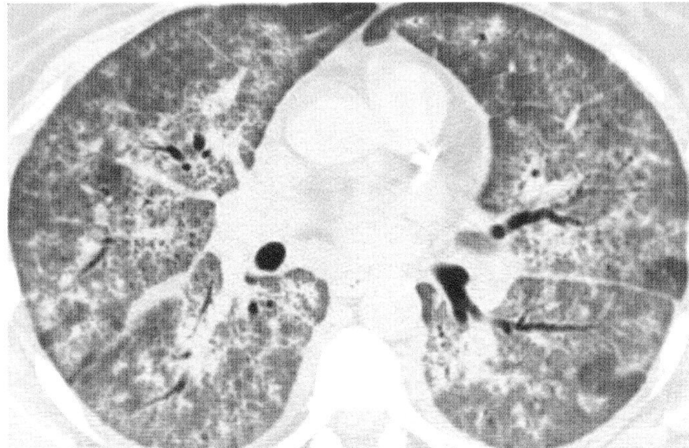

AIP (early or exudative phase):

Axial CT shows extensive geographic ground glass attenuation. This is a nonspecific pattern and may represent pulmonary edema, hemorrhage, infection, or ARDS/AIP.

Case courtesy Seth Kligerman, MD, University of Maryland.

- The **chronic (organizing) phase** features alveolar wall thickening due to granulation tissue. The chronic phase usually begins one week after the initial injury.

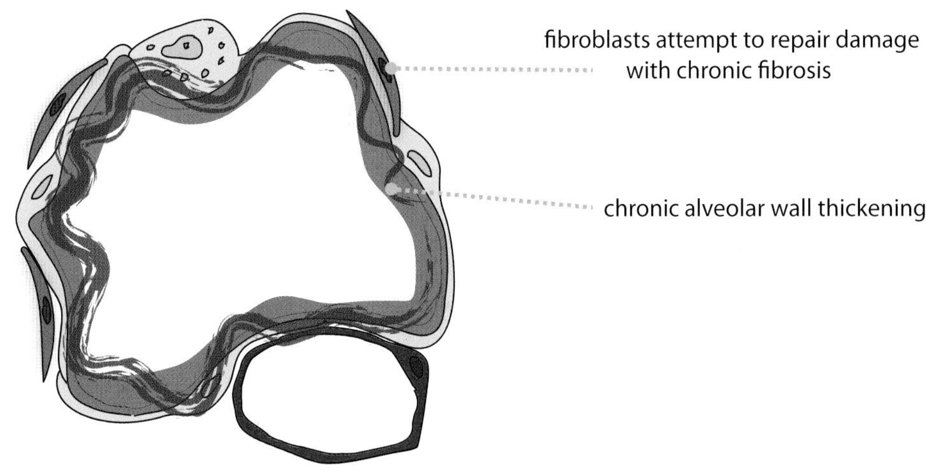
fibroblasts attempt to repair damage
with chronic fibrosis
chronic alveolar wall thickening

- Most inhalational lung diseases predominantly affect the upper lobes because the lower lobes have more robust blood flow and lymphatic drainage.

Hypersensitivity pneumonitis (HSP)

- Hypersensitivity pneumonitis (HSP) is a common lung disease caused by a hypersensitivity reaction to inhaled organic antigens, such as bird proteins or thermophilic actinomycetes, although a history of antigen exposure is not always elicited.
- HSP is characterized by three distinct phases, from acute to subacute to chronic.
- **Acute** HSP is characterized by inflammatory exudate filling the alveoli, which manifests on imaging as nonspecific groundglass or consolidation. Small, ill-defined centrilobular nodules may also be present.
- The imaging hallmark of **subacute** HSP is centrilobular ground glass nodules. Mosaic attenuation (geographic areas of relative lucency) and ground glass can also be seen.

    Mosaic attenuation can be secondary to mosaic perfusion on inspiration and air trapping on expiration.

    The abnormalities of subacute HSP involve the entire axial cross-section of lung.

    The *head-cheese* sign describes the combination of patchy ground glass and areas of lucency due to mosaic perfusion or air trapping.

- **Chronic** HSP, from long-term exposure to the offending antigen, leads to upper-lobe predominant pulmonary fibrosis. Often the findings of subacute disease, including centrilobular nodules, ground glass, and mosaic attenuation, may be superimposed.

    Unlike IPF, honeycombing is not common in HSP, but when present may involve the upper lobes.

    If there is relative sparing of the bases, chronic HSP is much more likely than IPF.

Pneumoconioses

- A pneumoconiosis is a lung disease secondary to *inorganic* dust inhalation. In contrast, hypersensitivity pneumonitis is caused by *organic* dust inhalation.
- **Silicosis** and **coal workers pneumoconiosis (CWP)** are the two most common pneumoconioses. They often have indistinguishable imaging findings even though they are due to different inhaled dusts and have different histologic findings.

    Silicosis is due to inhalation of silica dust, which miners may be exposed to.

    CWP is caused by inhalation of coal dust, which does not contain any silica.

    The most characteristic finding of *uncomplicated* disease is multiple upper lobe predominant centrilobular and subpleural nodules.

    Eggshell lymph node calcifications are commonly seen in silicosis, less commonly in CWP.

    Silicosis or CWP can become *complicated* with large conglomerate masses or progressive massive fibrosis.

    Both silicosis and CWP confer an increased risk of TB.

    Caplan syndrome is seen in patients with rheumatoid arthritis *and* either CWP or silicosis (more common in CWP) and represents necrobiotic rheumatoid nodules superimposed on the smaller centrilobular and subpleural nodules of the pneumoconiosis.

- **Asbestosis** is lung disease caused by inhalation of asbestos fibers. End-stage asbestosis can lead to pulmonary fibrosis with a UIP pathology.

    Unlike the other inhalational lung diseases, asbestosis predominantly affects the lower lobes because the asbestos particles are too large to be removed by the alveolar macrophages and lymphatic system.

    The radiographic/CT appearance and distribution of advanced asbestosis may be indistinguishable from IPF; however, an important clue seen in asbestosis is evidence of asbestos exposure, such as pleural thickening and plaques.

    Even though pleural plaques (which may or may not be calcified) are due to asbestos exposure, they are not a component of asbestosis, do not lead to fibrosis, and are usually asymptomatic.

Eosinophilic lung disease

- Eosinophilic lung disease is a spectrum of diseases that feature accumulation of eosinophils in the pulmonary airspaces and interstitium.

Simple pulmonary eosinophilia (Löffler syndrome)

- Simple pulmonary eosinophilia (also known as Löffler syndrome) is characterized by transient and *migratory* areas of focal consolidation, with an elevated eosinophil count in the peripheral smear.
- An identical appearance can be seen as a response to injury, especially with parasitic disease and drug reactions. The term *simple pulmonary eosinophilia* is reserved for idiopathic cases.

Chronic eosinophilic pneumonia

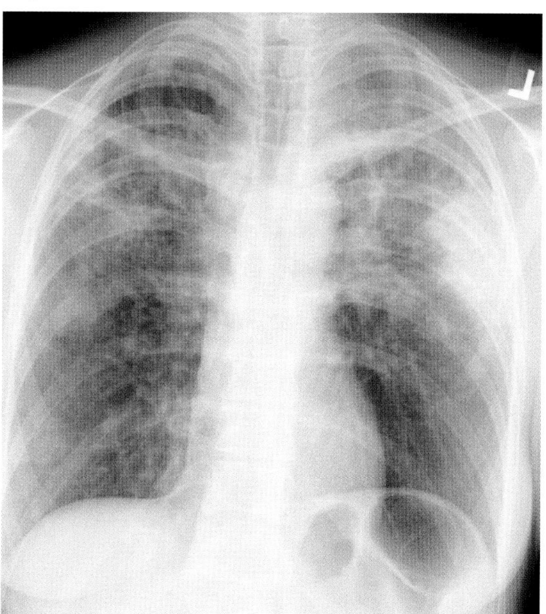
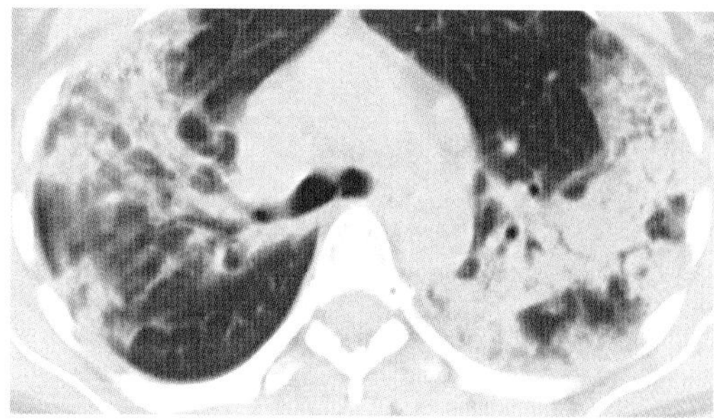
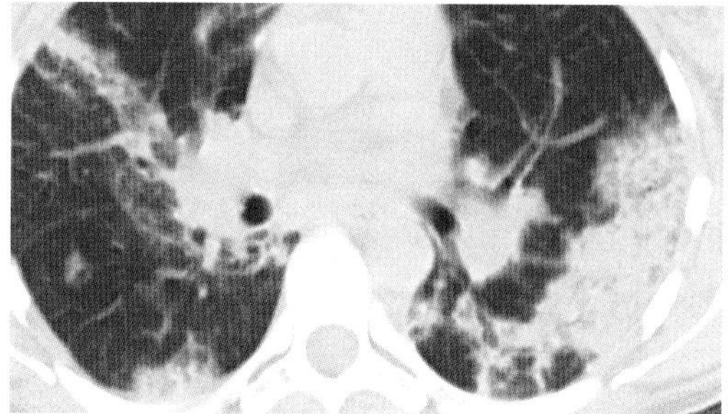

Chronic eosinophilic pneumonia: Chest radiograph demonstrates upper-lobe and peripheral consolidation. Axial CT shows bilateral patchy peripheral consolidative opacities. Although this is a nonspecific appearance, the appearance was unchanged over multiple priors, which suggests against bacterial pneumonia.

Case courtesy Ritu R. Gill, MD, MPH, Brigham and Women's Hospital.

- Chronic eosinophilic pneumonia is an important consideration in the differential diagnosis of chronic consolidation. Chronic eosinophilic pneumonia causes extensive alveolar filling and interstitial infiltration with inflammatory eosinophils.
- Consolidation is patchy and *peripheral*, with an *upper lobe* predominance. Unlike simple pulmonary eosinophilia, the pattern of consolidation can remain unchanged for months.
- Chronic eosinophilic pneumonia responds rapidly to steroids.

Pulmonary vasculitis

Churg–Strauss

- Also called allergic angiitis and granulomatosis, Churg–Strauss is a systemic small-vessel vasculitis associated with asthma and peripheral eosinophilia.
- P-ANCA is positive, which is not very specific. P-ANCA can also be positive in collagen vascular disease and microscopic polyangiitis (discussed below).
- Imaging findings of Churg–Strauss are varied. The most common appearance is peripheral consolidation or ground glass.

Microscopic polyangiitis

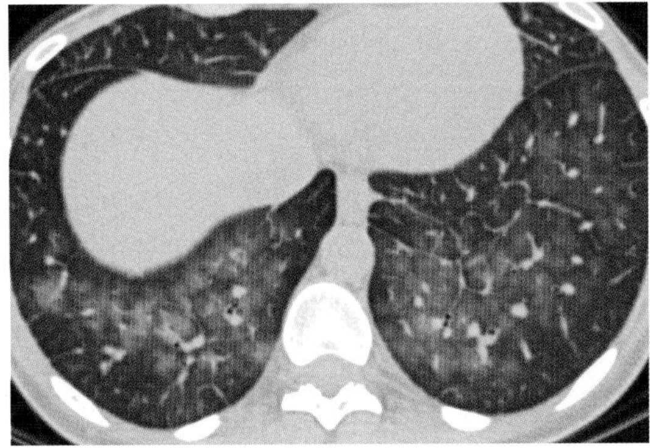

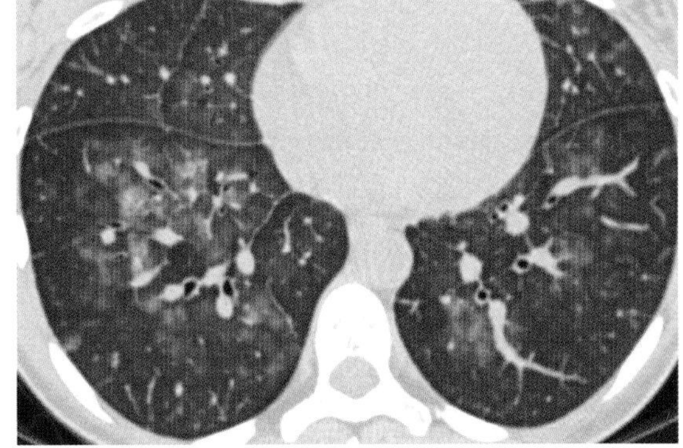

Alveolar hemorrhage due to microscopic polyangiitis: Axial CT shows basal predominant central ground glass with associated mild interlobular septal thickening. This patient had renal insufficiency and had a P-ANCA positive vasculitis with alveolar hemorrhage.

Case courtesy Ritu R. Gill, MD, MPH, Brigham and Women's Hospital.

- Microscopic polyangiitis is the most common cause of pulmonary hemorrhage with renal failure. P-ANCA is positive.
- Imaging shows diffuse central-predominant ground glass representing hemorrhage.

Wegener granulomatosis (WG)

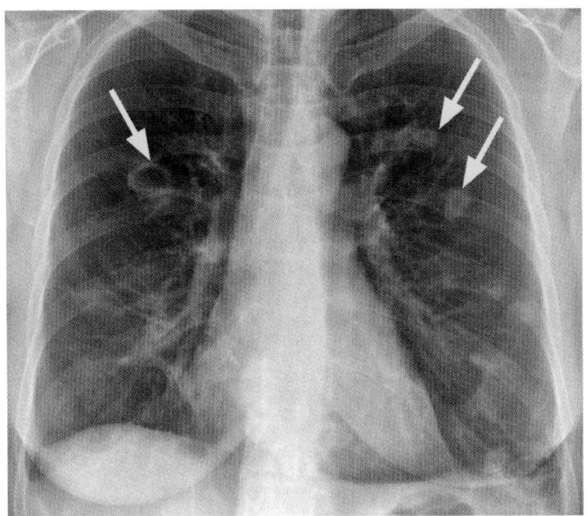

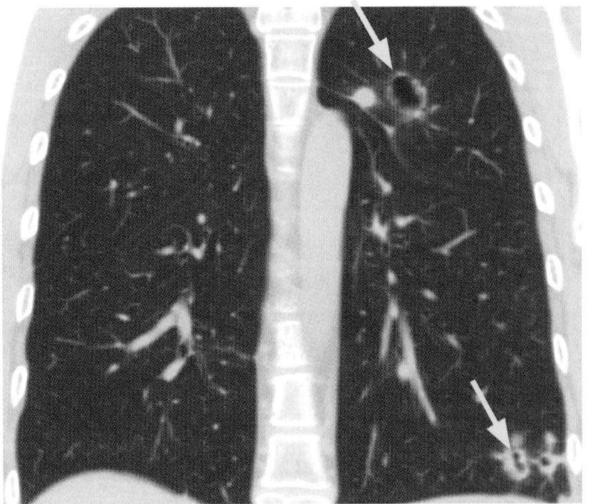

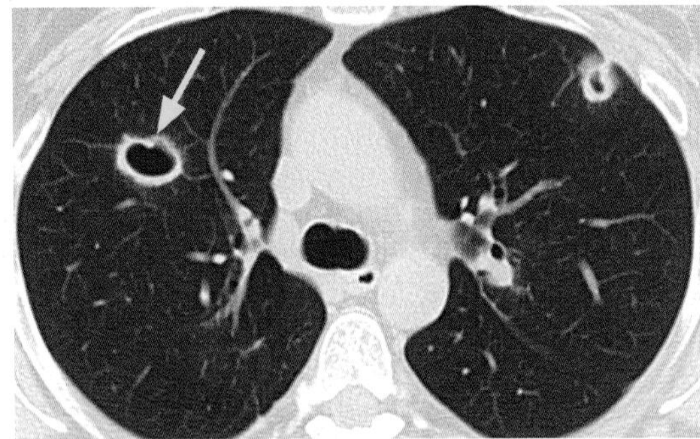

Wegener granulomatosis:

Chest radiograph shows numerous cavitary lesions bilaterally (arrows).

Coronal and axial CT confirms multiple thick-walled cavitary lesions (arrows). The primary differential consideration would be septic emboli; however, this patient was C-ANCA positive.

Case courtesy Ritu R. Gill, MD, MPH, Brigham and Women's Hospital.

- Wegener granulomatosis (WG) is a systemic small-vessel vasculitis with a classic clinical triad of sinusitis, lung involvement, and renal insufficiency.
- C-ANCA is positive, which is very specific for Wegener granulomatosis.
- In the upper airways, WG may cause nasopharyngeal and eustachian tube obstruction. Involvement of the larynx and bronchi is common, leading to airway stenosis.
- In the lungs, WG may cause **multiple cavitary nodules** that don't respond to antibiotic therapy. An intra-cavitary fluid level suggests superimposed infection.

Drug toxicity

- The lung has a diverse but finite repertoire of responses to injury, including pulmonary edema (due to increased capillary permeability), ARDS, organizing pneumonia, eosinophilic pneumonia, bronchiolitis obliterans, pulmonary hemorrhage, NSIP, and UIP.
- Pulmonary drug reaction, most commonly to cytotoxic drugs, may elicit any of these injury responses.

Radiation lung injury

- Up to 40% of patients develop radiographic abnormalities after external radiotherapy, although most patients are asymptomatic. The radiographic abnormality is largely confined to the radiation port, usually with non-anatomic linear margins.
- Radiation pneumonitis is the early stage of radiation injury, which can occur within 1 month of radiotherapy and is most severe 3–4 months after treatment. Radiation pneumonitis features ground glass centered on the radiation port, although extension out of the port is relatively common.

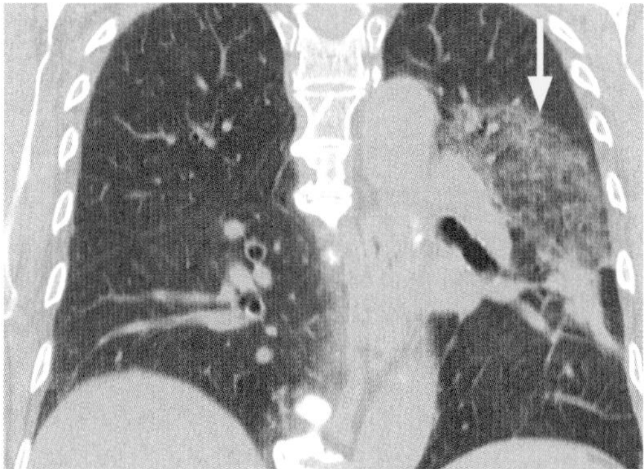
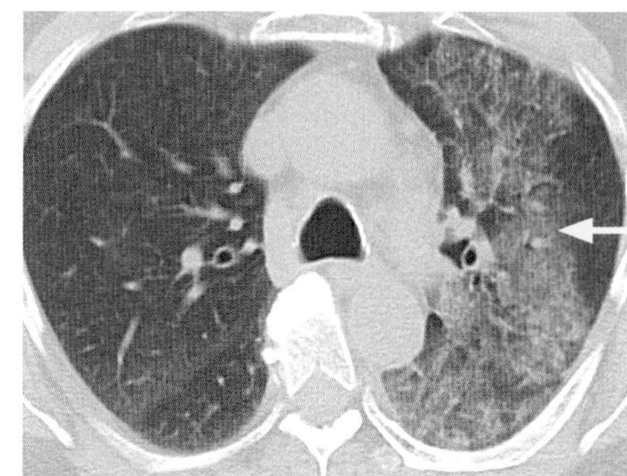

Acute radiation pneumonitis: Coronal and axial CT demonstrate geographic left upper lung ground glass (arrows) with non-anatomic superior and lateral linear margins.

Case courtesy Ritu R. Gill, MD, MPH, Brigham and Women's Hospital.

- Radiation fibrosis is the late stage of radiation injury. Fibrosis becomes apparent approximately 6–12 months after therapy. The key imaging finding is the distribution of fibrosis and traction bronchiectasis *within the radiation port*, although fibrosis may extend outside the port in 20%.

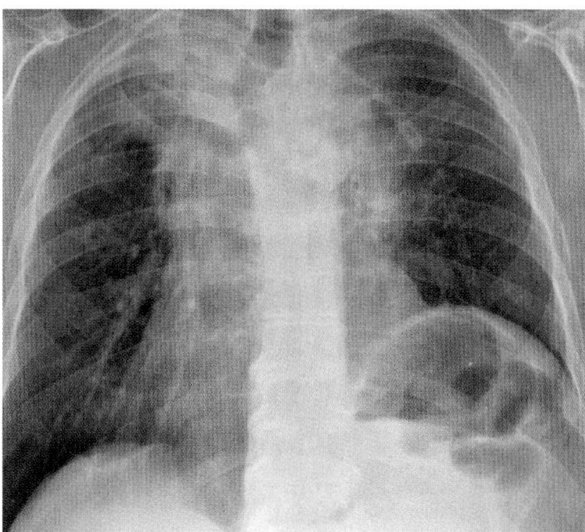
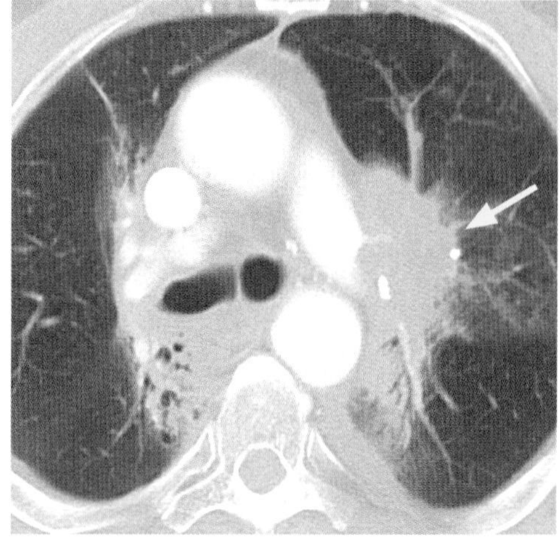

Radiation fibrosis: Chest radiograph and enhanced CT shows paramediastinal fibrotic changes within the radiation port. Despite radiation, the patient has persistent left mediastinal adenopathy (arrow).

Sarcoidosis

- Sarcoidosis is an idiopathic systemic disorder of noncaseating granulomas that become coalescent to form nodules and masses throughout the body.
- Pulmonary sarcoidosis may progress to pulmonary fibrosis with honeycombing. Unlike IPF (the most common cause of pulmonary fibrosis), the fibrotic changes of sarcoid have a mid and upper-lung predominance, similar to end-stage hypersensitivity pneumonitis.
- A historical staging system has been used for radiographic findings (not CT) in sarcoidosis; however, there is not always stepwise progression through the stages.

> **Stage 0**: Normal radiograph.
>
> **Stage 1**: Hilar or mediastinal adenopathy only, *without* lung changes.
>
> **Stage 2**: Adenopathy *with* lung changes.
>
> **Stage 3**: Diffuse lung disease *without* adenopathy.
>
> **Stage 4**: End-stage fibrosis.

- The most common radiographic finding in sarcoidosis is *symmetric adenopathy.* Lymph nodes may contain stippled or eggshell calcification in up to 50%.

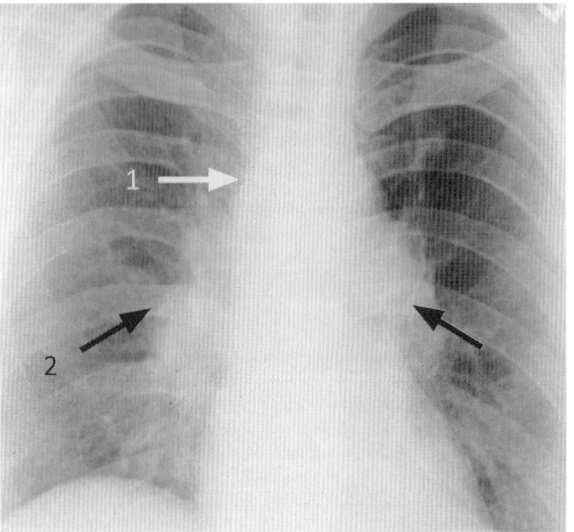

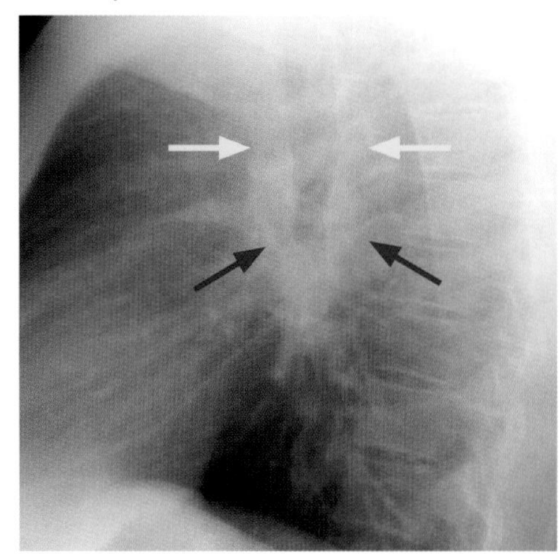

Stage 1 sarcoidosis: Frontal (left image) and lateral radiographs show symmetric adenopathy demonstrating the *1-2-3* sign:
Right paratracheal adenopathy (yellow arrows, "1")
Right hilar adenopathy (red arrow, "2")
Left hilar adenopathy (red arrow, "3")

The lateral radiograph demonstrates the *donut* sign with adenopathy circumferentially encircling the trachea (arrows).

The lung parenchyma is normal. *Case courtesy Ritu R. Gill, MD, MPH, Brigham and Women's Hospital.*

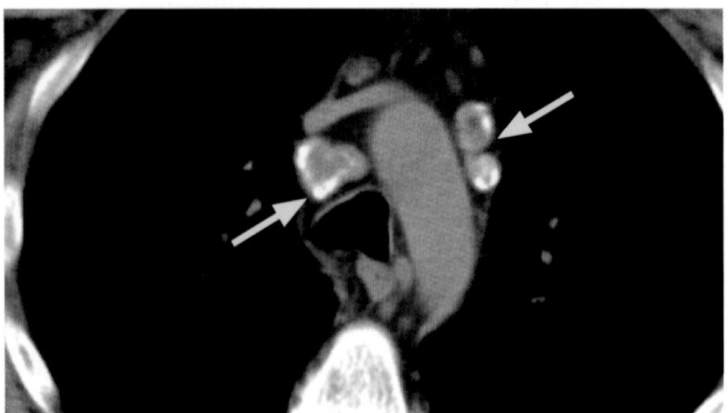

Sarcoidosis: Axial CT in a different patient shows peripherally-calcified ("eggshell") prevascular and paratracheal lymph nodes (arrows).

Case courtesy Ritu R. Gill, MD, MPH, Brigham and Women's Hospital.

- The most common CT finding in sarcoidosis, in addition to adenopathy, is upper-lobe predominant *perilymphatic* nodules of variable sizes, representing sarcoid granulomas.

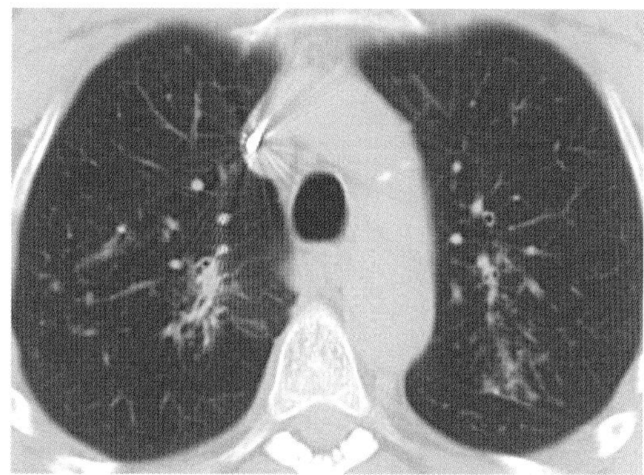

CT in a patient with sarcoidosis shows tiny peribronchovascular and fissural (subpleural) nodules in the bilateral upper lobes.

Case courtesy Darryl Sneag, MD, Brigham and Women's Hospital.

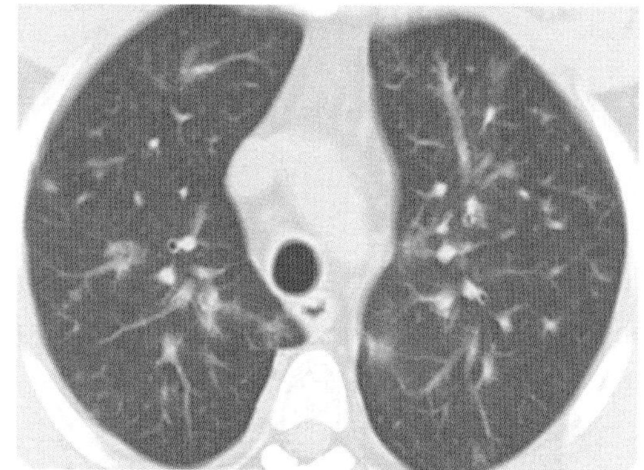

CT in a different patient with sarcoidosis shows slightly larger nodules in a peribronchovascular distribution.

Case courtesy Ritu R. Gill, MD, MPH, Brigham and Women's Hospital.

Perilymphatic nodules are found along the course of the pulmonary lymphatics, which are peribronchovascular, subpleural, and within the interlobular septa.

Perilymphatic nodules may coalesce into a mass up to several centimeters in diameter. The *galaxy* sign is seen when small nodules are peripheral to a confluent mass.

Nodules may occasionally be miliary.

Ground glass may also be present, superimposed upon the perilymphatic nodules.

- Bronchial involvement may cause mosaic perfusion due to air trapping.
- Sarcoidosis may involve other organs, including the spleen, brain, and rarely bone.

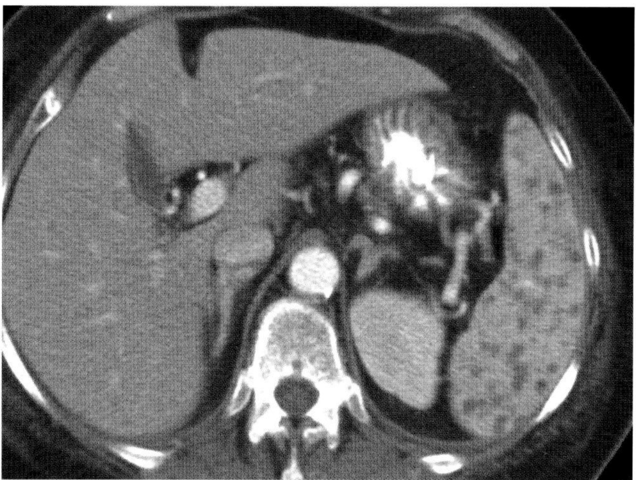

Axial contrast-enhanced CT through the liver and spleen in a patient with sarcoidosis shows innumerable small hypoattenuating splenic nodules.

Case courtesy Michael Hanley, MD, University of Virginia Health System.

Pulmonary Langerhans cell histiocytosis (PLCH)

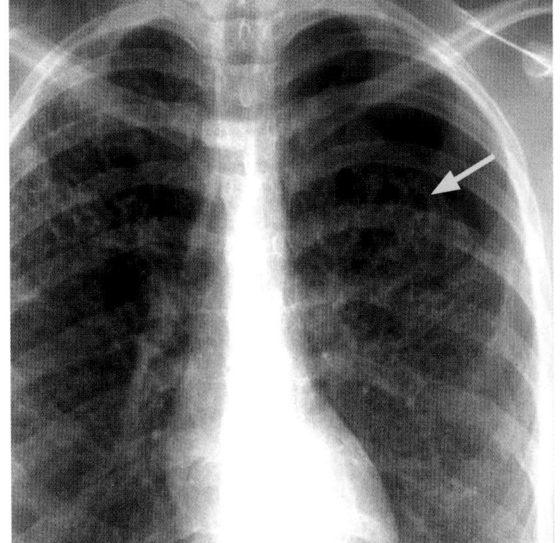

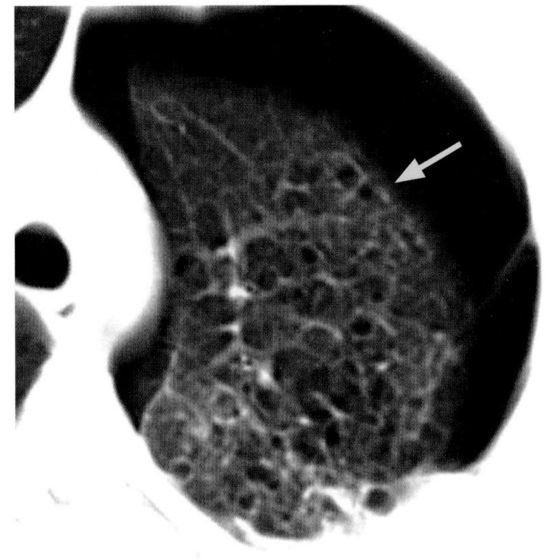

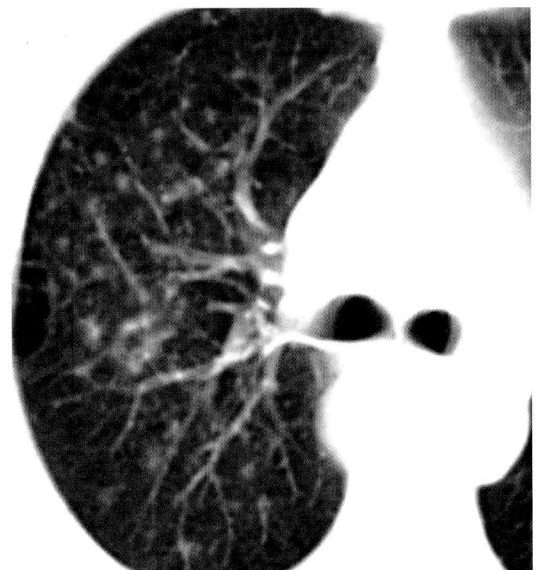

Pulmonary Langerhans cell histiocytosis: Chest radiograph shows multiple upper-lobe predominant cysts with the suggestion of multiple small nodules. There is a moderate left pneumothorax (yellow arrow).

CT confirms the pneumothorax (yellow arrow) but more clearly delineates the upper lobe predominant cysts (better seen in the top right image) and nodules (bottom left image, red arrows).

Case courtesy Ritu R. Gill, MD, MPH, Brigham and Women's Hospital.

- Pulmonary Langerhans cell histiocytosis (PLCH) is a smoking-related lung disease – nearly 100% of adults with PLCH are smokers.

  The other smoking-related interstitial lung diseases (aside from emphysema) are RB-ILD and DIP.

  Multiple smoking-related lung diseases may be present simultaneously.
- PLCH may present as a spontaneous pneumothorax.
- Disease is most often isolated to the lungs; however, lucent bone lesions, diabetes insipidus from inflammation of the pituitary stalk (hypophysitis), and skin involvement can occasionally be seen.

> In addition to LCH, the differential diagnosis for diseases affecting the lungs and bones includes **malignancy**, **tuberculosis**, **fungal disease** (including blastomycosis, histoplasmosis, and coccidiomycosis), **sarcoidosis**, and **Gaucher disease** (pulmonary involvement is rare and may resemble DIP).

- The first detectable abnormality is nodules associated with airways. As the disease progresses, the nodules cavitate and resultant irregular cysts predominate.
- The natural progression is from nodules → cavitary nodules → irregular cysts.
- Radiographic and CT findings include upper lobe predominant cysts and irregular peribronchovascular nodules, both sparing the costophrenic sulci.
- PLCH is generally steroid responsive and smoking cessation is critical.

Pulmonary alveolar proteinosis (PAP)

- Pulmonary alveolar proteinosis (PAP) is an idiopathic disease causing filling of the alveoli with a proteinaceous lipid-rich material.
- On chest radiography, PAP may resemble pulmonary edema with perihilar opacification; however, the heart is normal in size in PAP and pleural effusions are not typically seen.
- The CT hallmark of PAP is the *crazy paving* pattern of smooth interlobular septal thickening in areas of patchy or geometric ground glass. Although initially described for PAP, the *crazy paving* pattern is not specific for PAP, and can also be seen in *Pneumocystis* pneumonia, cryptogenic organizing pneumonia, bronchoalveolar carcinoma, and lipoid pneumonia, among others.

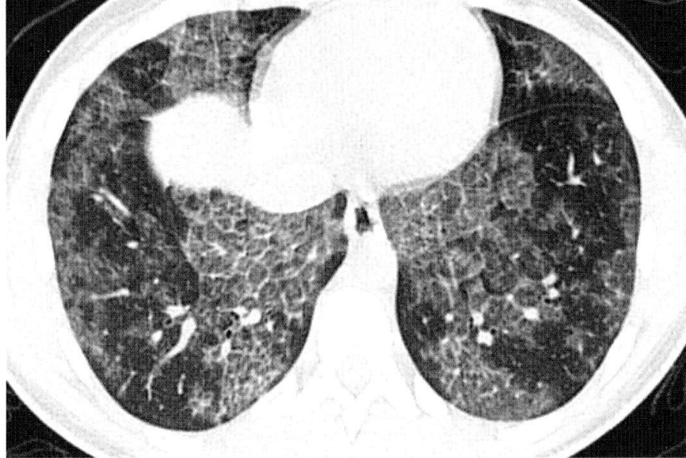

Pulmonary alveolar proteinosis:

CT shows predominantly central ground glass opacification with interlobular septal thickening representing the *crazy paving* pattern.

Case courtesy Ritu R. Gill, MD, MPH, Brigham and Women's Hospital.

- Patients with PCP are susceptible to superimposed infection, classically with *Nocardia*, which typically presents as a consolidation.

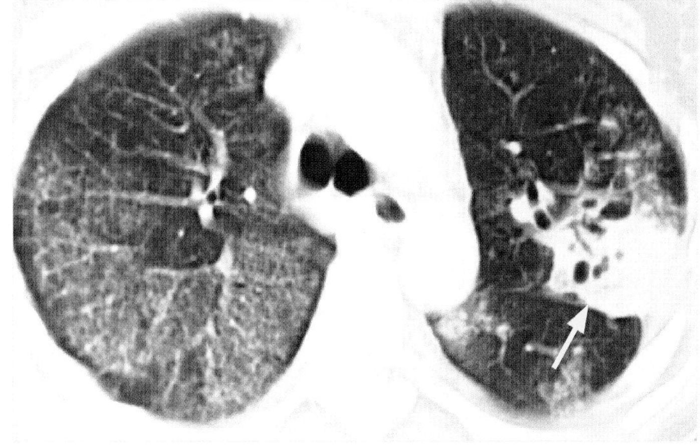

Pulmonary alveolar proteinosis with superimposed *Nocardia*:

CT shows bilateral *crazy paving* predominantly in the right lung, with a dense consolidative opacity in the left upper lobe (arrow) representing superimposed *Nocardia* pneumonia.

Case courtesy Ritu R. Gill, MD, MPH, Brigham and Women's Hospital.

- Treatment of PAP is bronchoalveolar lavage.

Lymphangioleiomyomatosis (LAM)

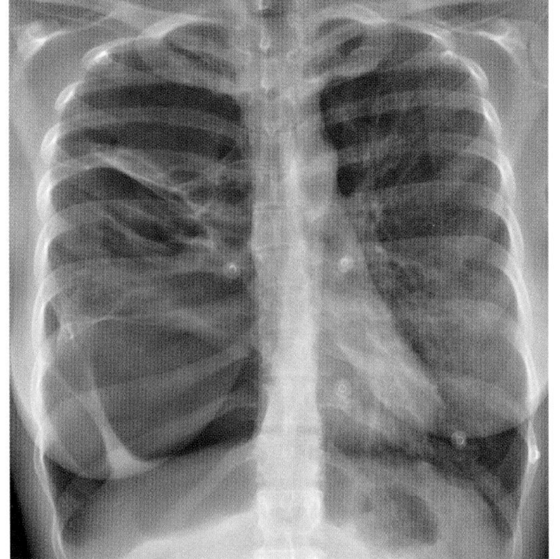

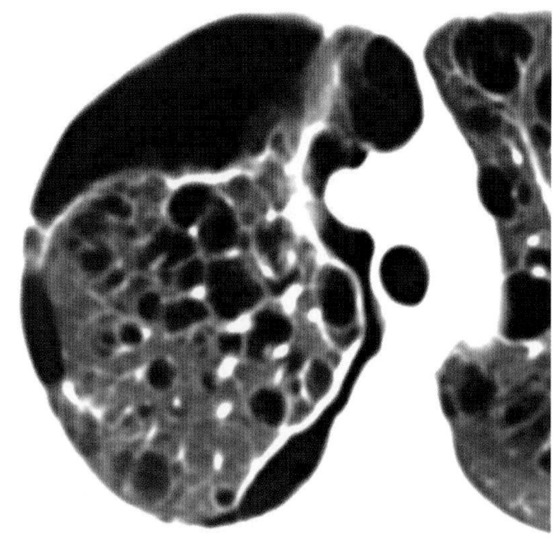

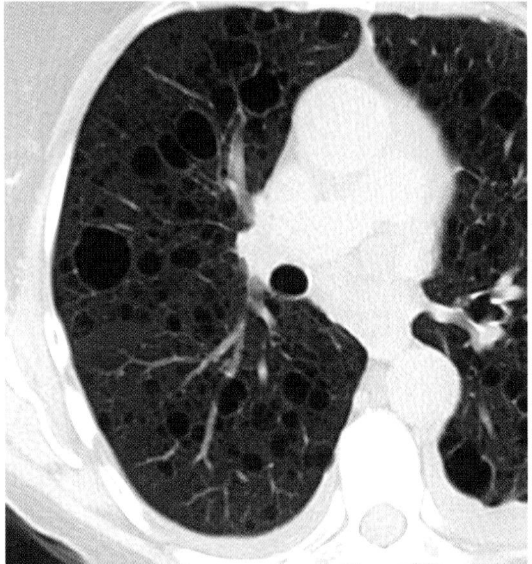

Two separate patients with lymphangioleiomyomatosis:

Patient 1 (top radiograph and top CT) has end-stage LAM with severe cystic change and moderate right apical and posterior pneumothoraces.

Patient 2 (bottom left CT) shows a less severe stage of disease, with multiple smooth-walled cysts and bilateral pleural effusions. Although the pleural fluid was not sampled in this case, there is an association of LAM with chylous effusion.

Cases courtesy Ritu R. Gill, MD, MPH, Brigham and Women's Hospital.

- Lymphangioleiomyomatosis (LAM) is a diffuse cystic lung disease caused by bronchiolar obstruction and lung destruction due to proliferation of immature smooth muscle cells in small vessels, lymphatics, and bronchioles.
- Approximately 1% of patients with tuberous sclerosis (triad of seizures, mental retardation, and adenoma sebaceum) have a lung disease that is nearly identical to LAM.
- Almost all cases of sporadic LAM are in women of childbearing age.
- Some cases respond to anti-estrogen therapy.
- LAM is associated with pneumothorax and chylous pleural effusion.
- CT of LAM shows numerous thin-walled lung cysts. In contrast to LCH, the cysts tend to be round and regular. Also, LAM affects all five lobes while LCH is upper-lobe predominant.

Mediastinum

Anatomy of the mediastinum

- The mediastinum is divided into three arbitrary compartments to aid in the differential diagnosis of a mediastinal mass. However, there are no anatomic planes separating these divisions and disease can spread from one "compartment" to another.

  Several methods have been proposed to divide the mediastinum, including the anatomical method, the Felson method, and others. This text follows the method proposed by Whitten et al. in Radiographics 2007.

- The three divisions are primarily used to aid in the differential diagnosis of a mass seen on radiography. For CT diagnosis of a mediastinal mass, it is often possible to be more precise and state exactly where a lesion is arising from.

Anterior mediastinum

- The anterior mediastinum is the space between the sternum and the pericardium inferiorly and ascending aorta and brachiocephalic vessels superiorly.
- The anterior mediastinum can be thought of as two compartments – the prevascular compartment superiorly and the precardiac compartment inferiorly.
- The contents of the **prevascular anterior mediastinum** include:

  Thymus.

  Lymph nodes.

  Enlarged thyroid gland, if it extends inferiorly into the mediastinum.

- The **precardiac anterior mediastinum** is a potential space.

Middle mediastinum

- The anterior border of the middle mediastinum is the anterior pericardium and the posterior borders are the posterior pericardium and posterior tracheal wall.
- The contents of the **middle mediastinum** include:

  Heart and pericardium. Some authors place the heart in the anterior mediastinum. However, for the purpose of differential diagnosis, diseases of the heart and pericardium have more in common with the other vascular structures of the middle mediastinum.

  Ascending aorta and aortic arch.

  Great vessels including SVC, IVC, pulmonary arteries and veins, and brachiocephalic vessels.

  Trachea and bronchi.

  Lymph nodes.

  Phrenic, vagus, and recurrent laryngeal nerves (all of which pass through the AP window).

Posterior mediastinum

- The anterior border of the posterior mediastinum is the posterior trachea and posterior pericardium. The posterior border is somewhat loosely defined as the anterior aspect of the vertebral bodies; however, paraspinal masses are generally included in the differential of a posterior mediastinal mass.
- The contents of the **posterior mediastinum** include:

Esophagus.	Thoracic duct.
Descending thoracic aorta.	Vagus nerves.
Azygos and hemiazygos veins.	Lymph nodes.

- Interfaces between anatomic structures in the lungs, mediastinum, and pleura may be displaced or thickened in the presence of a mediastinal mass or abnormality. With the exception of the right paratracheal stripe, it is generally uncommon to see these interfaces in the absence of pathology.

  A "line" is a thin interface formed by tissue (typically <1 mm in thickness) with air on both sides.

  A "stripe" is a thicker interface formed between air and adjacent soft tissue.

  An "interface" is formed by the contact of two soft tissue structures of different densities.

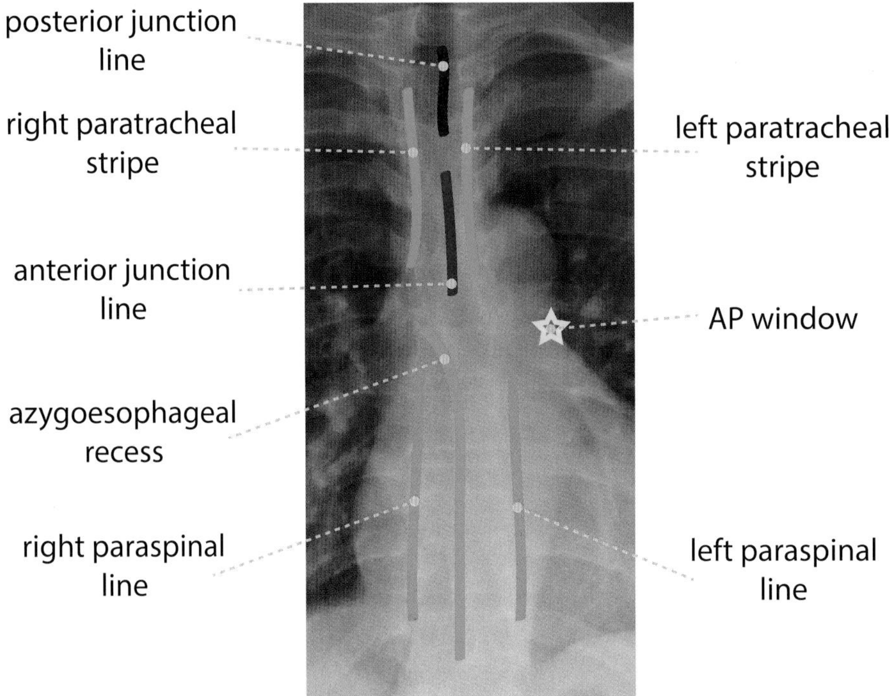

- The **anterior junction line** is formed by four layers of pleura (parietal and visceral pleura of each lung) at the anterior junction of the right and left lungs.

  On a frontal radiograph, the anterior junction line is a vertical line projecting over the superior two-thirds of the sternum.

  Abnormal convexity or displacement of this line suggests an anterior mediastinal mass.

- The **posterior junction line** is also formed by four layers of pleura (parietal and visceral pleura of each lung), but at the posterior junction of the right and left lungs.

  On a frontal radiograph, the posterior junction line is a vertical line projecting through the trachea on the frontal view, more superior than the anterior junction line. Unlike the anterior junction line, the posterior junction line is seen above the clavicles because the posterior lungs extend more superiorly than the anterior lungs.

  Abnormal convexity or displacement of this line suggests a posterior mediastinal mass or aortic aneurysm.

- The **right and left paratracheal stripes** are formed by two layers of pleura where the medial aspect of each lung abuts the lateral wall of the trachea and intervening mediastinal fat.

  The right paratracheal stripe is the most commonly seen of these landmarks, seen in up to 97% of normal PA chest radiographs.

  Thickening of the right paratracheal stripe is most commonly due to pleural thickening, although a paratracheal or tracheal mass (including adenopathy or thyroid or tracheal neoplasm) can also be a cause.

  Thickening of the left paratracheal stripe has a similar differential. In addition, however, a mediastinal hematoma should also be considered, especially in trauma.

- The **posterior tracheal stripe** is the only interface seen on the *lateral radiograph*, representing the interface of the posterior wall of the trachea with the two pleural layers of the medial right lung.

- The **right and left paraspinal lines** are actually interfaces but appear as lines due to Mach effect and are formed by 2 layers of pleura abutting the posterior mediastinum.

  In contrast to the posterior junction line, the paraspinal lines are located inferiorly in the thorax, typically from the 8th through 12th ribs.

  A paraspinal line abnormality suggests a posterior mediastinal mass lesion, including hematoma, neurogenic tumor, aortic aneurysm, extramedullary hematopoiesis, esophageal mass, and osteophyte.

- The **azygoesophageal recess** is an interface formed by the contact of the posteromedial right lower lobe and the retrocardiac mediastinum.

  The azygoesophageal recess extends from the subcarinal region to the diaphragm inferiorly.

  Distortion of the azygoesophageal recess may be due to esophageal mass, hiatal hernia, left atrial enlargement, and adenopathy.

Aortopulmonary (AP) window

- The aortopulmonary (AP) window is a mediastinal space nestled underneath the aortic arch (which forms the superior, anterior, and posterior boundaries) and the top of the pulmonary artery. The medial border of the AP window is formed by the esophagus, trachea, and left mainstem bronchus.
- On a normal frontal radiograph, the AP window is a shallow concave contour below the aortic knob and above the pulmonary artery.
- Abnormal convexity (outwards bulging) of the AP window suggests a mass arising from or involving structures that normally live within the AP window, including:

  Lymph nodes: Adenopathy is the most common cause of an AP window abnormality.

  Left phrenic nerve: Injury may cause paralysis of the left hemidiaphragm.

  Recurrent laryngeal nerve: The AP window should be carefully evaluated in new-onset hoarseness, especially if associated with diaphragmatic paralysis.

  Left vagus nerve.

  Ligamentum arteriosum.

  Left bronchial arteries.

- A thoracic aortic aneurysm may also cause convexity of the AP window.

Retrosternal clear space

- The retrosternal clear space is a normal area of lucency posterior to the sternum seen on the lateral radiograph only. It correlates to the prevascular space on CT.
- Obliteration of the retrosternal clear space suggests an anterior mediastinal mass, right ventricular dilation, or pulmonary artery enlargement.
- Increase in the retrosternal clear space can be seen in emphysema.

Left superior intercostal vein (LSIV)

- The left superior intercostal vein (LSIV) is a normal vein that is not often seen on radiography. When visible, the LSIV produces the *aortic nipple*, appearing as a small round shadow to the left of the aortic knob on the frontal radiograph.
- The LSIV may be dilated as a collateral pathway in SVC obstruction.

Radiographic localization of a mediastinal mass

Detection of an anterior mediastinal mass

- Deformation of the anterior junction line suggests an anterior mediastinal mass. However, since the anterior junction line is not always seen, it is more common to infer the anterior location of a mass by preservation of the posterior lines in the presence of a mass.
- The *hilum overlay* sign is present on the frontal view if hilar vessels are visualized through the mass. It indicates that the mass cannot be in the middle mediastinum. The mass may be in the anterior (most likely) or posterior mediastinum.

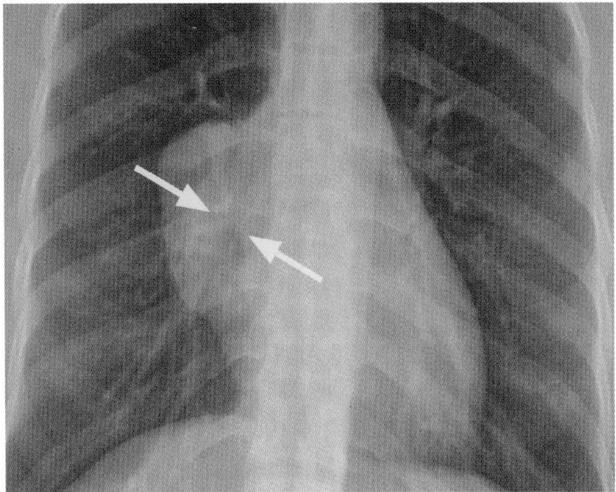
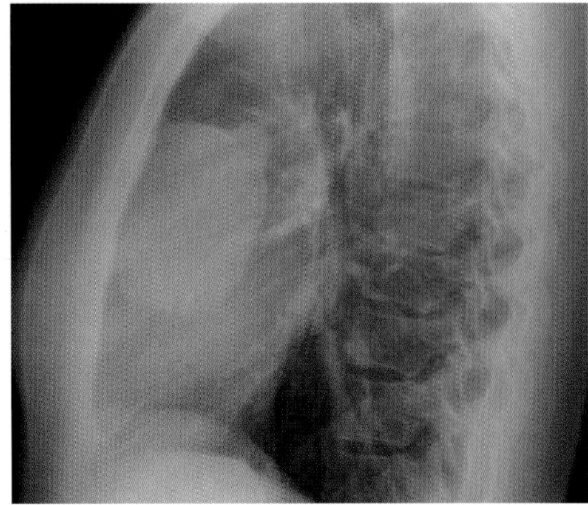

Anterior mediastinal mass: Frontal radiograph shows a right mediastinal mass with silhouetting of the right heart border. The right pulmonary artery is visible through the mass (arrows), representing the *hilum overlay sign* and indicating that the mass is not in the middle mediastinum. Lateral radiograph shows the mass in the retrosternal clear space, confirming its anterior mediastinal location. This was a teratoma.

- Obliteration of the retrosternal clear space on the lateral radiograph is a direct sign of anterior mediastinal location.

Detection of a middle mediastinal mass

- Distortion of the paratracheal stripes or convexity of the AP window suggests a middle mediastinal mass.

Detection of a posterior mediastinal mass

- Distortion of the azygoesophageal recess, distortion of the posterior junction line, or displacement of the paraspinal lines suggest paravertebral/posterior mediastinal disease.

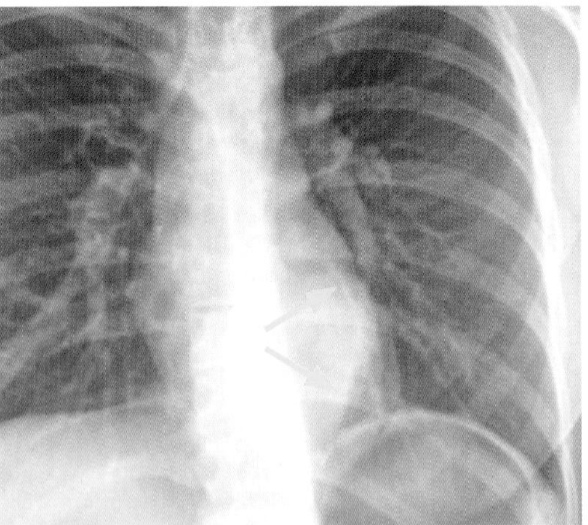
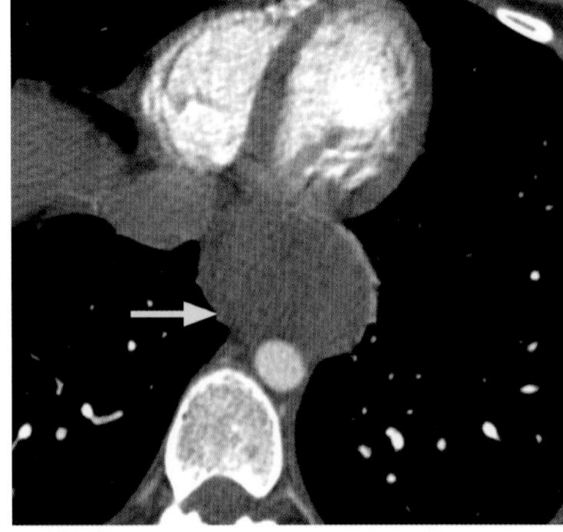

Displacement of the left paraspinal line: Frontal chest radiograph (left) shows lateral displacement and bowing of the left paraspinal line (arrows), suggestive of a posterior mediastinal mass. Axial contrast-enhanced CT shows a nonenhancing homogeneous mass (arrow) effacing the esophagus. Although extremely rare, this was a liposarcoma.

Overview of prevascular anterior mediastinal masses

- A mnemonic for prevascular anterior mediastinal masses often learned in medical school is the *four T's*: Thymoma, teratoma, thyroid lesion, and terrible lymphoma. However, a more sophisticated approach is necessary when communicating with subspecialized clinicians.
- A better (but considerably less catchy) differential for an anterior mediastinal mass includes:

> **Thymic epithelial neoplasm**, such as thymoma if the patient is middle aged or older, or has a history of myasthenia gravis. Less common would be thymic carcinoma.
>
> **Germ cell tumor**, including teratoma, if the patient is a young adult.
>
> **Thyroid lesion**, if there is extension of the mass above the thoracic inlet.
>
> **Lymphoma**.

Thymoma

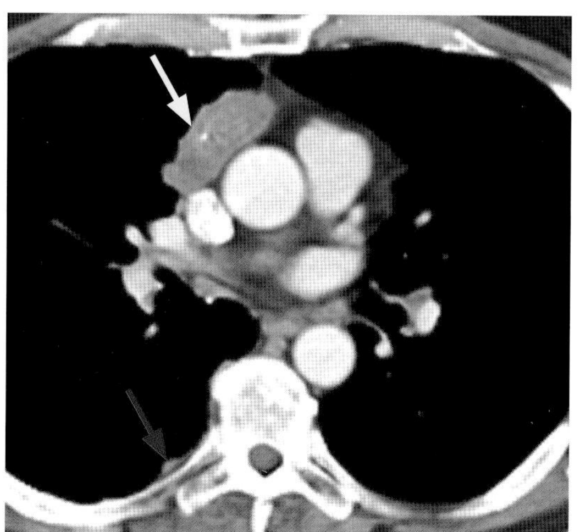

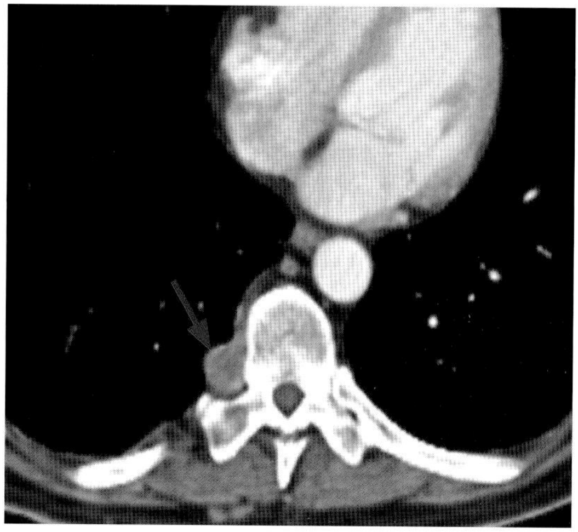

Invasive thymoma with drop metastasis: Contrast-enhanced CT shows a slightly heterogeneous mass (yellow arrow) anterior to the aorta and SVC, with two pleural-based metastases (red arrows).

Case courtesy Ritu R. Gill, MD, MPH, Brigham and Women's Hospital.

- Thymoma is the most common primary tumor of the anterior mediastinum and typically occurs in middle-aged or older individuals, between 45 and 60 years.
- Thymoma is associated with myasthenia gravis (MG). Approximately 33% of patients with thymoma have MG, and 10% of patients with MG have a thymoma.
- In addition to MG, thymomas are often associated with other diseases including red cell aplasia, hypogammaglobulinemia, paraneoplastic syndromes, and malignancies such as lymphoma or thyroid cancer.
- Thymoma can be pathologically classified as low-risk or high-risk based on histology, and non-invasive or invasive based on whether the capsule is intact.

  Approximately 30% of thymomas are invasive. If invasive, the tumor may invade adjacent structures including the airways, chest wall, great vessels, and phrenic nerves.

  Elevation of a hemidiaphragm is suggestive of phrenic nerve invasion.

  Invasive thymoma may spread along pleural and pericardial surfaces, called *drop metastases*. However, hematogenous metastases are exceedingly rare.

- Thymoma is histologically classified by the WHO system into A, AB, B1, B2, B3, and C subtypes, with progressively worse prognosis.

  Type A tumors are relatively uncommon, but are usually encapsulated.

  Type B tumors contain increasing number of epithelial cells, which represent the malignant component.

  Type C represents thymic carcinoma, which may metastasize hematogenously.

Less common thymic lesions

- **Thymic carcinoma**

  Unlike invasive thymoma, thymic carcinoma is histologically malignant, very aggressive, and often metastasizes hematogenously to lungs, liver, brain, and bone. Prognosis is poor.

  Distinction between invasive thymoma and thymic carcinoma is difficult on CT, unless there is evidence of distant metastatic disease.

- **Thymic carcinoid**

  Thymic carcinoid is of neural crest origin. 50% of thymic carcinoids are hormonally active, often secreting ACTH and causing Cushing syndrome.

  Thymic carcinoid is associated with multiple endocrine neoplasia (MEN) I and II.

  On imaging, thymic carcinoid is generally indistinguishable from thymoma and thymic carcinoma on CT.

  If carcinoid is suspected, a preoperative Indium-111 Octreotide scan can be performed.

- **Thymic cyst**

  A thymic cyst may be secondary to radiation therapy (e.g., administered to treat Hodgkin disease), may be associated with AIDS (especially when multilocular), or may be congenital. When congenital, thymic cysts arise from remnants of the thymopharyngeal duct. A congenital thymic cyst may occur anywhere along the course of thymic descent from the neck, but most commonly in the anterior mediastinum.

  Thymic cyst is typically evident on CT as a simple fluid-attenuation cyst in the anterior mediastinum.

- **Thymolipoma**

  Thymolipoma is a benign fat-containing lesion with interspersed soft tissue. It may become quite large and drape over the mediastinum.

Germ cell tumor (GCT)

- Several different types of germ cell tumors may arise in the anterior mediastinum from primitive germ cell elements, most of which are benign. Malignant GCT occurs more commonly in males.
- **Teratoma** is the most common anterior mediastinal germ cell tumor, usually encapsulated and predominantly cystic in nature, but fat and calcification are common. A fat/fluid level is specific for teratoma, but is not commonly seen. Teratoma can rarely be malignant, especially if large in size and irregular in shape.

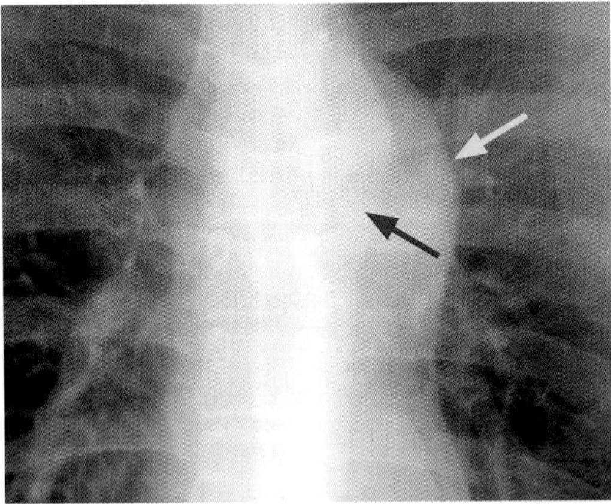

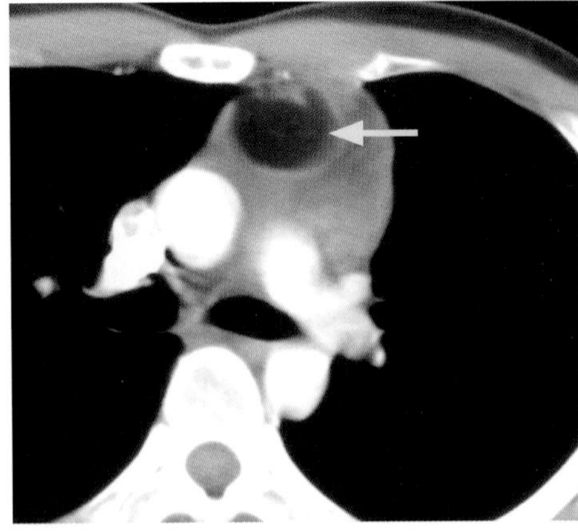

Teratoma: Chest radiograph shows an extra mediastinal contour (yellow arrow) lateral to the aortic arch (red arrow). Because the mass does not silhouette the aorta it cannot be in the posterior mediastinum. On CT there is an anterior mediastinal mass containing a large focus of fat (yellow arrow). The differential in this case would include a thymolipoma.

Case courtesy Ritu R. Gill, MD, MPH, Brigham and Women's Hospital.

- **Seminoma** is the most common *malignant* anterior mediastinal germ cell tumor. It occurs almost exclusively in men.

Thyroid lesion

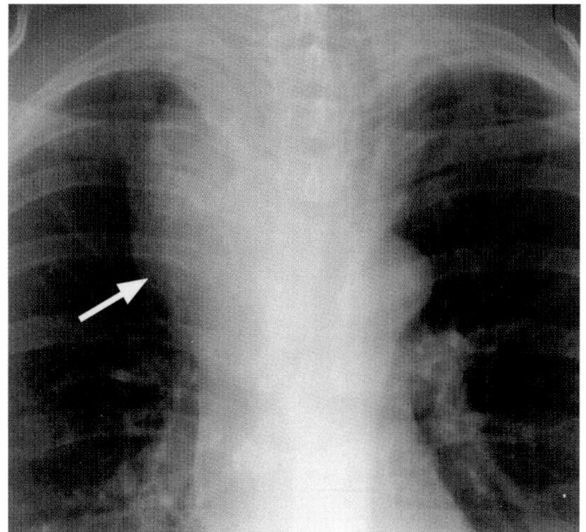

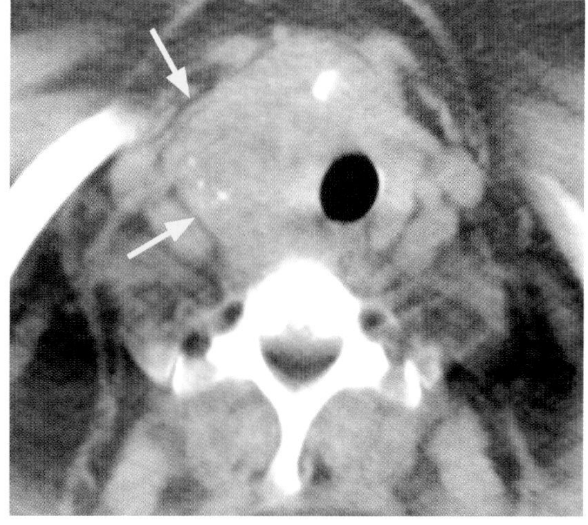

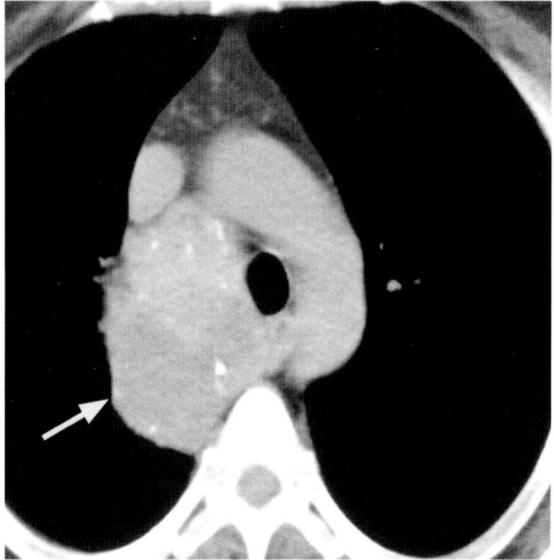

Inferior extension of a goiter into the mediastinum:

Chest radiograph demonstrates a right superior mediastinal mass (arrow) with obscuration of the superior border of the mass, representing the *cervicothoracic* sign, which implies that the mass is in continuity with the soft tissues of the neck.

Noncontrast CT shows a large heterogeneous mass (arrows) with coarse calcifications replacing the thyroid gland.

Although the thyroid is anterior, the goiter extends inferiorly into the posterior mediastinum due to an embryologic fascial plane created by the inferior thyroidal artery.

Case courtesy Ritu R. Gill, MD, MPH, Brigham and Women's Hospital.

- Benign and malignant thyroid masses may extend into the mediastinum, including goiter, thyroid neoplasm, and an enlarged gland due to thyroiditis.
- The key to diagnosis is to show continuity superiorly with the thyroid.

Lymphoma

- Both Hodgkin disease and non-Hodgkin lymphoma are important differential considerations for an anterior mediastinal mass.
- Hodgkin disease commonly involves the thorax, most often the superior mediastinal lymph nodes including prevascular, AP window, and paratracheal nodal stations.
- Non-Hodgkin lymphoma is a diverse group of diseases, which less commonly involve the thorax compared to Hodgkin disease.
- Calcification is rare in untreated lymphoma.

Non-lymphomatous adenopathy

- Lymph node calcification, low attenuation, and avid enhancement are unusual features for lymphoma. An alternative diagnosis should be considered if these imaging findings are seen.
- **Eggshell calcification** of lymph nodes is often present in silicosis and coal workers pneumoconiosis, less commonly in sarcoidosis. Given the greater prevalence of sarcoidosis, however, eggshell calcification may be seen more commonly in sarcoid overall.
- Dense calcification within a lymph node can be seen in sarcoidosis or as a sequela of prior granulomatous disease.

- Low attenuation lymph nodes, while nonspecific, should raise concern for active tuberculosis. Low attenuation lymph nodes can also be seen in fungal infection, lymphoma, and metastatic disease.
- Avid lymph node enhancement can be seen in Castleman disease, sarcoidosis, tuberculosis, and vascular metastases. Avidly enhancing vascular metastases include:

> Renal cell carcinoma.
> Thyroid carcinoma.
> Lung carcinoma.
> Sarcoma.
> Melanoma.

Castleman disease

- Castleman disease, also known as angiofollicular lymph node hyperplasia, is a cause of highly vascular thoracic lymph node enlargement, of uncertain etiology.
- Localized Castleman disease is seen in children or young adults. Surgical resection is usually curative.
- Multicentric Castleman disease manifests in older patients or in association with AIDS. Multicentric disease often results in systemic illness including fever, anemia, and lymphoma. It is typically treated with chemotherapy.
- The key imaging finding of Castleman disease is avidly enhancing adenopathy.

Anterior mediastinal mass - precardiac (inferior anterior mediastinum)

Overview of precardiac anterior mediastinal masses

- A precardiac anterior mediastinal mass is in contact with the diaphragm.

Epicardial fat pad

- A prominent epicardial fat pad silhouettes the cardiac border on a frontal radiograph and may simulate cardiomegaly.

Pericardial cyst

- A pericardial cyst is a benign cystic lesion thought to be congenital. Most are located at the right cardiophrenic angle (between the heart and the diaphragm).
- Imaging shows a cystic lesion abutting the pericardium, which may change in shape on subsequent studies.

Morgagni hernia

- Morgagni hernia is a diaphragmatic hernia through the foramen of Morgagni, containing omental fat and often bowel. A Morgagni hernia usually occurs on the right.
- An anterior mediastinal mass in contact with the diaphragm containing bowel gas is diagnostic for a Morgagni hernia.
- If bowel gas is absent, a key to diagnosis on CT is the detection of omental vessels in the mass which can be traced into the upper abdomen.

Middle mediastinal mass

Lymphadenopathy

- Lymphadenopathy is an important cause of a middle mediastinal mass on radiography.

Ascending aortic or aortic arch aneurysm

- An abnormality of the ascending aorta or aortic arch may appear as a middle mediastinal mass on radiography.

Enlarged pulmonary artery (PA)

- An enlarged pulmonary artery (PA) can simulate a mass on a chest radiograph. As previously discussed, the *hilum convergence* sign can help distinguish between an enlarged PA and a mediastinal mass. The hilum convergence sign shows the peripheral pulmonary arteries converging into the "mass" if the mass represents an enlarged pulmonary artery.

Foregut duplication cyst

- Foregut duplication cysts include bronchogenic cysts, esophageal duplication cysts, and neurenteric cysts. Foregut duplication cysts may occur in the middle or posterior mediastinum.

Posterior mediastinal mass

Neurogenic tumor

- A neurogenic tumor may arise from either a peripheral nerve or the sympathetic ganglia. Most adult tumors are peripheral nerve sheath tumors and the vast majority of tumors in children are of sympathetic ganglionic origin. Overall, neurogenic tumors are the most common posterior mediastinal masses.
- Peripheral nerve tumors (more common in adults) include:

> **Schwannoma** (most common), **neurofibroma**, and **malignant peripheral nerve sheath tumor**.

- Sympathetic ganglion tumors (more common in children/young adults) include:

> **Ganglioneuroma** (most common), a benign tumor of sympathetic ganglion cells.
>
> **Neuroblastoma**, a malignant tumor of ganglion cells seen in early childhood.
>
> **Ganglioneuroblastoma**, intermediate in histology between ganglioneuroma and neuroblastoma, seen in older children than neuroblastoma.

Hiatal hernia

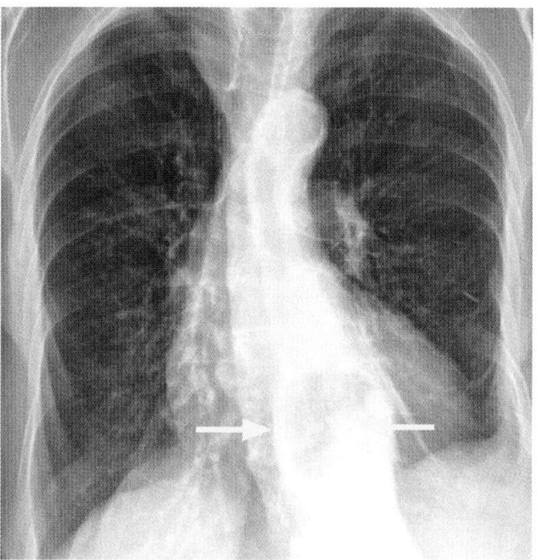
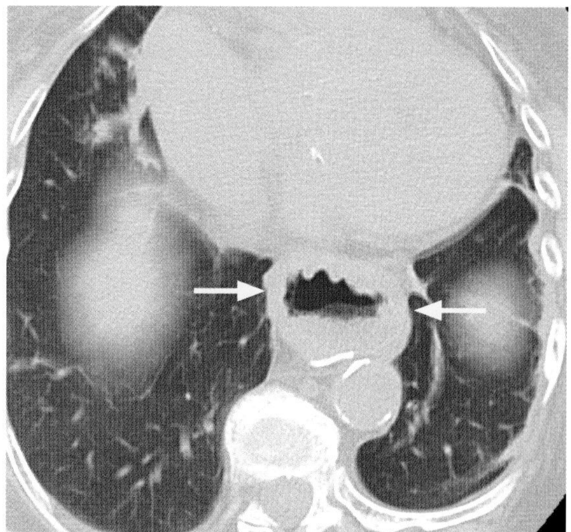

Hiatal hernia: Frontal radiograph shows a retrocardiac lucency (arrows), which was confirmed to be a moderate-sized hiatal hernia on CT (arrows).

- A hiatal hernia is protrusion of a portion of the stomach through the esophageal hiatus. The esophageal hiatus is an elliptical opening in the diaphragm just to the left of midline.
- On radiography, air or an air–fluid level is present above the diaphragm.

Descending thoracic aortic aneurysm

- Thoracic aortic aneurysm may appear as a posterior mediastinal mass on radiography.

Extramedullary hematopoiesis

- Extramedullary hematopoiesis causes soft tissue paravertebral masses in patients with severe hereditary anemias including thalassemia and sickle cell anemia. The masses are of uncertain origin but may represent herniation of vertebral marrow or may represent elements of the reticuloendothelial system.
- On imaging, lobulated soft tissue masses are typically bilateral and inferior to T6.

Lateral meningocele

- A lateral meningocele is lateral herniation of the spinal meninges through either an intervertebral foramen or a defect in the vertebral body. Lateral meningocele is associated with neurofibromatosis.

Esophageal neoplasm

- Esophageal carcinoma can present on radiography as abnormal convexity of the azygoesophageal recess, mediastinal widening, or a retrotracheal mass. Benign mesenchymal esophageal tumors, such as leiomyoma, fibroma, or lipoma may appear similar on radiography.

Foregut duplication cyst

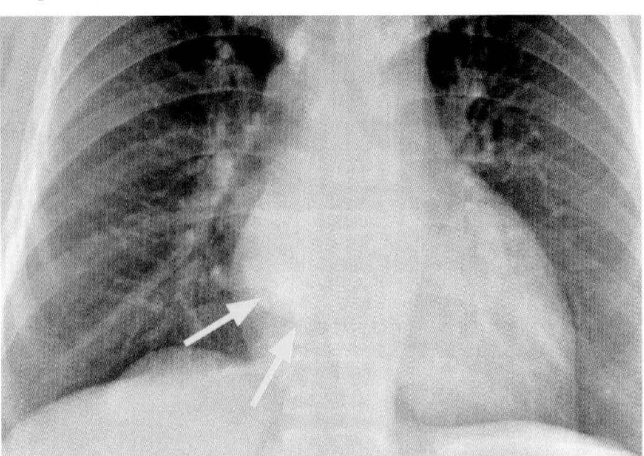

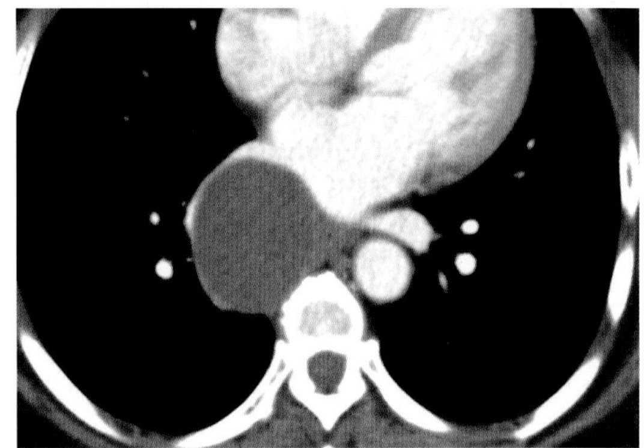

Foregut duplication cyst: Frontal radiograph shows a subtle opacity overlying the right heart (arrow), shown to be a fluid attenuation lesion adjacent to the esophagus on CT.

Case courtesy Darryl Sneag, MD, Brigham and Women's Hospital.

- A foregut duplication cyst, a remnant of the fetal foregut, may present as a middle or posterior mediastinal mass.

Paraspinal abscess

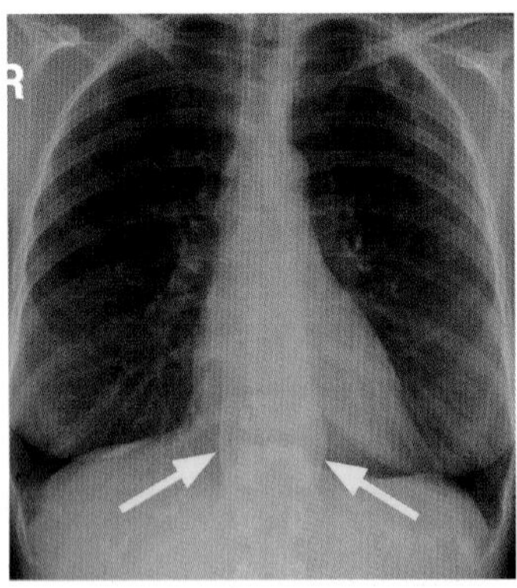

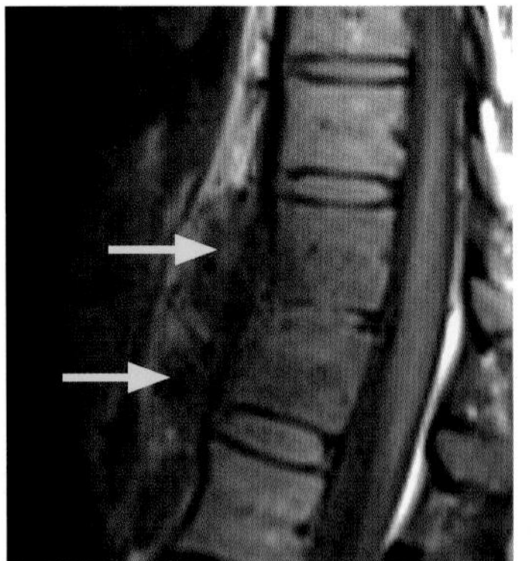

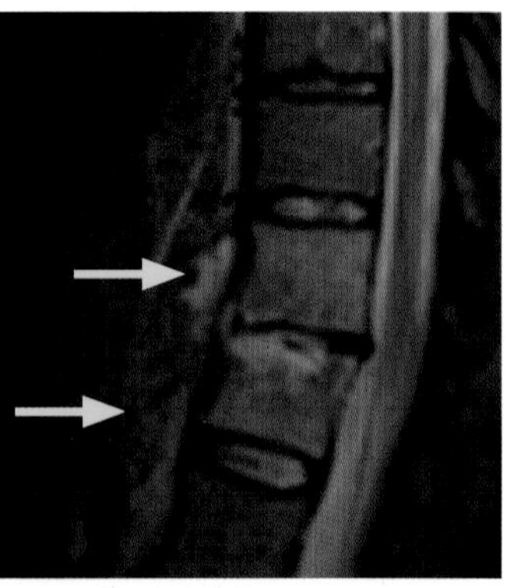

Osteomyelitis and paraspinal phlegmon: Radiograph shows displacement of the bilateral paraspinal lines (arrows). Sagittal T1 (middle image) and T2-weighted MRI (right image) shows loss of disk space height and marrow edema in two adjacent lower thoracic vertebral bodies. There is associated paraspinal phlegmonous change (arrows), which caused the paraspinal line displacement on radiography.

- A clue to vertebral body pathology on radiography may be paraspinal line displacement.

MULTIFOCAL OR DIFFUSE NON-NEOPLASTIC TRACHEAL STENOSIS/WALL THICKENING

Overview of non-neoplastic diffuse tracheal disease

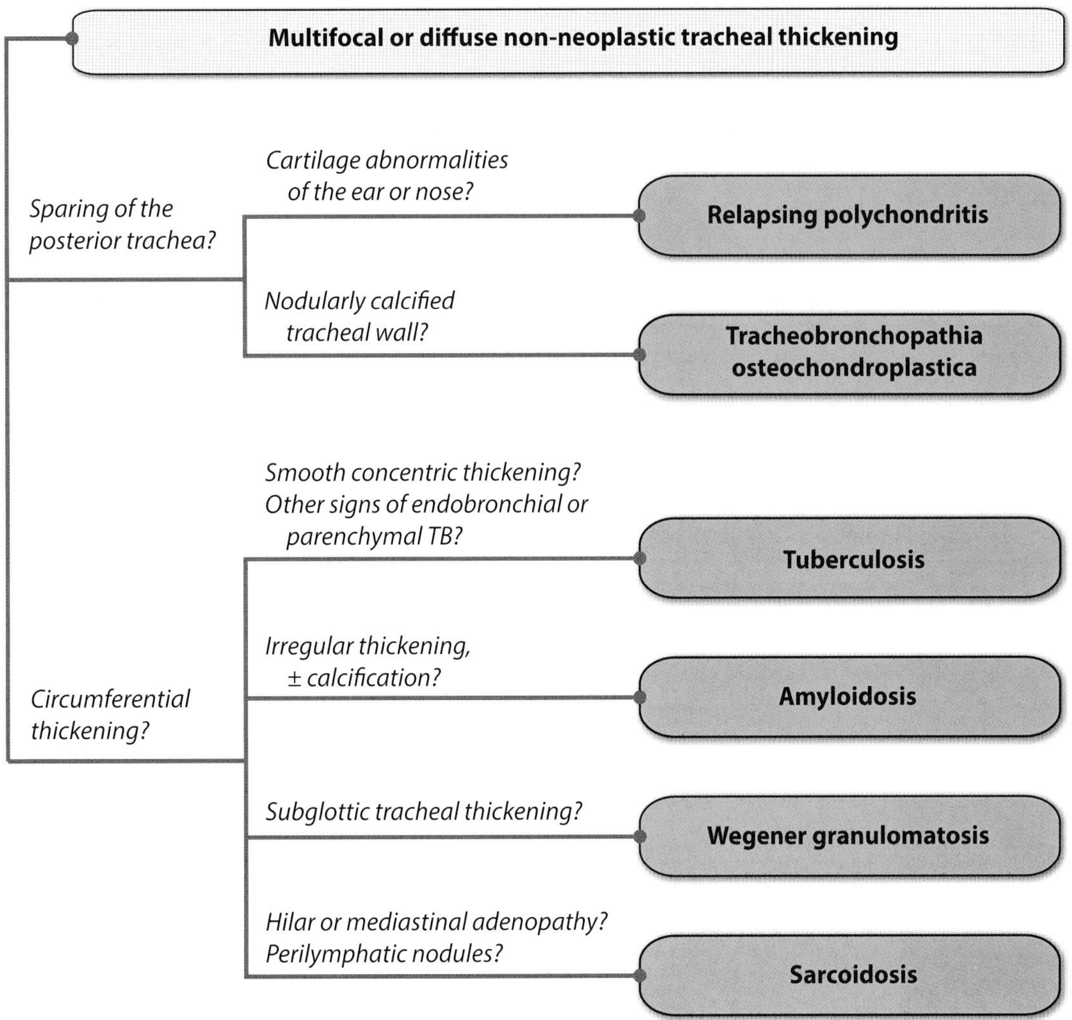

Relapsing polychondritis

- Relapsing polychondritis is a multisystemic disease of unknown etiology characterized by recurrent inflammation of cartilaginous structures. The nose, ear, joints, larynx, trachea, and bronchi can be affected, with airway involvement seen in 50% of patients.

  The larynx and subglottic trachea are the most common sites of airway involvement.
- Relapsing polychondritis usually occurs in middle-aged women.
- On cross-sectional imaging, there is smooth tracheal/bronchial wall thickening, with *sparing of the posterior membranous* trachea.

  The tracheal cartilage is an incomplete ring, with no cartilage in the posterior membranous portion.
- There is often increased attenuation of the airway wall, ranging from subtly increased attenuation to frank calcification.

Tracheobronchopathia osteochondroplastica (TPO)

- Tracheobronchopathia osteochondroplastica (TPO) is a benign condition of multiple submucosal calcified osteocartilaginous nodules along the tracheal walls.
- Similar to relapsing polychondritis, there is sparing of the posterior membranous trachea.

Tuberculosis

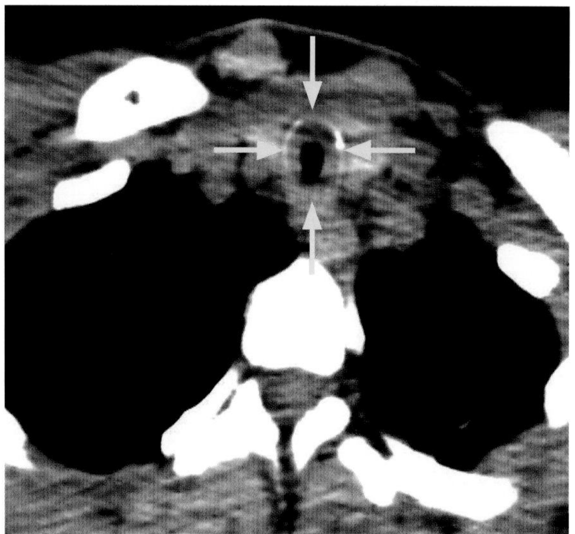

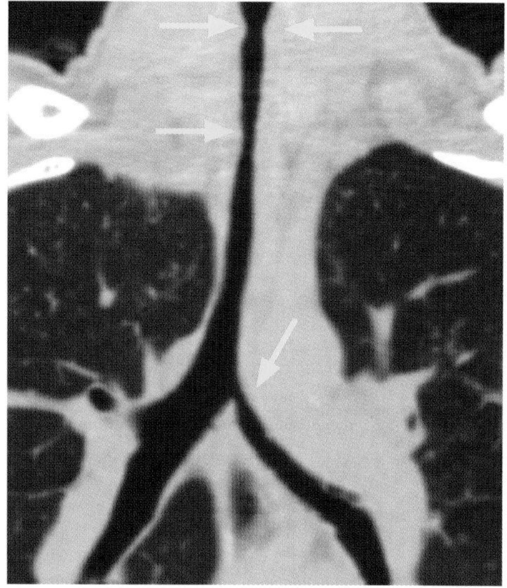

Tracheal tuberculosis: Axial CT in soft-tissue window through the upper trachea (left image) shows circumferential tracheal thickening (arrows). Coronal curved-multiplanar reformation (right image) shows multifocal tracheal stenosis (arrows) and left mainstem bronchus stenosis. These images were obtained approximately one month after treatment for active post-primary tuberculosis.

Case courtesy Ritu R. Gill, MD, MPH, Brigham and Women's Hospital.

- Endobronchial spread of tuberculosis occurs in a prominent minority of patients with pulmonary tuberculosis, most commonly involving the distal trachea and proximal bronchi.
- Imaging findings are nonspecific. There is usually smooth concentric narrowing of a relatively long airway segment (typically >3cm).

Amyloidosis

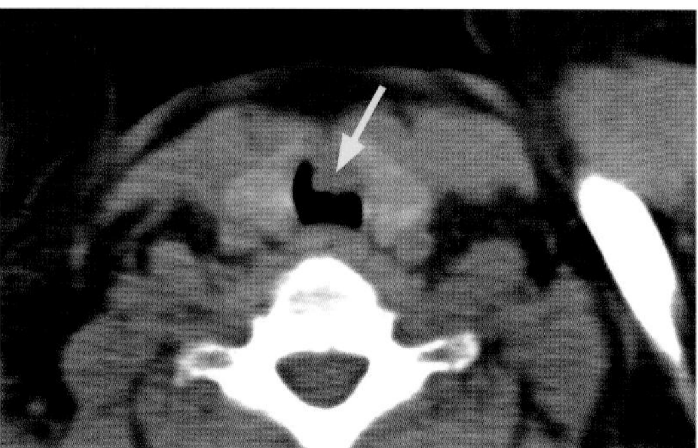

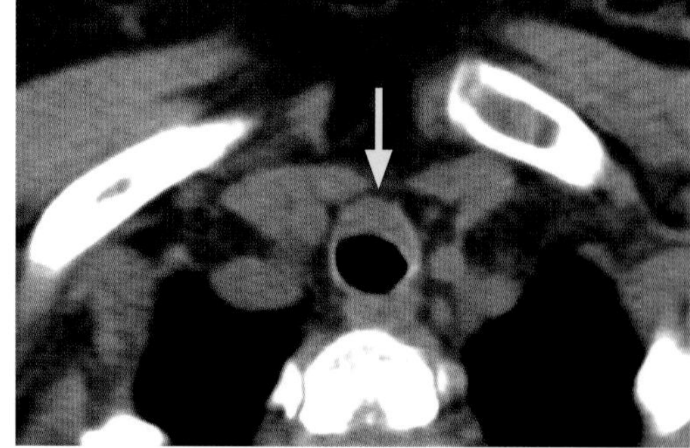

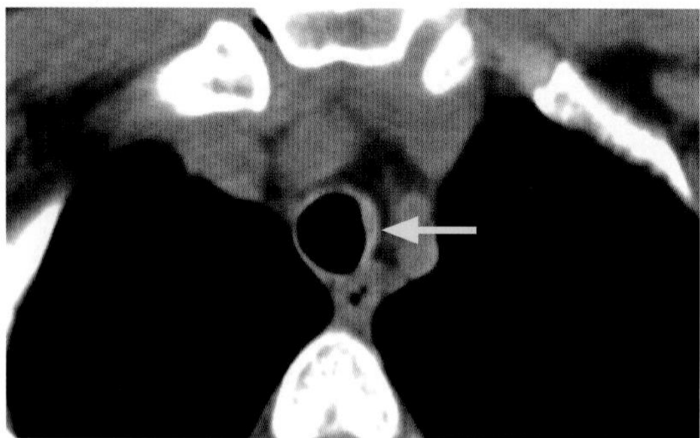

Tracheal amyloid: Axial CT images show nodular and irregular thickening of the trachea (arrows). This pattern is not specific, and the differential would include also include sarcoidosis, multifocal adenoid cystic carcinoma, and tracheal metastases.

Case courtesy Ritu R. Gill, MD, MPH, Brigham and Women's Hospital.

- Amyloidosis causes irregular narrowing of the airways due to submucosal amyloid deposition, which may be calcified. Tracheal amyloidosis is very rare.
- The posterior membranous trachea is not spared.

Wegener granulomatosis

- Large airway involvement is seen in approximately 20% of patients with Wegener granulomatosis, most commonly manifesting as subglottic tracheal stenosis with circumferential mucosal thickening.
- The posterior membranous trachea is not spared in Wegener granulomatosis.

Sarcoidosis

- Tracheal involvement by sarcoid is rare and usually seen in advanced disease. Tracheal sarcoid has a variable appearance ranging from smooth stenosis to a nodular or mass-like appearance.
- The posterior membranous trachea is not spared in tracheal sarcoidosis.

Focal non-neoplastic tracheal stenosis/wall thickening

Intubation/tracheostomy

- There is approximately 1% risk of tracheal stenosis after intubation, but approximately 30% risk of stenosis after long-standing tracheostomy.

Rare causes of focal tracheal stenosis

- Extremely uncommon causes of focal tracheal stenosis include Behçet and Crohn disease.

Large airways

Bronchiectasis

- Bronchiectasis is progressive, irreversible dilation of cartilage-containing bronchi.
- Three etiologies of bronchiectasis have been described, with a final common pathway of mucus plugging, superimposed bacterial colonization, and inflammatory response.

Bronchial wall injury, typically from infection or inflammation.

Bronchial lumen obstruction.

Traction from adjacent fibrosis.

- Specific causes of bronchiectasis include:

Ineffective clearing of secretions – **cystic fibrosis** and **Kartagener** (primary ciliary dyskinesia).

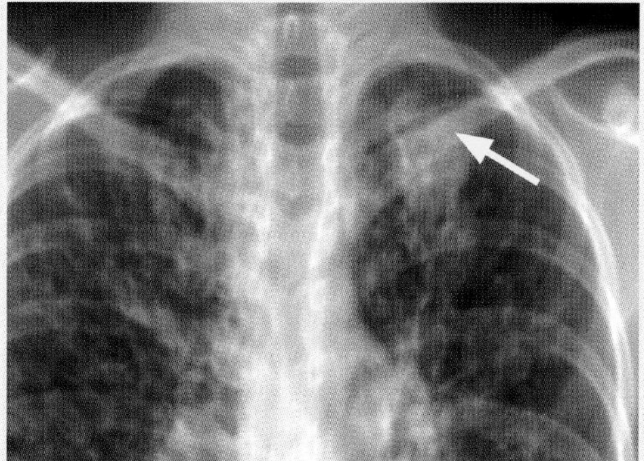

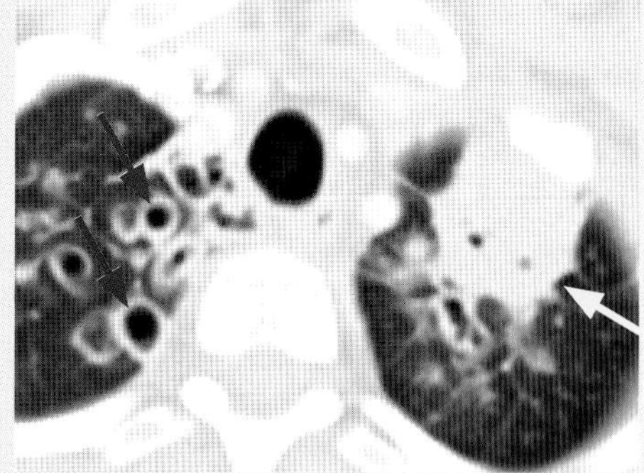

Bronchiectasis from cystic fibrosis with superimposed pneumonia: Radiograph shows upper-lobe bronchiectasis with a focal left upper lobe opacity (yellow arrow). CT confirms bronchiectasis (red arrows) and a left upper lobe consolidation (yellow arrow), representing pneumonia.

Case courtesy Ritu R. Gill, MD, MPH, Brigham and Women's Hospital.

Recurrent pneumonia.

Bronchocentric infections, such as **tuberculosis** and **atypical mycobacteria.**

Exaggerated immune response, as seen in **ABPA** and **vasculitis.**

Impaired immunity: **Congenital immunodeficiency**, **transplant recipients,** and **agammaglobulinemia.**

Congenital connective tissue disorders – **Mounier–Kuhn** (a connective tissue disorder causing tracheobronchomegaly leading to recurrent pneumonia), or **Williams–Campbell** (a rare disorder of the distal bronchial cartilage, which may be congenital or acquired as a sequela of viral infection).

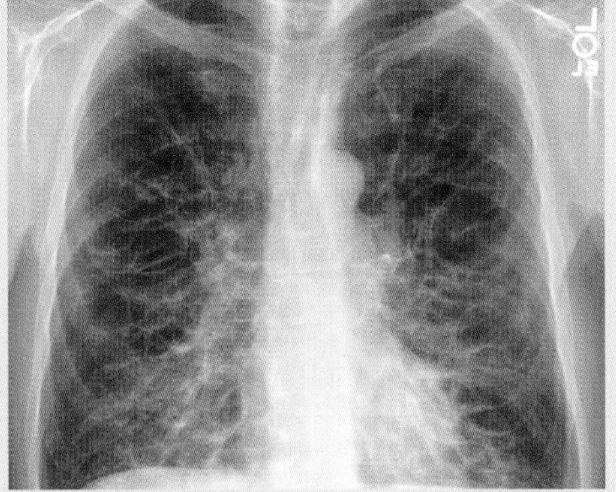

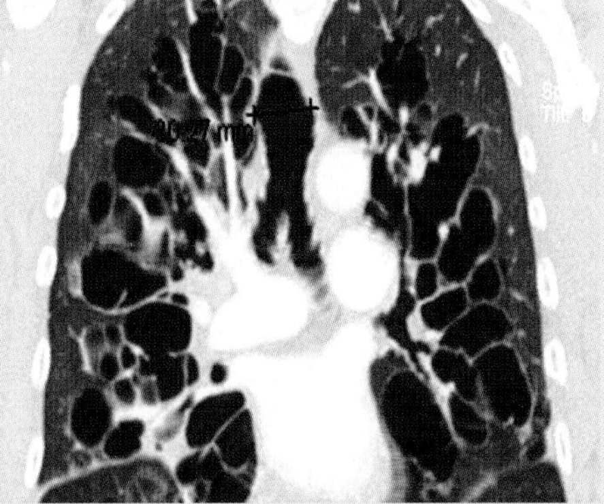

Mounier–Kuhn: Chest radiograph (left image) shows severe diffuse bronchiectasis. CT shows tracheal dilation (calipers) and severe cystic bronchiectasis.

Case courtesy Ritu R. Gill, MD, MPH, Brigham and Women's Hospital.

- ***CAPTAIn Kangaroo has Mounier–Kuhn*** is a mnemonic to remember the common causes of bronchiectasis.

Cystic fibrosis is one of the most common causes of bronchiectasis.

Allergic bronchopulmonary aspergillosis (ABPA).

Post infectious.

TB/atypical mycobacteria.

Agammaglobulinemia.

Immunodeficiency.

Kartagener.

Mounier–Kuhn.

- Cystic fibrosis tends to be upper lobe predominant. In contrast, post-infectious bronchiectasis tends to be lower-lobe predominant.
- Morphologic classification of bronchiectasis is most useful as a rough gauge of severity.

Cylindrical bronchiectasis (least severe): Mild bronchial dilation.

Varicose bronchiectasis (moderately severe): Bronchi may become beaded and irregular.

Cystic bronchiectasis (most severe): Bronchi are markedly enlarged and ballooned, with formation of multiple cysts that may not connect to the airways.

- Radiographic findings depend on severity. In mild cases only *tram tracks* may be visible, representing thickened bronchial walls causing parallel radiopaque lines resembling tram tracks. In more severe cases there can be extensive cystic change.
- CT findings include the *signet ring* sign, which describes a dilated bronchus adjacent to a normal pulmonary artery branch.

  Normally each bronchus should be approximately the same size as the adjacent pulmonary artery branch.

  Other CT findings of bronchiectasis include lack of bronchial tapering, bronchial wall thickening, and mucus-filled bronchi. Often, adjacent tree-in-bud nodules are present, likely representing associated small-airways infection.

Broncholithiasis

- Broncholithiasis is a rare disorder of calcified/ossified material within the bronchial lumen, most commonly caused by erosion of an adjacent calcified granulomatous lymph node.
- Broncholithiasis clinically presents with nonproductive cough, hemoptysis, and air trapping.

- Emphysema is the destruction of alveolar walls resulting in irreversible enlargement of the distal airspaces. Although emphysema initially does not involve fibrosis, end-stage emphysema may lead to a reparative response that ultimately leads to pulmonary fibrosis.
- Elastase is produced by alveolar macrophages and neutrophils, both of which are increased in smokers. Elastase is a powerful destructive enzyme which functions in the host defense mechanism, but excess elastase can be highly harmful to the native tissues. Alpha-1-antitrypsin normally neutralizes elastase. Either a surplus of elastase (in smoking-related emphysema) or a deficiency of neutralizing enzyme (in alpha-1-antitrypsin) can cause lung destruction and resultant emphysema.

Centrilobular emphysema

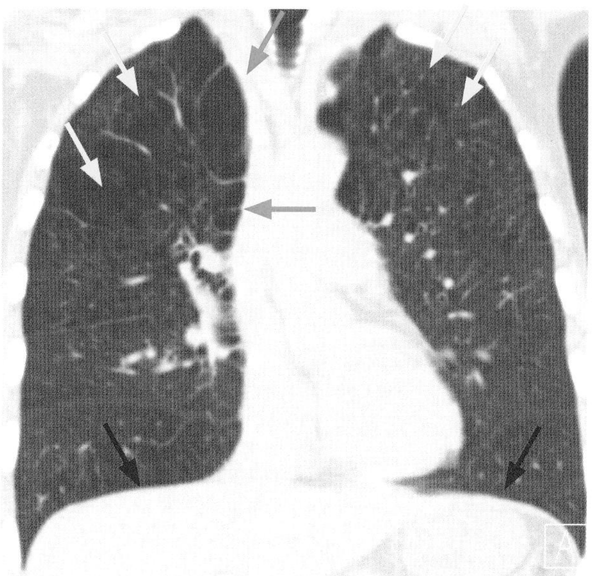
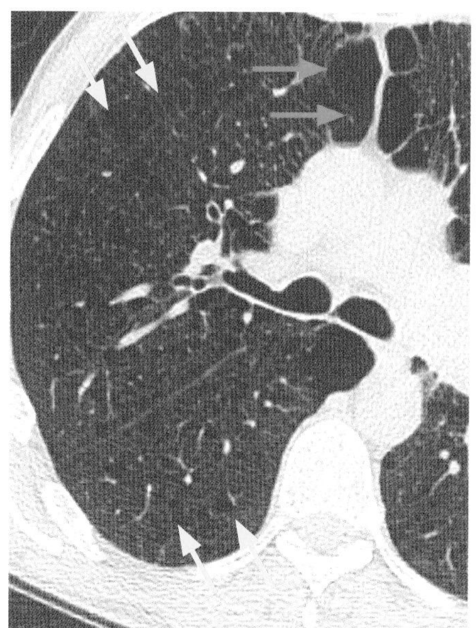

Centrilobular and paraseptal emphysema: Coronal (left image) and axial CT demonstrate both centrilobular and paraseptal emphysema. Centrilobular emphysema is predominant in the upper lobes (yellow arrows) and paraseptal emphysema is seen anteromedially (blue arrows).

Flattening of the diaphragms is seen on the coronal view (red arrows).

- Centrilobular emphysema is a smoking-related lung disease.
- Centrilobular emphysema predominantly affects the upper lobes. Like RB-ILD, another smoking-related lung disease, centrilobular emphysema primarily affects the center of the secondary pulmonary lobule.

  All smoking-related lung disease (RB, RB-ILD, DIP, PLCH, and emphysema) may be within the same spectrum of disease caused by macrophage-mediated inflammation in reaction to inhaled particles and toxins.

Paraseptal emphysema

- Paraseptal emphysema is usually seen in combination with other forms of emphysema. It is also usually smoking related.
- Paraseptal emphysema is subpleural in location and may predispose to pneumothorax.

Panacinar (panlobular) emphysema

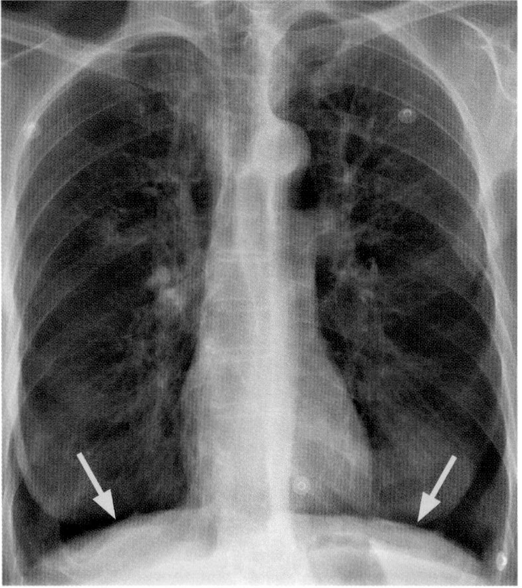

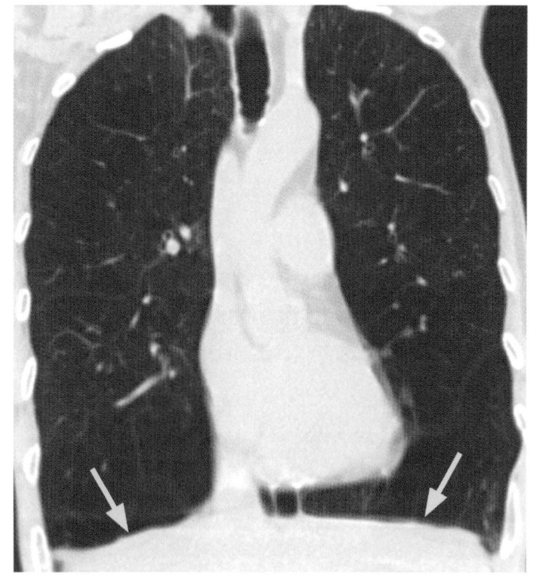

Panacinar emphysema due to alpha-1-antitrypsin deficiency: Frontal radiograph and coronal CT show diffuse emphysematous changes most severely affecting the lower lobes, with flattening of the diaphragms (arrows).

- Panacinar (also called panlobular) emphysema affects the entire acinus diffusely throughout the lung. The emphysematous changes are usually more severe at the lung bases.
- Alpha-1-antitrypsin deficiency is an important cause of panacinar emphysema.

Airway tumors

- Primary tumors of the trachea and central bronchi are rare. In adults, the vast majority of tumors are malignant, while in children most are benign.
- Squamous cell carcinoma and adenoid cystic carcinoma are by far the two most common primary central airway tumors in adults.

Squamous cell carcinoma (SCC)

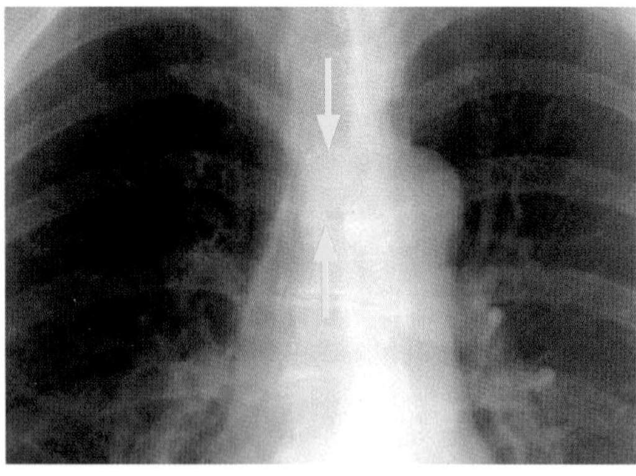

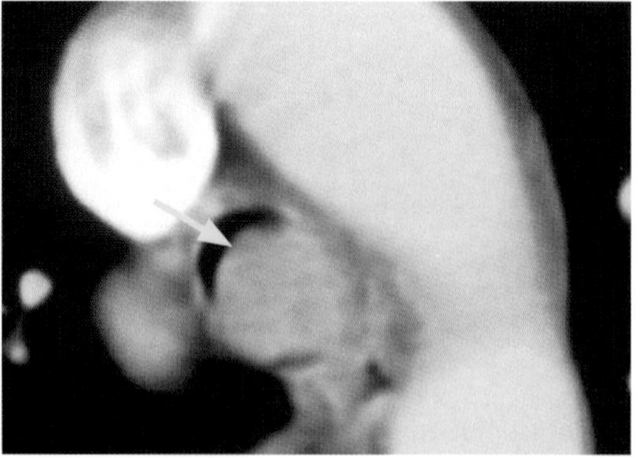

Endotracheal squamous cell carcinoma: Radiograph shows a subtle tracheal filling defect (arrows). On CT there is a heterogeneously enhancing, well-circumscribed mass markedly narrowing the tracheal lumen (arrow).

Case courtesy Ritu R. Gill, MD, MPH, Brigham and Women's Hospital.

- Squamous cell carcinoma is the most common primary tracheal malignancy. It is strongly associated with cigarette smoking.
- The typical CT appearance of tracheal squamous cell carcinoma is a polypoid intraluminal mass. The contours of the mass can be irregular, smooth, or lobulated. The tumor can occasionally invade into the esophagus, causing tracheoesophageal fistula.

Adenoid cystic carcinoma (ACC)

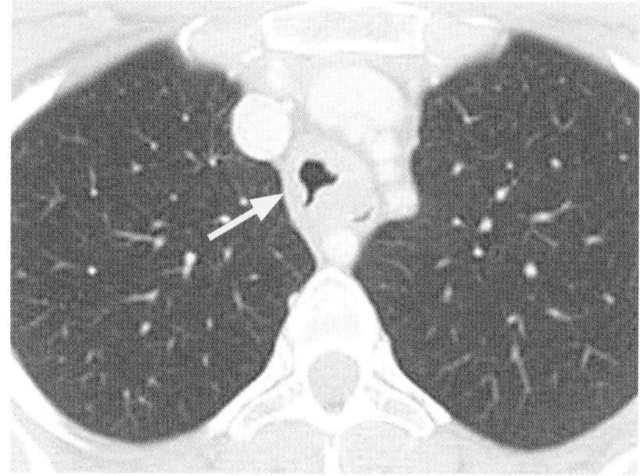

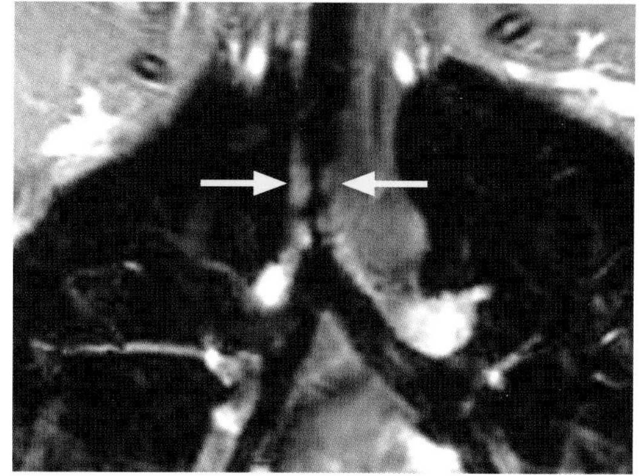

Tracheal adenoid cystic carcinoma: CT (left image) shows irregular circumferential tracheal thickening (arrow). Post-contrast coronal T1-weighted MRI (right image) shows an enhancing nodular mass extending into the tracheal lumen (arrows).

Case courtesy Ritu R. Gill, MD, MPH, Brigham and Women's Hospital.

- Adenoid cystic carcinoma (ACC) is a relatively low grade malignancy that usually affects patients in their forties, a decade or two younger than the typical SCC patient. It is not associated with cigarette smoking.
- ACC has a propensity for perineural and submucosal spread. Despite indolent growth, metastatic disease tends to have intense FDG uptake on PET imaging.
- The typical CT appearance of ACC is a submucosal mass that infiltrates the tracheal wall and surrounding mediastinal fat. ACC may also present as circumferential tracheal or bronchial thickening causing airway stenosis.

Carcinoid

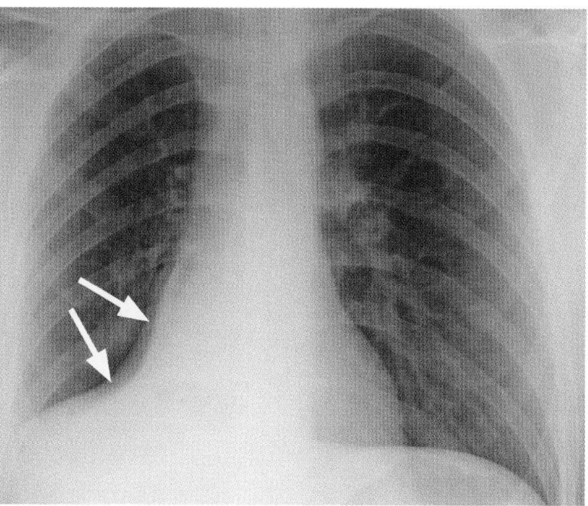

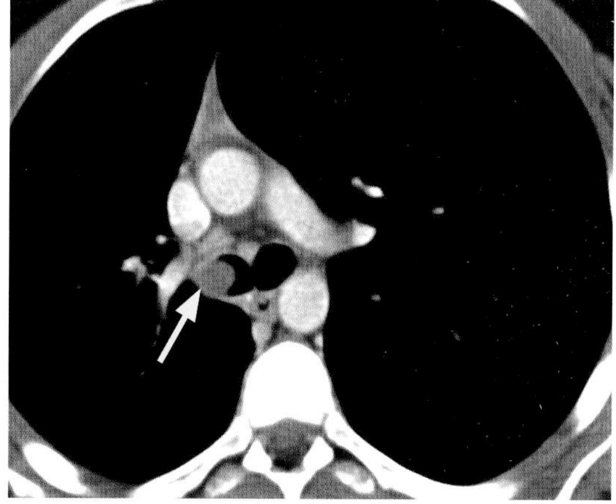

Endobronchial carcinoid: Chest radiograph shows right lower lobe atelectasis (arrows) and volume loss. Axial contrast-enhanced CT shows a mildly enhancing well-circumscribed endobronchial mass (arrow) in the right mainstem bronchus just distal to the carina.

- Carcinoid is a spectrum of neuroendocrine neoplasms including low-grade carcinoid, aggressive carcinoid, and small cell carcinoma, featuring a range of biologic behaviors. Carcinoid tumors may rarely secrete hormones such as ACTH. While endobronchial carcinoid is rare in adults, it is the most common bronchial tumor in children.
- Carcinoid almost always occurs distal to the carina.
- CT shows an endoluminal bronchial mass with homogeneous arterial enhancement.

> In addition to carcinoid, the differential diagnosis of an enhancing endobronchial mass includes **mucoepidermoid carcinoma** and very rare entities such as **hemangioma** and **glomus tumor**.

Mucoepidermoid carcinoma

- Mucoepidermoid carcinoma is a rare tumor that originates from tiny salivary glands lining the tracheobronchial tree.
- Mucoepidermoid carcinoma tends to affect younger patients than adenoid cystic carcinoma.
- CT appearance is a round or oval endobronchial mass, indistinguishable from carcinoid.

Tracheal lymphoma

- Tracheal lymphoma is rare. It is usually associated with mucosa-associated lymphoid tissue (MALT), a low-grade malignancy.

Endobronchial metastasis

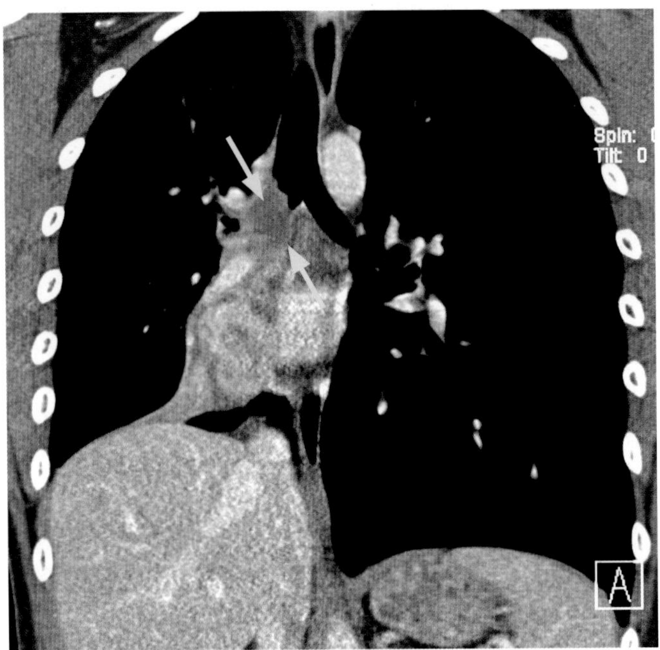

Endobronchial metastasis:

Coronal contrast-enhanced CT demonstrates a heterogeneously enhancing mass, which invades the right mainstem bronchus (arrows). This was a spindle-cell carcinoma, but the imaging appearance is nonspecific.

- Breast cancer, renal cell carcinoma, thyroid cancer, lung cancer, melanoma, and sarcoma are the most common malignancies to metastasize to the central airways.
- The mnemonic **BR**e**T**h **Lung** may be helpful to remember the four most common airway metastases (breast, renal cell, thyroid, and lung).

Direct invasion of the central airways by adjacent malignancy

- Direct central airway invasion occurs more commonly than endobronchial metastases. Aggressive laryngeal, thyroid, esophageal, and lung cancer may cause direct airway invasion.

Benign endobronchial lesions

- Papilloma is a benign but potentially pre-malignant lesion that may transform into carcinoma. Suspected papillomas are typically closely followed.

  A single papilloma is usually caused by chronic irritation.

  Multiple papillomas (laryngotracheal papillomatosis) are caused by HPV, which may be acquired at birth. Rarely (<1% of cases), papillomas spread to the lungs, where they may form multiple cavitary nodules.
- Chondroma is a benign cartilaginous tumor that rarely may occur in the airways.
- Other benign endobronchial lesions include schwannoma, adenoma, hamartoma, hemangioma, lipoma, and leiomyoma.

PLEURAL MALIGNANCY

Mesothelioma

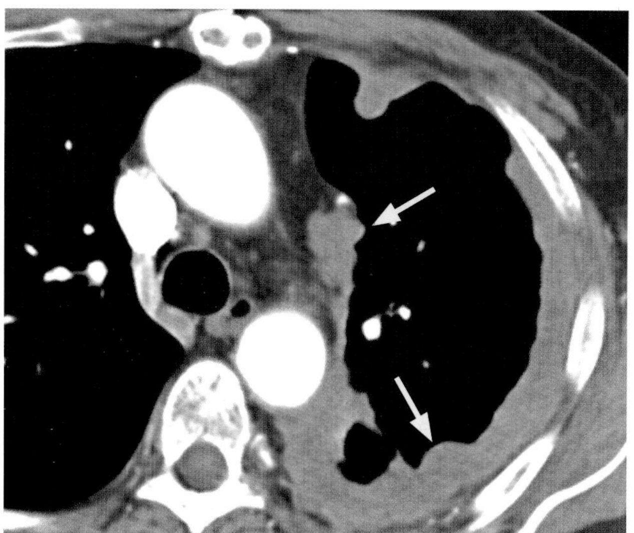
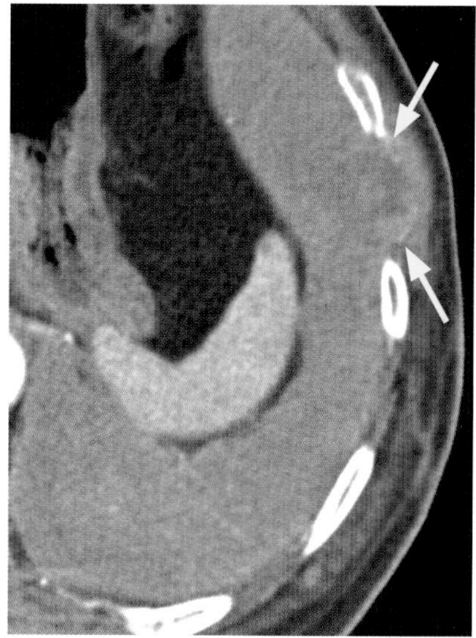

Mesothelioma: Contrast-enhanced CT through the thorax (left image) shows extensive nodular pleural thickening of the left hemithorax (arrows). Images through the upper abdomen show extensive soft tissue abnormality with invasion of the chest wall (arrows).

Case courtesy Ritu R. Gill, MD, MPH, Brigham and Women's Hospital.

- Mesothelioma is a highly aggressive neoplasm arising from the pleura. Most cases are due to prior asbestos exposure, with a latency of >20 years.
- The epithelial subtype is more common and has a slightly better prognosis. Sarcomatoid and mixed subtypes are more aggressive.
- CT of mesothelioma typically shows nodular concentric pleural thickening, often with an associated pleural effusion.
- The role of surgery is evolving, with the goal to resect all visible tumor.
- **Extrapleural pneumonectomy** is performed for patients with locally invasive disease.
- **Pleurectomy and decortication** is preferred for less advanced disease, where the lung and fissures are spared. Prognosis is equivalent to pleurectomy or pneumonectomy for the less aggressive epithelial subtype.
- Trimodality therapy involving surgery, intraoperative heated chemotherapy, and radiation has been shown to provide benefit for a subset of patients.

Metastases

- Lung cancer, gastrointestinal and genitourinary adenocarcinoma, and invasive thymoma can metastasize to the pleura.

Multiple myeloma/plasmacytoma

- Rib-based lesions may appear to be pleural-based, although the epicenter of a mass arising from a rib will be centered on the rib.

Fibrous tumor of the pleura (FTP)

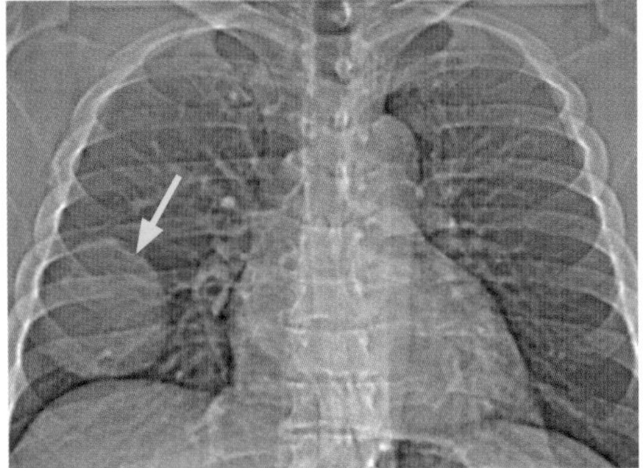

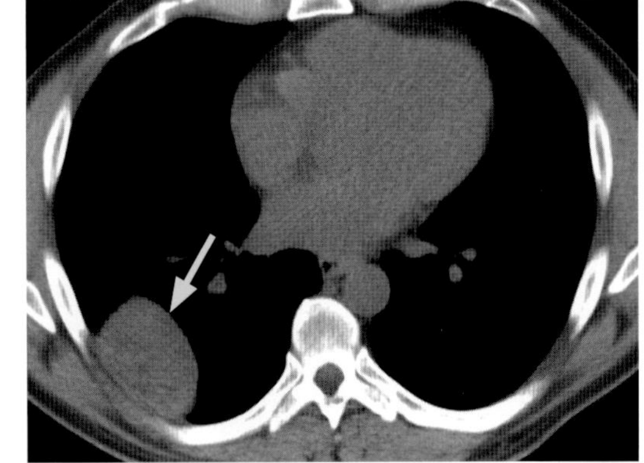

Fibrous tumor of the pleura: CT topogram (left image) shows a round opacity (arrow) with a circumscribed medial margin and indistinct lateral margin, suggesting a pleural-based mass. CT confirms that the mass (arrow) is pleural-based, with a broad attachment to the pleura.

Case courtesy Ritu R. Gill, MD, MPH, Brigham and Women's Hospital.

- Fibrous tumor of the pleura (FTP) is a focal pleural mass not related to asbestosis or mesothelioma. It is not mesothelial in origin.
- Approximately 20–30% of FTP are malignant, so all are excised. Malignant potential is determined by number of mitoses seen at pathology.
- FTP may be associated with hypoglycemia or hypertrophic pulmonary osteoarthropathy, although these associated conditions are uncommon (5%).
- FTP may be pedunculated. A pleural-based mass that changes position is suggestive of FTP. FTP tends to have low FDG uptake on PET.

PLEURAL EFFUSION

Transudate

- A transudative effusion is caused by systemic or local imbalances in hydrostatic and oncotic forces. Common causes include systemic low-protein states, heart failure, and nephrotic syndrome.

Exudate

- An exudative effusion is distinguished from a transudate by thoracentesis. There are no reliable imaging features to distinguish between transudative and exudative effusions.
- Analysis of the thoracentesis fluid by Light's criteria is the most reliable method to distinguish transudate from exudate. If **any** one of the following is present, the effusion is classified as an exudate:

> Ratio of pleural fluid protein to serum protein >0.5.
>
> Ratio of pleural fluid LDH to serum LDH >0.6.
>
> Pleural fluid LDH >2/3 upper limits of normal for serum.

- The presence of an exudate implies pleural disease causing increased permeability of pleural capillaries, which may be due to:

> **Pneumonia** with parapneumonic effusion, **empyema**, or **tuberculous** pleuritis.
>
> **Mesothelioma** or pleural **metastasis**.
>
> **Rheumatoid arthritis** or other collagen vascular diseases.

Chylothorax

- A chylothorax is a pleural effusion consisting of intestinal lymph, most commonly caused by neoplastic obstruction of the thoracic duct. Chylothorax is also associated with lymphangioleiomyomatosis (LAM).
- The thoracic duct originates at the cisterna chyli in the upper abdomen and drains into the left brachiocephalic or subclavian vein.

References, resources, and further reading

General references:

Webb, W.R. & Higgins, C.B. Thoracic Imaging - Pulmonary and Cardiovascular Radiology. Lung. Lippincott Williams & Williams. (2005).

Hansell, D.M., Lynch, D., McAdams, H.P. & Bankier, A.A. Imaging of Diseases of the Chest (5th ed.). Mosby. (2010).

Anatomy and basic concepts:

Eisenhuber, E. Signs in imaging - the tree in bud sign. Radiology 222, 771-2(2002).

Engoren, M. Lack of association between atelectasis and fever. Chest 107, 81-84(1995).

Gibbs, J.M. et al. Lines and stripes: where did they go? – From conventional radiography to CT. Radiographics 27, 33-48(2007).

Marshall, G.B. et al. Signs in thoracic imaging. Journal of Thoracic Imaging 21, 76-90(2006).

Pulmonary infection:

Franquet, T. et al. Spectrum of Pulmonary Aspergillosis: Histologic, Clinical, and Radiologic Findings. Radiographics 21, 825(2001).

Gotway, M.B. et al. The radiologic spectrum of pulmonary Aspergillus infections. Journal of Computer Assisted Tomography 26, 159-73(2002).

Systrom, D.M. & Wittram, C. Case 9-2005-A 67-Year-Old Man with Acute Respiratory Failure. New England Journal of Medicine 352, 1238(2005).

Tarver, R.D. et al. Radiology of community-acquired pneumonia. Radiologic Clinics of North America 43, 497-512, viii(2005).

Waite, S., Jeudy, J. & White, C.S. Acute lung infections in normal and immunocompromised hosts. Radiologic Clinics of North America 44, 295-315, ix(2006).

Pulmonary edema and ICU imaging:

Ely, E.W. Using the Chest Radiograph To Determine Intravascular Volume Status: The Role of Vascular Pedicle Width. Chest 121, 942-50(2002).

Martin, G.S. Findings on the Portable Chest Radiograph Correlate With Fluid Balance in Critically Ill Patients. Chest 122, 2087-2095(2002).

Lung cancer:

Hartman, T.E. Radiologic evaluation of the solitary pulmonary nodule. Radiologic Clinics of North America 43, 459-65, vii(2005).

MacMahon, H. et al. Guidelines for management of small pulmonary nodules detected on CT scans: a statement from the Fleischner Society. Radiology 237, 395-400(2005).

Travis, W.D. et al. International Association for the Study of Lung Cancer/American Thoracic Society/European Respiratory Society international multidisciplinary classification of lung adenocarcinoma. Journal of Thoracic Oncology 6, 244-85(2011).

UyBico, S.J. et al. Lung cancer staging essentials: the new TNM staging system and potential imaging pitfalls. Radiographics 30, 1163-81(2010).

Pulmonary vascular disease:

Agnelli, G. & Becattini, C. Acute Pulmonary Embolism. New England Journal of Medicine 363, 266-74(2010).

Durán-Mendicuti, A. & Sodickson, A. Imaging evaluation of the pregnant patient with suspected pulmonary embolism. International Journal of Obstetric Anesthesia 20, 51-9(2011).

Frazier, A. et al. From the Archives of the AFIP: Pulmonary Veno-occlusive Disease and Pulmonary Capillary Hemangiomatosis. Radiographics 27, 867-83(2007).

Kuriakose, J. & Patel, S. Acute pulmonary embolism. Radiologic Clinics of North America 48, 31-50(2010).

Patel, N.M. et al. Pulmonary hypertension in idiopathic pulmonary fibrosis. Chest 132, 998-1006(2007).

Wittram, C. et al. CT angiography of pulmonary embolism: diagnostic criteria and causes of misdiagnosis. Radiographics 24, 1219-38(2004).

Diffuse lung disease:

Attili, A.K. et al. Smoking-related interstitial lung disease: radiologic-clinical-pathologic correlation. Radiographics 28, 1383-96; discussion 1396-8(2008).

Gill, R., Matsusoka, S. & Hatabu, H. Cavities in the lung in oncology patients: imaging overview and differential diagnoses. Applied Radiology (June), 10–21(2010).

Gotway, M.B. et al. High-resolution CT of the lung: patterns of disease and differential diagnoses. Radiologic Clinics of North America 43, 513-42, viii(2005).

Kligerman, S.J. et al. Nonspecific interstitial pneumonia: radiologic, clinical, and pathologic considerations. Radiographics 29, 73-87(2009).

Medoff, B.D., Abbott, G.F. & Louissaint Jr, A. Case 16-2010–A 48-Year-Old Man with a Cough and Pain in the Left Shoulder. New England Journal of Medicine 362, 2013(2010).

Mueller-Mang, C., Grosse, C. & Schmid, K. What Every Radiologist Should Know about Idiopathic Interstitial Pneumonias. Radiographics 27, 595-616(2007).

Rossi, S.E. et al. "Crazy-Paving" Pattern at Thin-Section CT of the Lungs: Radiologic- Pathologic Overview. Radiographics 23, 1509-519(2003).

Webb, W.R. Thin-section CT of the secondary pulmonary lobule: anatomy and the image – the 2004 Fleischner lecture. Radiology 239, 322-38(2006).

Mediastinum:

Quint, L.E. Imaging of anterior mediastinal masses. Cancer Imaging 7 Spec No, S56-62(2007).

Tecce, P.M., Fishman, E.K. & Kuhlman, J.E. CT evaluation of the anterior mediastinum: spectrum of disease. Radiographics 14, 973(1994).

Whitten, C., Khan, S. & Munneke, G. A Diagnostic Approach to Mediastinal Abnormalities. Radiographics 27, 657-71(2007).

Airways:

Ferretti, G.R. et al. Imaging of tumors of the trachea and central bronchi. Radiologic Clinics of North America 47, 227-41(2009).

Javidan-Nejad, C. & Bhalla, S. Bronchiectasis. Radiologic Clinics of North America 47, 289-306(2009).

Martinez, S. et al. Mucoid impactions: finger-in-glove sign and other CT and radiographic features. Radiographics 28, 1369-82(2008).

Pleura:

Qureshi, N.R. & Gleeson, F.V. Imaging of pleural disease. Clinics in Chest Medicine 27, 193-213(2006).

Sugarbaker, D. & Wolf, A. Surgery for malignant pleural mesothelioma. Expert Review of Respiratory Medicine 4, 363-72(2010).

Wang, Z.J. et al. Malignant Pleural Mesothelioma: Evaluation with CT, MR Imaging, and PET. Radiographics 24, 105(2004).

2 Gastrointestinal imaging

Contents

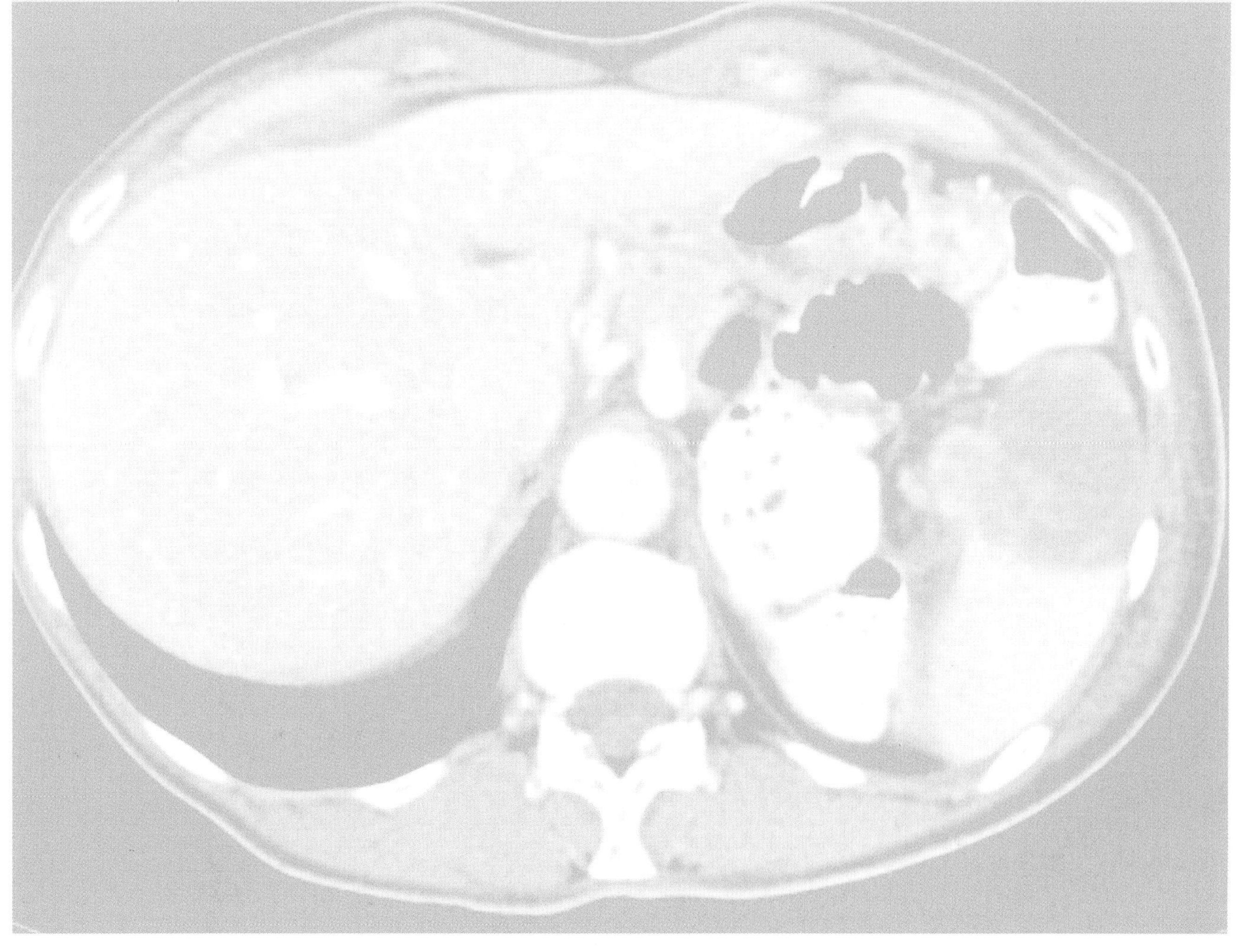

LIVER ANATOMY

- The Couinaud classification divides the liver into eight segments. Because each segment is self-contained, an individual segment can be completely resected without disturbing the other segments.
- Numbering of hepatic segments is clockwise when looking at a frontal/coronal view.

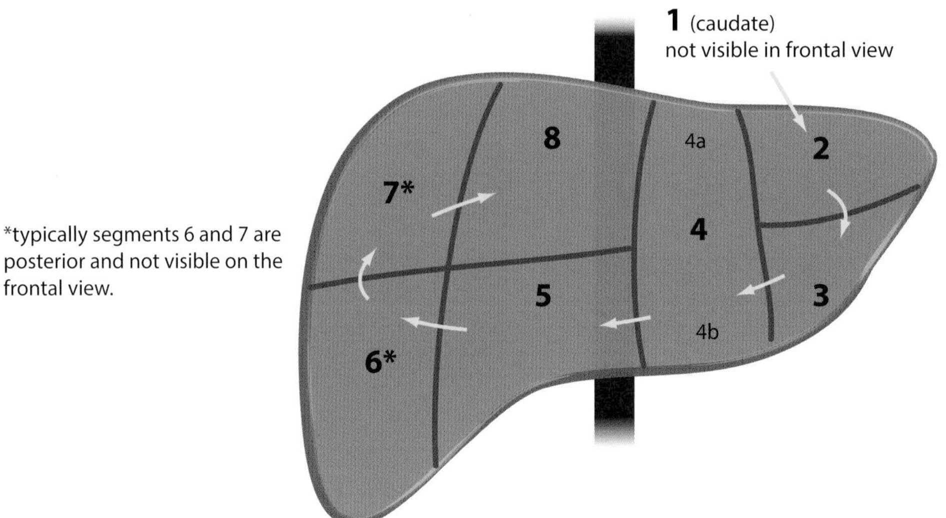

The portal veins divide the superior from inferior segments,
while the hepatic veins form the segmental borders in the axial plane.
The middle hepatic vein divides the left (2-4) from right (5-8) lobes of the liver.

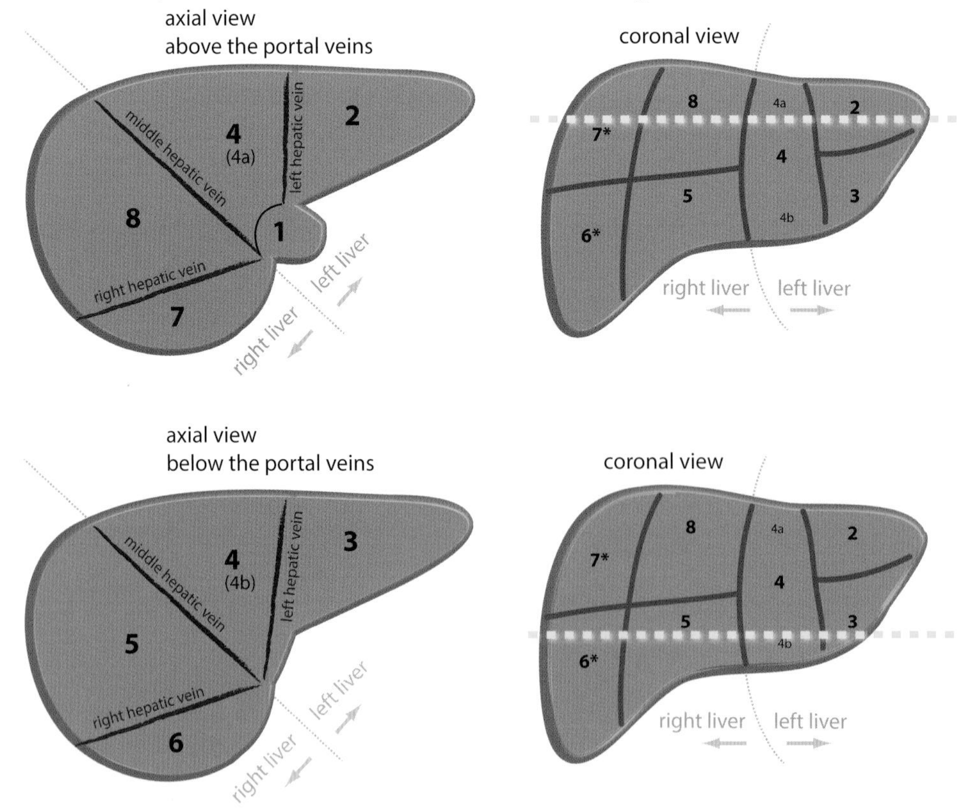

- Each hepatic segment features its own:
  - Central portal triad including branches of the portal vein, hepatic artery, and bile duct.
  - Peripheral venous drainage to the hepatic veins and ultimately the IVC.
- Mnemonic for remembering the segments:
  - Superior segments, from left to right: 2, 4, 8, 7, 1 (caudate). 2 doubled is 4; 4 doubled is 8; 8 minus 1 is 7.
  - Inferior segments, from left to right: 3, 4, 5, 6.
- Segments 2, 3, and 4 are in the left lobe of the liver.
- Segments 5, 6, 7, 8 are in the right lobe of the liver.
- The left and right main portal veins divide the superior from the inferior segments and continue to branch superiorly and inferiorly before terminating in the center of each segment.
- The branching of the portal veins is variable. The most common pattern is a bifurcation into right and left main portal veins, with the right main portal vein then branching into anterior and posterior branches.
- Small hepatic vein tributaries mark the peripheral margins of each segment.
- The caudate lobe drains directly to the IVC, not into the hepatic veins. The caudate lobe is spared in early cirrhosis since the direct drainage to the IVC spares the caudate from increased venous pressures due to portal hypertension. This leads to compensatory hypertrophy of the caudate lobe, which is a typical morphologic change of early cirrhosis.
  - Similarly, direct venous drainage to the IVC allows the caudate lobe to bypass the increased hepatic venous pressures seen in Budd–Chiari syndrome. Compensatory hypertrophy of the caudate lobe may preserve liver function in these patients.

CT and MRI of the liver

Liver CT

- A "routine" contrast-enhanced abdominal CT is acquired in the portal venous phase of enhancement, typically obtained 70 seconds following intravenous contrast administration.
- A portal venous phase CT reveals characteristic attenuation alterations and/or morphologic changes of diffuse liver disease, such as hepatic steatosis and cirrhosis. Most metastatic tumors are *not* hypervascular (although a few notable exceptions will be subsequently discussed) and can also generally be detected on the portal venous phase. Of note, rarely some breast cancers may be isoattenuating on the portal venous phase and more conspicuous on unenhanced CT.
- Most benign and malignant primary liver masses are hypervascular and thus most conspicuous in the arterial phase of enhancement. The arterial phase begins approximately 20–25 seconds after intravenous contrast injection. Many authors advocate that optimal conspicuity of a hypervascular liver lesion is obtained in the late arterial phase, which is between 9 and 16 seconds after abdominal aortic enhancement, or approximately 35 seconds after intravenous injection.

Liver MRI

- Compared to CT, MRI of the liver displays the same patterns of contrast enhancement but has superior lesion-to-liver contrast. MRI also does not impart ionizing radiation.
- MRI is able to obtain dynamic post-contrast images in multiple phases without any penalty in radiation exposure. In- and out-of-phase gradient imaging allows detection of intracytoplasmic lipid, which is seen in hepatic steatosis. Additionally, advanced techniques such as diffusion-weighted imaging may show potential for clinical use.

Fatty liver (hepatic steatosis)

- Nonalcoholic fatty liver disease can be divided into steatosis and steatosis with associated inflammatory activity (steatohepatitis). Overall, greater than 15% of the population is afflicted with nonalcoholic fatty liver disease (NAFLD), which is a component of the metabolic syndrome of obesity, insulin resistance, and dyslipidemia. Ultimately, steatohepatitis may progress to cirrhosis.
- CT can determine if steatosis is present and can provide a rough gauge as to its severity. In- and out-of-phase MRI imaging can more accurately quantify the degree of steatosis, although liver biopsy is the gold standard and best evaluates for the presence of inflammatory and early fibrotic change. By the time imaging can detect morphologic changes of cirrhosis, the changes may be irreversible.
- On unenhanced CT, the liver should be slightly hyperattenuating relative to the spleen. The traditional teaching is that steatosis is present if the liver attenuates at least 10 Hounsfield units (HU) less than the spleen, although new work suggests that even a single HU of relative hypoattenuation compared to the spleen may represent hepatic steatosis.
- On contrast-enhanced CT, evaluation of hepatic steatosis is much less reliable compared to unenhanced CT due to different contrast uptake rates of the liver and the spleen. However, the liver is considered diffusely hypoattenuating if it attenuates at least 25 HU less than the spleen in the portal venous phase.
- In- and out-of-phase GRE MRI is a sensitive imaging technique to evaluate for the presence of (and to quantify the degree of) hepatic steatosis.

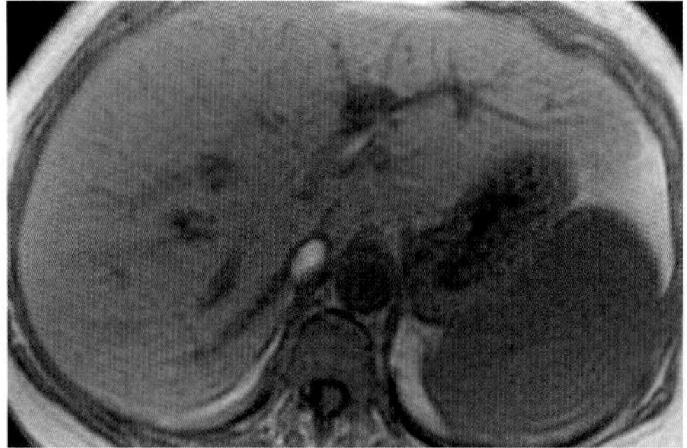
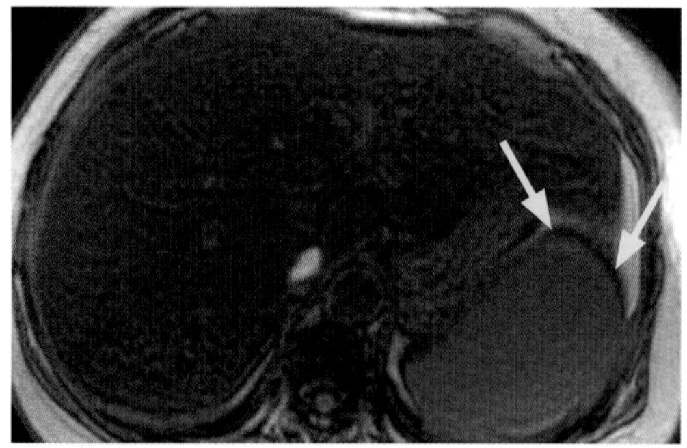

Diffuse hepatic steatosis: in- (left image) and out-of-phase (right image) images demonstrate near complete signal loss of the entire liver on out-of-phase images. Note the India-ink artifact at the periphery of organs that abut fat (e.g., spleen; arrows) in the out-of-phase images.

Case courtesy Cheryl Sadow, MD, Brigham and Women's Hospital.

When water-protons and fat-protons are present in the same MR voxel, the fat and water signals are summed in the in-phase images and subtracted in the out-of-phase images.

Relatively decreased signal on *in-phase* images suggests hepatic iron overload due to the longer TE of the in-phase images, which allows a longer dephasing time, exaggeration of T2* effect, and loss of signal.

- Variations in portal venous supply may cause geographic regions that are more or less affected by fatty change. Focal fat does not have any mass effect, vessels characteristically run through it, and it tends to occur in the following typical locations and distributions:

Gallbladder fossa (drained by gallbladder vein).

Subcapsular (along the falciform ligament).

Periportal.

Focal fat may also be nodular throughout the liver. Ultrasound would demonstrate multiple hyperechoic lesions which would be hypoattenuating on CT. MRI shows pseudolesions drop in signal intensity on out-of-phase dual-phase GRE, consistent with nodular focal fat.

Amyloid

- Abnormal extracellular deposition of amyloid protein in the liver can cause focal or diffuse areas of decreased attenuation on CT imaging.

Wilson disease

- Wilson disease causes high levels of copper to accumulate in the basal ganglia, cornea, and liver due an autosomal recessive genetic defect. The liver may be hyperattenuating on CT with multiple nodules, eventually leading to hepatomegaly and cirrhosis.

Hepatic iron overload

- There are two pathways to excess hepatic iron accumulation. Accumulation within hepatocytes is seen in hemochromatosis. Uptake within the reticuloendothelial system (RES) causes hepatic Kupffer cell iron overload, as seen in hemosiderosis.
- Regardless of the etiology, the iron-overloaded liver is hypointense on all MRI sequences, relative to the paraspinal muscles as an internal control.
- Hemochromatosis is the most common cause of iron overload, due to a genetic defect causing increased iron absorption. Excess iron is *unable* to be stored in the RES, so the spleen and bone marrow are not affected. Treatment of hemochromatosis is phlebotomy.

  Excess iron is deposited in **hepatocytes** (not the Kupffer cells that make up the intrahepatic RES), pancreas, myocardium, skin, and joints. Excess iron in hepatocytes can cause cirrhosis.

  The spleen and bone marrow are normal since the RES is not involved.
- Hemosiderosis is excess iron stored within the reticuloendothelial system, which may be due to frequent blood transfusions or defective erythrocytosis. Treatment of hemosiderosis is with iron chelators, not phlebotomy.

  The RES has a large capacity for iron. Iron stored in the RES is generally not harmful and the liver is normal in morphology, without cirrhosis.

  MRI imaging of hemosiderosis demonstrates hypointense liver on conventional MRI sequences, similar to hemochromatosis. Additionally, the spleen and bone marrow will also appear hypointense due to increased iron stores throughout the entire reticuloendothelial system.
- Hemosiderosis is a precursor to secondary hemochromatosis. Secondary hemochromatosis is hepatic damage from iron overload after the RES system becomes saturated from prolonged hemosiderosis.

  When the RES becomes overwhelmed with iron, the hepatocytes begin to store the excess. Similar to hemochromatosis, hepatocyte iron uptake may lead to cirrhosis.
- In clinical practice, the distinction between hemosiderosis and secondary hemochromatosis often overlaps. Many authors recommend against the term "secondary hemochromatosis" in favor of describing the primary disease (e.g., thalassemia) with secondary iron overload.

Differential based on CT attenuation

- **Hypoattenuating** liver: The liver is considered hypoattenuating if it attenuates less than the spleen on an unenhanced CT.

  Fatty liver (hepatic steatosis) is by far the most common cause of a diffusely hypoattenuating liver.

  Hepatic amyloid is rare and may cause either focal or diffuse hepatic hypoattenuation.
- **Hyperattenuating** liver: The normal unenhanced attenuation of the liver is 30 to 60 HU. An absolute attenuation greater than 75 HU is considered hyperattenuating.

  Iron overload is by far the most common cause of a hyperattenuating liver.

  Medications (e.g., amiodarone, gold, and methotrexate).

  Copper overload (Wilson disease).

  Glycogen excess.

Hepatic infection

Viral hepatitis

- Patients with viral hepatitis often have a normal CT scan. Viral hepatitis may cause nonspecific CT findings, such as gallbladder wall thickening or periportal edema (fluid on both sides of the portal veins).

Candidiasis

- Systemic fungal infection may seed the liver (and commonly the spleen as well) due to portal venous drainage of infected bowel.
- CT shows multiple tiny hypoattenuating microabscesses in the liver and the spleen, which may be rim-enhancing.
- Candidiasis is almost always seen in immunocompromised patients.
- The differential diagnosis for multiple tiny hypoattenuating hepatic lesions includes metastatic disease, lymphoma, biliary hamartomas, and Caroli disease.

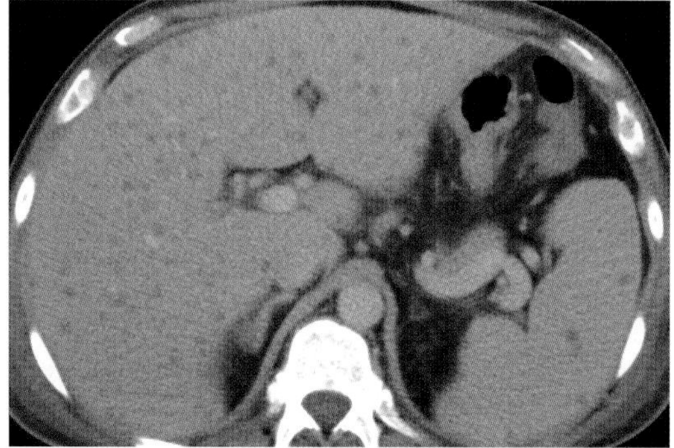

Candidiasis: Noncontrast CT shows innumerable tiny hypoattenuating lesions scattered throughout the liver and spleen, representing candidal microabscesses in a bone marrow transplant patient with fungemia.

Abscess

- Hepatic abscess is most commonly caused by a bowel process and resultant infectious nidus carried through the portal system to the liver. Common causes include diverticulitis, appendicitis, Crohn disease, and bowel surgery. *E. coli* is the most common organism. A primary hepatobiliary infection, such as ascending cholangitis, may be a less common cause.
- Imaging features of hepatic abscess may mimic metastasis, appearing as a ring-enhancing mass on CT. On MRI, there is typically central hyperintensity on T2-weighted images with an irregular wall that enhances late. Perilesional enhancement may be present.

Echinococcal disease

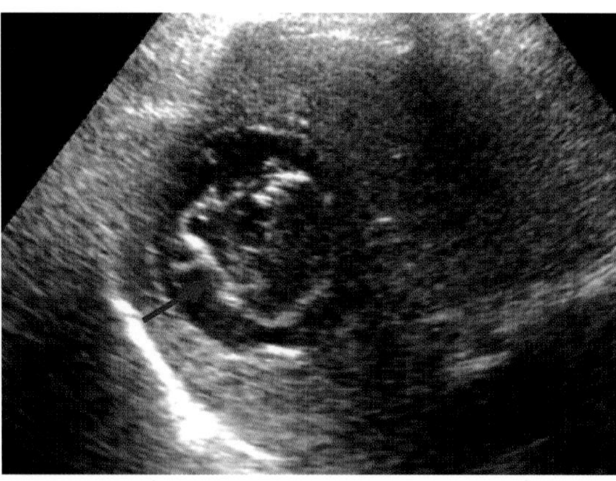

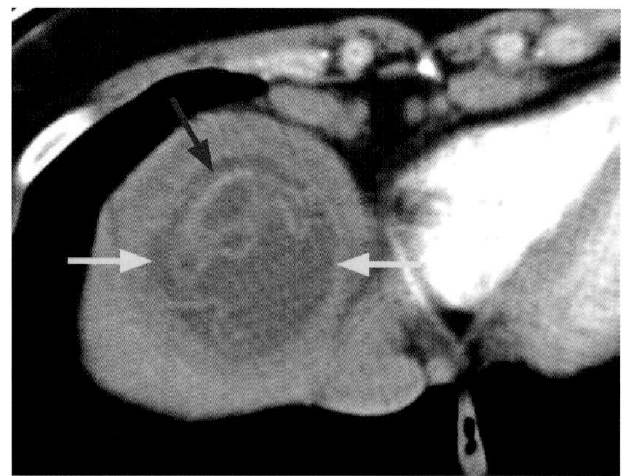

Hepatic echinococcus: Ultrasound (left image) shows a complex, primarily hypoechoic mass in the superior aspect of the liver containing a hyperechoic undulating membrane (red arrow). Contrast-enhanced CT (right image) shows a fluid-attenuating cystic mass (yellow arrows) containing an undulating membrane (red arrow).

Case courtesy Cheryl Sadow, MD, Brigham and Women's Hospital.

- Hepatic echinococcosis is caused by ingestion of the eggs of *Echinococcus granulosus*, which is endemic in the Mediterranean basin and associated with sheep-raising. Echinococcal eggs can develop into hydatid cysts.
- On CT, a hydatid cyst is a well-defined hypoattenuating mass featuring a characteristic floating membrane or an associated daughter cyst. Peripheral calcification may be present.

Cirrhosis

Etiology and pathology

- Cirrhosis is caused by repeated cycles of injury and repair, which can be due to metabolic (alcohol, steatohepatitis, hemochromatosis, or Wilson disease), infectious (chronic hepatitis B or C), or inflammatory (primary biliary cirrhosis or primary sclerosing cholangitis) etiologies. The hallmarks of cirrhosis are fibrosis and attempted, disorganized regeneration.
- The micronodular form of cirrhosis is most often due to metabolic causes.
- The macronodular form of cirrhosis is most often post-viral (hepatitis B or C).

Early signs of cirrhosis

- One of the earliest signs of cirrhosis is expansion of the preportal space. Atrophy of the medial segment of the left hepatic lobe in early cirrhosis causes increased fat anterior to the right main portal vein.
- Enlargement of the caudate lobe is a specific sign of cirrhosis. Specifically, a caudate to right lobe size ratio of >0.65 highly suggests cirrhosis. As previously discussed, the caudate drains directly to the IVC, not via the hepatic veins, which results in compensatory caudate hypertrophy.
- The *empty gallbladder fossa* sign results when hepatic parenchyma surrounding the gallbladder is replaced with periportal fat.

Secondary manifestations of cirrhosis

- Portal hypertension causes splenomegaly, portosystemic collaterals, and varices.
- Gallbladder wall thickening is due to hypoalbuminemia and resultant edema.
- **Gamna–Gandy bodies** are splenic microhemorrhages, which appear hypointense on GRE.

Malignant hepatic masses

Pathway to hepatocellular carcinoma

- In the setting of cirrhosis, hepatocellular carcinoma (HCC) is thought to develop in a sequence from regenerative nodule to dysplastic nodule to HCC. Regenerative and dysplastic nodules cannot be reliably differentiated on imaging; and high-grade dysplastic nodules cannot be reliably differentiated from low-grade HCC.
- **Regenerative nodule**: A regenerative nodule is completely supplied by the portal vein and is not premalignant. A regenerative nodule should *not* enhance in the arterial phase.

  Most regenerative nodules show low signal intensity on T2-weighted images, with variable signal intensity on T1-weighted images. Rarely, a regenerative nodule may be hyperintense on T1-weighted images due to glycogen deposition.

  On contrast-enhanced MRI, most regenerative nodules enhance to the same (or slightly less) degree as the adjacent hepatic parenchyma.
- **Dysplastic nodule**: Unlike a regenerative nodule, a dysplastic nodule is premalignant. However, most dysplastic nodules do not demonstrate arterial phase enhancement (unless high grade), since blood supply is still from the portal vein.

  Dysplastic nodules are variable in signal intensity on T1-weighted images. Most dysplastic nodules are hypointense on T2-weighted images, although high-grade dysplastic nodules may be T2 hyperintense.

  Contrast-enhanced MRI shows low-grade dysplastic nodules to be iso-enhancing relative to liver and thus indistinguishable from regenerative nodules. High grade dysplastic nodules may demonstrate arterial enhancement and be indistinguishable from well-differentiated hepatocellular carcinoma.
- A siderotic nodule is an iron-rich regenerative or dysplastic nodule. A siderotic nodule is hypointense on T1 and T2*-weighted images and hyperattenuating on CT. A siderotic nodule is rarely, if ever, malignant.

Hepatocellular carcinoma (HCC)

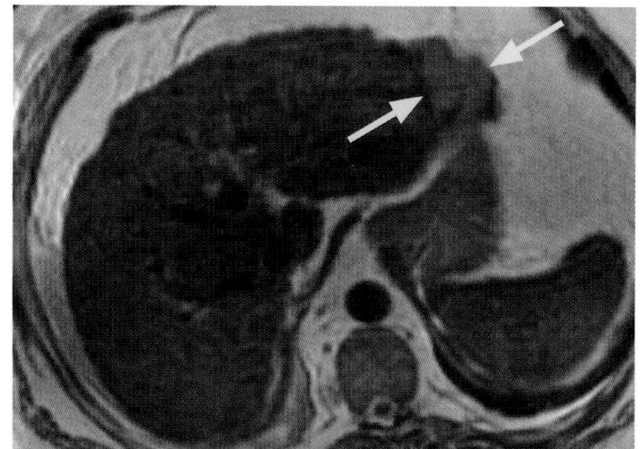

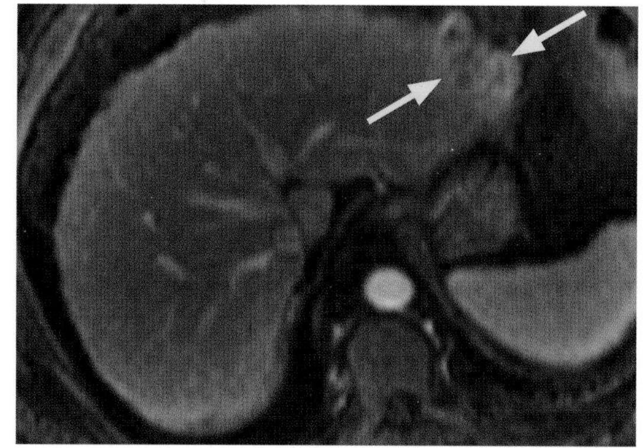

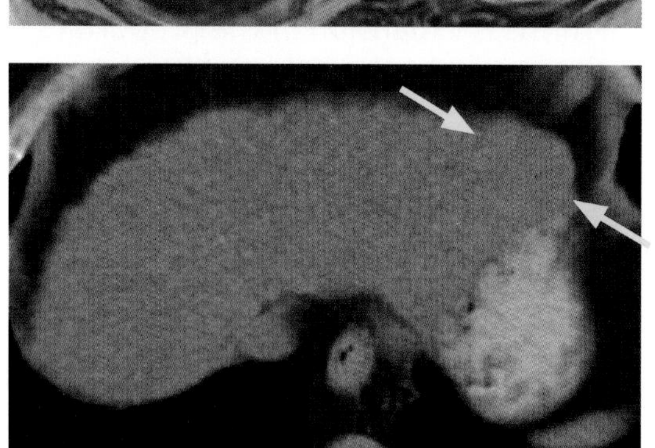

HCC in a cirrhotic liver: T2-weighted (top left image) and T1-weighted post-contrast late arterial phase (top right image) MRI shows a nodular external contour of the liver, consistent with cirrhosis. There is a T2 hyperintense, hypervascular mass in hepatic segment 2 (arrows), representing hepatocellular carcinoma.

Unenhanced CT (left image) shows the mass to be isoattenuating and barely perceptible (arrows).

Case courtesy Cheryl Sadow, MD, Brigham and Women's Hospital.

- Hepatocellular carcinoma (HCC) is the most common primary liver tumor. Cirrhosis is the major risk factor for development of HCC. A hypervascular liver mass in a patient with cirrhosis or chronic hepatitis is an HCC until proven otherwise.
- Alpha-feto protein (AFP) is elevated in approximately 75% of cases of HCC.
- Arterial phase enhancement is the characteristic imaging feature of HCC. However, between 10 and 20% of HCCs are hypovascular and thus slightly hypoenhancing relative to surrounding liver on arterial phase imaging.
- The classic CT or MRI appearance of HCC is an encapsulated mass that enhances on arterial phase and washes out on portal venous phase. HCC may be difficult to detect on non-contrast or portal venous phase CT. On unenhanced MRI, HCC is characteristically slightly hyperintense on T2-weighted images relative to surrounding liver.

  The nodule in a nodule appearance describes an enhancing nodule within a dysplastic nodule and represents an early HCC.
- HCC is locally invasive and tends to invade into the portal and portal veins, IVC, and bile ducts. In contrast, metastases to the liver are much less likely to be locally invasive.
- Treatment options for HCC include partial hepatectomy, orthotopic liver transplantation, percutaneous ablation, and transcatheter embolization.

Fibrolamellar HCC

- Fibrolamellar carcinoma is a subtype of HCC that occurs in young patients without cirrhosis.
- The tumor tends to be large when diagnosed, but has a better prognosis than typical HCC. Unlike in HCC, AFP is not elevated.
- On MRI, fibrolamellar HCC is a large, heterogeneous mass. A fibrotic central scar is classic, which is hypointense on T1- and T2-weighted images (in contrast, focal nodular hyperplasia features a T2 hyperintense scar that enhances late). Capsular retraction may be seen in 10%.
- Unlike HCC, the fibrolamellar subtype does not have a capsule, although there may be a pseudocapsule of peripherally compressed normal hepatic tissue.

Hepatic metastases

- Although metastases are supplied by branches of the hepatic artery induced by tumoral angiogenesis, most metastases are hypovascular and best appreciated on portal venous phase (in contrast to HCC, which is hypervascular and best visualized on late arterial phase).
- Hypervascular metastases (best seen on arterial phase) classically include:

Neuroendocrine tumors, including pancreatic neuroendocrine tumors and carcinoid.	**Renal cell** carcinoma. **Thyroid** carcinoma.	**Melanoma.** **Sarcoma.**

- Colorectal and pancreatic adenocarcinoma metastases are typically hypovascular and can usually be diagnosed on portal venous imaging.
- Calcifications can be seen in mucinous colorectal tumors or ovarian serous tumors Calcification within a metastatic lesion may imply a better prognosis.
- On MRI, metastatic lesions tend to be hypointense on T1-weighted images and hyperintense on T2-weighted images. Blood products and melanin (as in melanoma) are T1 hyperintense.
- *Pseudocirrhosis* describes the macronodular liver contour resulting from multiple scirrhous hepatic metastases, which may mimic cirrhosis. Treated breast cancer is the most common cause of this appearance. Capsular retraction, although not always seen, is characteristic of pseudocirrhosis, and when present suggests pseudocirrhosis over cirrhosis.

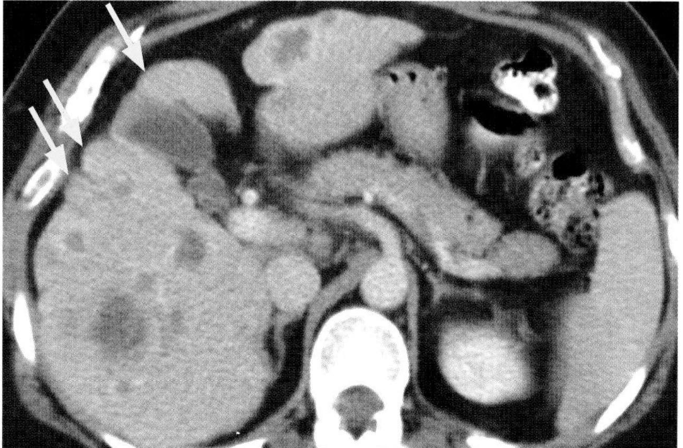

Pseudocirrhosis due to multiple treated breast cancer metastases: Contrast-enhanced CT shows numerous hypoattenuating hepatic lesions with a markedly nodular external hepatic contour (arrows) that resembles cirrhosis.

Liver function in this patient remained normal.

Hepatic lymphoma

- Primary hepatic lymphoma is very rare. Lymphomatous involvement of the liver tends to be secondary to systemic disease, with associated splenomegaly and lymphadenopathy.

Epithelioid hemangioendothelioma

- Epithelioid hemangioendothelioma is a rare vascular malignancy that characteristically causes multiple spherical subcapsular masses than can become confluent. The individual masses may have a *halo* or *target* appearance.
- Epithelioid hemangioendothelioma is one cause of capsular retraction.

Hepatic capsular retraction

- Capsular retraction is a focal concavity of the normally convex external liver contour.

Differential diagnosis of capsular retraction

- **Metastatic tumor** (more commonly post-treatment).
- **Fibrolamellar hepatocellular carcinoma** (10% of cases of fibrolamellar HCC).
- **Hepatocellular carcinoma** (capsular retraction has been reported but is uncommon).
- **Epithelioid hemangioendothelioma**.
- **Intrahepatic cholangiocarcinoma**.
- **Confluent hepatic fibrosis** (wedge-shaped fibrosis seen in cirrhosis, most commonly the medial segment of the left hepatic lobe or the anterior segment of the right hepatic lobe).

Focal nodular hyperplasia (FNH)

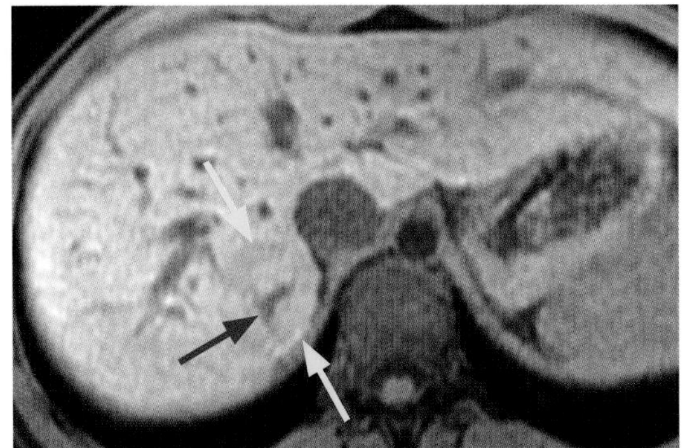

T1-weighted fat-saturated MRI

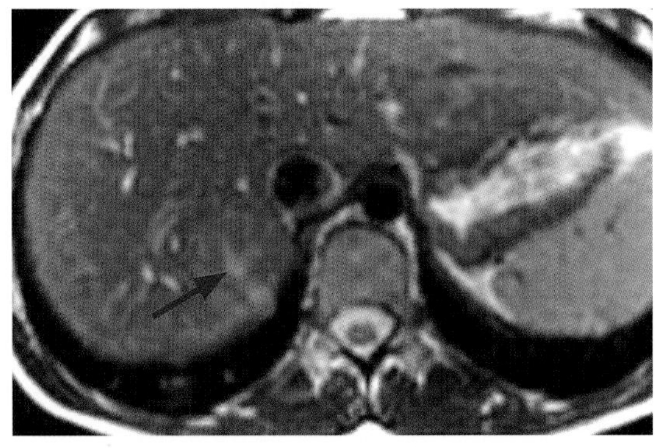

T2-weighted MRI

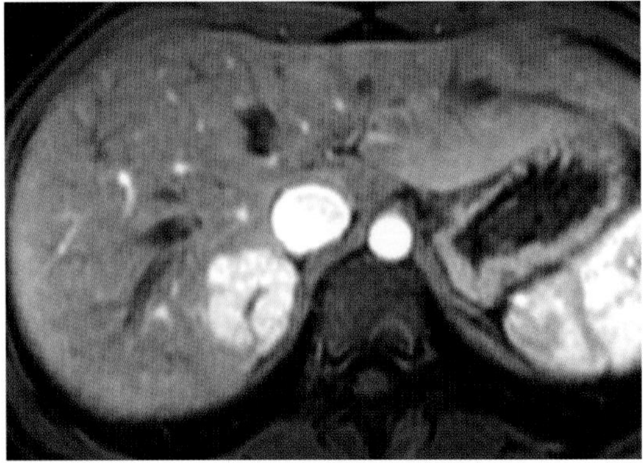

Late arterial post-contrast T1-weighted fat-sat MRI

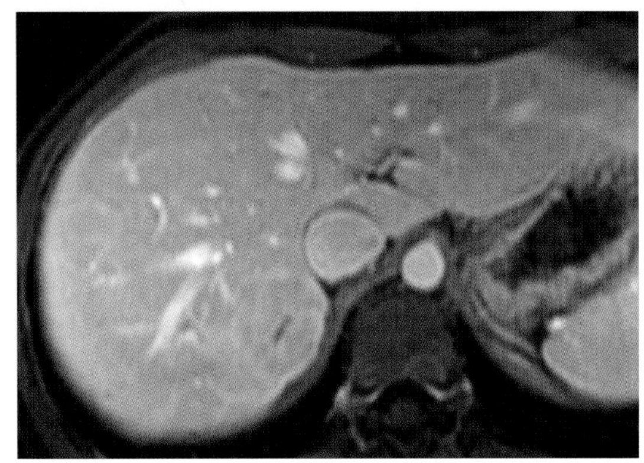

Portal venous post-contrast T1-weighted fat-sat MRI

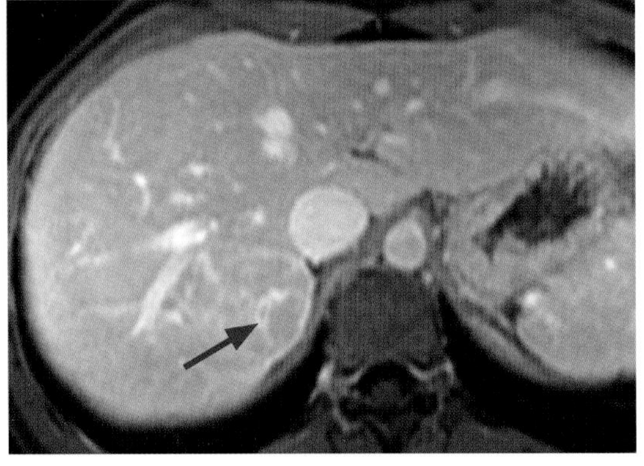

Delayed post-contrast T1-weighted fat-sat MRI

Focal nodular hyperplasia: T1-weighted MRI shows a barely perceptible mass in the right liver (yellow arrows) with a central low intensity scar (red arrow).

The mass is T2 isointense with the subtle suggestion of T2 hyperintense central scar (red arrow).

Arterial phase of enhancement shows avid enhancement with non-enhancement of the scar.

The mass washes out immediately on portal venous phase, with no change in intensity of the scar.

Delayed T1-weighted image shows late enhancement of the central scar (red arrow).

Case courtesy of Cheryl Sadow, MD, Brigham and Women's Hospital

- Focal nodular hyperplasia (FNH) is disorganized liver tissue with no malignant potential. It is primarily seen in asymptomatic women and is not associated with oral contraceptives.
- FNH has a characteristic central "scar" which does not contain fibrotic tissue and is therefore not a true scar. Instead, the central area consists of T2-hyperintense ductules and venules, and demonstrates delayed enhancement. FNH does not have a capsule.
- FNH can be difficult to see without contrast on CT and T1- and T2-weighted MRI sequences. FNH avidly enhances during the arterial phase, then washes out very quickly. The portal venous phase will often show just the unenhanced scar, which enhances late.
- Kupffer cells and bile duct epithelium are both present. Kupffer cells may be confirmed by a sulfur colloid study (1/3 of the time) and bile duct cells can be seen on a HIDA scan.

Hemangioma

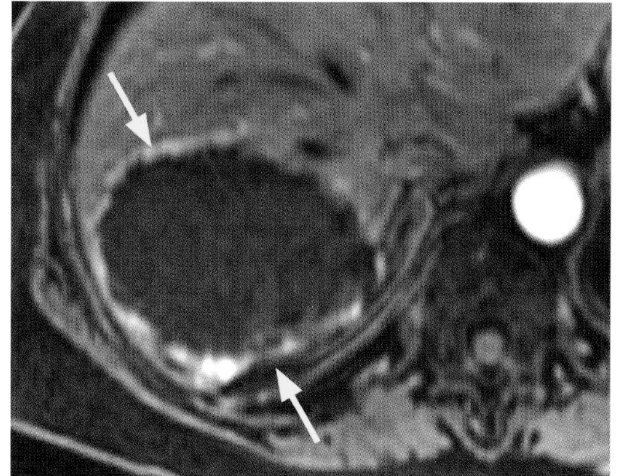

Early arterial post-contrast T1-weighted image

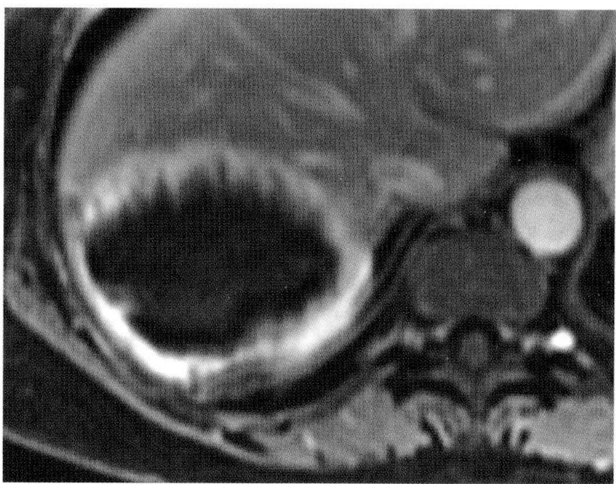

Portal venous post-contrast T1-weighted image

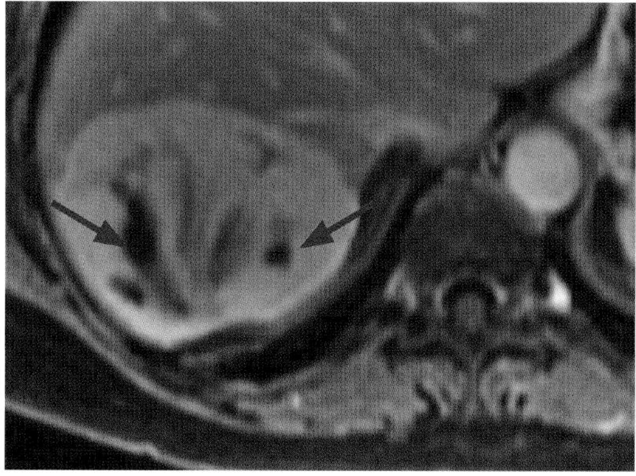

Delayed post-contrast T1-weighted image

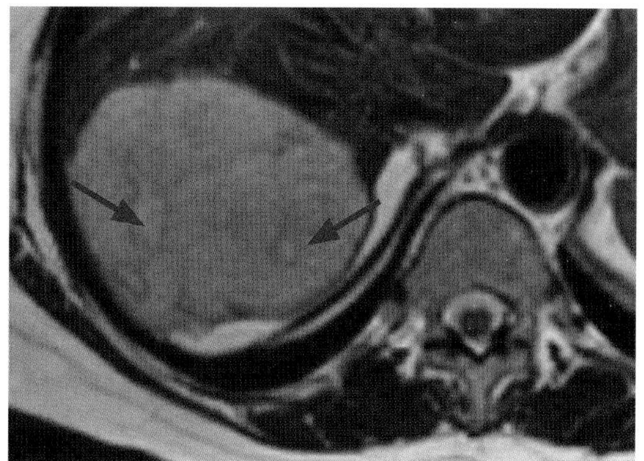

T2-weighted image

Hemangioma: Dynamic contrast-enhanced T1-weighted MRI (early arterial top left image to delayed bottom left image) shows a large mass (yellow arrows) in hepatic segment 7 demonstrating peripheral discontinuous nodular enhancement. There is progressively increasing centripetal enhancement towards the center of the lesion on delayed images. The signal intensity of the peripheral enhancement is similar to that of the aorta. On delayed images, there are a few central foci of nonenhancement (red arrows), consistent with cystic degeneration.

The hemangioma is hyperintense on the T2-weighted image (bottom right image) with subtle central areas of even higher signal centrally (red arrows), corresponding to the areas of cystic degeneration.

Case courtesy of Cheryl Sadow, MD, Brigham and Women's Hospital.

- A hepatic hemangioma is a benign mass composed of disorganized endothelial-lined pockets of blood vessels, supplied by a branch of the hepatic artery at the periphery.
- Hemangioma is more common in females and uncommon in cirrhosis. When a known hemangioma is sequentially followed in a patient with early cirrhosis, the hemangioma involutes as the liver becomes more cirrhotic.
- Hemangiomas may range in size from <1 cm to >10 cm. Giant hemangiomas tend to have a nonenhancing central area representing cystic degeneration.
- A virtually pathognomonic imaging feature is peripheral, discontinuous, progressive, nodular enhancement. The attenuation (or signal intensity on MR) of the enhancement is identical to the aorta and features gradual centripetal fill-in on later phases.
- The unenhanced CT appearance of a hemangioma is a nonspecific hypoattenuating liver mass.

Hepatic adenoma

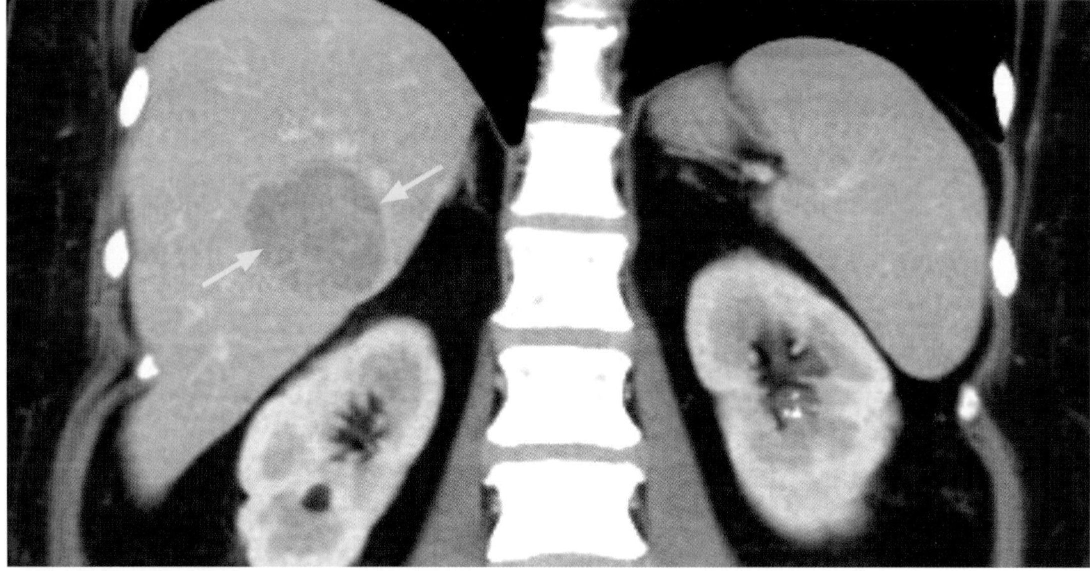

Hepatic adenoma: Coronal portal venous phase contrast-enhanced CT demonstrates a heterogeneously enhancing hypoattenuating mass (arrows) in the liver, which is a nonspecific appearance.

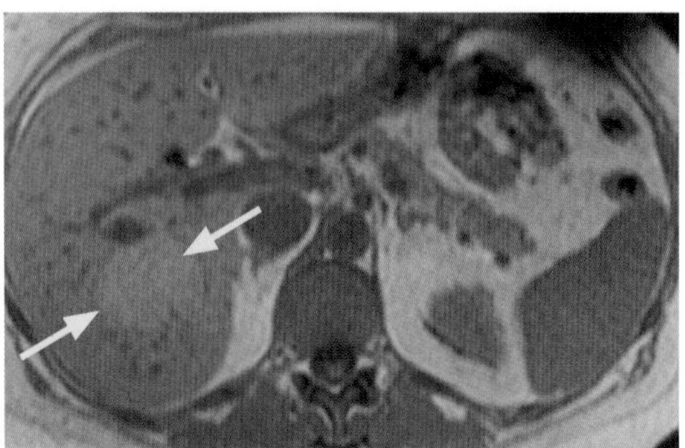

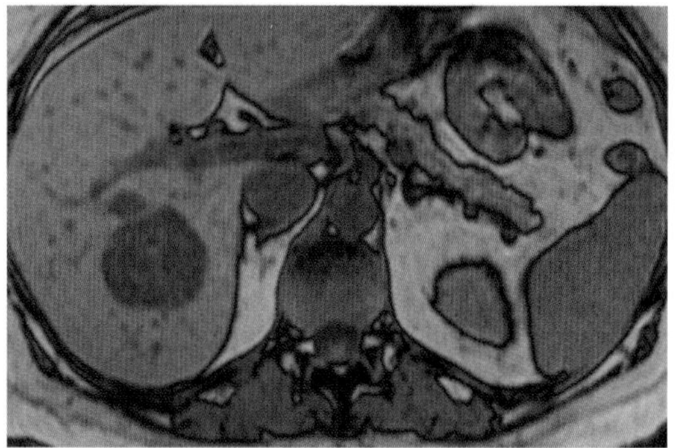

In- (left image) and out-of-phase (right image) MRI shows a mass in the right lobe of the liver (arrows) that demonstrates signal loss on out-of-phase images, consistent with a lesion containing intracellular lipid.

Case courtesy Cheryl Sadow, MD, Brigham and Women's Hospital.

- Hepatic adenoma is a benign hepatic neoplasm containing hepatocytes, scattered Kupffer cells, and no bile ducts.

  The absence of bile ducts makes a nuclear medicine HIDA scan a useful test to distinguish between focal nodular hyperplasia (which contains bile ducts and would be positive on HIDA) and a hepatic adenoma, which does not contain bile ducts.

- Adenomas are much more common in females, especially with prolonged oral contraceptive use. When seen in males, adenoma may be associated with anabolic steroids.
- Adenomas have a relatively high risk of hemorrhage, which is often the presenting symptom. For this reason, incidentally discovered adenomas are usually resected.
- Multiple hepatic adenomas are seen in von Gierke disease (type I glycogen storage disease).
- A pseudocapsule may be present, which tends to enhance late.
- Adenomas lack portal venous drainage and thus are hypervascular on arterial phase. The presence of microscopic fat, when present, is best seen on in- and out-of-phase MRI. Intralesional hemorrhage may cause T1 hyperintensity. Adenomas may be difficult to differentiate from other hypervascular liver lesions in the absence of fat or hemorrhage.

Vascular liver disease

Budd-Chiari

- Budd–Chiari is hepatic venous outflow obstruction, which can be thrombotic or non-thrombotic. Budd–Chiari may be due to hypercoagulative states including hematological disorders, pregnancy, oral contraceptives, malignancy, infection, and trauma. It is very rare to have primary Budd–Chiari due to congenital hepatic vein anomaly, as pictured below.
- Acute Budd–Chiari presents with a clinical triad of hepatomegaly, ascites, and abdominal pain.
- Direct vascular findings include lack of flow within hepatic veins, thrombus in the hepatic veins/IVC, and the formation of collateral vessels.
- Acute intraparenchymal findings include an edematous peripheral liver with sparing of the caudate lobe. The caudate is spared as it drains directly into the IVC.
- Progressive liver failure may result in chronic disease, producing caudate lobe hypertrophy and atrophy of peripheral liver with prominent regenerative nodules.

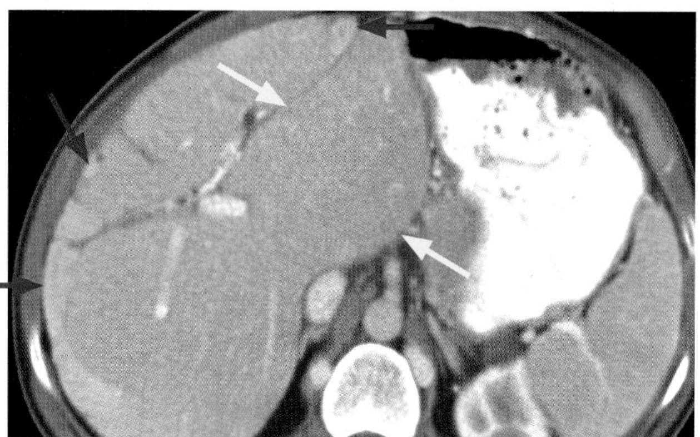

Congenital Budd–Chiari: Axial contrast-enhanced CT shows massive enlargement of the caudate lobe (yellow arrows) and the right posterior segment. There is atrophy of the left lobe and right anterior segments of the liver. Collateral venous drainage in the periphery of the liver is seen as geographic peripheral hyperenhancement (red arrows). The causative congenital hepatic vein anomaly is not visualized at this level.

Case courtesy Cheryl Sadow, MD, Brigham and Women's Hospital.

Veno-occlusive disease

- Veno-occlusive disease (VOD) is destruction of post-sinusoidal venules, with patent hepatic veins. VOD is seen in bone marrow transplant patients, possibly due to chemotherapy.
- Imaging findings are nonspecific. Periportal edema, narrowing of the hepatic veins, hepatomegaly, and heterogeneous hepatic enhancement have been reported. In contrast to Budd–Chiari, the caudate lobe is not spared.

Cardiac hepatopathy

- Cardiac hepatopathy is passive hepatic congestion from heart failure, constrictive pericarditis, or right-sided valvular disease, which ultimately may lead to cirrhosis.
- Imaging clues are enlarged hepatic veins and IVC, with reflux of intravenous contrast from the right atrium into the IVC and hepatic veins. The liver is typically enlarged and demonstrates mottled enhancement. Ascites is usually present.

Congenital cystic liver disease

Biliary hamartomas (von Meyenburg complexes)

- Biliary hamartomas are incidental small cystic hepatic lesions that do not communicate with the biliary tree, caused by embryologic failure of normal bile duct formation.
- Biliary hamartomas tend to be smaller and more irregularly shaped than simple cysts.

Autosomal dominant polycystic liver disease (ADPLD)

- 40% of patients with autosomal dominant polycystic kidney disease (ADPKD) have a similar disease process in the liver, called ADPLD. Even in severe disease, hepatic failure is rare.
- On imaging, there are innumerable nonenhancing simple cysts throughout the liver.

LIVER TRAUMA

Overview of liver trauma

- The liver is the second most commonly injured solid organ due to blunt trauma, second to the spleen. The CT description and grading of liver injury is similar to splenic injury.
- The American Association for the Surgery of Trauma (AAST) classification describes hepatic injury based on findings at laparotomy.
- The MDCT hepatic injury grading scale is based on CT findings and is more commonly used by radiologists. It is similar to the MDCT grading scale for splenic trauma.

MDCT grading of hepatic injury

MDCT hepatic trauma

- Grade I: Superficial laceration or subcapsular hematoma <1 cm in size.
- Grade II: Laceration or subcapsular/intraparenchymal hematoma >1 and <3 cm in size.
- Grade III: Laceration or subcapsular/intraparenchymal hematoma >3 cm in diameter.
- Grade IV: Massive hematoma >10 cm, or destruction/devascularization of one hepatic lobe.
- Grade V: Destruction or devascularization of both hepatic lobes.

BILIARY IMAGING

INTRODUCTION TO MRCP

Magnetic resonance cholangiopancreatography (MRCP) overview

- Magnetic resonance cholangiopancreatography (MRCP) is an abdominal MRI acquired with heavily T2-weighted sequences that increase the contrast between T2 hyperintense stationary fluid in the biliary tract and surrounding structures.
- Fast spin echo sequences are most commonly used for MRCP acquisition. Various techniques can be employed to optimize imaging including breath-hold sequences and respiratory-triggered sequences.
- Heavily T2-weighted sequences primarily image the biliary tree.
- Sequences with intermediate T2 (TE 80–100 ms) are best suited for visualization of the biliary ductal system *and* surrounding tissue, in particular to evaluate extraluminal structures.
- Advantages of MRCP over ERCP include:

  MRCP has the ability to see extra-luminal findings.

  MRCP can visualize excluded (obstructed) ducts.

  MRCP is non-invasive.

- Disadvantages of MRCP compared to ERCP include:

  MRCP does not allow for concurrent therapeutic intervention.

  MRCP does not actively distend the biliary ductal system with contrast.

  MRCP has worse spatial resolution compared to ERCP.

- Contrast-enhanced MRCP can also be performed with fat-saturated T1-weighted imaging after injection of gadolinium contrast agents that have biliary excretion, such as gadoxetic acid disodium (Eovist, Bayer Healthcare, Germany) and gadobenate dimeglumine (Multihance, Bracco Diagnostics). These agents shorten T1 relaxation, resulting in T1 hyperintense biliary fluid, but require a 20–45 minute delay prior to imaging to allow time for biliary excretion.

Overview and Todani classification of choledochal cysts

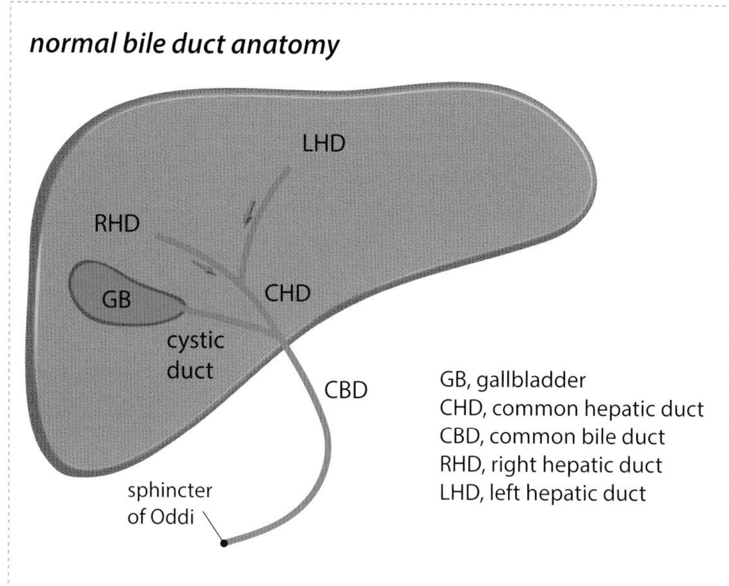

Type I choledochal cyst:
Fusiform common bile duct dilation

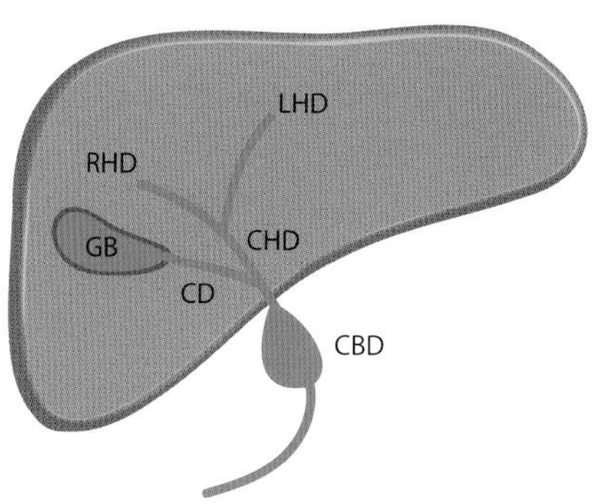

Most common, makes up ~50% of choledochal cysts

Type II choledochal cyst:
Extrahepatic saccular dilation

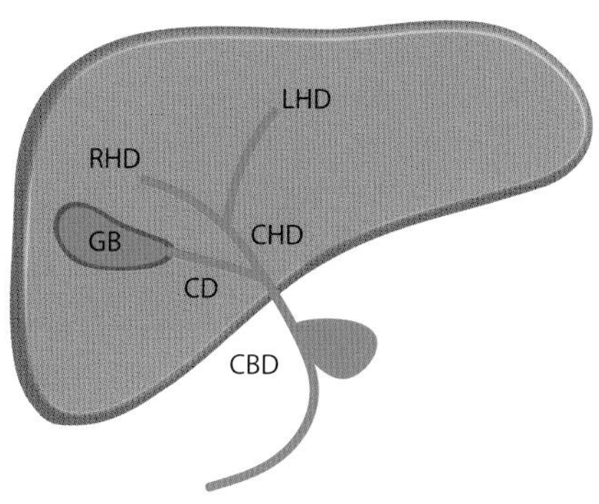

Type III choledochal cyst:
Dilation of intraduodenal bile duct

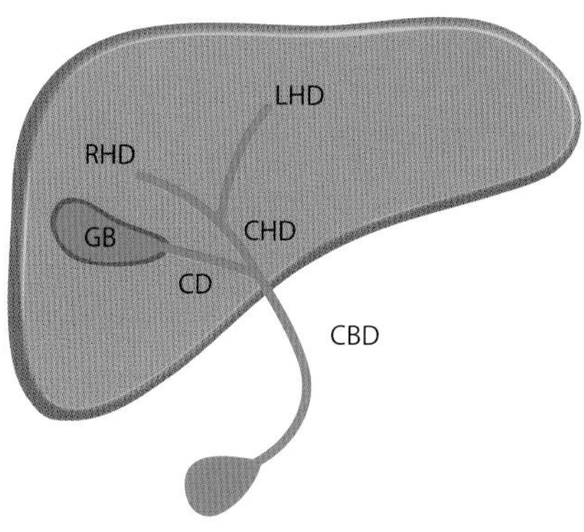

Type IV choledochal cyst:
Multiple segments dilated

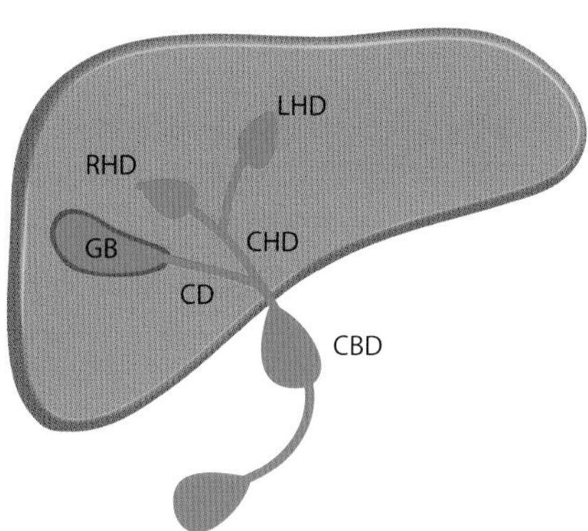

Type IVA: Intra and extrahepatic dilation (pictured)
Type IVB: Extrahepatic dilation only

Type V choledochal cyst:
Intrahepatic dilation = Caroli disease

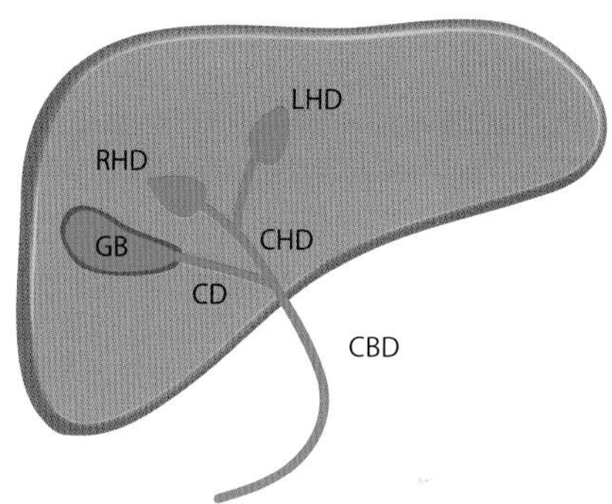

- Choledochal cysts are thought to represent a heterogeneous group of diseases with a common end pathway of intrahepatic or extrahepatic biliary ductal dilation.
- The Todani system divides the cysts into types I–V based on their number, distribution, and morphology.
- Most choledochal cysts are diagnosed in childhood, but less commonly may be a new diagnosis for an adult. Clinically, choledochal cysts can present with nonspecific abdominal pain or may be found incidentally.
- Choledochal cysts are often resected due to increased cholangiocarcinoma risk, which can be as high as 25%.
- In contrast to biliary hamartomas, choledochal cysts *do* communicate with the biliary tree.

Type I choledochal cyst

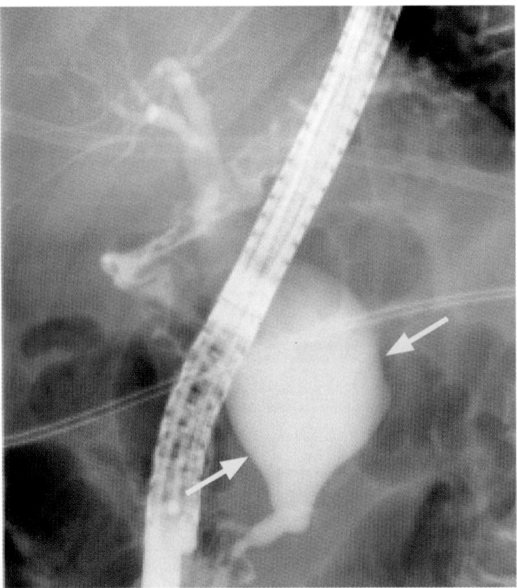

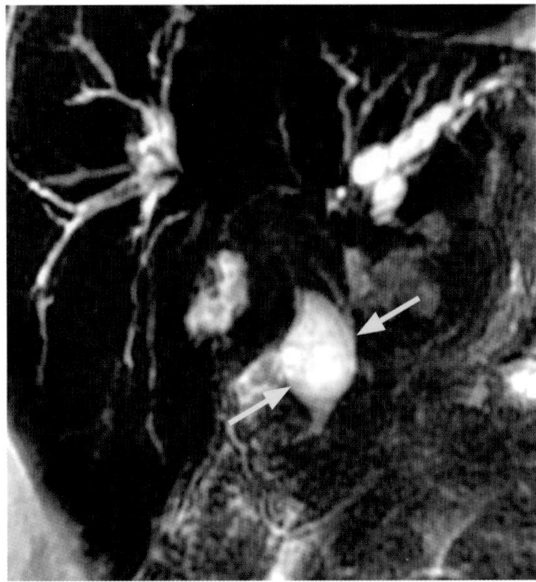

Type I choledochal cyst: ERCP (left image) and thick-slab coronal MRCP heavily T2-weighted sequence (right image) shows a fusiform dilation of common bile duct (arrows).

Case courtesy Cheryl Sadow, MD, Brigham and Women's Hospital.

- A type I choledochal cyst, representing extrahepatic dilation of the common bile duct, is the most common type of extrahepatic cyst.

Caroli disease (Type V choledochal cysts)

- Caroli disease represents saccular dilation of the intrahepatic bile ducts, which may be segmental or diffuse. Caroli disease may be associated with polycystic kidneys.
- Caroli *syndrome* is Caroli disease plus hepatic fibrosis.
- The *central-dot* sign describes the small branches of the portal vein and hepatic artery bridging the dilated bile ducts, which look like a central dot on contrast-enhanced CT.

Biliary anatomical variants

Low insertion of cystic duct

- With a low insertion of the cystic duct, the surgeon may misidentify the common duct as the cystic duct if the patient undergoes cholecystectomy, possibly leading to inadvertent common duct ligation.

Aberrant right posterior duct

- An aberrant right posterior duct is only important if the patient is a right hepatic lobe liver donor, as the two right hepatic ducts need to be anastomosed separately in the recipient.

- Gallbladder pathology is further discussed in the ultrasound section.

Acute cholecystitis

- Cholecystitis is inflammation and localized infection secondary to obstruction of the gallbladder neck or cystic duct.
- Calculous cholecystitis is caused by a gallstone which blocks the cystic duct.
- Acalculous cholecystitis is a functional obstruction of the cystic duct without a culprit stone. It is typically seen in ICU patients.
- Acute cholecystitis is typically diagnosed by ultrasound, but similar criteria can be applied to CT:

> **Gallbladder wall thickening** >3 mm (a nonspecific finding).
>
> **Pericholecystic fluid** or inflammatory changes in the pericholecystic fat.
>
> **Gallbladder hyperemia**.
>
> **Gallbladder calculi** (although not all gallstones are radiopaque; ultrasound is more sensitive).

- Complications of acute cholecystitis include gangrenous cholecystitis, gallbladder perforation, and emphysematous cholecystitis.
- **Gangrenous cholecystitis** is due to increased intraluminal pressure, leading to gallbladder wall ischemia. On imaging, the gallbladder wall thickening may be notably asymmetric and intraluminal membranes may be present. Due to the increased risk of perforation, treatment is emergent cholecystectomy or cholecystostomy.
- **Acute gallbladder perforation** has a very high mortality due to generalized bile peritonitis. Subacute perforation may lead to a pericholecystic abscess and chronic perforation may cause a cholecystoenteric fistula.
- **Emphysematous cholecystitis** is a severe complication of acute cholecystitis caused by gas-forming bacteria. Gas may be present either within the lumen or the wall of the gallbladder. The typical patient susceptible to emphysematous cholecystitis is an elderly diabetic. Treatment of emphysematous cholecystitis is most often emergent cholecystectomy or cholecystostomy, although treatment can be conservative in patients with a very high surgical risk.

Porcelain gallbladder

- Porcelain gallbladder describes a peripherally calcified gallbladder wall, thought to be a sequela of chronic cholecystitis.
- Porcelain gallbladder is associated with a (somewhat controversial) increased risk of gallbladder carcinoma. Typically, a porcelain gallbladder is an indication for non-emergent cholecystectomy.

Ascending cholangitis

- Obstruction of the biliary tree, most commonly due to choledocholithiasis, may cause ascending cholangitis, which presents with the clinical triad of fever, abdominal pain, and jaundice (Charcot's triad).
- On imaging, the key finding is hyperenhancement and thickening of the walls of the bile ducts, often with a common bile duct stone present. On ultrasound, debris within the biliary system may be apparent.
- Initial treatment is antibiotics and fluid resuscitation. Endoscopic biliary intervention may be necessary if the patient does not respond to conservative management.

Primary sclerosing cholangitis (PSC)

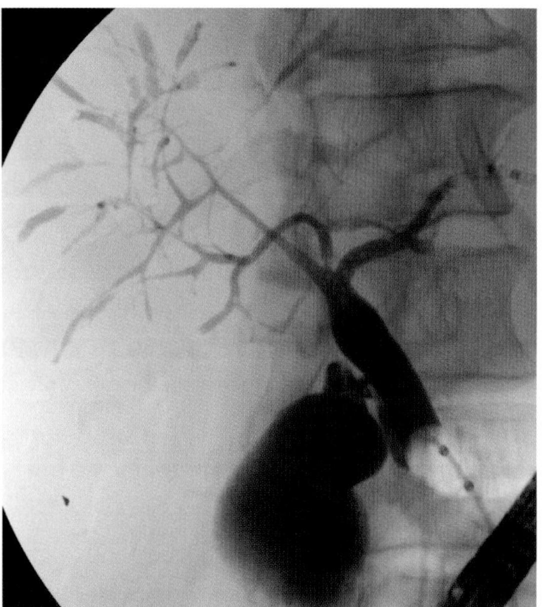
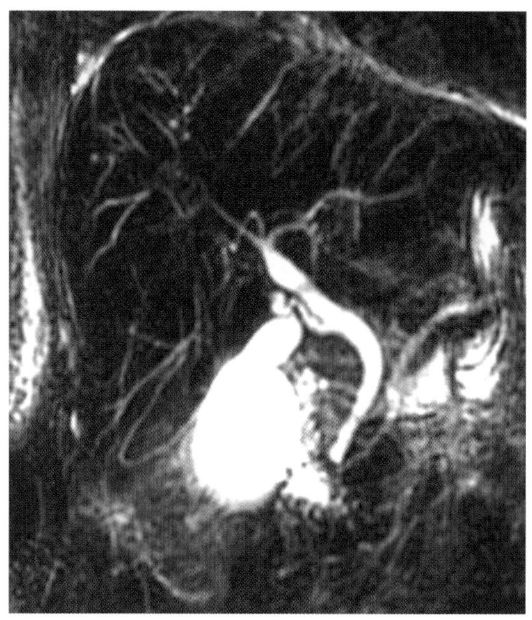

Primary sclerosing cholangitis: ERCP (left image) and thick-slab coronal MRCP heavily T2-weighted sequence (right image) show a beaded, irregular appearance to the intrahepatic bile ducts.

Case courtesy Cheryl Sadow, MD, Brigham and Women's Hospital.

- Primary sclerosing cholangitis (PSC) is idiopathic inflammation and destruction of bile ducts.
- PSC is associated with ulcerative colitis (UC) and is more common in males.
  Most (75%) patients with PSC have UC, while only a few (4–5%) of patients with UC have PSC.
- Biliary imaging shows a characteristic beaded, irregular appearance of the common bile duct and intrahepatic bile ducts.
- PSC appears similar to HIV-cholangiopathy, although cholangitis in HIV patients is more commonly associated with papillary stenosis.
- Long-term complications of PSC include cirrhosis, cholangiocarcinoma, and recurrent biliary infections. Cross-sectional imaging is better at evaluating for these complications compared to ERCP.

Primary biliary cirrhosis (PBC)

- Primary biliary cirrhosis (PBC) is inflammation and destruction of smaller bile ducts compared to PSC. PBC affects middle-aged women and often initially presents with pruritus.
- Similar to PSC, chronic PBC can lead to hepatic cirrhosis.

AIDS cholangitis (AIDS cholangiopathy)

- Patients with acquired immunodeficiency syndrome are susceptible to biliary infection with *Cryptosporidium* and CMV, which clinically present with right upper quadrant pain, fever, and elevated LFTs.
- The imaging of AIDS cholangitis appears nearly identical to primary sclerosing cholangitis, with multiple strictures and a beaded appearance of the bile ducts. A distinguishing feature of AIDS cholangitis is papillary stenosis, which is not typically seen in PSC.

Recurrent pyogenic cholangitis (Oriental cholangiohepatitis)

- Recurrent pyogenic cholangitis, also known as Oriental cholangiohepatitis, is thought to be caused by the parasite *Clonorchis sinensis*, which leads to pigment stone formation, biliary stasis, and cholangitis. Nutritional deficiency may also play a role. The disease typically affects patients indigenous to Southeast Asia. Clinically, patients present with recurrent jaundice and fevers.
- Recurrent pyogenic cholangitis features an imaging triad of:
  1) Pneumobilia.
  2) Lamellated bile duct filling defects.
  3) Intrahepatic and extrahepatic bile duct dilation and strictures.
- Patients with recurrent pyogenic cholangitis have an increased risk of cholangiocarcinoma.

Biliary neoplasia

Biliary cystadenoma

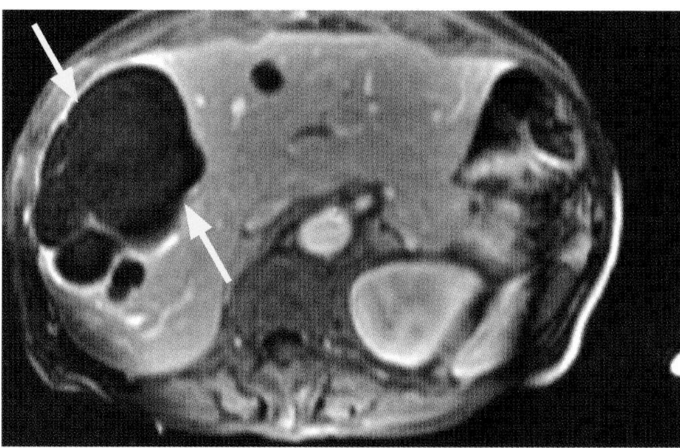
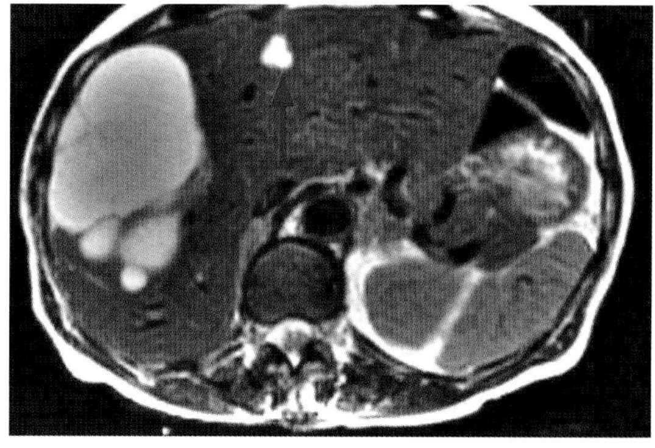

Biliary cystadenoma: T1-weighted post-contrast (left image) and T2-weighted (right image) MRI shows a large multiloculated cystic mass (arrows) in the right lobe of the liver, with enhancing septations. There are no enhancing nodules. There is also a small simple-appearing cyst in the left liver (segment 4; red arrow).

Case courtesy Cheryl Sadow, MD, Brigham and Women's Hospital.

- Biliary cystadenoma is a benign cystic neoplasm, occurring predominantly in middle-aged women. Biliary cystadenoma may be quite large at presentation and cause nonspecific symptoms such as abdominal pain, nausea, vomiting, and obstructive jaundice.
- Biliary cystadenoma does not communicate with the biliary system.
- On imaging, biliary cystadenoma appears as a large, multiloculated, cystic mass. The presence of septations distinguishes cystadenoma from a simple cyst. The septations may mimic an echinococcal cyst. In contrast to hepatic abscess or necrotic metastasis, a thick enhancing wall is not a feature of cystadenoma.
- Although benign, cystadenoma may uncommonly recur after resection.
- Malignant degeneration to biliary cystadenocarcinoma has been reported but is rare. The presence of a large solid component or thick calcification should raise concern for cystadenocarcinoma.

Cholangiocarcinoma

- Cholangiocarcinoma is a highly malignant tumor of the biliary ductal epithelium.
- A hilar tumor (at the confluence of the right and left intrahepatic biliary ducts), known as a **Klatskin tumor**, is the most common form of cholangiocarcinoma. In contrast, peripheral cholangiocarcinoma is rare.
- Cholangiocarcinoma tends to obstruct bile ducts and cause intrahepatic ductal dilation. Eventually, the obstruction may lead to lobar atrophy.
- Risk factors for development of cholangiocarcinoma include:

> Choledochal cyst(s).
>
> Primary sclerosing cholangitis.
>
> Familial adenomatous polyposis syndrome.
>
> *Clonorchis sinensis* infection.
>
> Thorium dioxide (alpha-emitter contrast agent), not used since the 1950s. Thorium dioxide is also associated with angiosarcoma and HCC.

- On cross-sectional imaging, cholangiocarcinoma typically presents as an intrahepatic mass at the confluence of the central bile ducts (Klatskin tumor), with resultant bile duct dilation and capsular retraction. Tumor fingers often extend into the bile ducts.

Gallbladder carcinoma

- Gallbladder carcinoma is rare and is usually due to chronic gallbladder inflammation.
- Gallstones and concomitant chronic cholecystitis are typically present. Porcelain gallbladder, a result of chronic cholecystitis, is thought to be a risk factor for gallbladder cancer, although this is controversial.
- Gallbladder carcinoma most commonly presents as a scirrhous infiltrating mass that invades through the gallbladder wall into the liver. Less commonly, gallbladder carcinoma may appear as a polypoid mass. Very rarely it can present as mural thickening.
- Tumor spread is via direct extension into the liver, although lymphatic and hematogenous metastases are also common.
- Prognosis is generally poor, although small polypoid lesions may undergo curative resection.

Gallbladder metastasis

- Melanoma has a propensity to metastasize to the gallbladder.

OVERVIEW OF PANCREATIC NEOPLASMS

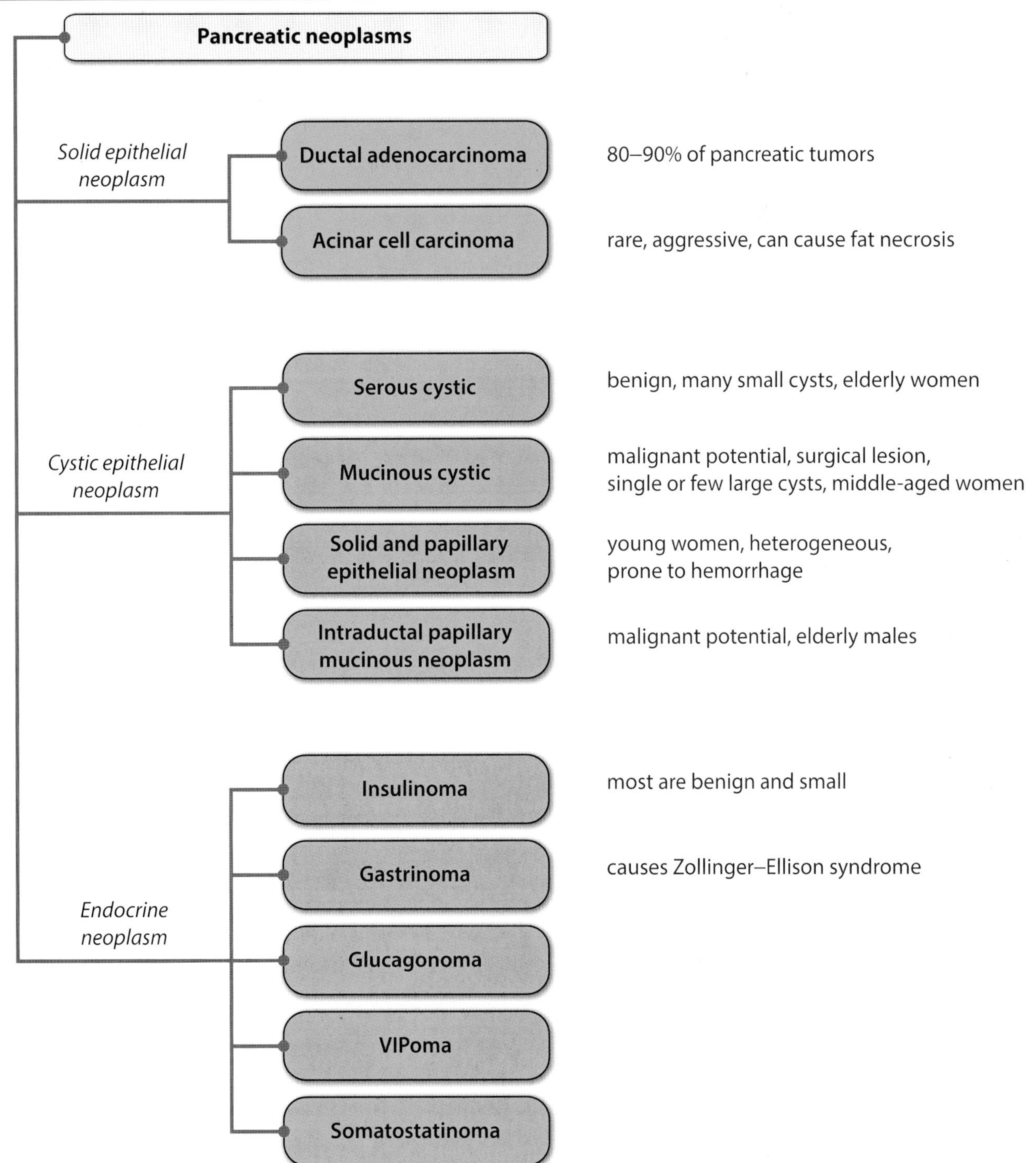
Pancreatic neoplasms
Solid epithelial neoplasm
Ductal adenocarcinoma
80–90% of pancreatic tumors
Acinar cell carcinoma
rare, aggressive, can cause fat necrosis
Cystic epithelial neoplasm
Serous cystic
benign, many small cysts, elderly women
Mucinous cystic
malignant potential, surgical lesion, single or few large cysts, middle-aged women
Solid and papillary epithelial neoplasm
young women, heterogeneous, prone to hemorrhage
Intraductal papillary mucinous neoplasm
malignant potential, elderly males
Endocrine neoplasm
Insulinoma
most are benign and small
Gastrinoma
causes Zollinger–Ellison syndrome
Glucagonoma
VIPoma
Somatostatinoma

Adenocarcinoma (ductal adenocarcinoma)

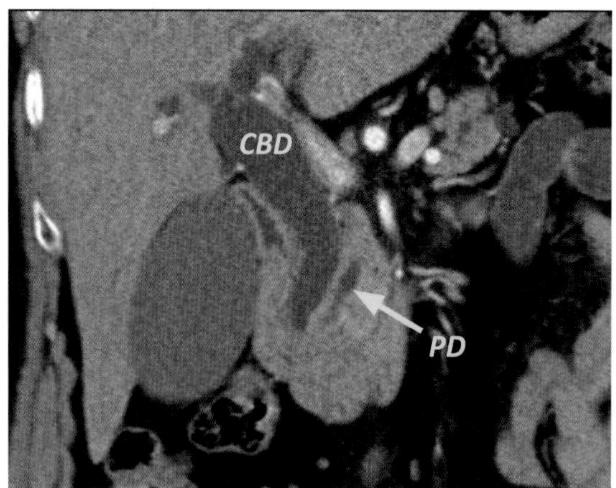

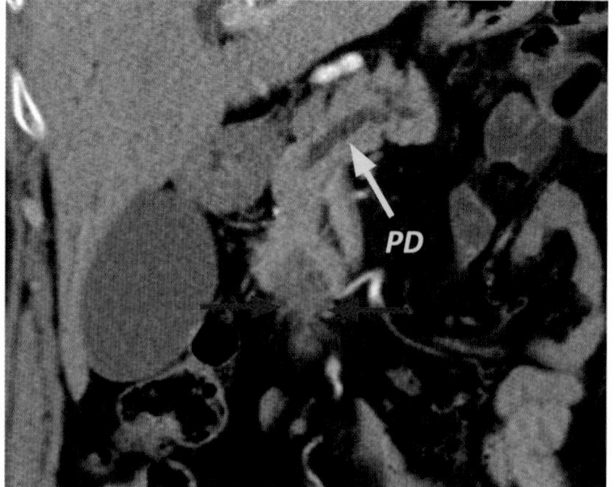

Pancreatic adenocarcinoma causing the *double duct* sign: Two coronal images from a contrast-enhanced CT show marked dilation of the common bile duct (CBD), moderate dilation of the pancreatic duct (PD), and an ill-defined hypoattenuating mass in the pancreatic head (red arrows).

Case courtesy Cheryl Sadow, MD, Brigham and Women's Hospital.

- Pancreatic ductal adenocarcinoma makes up 80–90% of all pancreatic tumors. It is typically seen in patients over age 60, with a slight male predominance. Risk factors include smoking, alcohol, and chronic pancreatitis.
- A pancreatic-mass CT includes unenhanced, late arterial phase, and portal venous phase images. The late arterial phase (pancreatic parenchymal phase) has the greatest conspicuity for detecting the hypoenhancing tumor against the background enhancing pancreas.
- The most common location of ductal adenocarcinoma is the pancreatic head.
- The classic appearance is a hypodense (CT), T1 hypointense (MR), ill-defined, hypovascular mass causing ductal obstruction and atrophy of the pancreatic tail. The *double duct* sign describes dilation of both the pancreatic duct and the common bile duct.
- Since pancreatic adenocarcinoma is almost always associated with a dilated pancreatic duct, an alternative diagnosis should be strongly considered if there is a pancreatic mass with no ductal dilation, such as:

Autoimmune pancreatitis.	Duodenal gastrointestinal stromal tumor (GIST).
Groove pancreatitis.	Peripancreatic lymph node.
Cystic pancreatic tumor.	Pancreatic metastasis (e.g., renal cell, thyroid, or melanoma).
Neuroendocrine tumor.	Lymphoma.

- Conversely, if the *double duct* sign is present but no mass is visible, one should still be suspicious for pancreatic adenocarcinoma. Approximately 10% of cases will be isoattenuating relative to pancreas in the pancreatic parenchymal (late arterial) phase and thus extremely difficult to directly detect.
- Most cancers present at an advanced, unresectable stage. Unresectable tumors show encasement (>180° circumference) of the SMA, extensive venous invasion, or evidence of metastasis.
- For lower-stage tumors, complete surgical resection is the only chance for cure. A resectable tumor features no evidence of celiac, SMA, or portal venous invasion. Limited extension to the duodenum, distal stomach, or CBD does not preclude resection, as these structures are resected during the Whipple procedure. Limited venous extension may be resectable.

Acinar cell carcinoma

- Acinar cell carcinoma is a rare, aggressive variant of pancreatic adenocarcinoma, exclusively seen in elderly males.
- The malignant cells produce a large amount of lipase to cause the clinical triad of lipase hypersecretion syndrome: Subcutaneous fat necrosis; bone infarcts causing polyarthralgias; and eosinophilia.

CYSTIC PANCREATIC EPITHELIAL NEOPLASMS

Serous cystadenoma

- Serous cystadenoma is a benign tumor that occurs in elderly women and has been nicknamed the *grandmother* tumor.
- It consists of many small cysts (>6 cysts that are <2 cm) that may have a solid appearance on CT due to apposition of many cyst walls. MRI is useful to show the cystic nature of the lesion.
- Serous cystadenoma is hypervascular, unique among cystic pancreatic tumors.
- Unlike adenocarcinoma, serous cystadenoma does not cause pancreatic duct dilation or tail atrophy.
- A classic imaging feature is central stellate calcification.

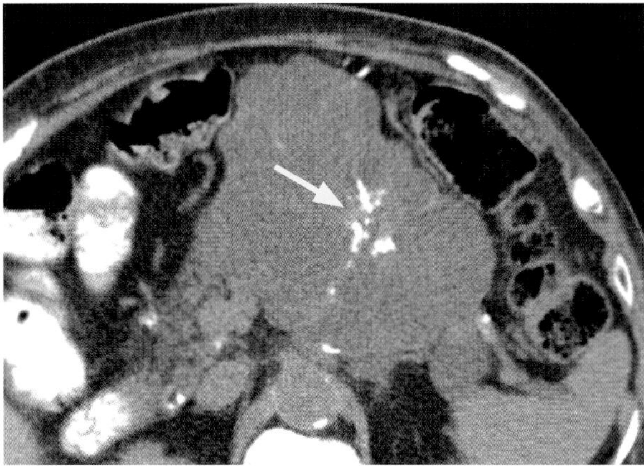

Serous cystadenoma: Axial oral-contrast-only CT shows a large multicystic pancreatic mass containing central stellate calcification (arrows).

Case courtesy Cheryl Sadow, MD, Brigham and Women's Hospital.

Mucinous cystic neoplasm

- Mucinous cystic neoplasm affects middle-aged women and has therefore been nicknamed the *mother* tumor.
- Mucinous cystic neoplasm is benign, but does have malignant potential. Treatment is typically resection due to malignant potential.
- The tumor consists of a single or a few large cysts (<6 cysts that are >2 cm) and typically occurs in the pancreatic body and tail.
- Mucinous cystic neoplasm has a capsule. The only other pancreatic tumor with a capsule is SPEN (below).

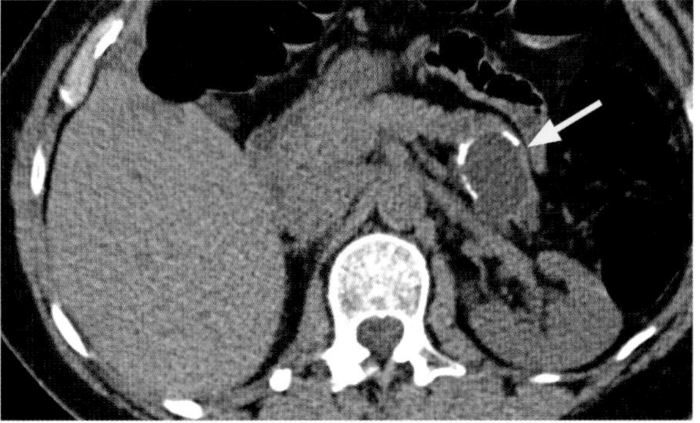

Mucinous cystic neoplasm: Axial noncontrast CT shows a cystic, peripherally calcified mass in the tail of the pancreas (arrow). Pathology at resection showed borderline malignancy.

Case courtesy Cheryl Sadow, MD, Brigham and Women's Hospital.

Solid and papillary epithelial neoplasm (SPEN)

- Solid and papillary epithelial neoplasm (SPEN) occurs in young women and children and is nicknamed the *daughter* tumor. It may be a rare cause of abdominal pain.
- It has a low malignant potential and is typically resected.
- On imaging, SPEN appears as a large mass with heterogeneous solid and cystic areas. Hemorrhage is typical. SPEN features a capsule, as does mucinous cystic neoplasm.

Intraductal papillary mucinous neoplasm (IPMN)

- Intraductal papillary mucinous neoplasm (IPMN) occurs most commonly in elderly males and is nicknamed the *grandfather* tumor, although these tumors exhibit the greatest age and sex variability of the cystic pancreatic neoplasms.
- IPMN features a spectrum of biological behavior from benign to indolent to aggressive carcinoma. IPMNs may arise from the main pancreatic duct or a sidebranch. The main duct IPMNs have greater malignant potential.
- The classic appearance on endoscopy is a *fish-mouth* papilla pouring out mucin. Cross-sectional imaging shows a cystic intrapancreatic lesion in contiguity with the duct or sidebranch. Any nodular or enhancing component should raise concern for malignancy.
- The recommended imaging follow-up and criteria for resectability are controversial. Current guidelines published in 2006 recommend following simple pancreatic cysts <1 cm annually by imaging (typically MR). However, up to 40% of elderly males have a pancreatic cyst, suggesting that they may be an acquired condition of aging rather than a premalignancy.
- In general, a suspected IPMN is resected if it is >3 cm in size, if there is a mural nodule, or if there is associated dilation of the pancreatic duct to >10 mm.

PANCREATIC ENDOCRINE NEOPLASMS

Overview

- Pancreatic neuroendocrine tumors may be hyperfunctioning or non-hyperfunctioning.
- Hyperfunctioning tumors come to clinical attention due to symptoms of endocrine excess.
- Non-hyperfunctioning tumors tend to be larger at diagnosis. These tumors may undergo cystic change and should be considered in the differential of a cystic pancreatic neoplasm. There is often central necrosis and calcification in these large tumors as well.
- Pancreatic endocrine tumors tend to be hypervascular and are best seen in the late arterial phase. Most are solid unless large. A hypervascular liver mass with an associated pancreatic mass is most likely a metastatic pancreatic endocrine neoplasm.

Insulinoma

- Insulinoma is the most common pancreatic endocrine tumor. Due to symptoms of hypoglycemia, insulinomas tend to present early and have the best prognosis of all neuroendocrine tumors, with only 10% demonstrating malignant behavior.
- The Whipple triad describes the clinical symptoms of insulinoma: Hypoglycemia, clinical symptoms of hypoglycemia, and alleviation of symptoms after administration of glucose.

Gastrinoma

- Gastrinoma causes hypersecretion of gastric acid resulting in Zollinger–Ellison syndrome. Gastrinoma is the second most common pancreatic endocrine tumor. Gastrinoma is associated with multiple endocrine neoplasia (MEN) type 1. When associated with MEN-1, gastrinomas tend to be multiple and located in the duodenum rather than the pancreas.
- The gastrinoma triangle describes the typical location of gastrinomas, in an area bounded by the junction of the cystic duct and CBD, the duodenum inferiorly, and the neck/body of the pancreas medially.
- High gastrin levels may cause formation of carcinoid tumors in the stomach, which may regress after the gastrinoma is resected.

Other pancreatic endocrine tumors

- Glucagonoma is the third most common pancreatic endocrine tumor. Prognosis is poor. VIPoma and somatostatinoma are very rare and also have poor prognoses.

Normal ductal anatomy

- Normally , the main pancreatic duct drains to the major papilla (the ampulla of Vater) through the duct of Wirsung, while the duct of Santorini drains to the minor papilla.

  The sphincter of Oddi is a circular band of muscle encircling the ampulla of Vater.

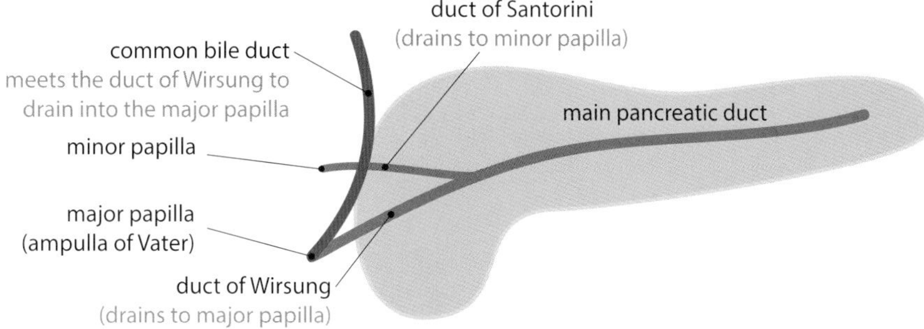

- Mnemonic for normal anatomy: Santorini is superior and drains to small (minor) papilla.
- The following anatomy is *always* constant, regardless of whether an anomaly is present:

  1) The common bile duct always drains to the major papilla where it meets the duct of Wirsung.

  2) The main pancreatic duct always drains the pancreatic tail.

  3) The duct of Santorini always drains to the minor papilla.

Pancreas divisum

- Pancreas divisum is the most common congenital pancreatic anomaly. It is caused by failure of fusion of ventral and dorsal pancreatic ducts. The ventral duct (Wirsung) only drains a portion of the pancreas while the majority of the pancreatic exocrine gland output is drained through the smaller duct of Santorini into the minor papilla.

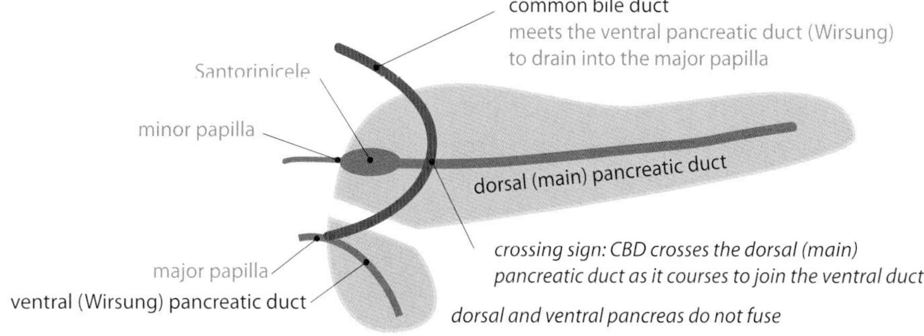

- Pancreas divisum may be a cause of pancreatitis due to obstruction at the minor papilla from a Santorinicele. A Santorinicele is a focal dilation of the terminal duct of Santorini.
- The *crossing* sign describes the CBD crossing over the main duct to join the duct of Wirsung.

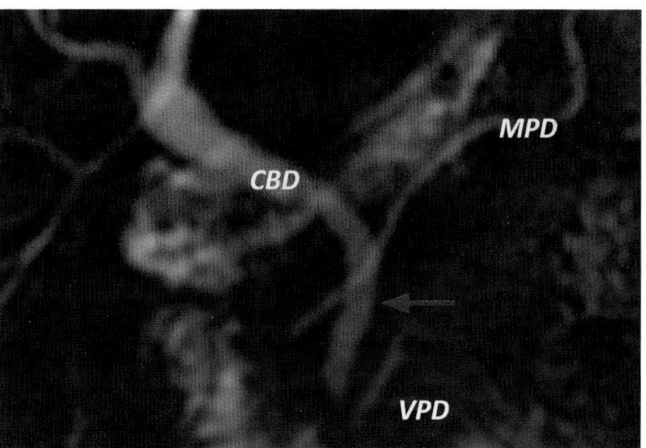

Crossing sign of pancreas divisum: Thick-slab coronal MRCP heavily T2-weighted sequence shows the common bile duct (CBD) crossing the main pancreatic duct (MPD) at the arrow. The CBD courses towards the ventral pancreatic duct (VPD) to empty into the major papilla. The main/dorsal pancreatic duct drains separately into the minor papilla.

Case courtesy Cheryl Sadow, MD, Brigham and Women's Hospital.

Annular pancreas

- Annular pancreas is a rare congenital anomaly where a portion of the pancreas wraps completely around the duodenum, secondary to incomplete rotation of the ventral pancreatic bud.

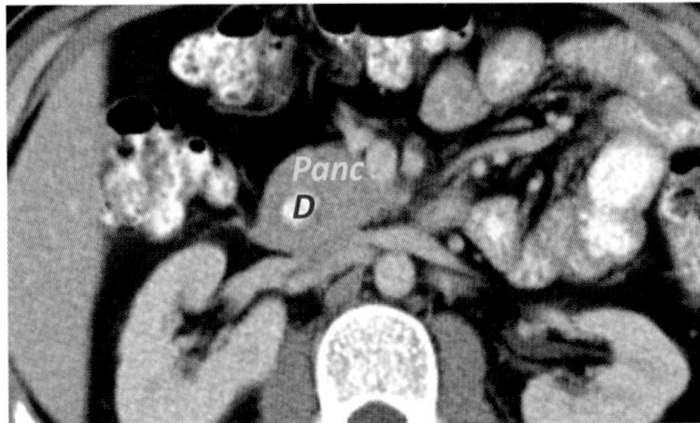

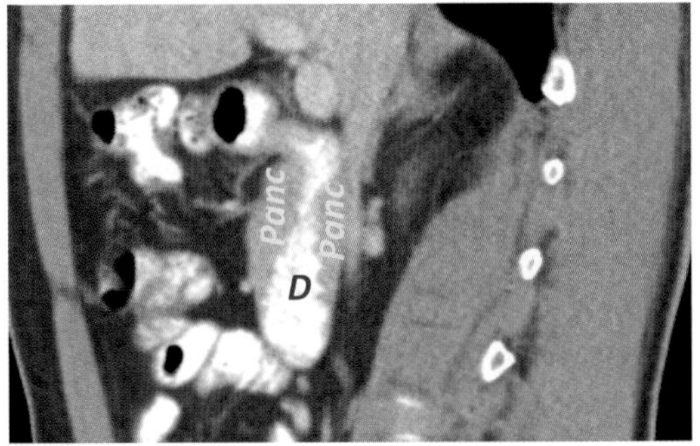

Annular pancreas: Axial (left image) and sagittal (right image) contrast-enhanced CT shows circumferential encircling of the pancreas (Panc) around the duodenum (D), which is filled with oral contrast.

Case courtesy Cheryl Sadow, MD, Brigham and Women's Hospital.

- In an adult, annular pancreas can cause pancreatitis, peptic ulcer disease, and duodenal obstruction. In a neonate, it can cause duodenal obstruction and is in the differential for the *double bubble* sign.

Common channel syndrome/pancreaticobiliary maljunction

- Normally the common bile duct and duct of Wirsung both drain to the major papilla, where there is usually a thin septum separating these two systems.
- In common channel syndrome, also known as pancreaticobiliary maljunction, the distal CBD and pancreatic duct are missing the septum, allowing reflux between the two systems.
- Common channel syndrome may be in the spectrum of choledochal cyst disease with the common channel representing a very mild form of choledochocele. Common channel syndrome may predispose to cholangiocarcinoma, but this is rare and controversial.

SYSTEMIC DISEASES THAT AFFECT THE PANCREAS

Pancreatic manifestations of von Hippel–Lindau

- von Hippel–Lindau is an inherited multisystemic disease with increased risk of multiple malignancies and formation of cysts in various organs including the pancreas.
- Pancreatic neoplasms seen in von Hippel–Lindau include serous cystadenoma and pancreatic neuroendocrine tumors.

Cystic fibrosis (CF)

- Cystic fibrosis (CF) is the most common cause of childhood pancreatic atrophy.
- CF can cause either fatty atrophy of the pancreas or pancreatic cystosis (diffuse replacement of the pancreas with innumerable cysts).

Schwachman–Diamond

- Schwachman–Diamond is a rare inherited disorder characterized by diffuse fatty replacement of the pancreas, resultant pancreatic exocrine insufficiency, neutropenia, and bone dysplasia.
- Schwachman–Diamond is the second-most common cause of childhood pancreatic atrophy.

Obesity and exogenous steroid use

- Both obesity and steroids can cause fatty atrophy of the pancreas.

Miscellaneous pancreatic lesions

Intrapancreatic accessory spleen

- Intrapancreatic accessory spleen is a benign mimic of a hypervascular pancreatic neoplasm.
- On imaging, an intrapancreatic spleen typically is a small (1–3 cm), well-defined mass usually found in the pancreatic tail. It follows the density, signal intensity, and enhancement of the spleen on all CT and MRI sequences.

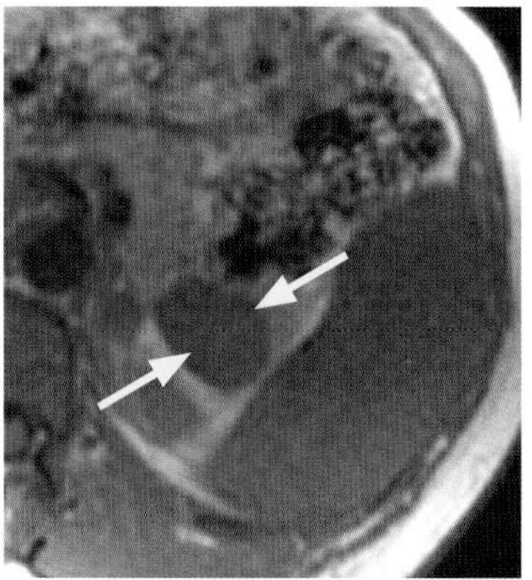
In-phase MRI

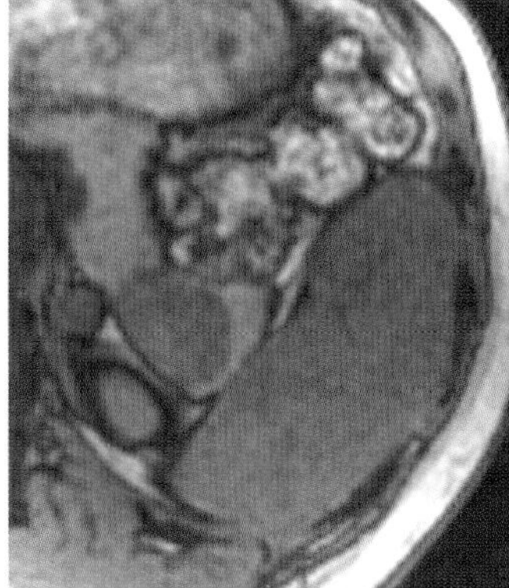
Out-of-phase MRI

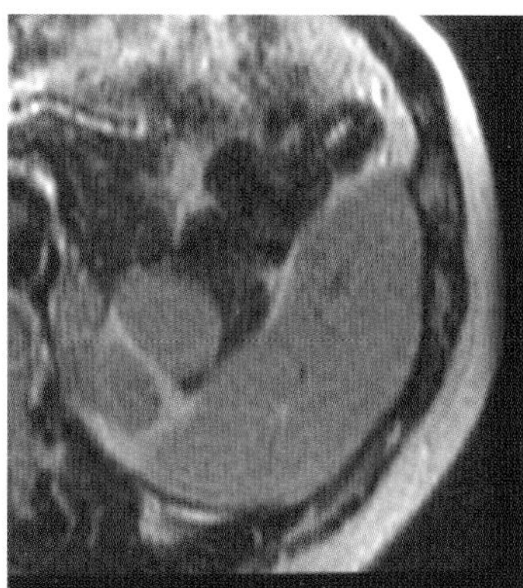
T2-weighted MRI

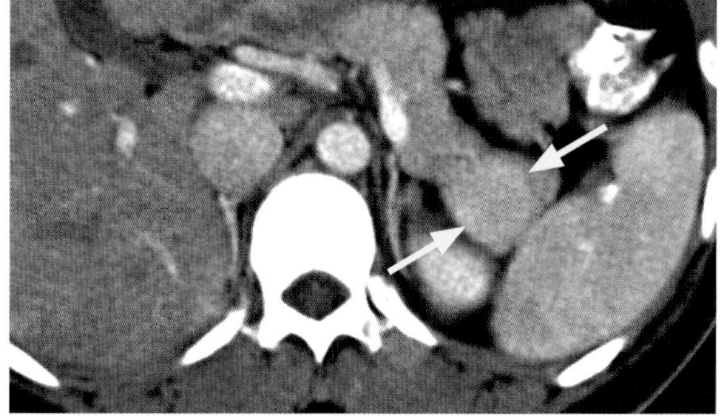
Contrast-enhanced CT

Intrapancreatic spleen: MRI images show a mass in the tail of the pancreas (arrows) that completely follows splenic signal intensity on all sequences. CT of the same areas (bottom left image) shows identical enhancement pattern of this mass compared to the spleen.

Case courtesy of Cheryl Sadow, MD, Brigham and Women's Hospital

- MRI is usually diagnostic. Either technetium-99m sulfur colloid or technetium-99m RBC scintigraphy can confirm the diagnosis in ambiguous cases.

Pancreatitis

- Pancreatitis is inflammation of the pancreas, which may be due to a wide variety of etiologies that share a final common pathway of premature activation of pancreatic enzymes and resultant autodigestion of pancreatic parenchyma.
- Pancreatitis may range in severity from mild self-limited disease to necrotizing pancreatitis resulting in multi-organ failure and death.

CT protocol and role of imaging

- Imaging of pancreatitis is optimally performed in the pancreatic parenchymal phase (late arterial; ~40 seconds after contrast injection), which is the most sensitive timing to detect subtle areas of decreased enhancement suggestive of necrosis.
- CT is key for pancreatitis imaging. In addition to often identifying an etiology of the pancreatitis, CT can grade severity, detect complications, and guide possible percutaneous interventions.
- CT imaging is *not* indicated in patients with clinical diagnosis of mild acute pancreatitis, especially if they are improving. CT imaging may be negative or show a mildly edematous pancreas in these cases.

Acute pancreatitis

- Acute pancreatitis is most commonly caused by alcohol or an obstructing gallstone.
- Acute pancreatitis can be classified either with the Balthazar grading system or by the CT severity index.
- **Balthazar** grading system:

> A: Normal-appearing pancreas
>
> B: Focal or diffuse pancreatic enlargement
>
> C: Mild peripancreatic inflammatory changes
>
> D: Single fluid collection
>
> E: Two or more fluid collections

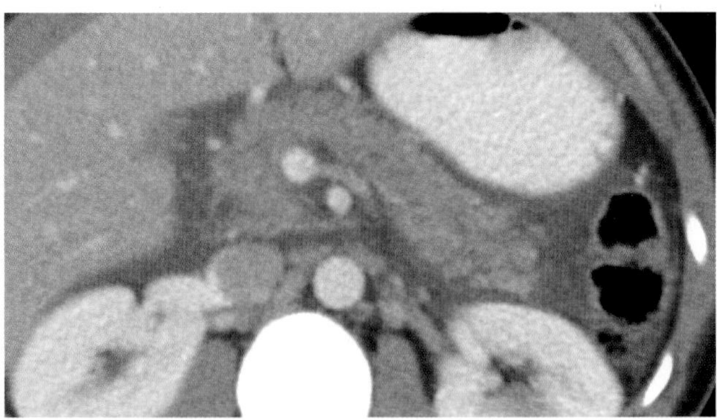

Acute pancreatitis: Contrast-enhanced axial CT demonstrates diffuse pancreatic enlargement and peripancreatic edema. The pancreatic parenchyma enhances uniformly, without evidence for necrosis. This would be a Balthazar grade B, with 0 points added for necrosis, for a CT severity index of 2.

0% mortality, 4% morbidity for grades A, B, and C.

14% mortality, 54% morbidity for grades D and E (a fluid collection is a poor prognostic indicator).

- **CT severity index (CTSI)** integrates the Balthazar grading system with the degree of necrosis:

> Assigns 0–4 points for Balthazar A–E, with 0 points for Balthazar A and 4 points for Balthazar E.
>
> Adds 0–6 points for necrosis to create a total score from 0-10.
>
> 0 points: 0% necrosis
>
> 2 points: <30% necrosis
>
> 4 points: 30–50% necrosis
>
> 6 points: >50% necrosis

CTSI 0–3: 3% mortality, 8% morbidity

CTSI 7–10: 17% mortality, 92% morbidity

- Pancreatic and peripancreatic complications:

Pancreatic necrosis: On imaging, pancreatic necrosis appears as a focal or diffuse area of nonenhancing pancreatic parenchyma. Evaluation of necrosis is best performed 48–72 hours after onset of acute pancreatitis. Late arterial phase imaging has the highest sensitivity for detecting pancreatic necrosis. Patients with pancreatic necrosis are at increased risk for infection and severe morbidity.

Fluid collections: Peripancreatic fluid may resolve or may evolve either into peripancreatic abscess or pseudocyst.

Pseudocyst: A pancreatic pseudocyst is a collection of pancreatic enzymes and fluid enclosed by a fibrous wall lacking an epithelial lining. The fibrous wall usually takes about 4–6 weeks to mature.

Pancreatic abscess: Pancreatic abscess is a purulent collection featuring thicker, more irregular walls compared to a pseudocyst. Gas locules may be present within the abscess.

- Extrapancreatic complications:

Extrapancreatic pseudocyst may occur nearly anywhere below the diaphragm and should always be considered in the differential of a cystic structure in a patient with history of pancreatitis. In particular, an intrasplenic pseudocyst may lead to intrasplenic hemorrhage.

Perihilar renal inflammation, which may lead to venous compression or thrombosis.

Bowel involvement, especially of the transverse colon.

- Secondary inflammation of adjacent vessels can cause vascular complications:

Arterial bleeding, most commonly due to erosion into the splenic artery.

Pseudoaneurysm, most commonly of the splenic artery.

Venous thrombosis, most commonly splenic vein thrombosis, which may lead to portal hypertension.

Chronic pancreatitis

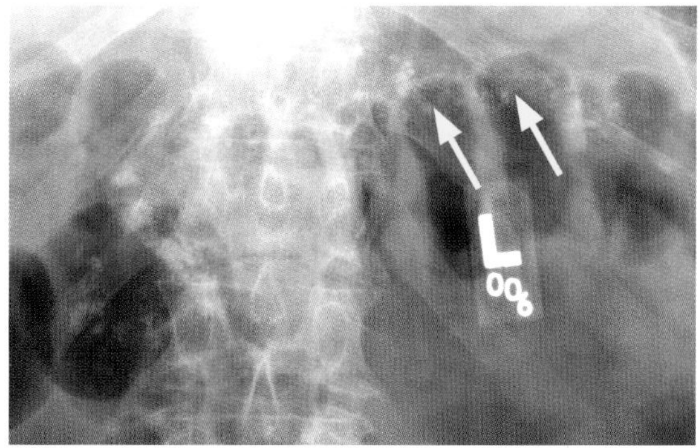

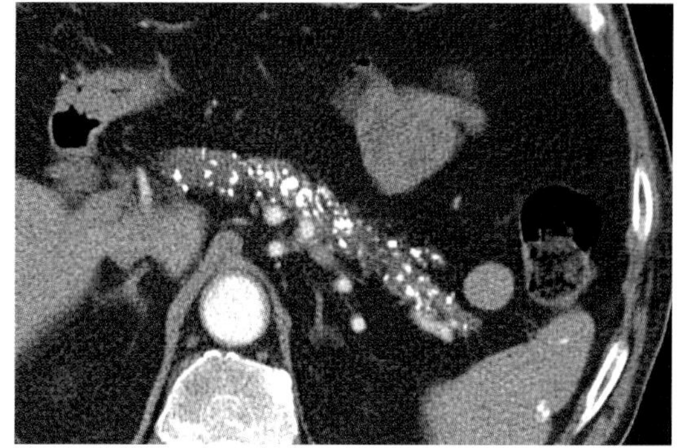

Chronic pancreatitis: Abdominal radiograph (left image) and contrast-enhanced axial CT (right image) show numerous coarse calcifications in the pancreas (arrows).

Case courtesy Cheryl Sadow, MD, Brigham and Women's Hospital.

- Chronic pancreatitis, most commonly from long-term alcohol abuse, causes irreversible pancreatic damage.

  A much less common cause of chronic pancreatitis is pancreas divisum.

- Calcifications in the distribution of the pancreatic duct are pathognomonic for chronic pancreatitis.

Autoimmune pancreatitis

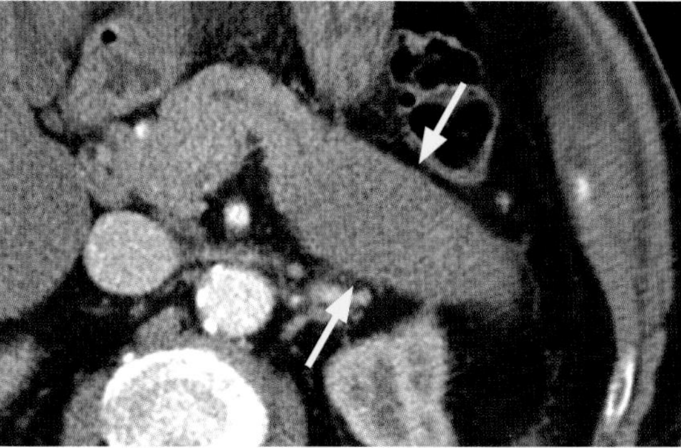

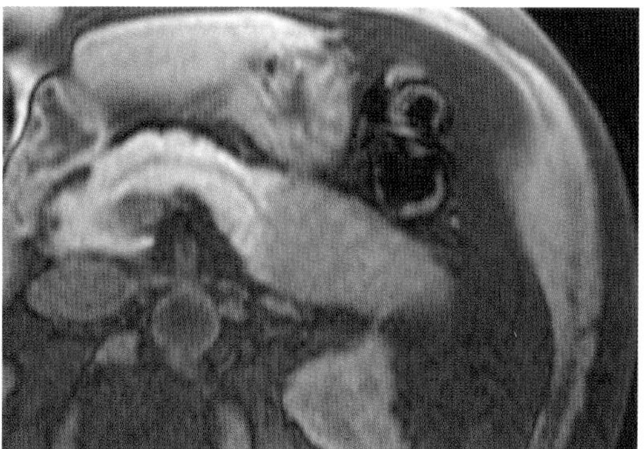

Segmental autoimmune pancreatitis: Contrast-enhanced axial CT (left image) shows a segmental region of low attenuation enlargement of the pancreatic tail and body (arrows), with loss of the normal ductal architecture.

T1-weighted unenhanced MRI (right image) shows a corresponding segmental loss of the normal T1-hyperintense pancreatic signal, with effacement of the pancreatic duct in the affected body and tail.

The differential diagnosis for this appearance would include pancreatic lymphoma, less likely pancreatic adenocarcinoma as there is no ductal dilation.

Case courtesy Cheryl Sadow, MD, Brigham and Women's Hospital.

- Autoimmune pancreatitis is caused by an inflammatory lymphoplasmacytic infiltrate. It is associated with Sjögren syndrome and causes elevated serum IgG-4 levels.
- The typical imaging appearance of autoimmune pancreatitis is diffuse "sausage-shaped" enlargement of the entire pancreas; however, a focal or segmental form may mimic a pancreatic mass.
- Treatment is with steroids, which can lead to a complete resolution.

Groove pancreatitis

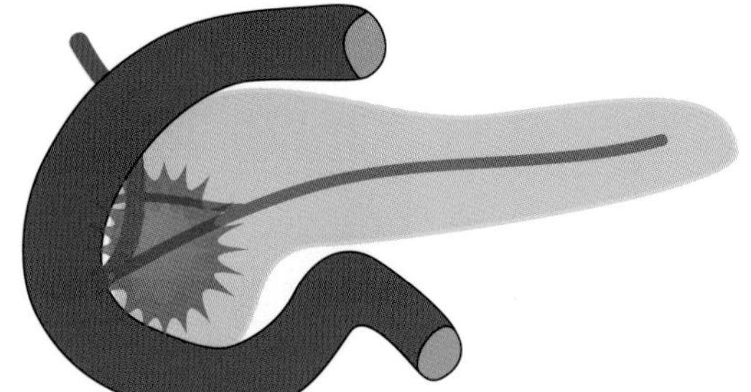

Diagram demonstrates inflammation within the groove between the head of the pancreas, duodenum, and common bile duct.

- Groove pancreatitis is an uncommon form of focal pancreatitis of the groove between the head of the pancreas, duodenum, and common bile duct. Groove pancreatitis usually affects young men who are heavy drinkers.
- The histopathologic hallmark is fibrosis in the pancreaticoduodenal groove. Chronic inflammation of the duodenum can cause varying levels of duodenal stenosis or cystic change of the duodenal wall. Imaging reflects these findings, with duodenal thickening and cystic change often apparent. The cystic change is best appreciated on MR.
- The main differential consideration is adenocarcinoma of the head of the pancreas.

Spleen

Congenital splenic variations and anomalies

Splenule (accessory spleen)

- Also called an accessory spleen, a splenule is a focus of normal splenic tissue separate from the main body of the spleen, due to embryologic failure of fusion of the splenic anlage. The most common location is the splenic hilum.
- Although usually an incidental finding, the presence of a splenule does have significance in certain clinical settings. For instance, splenectomy for consumptive thrombocytopenia may not be curative if there is sufficient unresected accessory splenic tissue present. A splenule may be mistaken for a lymph node or mass when in an unusual location. As previously discussed, an intrapancreatic splenule may be mistaken for a hypervascular pancreatic mass.
- A splenule should follow splenic tissue on all MRI sequences. If in doubt, a Tc-99m sulfur colloid scan or a heat-damaged Tc-99m RBC scan can be confirmatory.

Polysplenia syndrome

- Polysplenia syndrome is a spectrum of anatomic disorders characterized by some degree of visceral heterotaxia in addition to multiple discrete foci of splenic tissue. Multiple spleens may be on the right or left, but are always on the same side as the stomach.
- Polysplenia is usually associated with severe congenital cardiac anomalies. Most patients die in early childhood, but a few may have only minor cardiac defects and may be incidentally discovered as adults.
- Polysplenia is associated with venous anomalies including interruption of the IVC with azygos or hemiazygos continuation. A less common association is a preduodenal portal vein.

Wandering spleen

- A wandering spleen is a normal spleen with abnormal laxity or absence of its fixed ligamentous attachments.
- Wandering spleen may present clinically as an abdominal mass or may cause acute abdominal pain secondary to torsion.

Hemangioma

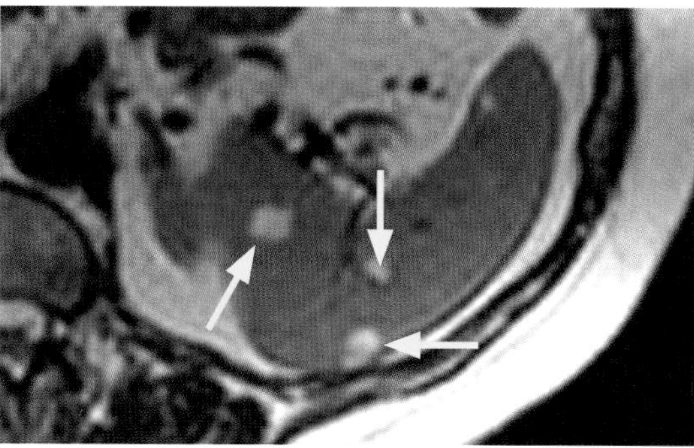
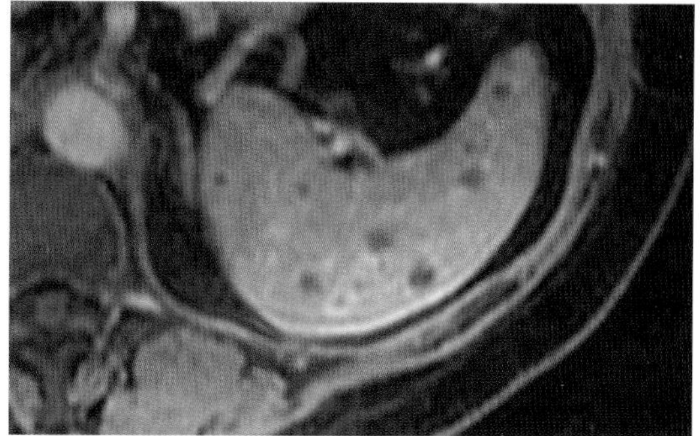

Multiple splenic hemangiomas: T2-weighted (left image) and post-contrast T1-weighted (right image) MRI shows multiple T2 hyperintense splenic lesions (arrows) that demonstrate subtle peripheral enhancement.

Case courtesy Cheryl Sadow, MD, Brigham and Women's Hospital.

- Hemangioma is the most common benign splenic neoplasm. Hemangioma may be solitary or multiple, and lesions tend to be small.
- Splenic hemangiomas are associated with **Kasabach–Merritt** syndrome (anemia, thrombocytopenia, and consumptive coagulopathy) and **Klippel–Trenaunay–Weber** syndrome (cutaneous hemangiomas, varicose veins, and extremity hypertrophy). These visceral hemangiomatosis syndromes are usually associated with phleboliths.
- On CT, hemangiomas are typically iso- or hypoattenuating pre-contrast and hyperenhancing. On MR, hemangiomas are typically hyperintense on T2-weighted images and may enhance peripherally or homogeneously. However, the classic pattern of discontinuous nodular enhancement seen in hepatic hemangiomas is uncommon.
- Nuclear medicine scintigraphy with Tc-99m labeled red blood cells would show increased activity within the lesion on delayed images. In contrast, Tc-99m sulfur colloid scanning may show either increased or decreased activity.

Hamartoma

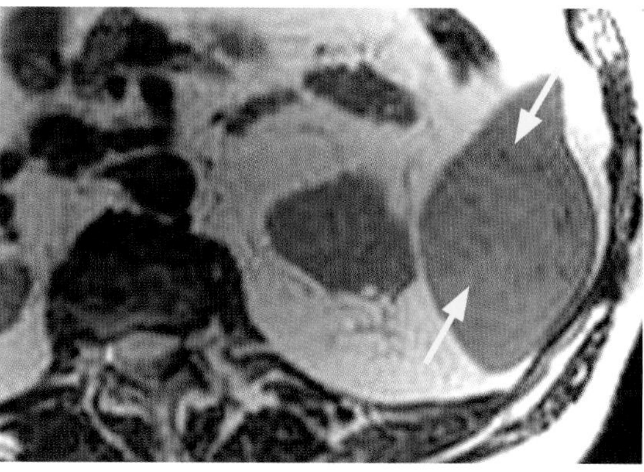
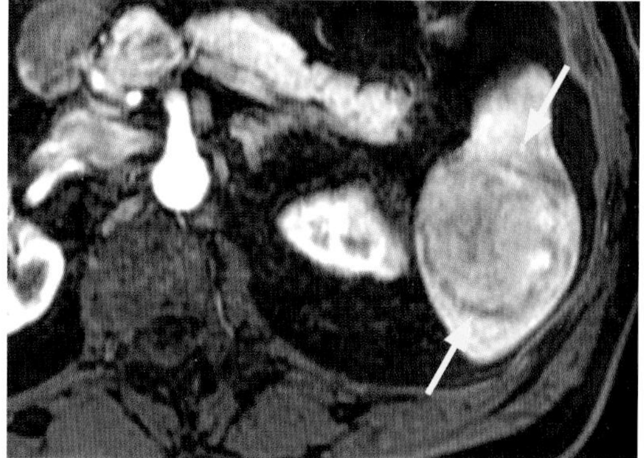

Splenic hamartoma: T2-weighted (left image) and arterial-phase enhanced T1-weighted (right image) MRI shows a vague T2 isointense splenic mass (arrows) that enhances heterogeneously.

Case courtesy Cheryl Sadow, MD, Brigham and Women's Hospital.

- Splenic hamartoma is a rare, benign lesion composed of malformed red pulp elements. It may be associated with tuberous sclerosis.
- Splenic hamartoma is typically a well-circumscribed, iso- or hypoattenuating mass on unenhanced CT that enhances heterogeneously after contrast administration. On MR, a hamartoma is iso- to slightly hyperintense on T2-weighted images, featuring heterogeneous early enhancement and relatively homogeneous delayed enhancement.

Benign cystic splenic lesions

Congenital true (epithelial) cyst

- A congenital true cyst is defined as having an epithelial lining. Interestingly, a splenic epithelial cyst may cause elevation of tumor markers including CA19-9, CA125, and CEA, despite its completely benign nature.
- Unlike a post-traumatic pseudocyst, a true cyst may have septations, but mural calcification is uncommon.

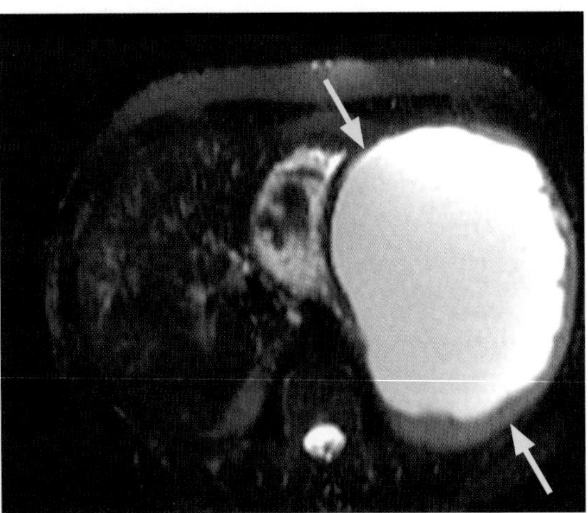
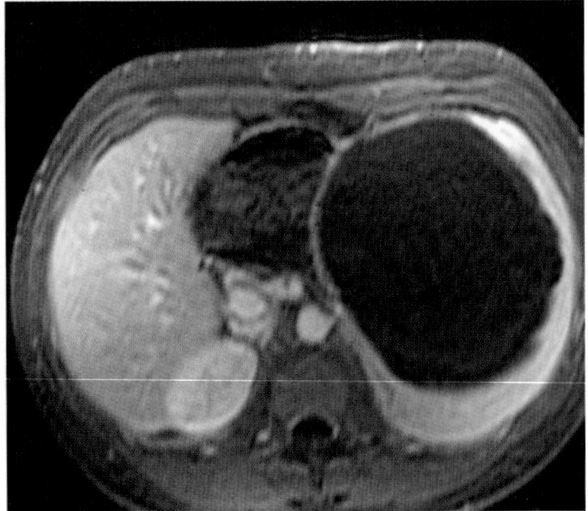

Splenic epithelial cyst: T2-weighted MRI with fat saturation (left image) and enhanced T1-weighted MRI (right image) shows a large T2 hyperintense, T1 hypointense, nonenhancing structure (arrows) replacing nearly the entire splenic parenchyma.

Case courtesy Cheryl Sadow, MD, Brigham and Women's Hospital.

Post-traumatic pseudocyst

- A post-traumatic pseudocyst is the end result of evolution of a splenic hematoma.
- Unlike a true (epithelial) splenic cyst, the periphery of a pseudocyst is not cellular but made of fibrotic tissue.
- On imaging, a post-traumatic pseudocyst appears as a well-circumscribed, fluid-density lesion, with no peripheral enhancement.
- In contrast to a true cyst, septations are uncommon but there may be mural calcification.

Intrasplenic pancreatic pseudocyst

- A post-pancreatitis pseudocyst involving the tail of the pancreas may extend into the spleen. There is almost always a history of pancreatitis.
- Unlike a true congenital cyst, an epithelial lining is lacking and histology more closely resembles a post-traumatic pseudocyst.
- Splenic rupture has been reported in some cases of intrasplenic post-pancreatitis pseudocysts.

Lymphangioma

- Splenic lymphangioma is a rare, benign neoplasm usually diagnosed in childhood, which may be solitary or multiple.
- Lymphangioma features a classic imaging appearance of a multilocular cystic structure with thin septations. Post-contrast images may show septal enhancement.

Inflammatory splenic lesions

Sarcoidosis

- Sarcoidosis is a systemic disease of unknown etiology characterized histologically by multiple nodules composed of noncaseating granulomas.
- When sarcoidosis involves the spleen, splenomegaly is the most common presentation, often associated with hepatomegaly and lymphadenopathy.
- Less commonly, sarcoidosis may involve the spleen in a multinodular pattern with numerous hypoattenuating 1–3 cm lesions demonstrating essentially no enhancement.

  These nodules are formed by coalescent sarcoid granulomas and have low signal on all MRI sequences.

  Sarcoid nodules are most conspicuous on T2-weighted images and early-phase post-contrast T1-weighted images. On the post-contrast images the nonenhancing nodules will stand out against the avidly enhancing splenic parenchyma.
- Imaging appearance is generally indistinguishable from splenic lymphoma.

Inflammatory pseudotumor

- Splenic inflammatory pseudotumor is a rare focal collection of immune cells and associated inflammatory exudate, of unclear etiology. Patients often have constitutional symptoms including fever and malaise.
- Inflammatory pseudotumor has a variable and nonspecific imaging appearance, but a typical presentation is of a well-circumscribed, heterogeneously enhancing mass.

Splenic infection

Pyogenic abscess

- Splenic bacterial abscesses are uncommon and usually seen in immunocompromised patients. A solitary abscess is much more likely to be bacterial. In contrast, multifocal small abscesses are more likely to be fungal.
- On CT, a bacterial abscess usually has an irregular, enhancing wall. Gas is not usually seen, but is highly specific for a bacterial abscess when present.
- A characteristic ultrasound finding is the *wheel within a wheel* or *bull's-eye* appearance, which describes concentric hyperechoic and hypoechoic rings surrounding the abscess.
- Treatment is CT- or ultrasound-guided percutaneous drainage in addition to antibiotics.

Fungal abscess

- Splenic fungal abscesses are typically multiple and small, usually <1 cm in size. Almost all patients with splenic fungal abscesses are immunocompromised.
- The most common causative agents include *Candida*, *Aspergillus*, and *Cryptococcus*, which all appear as multiple tiny hypoattenuating foci on CT.
- Splenic *Pneumocystis jiroveci* (formerly known as *Pneumocystis carinii*) infection is rare, almost always seen in advanced AIDS, and has a classic appearance of multiple calcified splenic lesions.

Echinococcal cyst

- Splenic involvement of *Echinococcus granulosus* infection is unusual, seen in only 1 to 3% of echinococcal infections, and is almost always associated with infection of other organs as well.
- An echinococcal cyst is a true cyst with a cellular lining. As with echinococcal abscess elsewhere, characteristic imaging findings are a cystic lesion with internal undulating membrane and daughter cysts.

Malignant splenic lesions

Splenic lymphoma

- Splenic lymphoma is the most common splenic malignancy.
- Primary splenic lymphoma is rare, accounting for less than 1% of all cases of lymphoma, and usually presents as a solitary hypovascular mass. In contrast to splenic hamartoma or metastatic disease, primary splenic lymphoma may extend beyond the splenic capsule and involve adjacent organs.
- Secondary splenic involvement of systemic lymphoma is much more common. Four imaging presentations have been described, depending on the size of the lymphomatous masses:

  Miliary masses, in which discrete tiny masses may be difficult to see.

  Multiple small to moderate sized masses.

  One large mass.

  Splenomegaly without discrete mass.
- Conspicuity is highest on post-contrast T1-weighted images, where the involved portion of the spleen tends to be *hypoenhancing.*
- On ultrasound, lymphoma may appear cystic but color Doppler shows internal flow.

Splenic metastasis

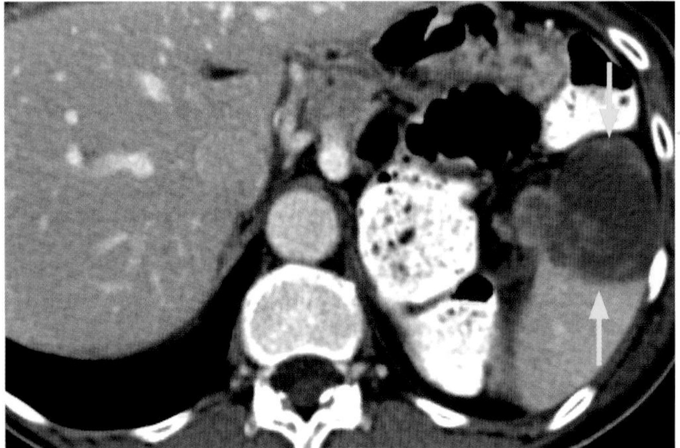

Splenic metastasis from lung cancer: Contrast-enhanced axial CT shows a hypoattenuating, irregular mass in the inferior anterior aspect of the spleen (arrows) demonstrating wispy, heterogeneous enhancement.

Case courtesy Cheryl Sadow, MD, Brigham and Women's Hospital.

- Splenic metastases may be solitary or multiple, cystic or solid. However, metastases to the spleen are rare, occurring in 2–9% of cancer patients. Most patients with splenic metastases already have known widespread disease.

  Isolated splenic metastases are seen in only 5% of patients with metastatic involvement of the spleen.
- Several theories for the low rate of splenic metastases have been proposed, which is thought to be due to the antineoplastic properties of lymphoid-rich splenic tissue and lack of afferent lymphatics to bring tumor cells into the spleen.
- The most common primary tumors known to metastasize to the spleen include breast, lung, ovarian, and melanoma. Ovarian cancer and melanoma typically cause cystic metastasis.
- Calcification is rare unless the primary is a mucinous adenocarcinoma.

Angiosarcoma

- Angiosarcoma is a rare, extremely aggressive malignancy, with 20% 6-month survival.
- Unlike hepatic angiosarcoma, the association with Thorotrast, vinyl chloride, and arsenic has not been well established.
- Angiosarcoma usually presents as enlarged, heterogeneous mass that may completely replace the normal spleen. Enhancement is variable and heterogeneous.

Miscellaneous splenic lesions

Splenic infarct

- Splenic infarcts are most commonly due to emboli (in older patients) and thrombosis (in younger patients with hematologic disease).
- Splenic infarct classically manifests as a wedge-shaped peripheral region of nonenhancement, but a more heterogeneous, mass-like appearance can also be seen.
- On MR, the affected regions may be T1 hyperintense if acute and hemorrhagic, while chronic infarcts are T1 hypointense and T2 hyperintense.
- Lack of enhancement of the entire spleen should raise the concern for complete infarction, possibly due to a wandering spleen with torsion.

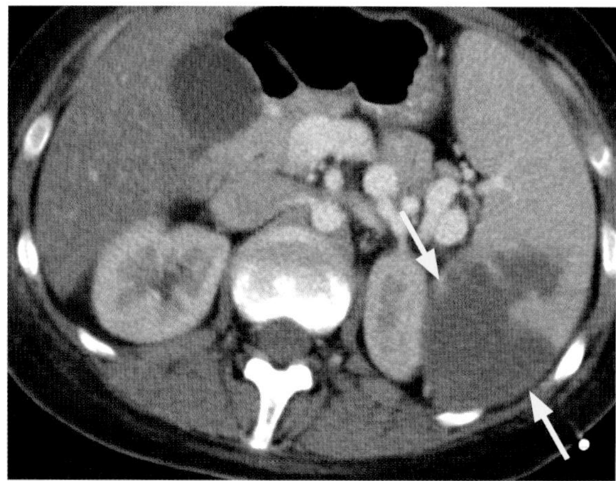

Splenic infarct: Axial contrast-enhanced CT shows a posterior peripheral region of splenic nonenhancement (arrows).

Case courtesy Cheryl Sadow, MD, Brigham and Women's Hospital.

Gamna-Gandy bodies

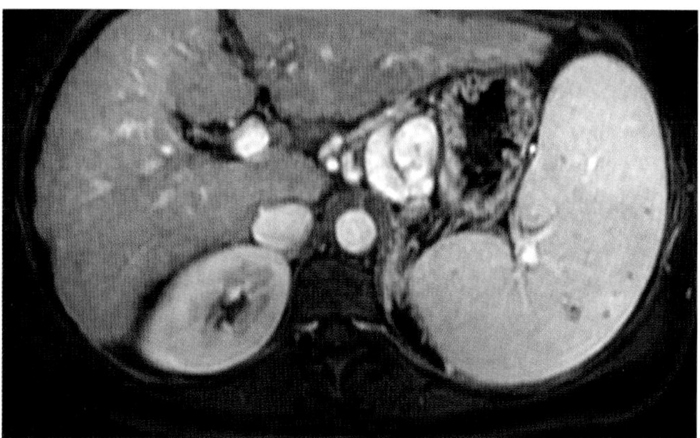

Gamna–Gandy bodies: Contrast-enhanced T1-weighted MRI shows numerous hypointense foci scattered throughout the spleen in a patient with evidence of cirrhosis (nodular liver contour, splenomegaly, and varices).

Case courtesy Cheryl Sadow, MD, Brigham and Women's Hospital.

- Gamna–Gandy bodies are multiple tiny foci of hemosiderin deposition resulting from portal hypertension.
- Usually, other signs of portal hypertension and cirrhosis are apparent on imaging, such as splenomegaly, varices, recanalized umbilical vein, ascites, and nodular liver contour.
- The hemosiderin deposits demonstrate low signal on all sequences. On in- and out-of-phase gradient-echo sequences, the longer TE of the in-phase images demonstrate blooming (relatively decreased signal on in-phase images), due to longer dephasing time and exaggeration of T2* effect.

Gaucher disease

- Gaucher disease is an autosomal recessive deficiency of glucocerebrosidase, leading to accumulation of glucocerebrosides in the reticuloendothelial system.
- Splenic manifestations of Gaucher disease include splenomegaly (almost always) and multiple splenic nodules (seen in one third of Gaucher patients).
- Associated bony findings seen in Gaucher disease include the characteristic Erlenmeyer flask deformity of the distal femurs, femoral head avascular necrosis, and H-shaped vertebral bodies from endplate avascular necrosis.

SPLENIC TRAUMA

Overview of splenic trauma

- The spleen is the most commonly injured abdominal organ from blunt trauma.
- Splenectomy dramatically increases the risk of subsequent sepsis, which has driven the trend towards splenic preservation and conservative management of splenic trauma.
- The spleen must be evaluated for injury in the portal venous phase, as physiologic heterogeneous enhancement in the arterial phase can both mask and mimic injury.
- A splenic hematoma is a focal collection of blood (hypoattenuating relative to enhanced spleen and hyperattenuating relative to unenhanced spleen), most commonly subcapsular. Less commonly, a hematoma may be intraparenchymal, where it may assume an irregular shape.
- A splenic laceration can only be well seen on a contrast-enhanced study, where it appears as a linear or branching area of decreased attenuation.
- Active contrast extravasation due to vessel injury appears as an area of increased attenuation (initially iso-enhancing to the arterial blood pool), which further increases in size on delayed scanning due to ongoing bleeding.
- In contrast to active extravasation, pseudoaneurysm and arteriovenous fistula are contained vascular injuries that also initially appear as a well-circumscribed area of increased attenuation, but do not increase on delayed scanning.

  A pseudoaneurysm is caused by injury to the intima and media of the arterial wall, and is essentially a rupture contained only by the adventitia. There is a high chance of rupture without treatment.

  A traumatic arteriovenous fistula is indistinguishable from pseudoaneurysm by CT and is due to injury of an artery and the adjacent vein. Splenic arteriography is the only way to differentiate pseudoaneurysm from arteriovenous fistula.

American Association for the Surgery of Trauma (AAST) grading scale

- The American Association for the Surgery of Trauma (AAST) splenic injury grading scale is based on the extent of injury seen at laparotomy, and is therefore limited in practicality as many splenic injuries are now managed conservatively.
- An additional limitation of the AAST grading scale is the exclusion of vascular injury.

MDCT-based splenic injury grading system.

- The most widely used CT grading system is the MDCT-based splenic injury grading system, which is similar to the AAST grading scale but incorporates vascular injury.

MDCT grading of splenic trauma

- MDCT grade I: Small (<1 cm) subcapsular hematoma, laceration, or parenchymal hematoma.
- MDCT grade II: Medium (>1 and <3 cm) subcapsular hematoma, laceration, or parenchymal hematoma.
- MDCT grade III: Splenic capsular disruption; or large (>3 cm) laceration or parenchymal hematomas.
- MDCT grade IVA: Active extravasation, vascular injury (pseudoaneurysm or arteriovenous fistula), or shattered spleen.
- MDCT grade IVB: Active intraperitoneal bleeding.

ESOPHAGUS

ANATOMY

Pharynx

- **Nasopharynx**: Extends from the base of the skull to the soft palate.
- **Oropharynx**: Located behind the mouth and extends from the uvula to the hyoid bone.
- **Hypopharynx**: Extends from the hyoid bone to the cricopharyngeus muscle, which is located at the lower end of the cricoid cartilage.

Esophagus

- The cricopharyngeus muscle, located at C5–6, is the upper esophageal sphincter and demarcates the transition between the pharynx superiorly and the cervical esophagus.
- The esophagus extends from the neck to the gastroesophageal junction. The distal esophagus passes through the diaphragmatic hiatus at approximately T10.
- The three anatomic rings of the distal esophagus are the A (muscular), B (mucosal), and C (diaphragmatic impression) rings.

ESOPHAGEAL RINGS AND WEBS

Esophageal web

- An esophageal web is a thin anterior infolding/indentation of the upper esophagus, which is usually asymptomatic but may be a cause of dysphagia. There is a controversial association with anemia (Plummer–Vinson syndrome) and upper esophageal carcinoma.

Schatzki ring

- A Schatzki ring is a focal narrowing of the B (mucosal) ring of the distal esophagus, causing intermittent dysphagia.
- A true Schatzki ring requires clinical symptoms of dysphagia in addition to esophageal narrowing seen on imaging.

  Asymptomatic narrowing of the B ring is referred to as a lower esophageal ring.
- An upper GI study is more sensitive than endoscopy. The key imaging feature is focal circumferential constriction near the gastroesophageal junction, almost always associated with a hiatal hernia.

  On an upper GI study, most symptomatic rings do not allow passage of a 12 mm tablet.
- The differential of circumferential esophageal constriction includes:

  Focal stricture.

  Muscular esophageal ring above the GE junction (also known as an *A ring*).

  Esophageal cancer.

  Esophageal web (rarely circumferential, usually in cervical esophagus).

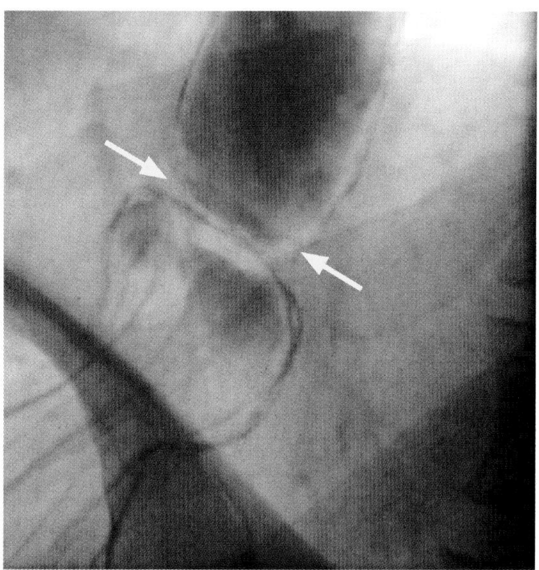

Schatzki ring: Double-contrast barium swallow in a patient with dysphagia shows a circumferential narrowing (arrows) at the gastroesophageal junction, which is slightly superiorly displaced in a hiatal hernia.

Case courtesy of Cheryl Sadow, MD, Brigham and Women's Hospital.

Esophagitis

Reflux (peptic) esophagitis

- Reflux (peptic) esophagitis is caused by exposure of the esophageal mucosa to acidic gastric secretions, which leads to distal ulcerations and eventual stricture.
- Peptic esophagitis is most commonly caused by gastroesophageal reflux, but is also seen in:
  - Zollinger–Ellison, due to increased acid production.
  - Scleroderma, due to gastroesophageal sphincter fibrosis and resultant incompetence.
- Reflux esophagitis appears as thickened distal esophageal folds.
- Chronic esophagitis and scarring develops after prolonged exposure to acid, which causes a smoothly tapered stricture above the GE junction.

Barrett esophagus

- An important long-term sequela of peptic esophagitis is Barrett esophagus, which is metaplasia of normal squamous epithelium to gastric-type adenomatous mucosa. Barrett esophagus is a precursor lesion to esophageal carcinoma.
- Nearly 10% of patients with reflux esophagitis may have some adenomatous metaplasia.
- On imaging, Barrett demonstrates a featureless distal esophagus, with signs of active reflux esophagitis (mucosal granularity and superficial erosions) more proximally.
- Barrett esophagus is often associated with esophageal stricture, which is abnormally high in location compared to a peptic stricture.

Infectious esophagitis

- Although radiographic distinction between types of infections has been described, endoscopy and biopsy are typically performed in clinical practice.
- **Esophageal candidiasis** can present as a spectrum from scattered plaque-like lesions in mild disease to very shaggy esophagus in severe cases.
- **Herpes esophagitis** typically causes discrete small ulcerations scattered randomly throughout esophagus.
- **CMV/HIV esophagitis** characteristically causes a large, flat, ovoid ulcer.

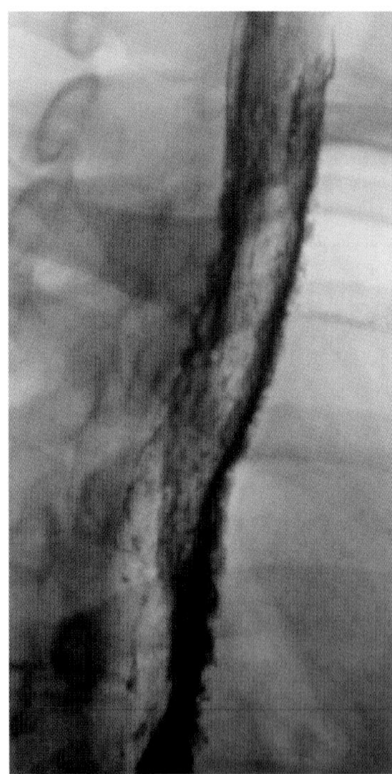

Candida esophagitis: Spot image from double-contrast esophagram shows a diffuse, shaggy appearance to the entire visualized esophagus, consistent with severe candida esophagitis.

Case courtesy of Cheryl Sadow, MD, Brigham and Women's Hospital.

Medication esophagitis

- Medication-induced esophagitis typically causes an ulcer at the level of the aortic arch or distal esophagus, which are areas of relative narrowing that may predispose to temporary hold-ups in passage.

Crohn esophagitis

- Crohn esophagitis is very rare and is usually seen in the setting of severe disease in the small bowel and colon.
- Aphthous ulcers (discrete ulcers surrounded by mounds of edema) may become confluent.

Esophageal strictures

Peptic stricture

- As previously discussed, a peptic stricture is secondary to chronic reflux.
- Peptic strictures are located distally, usually just above the GE junction.
- A peptic stricture may be focal or involve a longer segment of esophagus.
- Fibrosis can cause esophageal shortening, leading to a hiatal hernia as the stomach is pulled into the thorax.

Barrett esophagus stricture

- A Barrett stricture typically occurs in the mid-esophagus, above the metaplastic adenomatous transition. Barrett strictures occur higher than peptic strictures because adenomatous tissue is acid-resistant and therefore unaffected by gastric secretions.

Malignant stricture (due to esophageal carcinoma)

- Key imaging finding is shouldered margins, which suggests circumferential luminal narrowing by a mass.

Caustic stricture/nasogastric (NG) tube stricture

- Both caustic strictures and strictures secondary to nasogastric tube placement are typically long, smooth, and narrow.
- Strictures develop 1–3 months after the caustic ingestion or NG tube placement.
- Caustic strictures are associated with an increased risk of cancer, with a long lag time of up to 20 years after the initial insult. Caustic strictures are usually longer than peptic strictures.

Radiation stricture

- Radiation strictures are long, smooth and narrow, similar to caustic strictures. However, in contrast to strictures from an NG tube, caustic ingestion, and reflux, radiation strictures usually spare the GE junction.
- It generally requires more than 50 Gy of radiation to cause an esophageal stricture.
- Acute radiation esophagitis occurs 1–4 weeks after radiation therapy. Radiation strictures develop later, occurring 4–8 months after radiation.

Extrinsic compression from mediastinal adenopathy

- Cross-sectional imaging would best evaluate if extrinsic compression is suspected.

Evaluation of esophageal masses

- Masses arising from the mucosa, submucosa, and extrinsic to the esophagus produce characteristic effects on the esophagus, which are usually able to be seen on imaging.

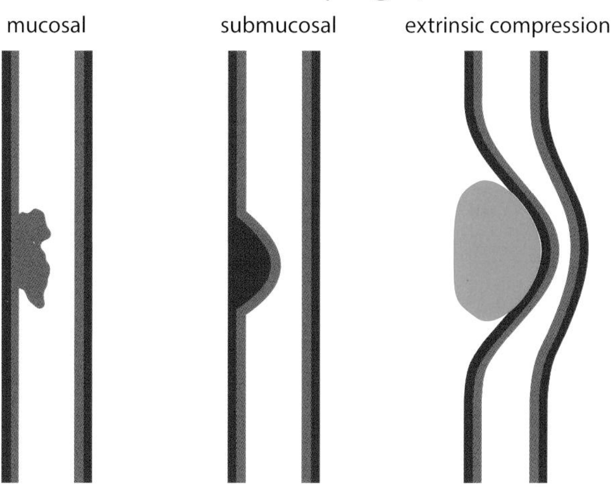

BENIGN ESOPHAGEAL MASSES

Mesenchymal tumor

- Benign mesenchymal tumors are the most common submucosal tumors and include gastrointestinal stromal tumor (GIST), leiomyoma, lipoma, hemangioma, and others. The classification varies in the literature, with both GIST and leiomyoma described as the most common. On a barium swallow, a mesenchymal tumor typically appears as smooth, round, submucosal filling defect.

Adenoma

- An esophageal adenoma is a benign mucosal lesion with malignant potential, usually arising within Barrett esophagus. Most are <1.5 cm in size and resected at endoscopy.

Inflammatory polyp

- An inflammatory polyp is a non-neoplastic, enlarged gastric fold that protrudes up into the lower esophagus. Inflammatory polyps are almost always associated with reflux and always contiguous with a gastric fold. They are mucosal in location.

Fibrovascular polyp

- A fibrovascular polyp is a pedunculated mass composed of mesenchymal elements with a significant fatty component. In contrast to an esophageal adenoma, there is no malignant potential. Fibrovascular polyps usually occur in the cervical esophagus. The clinical presentation can be dramatic, with regurgitation of a fleshy mass.
- CT is usually diagnostic, demonstrating intra-lesional fatty component.

Varices

- Esophageal varices are most commonly due to portal hypertension. Varices can usually be distinguished from a solid mass since varices change in size and shape with peristalsis. However, thrombosed varices may mimic a tumor.
- *Uphill* varices, due to portal hypertension, affect the distal esophagus.

  Blood flows "uphill" from the portal vein → left gastric (coronary vein) → periesophageal venous plexus → azygos/hemiazygos collaterals → SVC.
- *Downhill* varices are much less common, are caused by superior vena cava obstruction, and usually affect the proximal esophagus.

  Enlarged collateral vessels include the supreme intercostal veins (drain the first intercostal space), bronchial veins, and inferior thyroidal veins.

Foregut duplication cysts

- **Esophageal duplication cyst** is lined with squamous epithelium, has a smooth muscle wall, and is usually in the posterior mediastinum. It may be either extrinsic to the esophagus or submucosal; the latter is impossible to differentiate from a leiomyoma by esophagram.
- **Bronchogenic cyst** is lined by respiratory epithelium. It is generally indistinguishable from an esophageal duplication cyst on esophagram and CT.
- **Neurenteric cyst** is associated with vertebral body anomalies.

Esophageal foreign body

- A radiopaque esophageal foreign body is best visualized with a lateral radiograph or CT.
- Bony foreign objects usually get stuck in the cervical esophagus.
- Meat impaction usually occurs at the gastroesophageal junction. There is a risk of esophageal perforation from transmural ischemia if the food bolus is impacted for >24 hours. Most cases of food bolus impaction are treated with endoscopic removal of the impacted food. Historically, meat impaction was treated with effervescent granules and meat tenderizer, but this technique is no longer commonly performed.

MALIGNANT ESOPHAGEAL MASSES

Esophageal carcinoma

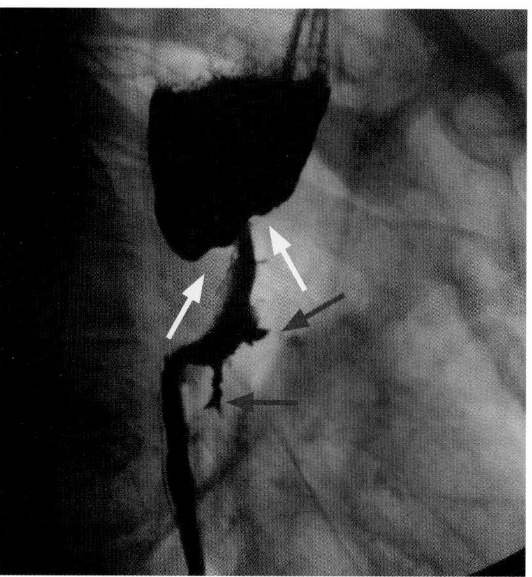

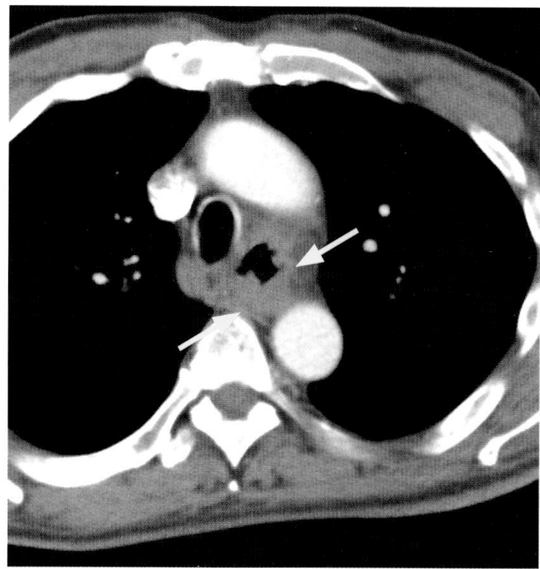

Esophageal carcinoma: Oblique photospot image from a barium swallow (left image) shows an irregular stricture in the proximal esophagus (yellow arrows) with proximal dilation of the esophagus. Two linear ulcerations (red arrows) project into the mural mass. Contrast-enhanced axial CT (right image) shows irregular thickening of the esophagus (arrows).

Case courtesy of Cheryl Sadow, MD, Brigham and Women's Hospital.

- Esophageal carcinoma has a broad range of appearances. Early esophageal cancer may be apparent on barium swallow as a plaque-like lesion, polypoid lesion, or focal irregularity of the esophageal wall. A classic appearance of advanced esophageal carcinoma is a mass causing a stricture with a "shouldered" edge and irregular contour. The uncommon varicoid appearance can be initially confused with varices, but the tumor does not change shape with peristaltic waves as varices typically do.
- Esophageal carcinoma may be squamous cell carcinoma (SCC) or adenocarcinoma, which cannot be reliably differentiated on barium studies. SCC tends to involve the upper or mid-esophagus and adenocarcinoma typically involves the distal esophagus and may extend into the stomach.
- Squamous cell carcinoma (SCC) is most commonly due to smoking and alcohol. Less common risk factors include celiac disease, Plummer–Vinson, achalasia, and human papilloma virus (which more commonly causes laryngeal squamous cell carcinoma).
- Adenocarcinoma is due to chronic reflux, arising from Barrett esophagus distally. Its incidence has been rising in recent years.

Metastasis

- Direct invasion of the esophagus is most commonly from gastric, lung, or breast primaries. Hematogenous spread is very rare.
- Most often, mediastinal lymph node metastases will be prominent. The mid-esophagus is most commonly affected due to its proximity to mediastinal lymph nodes.

Lymphoma

- Esophageal lymphoma is often indistinguishable from primary esophageal cancer.

Malignant GIST

- Malignant GIST tends to be bulkier and more irregular than the benign variant.

Esophageal motility disorders

Contraction waves

- A primary contraction wave is a normal, physiologic wave initiated by a swallow.
- A secondary contraction wave is a normal, physiologic wave initiated by a bolus in the esophagus.
- A tertiary wave is a nonpropulsive contraction that does not result in esophageal clearing. Tertiary contractions are seen more commonly in the elderly. They are not normal, but are also not thought to be clinically significant when seen.

Achalasia

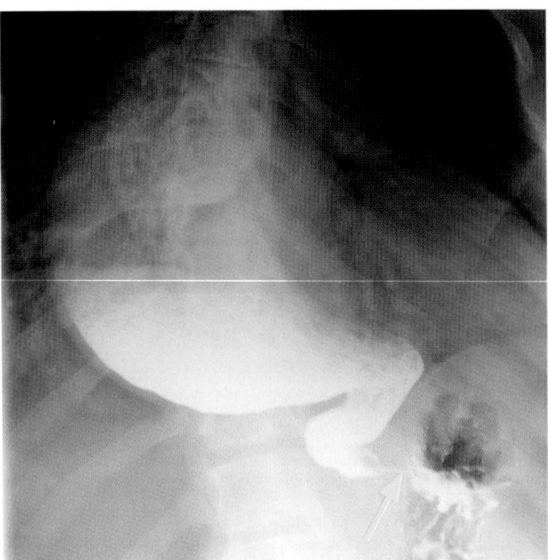

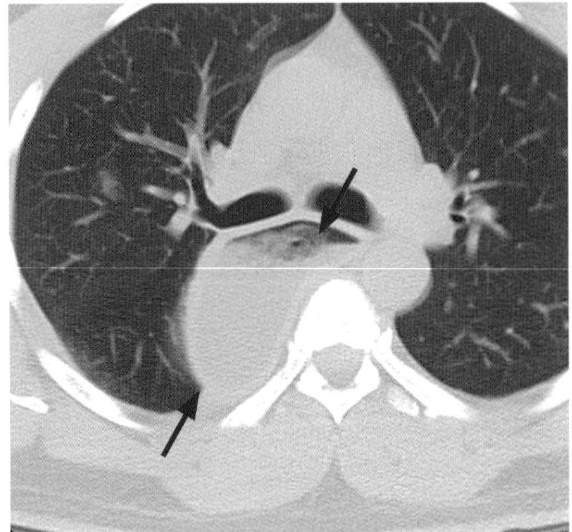

Achalasia: Photospot image from an upper GI series (left image) shows a markedly dilated esophagus terminating in a *bird's beak* (arrow) at the GE junction, due to failure of the distal esophageal sphincter to relax. Axial non-contrast CT confirms the markedly dilated, debris-filled esophagus (red arrows).

- Achalasia is a motility disorder of the distal esophagus, which is unable to relax due to an abnormality of myenteric ganglia in the Auerbach plexus. **Vigorous achalasia** is a less severe form of achalasia consisting of repetitive nonpropulsive contractions.
- Chagas disease causes a secondary achalasia that is indistinguishable radiographically from primary achalasia.
- Potential complications of chronic achalasia include esophageal cancer, which has a lag period of at least 20 years, and candidal infection from stasis.
- The classic imaging appearance of achalasia is a massively dilated esophagus with a *bird's beak* stricture near the gastroesophageal junction.
- Surgical treatment of achalasia is the Heller myotomy, which is an incision of the lower esophageal muscle fibers.
- **Pseudoachalasia** is caused by an obstructing gastroesophageal junction cancer. In achalasia, there is transient relaxation of the stricture when the patient stands. In pseudoachalasia, however, the fixed obstruction does not relax with standing.

Diffuse esophageal spasm (corkscrew esophagus; shish kebab esophagus)

- Diffuse esophageal spasm is a clinical syndrome of chest pain or dysphagia caused by repetitive, nonpropulsive esophageal contractions. The nonpropulsive contractions have a characteristic appearance on barium swallow, leading to the descriptive names of *corkscrew esophagus* and *shish kebab esophagus*.
- **Nutcracker esophagus** is a related disorder characterized by high-amplitude contractions on manometry in conjunction with chest pain, with normal radiological findings.

Esophageal diverticula

Types of diverticula

- **Pulsion diverticula** are caused by increased esophageal pressure and comprise nearly all diverticula seen in the USA.
- **Traction diverticula** are caused by traction of adjacent structures, typically resulting from tuberculous mediastinal adenopathy. They are rarely seen.

Zenker diverticulum

- Zenker diverticulum is an esophageal diverticulum caused by failure of the cricopharyngeus muscle to relax, leading to elevated hypopharyngeal pressure. Symptoms of a Zenker diverticulum include halitosis, aspiration, and regurgitation of undigested food.
- A Zenker diverticulum is posteriorly protruding. As a secondary finding, the cricopharyngeus muscle is usually hypertrophied.
- Treatment is with cricopharyngeal myotomy and diverticulopexy or diverticulectomy.
- A **pseudo-Zenker** diverticulum is barium trapped in a pharyngeal contraction wave.

Killian–Jamieson (KJ) diverticulum

- A Killian–Jamieson (KJ) diverticulum is located at the Killian–Jamieson space, which is an area of weakness below the attachment of the cricopharyngeus muscle.
- In contrast to Zenker diverticulum, KJ diverticula are more often bilateral.
- KJ diverticula protrude anteriorly, best seen on the lateral view.

Pseudodiverticulosis

- Pseudodiverticulosis is the imaging finding of multiple tiny outpouchings into the esophageal lumen caused by dilated submucosal glands from chronic reflux esophagitis.
- These submucosal glands are analogous to the Rokitansky–Aschoff sinuses of the gallbladder.
- Pseudodiverticulosis is often associated with a smooth stricture in mid/upper esophagus, which may cause symptoms.
- Candida is frequently cultured, but infection is not believed to be a causal factor.

Miscellaneous esophageal disorders

Feline esophagus

- Feline esophagus is thought to be a normal variant characterized by multiple transverse esophageal folds.
- There is a controversial association with esophagitis, where the incidence of esophagitis may be increased in the presence of feline esophagus.

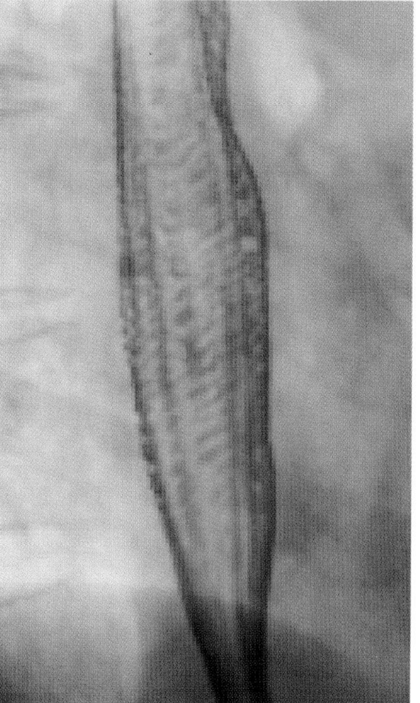

Feline esophagus: Spot image from double-contrast esophagram shows characteristic multiple transverse folds in the lower esophagus.

Case courtesy Cheryl Sadow, MD, Brigham and Women's Hospital.

Aberrant right subclavian artery

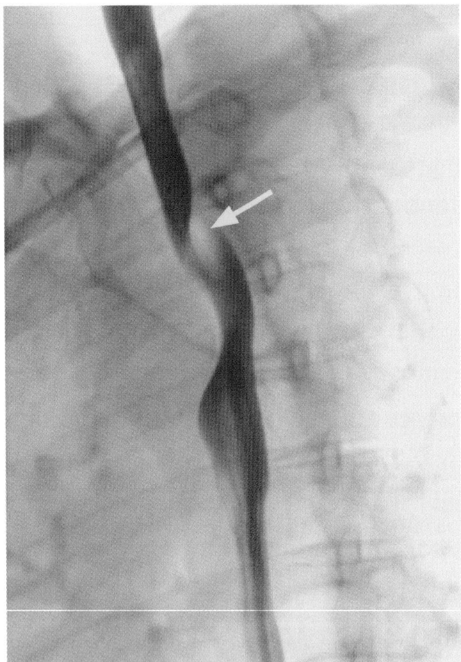

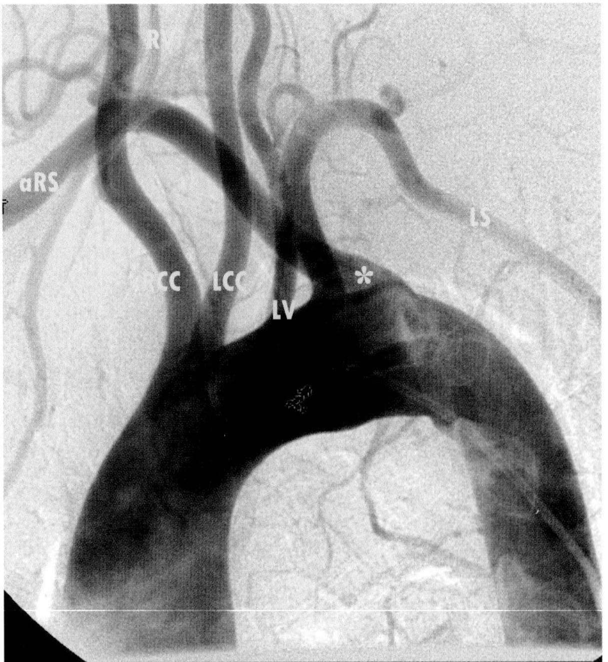

Aberrant right subclavian artery: Oblique single-contrast barium esophagram (left image) demonstrates a smooth posterior indentation of the proximal thoracic esophagus (arrow). Aortogram in the same patient (right image) demonstrates the aberrant right subclavian artery (aRS, * at origin) crossing the midline before heading towards the right arm. This patient has an additional aortic branching anomaly, with the left vertebral artery (LV) arising directly from the aorta. The right vertebral artery (RV), arising from the aberrant right subclavian, is hypoplastic. The right and left common carotid arteries (RCC and LCC), and left subclavian (LS) are normal.

Case courtesy Cheryl Sadow, MD, Brigham and Women's Hospital.

- Aberrant right subclavian artery (with a normal left arch) is seen in approximately 1% of patients and is almost always asymptomatic. The aberrant right subclavian artery travels posterior to the esophagus, where it may rarely produce dysphagia.
- On an upper GI study, the resultant posterior esophageal indentation is always smooth.

Scleroderma

- Scleroderma is a systemic disease involving excess collagen deposition in multiple tissues.
- The esophagus is involved in 80% of patients with scleroderma, producing lack of peristalsis of the distal 2/3 of the esophagus due to smooth muscle atrophy and fibrosis, which leads to marked esophageal dilation.
- Secondary candidiasis or aspiration pneumonia can result from prolonged esophageal stasis.
- The esophageal dilation is often apparent before the typical skin changes of scleroderma become evident.

Esophageal hernias

Hiatal hernia (HH)

- A hiatal hernia (HH) is present when gastric folds are seen above the diaphragm. A hiatal hernia may be sliding (most common) or short (secondary to chronic reflux esophagitis).

Paraesophageal hernia

- With a paraesophageal hernia, the GE junction is located normally below the diaphragm, but a portion of the stomach herniates into the thorax through the esophageal hiatus.
- Paraesophageal hernia is more prone to strangulation than HH. Most are surgically repaired.

STOMACH

THICKENED GASTRIC FOLDS

- Thickened gastric folds are most commonly due to inflammatory gastritis, which characteristically produces smooth fold thickening.
- Nodular fold thickening is suggestive of neoplasm, such as gastric lymphoma or submucosal carcinoma.

Helicobacter pylori gastritis

- *Helicobacter pylori* is a major cause of gastritis, gastric ulcers and duodenal ulcers.

Zollinger–Ellison (ZE)

- Zollinger–Ellison (ZE) is gastrin over-production from a gastrinoma, which is a pancreatic islet cell tumor that has a 50% rate of malignancy.

  ZE features elevated gastrin level and a paradoxical increase in gastrin after secretin administration.
- 25% of patients with gastrinoma have multiple endocrine neoplasia (MEN) type 1.

  MEN-1 consists of parathyroid adenoma, pituitary adenoma, and pancreatic islet cell tumors.

Eosinophilic gastritis

- Eosinophilic gastritis is characterized by thickened folds in the stomach and small bowel in a patient with a history of allergy.

Menetrier disease

- Menetrier disease is a protein-losing enteropathy that is often a diagnosis of exclusion. It usually affects the proximal stomach and is pathologically characterized by replacement of parietal cells by hyperplastic epithelial cells, leading to achlorhydria.
- Menetrier disease has a controversial association with gastric carcinoma.

Crohn disease

- Gastric Crohn disease is almost always associated with small bowel disease. Usually the distal half of the stomach is affected.
- The earliest pathologic change is the formation of aphthous ulcers.

Other causes of thickened gastric folds

- Gastric varices (from portal hypertension), gastric lymphoma, and submucosal carcinoma are non-inflammatory causes of thickened gastric folds.

GASTRIC POLYPS

Hyperplastic polyp (inflammatory polyp)

- A hyperplastic polyp, also known as an inflammatory polyp, is cystic dilation of a gastric gland that develops in response to chronic inflammation. Hyperplastic polyps are almost always benign, with very rare cases of malignant transformation having been reported.
- **Fundic gland polyposis syndrome** is a variant of familial adenomatous polyposis syndrome that also involves the stomach. In the stomach, most polyps are hyperplastic, but elsewhere in the GI tract the polyps are adenomatous.

Adenomatous polyp

- An adenomatous polyp is a neoplastic polyp with malignant potential. There is an elevated risk of malignant transforation to adenocarcinoma if >2 cm in size.
- Adenomatous polyps are usually treated with endoscopic biopsy and polypectomy.

Hamartomatous polyp

- Hamartomatous polyps are benign polyps usually associated with syndromes such as Peutz–Jeghers, juvenile polyposis, and Cronkhite–Canada syndromes.

BENIGN GASTRIC MASSES

Lipoma (benign)

- A lipoma is a benign, submucosal, mesenchymal neoplasm. At fluoroscopy, a gastric lipoma is indistinguishable from a GIST. Fatty attenuation on CT is diagnostic of a lipoma.

Gastrointestinal stromal tumor (GIST)

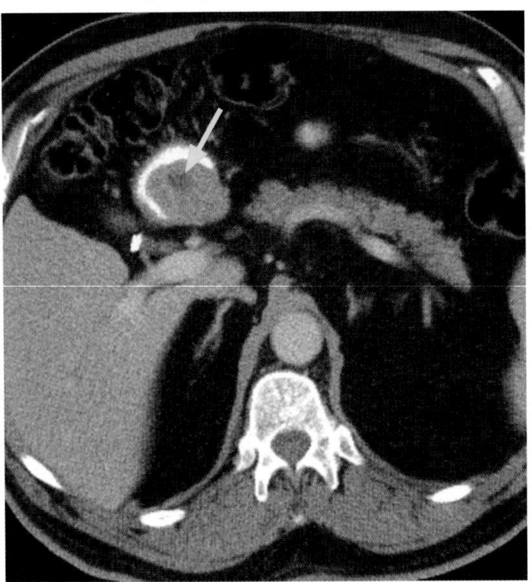

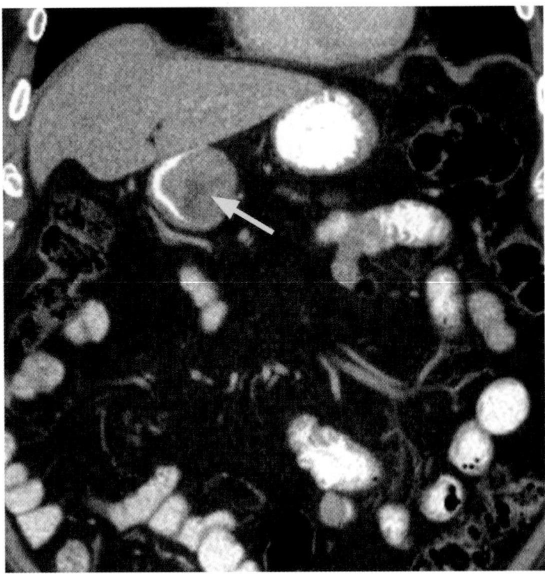

Submucosal GIST: Axial (left image) and coronal (right image) contrast-enhanced CT shows a well-circumscribed, relatively homogeneous mass with a central focus of necrosis (arrows), located in the submucosal posterior wall of the gastric antrum. Incidental cholecystectomy clips are seen on the axial CT.

Case courtesy Cheryl Sadow, MD, Brigham and Women's Hospital.

- Gastrointestinal stromal tumor (GIST) is the most common submucosal gastric tumor. The tumor arises from the interstitial cells of Cajal, which are pacemaker cells that drive peristalsis. GIST may occur anywhere in the gastrointestinal tract.
- GIST may be benign or malignant, with risk for malignancy determined by size and number of mitoses. Regardless of size and number of mitoses, gastric GIST is less likely to be malignant compared to similar-sized GISTs in the duodenum, jejunum/ileum, or rectum. Gastric tumors ≤2 cm in size are essentially always benign. Larger tumors carry a risk of malignancy as high as 86% for a gastric GIST >10 cm with an elevated mitotic rate.
- Small gastric GISTs are usually asymptomatic, but may be a cause of melena.
- On imaging, a smooth endoluminal surface is characteristic due to its submucosal location. Larger tumors have a tendency to become exophytic, or less commonly to invade the lumen.
- The differential diagnosis of a submucosal gastric mass includes mesenchymal tumors (GIST, fibroma, lipoma, neurofibromas, etc.), carcinoid, and ectopic pancreatic rest.

Ectopic pancreatic rest

- An ectopic pancreatic rest is a focus of heterotopic pancreas in the gastric submucosa. The ectopic pancreatic tissue is susceptible to pancreatic diseases, including pancreatitis and carcinoma. On imaging, the classic appearance is an umbilicated submucosal nodule, with the umbilication representing a focus of normal epithelium. The ulceration is not always seen, in which case the imaging is of a nonspecific submucosal gastric mass.

Malignant gastric masses

Gastric cancer

- Gastric adenocarcinoma may present either as a mass or as a gastric ulcer.
- Gastric cancer is generally caused by chronic inflammation, with specific risk factors including:

Ingestion of polycyclic hydrocarbons and nitrosamines (from processed meats). Atrophic gastritis.	Pernicious anemia. Post-subtotal gastrectomy.

- Gastric carcinoma may spread locally from the mucosal surface to the serosa, in which case 90% of patients will have omental involvement from trans-serosal spread.
- Lymphatic spread is along lesser curvature → gastrohepatic ligament and greater curvature.
- A Krukenberg tumor is classically described as metastatic spread of gastric carcinoma to the ovary; however, the term has also been used to describe any mucinous metastasis to the ovary.

GIST (malignant)

- Malignant GIST tends to be larger than benign GIST, often reaching sizes of greater than 10 cm, with central necrosis. Although the tumor begins in the submucosa, it can be difficult to determine the site of origin of large tumors.

Lymphoma

- Gastric lymphoma can have a wide variety of presentations. If solitary, lymphoma can mimic gastric carcinoma. To differentiate between lymphoma and gastric carcinoma, the pattern of adenopathy can be helpful. In gastric cancer, adenopathy at or below the level of the renal hila is unusual, but occurs more commonly in patients with lymphoma.
- The stomach is a common extranodal site for non-Hodgkin lymphoma.

Metastases

- Metastatic disease to the stomach is rare. Breast, lung, and melanoma are most common.

Gastric ulcers

Benign gastric ulcer

- Although less commonly encountered in the modern era of proton pump inhibitors and *Helicobacter pylori* treatment, benign gastric ulcers tend to have typical imaging findings:

Radiating gastric folds are smooth and symmetric. Ulcer extends beyond the normal contour of the gastric lumen. The *Hampton line* represents nonulcerated acid-resistant mucosa surrounding the ulcer crater. Most benign ulcers occur along the lesser curvature of the stomach, although benign ulcers associated with aspirin ingestion can occur in the greater curvature and antrum, which are dependent locations.

Gastric carcinoma

- Gastric carcinoma may present with malignant ulceration, which can usually be distinguished from a benign ulcer by the following features:

Asymmetric ulcer crater, with surrounding nodular tissue. Abrupt transition between normal gastric wall and surrounding tissue. Ulcer crater does *not* project beyond the expected location of gastric wall. The *Carman meniscus* sign is considered pathognomonic for tumor. It describes the splaying open of a large, flat malignant ulcer when compression is applied.

Overview of gastric bypass surgery

Postoperative anatomy of Roux-en-Y gastric bypass (RYGB)

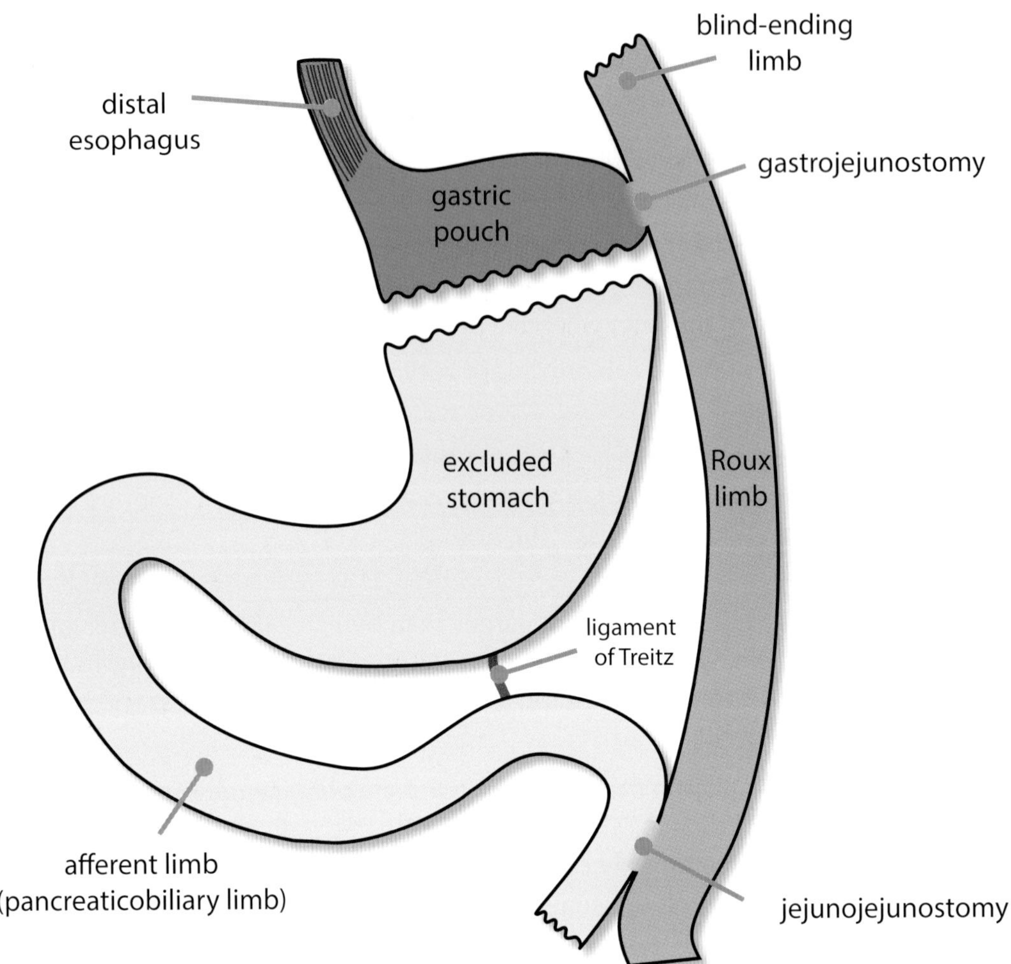

- In order to evaluate for and accurately describe complications of Roux-en-Y gastric bypass (RYGB) surgery, it is important to be familiar with the procedure and normal postsurgical anatomy.
- A small gastric pouch is created with a volume of approximately 15 to 30 cc by excluding the distal stomach from the path of food.
- The Roux limb is created by transecting the jejunum approximately 35–45 cm distal to the ligament of Treitz, then bringing it up to be anastomosed to the gastric pouch via a narrow gastrojejunostomy stoma.
- The current favored approach for placement of the Roux limb is antecolic (in front of the transverse colon). The Roux limb used to be placed retrocolic, which required the creation of a surgical defect through the transverse mesocolon (mesentery of the transverse colon). A retrocolic Roux limb has a higher risk of a transmesocolic hernia due to the defect in the transverse mesocolon.

  Although the antecolic approach is now more commonly performed, there are many patients who have previously undergone a retrocolic approach.
- A distal side-to-side jejunojejunostomy is created to connect the pancreaticobiliary limb to the jejunum.
- The RYGB leads to weight loss both from early satiety (due to small size of the gastric pouch) and malabsorption (due to surgical bypass of the proximal jejunum).

Complications of Roux-en-Y surgery

Postoperative leak

- Postoperative leak is usually diagnosed by 10 days after surgery.
- An upper GI study with water-soluble contrast is the study of choice if a leak is suspected.
- Leaks may arise from the distal esophagus, gastric pouch, or blind-ending jejunal limb. It is rare for a leak to arise from the distal jejunojejunostomy.

Gastrogastric fistula

- A gastrogastric fistula is a communication between the gastric pouch and the excluded stomach, which may be an early or late complication of RYGB.
- A gastrogastric fistula may be a cause of inadequate weight loss or recurrent weight gain.

Small bowel obstruction (SBO)

- Small bowel obstruction (SBO) in the acute postoperative period is most often due to edema or hematoma at the gastrojejunostomy or jejunojejunostomy.

  With a retrocolic Roux limb, edema at the transverse mesocolon defect may also cause obstruction.

  Treatment is usually conservative, with most cases resolving as the edema and/or hematoma resolves.
- A late presentation of small bowel obstruction may be due to internal hernia (more common with laparoscopic surgery) or adhesions (more common with open surgery).

Internal hernia

- Laparoscopic Roux-en-Y procedures are associated with a higher rate of internal hernias (seen in 2.5% of laparoscopic procedures) compared to open procedures (0.5%). Internal hernias can be difficult to diagnose, both clinically and by imaging.
- Internal hernias usually present within 2 years of bypass and are the most common cause of SBO after a laparoscopic Roux-en-Y.
- Most RYGB-associated internal hernias occur in three characteristic locations.
- The surgically created defect in the mesentery of the transverse colon is the most common site (the **transmesocolic** hernia), associated with a retrocolic Roux limb.
- Less common sites of internal hernia include **Peterson's space** (located between the mesentery of the Roux limb and the transverse mesocolon) and the **mesenteric defect created by the jejunojejunostomy**.
- Imaging features of internal hernia include swirling of the mesentery, a mushroom shape of the mesentery, and/or the presence of small bowel loops posterior to the superior mesenteric artery.

Stomal stenosis

- Narrowing of the gastrojejunostomy stoma may occur in up to 10% of patients, leading to dilation of the pouch and distal esophagus. Stomal stenosis is usually treated with endoscopic dilation.
- Narrowing of the distal jejunojejunostomy is much more rare and usually requires surgery.

Marginal ulcers

- The jejunal mucosa adjacent to the gastrojejunal anastomosis is susceptible to gastric secretions, which can cause marginal ulcers in up to 3% of patients.
- A marginal ulcer is diagnosed by upper GI as a thickening and small outpouching of a gastric fold.
- Treatment is conservative.

Small bowel

Small bowel anatomy

- The wall of the small intestine is made of four layers, from outside in:

Serosa.	**Submucosa.**
Muscularis (thin longitudinal and thick circumferential smooth muscle).	**Mucosa** (consists of intestinal villi, circular folds, glands, and lymphoid tissue).

- Valvulae conniventes create the characteristic small bowel fold pattern.
- The superior mesenteric artery (SMA) supplies both the jejunum and ileum. A common small bowel mesentery anchors the jejunum and ileum to the posterior abdominal wall. The jejunum features larger, more feature-full folds and larger villi compared to the ileum.

Small bowel obstruction (SBO)

- Small bowel obstruction (SBO) is common and most often due to adhesions from prior surgery or hernia. Neoplasm, stricture, and intussusception are less common causes.

Radiographic evaluation of small bowel obstruction

- An abdominal radiograph is often the initial imaging evaluation for suspected obstruction.
- Radiographic findings of SBO include small bowel distention and multiple air–fluid levels at different heights seen on the upright view. In addition, the lack of gas in the colon is especially suggestive of obstruction.

  An upright or decubitus view is generally necessary to confidently diagnose obstruction.
- Potential false positives for diagnosing SBO on plain radiographs include:

  Ileus with prior colectomy: Would not see gas in the colon.

  Ileus with ascites: Ascites often compresses the ascending and descending colon and rectum as these structures are not on a mesentery. However, gas in the transverse colon and sigmoid colon is still apparent.

CT imaging of small bowel obstruction

- CT is highly sensitive and specific for diagnosis of SBO. Small bowel distention ≥3 cm with a transition point to collapsed bowel is highly specific for a small bowel obstruction.
- In addition to diagnosing obstruction, CT can show the transition point, the cause of obstruction, and potential complications of obstruction such as ischemia or strangulation.
- It is important to approach the interpretation of an obstruction in a systematic way.
- **First**, look for the transition point to decompressed bowel to determine the cause.
- **Second**, always determine if the obstruction is *simple* or *closed-loop.* A closed-loop obstruction is a *never miss* lesion as there is very high risk for bowel ischemia and severe morbidity and mortality.
- **Third**, evaluate for signs of ischemia or impending ischemia, which include (in rough order of severity):

Engorged mesenteric vessels.
Ascites surrounding the bowel, due to increased capillary permeability.
Wall thickening, due to submucosal edema.
Lack of bowel wall enhancement, due to vasoconstriction or under-perfusion. Note that the presence or absence of bowel wall enhancement can only be assessed if positive oral contrast was not given.
Pneumatosis intestinalis, which is gas in the bowel wall due to necrosis. Pneumatosis produces multiple small locules of gas seen circumferentially in the bowel wall.

- In addition to small bowel distention >3 cm and a transition point to decompressed bowel, an additional helpful CT finding of SBO is the *small bowel feces sign,* which describes particulate feculent material mixed with gas bubbles in the small bowel that resembles the CT appearance of stool.

  The small bowel feces sign is often seen just proximal to the transition point and is helpful to localize the site of transition.

  The small bowel feces sign may be especially helpful in subacute or partial obstruction, which can otherwise be difficult to diagnose.

  The small bowel feces sign is thought to be due to bacterial overgrowth and undigested food.

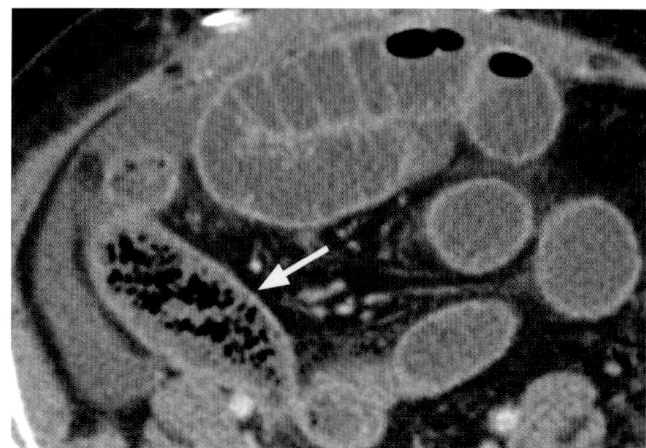

Small bowel feces sign: Axial CT shows an obstruction. A loop of small bowel in the right lower quadrant (arrow) demonstrates numerous gas locules and particulate material in the small bowel.

Closed loop obstruction

- Closed loop obstruction is a surgical emergency that may lead to bowel ischemia. Closed loop obstruction represents obstruction of both the efferent and afferent segments of a single loop of bowel.
- Closed loop obstruction may be secondary to adhesions or hernia. The formation of a narrow pedicle can lead to volvulus, which predisposes to ischemia.
- CT imaging features include a U-shaped distribution of the bowel loop with radially oriented vessels. If volvulus is present, the *whirl* sign may be seen, due to twisting of mesenteric vessels.

Obstruction due to adhesions

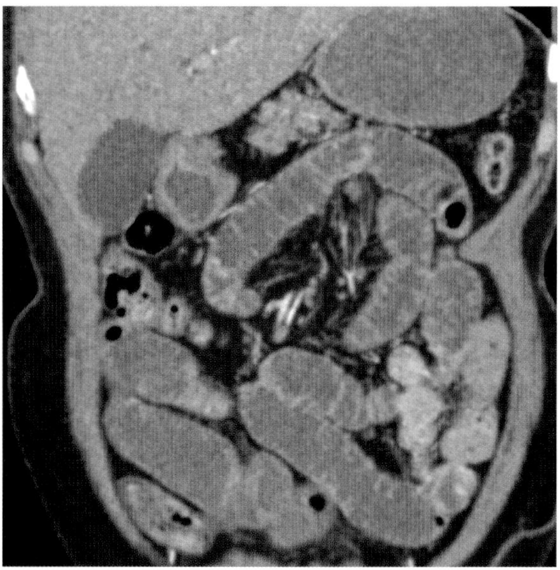

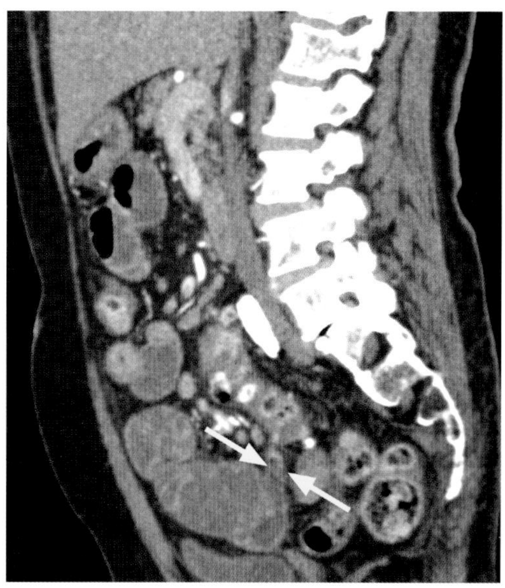

Small bowel obstruction due to adhesions: Coronal (left image) and sagittal CT (right image) shows multiple dilated, fluid-filled loops of small bowel. A transition point is located in the midline pelvis (arrows on sagittal image), with no obstructing mass or evidence of hernia.

- Adhesions from prior surgery or intra-peritoneal inflammatory process are the most common cause of small bowel obstruction.
- Adhesions are an imaging diagnosis of exclusion. On CT, a transition point is seen, but no obvious cause for the transition (e.g., no mass or hernia, etc.) is identified.
- The vast majority of patients with SBO due to adhesions have had prior abdominal surgery.

Obstruction due to external hernia

- Protrusion of bowel through the abdominal wall is the second most common cause of small bowel obstruction. Approximately 75% of external hernias occur in the groin, with the majority being inguinal hernias.
- An **inguinal hernia** may be either indirect or direct, depending on the relation of the hernia to the inferior epigastric vessels.

> **Indirect**: Indirect inguinal hernia is the most common type and is more common in males. The neck of the hernia is lateral to the inferior epigastric vessels. Hernia contents travel with the spermatic cord, often *into the scrotum.* Indirect inguinal hernias are considered a congenital lesion due to a patent processus vaginalis.
>
> **Direct**: The neck of an indirect inguinal hernia is medial to the inferior epigastric vessels, protruding through a weak area in the anterior abdominal wall. The hernia contents *do not go into scrotum.*

- In an **obturator hernia**, bowel herniates through the obturator canal. Obturator hernias are almost always seen in elderly women due to pelvic floor laxity.

  The key imaging finding is bowel located between the pectineus and obturator muscles.

  It is important to correctly diagnose an obturator hernia preoperatively. An obturator hernia requires a very different surgery from inguinal hernia, and has an especially high morbidity and mortality if incarcerated.

- **Ventral hernia** is often due to prior laparotomy.

Obstruction due to internal hernia

- Protrusion of bowel through the peritoneum or mesentery into a compartment in the abdominal cavity is a relatively uncommon cause of small bowel obstruction.
- **Transmesenteric hernia** is a broad category of bowel herniation through defects in any of the three true mesenteries (small bowel mesentery, transverse mesocolon, and sigmoid mesentery). The most common type of transmesenteric hernia is the **transmesocolic** hernia, due to a defect in the transverse mesocolon (mesentery of the transverse colon). Transmesocolic hernia is seen most commonly post Roux-en-Y gastric bypass or biliary-enteric anastomosis from liver transplant.

  The lack of confining hernia sac and variable imaging appearance make diagnosis difficult. A clue on imaging may be posterior displacement of the colon, with small bowel located anterior to the colon. The SMA and SMV may be displaced and engorged.

  Internal hernias carry a high rate of volvulus. If volvulus is present, the *whirl* sign may be visible.

  Transmesenteric hernias are also the most common type of hernia in children, not due to surgery but secondary to a congenital mesenteric defect thought to be from prenatal intestinal ischemia. In children, the mesenteric defect has a variable position.

- **Paraduodenal hernia** was previously the most common internal hernia (older literature states 53% of internal hernias were paraduodenal), prior to the rise in gastric bypass surgery. Paraduodenal hernias are congenital anomalies, due to embryologic failure of mesenteric fusion and resultant mesenteric defect. They more commonly occur on the left.

  Paraduodenal hernia is associated with abnormal rotation of the intestine.

  A common clinical complaint described by patients with paraduodenal hernia is chronic postprandial pain often relieved by massaging, which reduces the hernia.

  In the more common left paraduodenal hernia, the bowel can herniate through a mesenteric defect named Landzert's fossa, located behind the ascending (fourth) duodenum. The key imaging finding is a cluster of small bowel loops between the pancreas and stomach.

- **Foramen of Winslow hernia**: The foramen of Winslow is the communication between the lesser sac and the greater peritoneal cavity.

  The key imaging features of a foramen of Winslow hernia are dilated loops of bowel in the upper abdomen and presence of mesentery between the IVC and main portal vein.

Obstruction due to neoplasm

- A mass intrinsic to the bowel or external compression from an extrinsic mass may cause small bowel obstruction. An extrinsic mass is usually straightforward to diagnose by CT.
- Although the presence of an intraluminal mass may be more difficult to detect on CT, clues to the presence of an intrinsic mass include irregular bowel wall thickening and/or regional lymphadenopathy.
- Primary small bowel neoplasm causing intrinsic bowel obstruction may be due to adenocarcinoma, GIST, and carcinoid. Metastatic causes of intrinsic bowel neoplasm include melanoma, ovarian, and lung cancer. Melanoma is known to cause intussusception.
- Lymphoma is generally a "soft" tumor and rarely causes obstruction. *Aneurysmal* expansion of the small bowel wall is a classic appearance, but presentation is highly variable.

Obstruction due to intussusception

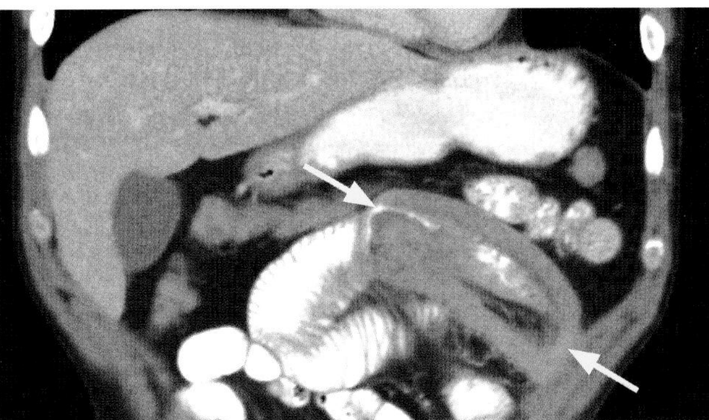

Intussusception causing small bowel obstruction: Coronal contrast-enhanced CT demonstrates a segmental jejunojejunal intussusception (arrows), causing an early or partial proximal small bowel obstruction. This was a case of metastatic melanoma (metastatic lesion not visualized on this image).

- While transient intussusceptions are a common incidental finding, an intussusception causing obstruction should raise suspicion for an underlying lesion and prompt surgery.

Obstruction due to Crohn disease

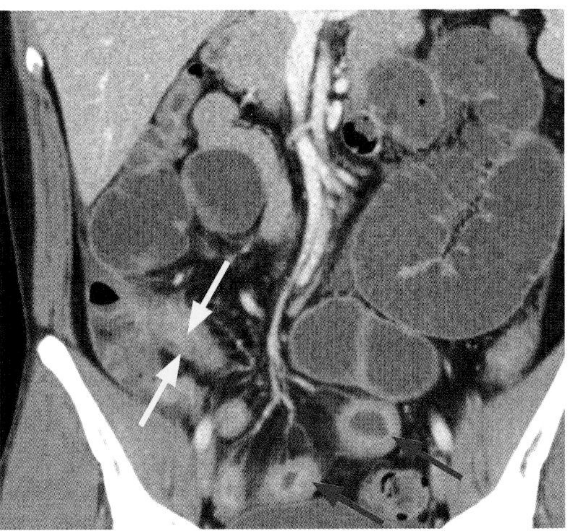

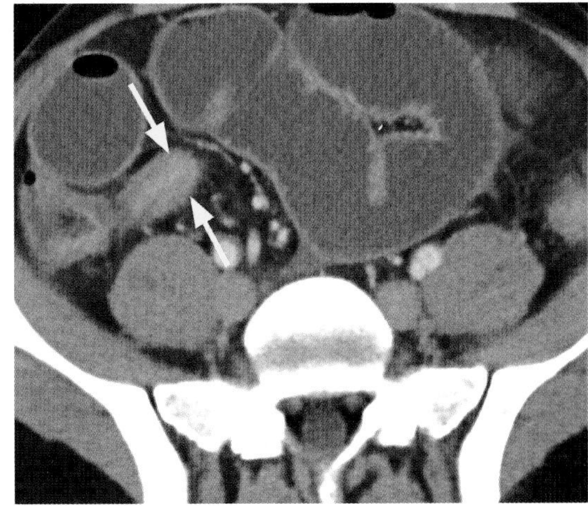

Obstruction due to Crohn ileitis: Coronal (left image) and axial contrast-enhanced CT shows dilated loops of proximal small bowel. The terminal ileum (yellow arrows) and several loops of distal ileum (red arrows) are thickened, reflecting enteritis.

- Stricture or active enteritis is an important cause of bowel obstruction in Crohn disease, especially the fibrostenotic subtype. Crohn disease is discussed on the following page.

Obstruction due to gallstone

- Gallstone ileus is due to a gallstone that has eroded through into the small bowel, causing the classic Rigler's triad of pneumobilia (from cholecystoduodenal fistula), small bowel obstruction, and ectopic gallstone within the small bowel.

- Enteritis is inflammation of the small bowel. The most common CT manifestation of enteritis is bowel wall thickening. Mesenteric stranding or free fluid may also be present.

Crohn disease

- Crohn disease is a chronic granulomatous inflammatory condition that may affect any part of the gastrointestinal tract from the mouth to the anus. Involvement is discontinuous, with characteristic skip lesions of intervening normal GI tract. The most common site of involvement is the small bowel, especially the terminal ileum.
- The earliest histologic changes occur in the submucosa, seen on imaging as aphthous ulcers due to lymphoid hyperplasia and lymphedema.
- Endoscopy and barium fluoroscopy (small bowel follow-through, enteroclysis, and barium enema) have historically been the modalities to evaluate Crohn disease. More recently, however, CT and MR enterography are emerging as the exams of choice.

  The advantages of CT and MRI are the ability to visualize beyond the bowel lumen to evaluate the bowel wall, presence of extraintestinal complications, and the vasculature.

  The disadvantages of CT and MRI compared to fluoroscopy and endoscopy are reduced spatial resolution and limited sensitivity for detecting subtle early signs of disease.
- The most common imaging finding on all modalities is wall thickening of the terminal ileum.
- Fluoroscopic findings include thickened, nodular folds in the affected regions of small bowel, luminal narrowing, mucosal ulceration, and separation of bowel loops. The typical *cobblestone* appearance seen on endoscopy and fluoroscopy is a result of crisscrossing deep ulcerations.

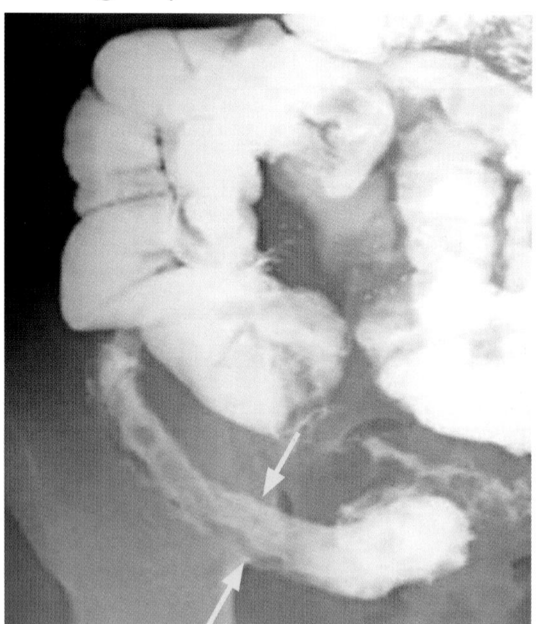

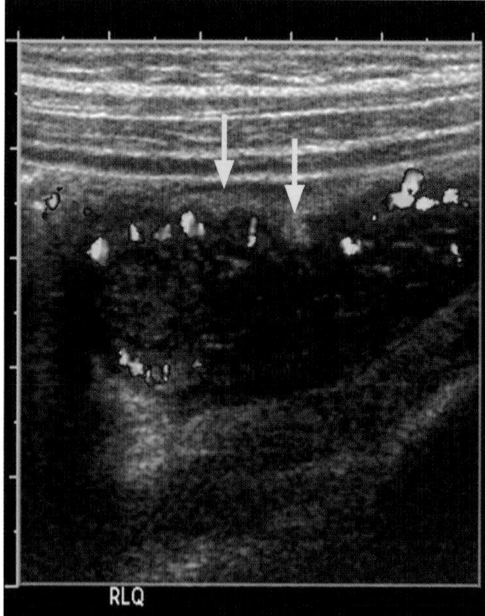

Crohn disease (terminal ileitis): Small bowel follow-through (left image) shows terminal ileum nodular fold thickening, mucosal ulceration, and separation of the terminal ileum (arrows) from adjacent loops of small bowel. Right lower quadrant color Doppler ultrasound (right image) in the same patient demonstrates the nodular fold thickening (arrows) and hyperemic wall.

Case courtesy Michael Callahan, MD, Boston Children's Hospital.

- The fibrostenotic subtype of Crohn disease may clinically present with bowel obstruction. Asymmetric bowel fibrosis from ulcerations of the mesenteric side of the bowel produces pseudosacculations on the antimesenteric side. The fibrosis can lead to a segmental stricture, called the *string* sign.

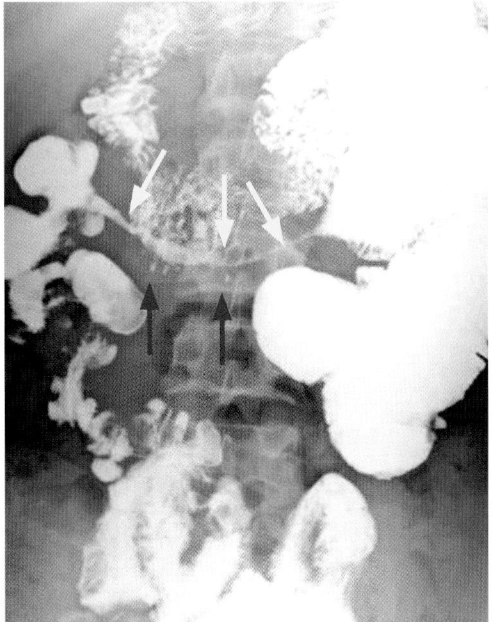
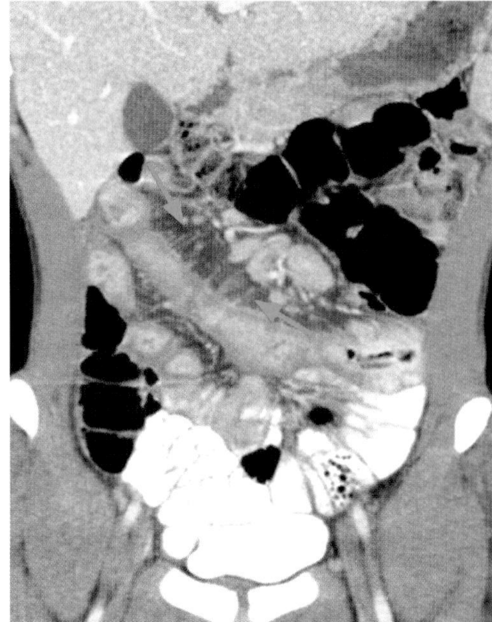

Crohn disease (fibrostenotic subtype): Small bowel follow-through (left image) shows the *string* sign of Crohn disease (yellow arrows) in a loop of distal ileum, with a few small antimesenteric pseudosacculations (red arrows). Contrast-enhanced CT (right image) shows bowel wall thickening and fibrofatty mesenteric changes (blue arrows), known by pathologists and surgeons as *creeping fat*.

Case courtesy Michael Callahan, MD, Boston Children's Hospital.

- Complications of Crohn disease include bowel strictures, fistulae, and abscesses.

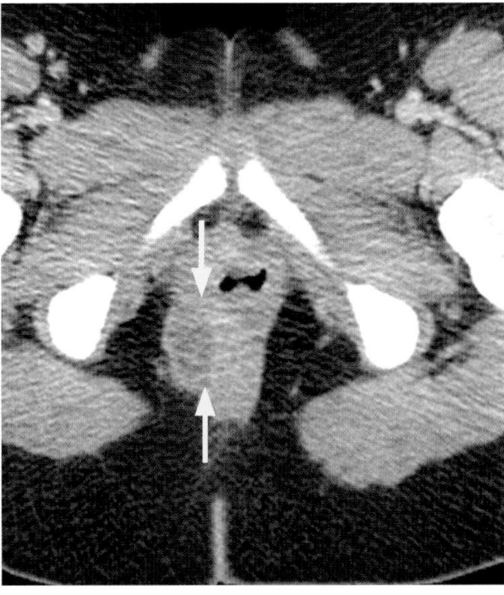
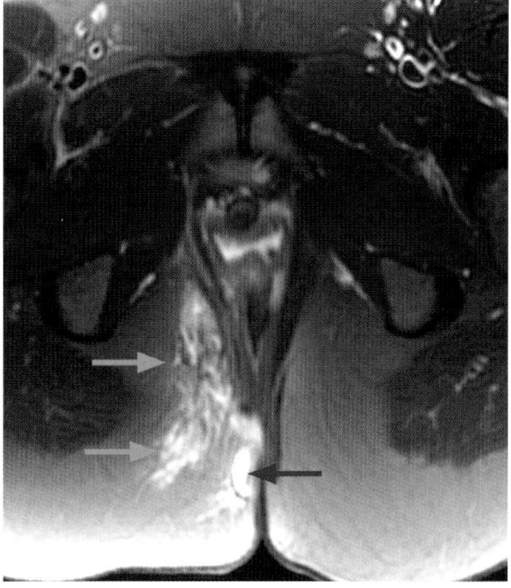

Perirectal abscess and enterocutaneous fistula secondary to Crohn disease: Contrast-enhanced CT (left image) shows a peripherally enhancing fluid collection to the right of the rectum (arrows). T2-weighted MRI (right image) shows the distal portion of an enterocutaneous fistula extending to the skin surface (red arrow). There is marked subcutaneous edema (blue arrows) extending into the subcutaneous tissues of the right buttock.

Case courtesy Michael Callahan, MD, Boston Children's Hospital.

Scleroderma

- Scleroderma is a systemic disease characterized by the deposition of collagen into multiple internal organs and the skin.
- The primary insult to the gastrointestinal tract in scleroderma is impaired motility due to replacement of the muscular layers with collagen, which leads to slowed transit and subsequent bacterial overgrowth, progressive dilation, and pseudo-obstruction.
- Radiographic findings are sacculations on the antimesenteric border (side opposite where the mesentery attaches) and a *hidebound* bowel due to thin, straight bowel folds stacked together.
- Treatment is with antibiotics for bacterial overgrowth and prokinetic drugs such as erythromycin or octreotide for bowel motility.

Celiac disease (sprue, gluten-sensitive enteropathy)

- Celiac disease, also known as sprue and gluten-sensitive enteropathy, is an autoimmune, proximal enteritis caused by a T-cell-mediated immune response triggered by antigens in ingested gluten.
- The primary sites of involvement are the duodenum and jejunum.
- The most characteristic imaging finding of celiac disease is reversal of jejunal and ileal fold patterns. Normally, the jejunum has more folds than the ileum. However, in celiac disease, the loss of jejunal folds causes a compensatory increase in the number of ileal folds.
- Villous atrophy causes the loss of jejunal folds and hypersecretion of intraluminal fluid that creates *flocculations* of barium due to lack of contrast adhesion to the bowel wall. The *moulage* (French for casting) sign is seen on a barium study and refers to a cast-like appearance of the featureless jejunum.
- The CT findings of celiac disease include dilated, fluid-filled bowels, often with intra-luminal flocculations of enteric contrast. Contrast can be seen both insinuated between the small bowel folds and centrally within the bowel, with a peripheral layer of low-attenuation secretions. Other CT findings of celiac disease include mesenteric adenopathy and engorgement of mesenteric vessels.
- Unlike other causes of enteritis, diffuse bowel wall thickening and ascites are less common.
- An important complication of celiac disease is small bowel **T-cell lymphoma**, which may manifest as an exophytic mass, circumferential bowel wall thickening, or enlarged mesenteric lymph nodes.
- Other complications of celiac disease include:

Intussusception, thought to be due to uncoordinated peristalsis, without a lead-point mass.

Pneumatosis intestinalis, thought to be due to dissection of intraluminal gas through the inflamed bowel wall. Pneumatosis in the setting of celiac disease is not thought to reflect bowel ischemia.

Splenic atrophy.

Increased risk of **venous thromboembolism**.

Lab abnormalities include anemia (secondary to malabsorption), leukopenia, and immunoglobulin deficiency. Skin abnormalities include the characteristic dermatitis herpetiformis rash.

Cavitating mesenteric lymph node syndrome (CMLNS) is a very rare complication of celiac disease, with only 36 reported cases in the literature. The central portion of affected lymph nodes shows low attenuation due to liquid necrosis. CMLNS is thought to be highly specific for celiac disease when seen in combination with villous atrophy and splenic atrophy. The differential diagnosis of low attenuation mesenteric lymph nodes includes tuberculosis, Whipple disease, treated lymphoma, and CMLNS.

Infectious enteritis

- Several bacterial, viral, and fungal organisms may cause enteritis.
- *Yersinia* and tuberculosis have a propensity to affect the terminal ileum, mimicking Crohn disease.
- *Salmonella* is the most common cause of food-borne gastroenteritis and causes segmental distal small bowel thickening on CT and segmental nodular thickened folds on fluoroscopy.

Radiation enteritis

- Long-term effects of radiation to the pelvis include adhesive and fibrotic changes to the mesentery and small bowel.
- Clues to the diagnosis of radiation enteritis include a history of radiation therapy and regional involvement of bowel loops not confined to a vascular territory.
- Imaging findings include mural thickening and mucosal hyperenhancement with narrowing of the lumen. Radiation enteritis may be a cause of small bowel obstruction.

Whipple disease

- Whipple disease is due to infection by *Tropheryma whippelii,* which manifests in the GI tract as malabsorption and abdominal pain. Whipple disease may cause arthralgias and increased skin pigmentation.
- Whipple disease characteristically causes low attenuation adenopathy that may appear similar to the cavitating mesenteric lymph node syndrome seen in celiac disease.
- Radiographically, Whipple disease causes thickening and nodularity of duodenal and proximal small bowel folds. In contrast to celiac disease, there is typically no hypersecretion.

Graft versus host disease (GVHD)

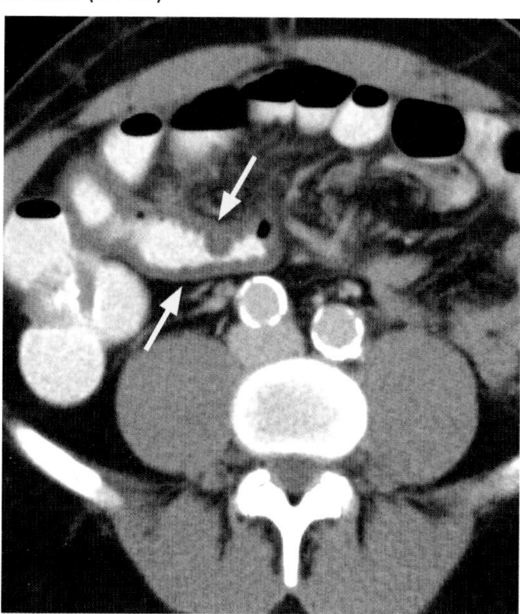

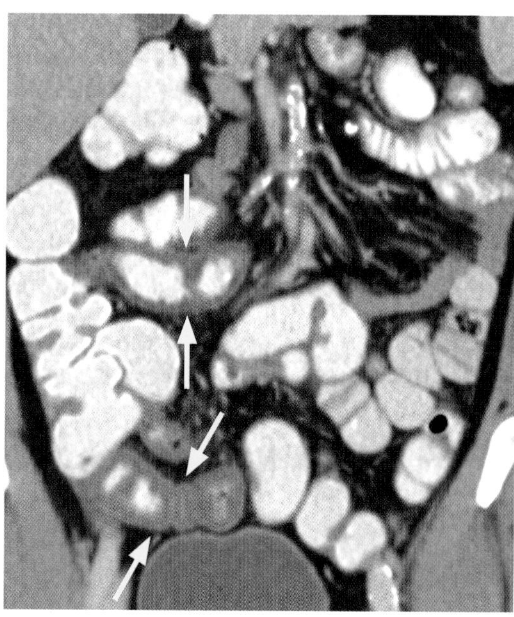

GVHD: Axial (left image) and coronal contrast-enhanced CT shows marked thickening of the wall of the distal ileum (arrows). This finding is not specific and may also represent Crohn disease; however, this patient has a history of stem cell transplant for a congenital immunodeficiency.

- Graft versus host disease is a complication of bone marrow transplantation. The skin, liver, and gastrointestinal tract are most commonly affected.
- Imaging findings of GVHD include nonspecific wall thickening and effacement of the normal small bowel fold pattern. While the classic barium finding is the *ribbon* bowel, this is not often seen.

COLITIS

Overview of colitis

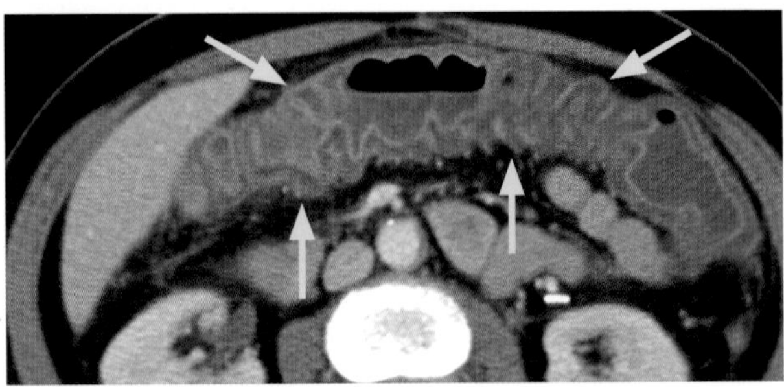

Pancolitis: Contrast enhanced CT shows severe mural thickening of the entire visualized colon (arrows) with mucosal hyperenhancement. Although nonspecific, this was a case of pseudomembranous colitis.

- Colitis is inflammation of the colon that may be caused by several unrelated etiologies, often with overlapping imaging findings.
- The primary imaging feature of colitis is bowel wall thickening. Generally, a full clinical evaluation, stool studies, and sometimes colonic biopsy are required for a definitive diagnosis.
- Incidental colonic wall thickening is found in as many as 10% of CT scans.

Ischemic colitis

- Colonic ischemia can be caused by acute arterial thrombus, chronic arterial stenosis, low-flow states (e.g., congestive heart failure), and venous thrombosis.
- The splenic flexure is the watershed region between the superior and inferior mesenteric arteries and is especially susceptible to ischemia in low-flow states.
- The rectum is supplied by a dual blood supply and is almost never affected by ischemia. The superior rectal artery (terminal branch of the IMA) and the inferior and middle rectal arteries (arising from the internal iliac artery anterior division) form perirectal collaterals.
- A suggestive CT finding of ischemic colitis is segmental, continuous thickening of the affected colon in a vascular distribution, with sparing of the rectum.

  If arterial thromboembolic disease is suspected, one should evaluate for the presence of aortic atherosclerotic disease or a left atrial thrombus in the setting of atrial fibrillation.

  If chronic arterial stenosis is suspected, one should evaluate for atherosclerosis of the mesenteric vessels.

Infectious colitis

- Infectious colitis can be bacterial, tubercular, viral, or amoebic. There is a large overlap in the clinical presentation and imaging findings of the various pathogens.
- In general, infectious colitis features pericolonic stranding and ascites in addition to the colonic wall thickening seen in all forms of colitis.
- *Yersinia*, *Salmonella*, and colonic tubercolosis affect the right colon. Tuberculosis is known to involve the ileocecal valve, resulting in a desmoplastic reaction that mimics Crohn disease.
- *E. coli*, CMV, and *C. difficile* colitis (discussed below) most commonly cause pancolitis.

Pseudomembranous colitis

- Pseudomembranous colitis is an especially prevalent form of infectious colitis caused by overgrowth of *Clostridium difficile*, most commonly due to alteration in colonic bacterial flora after antibiotic use. Pseudomembranous colitis may also occur without a history of antibiotics, especially in hospitalized or nursing home patients.
- A key imaging finding is marked thickening of the colonic wall, typically with involvement of the entire colon (pancolitis). The *accordion* sign describes severe colonic wall thickening combined with undulation of enhancing inner mucosa. It signifies severe colonic edema but is not specific to *C. difficile*. *Thumbprinting* is a fluoroscopic finding of thickened haustra and is also due to edema.

Ulcerative colitis (UC)

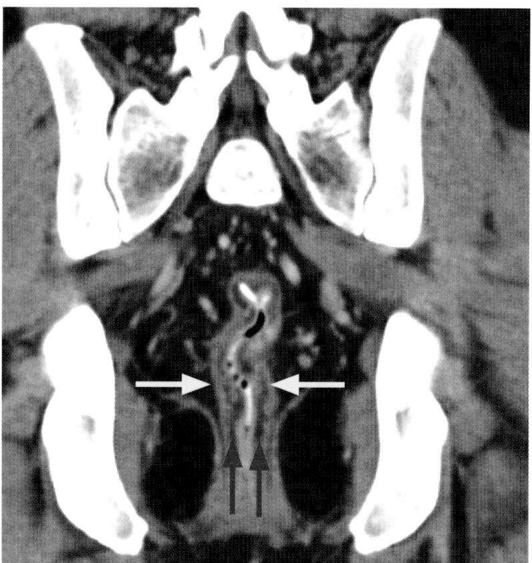
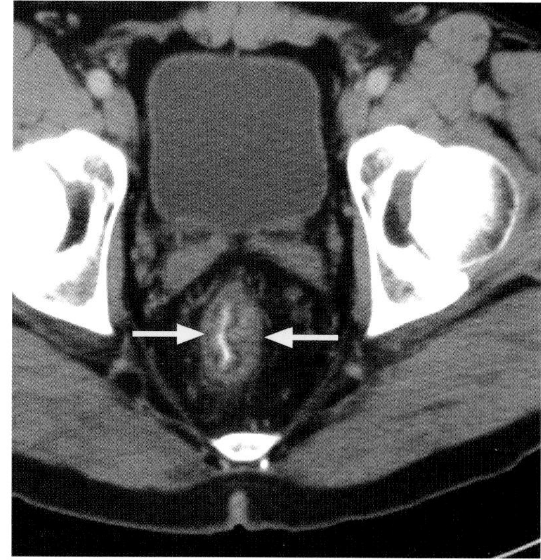

Chronic ulcerative colitis: Coronal (left image) and axial contrast-enhanced CT shows continuous thickening of the rectal wall (yellow arrows) with fat attenuation of the submucosa (red arrows).

- Ulcerative colitis (UC) is an idiopathic inflammatory bowel disease that begins distally in the rectum and spreads proximally in a continual manner (unlike Crohn disease, which features skip areas).

  Of note, it is possible for the rectum to appear normal with more proximal colonic involvement present if the patient has been treated with corticosteroid enemas.

- Patients with UC have an increased risk of primary sclerosing cholangitis, colon cancer, and cholangiocarcinoma.
- Extra-abdominal manifestations of UC include sacroiliitis, iritis, erythema nodosum (tender red subcutaneous nodules), and pyoderma gangrenosum (cutaneous ulcers).
- UC does not extend more proximally than the cecum; however, a *backwash ileitis* caused by reflux of inflammatory debris into the ileum may mimic Crohn disease.
- Imaging of ulcerative colitis features circumferential wall thickening with a granular mucosal pattern that is best seen on barium enema. Pseudopolyps may be present during acute inflammation, representing islands of normal mucosa surrounded by inflamed mucosa. A *collar-button* ulcer is nonspecific but represents mucosal ulceration undermined by submucosal extension.
- Chronic changes of ulcerative colitis include a featureless and foreshortened *lead pipe* colon. Similar to Crohn disease, fat-attenuation of the colonic wall suggests chronic disease, as seen in the case above.
- Toxic megacolon is a severe complication of ulcerative colitis (and less commonly, Crohn disease) caused by inflammation extending through the muscular layer. Imaging of toxic megacolon shows dilation of the colon to greater than 6 cm in association with an adynamic ileus. Colonic perforation may occur and colonoscopy is contraindicated in suspected toxic megacolon.

Typhlitis (neutropenic enterocolitis)

- Typhlitis is a right-sided colitis seen in immunocompromised patients.
- Treatment is with broad-spectrum antibiotics and antifungals.

Polyposis syndromes affecting the bowel

Familial adenomatous polyposis (FAP)

- Familial adenomatous polyposis (FAP) is an autosomal-dominant syndrome featuring innumerable premalignant adenomatous polyps in the colon and to a lesser extent the small bowel. Prophylactic colectomy is the standard of care to prevent colon cancer.
- Gastric polyps are also present, although the gastric polyps are hyperplastic and are not premalignant.
- **Gardner** syndrome is a variant of FAP. In addition to colon polyps, patients also have:

Desmoid tumors.	Papillary thyroid cancer.
Osteomas.	Epidermoid cysts.

Mnemonic: DOPE Gardner

- **Turcot** syndrome is another variant of FAP. In addition to colon polyps, patients also have CNS tumors (gliomas and medulloblastomas).

Hereditary nonpolyposis colon cancer syndrome (HNPCC) = Lynch syndrome

- Hereditary nonpolyposis colon cancer (HNPCC) syndrome (also called Lynch syndrome) is an autosomal dominant polyposis syndrome caused by DNA mismatch repair, leading to colon cancer from microsatellite instability on a molecular level.
- Similar to FAP, the colon polyps of HNPCC are adenomatous.
- HNPCC is associated with other cancers, including endometrial, stomach, small bowel, liver, and biliary malignancies.

Peutz–Jeghers

- Peutz–Jeghers is an autosomal dominant syndrome that features multiple hamartomatous pedunculated polyps, usually in the small bowel. These polyps may act as lead points and cause intussusception.
- Characteristic skin manifestations include perioral mucocutaneous blue/brown pigmented spots on the lips and gums.
- Peutz–Jeghers is associated with gynecologic neoplasms as well as gastric, duodenal, and colonic malignancies.

Cowden syndrome

- Cowden syndrome is an autosomal dominant syndrome of multiple hamartomatous polyps most commonly found in the skin and external mucous membranes, but also in the gastrointestinal tract.
- Cowden syndrome is associated with an increased risk of thyroid cancer (usually follicular), as well as skin, oral, breast, and uterine malignancies.

Cronkhite–Canada

- Cronkhite–Canada is a non-inherited disorder (the only polyposis syndrome in this list that is not autosomal dominant) consisting of hamartomatous polyps throughout the gastrointestinal tract.
- Cutaneous manifestations include abnormal skin pigmentation, alopecia, and onychodystrophy (malformation of the nails).

Appendicitis

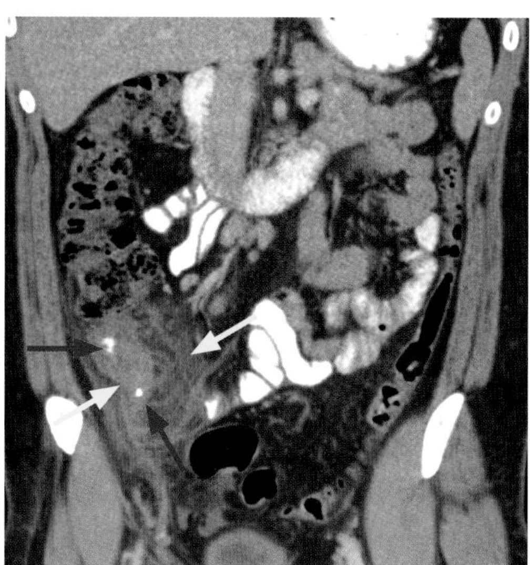

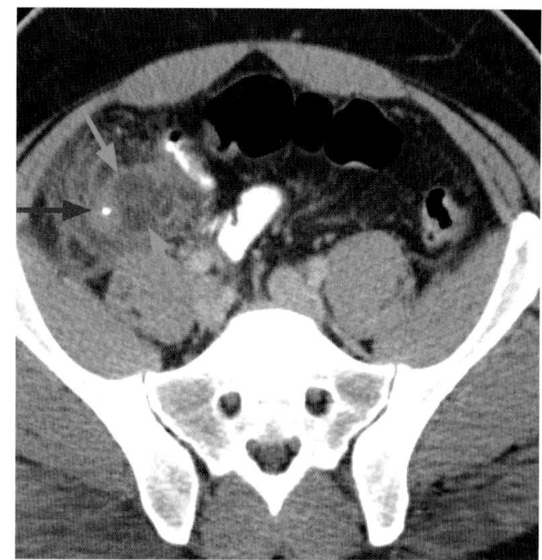

Appendicitis: Coronal (left image) and axial contrast-enhanced CT shows a large focus of inflammatory stranding centered around the appendix in the right lower quadrant (yellow arrows). The margins of the appendix itself are indistinct and there is the suggestion of an early fluid collection (blue arrows). Note the two appendicoliths within the appendix (red arrows).

- Appendicitis is the most common surgical cause of acute abdomen. Acute inflammation of the appendix is thought to be due to obstruction of the appendiceal lumen, leading to venous congestion, mural ischemia, and bacterial translocation.
- Appendicitis represents a spectrum of severity ranging from *tip appendicitis* (inflammation isolated to the distal appendix) to *gangrenous appendicitis* with abscess if the disease is not diagnosed until late.
- Greater than 97% of patients undergo a preoperative CT prior to appendectomy, with resultant decrease in negative appendectomy rate from 23% in 1990 to 1.7% in 2007.
- Imaging of appendicitis relies on direct and indirect imaging findings.
- **Direct findings of appendicitis** are due to abnormalities of the appendix itself:

Distended, fluid-filled appendix: 6 mm is used as cutoff for normal diameter of the appendix, although there is wide normal variability and 6 mm is from the ultrasound literature using compression. A normal appendix distended with air can measure >6 mm; therefore, some authors advocate using caution with a numeric cutoff in an otherwise normal-appearing appendix filled with air or enteric contrast.

Appendiceal wall-thickening.

Appendicolith, which may be a cause of luminal obstruction; however, appendicoliths are commonly seen without associated appendicitis.

- **Indirect findings of appendicitis** are due to the spread of inflammation to adjacent sites:

Periappendiceal fat stranding.	Hydroureter.
Cecal wall thickening.	Small bowel ileus.

- Appendicitis can also be evaluated by ultrasound, with the key sonographic finding a tubular, blind-ending, non-compressible right lower quadrant structure measuring >6 mm in diameter. Is is generally necessary to use graded compression to evaluate for compressibility.

    Secondary findings of appendicitis can be evaluated by ultrasound, including free fluid and periappendicular abscess.

Diverticulitis

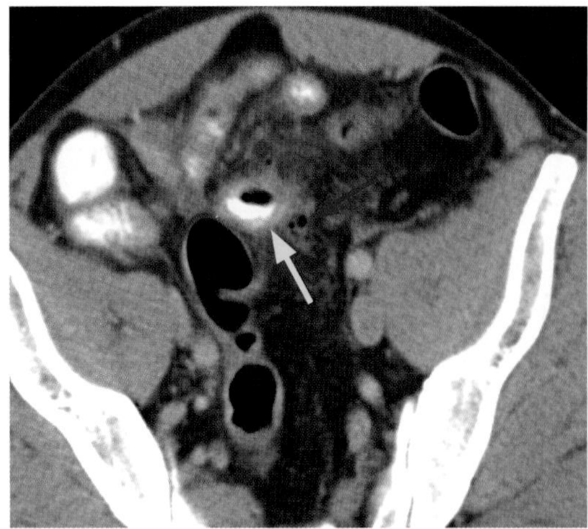

Complicated diverticulitis: Axial CT shows a large diverticulum arising from the sigmoid colon containing enteric contrast (yellow arrow), with surrounding mesenteric fat stranding. A few adjacent locules of extraluminal gas (red arrow) are present.

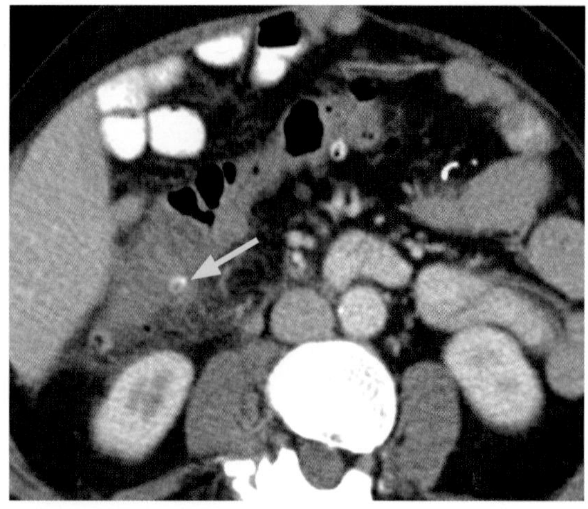

Uncomplicated diverticulitis: Axial CT in a different patient shows fat stranding surrounding a diverticulum at the hepatic flexure (arrow).

- Diverticulitis is microperforation and acute inflammation of a colonic diverticulum. CT is the primary modality for diagnosis, triage, and evaluation of severity and complications.
- The left colon is affected far more commonly than the right.
- It is often impossible to distinguish acute diverticulitis from microperforated colon cancer. Many authors recommend follow-up colonoscopy after the acute episode has resolved, although this recommendation is somewhat controversial and varies by institution.
- **Uncomplicated diverticulitis** does not have any imaging evidence of bowel perforation (even though histopathologically all diverticulitis is associated with bacterial translocation across the bowel wall). CT findings of uncomplicated diverticulitis include bowel wall thickening and pericolonic fat stranding, usually centered around a culprit diverticulum.
- **Complicated diverticulitis** implies the presence of an additional complication, including:

Pericolonic or hepatic abscess. Extraluminal air. Bowel obstruction.	Bowel fistula (colovesical fistula most common, apparent on imaging as gas in the bladder not explained by Foley catheter placement). Mesenteric venous thrombosis.

- Uncomplicated diverticulitis is typically treated conservatively.
- Abscesses can usually be drained percutaneously.
- Indications for surgery include the presence of a fistula or recurrent diverticulitis, with two prior episodes of diverticulitis treated conservatively.

Epiploic appendagitis

- Epiploic appendagitis is a benign, clinical mimic of diverticulitis caused by torsion of a normal fatty tag (appendage) hanging from the colon.
- Epiploic appendagitis has a pathognomonic imaging appearance of an oval fat-attenuation lesion abutting a normal colonic wall, with mild associated fat stranding. A central hyperdense dot in cross-section represents the thrombosed central vein of the epiploic appendage.
- Treatment is with anti-inflammatories, *not* antibiotics or surgery.

ANATOMY

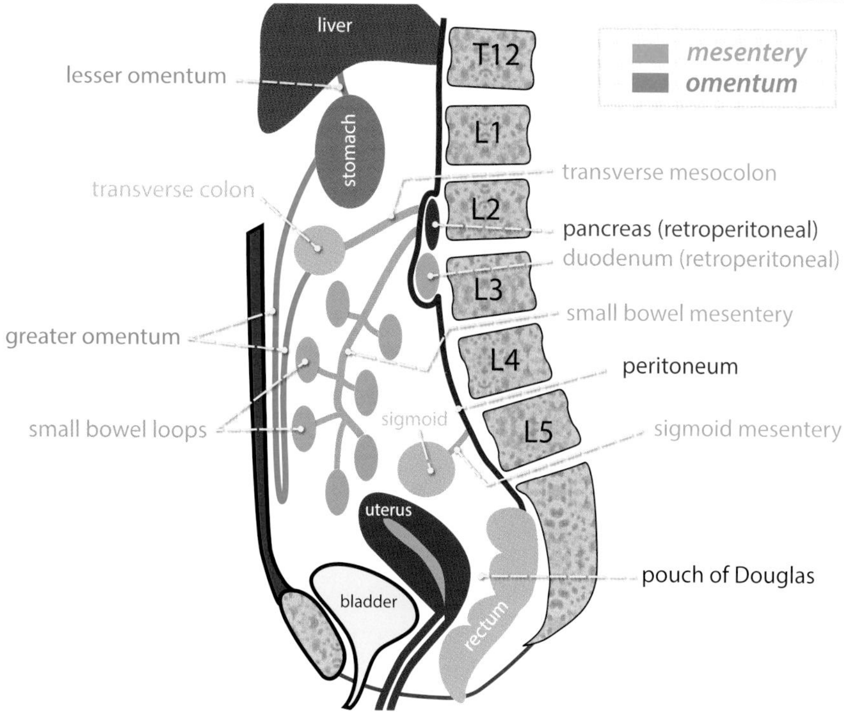

Peritoneum

- The peritoneum is a thin membrane consisting of a single layer of mesothelial cells that are supported by subserosal fat cells, lymphatic cells, and white blood cells.
- The visceral peritoneum lines the surface of all intraperitoneal organs, while the parietal peritoneum lines the outer walls of the peritoneal cavity.
- The most dependent portion of the peritoneal cavity (both supine and upright) is the pouch of Douglas in women and the retrovesical space in men.

Mesentery

- There are three true mesenteries, which each supply a portion of the bowel and connect to the posterior abdominal wall. Each mesentery consists of a network of blood vessels and lymphatics, sandwiched between the peritoneal layers. The three true mesenteries are:

Small bowel mesentery: Supplies both the jejunum and ileum. Oriented obliquely from the ligament of Treitz in the left upper quadrant to the ileocecal junction in the right lower quadrant.

Transverse mesocolon: Mesentery to the transverse colon, connecting the posterior transverse colon to the posterior abdominal wall

Sigmoid mesentery: Mesentery to the sigmoid colon.

- The greater and lesser omentum are specialized mesenteries that attach to the stomach. The greater and lesser omentum do not connect to the posterior abdominal wall.

Greater omentum: Large, drape-like mesentery in the anterior abdomen, which connects the stomach to the anterior aspect of the transverse colon.

Lesser omentum: Connects stomach to liver.

Flow of peritoneal fluid

- Peritoneal fluid is constantly produced, circulated, and finally resorbed around the diaphragm, where it eventually drains into the thoracic duct.

"MISTY" MESENTERY

Overview of the "misty" mesentery

- As previously discussed, the abdominal mesenteries are fatty folds through which the arterial supply and venous and lymphatic drainage of the bowel run.
- The mesenteries themselves are not seen on CT because they are made primarily of fat and blend in with intra-abdominal fat. However, the vessels which course through the mesentery are normally seen.
- Infiltration of the mesentery by fluid, inflammatory cells, tumor, or fibrosis may increase the attenuation of the mesentery and cause the mesenteric vasculature to appear indistinct. These findings are often the first clue to certain pathologies.

Mesenteric edema

- Edema of the mesentery may be secondary to either systemic or intra-abdominal etiologies.
- Systemic causes of edema include congestive heart failure, low protein states, and third-spacing, all of which can lead to diffuse mesenteric edema.
- Focal mesenteric edema may be secondary to an intra-abdominal vascular cause, such as mesenteric vessel thrombosis, Budd–Chiari syndrome, or IVC obstruction. Abdominal vascular insults may cause bowel ischemia, which manifest on imaging as bowel wall thickening, pneumatosis, or mesenteric venous gas.

Mesenteric inflammation

- The most common cause of mesenteric inflammation in the upper abdomen is acute pancreatitis. However, any focal inflammatory process such as appendicitis, inflammatory bowel disease, and diverticulitis may cause local mesenteric inflammation leading to the "misty" mesentery appearance.
- Mesenteric panniculitis is an idiopathic inflammatory condition, which may cause a diffuse "misty" mesentery.

Intra-abdominal hemorrhage

- Intra-abdominal hemorrhage tends to be localized, surrounding the culprit bleeding vessel unless large. Hemorrhage may be secondary to trauma, post-procedural, or due to anticoagulation.

Neoplastic infiltration

- Neoplastic infiltration of the mesentery may cause the "misty" mesentery. The most common tumor involving the mesentery is non-Hodgkin lymphoma, which typically also causes bulky adenopathy.
- Mesenteric involvement may be especially apparent after treatment, where the "misty" mesentery is limited to the portion of the mesentery that contained the treated lymph nodes.
- Other tumors that may involve the mesentery include pancreatic, colon, breast, gastrointestinal stromal tumor, and mesothelioma.

Mesenteric masses

Overview of mesenteric masses

- Primary mesenteric tumors are rare, although the mesentery is a relatively common site of metastasis.

Carcinoid

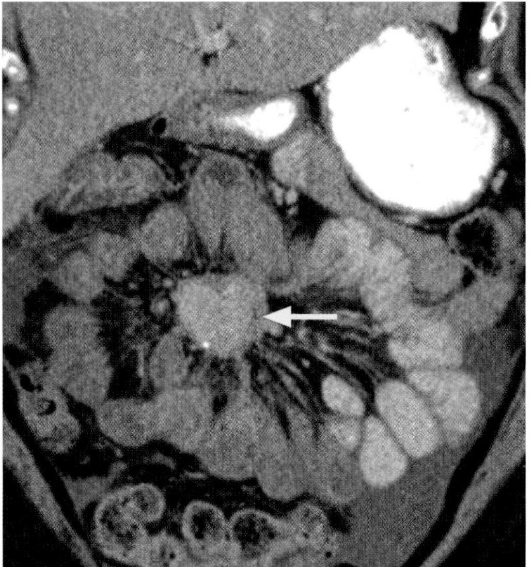
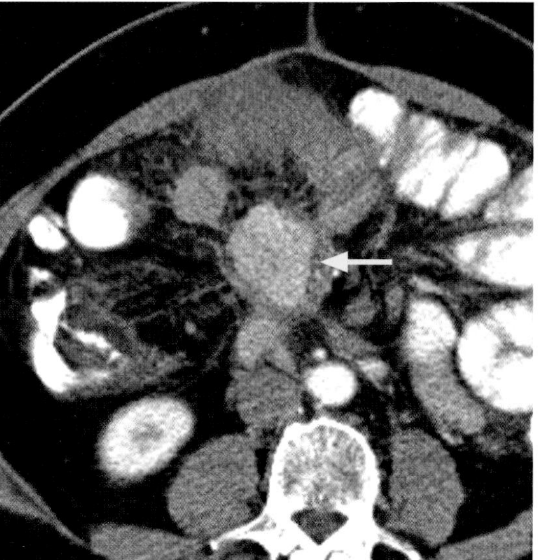

Carcinoid metastatic to the mesentery: Coronal (left image) and axial contrast-enhanced CT shows a hyperenhancing mesenteric mass (arrows) that contains a few tiny foci of calcification peripherally. There are numerous linear soft tissue strands radiating from the mass.

Case courtesy Cheryl Sadow, MD, Brigham and Women's Hospital.

- Gastrointestinal carcinoid is a relatively rare tumor compared to other gastrointestinal malignancies, but is the most common small bowel tumor. It typically occurs in the distal ileum.
- Carcinoid usually arises as an intraluminal mass and may secondarily spread to the mesentery either by direct extension or lymphatic spread. Up to 80% of carcinoids spread to the mesentery.
- A classic imaging appearance of carcinoid affecting the mesentery is an enhancing soft-tissue mass with radiating linear bands extending into the mesenteric fat. Calcification is common.

  The radiating linear bands do not represent infiltrative tumor but are the result of an intense desmoplastic reaction caused by the release of serotonin by the tumor.
- The differential diagnosis of a sclerosing mesenteric mass includes:

  Carcinoid.

  Desmoid tumor.

  Sclerosing mesenteritis.

Desmoid tumor

- Desmoid tumor is a benign, locally aggressive mass composed of proliferating fibrous tissue.
- Desmoid may be sporadic, but mesenteric desmoid tumors are more common in patients with Gardner syndrome (a variant of familial adenomatous polyposis).
- On CT, most desmoids are isoattenuating to muscle, but large tumors may show central necrosis. A characteristic imaging feature is strands of tissue radiating into the adjacent mesenteric fat, similar to mesenteric carcinoid and sclerosing mesenteritis.

Sclerosing mesenteritis

- Sclerosing mesenteritis is a rare inflammatory condition that leads to fatty necrosis and fibrosis of the mesenteric root.
- Imaging of sclerosing mesenteritis shows mesenteric masses with striations of soft tissue extending into the adjacent fat. Calcification may be present.
- Mesenteric panniculitis is a variant where inflammation predominates and presents as acute abdominal pain. On CT, there is a "misty" mesentery, sometimes with linear bands of soft tissue representing early fibrosis.

Mesenteric metastases and lymphoma

- Gastric, ovarian, breast, lung, pancreatic, biliary, colon cancer, and melanoma can metastasize to mesenteric lymph nodes.
- Mesenteric lymphoma can produce the *sandwich* sign, where the mesenteric fat and vessels (the sandwich filling) are engulfed on two sides by bulky lymphomatous masses (the bread).

Diffuse peritoneal disease

Peritoneal carcinomatosis

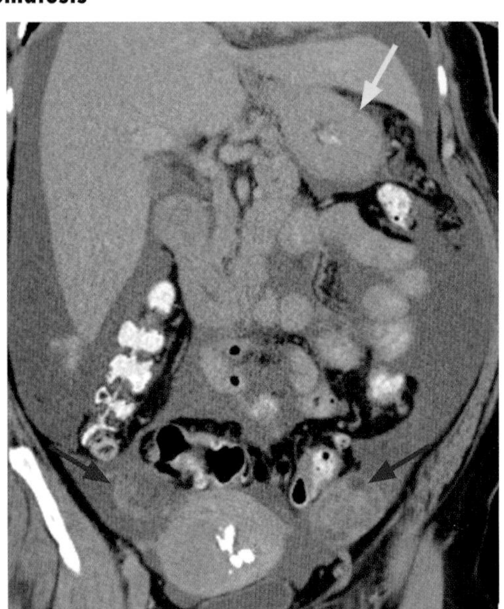
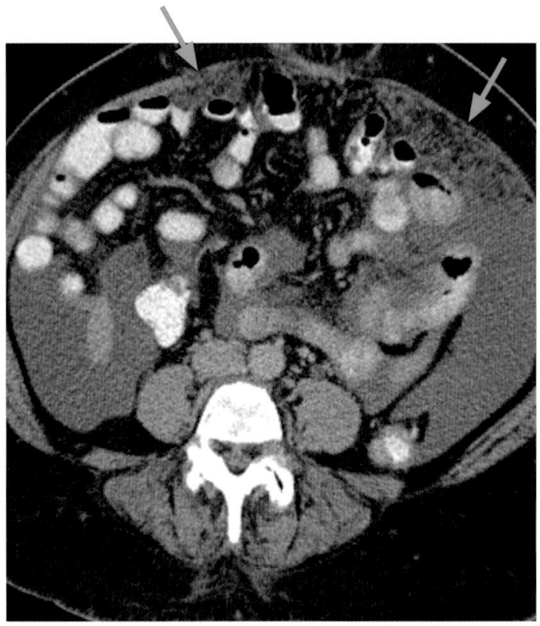

Peritoneal carcinomatosis due to gastric cancer, with Krukenberg tumors of the ovaries: Coronal contrast-enhanced CT (left image) shows marked thickening of the gastric wall (yellow arrow). There are bilateral adnexal masses (red arrows), representing ovarian metastases. Moderate ascites is present. Axial CT (right image) demonstrates peritoneal nodularity and thickening, especially in the left anterior abdomen (blue arrows), consistent with peritoneal carcinomatosis.

Case courtesy Cheryl Sadow, MD, Brigham and Women's Hospital.

- Peritoneal carcinomatosis represents disseminated metastases to the peritoneal surface.
- The term *omental caking* describes the replacement of omental fat by tumor and fibrosis.
- Mucinous adenocarcinoma is the most common tumor type to cause peritoneal carcinomatosis. Peritoneal carcinomatosis due to mucinous adenocarcinoma should not be confused with pseudomyxoma peritonei, discussed on the following page.

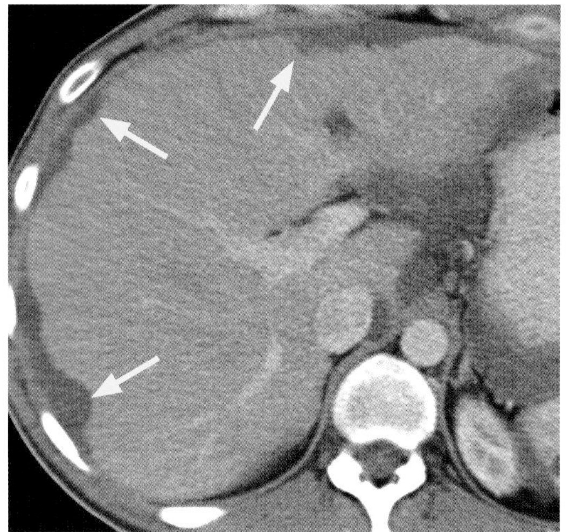

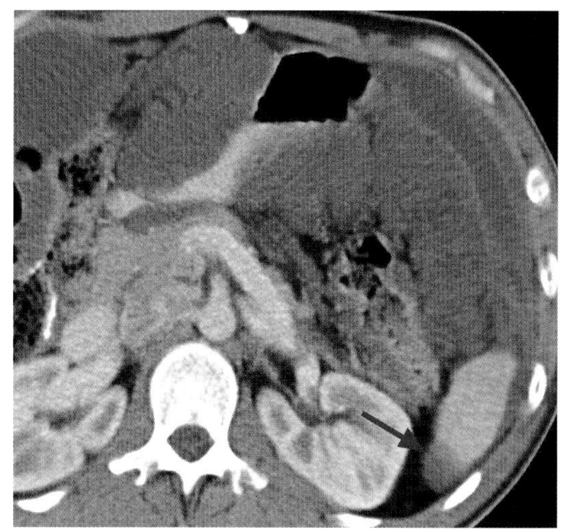

Pseudomyxoma peritonei: Axial contrast-enhanced CT through the liver (left image) shows scalloping of the hepatic capsule (arrows). A lower image through the kidneys shows the lobulated, mucinous ascites exerting mass effect on adjacent bowel loops. A splenic implant is also visible (red arrow).

Case courtesy Cheryl Sadow, MD, Brigham and Women's Hospital.

- Pseudomyxoma peritonei is a low-grade malignancy characterized by copious mucus in the peritoneal cavity.
- In general, pseudomyxoma peritonei is thought to be produced by a mucin-producing adenoma or adenocarcinoma of the appendix; however, there is some controversy as to whether the ovary or colon can be a primary site as well.

  Pseudomyxoma peritonei is often associated with an ovarian mass (up to 30% of female patients), but it is thought that these are most often metastatic deposits.
- Pseudomyxoma peritonei was previously thought to be produced by a benign appendiceal mucocele, which is now believed to occur much less commonly than originally thought.

  20% of all appendiceal adenomas or adenocarcinomas will cause pseudomyxoma peritonei.

  Only 2% of all appendiceal mucoceles (which occur slightly less commonly than appendiceal adenomatous lesions) will cause pseudomyxoma peritonei.
- Tumor deposits tend to be spread throughout the entire peritoneal cavity due to intraperitoneal fluid currents.
- Clinically, pseudomyxoma peritonei presents with recurrent mucinous ascites. The surgeons refer to the mucinous ascites as a "jelly belly."
- CT shows lobular ascites that is typically of slightly higher attenuation (5–20 Hounsfield units) compared to fluid ascites. Occasionally, mucus can be seen in the region of the appendix, but the flow of peritoneal contents tends to spread the mucinous ascites diffusely throughout the peritoneum.
- Advanced disease shows pathognomonic scalloping of the hepatic margin.
- Treatment continues to evolve, but the best outcomes are primarily with surgical treatment and hyperthermic intraperitoneal chemotherapy lavage.

References, resources, and further reading

General references:

Johnson, D.C. & Schmit, G.D. Mayo Clinic Gastrointestinal Imaging Review. Mayo Clinic Scientific Press. (2005).

Ros, P.R., Mortele K.J. CT and MRI of the Abdomen and Pelvis: A Teaching File. Lippincott Williams & Wilkins. (2006).

Roth, C.G. Fundamentals of Body MRI (1st ed.). Elsevier/Saunders. (2012).

Liver:

Alústiza, J.M. et al. Iron overload in the liver diagnostic and quantification. European Journal of Radiology 61, 499-506(2007).

Blachar, A., Federle, M.P. & Sosna, J. Liver Lesions With Hepatic Capsular Retraction. Seminars in Ultrasound, CT, and MRI 30, 426-35(2009).

Brancatelli, G. et al. Budd-Chiari Syndrome: Spectrum of Imaging Findings. American Journal of Roentgenology 188, 168-76(2007).doi:10.2214/AJR.05.0168

Chung, Y.E. et al. Varying appearances of cholangiocarcinoma: radiologic-pathologic correlation. Radiographics 29, 683-700(2009).

Elsayes, K.M. et al. Focal hepatic lesions: diagnostic value of enhancement pattern approach with contrast-enhanced 3D gradient-echo MR imaging. Radiographics 25, 1299-320(2005).

Hanna, R. et al. Cirrhosis-associated Hepatocellular Nodules: Correlation of Histopathologic and MR imaging features. Radiographics 28, 747-69(2008).

Kamaya, A. et al. Hypervascular Liver Lesions. Seminars in Ultrasound, CT, and MRI 30, 387-407(2009).

Kim, T., Hori, M. & Onishi, H. Liver Masses With Central or Eccentric Scar. Seminars in Ultrasound, CT, and MRI 30, 418-25(2009).

Martin, D. & Semelka, R. Magnetic Resonance Imaging of the Liver: Review of Techniques and Approach to Common Diseases. Seminars in Ultrasound, CT, and MRI 26, 116-31(2005).

Martin, D.R., Danrad, R. & Hussain, S.M. MR imaging of the liver. Radiologic Clinics of North America 43, 861-86, viii(2005).

Mortele, K.J. & Ros, P.R. Cystic Focal Liver Lesions in the Adult: Differential CT and MR Imaging Features. Radiographics 21, 895-910(2001).

Pancreaticobiliary:

Acar, M., Tatli, S. Cystic tumors of the pancreas: a radiological perspective. Diagnostic and Interventional Radiology (Ankara, Turkey), 17(2), 143-49(2011).

Blachar, A., Federle, M.P. & Brancatelli, G. Primary biliary cirrhosis: clinical, pathologic, and helical CT findings in 53 patients. Radiology 220, 329-36(2001).

Blasbalg, R. et al. MRI features of groove pancreatitis. AJR. American Journal of Roentgenology 189, 73-80(2007).

Fasanella, K.E. & McGrath, K. Cystic lesions and intraductal neoplasms of the pancreas. Best Practice & Research. Clinical Gastroenterology 23, 35-48(2009).

Kim, S.H. et al. Intrapancreatic accessory spleen: findings on MR Imaging, CT, US and scintigraphy, and the pathologic analysis. Korean Journal of Radiology 9, 162-74(2008).

Koo, B.C., Chinogureyi, A. & Shaw, A.S. Imaging acute pancreatitis. The British Journal of Radiology 83, 104-12(2010).

Levy, A.D. et al. From the Archives of the AFIP: Benign Tumors and Tumorlike Lesions of the Gallbladder and Extrahepatic Bile Ducts: Radiologic-Pathologic Correlation. Radiographics 22, 387-413(2002).

Mortele, K.J. et al. Multimodality Imaging of Pancreatic and Biliary Congenital Anomalies. Radiographics 26, 715-31(2006).

Nakajima, Y., Yamada, T. & Sho, M. Malignant potential of intraductal papillary mucinous neoplasms of the pancreas. Surgery Today 40, 816-24(2010).

Nishimori, I., Onishi, S. & Otsuki, M. Review of diagnostic criteria for autoimmune pancreatitis; for establishment of international criteria. Clinical Journal of Gastroenterology 1, 7-17(2008).

Pedrosa, I. & Boparai, D. Imaging considerations in intraductal papillary mucinous neoplasms of the pancreas. World Journal of Gastrointestinal Surgery 2, 324-30(2010).

Saokar, A., Rabinowitz, C.B. & Sahani, D.V. Cross-sectional imaging in acute pancreatitis. Radiologic Clinics of North America 45, 447-60, viii(2007).

Sawai, Y. et al. Development of pancreatic cancers during long-term follow-up of side-branch intraductal papillary mucinous neoplasms. Endoscopy 43, 79(2011).

Scaglione, M. et al. Imaging Assessment of Acute Pancreatitis: A Review. Seminars in Ultrasound, CT, and MRI 29, 322-40(2008).

Sidden, C.R., Mortele, K.J. Cystic Tumors of the Pancreas: Ultrasound, Computed Tomography, and Magnetic Resonance Imaging Features. Seminars in Ultrasound, CT, and MRI 28(5), 339-56(2007).

Spencer, L.A., Spizarny, D.L. & Williams, T.R. Imaging features of intrapancreatic accessory spleen. The British Journal of Radiology 83, 668-73(2010).

Triantopoulou, C. et al. Groove pancreatitis: a diagnostic challenge. European Radiology 19, 1736-43(2009).

Trout, A.T. et al. Imaging of acute pancreatitis: prognostic value of computed tomographic findings. Journal of Computer Assisted Tomography 34, 485-95(2010).

Vikram, R. et al. Pancreas: peritoneal reflections, ligamentous connections, and pathways of disease spread. Radiographics 29, e34(2011).

Spleen:

Boscak, A. & Shanmuganathan, K. Splenic trauma: what is new? Radiologic Clinics of North America, 50(1), 105-22(2012).

Elsayes, K.M. et al. MR imaging of the spleen: spectrum of abnormalities. Radiographics 25, 967-82(2005).

Gayer, G. et al. Congenital Anomalies of the Spleen. Seminars in Ultrasound, CT, and MRI 27, 358-369(2006).

Kamaya, A., Weinstein, S. & Desser, T. Multiple Lesions of the Spleen: Differential Diagnosis of Cystic and Solid Lesions. Seminars in Ultrasound, CT, and MRI 27, 389-403(2006).

Warshauer, D. & Hall, H. Solitary Splenic Lesions. Seminars in Ultrasound, CT, and MRI 27, 370-88(2006).

Esophagus and Stomach:

Carucci, L.R. & Turner, M.A. Imaging after bariatric surgery for morbid obesity: Roux-en-Y gastric bypass and laparoscopic adjustable gastric banding. Seminars in Roentgenology 44, 283-96(2009).

Blachar, A. et al. Radiographic manifestations of normal postoperative anatomy and gastrointestinal complications of bariatric surgery, with emphasis on CT imaging findings. Seminars in Ultrasound, CT, and MRI 25, 239-51(2004).

Oh, J.Y. et al. Benign submucosal lesions of the stomach and duodenum: imaging characteristics with endoscopic and pathologic correlation. European Journal of Radiology, 67(1), 112–24(2008).

Paroz, A., Calmes, J.M., Giusti, V. & Suter, M. Internal hernia after laparoscopic Roux-en-Y gastric bypass for morbid obesity: a continuous challenge in bariatric surgery. Obesity Surgery, 16(11), 1482-7(2006).

Patel, R.Y. et al. Internal hernia complications of gastric bypass surgery in the acute setting: spectrum of imaging findings. Emergency Radiology 16, 283-9(2009).

Sunnapwar, A. et al. Taxonomy and imaging spectrum of small bowel obstruction after Roux-en-Y gastric bypass surgery. AJR. American Journal of Roentgenology, 194(1), 120-8(2010).

Trenkner, S.W. Imaging of morbid obesity procedures and their complications. Abdominal Imaging, 34(3), 335-44(2009).

Small Bowel:

Dilauro, S. & Crum-Cianflone, N.F. Ileitis: when it is not Crohn's disease. Current Gastroenterology Reports 12, 249-58(2010).

Furukawa, A. et al. Cross-sectional Imaging in Crohn Disease 1. Radiographics 24, 689(2004).

Khurana, B. Signs in Imaging. The Whirl Sign. Radiology 1, 69-70(2003).

Khurana, B. et al. Bowel obstruction revealed by multidetector CT. AJR. American Journal of Roentgenology 178, 1139-44(2002).

Martin, L.C., Merkle, E.M. & Thompson, W.M. Review of internal hernias: radiographic and clinical findings. AJR. American Journal of Roentgenology 186, 703-17(2006).

Scholz F, Afnan J. CT Findings in Adult Celiac Disease. Radiographics 31, 977-93(2011).

Silva, A.C., Pimenta, M. & Guimarães, L.S. Small bowel obstruction: what to look for. Radiographics 29, 423-39(2009).

Soyer, P. et al. Celiac disease in adults: evaluation with MDCT enteroclysis. AJR. American Journal of Roentgenology 191, 1483-92(2008).

Takeyama, N. et al. CT of Internal Hernias. Radiographics 25, 997-1015(2005).

Colon:

Buckley, O. et al. Computed tomography in the imaging of colonic diverticulitis. Clinical Radiology 59, 977-83(2004).

Chintapalli, K.N. et al. Diverticulitis versus colon cancer: differentiation with helical CT findings. Radiology 210, 429-35(1999).

Cloutier, R.L. Neutropenic enterocolitis. Emergency Medicine Clinics of North America 27, 415-22(2009).

Kawamoto, S., Horton, K.M. & Fishman, E.K. Pseudomembranous colitis: spectrum of imaging findings with clinical and pathologic correlation. Radiographics 19, 887-97(1999).

Macari, M. & Balthazar, E.J. CT of bowel wall thickening: significance and pitfalls of interpretation. AJR. American Journal of Roentgenology 176, 1105-16(2001).

Macari, M., Balthazar, E.J. & Megibow, A.J. The accordion sign at CT: a nonspecific finding in patients with colonic edema. Radiology 211, 743-6(1999).

Moraitis, D. et al. Colonic wall thickening on computed tomography scan and clinical correlation. Does it suggest the presence of an underlying neoplasia? The American Surgeon 72, 269-71(2006).

Sarma, D. & Longo, W.E. Diagnostic imaging for diverticulitis. Journal of Clinical Gastroenterology 42, 1139-41(2008).

Taourel, P. et al. Imaging of ischemic colitis. Radiologic Clinics of North America 46, 909-24, vi(2008).

Touzios, J.G. & Dozois, E.J. Diverticulosis and acute diverticulitis. Gastroenterology Clinics of North America 38, 513-25(2009).

Peritoneum and Mesentery:

Levy, A. & Shaw, J. Secondary Tumors and Tumorlike Lesions of the Peritoneal Cavity: Imaging Features with Pathologic Correlation 1. Radiographics 29, 4799(2009).

Lucey, B.C., Stuhlfaut, J.W. & Soto, J.A. Mesenteric Lymph Nodes Seen at Imaging: Causes and Significance. Radiographics 25, 351(2005).

Mindelzun, R.E. et al. The misty mesentery on CT: differential diagnosis. American Journal of Roentgenology 167, 61(1996).

Sheth, S. et al. Mesenteric Neoplasms: CT Appearances of Primary and Secondary Tumors and Differential Diagnosis. Radiographics 23, 457-73(2003).

Smeenk, R.M., Bruin, S.C., van Velthuysen, M.-L.F., & Verwaal, V.J. Pseudomyxoma peritonei. Current Problems in Surgery, 45(8), 527-75(2008).

3 Genitourinary imaging

Contents

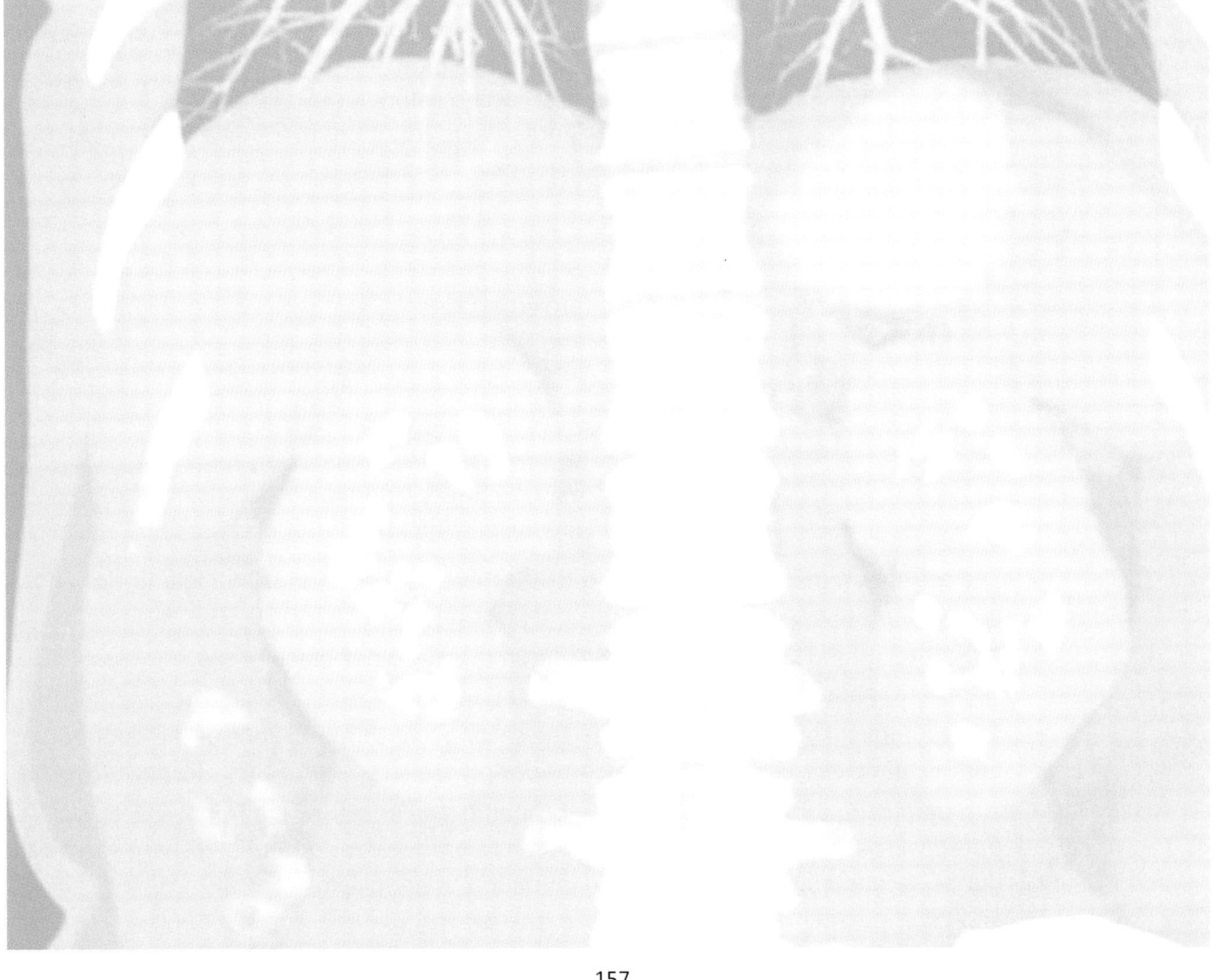

Retroperitoneum

Retroperitoneal anatomy

3 compartments of the retroperitoneum

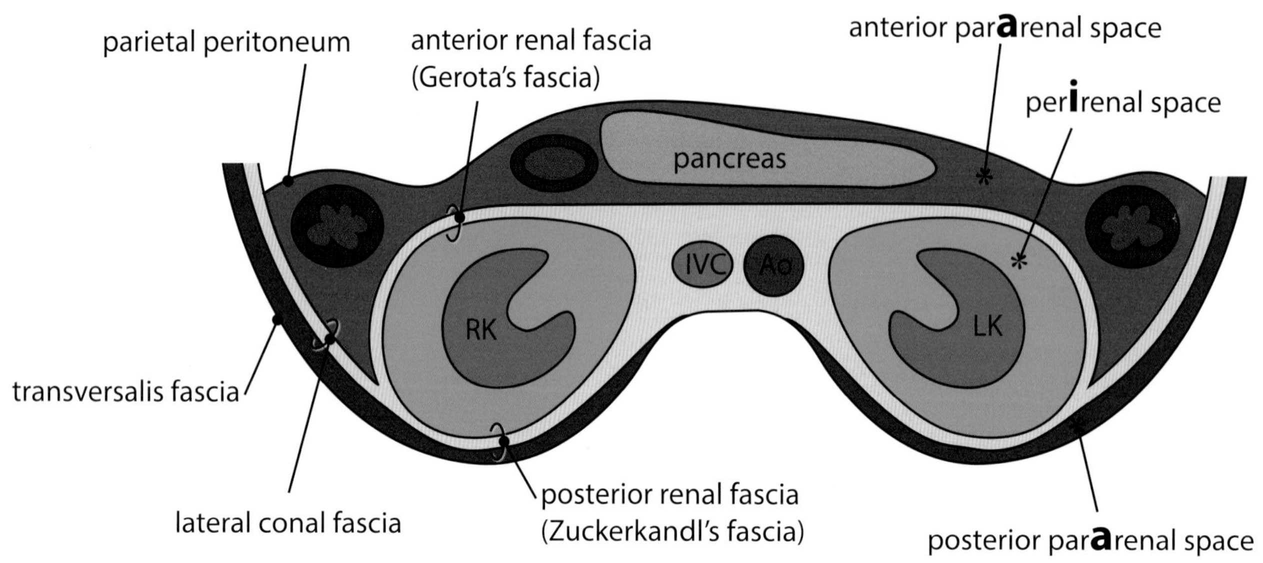

RK, right kidney
LK, left kidney
IVC, inferior vena cava
Ao, aorta

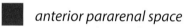

anterior pararenal space
- ascending colon
- descending colon
- (2nd and 3rd) duodenum
- pancreas

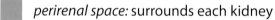

perirenal space: surrounds each kidney
- kidneys
- proximal ureter
- adrenals
- lots of fat

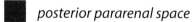

posterior pararenal space
- potential space, contains only fat
- may become secondarily involved in inflammatory processes

- The retroperitoneum can be separated into three compartments by the anterior and posterior renal fascia and the lateral conal fascia.
- The adrenals and kidneys are located within the perirenal space of the retroperitoneum.
- The ascending and descending colon, the second and third portions of the duodenum, and the pancreas are located in the anterior pararenal space of the retroperitoneum.
- The third compartment of the retroperitoneum, the posterior pararenal space, is a potential space that is clinically important as a pathway for potential disease spread due to secondary involvement of inflammation or neoplasm.

Liposarcoma

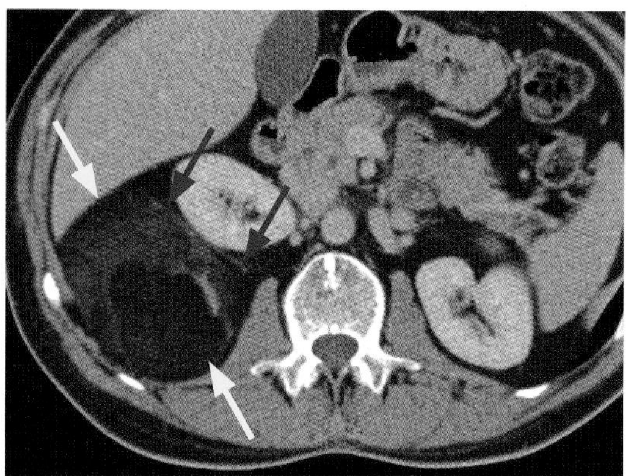
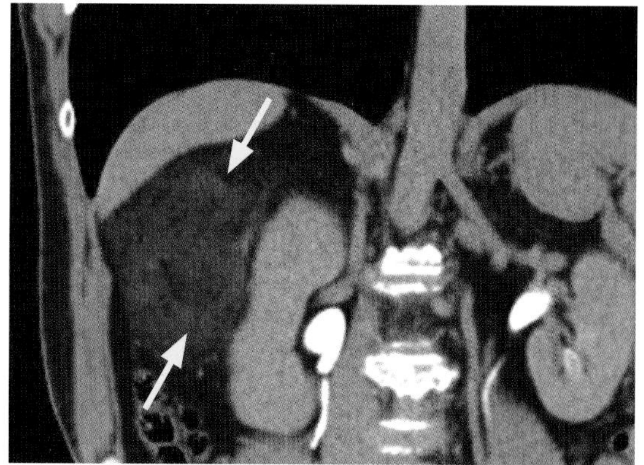

Retroperitoneal liposarcoma: Axial contrast-enhanced nephrographic phase (left image) and coronal pyelographic phase CT shows a predominantly fat-attenuation mass (yellow arrows) in the right posterior pararenal space, with Zuckerkandl's fascia (red arrows) separating the mass from the perirenal space. Pathology showed a well-differentiated adipocytic liposarcoma.

Case courtesy of Cheryl Sadow, MD, Brigham and Women's Hospital.

- Liposarcomas are a diverse group of neoplasms that make up the most common primary retroperitoneal tumors. 10–15% of all liposarcomas arise from the retroperitoneum.
- The most common type of liposarcoma is the well-differentiated group, which is composed of adipocytic, sclerosing, and inflammatory subtypes. Adipocytic liposarcoma resembles a lipoma, predominantly composed of fat with strands of tissue representing collagen bands.
- In order of increasing malignancy, liposarcomas may also be myxoid, round-cell, pleomorphic, or dedifferentiated. The more aggressive subtypes may have minimal or no areas of macroscopic fat and may be indistinguishable from other malignant soft-tissue masses.

Retroperitoneal fibrosis

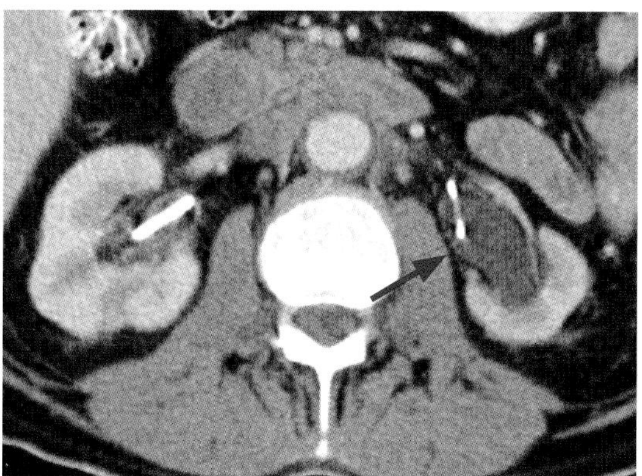
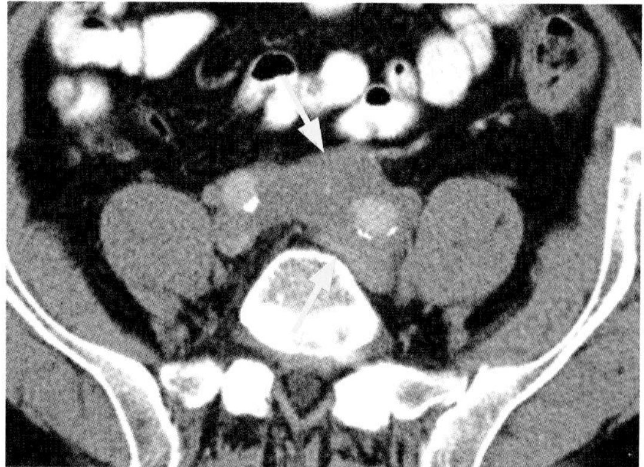

Retroperitoneal fibrosis: Axial contrast enhanced CT through the kidneys (left image) shows bilateral nephroureteral stents and left hydronephrosis (red arrow). Axial image through the lower abdomen shows a soft tissue mass (yellow arrows) surrounding the common iliac arteries, with no significant narrowing of the vessels.

Case courtesy of Cheryl Sadow, MD, Brigham and Women's Hospital.

- Retroperitoneal fibrosis is a rare inflammatory disorder causing increased fibrotic deposition in the retroperitoneum, often leading to ureteral obstruction.
- Unlike malignant retroperitoneal adenopathy, retroperitoneal fibrosis tends *not* to elevate the aorta off the spine.

Adrenal glands

Anatomy

- The adrenal glands are inverted Y-shaped endocrine glands, which primarily mediate the stress response by releasing cortisol and catecholamines. The adrenals are also a site of secondary sex hormone synthesis and blood pressure regulation (with aldosterone).
- The two distinct components to the adrenal glands are the cortex and the medulla, which are derived from completely different embryological origins (the cortex is derived from mesothelium; the medulla is derived from neural crest) and are susceptible to different diseases.

Adrenal cortex

- The adrenal cortex synthesizes the steroid hormones aldosterone, glucocorticoids, and androgens, which are all biochemical derivatives of cholesterol.
- Each of the three layers of the adrenal cortex synthesizes one type of hormone:

> **Zona glomerulosa** (most superficial): Produces aldosterone.
>
> **Zona fasciculata**: Produces glucocorticoids in response to pituitary adrenocorticotropic hormone (ACTH).
>
> **Zona reticularis** (deepest; closest to the adrenal medulla): Produces androgens.

- Pathology of the adrenal cortex that can be diagnosed on imaging includes adrenal hyperplasia, adrenal adenoma, and adrenal cortical carcinoma.

Adrenal medulla

- The adrenal medulla is the central portion of the adrenal gland and produces the catecholamines norepinephrine and epinephrine, which are derived from tyrosine.
- Pathology of the adrenal medulla includes pheochromocytoma and the neuroblastic tumors (ganglioneuroma, ganglioneuroblastoma, and neuroblastoma). Neuroblastoma is the most common extracranial solid tumor of childhood and is discussed in the pediatric imaging section.

Biochemical approach to adrenal lesions

- A patient may be suspected of having a hyperfunctioning adrenal lesion based on clinical symptoms or lab abnormalities. However, not all adrenal lesions produce adrenal hyperfunction.

Adrenal hyperfunction

- **Cushing syndrome** is excess cortisol production from non-pituitary disease, such as idiopathic adrenal hyperplasia, adrenal adenoma, or ectopic/paraneoplastic ACTH (e.g., from small cell lung cancer).
- **Cushing disease** is excess cortisol production driven by excessive *pituitary* ACTH.
- **Conn syndrome** is excess aldosterone production, most commonly from an adrenal adenoma, which causes hypertension and hypokalemia. The adenomas implicated in Conn syndrome are typically small and may be difficult to detect on CT. Localizing the side of excess hormone production with venous sampling may be a helpful diagnostic adjunct.
- **Adrenal cortical carcinoma** is a very rare adrenal malignancy that arises from the cortex and typically causes a disordered increase in all cortical adrenal hormones and precursors.
- **Pheochromocytoma** is a usually benign tumor of the adrenal medulla that causes an increase in catecholamines.

Adrenal hypofunction

- Significant destruction of the adrenals is required to produce adrenal insufficiency.
- Although usually not an imaging diagnosis, Addison disease represents chronic adrenocortical insufficiency and may be caused by autoimmune destruction of the adrenal glands or as a sequela of infection.
- Waterhouse–Friderichsen syndrome is post-hemorrhagic adrenal failure secondary to *Neisseria meningitidis* bacteremia.
- Idiopathic adrenal hemorrhage is usually unilateral and rarely causes adrenal hypofunction.

IMAGING OF ADRENAL ADENOMA AND THE INDETERMINATE ADRENAL MASS

Adrenal adenoma

- Adrenal adenoma is a benign tumor of the adrenal cortex. Adenomas are usually incidental, but they may occasionally produce excess aldosterone to cause secondary hypertension (Conn syndrome). Non-contrast imaging of the adrenal glands is the best test to evaluate for the presence of an adrenal adenoma in the presence of suspicious clinical symptoms or lab values.
- A common clinical scenario is the need to differentiate between an adrenal adenoma and an adrenal metastasis in the staging of a patient with known malignancy. The diagnosis of an adenoma is made by the detection of intracellular lipid.
- An adrenal nodule attenuating ≤10 Hounsfield units (HU) can be reliably diagnosed as an adenoma with no further imaging or follow-up needed. Most (80%) adenomas are lipid-rich and will attenuate below this cutoff. Up to 20% may be lipid-poor adenomas, which attenuate >10 HU and are not able to be diagnosed on a noncontrast CT.

  An indeterminate (>10 HU), small, homogeneous adrenal lesion in a patient without a known malignancy is overwhelmingly likely to represent a lipid-poor adenoma, and advanced imaging is usually not required in such cases.

- If the nodule in question attenuates >10 HU and clinical confirmation of an adenoma is necessary for clinical management (for instance, in a patient with lung cancer and no evidence of metastatic disease but with an indeterminate adrenal nodule), then an adrenal washout CT or in- and out-of-phase MRI may be helpful to characterize the lesion.
- A *collision tumor* represents metastasis into an adrenal gland with a pre-existing adenoma.

  If an "adenoma" appears heterogeneous or has shown an interval increase in size, then a collision tumor should be considered in a patient with a known primary even if a region attenuates <10 HU.

MRI adrenal imaging: Chemical shift imaging = in- and out-of-phase imaging

- Adenomas contain intracytoplasmic lipid due to steroid production. MRI is able to detect even a small amount of intracytoplasmic lipid that may be undetectable on CT by taking advantage of the fact that protons resonate at different frequencies in fat and in water.

  Chemical shift imaging consists of images obtained both in-phase and out-of-phase. When fat and water are contained within the same voxel, out-of-phase images show fat drop-out of signal because fat protons are more shielded and resonate at a slower frequency. Chemical shift imaging is based on T1 images.

- Adenomas suppress on out-of-phase images, while metastases generally do not.
- A short list of malignancies do contain intracytoplasmic lipid and thus would *also* lose signal on out-of-phase images:

  Well-differentiated adrenocortical carcinoma (very rare).

  Clear cell renal cell carcinomas metastatic to the adrenal gland.

  Hepatocellular carcinoma metastatic to the adrenal gland.

  Liposarcoma (typically a predominantly fatty mass that is rarely confused with adrenal adenoma).

- Adrenal adenomas demonstrate more rapid contrast washout than metastases do. The more rapid contrast washout of benign adenomas appears to be true even compared to adrenal metastases of hypervascular primaries.
- The timing of the washout phase remains controversial, with recent evidence suggesting 15-minute washout has greater sensitivity than 10 minutes.
- **>60% absolute washout is diagnostic of adenoma**.

$$\textbf{\% washout} = \frac{\mathbf{E-D}}{\mathbf{E-U}} = \frac{\text{enhanced attenuation} - \text{delayed attenuation}}{\text{enhanced attenuation} - \text{unenhanced attenuation}}$$

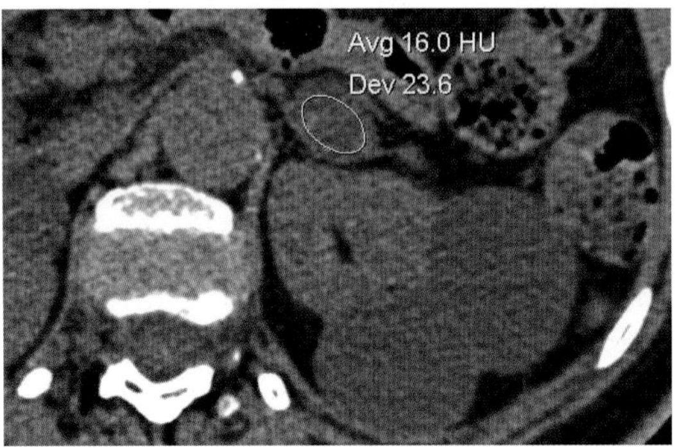

Precontrast

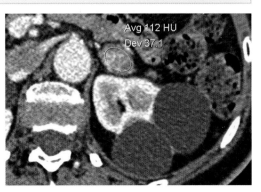

60-second post-contrast (adrenal parenchymal phase)

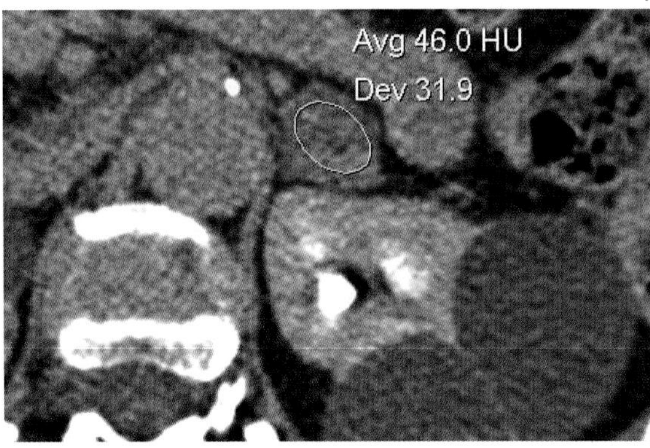

15-minute delay washout

Adrenal adenoma. Axial images from adrenal washout-protocol CT show an adrenal nodule measuring 16 HU precontrast, 112 HU at 60 seconds, and 46 HU on 15 minute washout.

Using the washout formula E – D/E – U:
(112 – 46) / (112 – 16) = 69% washout
>60% washout is diagnostic of an adenoma.

Note is made of two large simple cysts of the left kidney.

Case courtesy of Cheryl Sadow, MD, Brigham and Women's Hospital.

- If unenhanced CT is not available or not performed due to concern for radiation exposure,
>40% relative washout is diagnostic of adenoma:

$$\textbf{\% relative washout} = \frac{\mathbf{E-D}}{\mathbf{E}} = \frac{\text{enhanced attenuation} - \text{delayed attenuation}}{\text{enhanced attenuation}}$$

- In a patient with a known primary malignancy, lesions that do not demonstrate benign washout kinetics are suspicious for, but not diagnostic of, metastasis.

Role of biopsy of an adrenal mass

- Adrenal mass biopsy is indicated for an indeterminate adrenal mass after full imaging workup remains nondiagnostic.
- Biopsy is safe and generally very accurate.

Myelolipoma

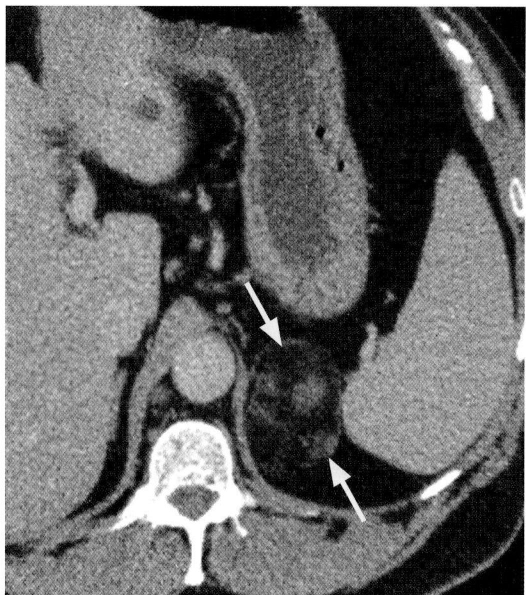
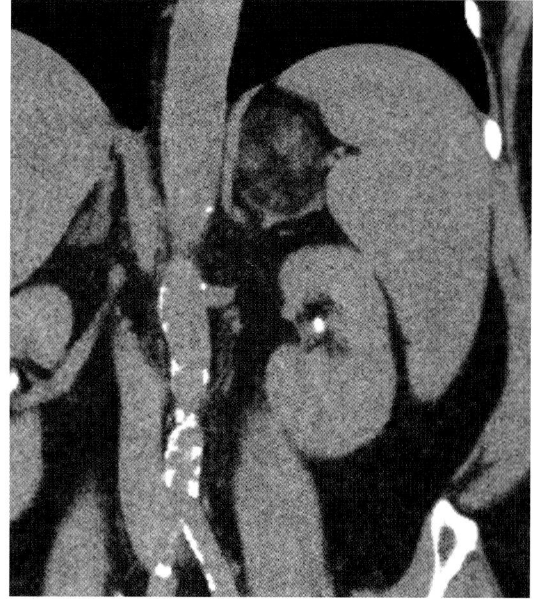

Adrenal myelolipoma. Axial (left image) and coronal (right image) CT shows a predominantly fatty mass with a few circumscribed foci of soft-tissue attenuation in the left adrenal (arrows). The mass is clearly distinct from the kidney, as best seen on the coronal image.

Case courtesy of Cheryl Sadow, MD, Brigham and Women's Hospital.

- An adrenal myelolipoma is a benign neoplasm consisting of myeloid cells (i.e., erythrocyte precursors – *not* "myo" as in muscle) and fat cells.
- An adrenal mass with any discrete focus of macroscopic fat is virtually diagnostic of a myelolipoma. Exceedingly rare cases of adrenocortical carcinoma and metastatic carcinoma have been reported to contain macroscopic fat. A retroperitoneal liposarcoma may mimic a myelolipoma, although liposarcoma typically presents as a large mass that may displace, rather than arise from, the adrenal.
- An adrenal myelolipoma should not be confused with a *renal angiomyolipoma (AML).* These two entities are unrelated, although they do have similar names, are located in adjacent organs, and are both diagnosed by the presence of macroscopic fat.

Adrenal cyst

- Adrenal cysts are uncommon but have imaging characteristics typical of cysts elsewhere (thin, smooth, nonenhancing wall, and water-attenuation internal contents).
- Endothelial adrenal cysts are the most common (45%) type and may be lymphatic or angiomatous in origin.
- Pseudocysts secondary to adrenal hemorrhage represent 39% of adrenal cysts and lack an epithelial lining. Peripheral calcification may be present.
- Epithelial cysts are rare, comprising only 9% of adrenal cysts.
- Occasionally an adrenal cyst may have a complex appearance that may be difficult to differentiate from a cystic/necrotic neoplasm. In such a case, percutaneous aspiration or surgical resection may be considered.
- Small, asymptomatic, simple cysts can be ignored. A cyst may rarely grow so large as to cause symptoms, such as dull pain or compression of the stomach/duodenum, in which case surgery may be indicated.
- Very rarely, hydatid disease may affect the adrenal glands, typically producing a complex cystic lesion with an internal membrane.

Pheochromocytoma: Potentially malignant

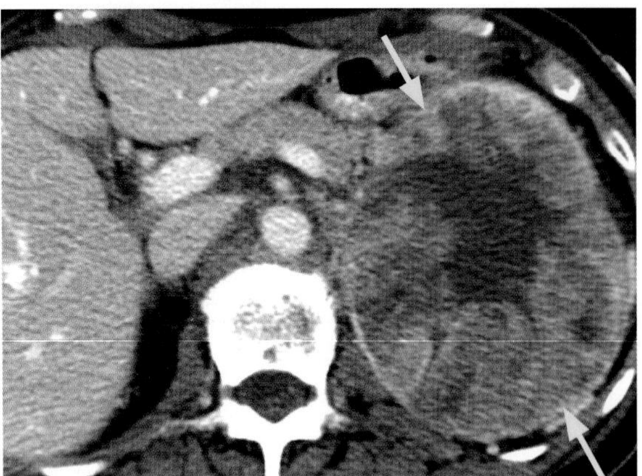
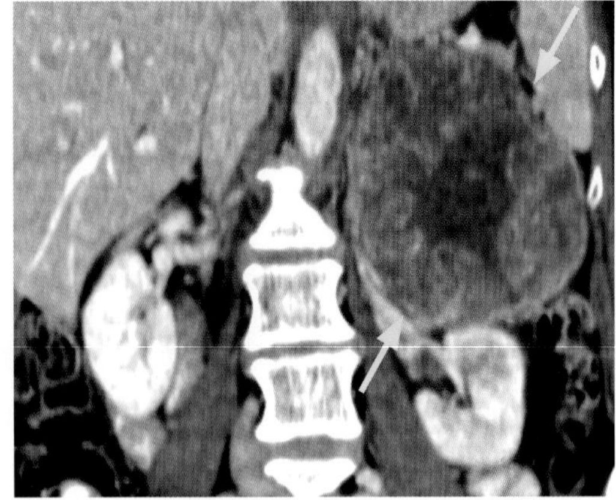

Pheochromocytoma: Contrast enhanced axial (left image) and coronal (right image) CT shows a large, heterogeneous mass (arrows) with central necrosis arising superior to the left kidney. The extra-renal origin is best seen on the coronal image.

- Pheochromocytoma is a neoplasm of chromaffin cells, usually arising from the adrenal medulla. Pheochromocytoma may cause hypertension and episodic headaches/ diaphoresis.
- The "rule of 10's" is a general rule characterizing the features of pheochromocytomas:

> 10% are extra-adrenal.
>
> 10% are bilateral.
>
> 10% are malignant.
>
> 10% are familial or syndromic.

- Pheochromocytoma is associated with several syndromes:

> **Multiple endocrine neoplasia** (MEN) 2A and 2B: Typically bilateral intra-adrenal pheochromocytomas.
>
> **von Hippel–Lindau**.
>
> **Neurofibromatosis type 1**.
>
> **Carney's triad** (gastric leiomyosarcoma, pulmonary chondroma, and extra-adrenal pheochromocytoma).

- An extra-adrenal pheochromocytoma is a paraganglioma. The most common intra-abdominal location of a paraganglioma is the organ of Zuckerkandl, located at the aortic bifurcation. A rare intra-abdominal location of a paraganglioma is the bladder, producing the distinctive clinical presentation of post-micturition syncope (syncope after urination).
- Paragangliomas occur in the head and neck in characteristic locations. Paragangliomas of the head and neck are generally called glomus tumors and may be associated with the tympanic membrane (glomus tympanicum), the jugular foramen (glomus jugulare), the carotid body (called a carotid body tumor), or the vagus nerve (glomus vagale).
- Nuclear medicine studies can be used in the workup of pheochromocytoma. Of note, I-123 MIBG is used for metastatic workup of adrenal pheochromocytoma and Indium-111 pentetreotide (an analog of octreotide) is used as tracer for localization of a paraganglioma.
- In theory, pheochromocytoma should be diagnosed by urine/plasma metanephrines before imaging is performed, with imaging used for localization and staging. In clinical practice, CT is often employed based on suspicious symptoms (such as episodic hypertension or other symptoms of catecholamine excess).

- The classic MRI appearance of pheochromocytoma is a hyperintense mass on T2-weighted images. When large, pheochromocytoma may appear heterogeneous on MRI and CT.

Adrenal cortical carcinoma

- Adrenal cortical carcinoma is a very rare malignancy, with a prevalence of approximately 1/1,000,000. Approximately 66% are functional, producing a disordered array of hormones that may manifest as Cushing syndrome, hyperaldosteronism, and virilization.
- Adrenal cortical carcinoma usually presents on imaging as a large, heterogeneous mass. Central necrosis and hemorrhage are typical.

Metastasis

- Autopsy studies show adrenal metastases are present in >25% of patients with a known primary. Lung cancer and melanoma are the most common adrenal metastases.

Lymphoma

- Primary adrenal lymphoma is rare.

Diffuse adrenal disorders

Adrenal hyperplasia

- Adrenal hyperplasia is caused by prolonged stress response or ectopic ACTH secretion.

Adrenal hemorrhage

- Adrenal hemorrhage can be spontaneous or due to anticoagulation. When secondary to anticoagulation, the hemorrhage typically occurs within the first few weeks of beginning anticoagulation. Hemorrhage involves the right adrenal gland more commonly than the left.
- Hemorrhage may appear mass-like and is often of heterogeneous attenuation on CT. The most important clue is a new adrenal mass within a short time interval if priors are available.
- Hemorrhage does not enhance and decreases in size on follow-up studies.

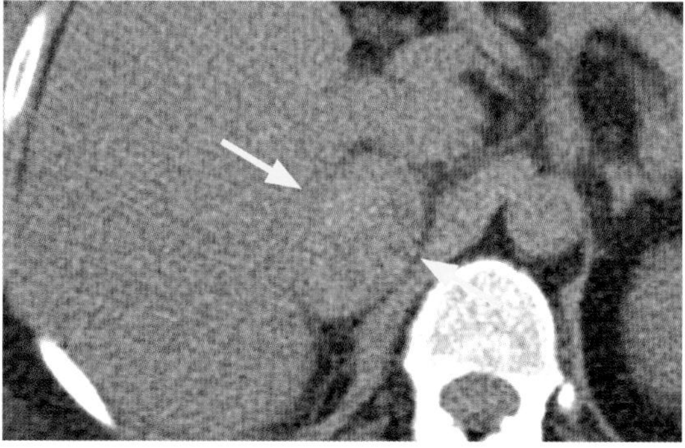

Noncontrast axial CT

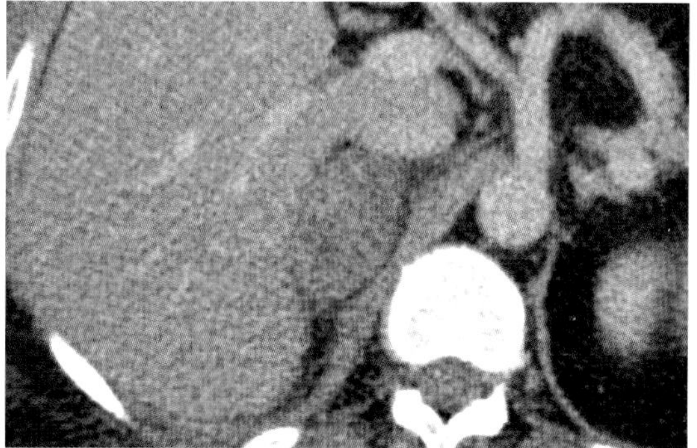

60-second delay post-contrast axial CT

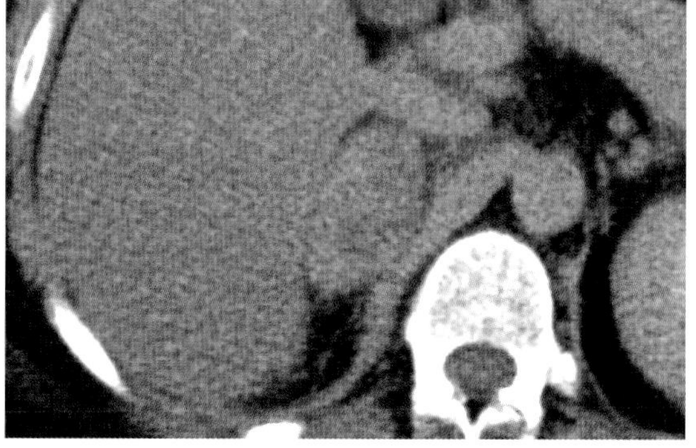

15-minute delay washout axial CT

Adrenal hemorrhage:

Multiphase adrenal mass CT demonstrates a nonenhancing right adrenal mass (arrows) that attenuates 46 Hounsfield units on all three phases.

The mass is new compared to imaging from two weeks prior (not shown).

Adrenal calcification

- Adrenal calcification rarely causes adrenal hypofunction. Adrenal calcification can be due to Wegener granulomatosis, tuberculosis, histoplasmosis, or old hemorrhage.

DIAGNOSTIC APPROACH TO A RENAL MASS

Renal mass protocol multiphase CT

- A renal mass protocol CT consists of at least three phases of data acquisition, with each phase providing important information to aid in the diagnosis of a renal mass.
- **Unenhanced** phase: Necessary as a baseline to quantify enhancement.
- **Nephrographic** phase (100 second delay): The nephrographic phase is the critical phase for evaluating for enhancement, comparing to the unenhanced images.
- **Pyelographic** phase (15 minute delay; also called the excretory phase): The pyelographic phase is helpful for problem solving and to diagnose potential mimics of cystic renal masses.

  The pyelographic phase can distinguish between hydronephrosis (will show dense opacification in the pyelographic phase) and renal sinus cysts (will not opacify).

  Reflux nephropathy may cause a dilated calyx that can simulate a cystic renal mass on the nephrographic phase. The pyelographic phase would show opacification of the dilated calyx.

  The pyelographic phase is also useful to demonstrate a calyceal diverticulum and to show the relationship of a renal mass to the collecting system for surgical planning.
- Optionally, a vascular phase can be performed for presurgical planning.

Evaluating enhancement (CT and MRI)

- The presence of enhancement is the most important characteristic to distinguish between a benign and malignant non-fat-containing renal mass (a lesion containing intralesional fat is almost always a benign angiomyolipoma, even if it enhances).
- On CT, enhancement is quantified as the *absolute* increase in Hounsfield units on post-contrast images, compared to pre-contrast:

<10 HU: No enhancement.	10–19 HU: Equivocal enhancement.	≥20 HU: Enhancement.

- On MRI, enhancement is quantified as the *percent* increase in signal intensity as measured on post-contrast images:

<15%: No enhancement.	15–19%: Equivocal enhancement.	≥20%: Enhancement.

- Lesions are considered "too small to characterize" if the lesion diameter is smaller than twice the slice thickness. For instance, using 3 mm slices, a lesion less than 6 mm cannot be accurately characterized based on attenuation or enhancement.

Renal mass biopsy

- After full imaging workup is complete, there are several well-accepted indications for percutaneous renal mass biopsy:

Indications for renal mass biopsy

- To distinguish renal cell carcinoma from metastasis in a patient with a known primary.
- To distinguish between renal infection and cystic neoplasm.
- To definitively diagnose a hyperdense, homogeneously enhancing mass (after MRI has been performed), which may represent a benign angiomyolipoma with minimal fat versus a renal cell carcinoma.
- To definitively diagnose a suspicious renal mass in patient with multiple comorbidities for whom nephrectomy would be high risk.
- To ensure correct tissue diagnosis prior to renal mass ablation.

Renal cell carcinoma (RCC)

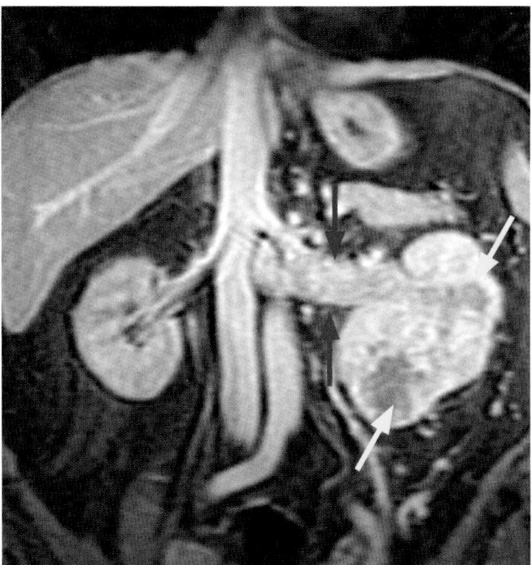

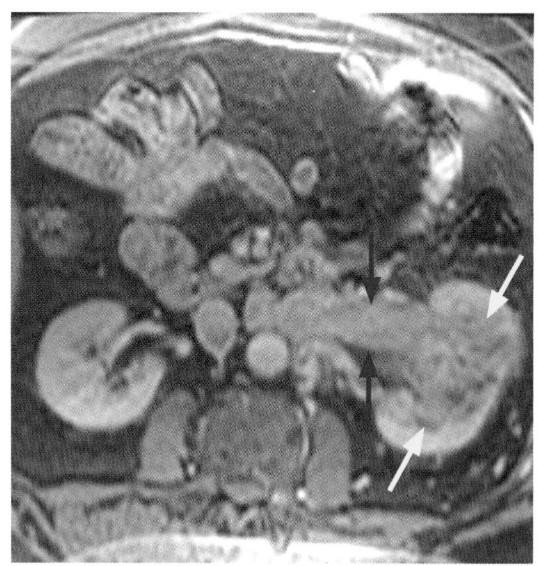

Renal cell carcinoma, stage 3A: Coronal (left image) and axial post-contrast fat-suppressed T1-weighted MRI shows a heterogeneously enhancing mass (yellow arrows) replacing and expanding most of the left kidney. Contiguous to the mass there is expansion and heterogeneous enhancement of the left renal vein (red arrows), representing tumor thrombus and extension of the renal carcinoma into the renal vein.

Case courtesy of Cheryl Sadow, MD, Brigham and Women's Hospital.

- Renal cell carcinoma (RCC) is a relatively uncommon tumor that arises from the renal tubular cells. It represents 2–3% of all cancers. Risk factors for development of RCC include smoking, acquired cystic kidney disease, von Hippel–Lindau (VHL), and tuberous sclerosis.
- **Clear cell** is the most common RCC subtype (~75%), with approximately 55% 5-year survival.

  Clear cell RCC tends to enhance more avidly than the less common subtypes.

  Clear cell can be sporadic or associated with von Hippel–Lindau.
- **Papillary** RCC is a hypovascular subtype, with a 5-year survival of 80–90%.

  Papillary RCC tends to enhance only mildly due to its hypovascularity.

  A renal "adenoma" is frequently seen on autopsy specimens and is a papillary carcinoma ≤5 mm.
- **Chromophobe** is the subtype with the best prognosis, featuring a 90% 5-year survival.
- **Collecting duct carcinoma** is rare and has a poor prognosis.
- **Medullary carcinoma** is also rare, but is known to affect mostly young adult males with sickle cell trait. Medullary carcinoma is an extremely aggressive neoplasm, with a mean survival of 15 months, not helped by chemotherapy.
- Staging of renal cell carcinoma is based on the Robson system, which characterizes fascial extension and vascular/lymph node involvement. Stages I–III are usually resectable, although the surgical approach may need to be altered for venous invasion (stages IIIA and IIIC).

Stage I: Tumor confined to within the renal capsule.

Stage II: Tumor extends out of the renal capsule but remains confined within Gerota's fascia.

Stage III: Vascular and/or lymph node involvement.

IIIA: Renal vein involvement or IVC involvement.

IIIB: Lymph node involvement.

IIIC: Venous *and* lymph node involvement.

Stage IVA: Tumor growth through Gerota's fascia; **Stage IVB**: Distant metastasis.

Angiomyolipoma (AML)

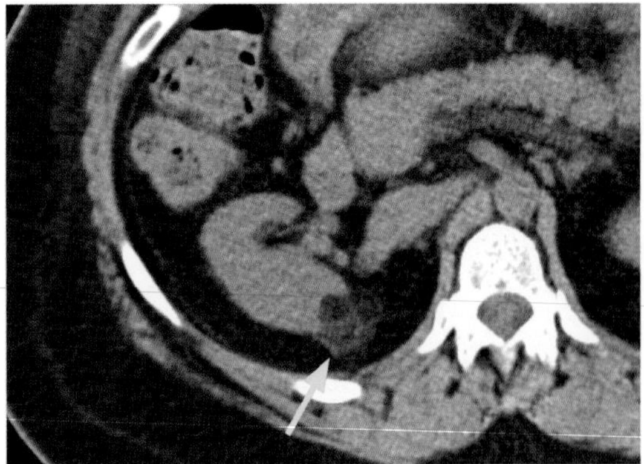

Axial non-contrast CT shows an exophytic mass (arrow) in the right kidney containing macroscopic fat. There are a few linear strands of soft tissue within the lesion.

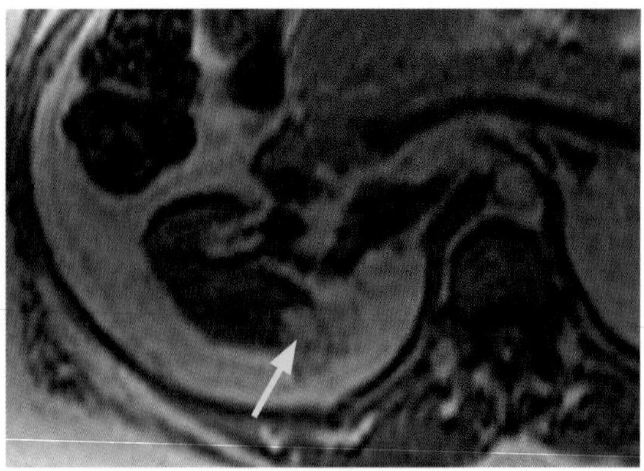

Axial T1-weighted MRI shows that the lesion is predominantly isointense to intra-abdominal fat.

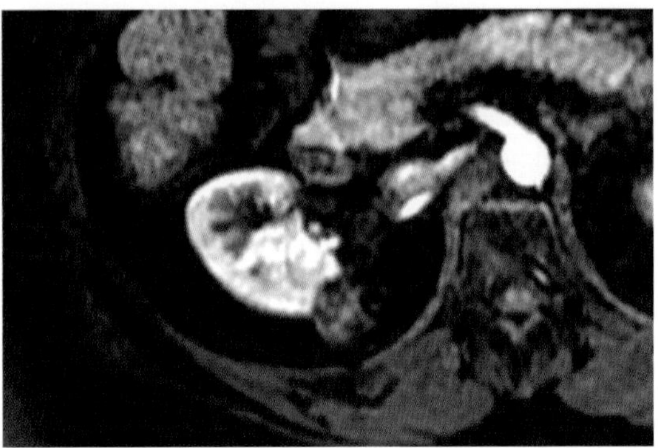

Axial early arterial post-contrast T1-weighted fat suppressed image shows slight enhancement of the soft tissue components.

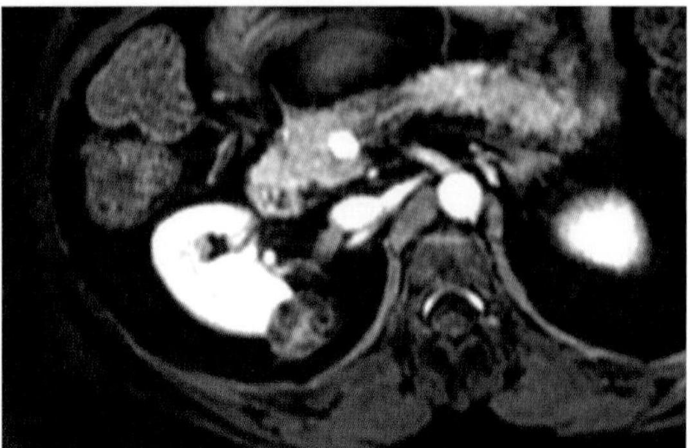

Late arterial post-contrast T1-weighted fat suppressed image shows more prominent enhancement of the soft tissue components of the lesion.

Case courtesy of Cheryl Sadow, MD, Brigham and Women's Hospital.

- Angiomyolipoma (AML) is the most common benign renal neoplasm, composed of fat, smooth muscle, and disorganized blood vessels. The majority are sporadic, but 40% are associated with tuberous sclerosis (where AMLs are bilateral, with multiple renal cysts).
- AML has a risk of hemorrhage when large (≥4 cm), thought to be due to aneurysmal change of the vascular elements. Small, asymptomatic AMLs are not typically followed or resected.
- A early pathognomonic imaging finding is the presence of macroscopic fat in a non-calcified renal lesion. The non fat-containing portion enhances avidly and homogeneously. Calcification is almost never present.
- On MRI, the fat component will follow retroperitoneal fat on all sequences and will saturate out on fat-saturated sequences. Intracytoplasmic lipid is not a feature of AML, so there should be no significant signal drop-out on dual-phase MRI.
- Approximately 4% of AMLs will not contain visible macroscopic fat and will appear as a hyperdense enhancing mass. MRI is the next step, with the T2-weighted images the most useful to distinguish from renal cell carcinoma in some cases.

  A T2 hyperintense mass suggests RCC (clear cell subtype) and the patient can proceed to surgery.

  A T2 hypointense mass is nonspecific and can represent either RCC (papillary type) or AML with minimal fat. Although an AML typically would enhance more avidly than a papillary RCC, biopsy is warranted for definitive diagnosis.
- AML appears hyperechoic on ultrasound, although up to 1/3 of renal cell carcinomas may also be hyperechoic and ultrasound is thus unreliable to distinguish AML from RCC.

Oncocytoma

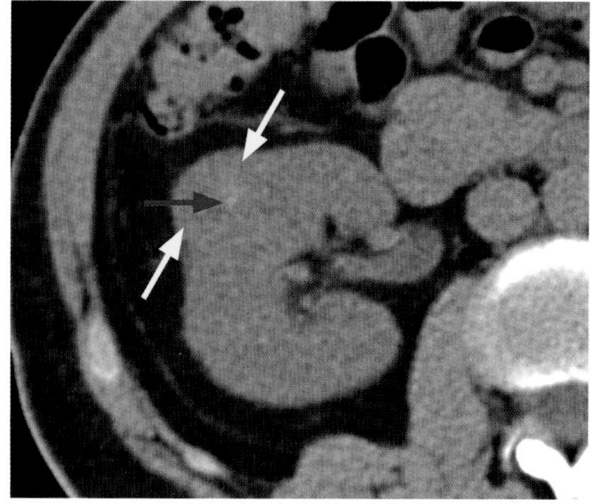

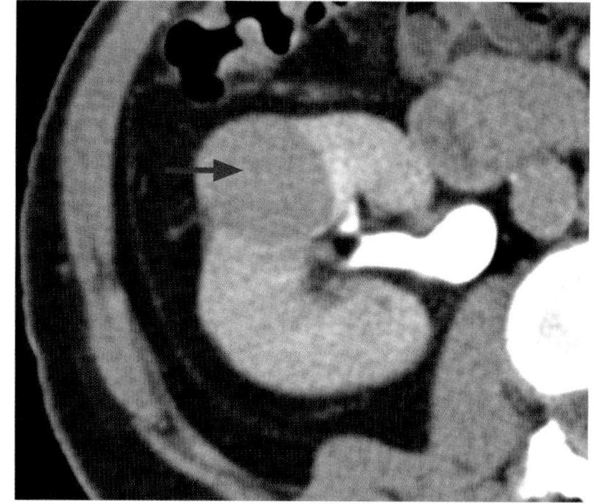

Oncocytoma. Noncontrast CT (left image) shows an isodense renal mass (yellow arrows) containing a central punctate focus of hyperattenuation (red arrow). The contrast-enhanced pyelographic phase CT (right image)demonstrates that the mass enhances. There is a faint suggestion of a central focus of non-enhancement (red arrow), corresponding to a central scar.

- Oncocytoma is the most commonly resected benign renal mass and has overlapping imaging findings with renal cell carcinoma.
- Imaging features can *suggest* oncocytoma, but imaging features are not specific and cannot be reliably differentiated from RCC. The imaging features suggestive of oncocytoma are homogeneous enhancement and a central scar.
- Complicating the pathologic diagnosis, oncocytic cells can sometimes be found in the rare chromophobe RCC subtype. The pathologist can usually distinguish oncocytoma from the more common clear cell and papillary renal cell carcinoma subtypes.

Renal lymphoma

- Primary renal lymphoma is rare, as the kidneys do not contain native lymphoid tissue. However, the kidneys may become involved from hematogenously disseminated disease or spread from the retroperitoneum.
- Renal involvement of lymphoma has several patterns of disease:

> Multiple lymphomatous masses (most common pattern; seen in 50% of cases of renal lymphoma).
>
> Solitary renal mass.
>
> Diffuse lymphomatous infiltration, causing nephromegaly.
>
> Direct extension of retroperitoneal disease.

Non-neoplastic solid renal masses

- When evaluating a potential renal mass, it's important to always consider that an apparent solid renal mass may represent a non-neoplastic lesion.
- **Infection**, especially focal pyelonephritis, can masquerade as a solid renal mass. Renal abscess may be difficult to differentiate on imaging from a cystic renal cell carcinoma.
- **Renal arteriovenous malformation** (AVM) will avidly enhance and can mimic a hypervascular renal mass. One clue to the presence of an AVM would be asymmetric enhancement of the renal vein on the affected side, due to early shunting of venous blood.

Renal pseudotumors

- Renal pseudotumors are normal variations of renal morphology that may mimic a renal mass.
- **Hypertrophied column of Bertin**: The columns (septa) of Bertin are normal structures that anchor the renal cortex to the hilum and create the separations between the renal pyramids. When hypertrophied, the columns of Bertin may mimic a renal mass.
- **Persistent fetal lobation/lobulation**: In normal fetal development, the fetal kidneys are divided into discrete lobes. Occasionally these lobulations persist in adulthood, producing an indentation of the renal cortex. This indentation can cause an adjacent focal bulge that simulates a renal mass. This pseudomass can usually be distinguished from a true mass by the presence of septa of Bertin on either side.

SYNDROMES WITH RENAL MASSES (ALL HAVE INCREASED RISK OF RCC)

von Hippel–Lindau (VHL)

- von Hippel–Lindau (VHL) is an autosomal dominant multiorgan syndrome caused by a mutation in the VHL tumor suppressor gene on chromosome 3, which leads to cysts and neoplasms in multiple organs.
- The primary manifestation of VHL in the genitourinary system is bilateral or multifocal renal cell carcinomas, most commonly the clear-cell subtype.
- Other genitourinary manifestations of VHL include multifocal pheochromocytoma and renal cysts.
- Central nervous system manifestations of VHL include hemangioblastoma of the brainstem, cerebellum, or spinal cord.
- Pancreatic and hepatic manifestations include malignant neuroendocrine pancreatic tumor, pancreatic serous cystadenoma (a benign neoplasm), and pancreatic/hepatic cysts.

Birt–Hogg–Dube

- Birt–Hogg–Dube is an autosomal dominant syndrome of dermatologic lesions, cystic lung disease, and multiple renal oncocytomas and renal cell carcinomas.

Tuberous sclerosis (TS)

- Tuberous sclerosis is an autosomal dominant neurocutaneous disease caused by a tumor suppressor gene mutation. It manifests clinically with seizures, developmental delay, and (mostly) benign tumors in multiple organ systems.
- The most common renal manifestation of tuberous sclerosis is multiple bilateral renal angiomyolipomas (AMLs). Approximately 50% of patients with TS will have at least one AML.
- Renal cysts can be seen in ~25%.
- The relative risk of renal cell carcinoma is increased in patients with TS, and occurs in approximately 2–3% of patients. Diagnosis of renal cell carcinoma is complicated by the abnormal kidneys that may have multiple cysts and/or AMLs.
- In the heart, the most common neoplasm is a rhabdomyoma. A cardiac rhabdomyoma may be present during fetal life and can be detected by fetal ultrasound.
- In the lung, a process of smooth muscle proliferation identical to lymphangioleiomyomatosis can occur, causing cystic replacement of lung parenchyma. It has been suggested that the abnormal smooth muscle in the lung in patients with TS represents genetically identical metastatic smooth muscle from a renal angiomyolipoma.

APPROACH TO A CYSTIC RENAL MASS

- A cystic renal mass may be neoplastic or infectious; the two most common entities to cause a cystic renal mass are renal cell carcinoma and renal abscess.

Neoplastic differential of a cystic renal mass

- **Cystic renal cell carcinoma.** Although renal cell carcinoma most commonly presents as a solid renal mass, it can also manifest as a cystic renal mass.
- **Multilocular cystic nephroma** is a benign cystic neoplasm with enhancing septa that occurs in a bimodal age distribution in baby boys and middle-aged women. A characteristic but nonspecific feature is the propensity to herniate into the renal pelvis, causing hydronephrosis.

  In adults, multilocular cystic nephroma can be indistinguishable from cystic renal cell carcinoma.

  In children, multilocular cystic nephroma can be indistinguishable from cystic Wilms tumor.
- **Mixed epithelial and stromal tumor (MEST)** is a benign neoplasm composed of epithelial and mesenchymal elements, typically found in middle-aged women. MEST may appear as either a solid or cystic mass.

Non-neoplastic differential of a cystic renal mass

- **Renal abscess** is a contained purulent collection within the kidney.
- **Hemorrhagic renal cyst**, which will not have any enhancing component.

Role of MRI in evaluation of a complex cystic renal mass

- MRI has a limited role in the evaluation of a cystic renal mass. The key advantage of MRI is more accurate enhancement characterization, as MRI does not suffer from the CT phenomenon of pseudoenhancement due to beam hardening from adjacent, densely enhancing renal parenchyma.

  The increased accuracy of MRI to characterize enhancement is most useful to distinguish a Bosniak IIF from a Bosniak III lesion. Thickening of a septation or cyst wall that shows measurable enhancement defines a Bosniak III lesion. The Bosniak classification is discussed on the following page.
- MRI is more sensitive for detecting septations compared to CT.
- Calcifications are more difficult to detect with MRI.

RENAL CYSTS AND CYSTIC RENAL MASSES

Simple renal cyst

- Simple renal cysts are extremely common, found in approximately 50% of patients over age 50. A simple renal cyst is an incidental lesion that requires no follow-up, even when large.
- On CT a simple cyst must attenuate close to 0 Hounsfield units, not contain any enhancing components, and have a thin imperceptible wall.
- On MRI, a simple cyst must be hypointense on T1-weighted images, hyperintense on T2-weighted images, and not contain any enhancing component.

Renal sinus cyst

- Cysts in the renal sinus may be classified as **parapelvic** and **peripelvic** cysts. A parapelvic cyst is a renal cortical cyst that herniates into the renal sinus. These cysts are usually large but solitary. Peripelvic cysts, in contrast, are lymphatic in origin and usually small and multiple.

Hyperdense cyst

- A homogeneous renal cyst with an attenuation of >70 Hounsfield units on noncontrast imaging represents a benign hyperdense cyst, likely secondary to prior hemorrhage.
- A hyperdense cyst cannot be diagnosed if only post-contrast imaging is available as there is no way to distinguish a hyperdense cyst from an enhancing renal mass.

Bosniak classification of cystic renal masses

- The Bosniak classification risk-stratifies cystic renal masses, with increasing risk for cystic renal cell carcinoma with increasing Bosniak category. Classification is based on morphology, not size (except for hyperdense cysts in categories II and IIF).

> **Category I and II**: No risk of malignancy. No follow-up necessary.
>
> **Category IIF**: Small risk of malignancy. Imaging follow-up is needed.
>
> **Category III and IV**: Surgical lesions, concerning for cystic renal cell carcinoma.

- Category I

  Water-attenuation cyst, with a hairline wall and no areas of enhancement. Practically, this classification is never used as such a lesion is simply called a simple renal cyst.

  Always benign. No follow-up needed.

- Category II

  Water-attenuation cyst containing a few (3 or fewer) hairline septa. May contain fine septal calcification. No enhancement.

  Also includes small (<3 cm) hyperattenuating cysts without enhancement.

  Essentially always benign.
  No follow-up needed.

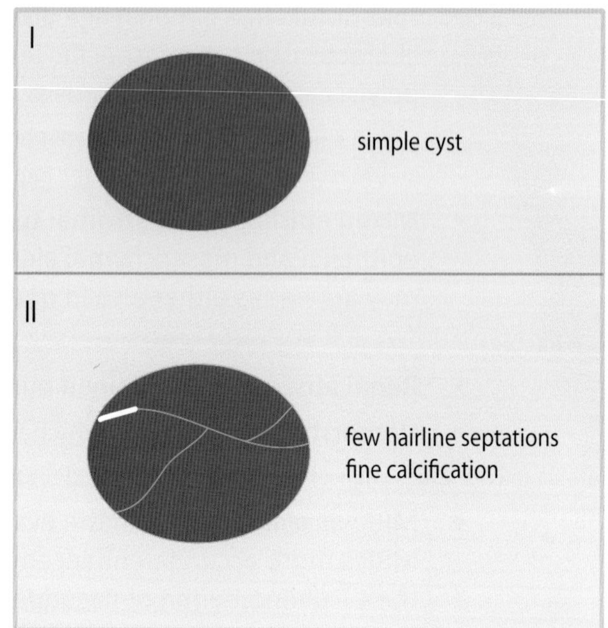

- Category IIF

  Multiple septa, with minimal smooth thickening (3 mm or less). May have thick and nodular mural calcification.

  Walls may slightly enhance.

  Also includes large (>3 cm) hyperattenuating cysts without enhancement.

  Usually benign. Radiographic follow-up is recommended, where morphologic change or new enhancement would be concerning for malignancy.

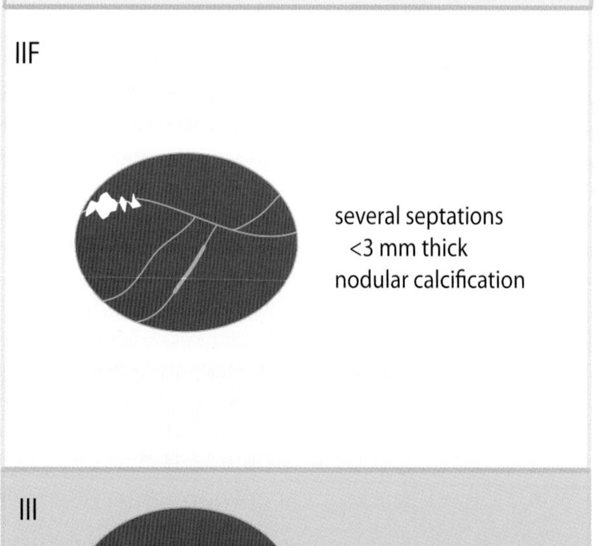

- Category III

  Thickened, irregular walls or septa, with measurable enhancement.

  Concern for malignancy, but may be benign (e.g., infection, multilocular cystic nephroma). Without comorbidities, treatment is surgical.

- Category IV

  Distinguishing feature is enhancing nodular component separate from the wall or septa.

  Clearly malignant. Surgical lesion unless significant comorbidities.

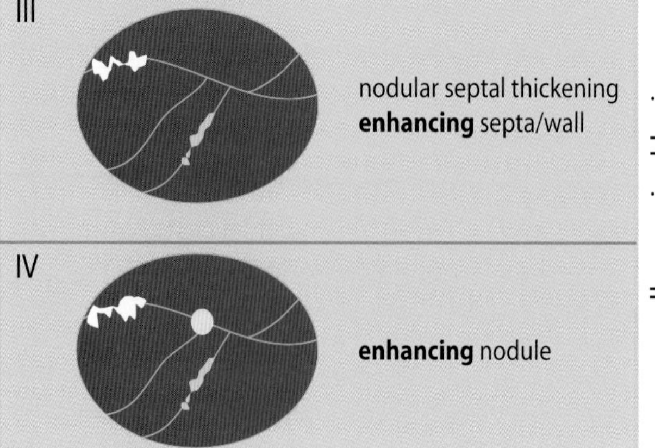

Multicystic renal disease and risk for renal neoplasm

Autosomal dominant polycystic kidney disease (ADPKD)

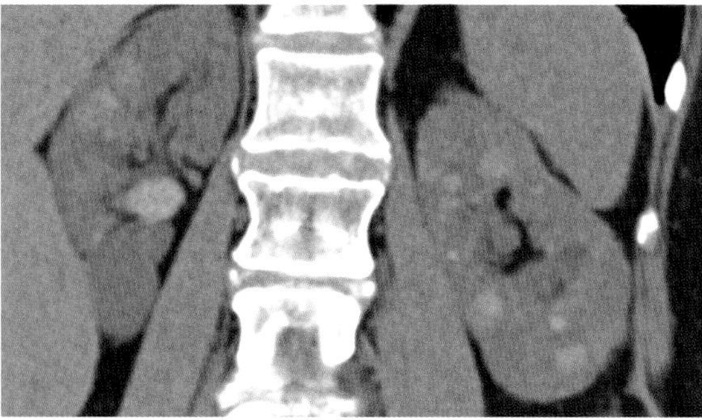
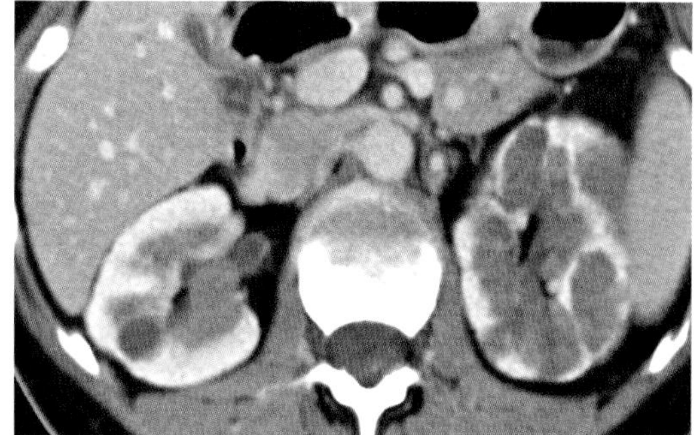

ADPKD: Coronal unenhanced (left image) and axial enhanced CT shows bilateral enlarged kidneys with innumerable renal cysts of mixed attenuation including several hyperdense cysts.

- Autosomal dominant polycystic kidney disease (ADPKD) is responsible for 10% of patients on long-term dialysis. Patients typically present in their third to fourth decades, initially presenting with upper abdominal pain and a clinical course of progressive renal failure. The kidneys may become so enlarged as to be palpable. Hypertension and hematuria (thought to be due nephrolithiasis or rupture of a renal cyst into the collecting system) are common. Approximately one half of patients will have a saccular aneurysm in the circle of Willis.
- On imaging, the kidneys are markedly enlarged and feature multiple cysts of varying attenuation or signal intensities due to hemorrhage.
- The traditional teaching is that ADPKD does not increase the risk of renal cell carcinoma. However, some authors propose that there is a slightly increased risk. Renal cell carcinoma associated with ADPKD tends to occur at a younger age and is more often bilateral, multifocal, and sarcomatoid. Diagnosis of renal malignancy is complicated by the presence of multiple (often hemorrhagic) cysts and frequently concomitant renal insufficiency, which may preclude the use of intravenous contrast.

Acquired cystic kidney disease (due to end-stage kidney disease)

- Dialysis-associated cystic renal disease does have an increased risk of renal cell carcinoma (~2–3% prevalence, compared to 1/10,000 prevalence in the general population).

Renal infection and inflammation

Pyelonephritis

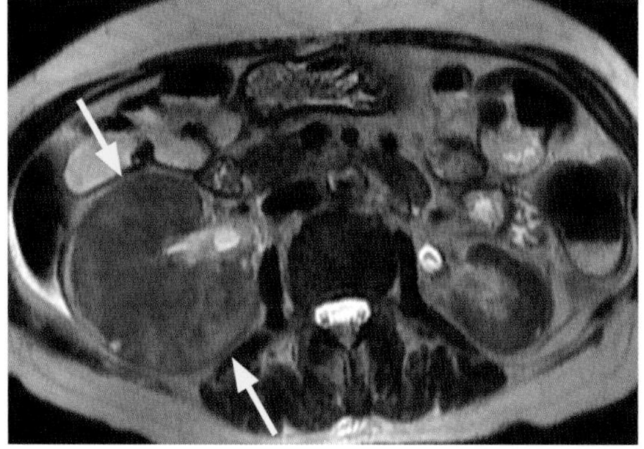
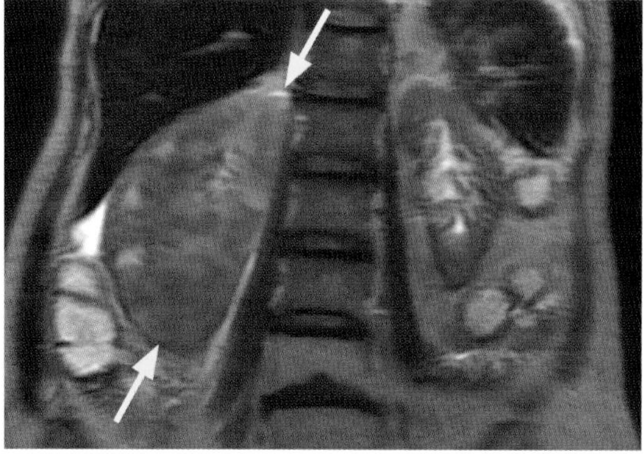

Pyelonephritis: Axial (left image) and coronal T2-weighted MRI shows a markedly enlarged, edematous right kidney, without hydronephrosis (arrows). Although a unilaterally enlarged kidney is a nonspecific finding, pyelonephritis is a primary concern in a patient with fever and costovertebral angle tenderness.

Case courtesy of Cheryl Sadow, MD, Brigham and Women's Hospital.

- Pyelonephritis is infection of renal parenchyma and is the most common bacterial infection of the kidney. The bacteria usually are ascending from the bladder.
- The imaging findings of pyelonephritis are nonspecific and imaging may be normal in up to 75%. Various patterns may be seen, including a unilaterally enlarged kidney, wedge-shaped or striated regions of decreased enhancement, and perinephric stranding. The urothelium may also be thickened and hyperenhancing.
- The differential diagnosis of a unilateral enlarged kidney includes pyelonephritis, acute ureteral obstruction, renal vein thrombosis, and compensatory hypertrophy.
- A striated nephrogram describes linear lucencies extending from the renal cortex to the medulla on a contrast-enhanced study. The differential diagnosis for a striated nephrogram is similar to that of a wedge-shaped perfusion defect and includes:

Pyelonephritis.	Acute urinary obstruction.
Renal infarct.	Renal tumor (especially lymphoma if infiltrative).
Renal vein thrombosis or vasculitis.	Radiation nephritis.
Renal contusion (typically focal).	

- Focal pyelonephritis (previously called *focal lobar nephronia*) may mimic a renal mass.
- Mild hydronephrosis can be seen on the affected side, thought to be due to a bacterial endotoxin causing reduced peristalsis, and should not be confused with obstructive uropathy.

Pyonephrosis

- Pyonephrosis is the infection of an obstructed collecting system and is colloquially referred to as "pus under pressure." Treatment is emergent percutaneous nephrostomy.

Renal abscess

- Renal abscess is a localized purulent collection within the kidney that most commonly results from coalescence of small microabscesses in the setting of acute bacterial pyelonephritis. An abscess may simulate a cystic renal mass.
- The treatment is conservative if <3 cm and percutaneous drainage if larger.

Emphysematous pyelonephritis

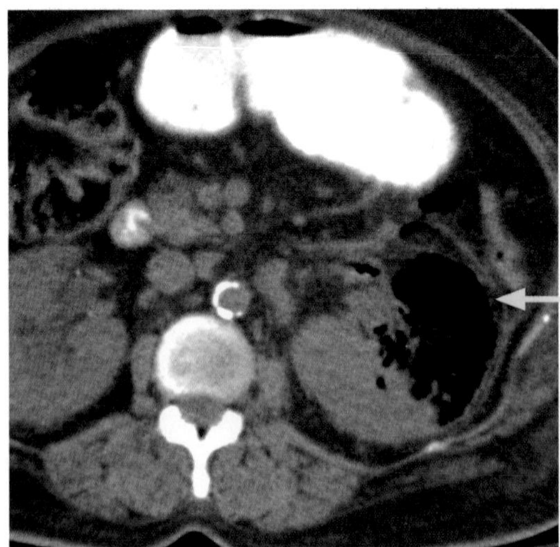

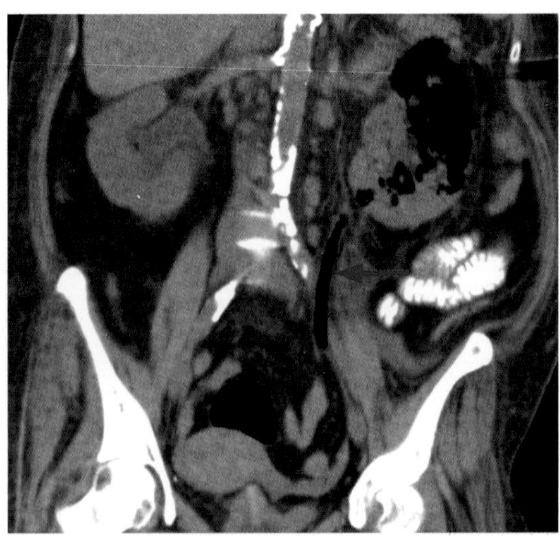

Emphysematous pyelonephritis: Axial (left image) and coronal CT with oral contrast only shows gas replacing the superior and lateral aspect of the left kidney (yellow arrow). There is gas extending into the left ureter, best seen on the coronal (red arrow).

- Emphysematous pyelonephritis is a severe renal infection characterized by gas replacing renal parenchyma, caused both by gas-forming organisms and renal infarction.

- Emphysematous pyelonephritis is seen almost exclusively in diabetic patients.
- Emphysematous pyelonephritis is a surgical emergency, requiring emergent nephrectomy.

Xanthogranulomatous pyelonephritis

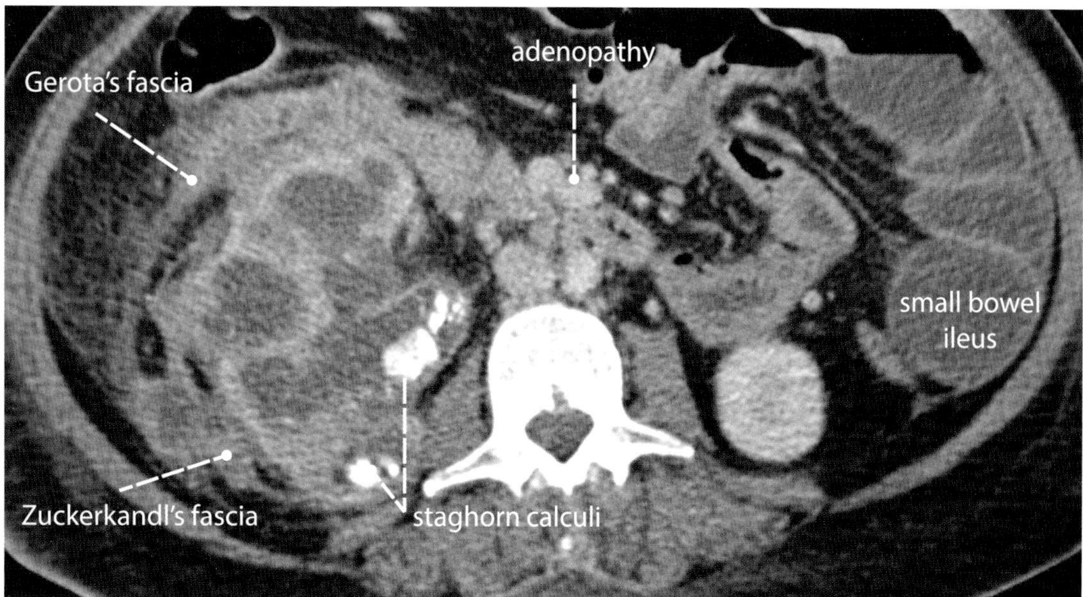

Xanthogranulomatous pyelonephritis: Contrast-enhanced CT shows a massively enlarged, poorly enhancing right kidney with dilated and distorted calyces. Several staghorn calculi are present. There is thickening of Zuckerkandl's and Gerota's fascia, perinephric stranding, and retroperitoneal adenopathy. The partially visualized small bowel in the left hemiabdomen is dilated secondary to ileus from perirenal inflammation.

Case courtesy of Shreya Sood, MD, Brigham and Women's Hospital.

- Xanthogranulomatous pyelonephritis (XGP) is a chronic renal infection due to obstructing calculi, leading to replacement of renal parenchyma with fibrofatty inflammatory tissue.
- *Proteus mirabilis* and *Escherichia coli* are the two most common organisms.
- The clinical presentation of XGP includes flank pain and nonspecific constitutional symptoms, such as fever and weight loss. Anemia and hematuria are also common.
- XGP can be diffuse (85%) or localized. The localized form, also known as "tumefactive XGP," may mimic a renal mass.
- CT is the primary modality for imaging, which demonstrates fatty replacement of the renal parenchyma, marked perinephric inflammatory standing, and staghorn calculi.
- The *bear paw* sign represents the configuration of the hypoattenuating fibrofatty masses arranged in a radial pattern, reminiscent of a bear's paw.
- Primary differential considerations include acute obstructing calculus with pyonephrosis or renal/transitional neoplasm with calcification.
- Treatment is nephrectomy.

Renal tuberculosis

- *Mycobacterium tuberculosis* infection of the renal parenchyma results from hematogenous dissemination. Active pulmonary TB is present in approximately 10%.
- Although initial renal TB infection typically involves both kidneys, chronic changes tend to be unilateral.
- Imaging findings include parenchymal calcification, scarring, papillary necrosis, and infundibular strictures. End-stage renal TB produces autonephrectomy and the characteristic *putty kidney* appearance, which represents an atrophic, calcified kidney.

Nephrolithiasis and ureterolithiasis

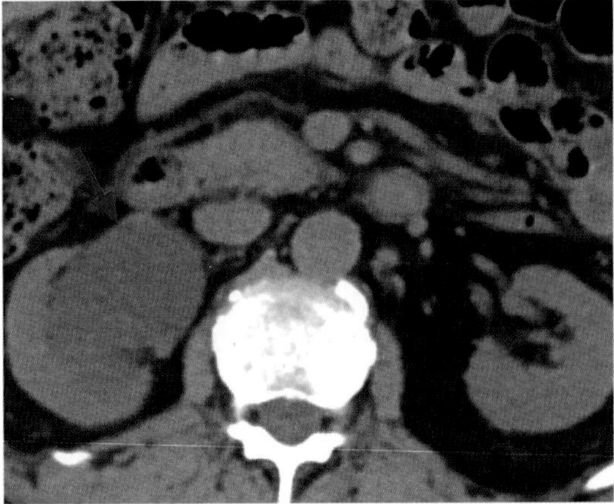

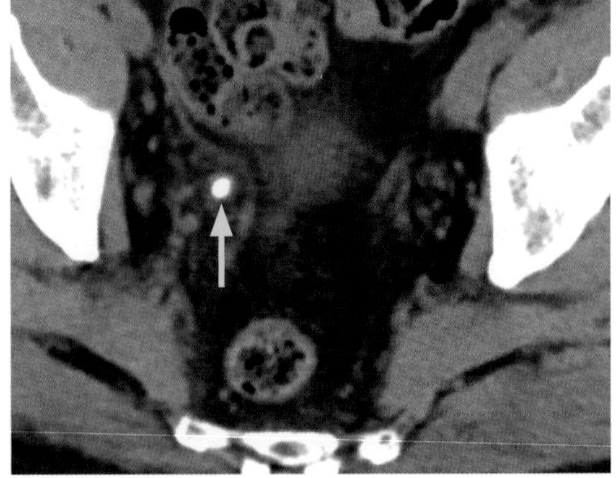

Right obstructive uropathy caused by a distal ureteral stone: Noncontrast axial CT through the kidneys (left image) shows unilateral right hydronephrosis (red arrow). Axial image through the pelvis shows a calcification along the expected course of the right ureter (yellow arrow) demonstrating the *soft tissue rim* sign, with a faint halo of soft tissue surrounding the calculus.

- Nephro/ureterolithiasis is a common problem that presents with renal colic. Hematuria is usually present, but may be absent if the stone is completely obstructing. Calcium-containing stones (comprised of calcium oxalate and phosphate, pure calcium oxalate, or the less common pure calcium phosphate stones) together represent 73% of urinary lithiasis.
- Uric acid, xanthine, matrix, pure struvite, and indinavir (seen in HIV patients on antiretroviral therapy) stones are lucent on radiographs. Virtually all renal stones are radiopaque on CT except for indinavir stones and the very rare uncalcified matrix stones made of mucin.
- Secondary signs of ureteral obstruction from a ureteral stone include ipsilateral hydronephrosis and perinephric stranding surrounding the affected kidney. The *soft tissue rim* sign helps to distinguish a phlebolith from a ureteral stone. The presence of a small amount of soft tissue surrounding the calcification, thought to represent the edematous ureteral wall, suggests a ureteral stone rather than a vascular calcification.

Papillary necrosis

- Papillary necrosis is necrosis and sloughing of renal papillary tissue, which clinically can cause gross hematuria and may lead to chronic renal insufficiency.
- There are numerous causes of papillary necrosis, most commonly NSAIDs, sickle cell anemia, diabetes, and renal vein thrombosis. The commonly used POSTCARD mnemonic may be helpful to remember all causes:

Pyelonephritis.	**C**irrhosis.
Obstruction.	**A**nalgesics (NSAIDS).
Sickle cell disease.	**R**enal vein thrombosis.
Tuberculosis.	**D**iabetes mellitus.

- On the delayed phase of CT urography, papillary necrosis causes multiple small poolings of extra-calyceal contrast adjacent to the renal calyces.
- Three classic uroradiologic signs of papillary necrosis include the *ball on tee* sign, *lobster claw* sign (not to be confused with the *bear paw* sign of xanthogranulomatous pyelonephritis), and *signet ring* sign, which describe patterns of papillary excavation.
- The *ball on tee* sign describes contrast filling a central papilla.
- The *lobster claw* sign describes contrast filling only the periphery of the papilla.
- The *signet ring* sign describes contrast surrounding the sloughed papilla.

Delayed (prolonged) nephrogram

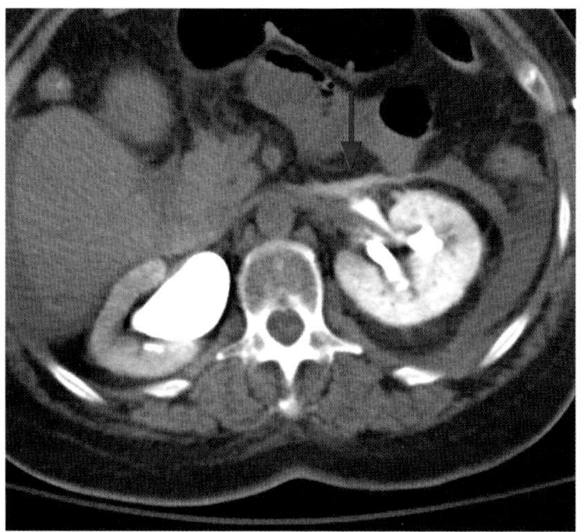

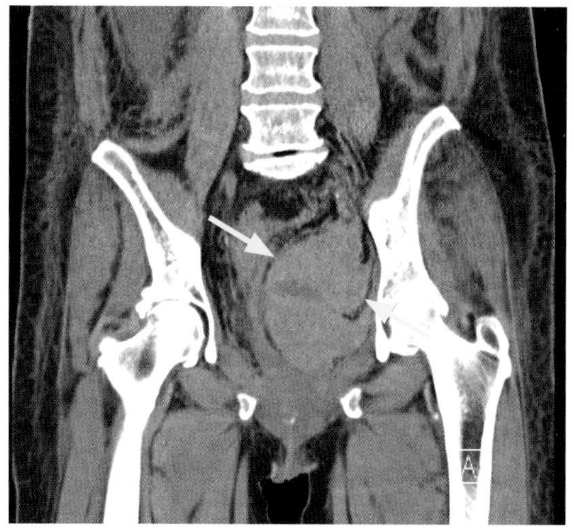

Bilateral delayed nephrogram due to obstruction: Unenhanced CT through the kidneys performed several hours after cardiac catheterization shows bilateral left > right persistent renal enhancement and densely opacified urine in the proximal collecting system. There is evidence of urine extravasation due to forniceal rupture (red arrow), consistent with distal obstruction. Coronal image from the same study shows the large left-sided pelvic hematoma (yellow arrows) compressing and displacing the bladder.

- A delayed (prolonged) nephrogram describes slow renal parenchymal uptake of intravenous contrast, prolonged enhancement, and delayed urine excretion.
- A unilateral prolonged nephrogram can be due to acute ureteral obstruction, renal vein thrombosis, and renal artery stenosis.
- Bilateral prolonged nephrograms can be seen in bilateral obstruction, contrast nephropathy, systemic hypotension, and myeloma kidney.

Medullary nephrocalcinosis

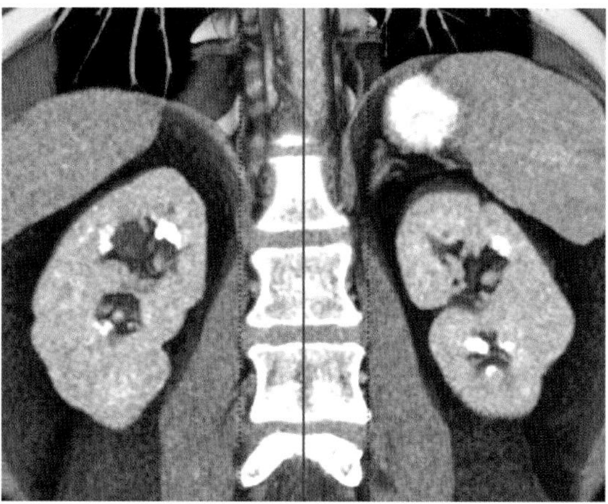

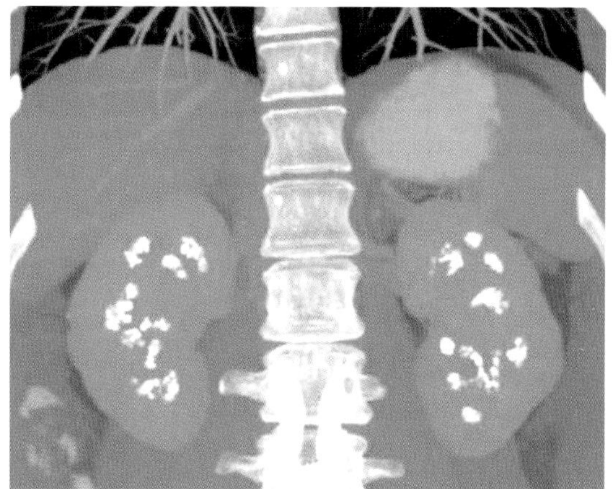

Medullary nephrocalcinosis: Thin and thick-slab coronal MIPs from a contrast-enhanced study show numerous amorphous calcifications within the renal medullary pyramids bilaterally.

- Medullary nephrocalcinosis represents calcification of the renal medullary pyramids, usually with preserved renal function. Medullary nephrocalcinosis can be caused by:

Hypercalcemic state (e.g., hyperparathyroidism, sarcoidosis, etc).

Medullary sponge kidney (cystic dilation of distal collecting ducts; may be unilateral or segmental).

Distal (type 1) **renal tubular acidosis** (RTA).

Furosemide therapy in a child.

Cortical nephrocalcinosis

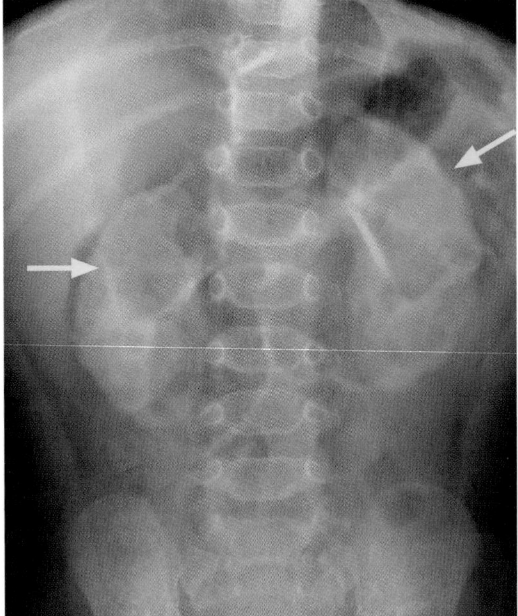

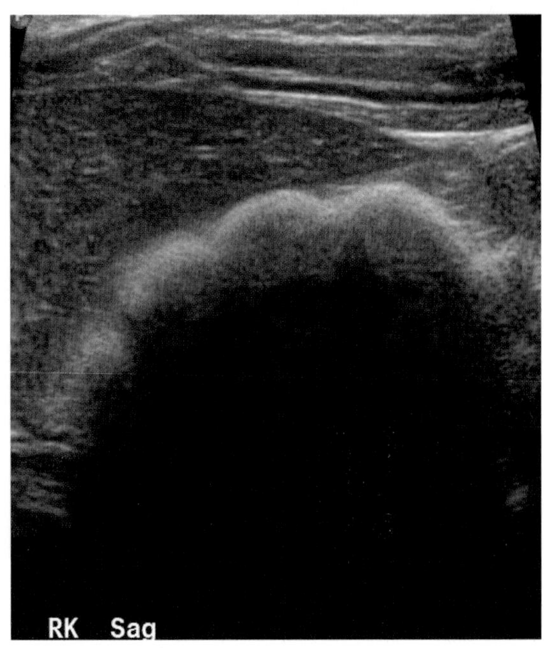

Cortical nephrocalcinosis in a child: Abdominal radiograph shows dense cortical calcification of the kidneys (arrows). Ultrasound shows densely calcified and shadowing renal cortex, obscuring the renal parenchyma.

Case courtesy of Michael Hanley, MD, University of Virginia Health System.

- Cortical nephrocalcinosis is dystrophic peripheral calcification of the renal cortex, with sparing of the medullary pyramids.
- Causes of cortical nephrocalcinosis include:

Acute cortical necrosis.	**Hyperoxaluria**.
Chronic glomerulonephritis.	**Alport syndrome** (hereditary nephropathy and deafness).
Chronic transplant rejection.	

Cortical necrosis

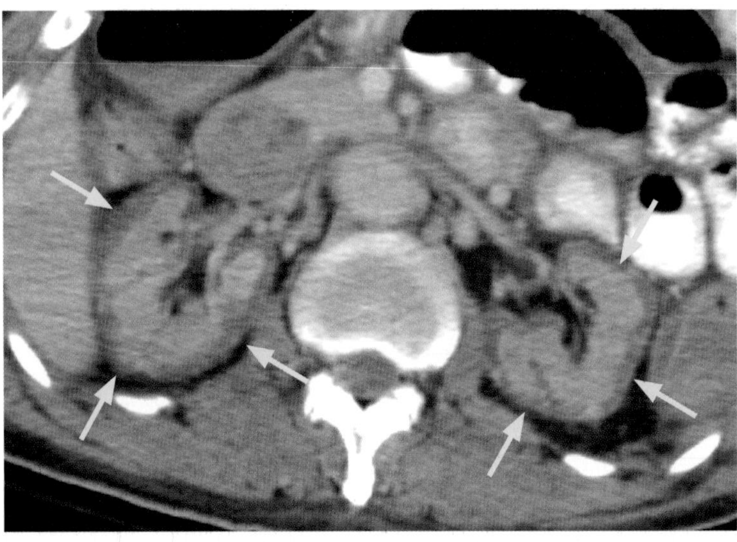

Cortical necrosis: Contrast-enhanced axial CT shows lack of enhancement of the renal cortices bilaterally (arrows).

- Cortical necrosis is a rare form of renal injury from acute ischemic necrosis of the renal cortex. Cortical necrosis may lead to cortical nephrocalcinosis. Chronic renal failure develops in up to 50% of patients.
- Ischemia may be due to small vessel vasospasm or systemic hypotension. Predisposing factors include hemolytic–uremic syndrome and thrombotic microangiopathy.

Extracalyceal contrast medium

- Contrast shouldn't normally be seen beyond the calyces on excretory urogram. Papillary necrosis, tubular ectasia, and calyceal diverticulum may cause this appearance.
- **Tubular ectasia** causes paintbrush-like streaks of contrast that extend from the papillae into the tubules on excretory urogram. **Medullary sponge kidney** is tubular ectasia with associated calcifications of the renal medullary pyramids.
- **Calyceal diverticulum** is an outpouching of the collecting system into the corticomedullary region. A dependent sediment or multiple small stones may be present.
- **Papillary necrosis**, previously discussed, may also cause extracalyceal contrast.

Renal trauma

Organ Injury Scale (OIS) - American Association for the Surgery of Trauma (AAST)

- The OIS scale from the AAST is the most commonly used system for classifying renal trauma. It is a surgical classification but correlates well with the CT findings.

OIS/AAST grading of renal trauma

- **Grade I** injury is by far the most common type of renal injury (95%) and describes a renal contusion or subcapsular hematoma. Treatment is conservative.
- **Grade II** injury is a superficial laceration (<1 cm) or confined perinephric hematoma, without urinary extravasation. Treatment is conservative.
- **Grade III** injury is a deeper laceration (>1 cm), without urinary extravasation. Treatment is typically conservative.

  A potential pitfall of a grade III injury is that a clot at the collecting system may prevent urinary extravasation initially, but urinary extravasation may occur later as the clot is lysed by urinary urokinase.
- **Grade IV** is a deep laceration that extends into the collecting system (causing urinary extravasation), or injury to the renal artery or vein with contained hemorrhage. Urinary extravasation is typically treated with surgical repair to prevent later development of urinoma or abscess formation. Vascular grade IV injury can be treated endovascularly.
- **Grade V** is a shattered kidney, or avulsion of the renal hilum. Treatment is variable but typically surgical.

CT description of renal trauma

- The OIS classification described above is somewhat limited as there are several important renal injuries, including traumatic renal artery thrombosis, renal artery pseudoaneurysm, and ureteral avulsion (most commonly occurring at the ureteropelvic junction) that are not included in the OIS classification but which can affect prognosis.
- Traumatic renal artery thrombosis is due to tearing of the intima, which initiates thrombosis. There is a permanent loss of renal function after approximately two hours of ischemia.
- Pseudoaneurysm is an arterial injury with a high risk of fatal rupture. On imaging, a pseudoaneurysm will be of similar density to the aorta, with arterial enhancement in the arterial phase and washout on delays. Treatment is endovascular embolization.

Page kidney

- A Page kidney (named after the doctor who performed experiments wrapping animal kidneys with cellophane) is a rare cause of secondary hypertension due to prior trauma.
- A subcapsular hematoma compresses the renal parenchyma and decreases its blood flow. These altered hemodynamics induce increased renin secretion, which can lead to hypertension. It usually takes several months for hypertension to develop.
- Imaging shows a subcapsular hematoma causing deformation and flattening of the kidney.
- Percutaneous drainage of the hematoma may be effective treatment.

Ureter

Overview of ureteral imaging

CT urography (CTU) indications and protocol

- The goal of CT urography (CTU) is to evaluate the kidneys, ureters, and bladder. The key to successful imaging is to maximally distend and opacify the ureters and bladder.
- One of the most common indications for CTU is for the evaluation of microscopic or macroscopic hematuria. Hematuria may be caused by a urinary tract calculus, renal mass (e.g., renal cell carcinoma), or urothelial tumor (e.g., transitional cell carcinoma).
- Protocols vary by institution. Typically, patients are given 900 mL of water PO and either 250 mL of IV saline or 10 mg of IV furosemide to optimally distend the ureters and bladder.
- In adults ≥40 years of age, CTU is performed as a three-phase exam:
  - Unenhanced CT of the abdomen and pelvis.
  - Nephrographic phase through the kidneys (100 seconds after IV contrast administration).
  - Excretory phase of the abdomen and pelvis (15 minutes after IV contrast).
- A split-bolus, dual-phase exam decreases radiation exposure in patients under age 40:
  - Unenhanced CT of the abdomen and pelvis.
  - Combined nephrographic/excretory phase (8 minutes delay after first IV contrast bolus and 100 seconds after the second bolus).

Malignant ureteral disease

Transitional cell carcinoma (TCC)

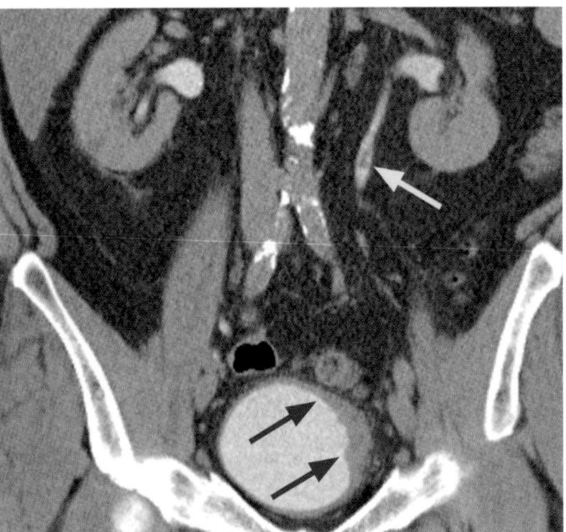
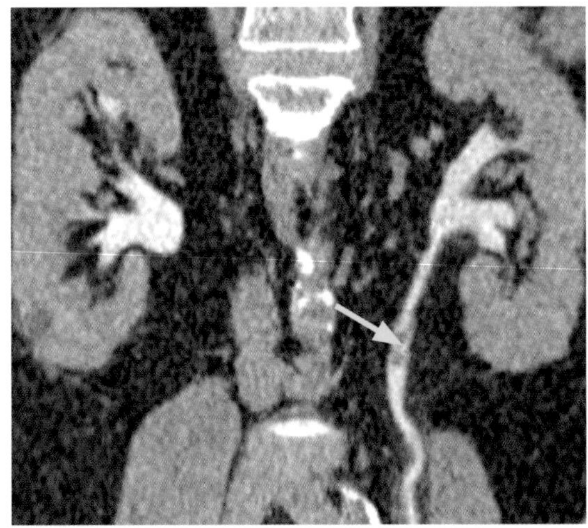

Multifocal transitional cell carcinoma: Coronal CT (left image) from the pyelographic phase of a CT urogram shows a sessile mass within the left lateral aspect of the bladder (red arrows) and a filling defect within the proximal left ureter (yellow arrow). Curved multiplanar reformation from the same study (right) better shows the proximal ureteral filling defect (arrow).

Case courtesy of Cheryl Sadow, MD, Brigham and Women's Hospital.

- Although upper-tract malignancy is rare, transitional cell carcinoma is the most common ureteral neoplasm.
- The typical imaging appearance is a single filling defect on CT urography; however, multiple filling defects may be seen in 40%. Less commonly, there may be focal thickening of the ureteral wall. Given the propensity of transitional cell carcinoma for multifocality, the bladder should be evaluated for a synchronous mass.

Benign ureteral masses

Fibroepithelial polyp

- Fibroepithelial polyp is the most common benign tumor of the ureter. It typically affects the proximal ureter. Fibroepithelial polyp features a long stalk and appears as an elongated smooth tubular lesion. CT urography best shows the lesion on the coronal images in the pyelographic phase.

Urothelial papilloma

- Urothelial papilloma is a rare benign neoplasm that may involve the bladder or ureter. The mass may become quite large and mimic a malignancy.

Inverted papilloma

- Inverted papilloma is a benign mass with a central core of urothelium.

Inflammatory and infectious ureteral disease

Ureteritis cystica

- Ureteritis cystica is a benign response to chronic urinary tract inflammation, such as chronic infection or stone disease. Several small subepithelial cysts are found unilaterally in the proximal third of the ureter and renal pelvis. Ureteritis cystica does not have any malignant potential.
- Imaging characteristically shows multiple tiny filling defects in the renal pelvis or ureter.
- The same disease entity affecting the bladder is called cystitis cystica, which shows multiple rounded contour defects at the base of the bladder.

Leukoplakia (squamous metaplasia)

- Leukoplakia, also known as squamous metaplasia, is a rare urothelial inflammatory condition named for the characteristic white patch that is produced. Leukoplakia is not thought to be premalignant when the renal collecting system is involved, although there is an association between squamous cell carcinoma and bladder leukoplakia.
- Imaging shows a flat mass or focal thickening of the renal pelvic or ureteral wall that may produce a characteristic *corduroy* appearance.

Malacoplakia

- Malacoplakia is an inflammatory condition associated with chronic urinary tract infection (usually *Escherichia coli*) that is typically seen in middle-aged women. It is not premalignant.
- Imaging shows multiple flat filling defects that characteristically involve the distal ureter.

Ureteral tuberculosis

- Multifocal ureteral stenoses are suggestive of ureteral tuberculosis, even more so if there is also evidence of renal tuberculosis (parenchymal calcification and scarring) and/or bladder tuberculosis (small capacity bladder with a thickened wall).

Differential diagnosis of a ureteral filling defect

- *The primary concern of a ureteral filling defect on CT urography is ureteral malignancy.*

Differential of ureteral filling defect		
	• **Ureteral malignancy**, of which transitional cell carcinoma is by far the most common. • Ureteral calculus, which is almost always visible on pre-contrast images. • Blood clot. • Malacoplakia (multiple flat defects).	• Leukoplakia. • Infectious debris (e.g., a mycetoma). • Sloughed renal papilla. • Benign ureteral mass (e.g., fibroepithelial polyp).

Ureteropelvic junction obstruction (UPJ obstruction)

- Obstruction of the ureteropelvic junction (UPJ) can be either primary or secondary to infection, stones, or prior surgery.
- Primary UPJ obstruction may be due to a congenital aperistaltic segment of ureter, high insertion of the ureter on the renal pelvis, or crossing vessels causing extrinsic compression.
- The key imaging finding is a dilated renal pelvis with a normal caliber ureter.

Ureterocele

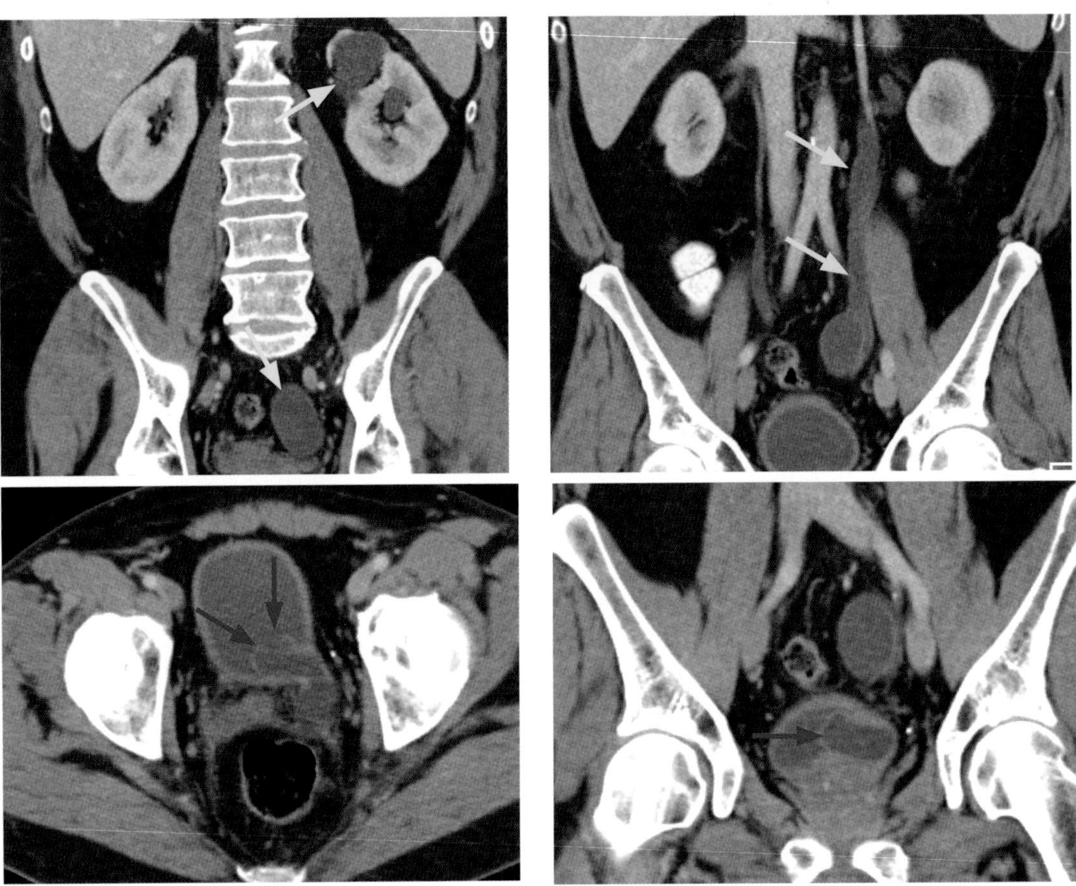

Duplicated ureter with ureterocele: Coronal contrast-enhanced CT (top images) shows a duplicated left ureter. There is hydronephrosis of the upper pole moiety and marked dilation of the upper pole ureter (yellow arrows). Axial (bottom left image) and coronal (bottom right image) CT shows the dilated ureter terminating within a ureterocele (red arrows). The dilated upper pole ureter inserts slightly posteriorly relative to the lower pole ureter (not shown) and represents an ectopic ureterocele.

Case courtesy of Cheryl Sadow, MD, Brigham and Women's Hospital.

- A ureterocele is a focal dilation of the most distal portion of the ureter that protrudes into the bladder. A ureterocele may be orthotopic or ectopic.
- An **orthotopic ureterocele** is seen with a normally inserting ureter, and is seen most commonly in adults. Orthotopic ureteroceles are also known as *simple*, *adult-type*, and *intravesicular* ureteroceles. Orthotopic ureteroceles are usually asymptomatic.
- An **ectopic ureterocele** is seen in the setting of a duplicated collecting system, with ectopic insertion of the upper pole ureter into the bladder, and is usually diagnosed in children.
- A **pseudoureterocele** represents intussusception of the distal ureter into the bladder, which may be due to tumor, radiation cystitis, or ureterovesicular junction stone.

Bladder stones

- Risk factors for bladder stones include urinary stasis (most commonly bladder outlet obstruction) and chronic inflammation (e.g., from infection or foreign body).
- An off-midline bladder stone should raise concern for displacement of the stone by a bladder mass or enlarged prostate, or a stone within a ureterocele or a bladder diverticulum.

Bladder transitional cell carcinoma (TCC)

- Transitional cell carcinoma is by far the most common bladder cancer. The bladder is the most common site of malignancy in the urinary tract.
- TCC is a disease of older adults with a male predominance. Risk factors include smoking and aromatic amines. It presents with painless hematuria.
- Bladder cancer spreads through the wall of the bladder. Organ-confined disease can be divided into non-muscle-invasive (70%; typically resected endoscopically) and invasive (25%; typically treated with radical cystectomy/nodal dissection).
- Metastatic bladder cancer (5%) is treated with systemic therapy.
- The presence of pelvic lymph nodes portends a poorer prognosis.
- If bladder cancer is clinically suspected, a negative CT urogram does not obviate the need for cystoscopy.

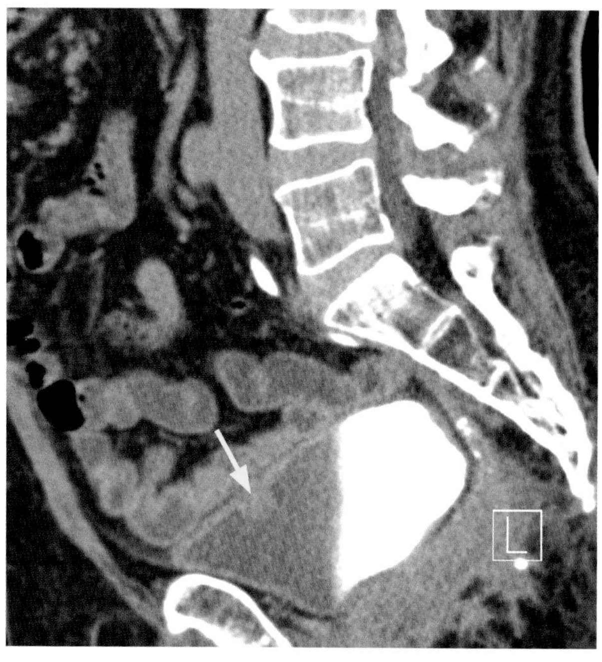

Transitional cell carcinoma of the bladder: Sagittal CT in the excretory phase shows excreted contrast opacifying the posterior half of the bladder. There is a mass (arrow) arising in the superior bladder wall in the unopacified portion of the bladder. This case emphasizes that bladder masses can be extremely subtle to detect without complete bladder opacification.

Bladder adenocarcinoma

- Adenocarcinoma of the bladder is rare but is associated with a urachal remnant.
- The fetal urachus extends from the bladder dome to the umbilicus. It should be obliterated after birth, but may persist as a urachal anomaly (discussed in the Pediatric Imaging section).

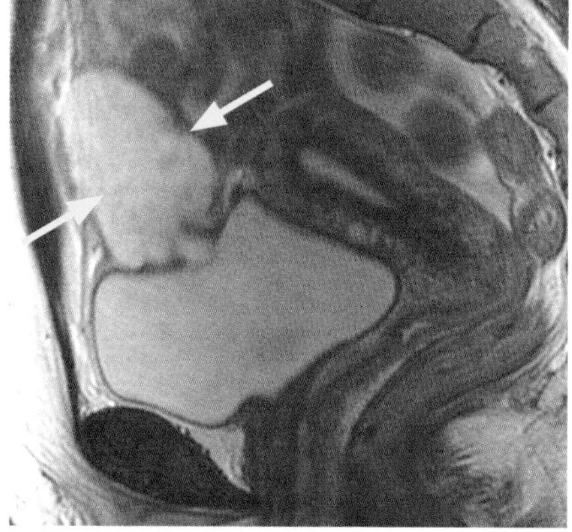

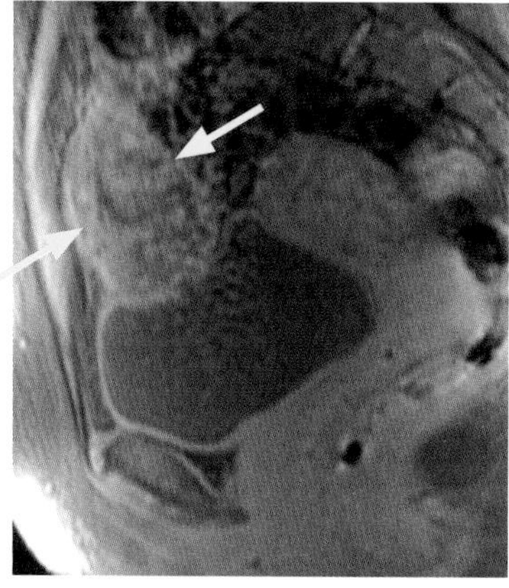

Urachal adenocarcinoma: Sagittal T2-weighted (left image) and sagittal post-contrast fat suppressed T1-weighted MRI (right image) shows an irregular, T2 hyperintense, avidly enhancing mass directly superior to the bladder (arrows). The mass connects to both the bladder and the umbilicus (not shown).

Case courtesy of Cheryl Sadow, MD, Brigham and Women's Hospital.

- CT cystography is the standard test to evaluate for suspected bladder rupture.
- Full distension of the bladder is necessary to evaluate for bladder rupture. Delayed imaging of an intravenous contrast study with opacification of excreted urine is *not* sensitive enough, and is not the standard of care.
- To perform a CT cystogram, a total volume of at least 350 mL (or as much as the patient can tolerate) of dilute water-soluble contrast (50 mL of IV contrast mixed in 500 mL of warm saline) is instilled into the bladder by gravity, with the bag raised 40 cm above the bladder.
- Male patients with bladder injury may have associated urethral injury. If there is blood at the urethral meatus or if there is gross hematuria, a retrograde urethrogram should be performed prior to Foley catheter placement.
- Bladder injury can be classified as extraperitoneal (most common), intraperitoneal, or combined.

Extraperitoneal bladder rupture

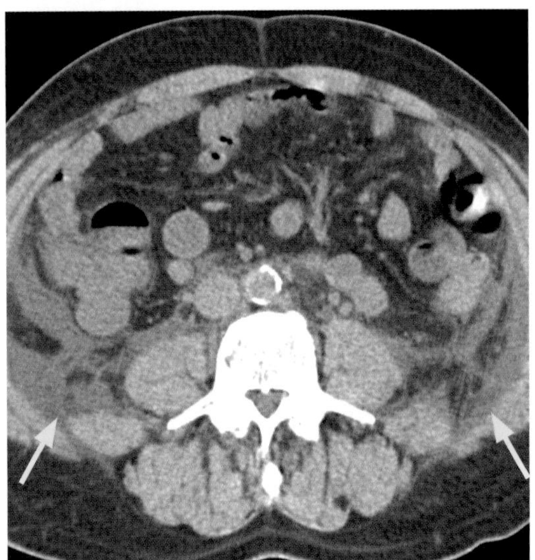

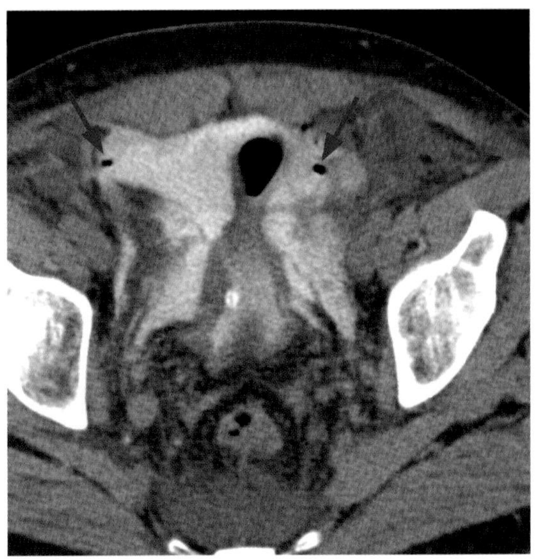

Extraperitoneal bladder rupture: Unenhanced CT (left image) shows fluid stranding within the retroperitoneum (yellow arrows). There is no fluid between loops of bowel. CT cystogram (right image) shows the *molar tooth* sign of extravasated contrast anterior and to and lateral to the bladder. There are few extra-luminal foci of gas (red arrows) within this extraperitoneal contrast collection.

Case courtesy of Cheryl Sadow, MD, Brigham and Women's Hospital.

- Extraperitoneal bladder rupture is defined as rupture of the bladder outside of the peritoneal space. Extraperitoneal bladder rupture is at least twice as common as intraperitoneal rupture.
- Extraperitoneal bladder rupture is more commonly associated with pelvic fractures compared to intraperitoneal rupture. Extraperitoneal bladder rupture is typically caused by direct laceration of the bladder by a bone fragment.
- The *molar tooth* sign describes the characteristic inverted U appearance of extravasated contrast in the extraperitoneal space of Retzius, which mimics a molar tooth.
- Extraperitoneal bladder rupture is typically managed conservatively, by placement of a urinary catheter.

Intraperitoneal bladder rupture

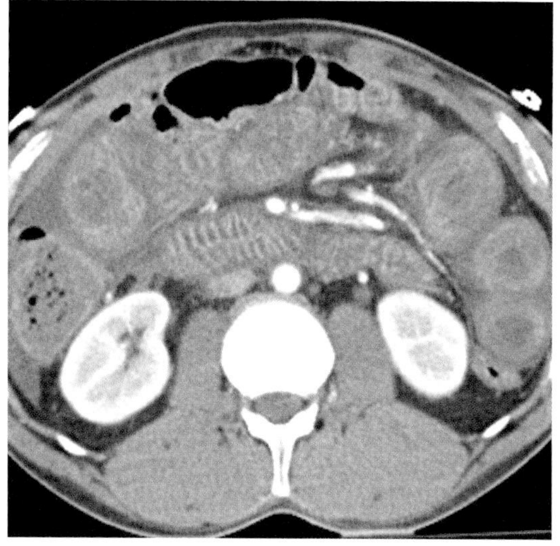

Contrast-enhanced axial CT shows marked hyperenhancing loops of small and large bowel with moderate wall thickening. There is fluid interdigitated between loops of bowel.

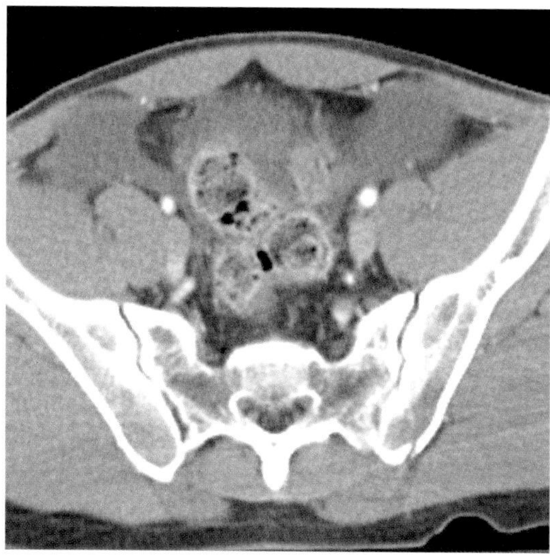

Axial CT through the lower abdomen also shows free fluid between the loops of bowel.

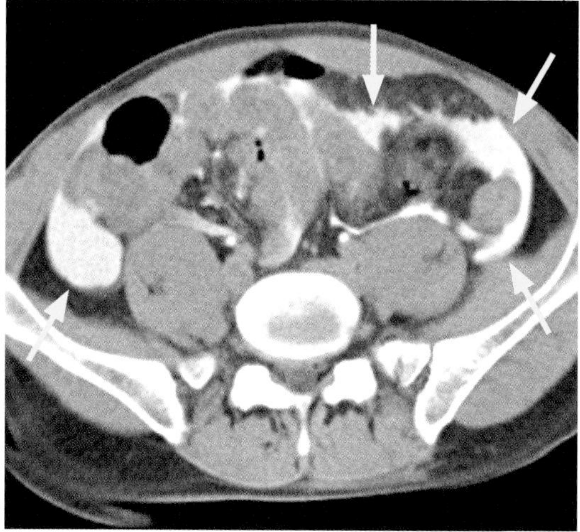

Axial CT cystogram shows intraperitoneal contrast extravasation (arrows) between numerous loops of bowel, diagnostic of an intraperitoneal bladder rupture.

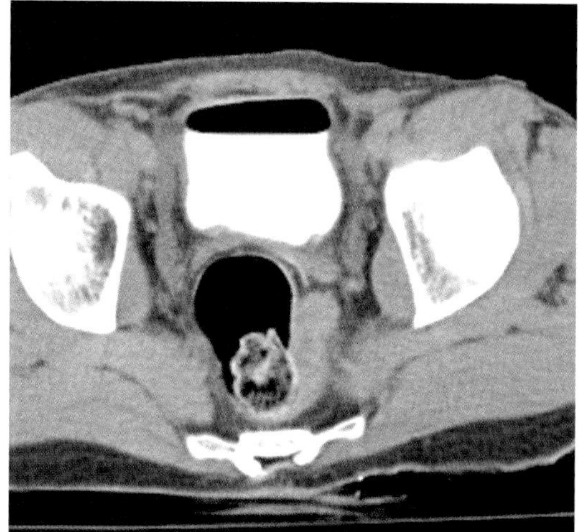

CT cystogram through the bladder shows that the bladder appears intact at this level, with no extra-peritoneal contrast extravasation.

In addition to clearly demonstrating an intraperitoneal bladder rupture, the abnormal mucosal hyperenhancement and wall thickening of the bowel in this case represent shock bowel due to acute hypovolemia in the setting of trauma.

Case courtesy of Cheryl Sadow, MD, Brigham and Women's Hospital.

- Intraperitoneal bladder rupture occurs with disruption of the bladder dome and peritoneum, causing resultant extravasation of urine into the peritoneal space.
- The mechanism of intraperitoneal bladder rupture is thought to be through pressure forces on a full bladder causing bursting at the dome into the peritoneum.
- The pathognomonic imaging finding on CT cystogram is intraperitoneal contrast interdigitating between loops of bowel.
- Intraperitoneal bladder rupture is typically treated surgically.

URETHRA

MALE URETHRAL ANATOMY

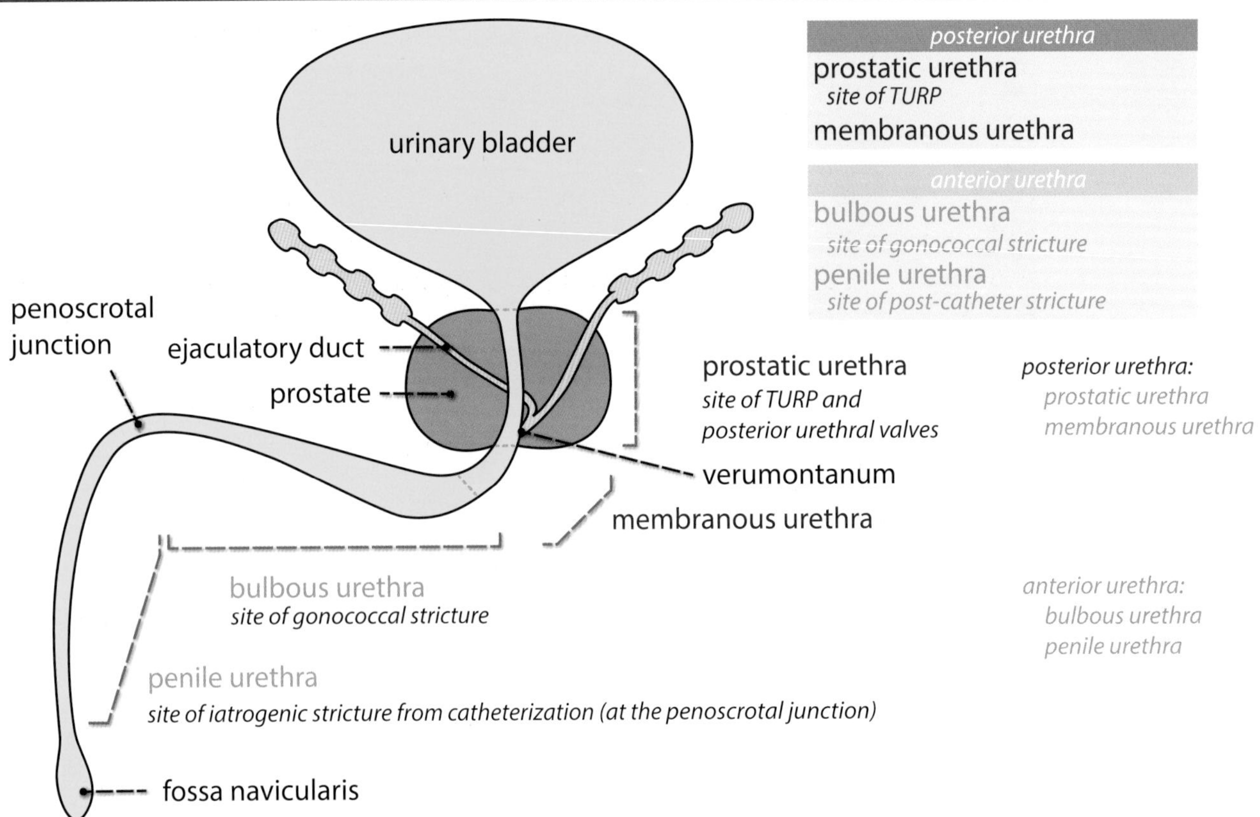

Prostatic urethra (posterior urethra)

- The prostatic urethra courses within the prostate and is lined with transitional epithelium.
- The verumontanum is a prominent ridge of smooth muscle in the posterior portion of the prostatic urethra, and is the site of the paired ejaculatory duct orifices. The verumontanum is also the site of obstruction in posterior urethral valves in children. The prostatic utricle is a Müllerian duct derivative and is the blind-ending male homologue of the uterus and vagina, which is also located at the verumontanum.

Membranous urethra (posterior urethra)

- The membranous urethra is the shortest, least mobile urethral segment.
- The membranous urethra is contained within the urogenital diaphragm, which contains the external urethral sphincter and the paired Cowper's glands.

Bulbous urethra (anterior urethra)

- The bulbar urethra is the site of drainage of Cowper's glands.

Penile urethra (anterior urethra)

- The penile urethra is the longest urethral segment. It is lined with squamous epithelium.
- The distal portion of the penile urethra is dilated at the glans penis. This dilation is called the fossa navicularis.
- The glands of Littré are small mucous glands of the penile urethra. Normally, small ducts would be occluded by balloon during a retrograde urethrogram, and therefore would not opacify with injected contrast. The glands of Littré tend to opacify more prominently when inflamed in the setting of urethritis.

Retrograde urethrogram (RUG)

- Retrograde urethrogram (RUG) provides excellent evaluation of the anterior urethra and may be performed to evaluate for suspected urethral injury, stricture, or fistula.
- To perform a RUG, the fossa navicularis is cannulated with a sterile balloon-tipped catheter that is inflated with 1–2 mL saline. Subsequently, approximately 10 mL of contrast is hand-injected under fluoroscopy.

Voiding cystourethrogram (VCUG)

- Voiding cystourethrogram (VCUG) best evaluates the posterior urethra and is typically performed for evaluation of bladder and voiding function.
- To perform a VCUG, a Foley catheter is sterilely placed in the bladder and subsequently contrast is instilled into the bladder. The patient initiates urination during fluoroscopy.

Urethral stricture

- Urethral strictures secondary to sexually transmitted disease (most commonly chronic urethritis from *Neisseria gonorrhoea*) occur most commonly in the bulbous urethra. A complication of chronic urethral infection is a periurethral abscess, which may result in a urethroperineal fistula.
- Post-traumatic saddle injury strictures also tend to occur in the bulbous urethra.
- In contrast, an iatrogenic stricture from a Foley catheter tends to occur in the penile urethra at the penile–scrotal junction.

Urethral trauma

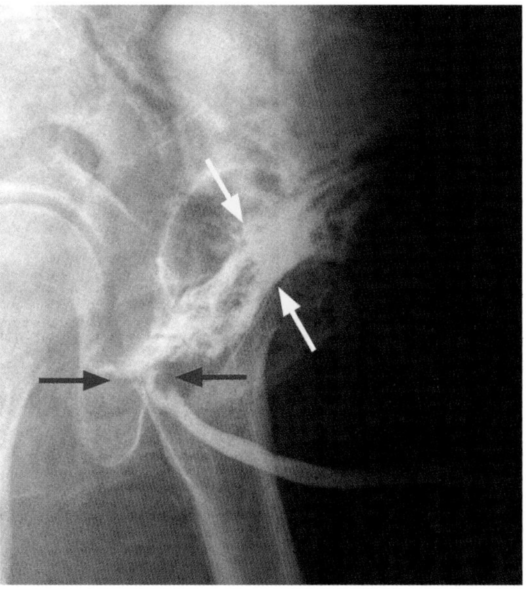

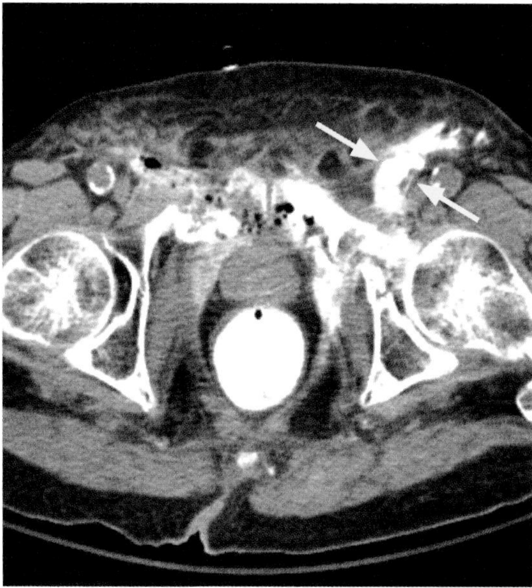

Type III urethral injury: Retrograde urethrogram (left image) shows free extravasation of contrast (yellow arrows) at the bulbomembranous urethra (red arrows). Post-RUG CT shows the extravasated contrast in the inguinal space (arrows) and the deep pelvis. Pelvic fractures and gas from a projectile tract are partially seen.

Case courtesy of Cheryl Sadow, MD, Brigham and Women's Hospital.

- In the setting of trauma, if there is blood at the meatus, painful urination, or inability to void, a RUG should be performed emergently. If the RUG shows evidence of urethral injury, a suprapubic catheter is typically placed.
- There are five types of urethral injury. Type III, pictured above, is the most common, with disruption of the urogenital diaphragm and rupture of the bulbomembranous urethra. Contrast extravasates both into the pelvis and out into the perineum in a type III injury.

Anatomy of the female urethra

- The female urethra is much shorter than the male urethra. Unlike the male urethra, the female urethra is not divided into discrete segments.
- The paraurethral glands of Skene are homologous to the male prostate and secrete mucus into the urethra. The proximal third of the urethra is lined by transitional epithelium, while the distal portion of the urethra is lined with a stratified squamous epithelium.

Urethral diverticulum

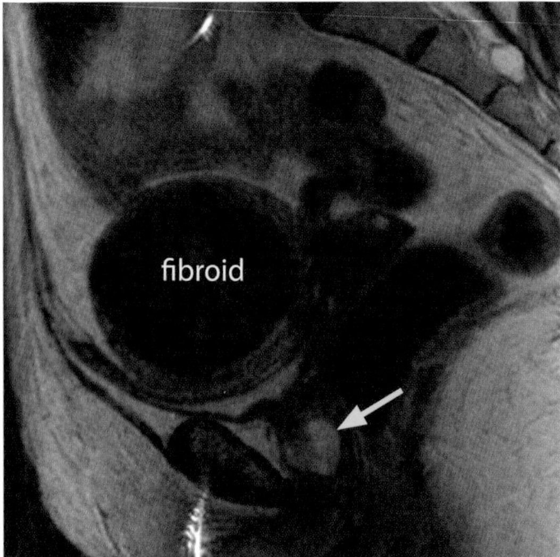

Midline sagittal T2-weighted MRI shows a rounded, hyperintense structure (arrow) in the region of the urethra, representing a urethral diverticulum. There is incidentally a large intramural fibroid.

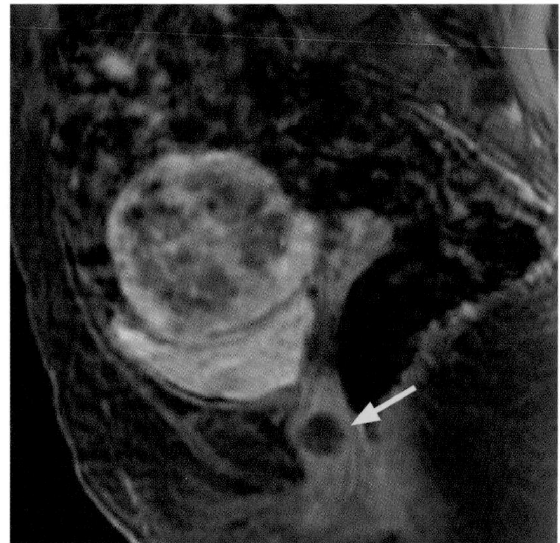

Post-contrast sagittal T1-weighted image shows no enhancement within or surrounding the diverticulum (arrow).

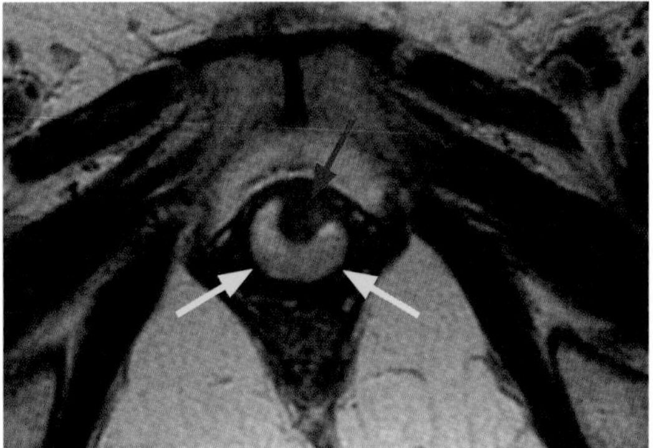

Axial T2-weighted image shows that the urethral diverticulum is U-shaped (yellow arrows) surrounding the normal decompressed urethra (red arrow).

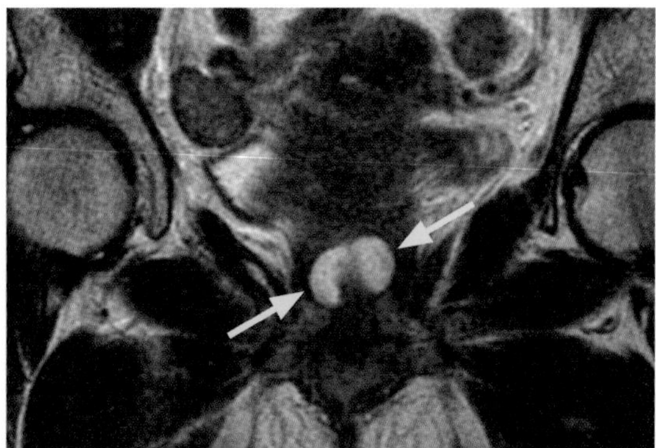

Coronal T2-weighted image again shows the urethral diverticulum as a lobulated focus of T2 hyperintensity (arrows) in the region of the urethra.

Case courtesy of Cheryl Sadow, MD, Brigham and Women's Hospital.

- Urethral diverticulum presents clinically with postvoid dribbling, urethral pain, and dyspareunia. Often, however, the symptoms may be vague and nonspecific.
- Diverticula are thought to arise from glandular dilation caused by inflammation and chronic infection of the paraurethral glands of Skene.
- Urethral diverticula are prone to develop calculi due to urinary stasis.
- Very rarely, adenocarcinoma may develop within a urethral diverticulum.

Prostate anatomy

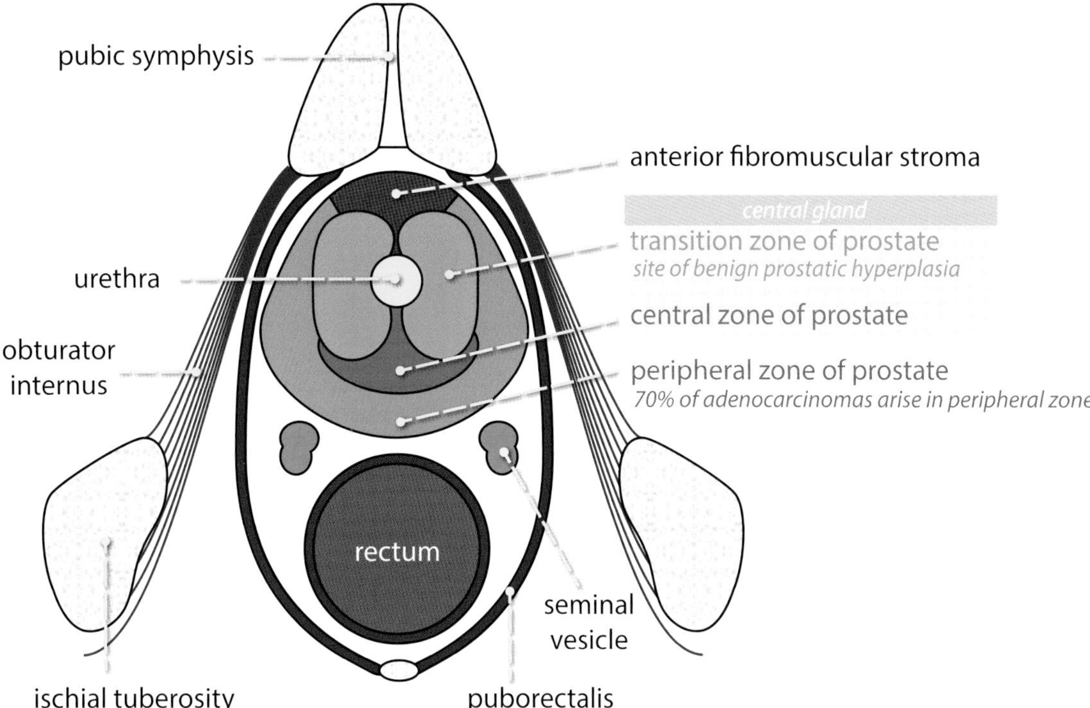

- From an imaging standpoint, there are two components to the prostate that can be resolved on MRI: The **peripheral zone** and the **central gland**. The central gland refers to both the central zone and the transition zone, as they cannot be distinguished on MRI.
- In younger men, the central gland is composed mostly of the central zone; however, the transition zone enlarges as benign prostatic hyperplasia develops. These changes result in the central gland becoming predominantly composed of transition zone in older males.

Prostate cancer

- MRI is able to clearly delineate the prostatic zonal anatomy (central gland versus peripheral zone) with T2-weighted sequences. Imaging is enhanced with an endorectal coil.
- MRI is inappropriate for screening due to cost and low sensitivity and specificity.
- The typical MRI appearance of prostate cancer is a T2 hypointense region within the T2 hyperintense peripheral zone.
- MRI may not detect all prostate cancer: Some cancer is not hypointense on T2-weighted images, central zone cancers are difficult to detect on T2-weighted images, and cancer conspicuity is decreased if the peripheral zone is not T2 hyperintense.
- MRI is also not specific: In addition to prostate cancer, the differential diagnosis of a region of peripheral zone T2 hypointensity includes prostatitis, hemorrhage, and involutional changes from androgen-deprivation therapy. Advanced MRI techniques, such as MRI spectroscopy, dynamic contrast-enhanced imaging, and diffusion imaging may increase specificity.
- MRI spectroscopy of prostate cancer may show elevated choline and depressed citrate peaks compared to normal prostate.
- Dynamic contrast-enhanced MRI typically shows prostate cancer to have early enhancement relative to the peripheral zone.
- Prostate cancer typically shows restricted diffusion.

- The most important goal of MRI is to distinguish between surgical and nonsurgical disease. Cancer that is contained within the gland (tumor stage T2) is generally amenable to radical prostatectomy, while cancer that has spread outside of the gland (T3 and above) is typically treated non surgically (e.g., anti-androgen and radiation therapy).
- T-staging:

> **T1**: Tumor apparent by biopsy only.
>
> **T2**: Tumor confined within the prostate.
> **T2a**: <50% of one lobe; **T2b**: >50% of one lobe; **T2c**: Tumor involves both lobes.
>
> **T3**: Tumor extends through the prostate capsule. May involve seminal vesicles.
>
> **T4**: Tumor invades adjacent structures other than seminal vesicles.

- N-staging: Any regional lymph node metastasis is N1; however, extra-pelvic nodes are M1a.
- M-staging:

> **M0**: No metastases.
>
> **M1a**: Nonregional lymph nodes; **M1b**: Bone metastasis; **M1c**: Other metastasis.

- Staging example: T2a prostate cancer, which can be treated with radical prostatectomy.

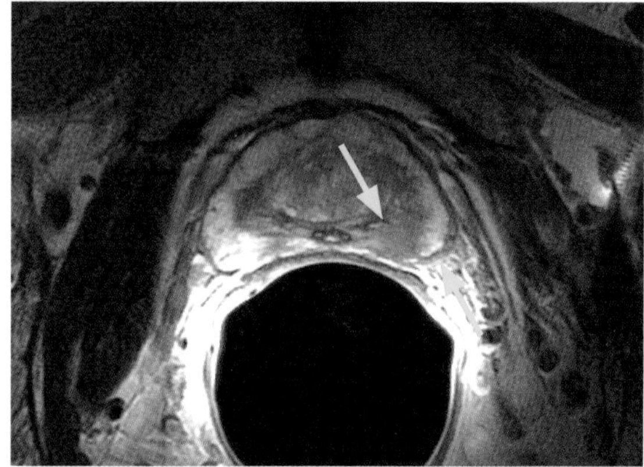

Axial T2-weighted MRI with an endorectal coil in place shows a focus of hypointensity within the posterior left peripheral zone (arrows), representing the site of cancer. There is no extraglandular extension.

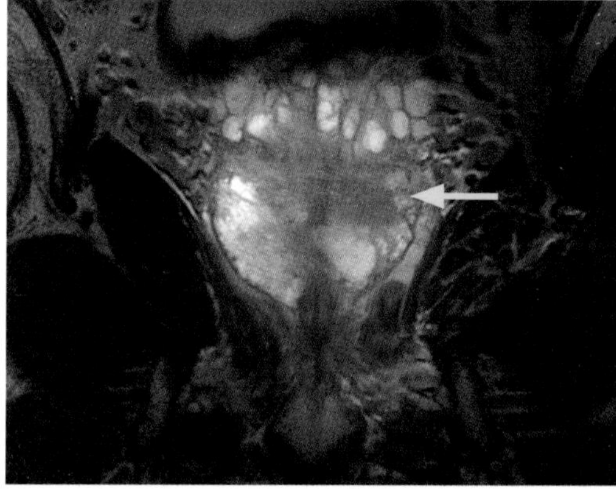

Coronal T2-weighted image through the posterior portion of the gland shows the tumor as a focal region of T2 hypointensity (arrow) in the peripheral zone.

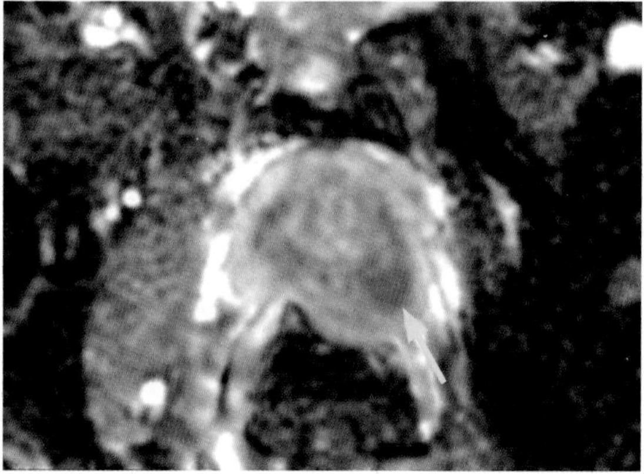

Axial ADC map shows that the tumor features restricted diffusion (arrow; dark on the ADC map).

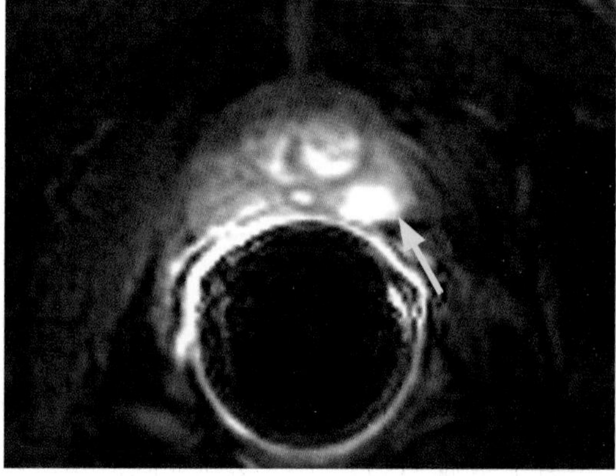

Axial early-phase dynamic gradient-echo contrast-enhanced MRI shows relative hyperenhancement of the prostate cancer (arrow).

In this case, the focus of prostate cancer is entirely confined within the gland. The tumor involves less than one half of one lobe for a stage of T2a. Because the tumor is so small, the advanced techniques of diffusion and dynamic contrast enhancement are helpful to increase specificity.

Case courtesy of Cheryl Sadow, MD, Brigham and Women's Hospital.

- Staging example: T3b N1 prostate cancer, which is typically treated non surgically.

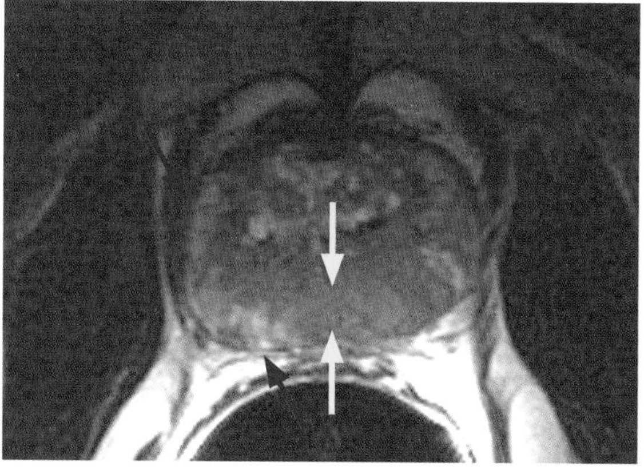

Axial T2 (with endorectal coil) of the prostate mid-gland shows near-complete replacement of the normal T2 hyperintense peripheral zone with a T2 hypointense mass (yellow arrows). There is some residual normal peripheral zone on the right (red arrows).

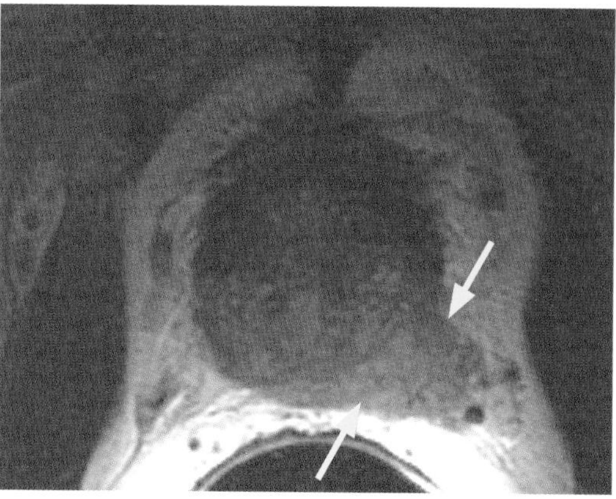

Axial T2 slightly more inferiorly shows left extra-glandular spread (arrows) with engulfment of the left seminal vesicle.

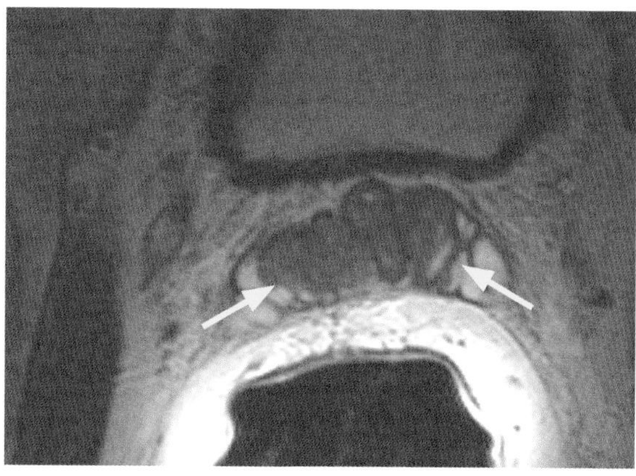

Axial T2 through the base of the bladder superior to the prostate shows abnormal T2 hypointensity in the medial aspect of both seminal vesicles (arrows).

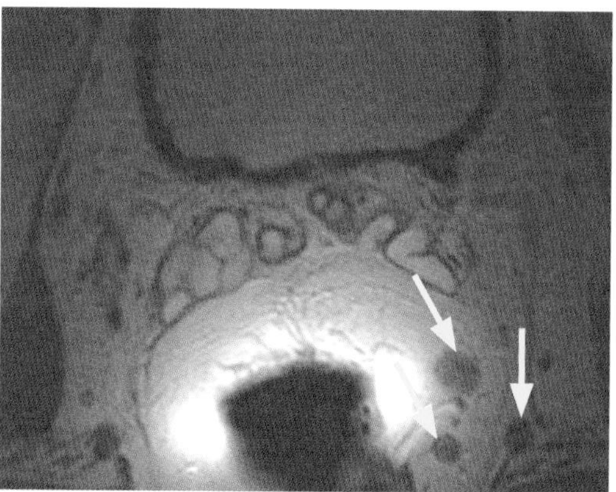

Superiormost axial T2 demonstrates several regional lymph nodes (arrows).

In this case, the tumor involves most of the peripheral zone of both lobes and clearly demonstrates extra-glandular spread, making the tumor T3. Because the tumor invades the seminal vesicles it is T3b: If it only extended out of the capsule, but the seminal vesicles were preserved, it would be T3a.

The presence of regional lymph nodes is N1.

Advanced MRI techniques would not add much in this case because the anatomic imaging demonstrates malignant behavior.

Case courtesy of Cheryl Sadow, MD, Brigham and Women's Hospital.

Uterine anatomy

Normal T2 zonal anatomy

- T2-weighted MRI can distinguish the three layers of the uterus.
- **Endometrial stripe:** Hyperintense on T2.
- **Junctional zone** (first zone of myometrium): T2 hypointense.
  - The hypointense T2 signal is due to the extremely compact smooth muscle.
  - The junctional zone should measure ≤12 mm: Thickening of the junctional zone is seen in adenomyosis.
- **Outer myometrium:** Relatively T2 hypointense, although less so than junctional zone.

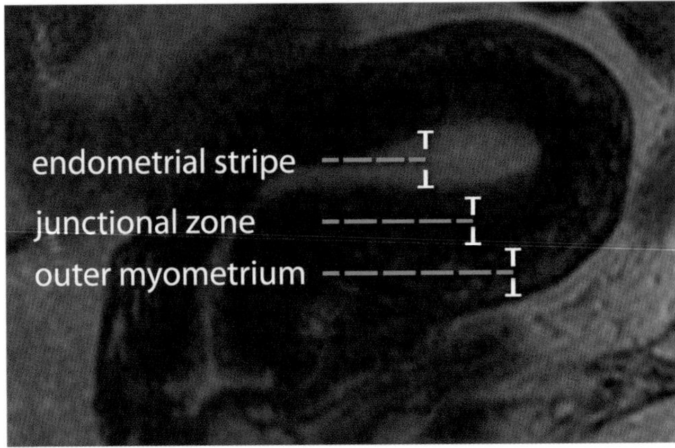

Normal sagittal T2 zonal anatomy of the uterus.

Case courtesy of Cheryl Sadow, MD, Brigham and Women's Hospital.

Benign uterine disease

Adenomyosis

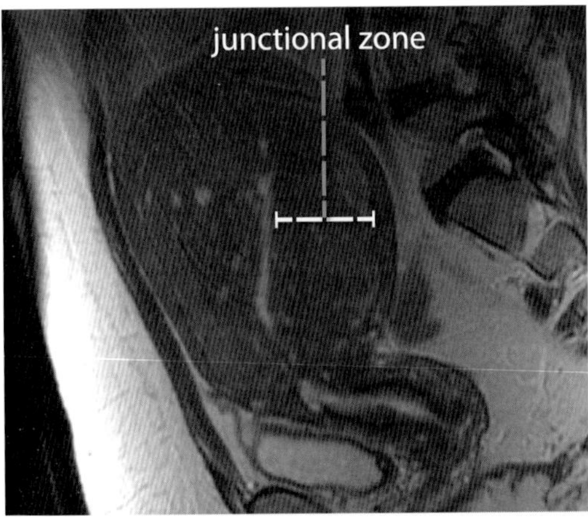

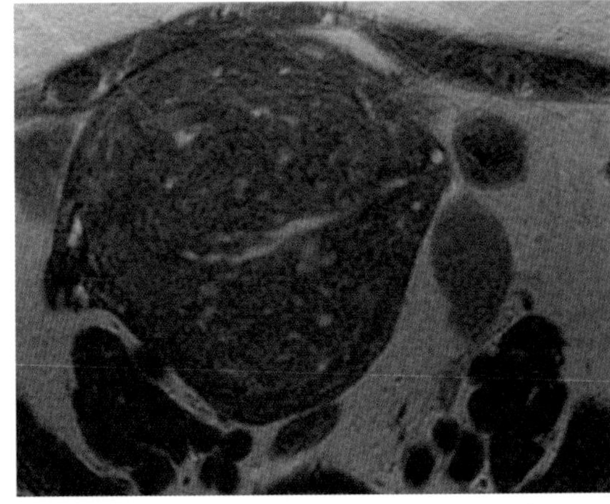

Adenomyosis: Sagittal (left) and axial T2-weighted MRI of the uterus shows a markedly thickened junctional zone containing numerous foci of T2 hyperintensity.

Case courtesy of Cheryl Sadow, MD, Brigham and Women's Hospital.

- Adenomyosis represents ectopic endometrial glands within the myometrium. In contrast to endometriosis, the ectopic endometrial tissue seen in adenomyosis is nonfunctioning.
- Adenomyosis can present with similar symptoms to leiomyomas, with pain and bleeding.
- Adenomyosis is best seen on T2-weighted images as a thickened junctional zone (>12 mm), often with multiple small foci of T2 hyperintensity. Borderline thickening of the junctional zone (8–12 mm) may be due to adenomyosis, but is not diagnostic of the condition.
- Focal adenomyosis may mimic a leiomyoma, appearing as a localized low-signal mass on T1- and T2-weighted images. Typically, adenomyosis features indistinct margins, in contrast to the characteristically sharp margins of a leiomyoma. However, the imaging features between these two entities do sometimes overlap.

Leiomyoma (fibroid)

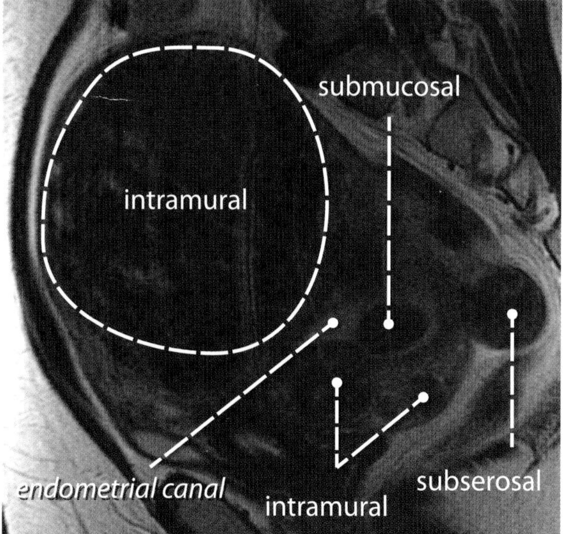

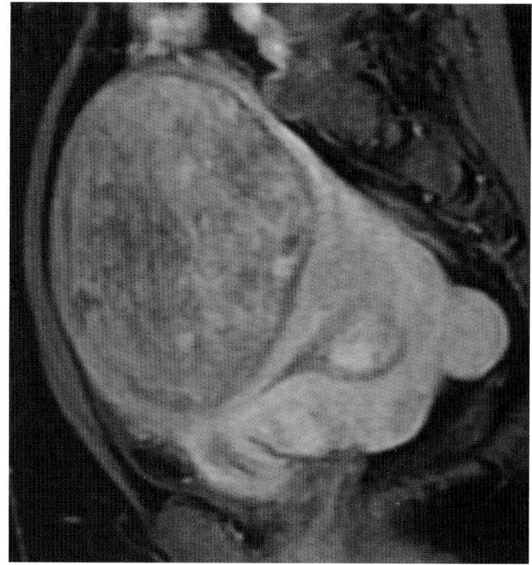

Submucosal, subserosal, and intramural fibroids: Sagittal T2-weighted (left image) and post-contrast sagittal T1-weighted fat suppressed MRI shows numerous fibroids, with the largest a dominant intramural fibroid. There are other smaller intramural fibroids, in addition to single submucosal and subserosal fibroids.

Case courtesy of Cheryl Sadow, MD, Brigham and Women's Hospital.

- A leiomyoma, commonly known as a fibroid, is an extremely common benign tumor of smooth muscle, which affects up to 40% of reproductive-age women.
- Fibroids are often multiple and may be intramural (within the myometrial wall), submucosal (directly underneath the endometrial mucosa), or subserosal (directly underneath the outer uterine serosa).
- Small leiomyomas are hypointense on T2-weighted images due to compact smooth muscle. However, cystic or myxoid degeneration may increase T2 signal heterogeneously. Carneous or hemorrhagic degeneration may appear hyperintense on T1-weighted images.
- Malignant leiomyosarcoma is very rare and may arise de-novo or from malignant degeneration of a fibroid. Imaging cannot reliably differentiate between leiomyoma and leiomyosarcoma unless clearly malignant behavior is identified (such as invasion of adjacent structures or metastases). In the absence of obvious malignant imaging findings, an unusual-looking fibroid is overwhelmingly likely to represent a degenerating benign fibroid rather than a leiomyosarcoma.
- MRI is often performed for treatment planning prior to uterine artery embolization (UAE). Hemorrhagic or necrotic leiomyomas are not treated effectively by UAE. Surgical myomectomy or hysterectomy would be the preferred treatment in these cases. Additionally, there is less chance of UAE success if an ovarian–uterine artery anastomosis is present.
- A uterine contraction may mimic a leiomyoma.

Endometrial carcinoma

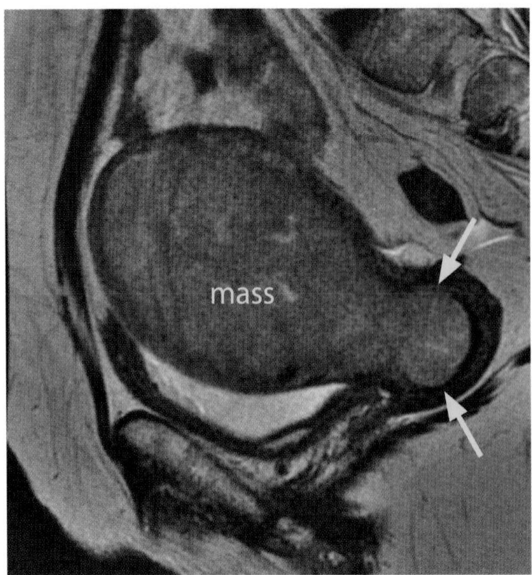

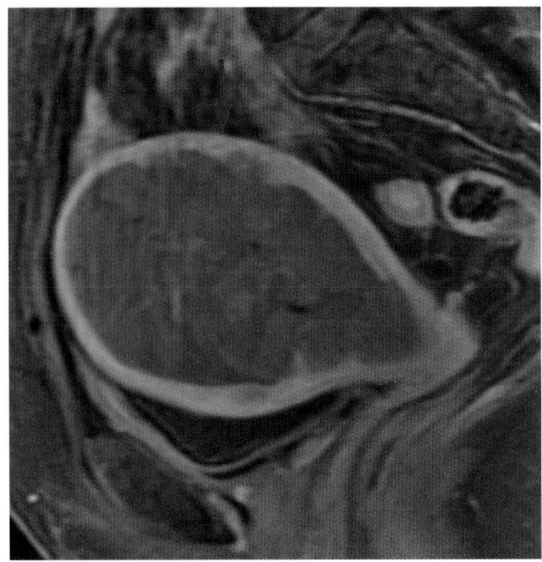

Endometrial carcinoma, stage IB: Sagittal T2-weighted MRI (left image) shows a large mass distending the endometrial canal and invading into the myometrial wall. The mass protrudes into the cervix (yellow arrows), without invasion of the cervical stroma.

Sagittal post-contrast fat-suppressed T1-weighted MRI (right image) shows that the mass is relatively hypoenhancing relative to the myometrium. The extent of myometrial invasion is better appreciated on this post-contrast image, where there are foci of invasion (red arrow) of the myometrial wall of >50% wall thickness.

Case courtesy of Cheryl Sadow, MD, Brigham and Women's Hospital.

- Endometrial carcinoma is the most common female gynecologic malignancy and is thought to be caused by prolonged estrogen exposure. Specific risk factors include nulliparity, hormone replacement, and Tamoxifen therapy.
- Endometrial carcinoma typically presents with post-menopausal bleeding.
- MRI can be used for staging once carcinoma is confirmed by histologic sampling.
- The presence and extent of myometrial invasion is key for staging. In a premenopausal patient, an intact junctional zone confirms that there is no myometrial invasion. The junctional zone cannot be distinguished in post-menopausal patients, however. The depth of myometrial invasion highly correlates with the presence of lymph node metastasis.
- Post-contrast images demonstrate the tumor with the highest conspicuity, as endometrial cancer enhances less avidly than the surrounding myometrium.
- The FIGO (International Federation of Gynecology and Obstetrics) staging of endometrial carcinoma was revised in 2010.

Stage I: Tumor confined to the uterus. Stage IA: <50% of myometrial invasion; stage IB: >50% myometrial invasion.

Stage II: Spread to the cervical stroma, but tumor still contained within the uterus. Involvement of the endocervical glands only is stage I.

Stage III: Spread to adnexa or uterine serosa (IIIA), vagina (IIIB), pelvic lymph nodes (IIIC1), or para-aortic lymph nodes (IIIC2). Prognosis is worse with para-aortic nodes, even in the absence of pelvic adenopathy.

Stage IVA: Spread to bladder or bowel mucosa.

Stage IVB: Distant metastases or inguinal lymph node spread.

Normal cervical T2 zonal anatomy

- **Endocervical canal**: T2 hyperintense due to mucin, analogous to uterine endometrium.
- **Cervical mucosa:** Intermediate T2 signal intensity.
- **Inner cervical stroma**: Very hypointense on T2, analogous to the uterine junctional zone. Unlike the uterine junctional zone, however, the decreased T2 signal is due to compact fibrous tissue, not smooth muscle. The superior aspect of the inner cervical stroma is continuous with junctional zone of the uterus.

Cervical carcinoma

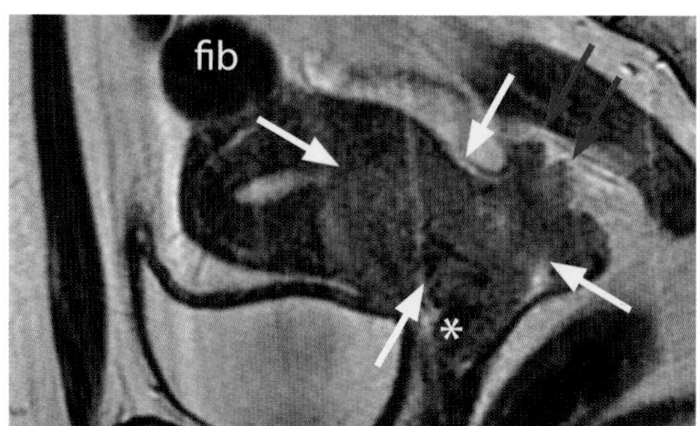

Sagittal T2-weighted MRI

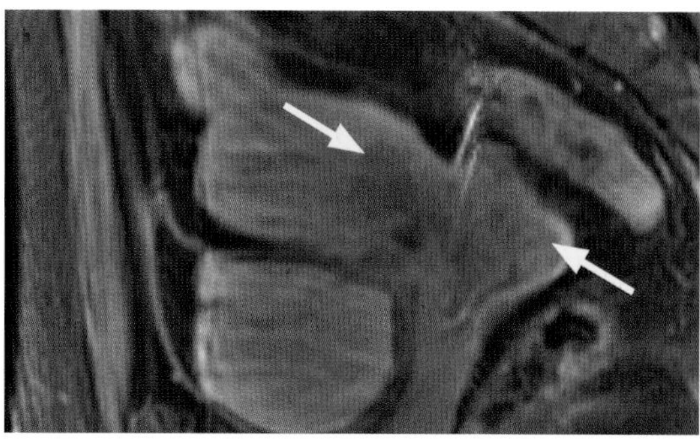

Post-contrast sagittal T1-weighted MRI with fat supp.

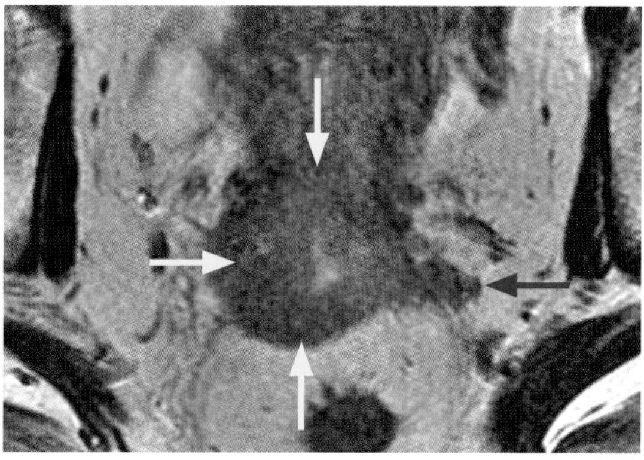

Axial T2-weighted MRI

Cervical carcinoma, stage IIB: Sagittal T2-weighted image (top left image) shows an ill-defined, hyperintense mass (yellow arrows) centered at the cervix, with invasion into the lower uterine segment and the anterior vaginal fornix (*). There is nodular parametrial invasion (red arrows). A subserosal fibroid (fib) is present. The mass enhances heterogeneously (top right image). The axial (left image) shows near complete circumferential cervical involvement (yellow arrows) and left parametrial spread (red arrow).

Case courtesy of Cheryl Sadow, MD, Brigham and Women's Hospital.

- Cervical carcinoma is the third most common gynecologic malignancy, with a steep decline in prevalence over the past 50 years due to screening with Pap smears.
- A cervical mass >1.5 cm should be evaluated by MRI for staging. The cervical stroma is the key landmark in the staging of cervical cancer: If tumor extends through the cervical stroma into the **parametrium**, the cancer is stage **IIB** and treatment is typically non-surgical. Other key findings to note are involvement of bladder or rectum, which denotes stage IV disease (if shown to extend to the mucosal surface with cystoscopy or endoscopy).
- The FIGO (International Federation of Gynecology and Obstetrics) staging of cervical cancer was revised in 2010. The new staging takes into account lymph node involvement.

> **Stage I**: Confined to cervix or uterus. IA: Microscopic lesion. IB: Clinically visible lesion.
>
> **Stage IIA**: Spread to upper 2/3 vagina, without parametrial invasion. Typically treated surgically.
>
> **Stage IIB**: Parametrial invasion. Typically treated non-surgically (e.g., brachytherapy).
>
> **Stage IIIA**: Spread to lower vagina.
>
> **Stage IIIB**: Pelvic sidewall extension, hydronephrosis, or pelvic nodal involvement.
>
> **Stage IVA**: Spread to bladder or rectum; **Stage IVB**: Distant metastasis.

- Müllerian duct anomalies may be a cause of infertility or recurrent pregnancy loss (most commonly in septate uterus). Septate and bicornuate uterus are the most common uterine anomalies, which may be differentiated by MRI. The American Fertility Society classification of Müllerian duct anomalies is discussed in the ultrasound section.

Septate uterus

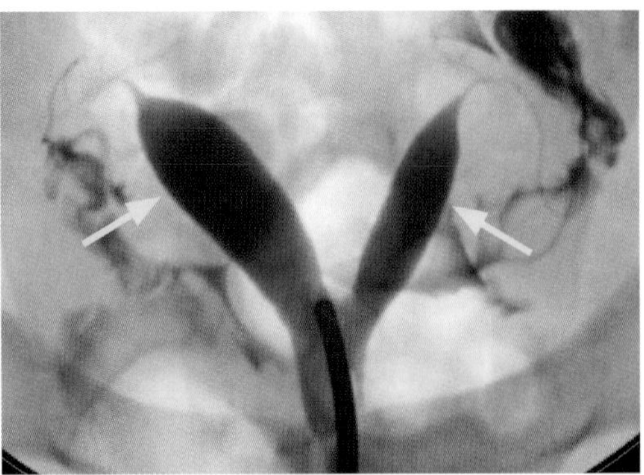

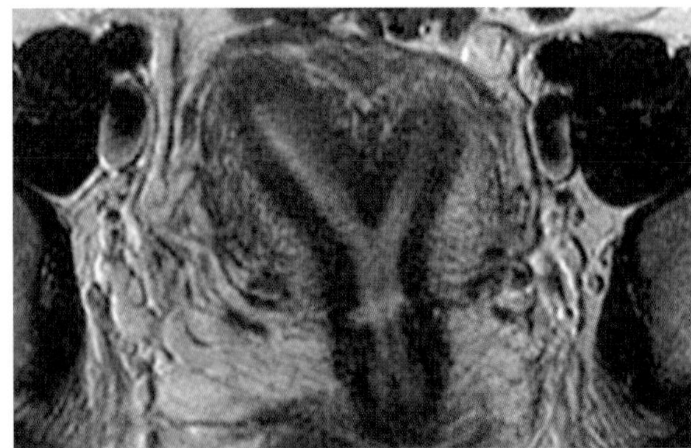

Septate uterus: Hysterosalpingogram (left image) shows a common lower endometrial cavity that splits to form two separate endometrial cavities (yellow arrows). This appearance on HSG is nonspecific and may represent either a septate or bicornuate uterus. There is bilateral intraperitoneal spillage of contrast, confirming normal patent fallopian tubes. Axial T2 MRI (right image) also shows the split endometrial canal; however, the outer myometrium has fused, yielding a continuous convex fundus.

Case courtesy of Cheryl Sadow, MD, Brigham and Women's Hospital.

- Septate uterus is caused by incomplete resorption of the septum of fused Müllerian ducts.
- A septate uterus has a single external fundus but a fibrous or muscular septation dividing two endometrial canals. Infertility is more common in women with septate uterus compared to bicornuate uterus. Metroplasty (resection of the septum) can be performed hysteroscopically if the septum is fibrous, or via an open approach if the septum is muscular.

Bicornuate uterus

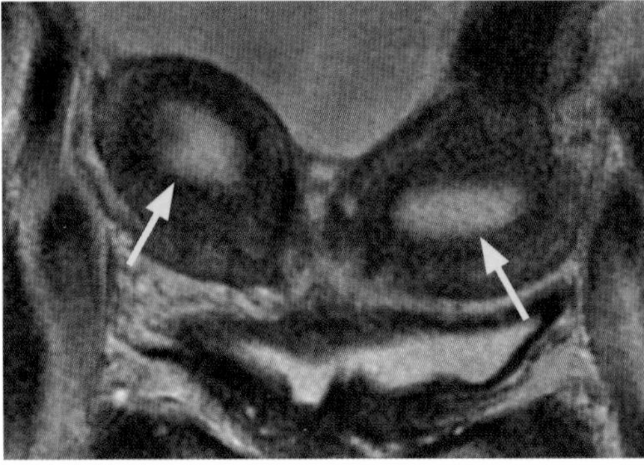

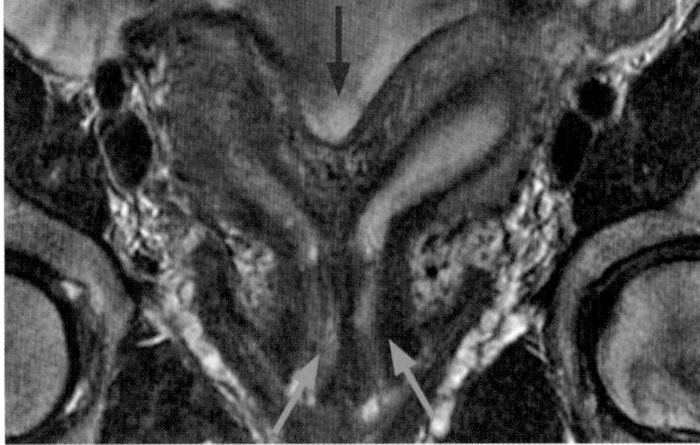

Bicornuate, bicollis uterus: Axial (left image) and coronal T2-weighted MRI (right image) shows two separate endometrial canals (yellow arrows) with a definite external fundal cleft (red arrow). There are two separate cervices (bicollis; blue arrows), which share a common myometrium.

Case courtesy of Cheryl Sadow, MD, Brigham and Women's Hospital.

- Bicornuate uterus is due to incomplete fusion of the Müllerian ducts.
- A bicornuate uterus describes a partially split uterus with two separate uterine fundi. In contrast to a septate uterus, the fundus of a bicornuate uterus pinches inwards >15 mm.
- If treated, metroplasty must be performed transabdominally, which is a more invasive procedure compared to hysteroscopic metroplasty.

- MRI can provide additional specificity for adnexal lesions that are indeterminate on ultrasound. Fat and hemorrhage are both hyperintense on T1-weighted images, but fat-suppressed T1-weighted imaging can distinguish between lesions containing fat (such as a mature cystic teratoma) and containing hemorrhage (such as an endometrioma).

Endometriosis

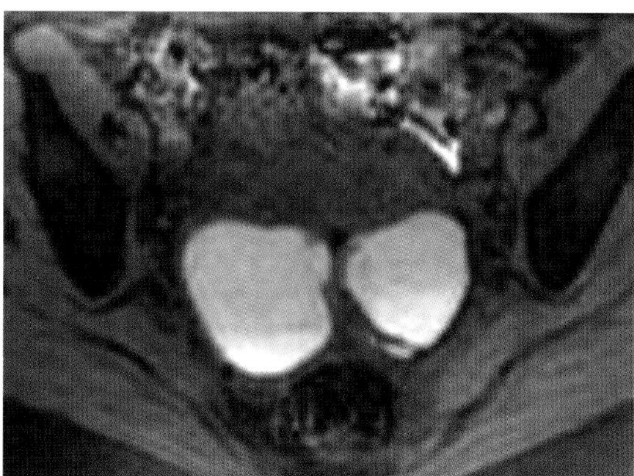
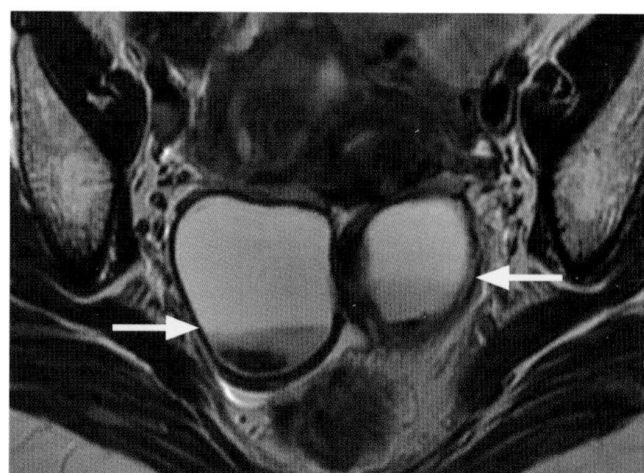

Endometriosis: Axial fat-suppressed T1-weighted MRI (left image) shows bilateral T1 hyperintense ovarian lesions. The T2-weighted axial MRI (right image) demonstrates characteristic dependent shading (arrows).

Case courtesy of Cheryl Sadow, MD, Brigham and Women's Hospital.

- Endometriosis represents ectopic foci of endometrial tissue that are hormonally responsive and therefore may be composed of blood products of varying ages.
- The typical MRI appearance of endometriosis is multiple hyperintense masses on T1-weighted images, which demonstrate shading (a gradient of signal intensity) on T2-weighted images. Endometriosis does not suppress on fat-saturated sequences. Less commonly, endometriosis may appear hyperintense on both T1- and T2-weighted images.
- Tiny hemorrhagic endometrial implants may only be apparent as tiny hyperintense foci on T1-weighted images.
- A ruptured endometrioma may be a cause of acute pelvic pain and may produce free fluid that is hyperintense on both T1- and T2-weighted images.
- Laparoscopy is the gold standard for evaluation of suspected endometriosis.

Mature cystic teratoma

- Also known as a dermoid cyst, mature cystic teratoma is the most common benign ovarian neoplasm in young women. It is composed of differentiated tissue from at least two embryonic cell layers.
- A mature cystic teratoma is typically a unilocular cystic structure filled with sebaceous material, hair follicles, and other tissues. Less commonly, a mature teratoma may appear as a heterogeneous mass or may be a solid fat-containing mass.
- A Rokitansky nodule is a solid nodule projecting into the cyst cavity, from which hair or teeth may arise.
- On imaging, the sebaceous intracystic component is typically hyperintense on T1- and T2-weighted images, matching fat intensity. Since both an endometrioma and a teratoma are predominantly hyperintense on T1-weighted images, the fat-suppressed sequences are key to differentiation. Teratoma will show signal loss on the fat suppressed images.
- Ovaries containing a dermoid cyst are predisposed to torsion.

Ovarian cancer

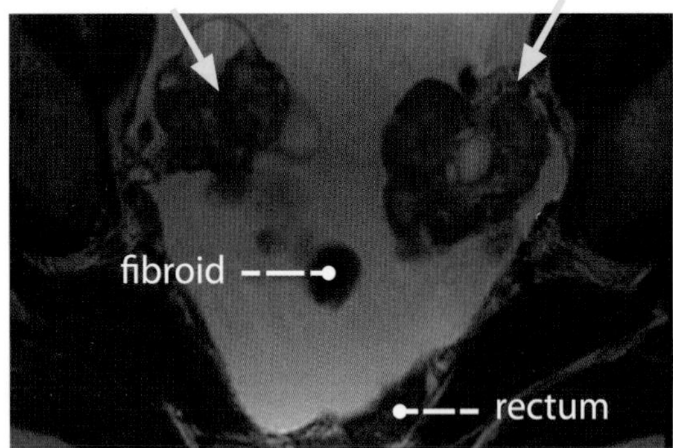

Axial T2-weighted fat suppressed MRI

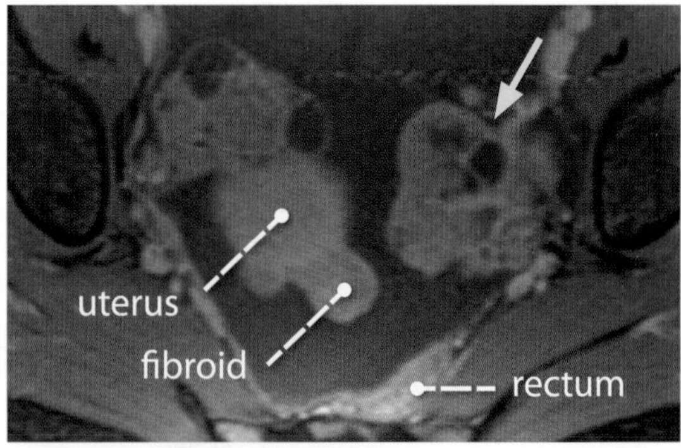

Axial post-contrast T1-weighted fat suppressed MRI

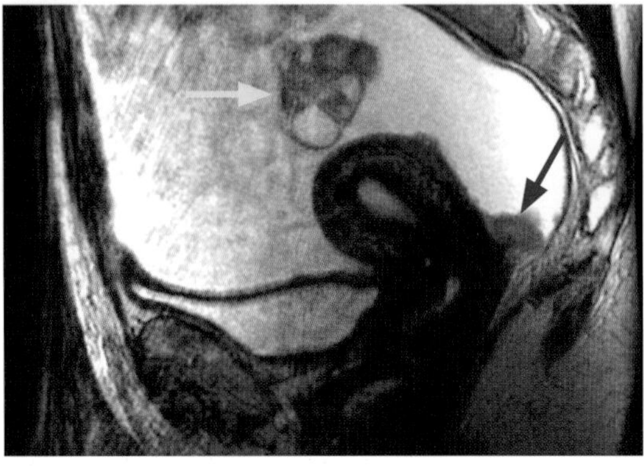

Sagittal T2-weighted fat suppressed MRI

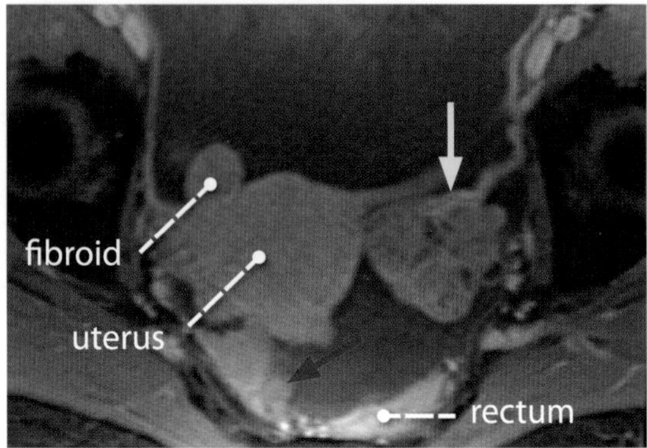

Axial post-contrast T1-weighted fat suppressed MRI

Ovarian cancer with peritoneal carcinomatosis: MRI shows bilateral enhancing adnexal masses (yellow arrows). There are enhancing peritoneal implants in the pouch of Douglas posterior to the uterus (red arrows). The uterus contains several T2 hypointense enhancing fibroids. This histology was papillary serous.

Case courtesy of Cheryl Sadow, MD, Brigham and Women's Hospital.

- Ovarian cancer is the second most common female pelvic malignancy but is one of the most lethal malignancies as 65% of patients present with advanced disease.
- MRI is used to characterize indeterminate adnexal masses, rather than for staging.
- The presence of a solid enhancing component, intra-lesional necrosis, ascites, or peritoneal nodularity suggests a malignant lesion, although no finding is 100% specific.
- MRI is highly sensitive to detect peritoneal implants, which occur most commonly in the pouch of Douglas, paracolic gutters, bowel surface, greater omentum, and liver surface.
- Ovarian cancer may be **epithelial**, **germ cell**, **sex-cord stromal**, or **metastatic** in origin.
- Approximately 90% of malignant tumors are of epithelial origin. Serous tumors are the most common epithelial subtype, followed by mucinous, endometrioid, and clear cell.

  Serous cystadenocarcinomas are frequently bilateral and typically appear as mixed solid and cystic masses. The solid portions demonstrate avid enhancement. There is often concomitant ascites.

  Mucinous cystadenocarcinomas are large, most commonly unilateral, and occur in older patients compared to serous cystadenocarcinomas. Mucinous cystadenocarcinomas typically present as a multiloculated cystic mass containing mucin-rich T1 hyperintense fluid.

  Clear cell carcinoma and less commonly **endometrioid carcinoma** are associated with endometriosis.

- Malignant **germ cell** tumors occur in younger patients and include dysgerminoma, endodermal sinus tumor, and immature teratoma.
- **Sex-cord stromal** tumors include granulosa cell (hormonally active) and Sertoli–Leydig (rare).
- **Metastases** are uncommon but may result from gastric cancer (Krukenberg tumor), colon cancer, pancreatic cancer, breast cancer, and melanoma. Metastases are often bilateral.

References, resources, and further reading

General Reference:

Dunnick, N.R., Sandler, C.M., Newhouse, J.H. & Amis, E.S. Textbook of Uroradiology (4th ed.). Philadelphia: Lippincott Williams & Wilkins. (2008).

Renal:

Bonsib, S.M. Renal cystic diseases and renal neoplasms: a mini-review. Clinical Journal of the American Society of Nephrology: CJASN 4, 1998-2007(2009).

Dwivedi, U.S. et al. Xanthogranulomatous pyelonephritis: our experience with review of published reports. ANZ Journal of Surgery 76, 1007-9(2006).

Israel, G.M. & Bosniak, M.A. Calcification in Cystic Renal Masses: Is It Important in Diagnosis? Radiology 226, 47-52(2003).

Israel, G.M. & Bosniak, M.A. An update of the Bosniak renal cyst classification system. Urology 66, 484-8(2005).

Israel, G.M. & Bosniak, M.A Pitfalls in renal mass evaluation and how to avoid them. Radiographics 28, 1325-38(2008).

Israel, G.M., Hindman, N. & Bosniak, M.A. Evaluation of cystic renal masses: comparison of CT and MR Imaging by using the Bosniak classification system. Radiology 231, 365-71(2004).

Jinzaki, M. et al. Evaluation of Small (≤3 cm) Renal Masses with MDCT: Benefits of Thin Overlapping Reconstructions. American Journal of Roentgenology 183, 223-8(2004).

Jonisch, A.I., Rubinowitz, A.N. & Israel, G.M. Can High-Attenuation Renal Cysts Be Differentiated from Renal Cell Carcinoma at Unenhanced CT? Radiology 243, 445-50(2007).

Kekelidze, M. et al. Kidney and Urinary Tract Imaging: Triple-Bolus Multidetector CT Urography as a One-Stop Shop. Radiology 255, 508-16(2010).

Kim, J.K. et al. Differentiation of subtypes of renal cell carcinoma on helical CT scans. AJR. American Journal of Roentgenology 178, 1499-506(2002).

Kim, J.K. et al. Angiomyolipoma with minimal fat: differentiation from renal cell carcinoma at biphasic helical CT. Radiology 230, 677-84(2004).

Meister, M. et al. Radiological evaluation, management, and surveillance of renal masses in Von Hippel-Lindau disease. Clinical Radiology 64, 589-600(2009).

Sadow, C.A. et al. Bladder Cancer Detection with CT Urography in an Academic Medical Center. Radiology 249, 195(2008).

Silverman, S.G. et al. Renal masses in the adult patient: the role of percutaneous biopsy. Radiology 240, 6-22(2006).

Silverman, S.G. et al. Management of the incidental renal mass. Radiology 249, 16-31(2008).

Silverman, S.G. et al. Hyperattenuating Renal Masses: Etiologies, Pathogenesis, and Imaging Evaluation. Radiographics 1131-44(2007).

Smith, J.K. & Kenney, P.J. Imaging of renal trauma. Radiologic Clinics of North America 41(5), 1019-35(2003).

Yan, B.C., Mackinnon, A.C. & Al-Ahmadie, H.A. Recent developments in the pathology of renal tumors: morphology and molecular characteristics of select entities. Archives of Pathology & Laboratory Medicine 133, 1026-32(2009).

Yuh, B.I. & Cohan, R.H. Different phases of renal enhancement: role in detecting and characterizing renal masses during helical CT. American Journal of Roentgenology 173, 747(1999).

Zugor, V., Schott, G.E. & Labanaris, A.P. Xanthogranulomatous pyelonephritis in childhood: a critical analysis of 10 cases and of the literature. Urology 70, 157-60(2007).

Retroperitoneal:

Cronin, C.G. et al. Retroperitoneal fibrosis: a review of clinical features and imaging findings. AJR. American Journal of Roentgenology, 191(2), 423-31(2008).

Sanyal, R. & Remer, E.M. Radiology of the retroperitoneum: case-based review. AJR. American Journal of Roentgenology, 192(6 Suppl), S112-7 (Quiz S118-21)(2009).

Adrenal:

Blake, M.A. et al. Pheochromocytoma: An Imaging Chameleon. Radiographics 24, S87(2004).

Elsayes, K.M. et al. Adrenal Masses: MR Imaging Features with Pathologic Correlation. Radiographics 24, S73(2004).

Krebs, T.L. & Wagner, B.J. MR Imaging of the adrenal gland: radiologic-pathologic correlation. Radiographics 18, 1425(1998).

Lockhart, M.E., Smith, J.K. & Kenney, P.J. Imaging of adrenal masses. European Journal of Radiology 41, 95-112(2002).

Sangwaiya, M., Boland, G. & Cronin, C. Incidental Adrenal Lesions: Accuracy of Characterization with Contrast-enhanced Washout Multidetector CT—10-minute Delayed Imaging Protocol Revisited. Radiology 256, 504-510(2010).

Ureter and Bladder:

Chavhan, G.B. Signs in Imaging Radiology The Cobra Head Sign 1. Radiology, 781-82(2002).

Daniels, R.E. III. Signs in Imaging the Goblet Sign. Radiology 210, 737-8(1999).

Dillman, J.R., Caoili, E.M. & Cohan, R.H. Multi-detector CT urography: a one-stop renal and urinary tract imaging modality. Abdominal Imaging 32(4), 519-29(2007).

Dyer, R.B., Chen, M.Y. & Zagoria, R.J. Classic Signs in Uroradiology. Radiographics, 24(suppl 1), S247-80(2004).

Joffe, S.A., Servaes, S., Okon, S. & Horowitz, M. Multi-detector row CT urography in the evaluation of hematuria. Radiographics 23(6), 1441-55; discussion 1455-6(2003).

Kawashima, A. et al. CT urography. Radiographics, 24 Suppl 1, S35-54; discussion S55-8(2004).

Sadow, C.A. et al. Positive predictive value of CT urography in the evaluation of upper tract urothelial cancer. AJR. American Journal of Roentgenology, 195(5), W337-43(2010).

Yu, J.S. et al. Urachal Remnant Diseases: Spectrum of CT and US Findings. Radiographics, 21(2), 451(2001).

Urethra:

Kawashima, A. et al. Imaging of Urethral Disease: A Pictoral Review. Radiographics, 24, 195-216(2004).

Kim, B., Kawashima, A. & LeRoy, A.J. Imaging of the Male Urethra. Seminars in Ultrasound, CT, and MRI, 28(4), 258-73(2007).

Levin, T.L., Han, B. & Little, B.P. Congenital anomalies of the male urethra. Pediatric Radiology, 37(9), 851-62; quiz 945(2007).

Pavlica, P., Barozzi, L. & Menchi, I. Imaging of male urethra. European radiology, 13(7), 1583-96(2003).

Prasad, S. et al. Cross-sectional Imaging of the Female Urethra: Technique and Results. Radiographics, 25, 749-61(2005).

Rovner, E.S. Urethral Diverticula: A Review and an Update. Neurourology and Urodynamics, 26, 972-7(2007).

Prostate MRI:

Akin, O. & Hricak, H. Imaging of prostate cancer. Radiologic Clinics of North America, 45(1), 207-22(2007).

Choi, Y.J. et al. Functional MR Imaging of Prostate Cancer 1. Radiographics, 27, 63-76(2007).

Coakley, F.V. & Hricak, H. Radiologic anatomy of the prostate gland: a clinical approach. Radiologic Clinics of North America, 38(1), 15–30(2000).

Yu, K.K. & Hricak, H. Imaging prostate cancer. Radiologic Clinics of North America, 38(1), 59–85(2000).

Female Pelvis MRI:

Beddy, P. et al. FIGO Staging System for Endometrial Cancer: Added Benefits of MR Imaging. Radiographics, 32(1), 241-54(2012).

Creasman, W. Revised FIGO staging for carcinoma of the endometrium. International Journal of Gynaecology and Obstetrics: the official organ of the International Federation of Gynaecology and Obstetrics, 105(2), 109(2009).

Pecorelli, S., Zigliani, L. & Odicino, F. Revised FIGO staging for carcinoma of the cervix. International Journal of Gynaecology and Obstetrics, 105(2), 107-8(2009).

Sala, E. Magnetic resonance imaging of the female pelvis. Seminars in Roentgenology, 43(4), 290-302(2008).

4 Neuroimaging

Contents

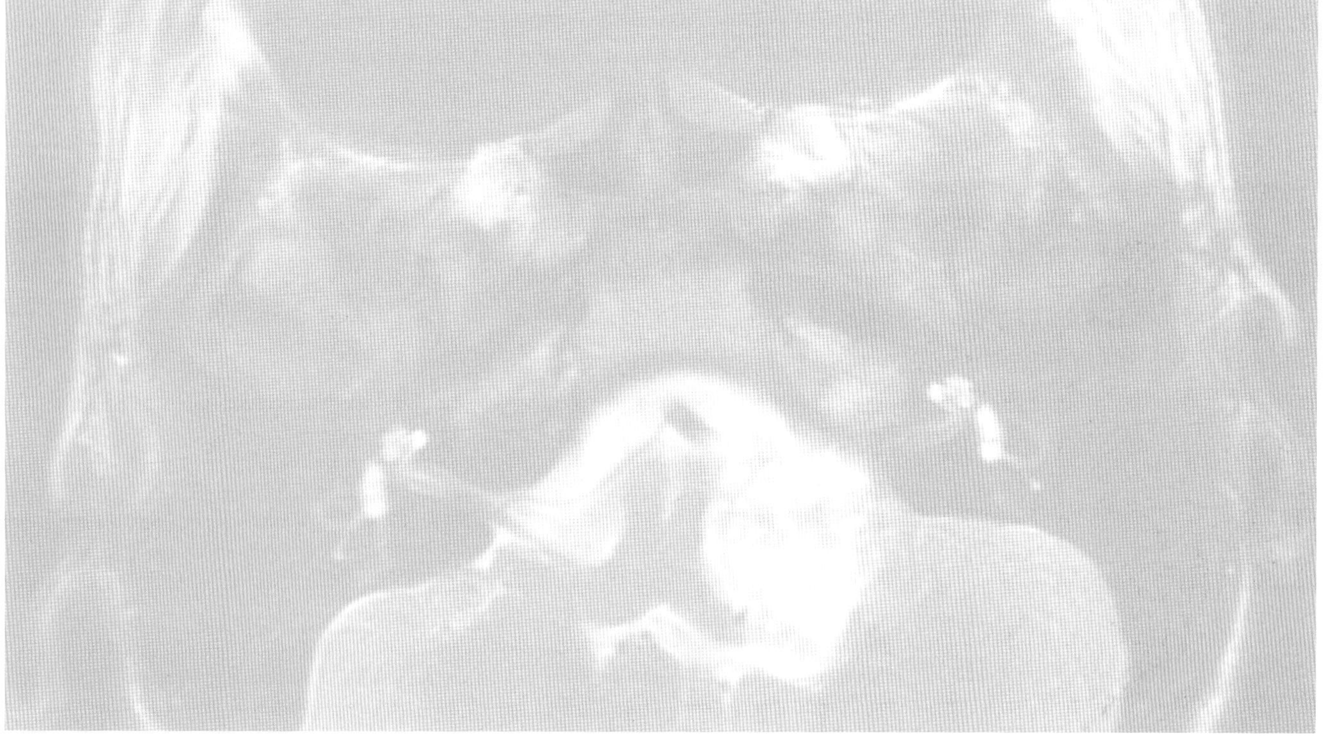

VENTRICULAR ANATOMY

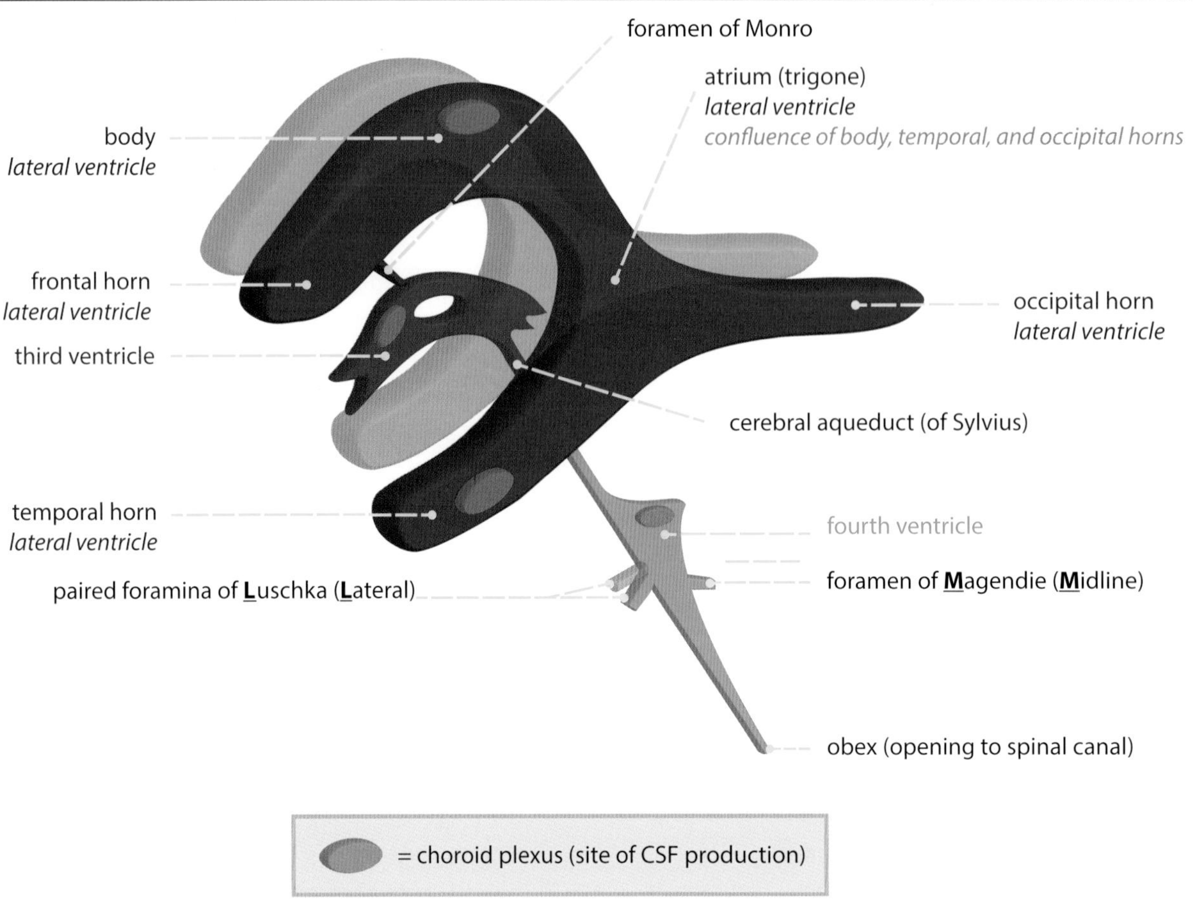

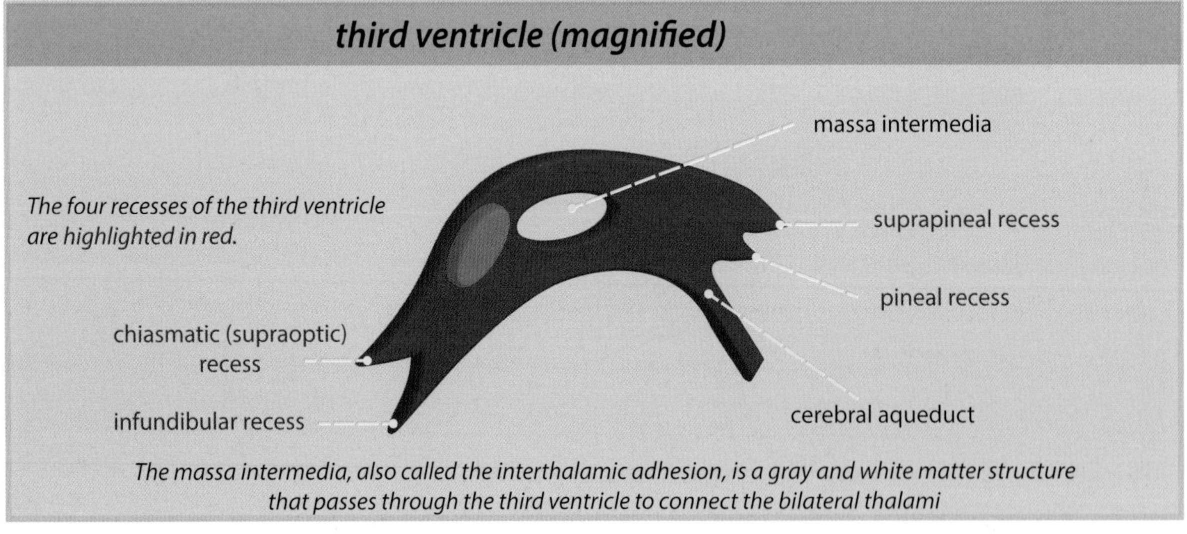

Cerebrospinal fluid (CSF)

Ventricular anatomy

- The ventricular system consists of two lateral ventricles and midline third and fourth ventricles.
- The foramen of Monro connects the lateral ventricles with the third ventricle.
- The cerebral aqueduct (of Sylvius) connects the third ventricle with the fourth ventricle.
- The fourth ventricle continues inferiorly as the central canal of the spinal cord. The fourth ventricle also drains into the subarachnoid space and basal cisterns via three foramina:

  Paired foramina of Luschka (Luschka is lateral).

  Single foramen of Magendie (Magendie is medial).

CSF dynamics

- Cerebrospinal fluid is produced by the choroid plexus, which is located in specific locations throughout the ventricular system:

  Body and temporal horn of each lateral ventricle.

  Roof of third ventricle.

  Roof of fourth ventricle.

  There is NO choroid plexus in the cerebral aqueduct or occipital or frontal horns of the lateral ventricles.

- The ventricular volume is approximately 25 mL. The volume of the subarachnoid space is approximately 125 mL, for a total CSF volume of approximately 150 mL.
- CSF production is 500 mL/day, which completely replenishes the total CSF volume 3–4 times per day.
- CSF is absorbed primarily by the arachnoid granulations (leptomeningeal evaginations extending into the dural venous sinuses) and to a lesser extent by the lymphatic system and cerebral veins.

Cerebral edema

- Edema within the brain can be caused by cell death, altered capillary permeability, or hemodynamic forces.

Cytotoxic edema

- Cytotoxic edema is cell swelling caused by damaged molecular sodium–potassium ATPase ion pumps. It can affect both gray and white matter.
- Cytotoxic edema is caused by cell death, most commonly due to infarct. Water ions trapped inside swollen cells feature reduced diffusivity.

Vasogenic edema

- Vasogenic edema is interstitial edema caused by increased capillary permeability. It is seen primarily in the white matter, as there is more interstitial space.
- Vasogenic edema is caused most commonly by neoplasm, infection, or infarct.

Interstitial edema

- Interstitial edema is caused by imbalances in CSF flow, most commonly due to obstructive hydrocephalus.
- Interstitial edema presents on imaging as periventricular fluid, often called "transependymal flow of CSF," even though it is unlikely that the CSF actually flows across the ependymal cells lining the ventricles.

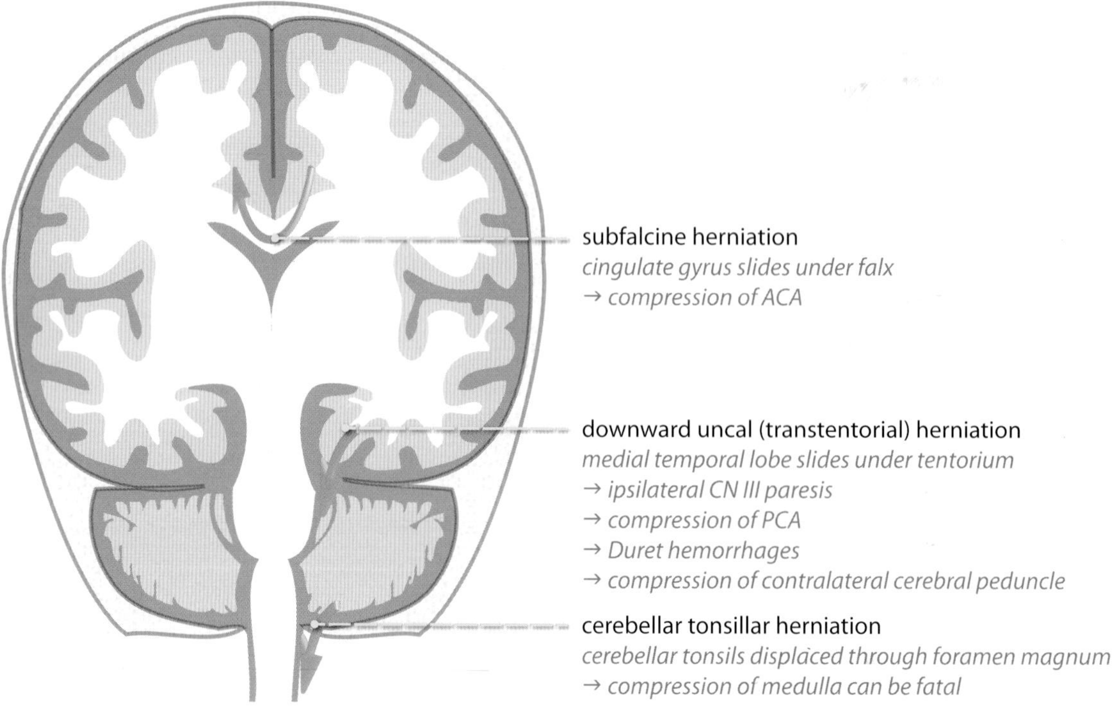
subfalcine herniation
cingulate gyrus slides under falx
→ compression of ACA
downward uncal (transtentorial) herniation
medial temporal lobe slides under tentorium
→ ipsilateral CN III paresis
→ compression of PCA
→ Duret hemorrhages
→ compression of contralateral cerebral peduncle
cerebellar tonsillar herniation
cerebellar tonsils displaced through foramen magnum
→ compression of medulla can be fatal

- The total volume in the skull is fixed. Increases in intracranial pressure may lead to herniation across a dural fold.
- Herniation may be due to a mass lesion (such as a neoplasm or hematoma) or may be due to edema secondary to a large stroke. Because the volume of the posterior fossa is especially limited, cerebellar infarcts are prone to herniation.

Subfalcine herniation

- Subfalcine herniation is seen when the cingulate gyrus slides underneath the falx.
- Subfalcine herniation may rarely cause compression of the anterior cerebral artery (ACA) against the falx, resulting in infarction.
- Contralateral hydrocephalus may result from foramen of Monro obstruction, resulting in ventricular entrapment.

Transtentorial (uncal) herniation

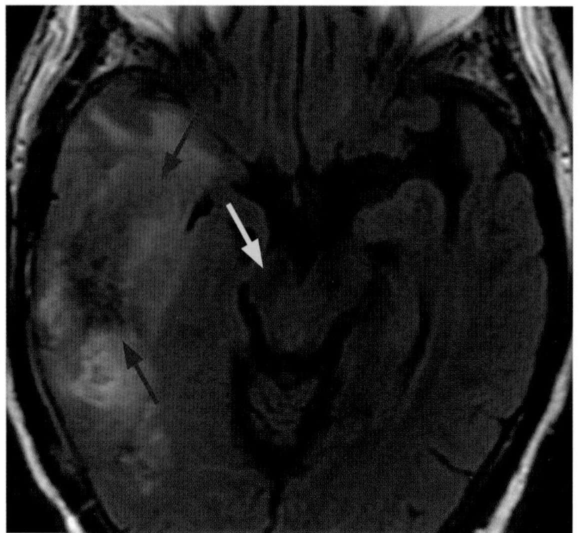

Early uncal herniation: Axial FLAIR MRI shows a heterogeneous mass in the right temporal lobe (red arrows), with effacement of the right lateral ventricle temporal horn. The mass effect causes mild downward uncal herniation with flattening of the right cerebral peduncle (yellow arrow).

- *Downward* transtentorial herniation results in inferomedial displacement of the medial temporal lobe (uncus) through the tentorial notch, causing compression on the brainstem and adjacent structures.

  > The ipsilateral cranial nerve III (oculomotor nerve) may be compressed, leading to pupillary dilation and CN III palsy (eye is "down and out").
  >
  > Compression of the ipsilateral posterior cerebral artery (PCA) may cause medial temporal/occipital infarct.
  >
  > Upper brainstem **Duret hemorrhages** are caused by shearing of perforating vessels due to downward force on the brainstem.
  >
  > Compression of the contralateral cerebral peduncle against Kernohan's notch causes a hemiparesis ipsilateral to the herniated side.

- *Upward* transtentorial herniation is superior transtentorial herniation of the cerebellar vermis due to posterior fossa mass effect. The main complication of upward transtentorial herniation is obstructive hydrocephalus from aqueductal compression.

Cerebellar tonsillar herniation

- Downward displacement of the cerebellar tonsils through foramen magnum causes compression of the medulla.
- Compression of medullary respiratory centers is often fatal.

Hydrocephalus

- **Communicating hydrocephalus** is ventricular enlargement without an obstructing lesion.

  Subarachnoid hemorrhage can cause communicating hydrocephalus by impeding arachnoid granulation reabsorption of CSF.

  Normal pressure hydrocephalus (NPH) is a form of communicating hydrocephalus characterized by normal mean CSF pressure and the clinical triad of dementia, ataxia, and incontinence. NPH is an important diagnosis as it is a treatable and potentially reversible cause of dementia. Imaging typically shows enlargement of the lateral and third ventricles.

- **Noncommunicating hydrocephalus** is hydrocephalus due to an obstructing lesion, such as a third ventricular colloid cyst or a posterior fossa mass obstructing the fourth ventricle.

Intra-axial and extra-axial compartments

- An intra-axial lesion is within the brain parenchyma itself, underneath the pial membrane.
- An extra-axial lesion is external to the pial membrane. The meninges and subarachnoid space are extra-axial.

Basal cisterns

- The basal cisterns, also known as the perimesencephalic cisterns, are CSF-filled spaces surrounding the midbrain and pons.
- Compression or effacement of the basal cisterns may be a sign of impending or actual herniation.
- The diagram to the right is highly schematic. In actuality, not all of the cisterns can be visualized on the same axial slice.

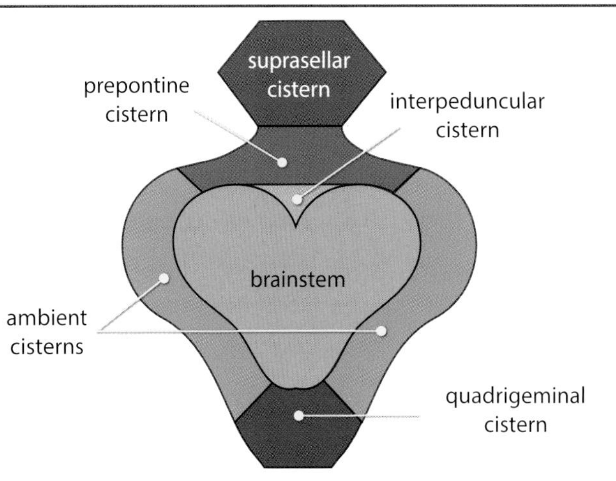

- As discussed in the physics section, inherent tissue T1 and T2 characteristics depend on the longitudinal recovery/relaxation (T1) and transverse relaxation (T2) times of the protons in that tissue. Any tissue signal abnormality is produced by alterations (prolongation or shortening) of the transverse or longitudinal relaxation.

  T1 shortening is hyperintense (bright) on T1-weighted images and T1 prolongation is hypointense (dark). Conversely, T2 shortening is hypointense on T2-weighted images and T2 prolongation is hyperintense.

- It is technically incorrect to refer to image signal abnormality as "T2 hypo/hyperintense" or "T1 hypo/hyperintense" as it is the *MR image* that may exhibit signal abnormalities, rather than the proton relaxation times. Correct terminology would include, "a lesion is hyperintense on T2-weighted images" or "a lesion demonstrates T2 prolongation."

Conventional spin-echo T1

- Most brain lesions are hypointense on T1-weighted images due to pathologic prolongation of the longitudinal recovery. The presence of hyperintensity on T1-weighted images (caused by T1 shortening) can be an important clue leading to a specific diagnosis.
- Causes of **T1 shortening (hyperintensity)** include:

Most commonly: **Gadolinium**, **fat**, and **proteinaceous** substance.

Some **paramagnetic stages of blood** (both intra- and extracellular methemoglobin).

Melanin.

Mineralization (copper, iron, manganese).

Slowly-flowing blood.

Calcium (rarely; when dispersed, not in bone). It is much more common for calcium to be hypointense.

Conventional spin-echo T2

- Most brain lesions are hyperintense on T2-weighted images. Water has a very long T2 relaxation constant (water is very "bright" on T2-weighted images). Edema is a hallmark of many pathologic processes and causes T2 prolongation.
- Since most pathologic lesions are hyperintense on T2-weighted images, the clue to a specific diagnosis may be obtained when a lesion is hypointense.
- Causes of **hypointensity** on T2-weighted images include:

Most **paramagnetic stages of blood** (except hyperacute blood and extracellular methemoglobin).

Calcification.

Fibrous lesion.

Highly cellular tumors with a high nucleus:cytoplasm ratio producing low lesional water content (for instance, lymphoma and medulloblastoma).

Vascular flow-void.

Mucin. Desiccated mucin, as seen in desiccated sinus secretions, is hypointense on T2-weighted images. Conversely, mucinous lesions in the pelvis tend to be hydrated and thus hyperintense.

Fluid attenuation inversion recovery (FLAIR)

- The FLAIR sequence is the workhorse of neuroradiology. FLAIR is a T2-weighted image with suppression of water signal based on water's T1 characteristics.
- A normal FLAIR image may appear similar to a T1-weighted image since the CSF is dark on both. However, the signal intensities of the gray and white matter are different.

  T1: Normal white matter is brighter than gray matter because the fatty myelinated white matter has a shorter T1 time.

  FLAIR: White matter is darker than gray matter.

Conventional spin-echo proton density (PD)

- Proton density (PD) images are not used in many neuroradiology MRI protocols, but they do have the highest signal to noise ratio of any MRI sequence.
- PD sequences are useful in the evaluation of multiple sclerosis (MS), especially for visualization of demyelinating plaques in the posterior fossa.

Diffusion weighted images and apparent diffusion coefficient (DWI and ADC)

- Diffusion MRI is based on the principal that the Brownian motion of water protons can be imaged. Signal is lost with increasing Brownian motion. Free water (CSF) experiences the most signal attenuation, while many pathologic processes (primarily ischemia) cause reduced diffusivity and less signal loss.
- Diffusion MRI consists of two separate sequences — DWI (diffusion weighted imaging) and ADC (apparent diffusion coefficient), which are interpreted together to evaluate the diffusion characteristics of tissue.
- Diffusion imaging has revolutionized evaluation of cerebral infarct and is approximately 95% sensitive and specific for infarct within minutes of symptom onset. In the setting of stroke imaging, diffusion restricted tissue represents infarction.
- **DWI** is an inherently T2-weighted sequence (obtained with an echo-planar technique). On DWI, reduced diffusivity will be **hyperintense** (less Brownian motion → less loss of signal) and lesions are very conspicuous.
- The **ADC** map shows pure diffusion information without any T2 weighting. In contrast to DWI, reduced diffusivity is **hypointense** on the ADC map. Because studies have shown that readers are less sensitive to detecting reduced diffusivity using the ADC map alone, DWI is the primary sequence used to detect diffusion abnormalities.
- An important pitfall to be aware of is the phenomenon of *T2 shine through*. Because DWI images are T2-weighted, lesions that are inherently hyperintense on T2-weighted images may also be hyperintense on DWI even without restricted diffusion. This phenomenon is called *T2 shine through*. Correlation with the ADC map for a corresponding dark spot is essential before concluding that diffusion is restricted.
- In the brain, diffusion images are obtained in three orthogonal gradient planes to account for the inherent anisotropy of large white matter tracts.

  Anisotropy is the tendency of water molecules to diffuse directionally along white matter tracts.
- The b-value is an important concept that affects the sensitivity for detecting diffusion abnormalities. The higher the b-value, the more contrast the image will provide for detecting reduced diffusivity. The downside to increasing the b-value is a decrease in the signal to noise ratio, unless scan time is proportionally increased for additional acquisitions.

  The previously described ADC map is calculated from a set of at least two different b-value images.
- Although diffusion MRI is most commonly used to evaluate for infarct, the differential diagnosis for reduced diffusion includes:

> **Acute stroke**.
>
> **Bacterial abscess**.
>
> **Cellular tumors**, such as lymphoma and medulloblastoma.
>
> **Epidermoid cyst**.
>
> **Herpes encephalitis**.
>
> **Creutzfeldt–Jakob disease**.

Gradient recall echo (GRE)

- Gradient recall echo (GRE) captures the T2* signal. Because the 180-degree rephasing pulse is omitted, GRE images are susceptible to signal loss from magnetic field inhomogeneities.
- Hemosiderin and calcium produce inhomogeneities in the magnetic field, which creates *blooming* artifacts on GRE and makes even small lesions conspicuous.
- The differential diagnosis of multiple dark spots on GRE includes:

> **Hypertensive microbleeds** (dark spots are primarily in the basal ganglia, thalami, cerebellum, and pons).
>
> **Cerebral amyloid angiopathy** (dark spots are in the subcortical white matter, most commonly the parietal and occipital lobes).
>
> **Familial cerebral cavernous malformations** (an inherited form of multiple cavernous malformations).
>
> **Axonal shear injury**.
>
> **Multiple hemorrhagic metastases.**

Magnetic resonance spectroscopy

- MR spectroscopy describes the chemical composition of a brain region. In some circumstances, spectroscopy may help distinguish recurrent tumor from radiation necrosis, or may be helpful to differentiate between glioblastoma and metastasis.

  Glioblastoma is an infiltrative tumor that features a gradual transition from abnormal to normal spectroscopy. In contrast, a metastasis would be expected to have a more abrupt transition.

- The ratios of specific compounds may be altered in various disease states. *N*-acetylaspartate (NAA) is a normal marker of neuronal viability that decreases in most abnormalities. In tumors, NAA decreases and choline increases, although this pattern is nonspecific. Creatine provides information about cellular energy stores. The peaks of the three principle compounds analyzed occur in alphabetical order: Choline (cho), creatine (cr), and NAA.

  Canavan disease is a dysmyelinating disorder known for being one of the few disorders with elevated NAA.

- A lactate "doublet" may be seen in high-grade tumors indicating anaerobic metabolism.
- "Hunter's angle" is a quick way to see if a spectrum is close to normal. A line connecting the tallest peaks should point up like a plane taking off.

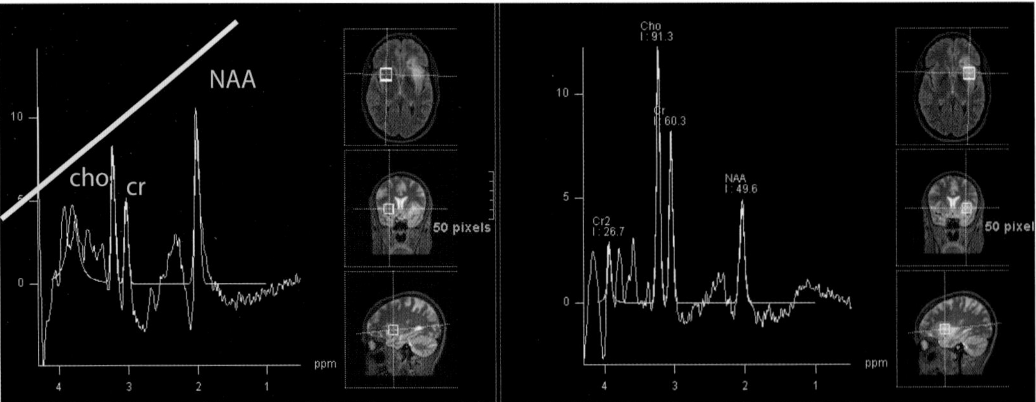

Left panel: Normal spectrum. Hunter's angle (yellow line) is pointing up like a plane at takeoff.

Right panel: Abnormal spectrum due to oligoastrocytoma, with elevated choline and decreased NAA. A line connecting the tallest peaks would point down, which is a clue that the spectrum is abnormal.

Perfusion

- Perfusion MR is an advanced technique where the brain is imaged repeatedly as a bolus of gadolinium contrast is injected. The principle of perfusion MR is based on the theory that gadolinium causes a magnetic field disturbance, which (counterintuitively) transiently *decreases* the image intensity.

- Perfusion images are echo-planar T2* images, which can be acquired very quickly.
- Perfusion MR may be used for evaluation of stroke and tumors.

Patterns of enhancement in the brain

Blood brain barrier (BBB) and enhancement

- Micro or macro disruption of the blood brain barrier (BBB) produces *parenchymal* enhancement after contrast administration, which may be secondary to infection, inflammation, neoplasm, trauma, and vascular etiologies.
- The BBB is formed by astrocytic foot processes of brain capillary endothelial cells and prevents direct communication between the systemic capillaries and the protected extracellular fluid of the brain.
- Several CNS regions do not have a blood brain barrier, and therefore normally enhance:

  Choroid plexus.

  Pituitary and pineal glands.

  Tuber cinereum (controls circadian rhythm, located in the inferior hypothalamus).

  Area postrema (controls vomiting, located at inferior aspect of 4th ventricle).

  The dura also lacks a blood brain barrier, but does not normally enhance. This phenomenon is subsequently explained in the section on pachymeningeal (dural) enhancement.

- *Vascular* enhancement is due to a localized increase in blood flow, which may be secondary to vasodilation, hyperemia, neovascularity, or arteriovenous shunting.

  On CT, the arterial phase of contrast injection (for instance a CT angiogram) mostly shows intravascular enhancement. Parenchymal enhancement, including the dural folds of the falx and tentorium, is best seen several minutes after the initial contrast bolus.

  On MRI, routine contrast-enhanced sequences are obtained in the parenchymal phase, several minutes after injection. Most intracranial vascular MRI imaging is performed with a noncontrast time of flight technique.

- Intracranial enhancement may be intra- or extra-axial. Extra-axial structures that may enhance in pathologic conditions include the dura (pachymeninges) and arachnoid (leptomeninges).

Periventricular enhancement (intra-axial)

- Enhancement of the subependymal surface can be either neoplastic, infectious, or demyelinating in etiology.

Differential diagnosis of periventricular enhancement

- **Primary CNS lymphoma** is a malignant B-cell neoplasm that can have diverse presentations including periventricular enhancement, solitary brain mass, or multiple brain masses.

  Primary CNS lymphoma is hyperattenuating on CT and demonstrates low ADC and low signal intensity on T2-weighted MRI due to hypercellularity.

  Primary CNS lymphoma rarely involves the meninges. In contrast, the meninges (both pachymeninges and leptomeninges) are commonly involved when systemic lymphoma spreads to the brain.

  CNS lymphoma tends to be centrally necrotic in immunocompromised patients, but usually enhances homogeneously in immunocompetent patients.

- **Infectious ependymitis** is most commonly caused by cytomegalovirus. Infectious ependymitis usually features thin linear enhancement along the margins of the ventricles.
- **Primary glial tumor** may cause periventricular enhancement.
- **Multiple sclerosis** may affect the subependymal surface. Although the majority of demyelinating lesions do not enhance, an active plaque may demonstrate enhancement.

Gyriform enhancement (intra-axial)

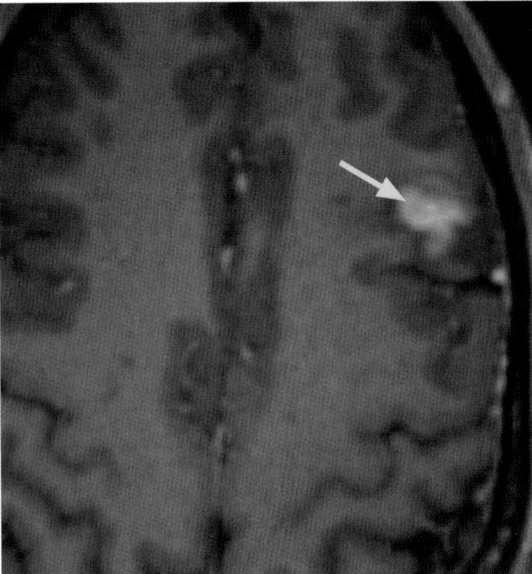

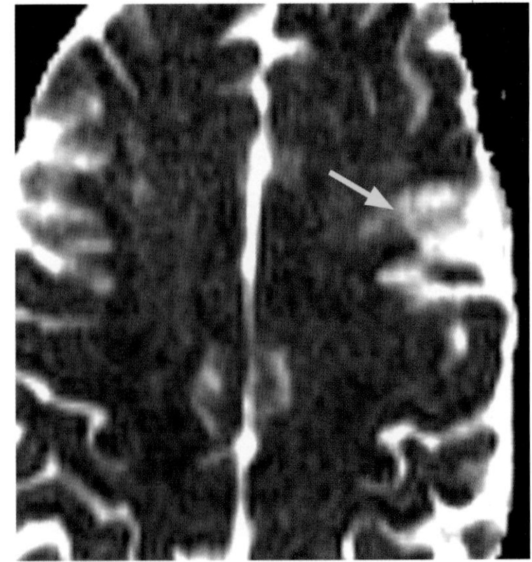

Gyriform enhancement: Axial T1-weighted postcontrast MRI (left image) shows a focus of enhancement along the gyral surface of the left frontal lobe (arrow) in a pattern typical of gyriform enhancement. This region is hyperintense on the ADC map (arrow on right image), consistent with increased diffusivity. There is no significant mass effect. This was a late subacute infarct.

- Superficial enhancement of the cortical (gyral) surface of the brain can be due to either cerebral infection, inflammation, or ischemia.

Differential diagnosis of gyriform enhancement

- **Herpes encephalitis** is a serious necrotizing infection of the brain parenchyma due to reactivation of latent HSV-1 infection within the trigeminal ganglion. The medial temporal lobes and cingulate gyrus are usually affected first and demonstrate gyral enhancement due to inflammation, petechial hemorrhage, and resultant BBB breakdown. The involved areas typically also demonstrate reduced diffusivity.
- **Meningitis** may cause gyral enhancement in addition to the more typical leptomeningeal enhancement (subsequently discussed).
- **Subacute infarct** can demonstrate gyriform enhancement lasting approximately 6 days to 6 weeks after the initial ischemic event.

  In contrast to the gyriform enhancement of subacute infarct, an acute infarct may demonstrate vascular enhancement due to reactive collateral vasodilation and resultant hyperemia.
- **Posterior reversible encephalopathy syndrome** (PRES) is a syndrome of vasogenic white matter edema triggered by altered autoregulation that may demonstrate gyral enhancement. PRES may rarely exhibit restricted diffusion.

Nodular subcortical enhancement (intra-axial)

- Nodular intra-axial enhancement is most commonly due to metastatic disease.
- **Hematogenously disseminated metastatic disease** is commonly found at the subcortical gray–white junctions. Tumor emboli become "stuck" at the junction between the simple vasculature of the white matter and the highly branching vasculature of the gray matter.
- Edema is almost always present with metastatic disease of the gray–white junction, although slightly more distal cortical metastases may not show any edema and may be detectable only on the post-contrast images.
- In contrast to the subcortical pattern seen with arterial metastases, venous dissemination of metastasis (e.g., pelvic malignancy spread via the Batson prevertebral venous plexus) leads to posterior fossa disease by transit through the retroclival venous plexus.

Ring enhancement (intra-axial)

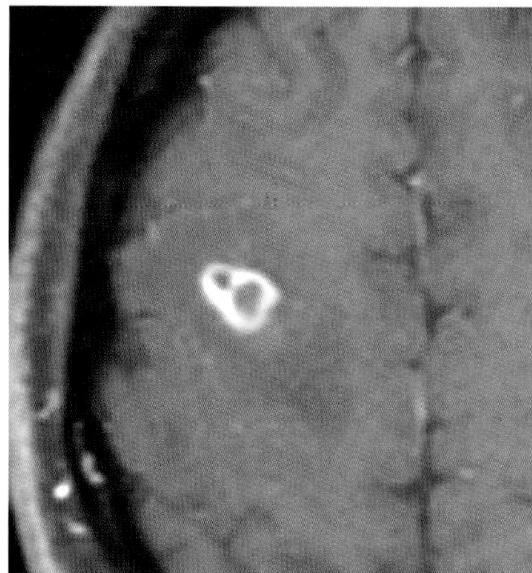

Patient 1: Axial post-contrast T1-weighted image shows a bilobed ring-enhancing lesion in the right frontal cortex. This was due to neurocysticercosis.

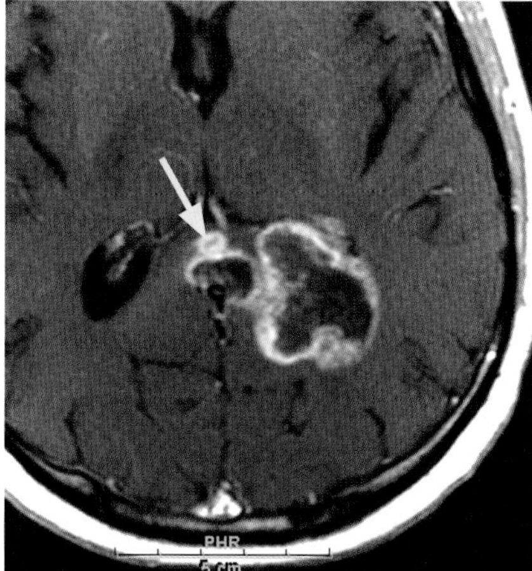

Patient 2: Axial post-contrast T1-weighted image shows an irregular ring enhancing lesion effacing the atrium of the left ventricle and extending across the splenium of the corpus callosum (arrow). This was a glioblastoma.

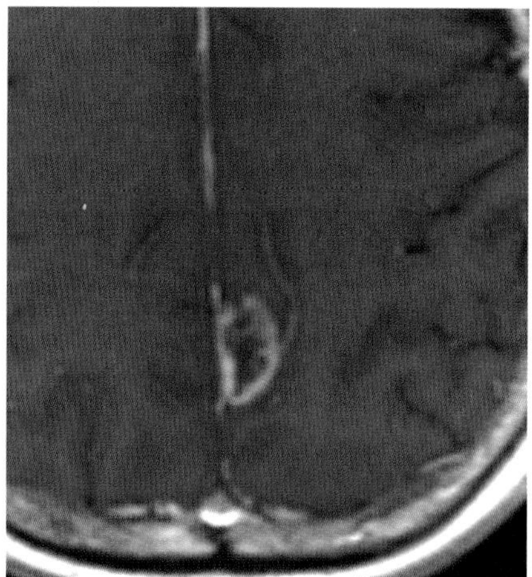

Patient 3: Axial post-contrast T1-weighted image shows a ring enhancing lesion in the left parietal lobe abutting the falx. This was a breast cancer metastasis.

- Peripheral (ring) enhancement is a common presentation with a broad range of differential diagnoses. The two most common causes are high-grade neoplasm and cerebral abscess.
- The mnemonic **MAGIC DR** (**m**etastasis, **a**bscess, **g**lioma, **i**nfarct, **c**ontusion, **d**emyelination, and **r**adiation) may be helpful to remember the wide range of etiologies for ring enhancement, although it is usually possible to narrow the differential based on the pattern of ring enhancement combined with additional MRI sequences and clinical history.

Differential diagnosis of ring enhancement

- **Metastasis**: Hematogenous metastases are typically found at the subcortical gray–white junction. Metastases are often multiple, but smaller lesions may not be ring-enhancing.
- **Abscess**: A pyogenic abscess is formed as a result of organization and sequestration of an infection, featuring a central region of viscous necrosis.

  The key imaging findings of abscess are reduced diffusivity (bright on DWI and dark on ADC) caused by high viscosity of central necrosis and a characteristic smooth, hypointense rim on T2-weighted images.
- **Glioma**: High grade tumors such as glioblastoma typically have a thick and irregular wall.

  Multivoxel MRI spectroscopy will be abnormal outside the margin of an enhancing high grade glial neoplasm secondary to nonenhancing infiltrative tumor. This is in contrast to a demyelinating lesion, abscess, and metastasis, where the spectral pattern returns to normal at the margin of the lesion.

  Perfusion MRI demonstrates elevated perfusion in a high grade glioma.
- **Infarct**: Although subacute cortical infarcts often demonstrate gyral enhancement, ring enhancement can be seen in subacute basal ganglia infarcts.

  In contrast to neoplasm and infection, a subacute infarct does not have significant mass effect.
- **Contusion**: Both traumatic and nontraumatic intraparenchymal hemorrhage can show ring enhancement in the subacute to chronic stage.
- **Demyelinating** disease: The key finding in ring-enhancing demyelinating disease is lack of significant mass effect. The "ring" of enhancement is often incomplete and "C" shaped.

  Multiple sclerosis is the most common demyelinating disease. Enhancement suggests active disease.

  Although the typical finding is an incomplete rim of enhancement, tumefactive demyelinating disease can look identical to a high-grade tumor.
- **Radiation** necrosis may look identical to a high-grade tumor. On perfusion, cerebral blood volume is generally low in radiation necrosis and typically increased in a high grade glioma.

Pachymeningeal (dural) enhancement (extra-axial)

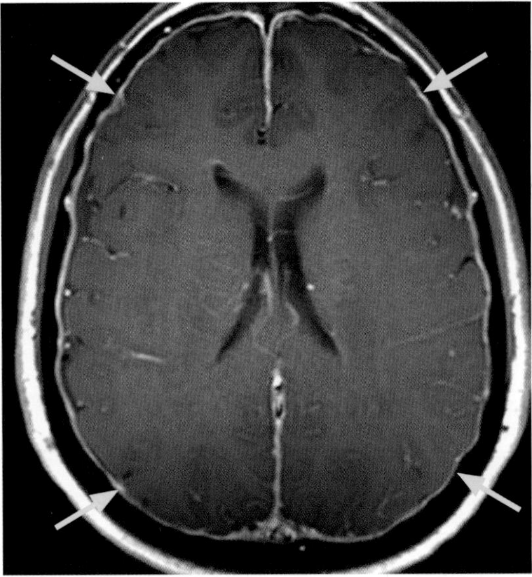

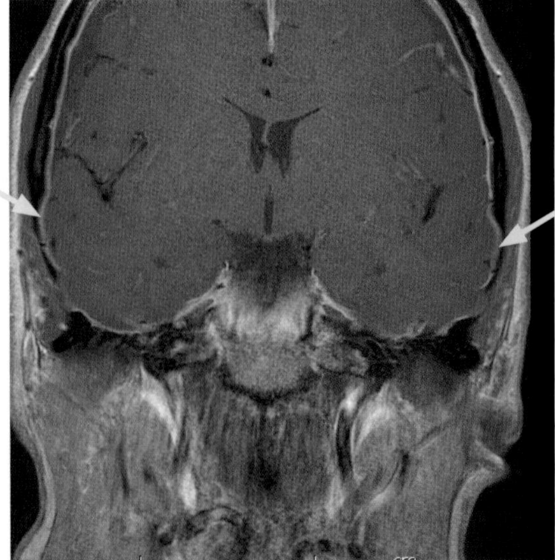

Diffuse dural enhancement: Axial (left image) and coronal post-contrast T1-weighted MRI (right image) shows diffuse dural enhancement (arrows). This was a case of intracranial hypotension.

- The pachymeninges (*pachy* means thick – a "thick-skinned" elephant is a pachyderm) refers to the dura mater, the thick and leather-like outermost covering of the brain.
- In addition to surrounding the surface of the brain, the dura forms several reflections, including the falx, tentorium, and cavernous sinus.
- The dura does not have a blood brain barrier. Although contrast molecules normally diffuse into the dura on enhanced CT or MRI, dural enhancement is never visualized on CT and is only visualized on MRI in pathologic situations.

  Dural enhancement is not seen on CT because both the skull and adjacent enhancing dura appear white.

  Enhancement of normal dura is not visible on MRI because MRI visualization of enhancement requires both water protons and gadolinium. Although gadolinium is present in the dura, there are normally very few water protons. However, dural pathology often causes dural edema, which provides enough water protons to make the gadolinium visible. Therefore, **dural enhancement on MRI is an indication of dural edema rather than BBB breakdown.**

Differential diagnosis of pachymeningeal enhancement

- **Intracranial hypotension**: Prolonged decrease in cerebrospinal fluid pressure can lead to vasogenic edema in the dura.

  Intracranial hypotension clinically presents as a postural headache exacerbated by standing upright.

  Intracranial hypotension may be idiopathic or secondary to CSF leak from surgery or lumbar puncture.

  Imaging shows thick, linear dural enhancement, enlargement of the pituitary gland, and "sagging" of the cerebellar tonsils. There may also be subdural hemorrhage due to traction effect on the cerebral veins.
- **Postoperative**: Dural enhancement may be seen postoperatively.
- **Post lumbar puncture**: Diffuse dural enhancement is occasionally seen (<5% of the time) after routine lumbar puncture.
- **Meningeal neoplasm**, such as meningioma, can produce a focal area of dural enhancement called a *dural tail*, due to reactive changes in the dura. Metastatic disease to the dura, most commonly breast cancer in a female and prostate cancer in a male, can cause irregular dural enhancement.
- **Granulomatous disease**, including sarcoidosis, tuberculosis, and fungal disease, can produce dural enhancement, typically of the basal meninges (meninges of the skull base).

Leptomeningeal (pia–arachnoid) enhancement (extra-axial)

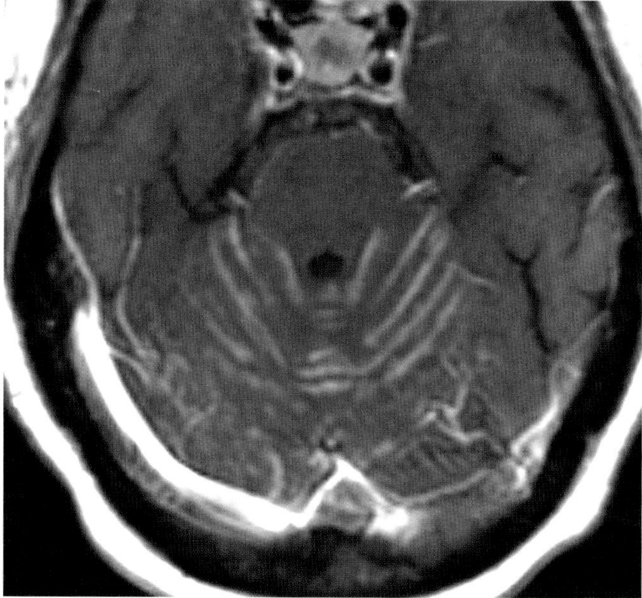

Cerebellar leptomeningeal enhancement: Contrast-enhanced T1-weighted MRI shows enhancement along the cerebellar folia. This patient had lymphoma causing leptomeningeal carcinomatosis.

- The leptomeninges (*lepto* means thin or narrow) include the pia and arachnoid.
- Leptomeningeal enhancement follows the undulating contours of the sulci as it includes enhancement of both the subarachnoid space and the pial surface of the brain.

Differential diagnosis of leptomeningeal enhancement

- **Meningitis** (either bacterial, viral, or fungal) is the primary consideration when leptomeningeal enhancement is seen.

  Leptomeningeal enhancement in meningitis is caused by BBB breakdown due to inflammation or infection.

  Fine, linear enhancement suggests bacterial or viral meningitis.

  Thicker, nodular enhancement suggests fungal meningitis.
- **Leptomeningeal carcinomatosis**, also called carcinomatous meningitis, is spread of neoplasm into the subarachnoid space, which may be due to primary brain tumor or metastatic disease.

  CNS neoplasms known to cause leptomeningeal carcinomatosis include medulloblastoma, oligodendroglioma, choroid plexus tumor, lymphoma, ependymoma, glioblastoma, and germinoma. Mnemonic: **MOCLEGG** or **GEMCLOG** (courtesy W. Stephen Poole, MD).

  Metastatic tumors known to cause carcinomatosis include lymphoma and breast cancer.
- **Viral encephalitis** may produce cranial nerve enhancement within the subarachnoid space.
- **Slow vascular flow** may mimic leptomeningeal enhancement at first glance, but a careful examination shows the distinction. Slow flow appears as an *intravascular* distribution of FLAIR hyperintensity due to "unmasking" of the inherent high signal of blood, which remains in the plane of imaging as the entire pulse sequence is obtained.

  Slow flow of peripheral vessels in moyamoya disease causes the *ivy* sign.

- The differential diagnosis of FLAIR hyperintensity in the subarachnoid space overlaps with the differential for leptomeningeal enhancement. Subarachnoid FLAIR hyperintensity may be due to:

  Meningitis and leptomeningeal carcinomatosis both have increased subarachnoid FLAIR signal and leptomeningeal enhancement.

  Subarachnoid hemorrhage manifests as increased subarachnoid FLAIR signal, without leptomeningeal enhancement. Blooming artifact on GRE or SWI from blood products will help differentiate subarachnoid hemorrhage from carcinomatosis.

  Subarachnoid FLAIR signal is artifactually increased when the patient is on **oxygen** or **propofol** therapy, without abnormal enhancement.

Brain Tumors

Approach to evaluation of a focal brain lesion

Are there any tumor-related complications?

- The three emergent complications of a brain tumor are the three H's: Hemorrhage, Hydrocephalus, and Herniation. CT is a good screening method to evaluate for these complications.
- **Hemorrhage**: Primary or metastatic brain tumors are often associated with neovascularity and tumoral vessels are more prone to hemorrhage than normal vasculature.

  The most common primary brain tumor to hemorrhage is a glioblastoma.

  Hemorrhagic metastases include melanoma, renal cell carcinoma, thyroid carcinoma, and choriocarcinoma. Although breast and lung cancer metastases are less frequently hemorrhagic on a case-by-case basis, these two malignancies are so common that they should also be considered in the differential of a hemorrhagic metastasis.
- **Hydrocephalus**: A tumor can cause hydrocephalus by blocking the flow of CSF.

  Posterior fossa tumors have increased risk of causing hydrocephalus by effacing the fourth ventricle.
- **Herniation**: The overall mass effect from tumor is a combination of the tumoral mass and associated vasogenic edema, which may contribute to brain herniation.

Is the mass intra- or extra-axial?

- After evaluation for emergent complications, the next step is to determine if the lesion is *intra*- or *extra*-axial. This distinction can sometimes be quite tricky.
- Although metastases may be either intra- or extra-axial, the differential diagnosis for each space is otherwise completely different.
- Findings of an extra-axial mass include a CSF cleft between the mass and the brain, buckling of gray matter, and gray matter interposed between the mass and white matter.

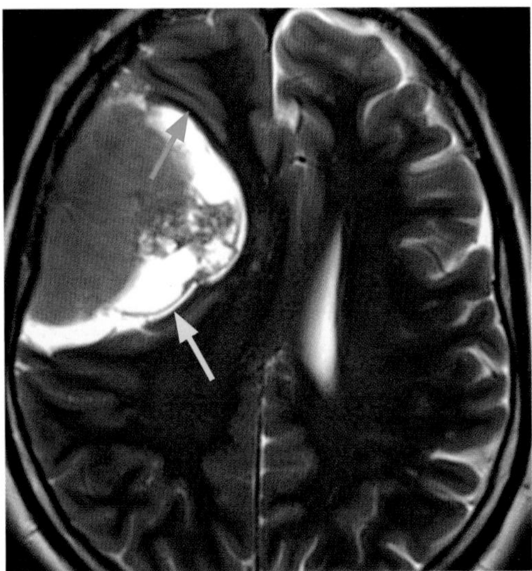
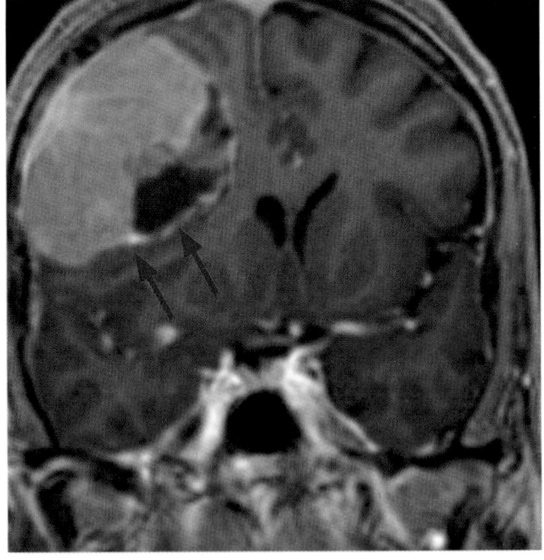

Extra-axial mass: Axial T2-weighted MRI (left image) shows a large, partially hypercellular and partially cystic mass adjacent to the right frontal lobe. A thin CSF cleft (yellow arrow) separates the mass from the brain parenchyma and there is adjacent gray matter buckling (blue arrow), confirming the mass's extra-axial location. Coronal post-contrast T1-weighted image (right image) shows gray matter interposed between the mass and the white matter (red arrows). The mass homogeneously enhances and invades the adjacent bony calvarium

This mass was a cystic meningioma. *Case courtesy Gregory Wrubel, MD, Brigham and Women's Hospital.*

- Findings of an intra-axial mass include absence of intervening gray matter between the mass and the white matter.

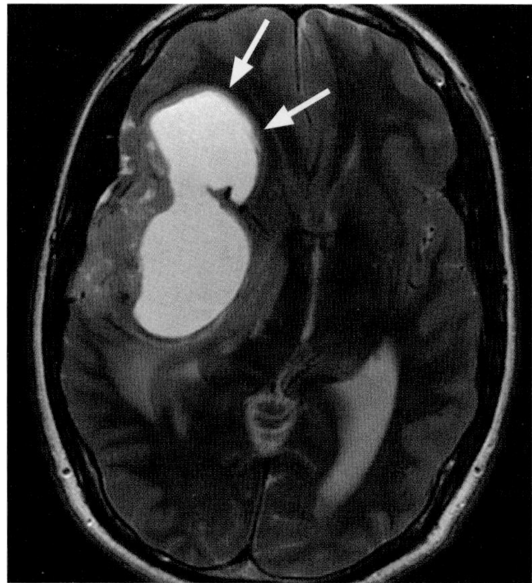
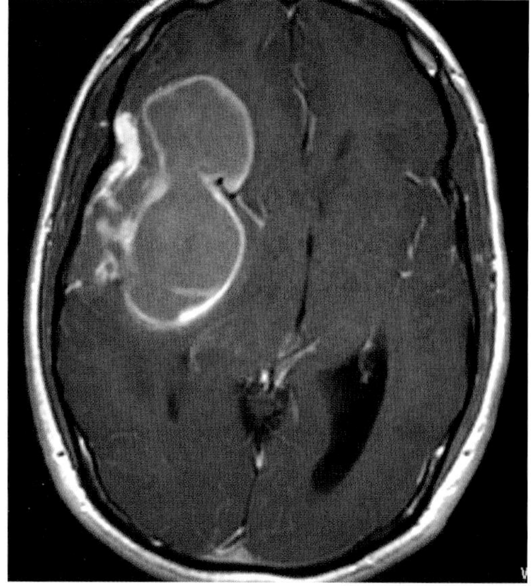

Intra-axial mass: Axial T2-weighted image (left image) shows a large, predominantly cystic mass with enhancing components laterally. The mass is located in the right frontal/temporal lobe and causes effacement of the right lateral ventricle and mild midline shift to the left. The mass directly abuts the white matter (yellow arrows), without intervening gray matter. Axial post-contrast T1-weighted image (right image) again shows that the mass directly abuts the white matter, confirming intra-axial location. This was a pleomorphic xanthoastrocytoma.

Case courtesy Raymond Huang, MD and David Lee, MD, Brigham and Women's Hospital.

- The presence of white matter edema is not specific to intra-axial masses. In particular, meningioma (an extra-axial dural neoplasm) is known to cause white matter edema of underlying brain.
- Meningeal enhancement is seen more commonly in extra-axial masses (most commonly meningioma), but can also be seen in intra-axial masses.

Where specifically is the lesion located?

- The differential can often be narrowed depending on the location. For instance, temporal lobe, posterior fossa, pineal, or suprasellar location may help point to a specific diagnosis.

Does the lesion enhance?

- Metastases always enhance due to tumoral neo-vessels, which lack a blood brain barrier.
- Low-grade primary infiltrating tumors may not enhance. Primary brain tumors may form near-normal CNS capillaries with an intact BBB.
- The degree of enhancement does not correlate with the histologic grade. Even large high grade primary brain tumors may enhance only slightly. Conversely, benign juvenile pilocytic astrocytoma features an avidly enhancing nodule, typically associated with an adjacent cyst.

Is there more than one lesion?

- If there is more than one lesion, the diagnosis is overwhelmingly likely to be metastases.

Are there any distinctive MRI signal characteristics?

- As previously described, most brain lesions are hyperintense on T2-weighted images and hypointense on T1-weighted images. MRI signal characteristics are most helpful if a lesion is either hypointense with T2 weighting or hyperintense with T1 weighting.

- Tumors **hypointense on T2-weighted** images include:

> **Metastases containing desiccated mucin**, such as some gastrointestinal adenocarcinomas. Note that mucinous metastases to the brain can have variable signal intensities on T2-weighted images, depending on the water content of the mucin. Hydrated mucin is hyperintense on T2-weighted images.
>
> **Hypercellular tumors**, including lymphoma, medulloblastoma, germinoma, and some glioblastomas.

- Tumors **hyperintense on T1-weighted** images include:

> Metastatic **melanoma** (melanin is hyperintense on T1-weighted images).
>
> Fat-containing tumors, such as **dermoid** or **teratoma**.
>
> **Hemorrhagic metastasis** (including renal cell, thyroid, choriocarcinoma, and melanoma).

- Some tumors contain cystic components, which are isointense to CSF on all sequences.

  Note that cysts tend to be at the periphery of enhancing low-grade tumors. In contrast, although intra-tumoral necrosis of a high-grade tumor may also follow CSF signal, necrosis tends to be surrounded by enhancing tumor.

Glial cells

Overview of glial cells

- A glioma is a primary CNS tumor that arises from a glial cell. Glial cells include astrocytes, oligodendrocytes, ependymal cells, and choroid plexus cells.
- Glioma is not a synonym for a "brain tumor." Only a tumor that arises from one of the aforementioned glial cells can accurately be called a glioma.

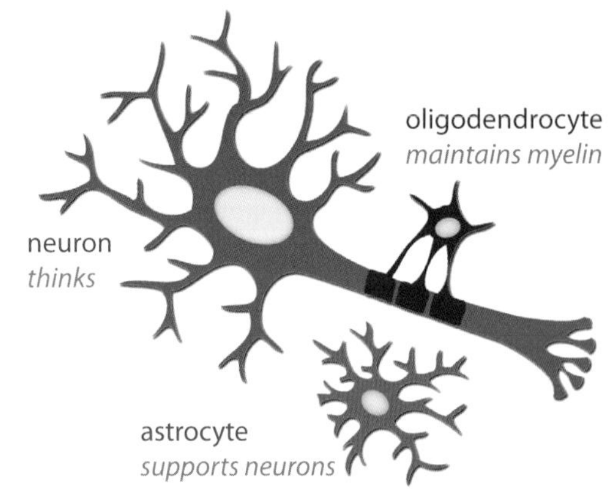

Astrocyte

- The normal functions of an astrocyte are to provide biochemical support to the endothelial cells that maintain the blood brain barrier, to maintain extracellular ion balance, and to aid in repair after a neuronal injury.
- Astrocytes are normally located throughout the entire brain (primarily in the white matter) and spinal cord.

Oligodendrocyte

- The normal function of an oligodendrocyte is to maintain myelin around CNS axons. A single oligodendrocyte can maintain the myelin of dozens of axons.

  The counterpart in the peripheral nervous system is the Schwann cell, which maintains myelin around a single peripheral nerve. Unlike the oligodendrocyte, each Schwann cell is in charge of only a single axon.

- Oligodendrocytes are normally located throughout the entire brain and spinal cord.

Ependymal cells

- The normal function of an ependymal cell is to circulate CSF with its multiple cilia.
- Ependymal cells line the ventricles and central canal of the spinal cord.

Choroid plexus cells

- The normal function of a choroid plexus cell is to produce CSF. A choroid plexus cell is a modified ependymal cell.
- Choroid plexus cells are located intraventricularly, in the body and temporal horn of each lateral ventricle, roof of the third ventricle, and roof of the fourth ventricle.

Grade I astrocytoma

Juvenile pilocytic astrocytoma (JPA)

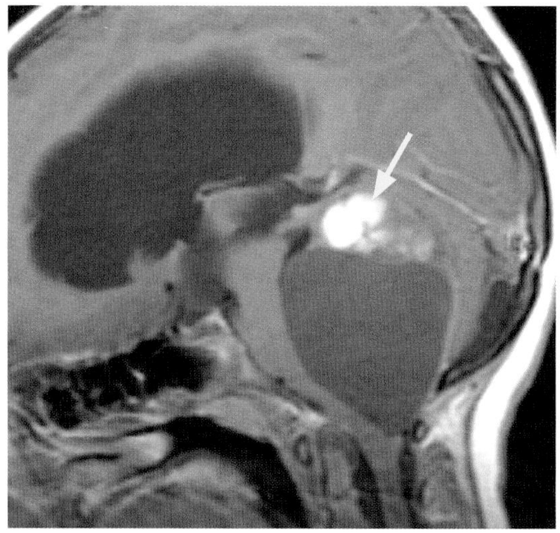

Juvenile pilocytic astrocytoma: Sagittal post-contrast T1-weighted MRI shows a large posterior fossa cystic lesion with a superior heterogeneously enhancing solid component (arrow). The fourth ventricle is completely effaced, the brainstem is deformed, and there is severe hydrocephalus.

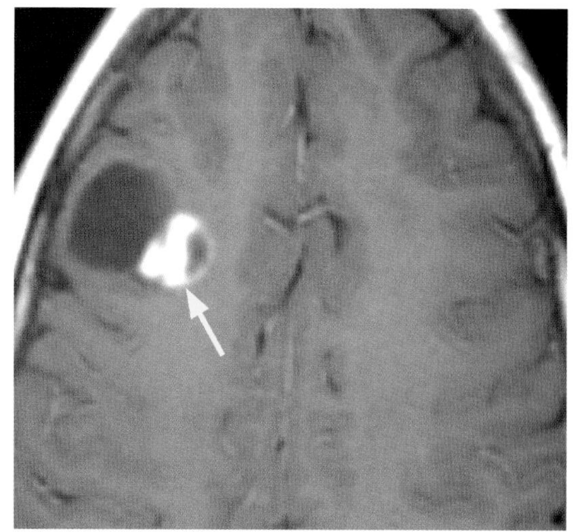

Juvenile pilocytic astrocytoma (JPA) in a different patient: Axial post-contrast T1-weighted MRI shows a cystic lesion in the right frontal lobe with an avidly enhancing solid nodule (arrow). Although the cyst and nodule appearance is typical for JPA, this supratentorial location is relatively uncommon.

- Juvenile pilocytic (hair-like) astrocytoma (JPA) is a benign World Health Organization (WHO) grade I tumor seen typically in the posterior fossa in children.
- Imaging shows a well-circumscribed cystic mass with an enhancing nodule and relatively little edema. When in the posterior fossa, JPA may compress the fourth ventricle.
- JPA can also occur along the optic pathway, with up to 1/3 of optic pathway JPA associated with neurofibromatosis type 1. Posterior fossa JPA is not associated with NF1.

Fibrillary astrocytoma

- Fibrillary astrocytomas are infiltrative tumors that include low-grade astrocytoma, anaplastic astrocytoma, and glioblastoma multiforme (GBM).
- Astrocytomas can occur in the brain or the spinal cord.

Low-grade astrocytoma

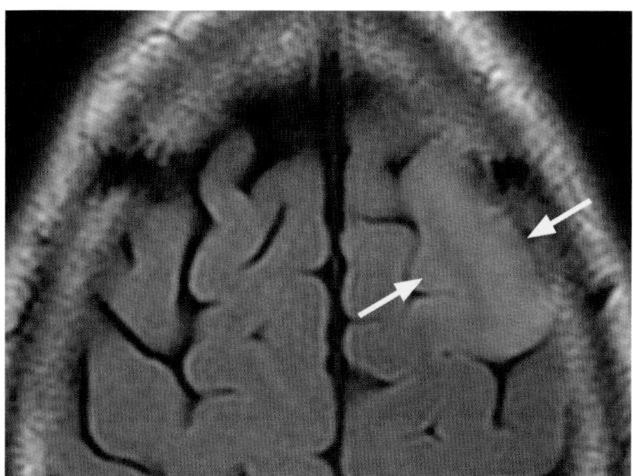

Low-grade astrocytoma: Axial FLAIR MRI shows subtle thickening and mild T2 prolongation in a single gyrus in the left frontal lobe (arrows). This lesion did not demonstrate any enhancement (post-contrast images not shown).

- Low-grade astrocytoma is a WHO grade II tumor that typically presents as a hyperintense mass on T2-weighted images, *without enhancement*. Imaging findings may be subtle.

Anaplastic astrocytoma

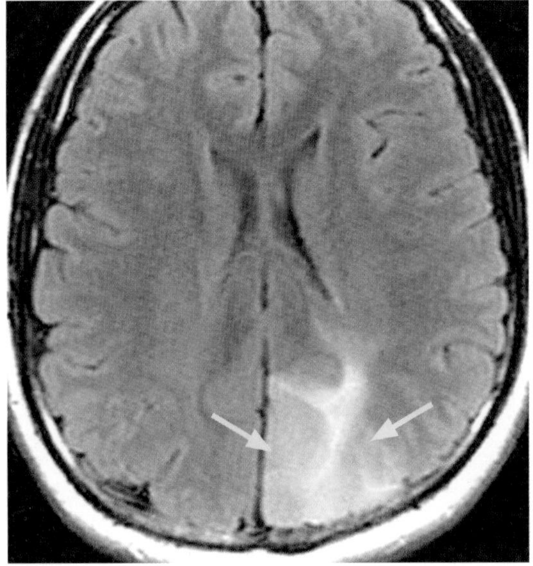

Anaplastic astrocytoma: Axial FLAIR image shows a geographic region of T2 prolongation in the left occipital white matter and cortex (arrows). There was no enhancement (not shown). This appearance is not specific and may also represent a low-grade astrocytoma.

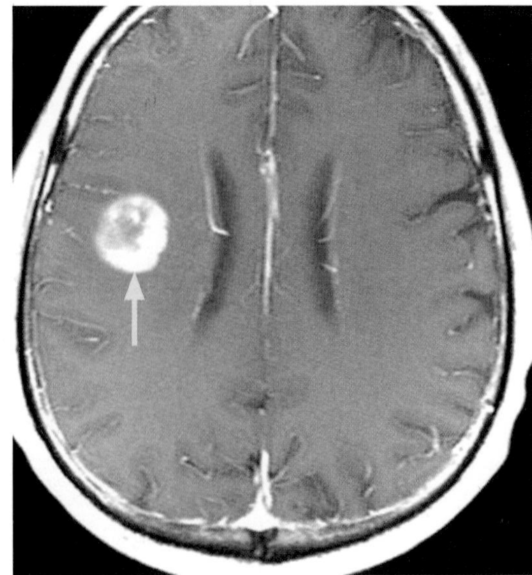

Anaplastic astrocytoma in a different patient: Axial post-contrast T1-weighted MRI shows an enhancing lesion in the right temporal lobe (arrow). This appearance is not specific and may represent a glioblastoma or metastatic disease.

Cases courtesy Amir Zamani, MD, Brigham and Women's Hospital.

- Anaplastic astrocytoma is a WHO grade III tumor. It features a range of appearances from thickened cortex (similar to low-grade astrocytoma) to an irregularly enhancing mass that may appear identical to glioblastoma. The natural history of the disease is eventual progression to glioblastoma.

Glioblastoma multiforme (GBM)

- Glioblastoma multiforme (GBM) is an aggressive WHO grade IV tumor of older adults. It is the most common primary CNS malignancy. GBM has a highly variable appearance ("multiforme") but typically presents as a white matter mass with heterogeneous enhancement and surrounding nonenhancing T2 prolongation.

  Most of the surrounding T2 prolongation is thought to represent infiltrative tumor.

- GBM is an infiltrative disease that spreads through white matter tracts, through the CSF, and subependymally.

  Subependymal spread describes spread within the walls of the ventricles under the ependymal cells, as shown in the case to the right.

- A GBM that crosses the midline via the corpus callosum is called a *butterfly glioma.* The differential diagnosis of a transcallosal mass includes glioblastoma, lymphoma, and demyelinating disease.

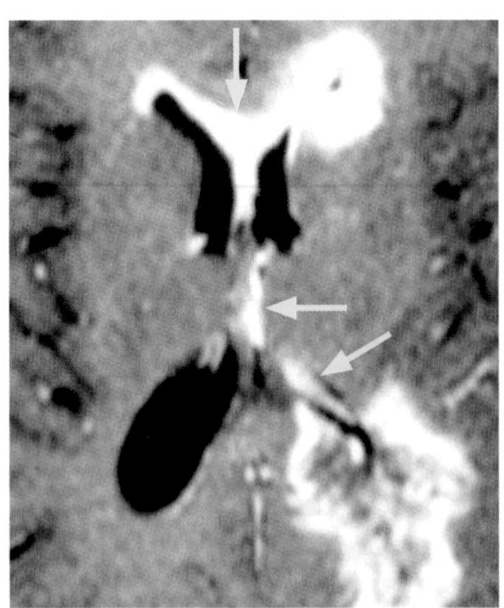

Transependymal spread of GBM: Post-contrast T1-weighted MRI shows extensive abnormal enhancement primarily in the left occipital lobe but extending into the bilateral periventricular frontal lobes via the subependymal surface (arrows).

Case courtesy Amir Zamani, MD, Brigham and Women's Hospital.

Other gliomas

Gliomatosis cerebri

- Gliomatosis cerebri is a diffuse infiltrative mid-grade (WHO II or III) astrocytoma that affects multiple lobes.
- Diagnostic criteria include involvement of at least two lobes plus extra-cortical involvement of structures such as the basal ganglia, corpus callosum, brainstem, or cerebellum.
- Gliomatosis has a poor prognosis and may degenerate into GBM.
- The typical imaging appearance is diffuse T2 prolongation throughout the involved brain.

  Diffuse T2 prolongation can be seen in several entities, typically in immunocompromised patients, including lymphoma, progressive multifocal leukoencephalopathy (demyelination caused by JC virus), and AIDS encephalopathy.
- Gliomatosis exerts mass effect but typically does not enhance.

Gliomatosis cerebri: Axial FLAIR shows diffuse confluent T2 prolongation involving the right medial temporal lobe, basal ganglia, and frontal lobe white matter (arrows). There is mild mass effect and shift to the left.

Case courtesy Gregory Wrubel, MD, Brigham and Women's Hospital.

Oligodendroglioma

- Oligodendroglioma is a WHO grade II tumor that usually presents as a slow-growing cortical-based mass.
- The typical patient is a young to middle-aged patient presenting with seizures.
- Oligodendrogliomas have a propensity to calcify (approximately 75% calcify). Variants such as oligoastrocytoma and anaplastic oligodendroglioma are much more aggressive.

  Oligoastrocytoma is a mixed tumor with an astrocytic component. Although oligoastrocytoma can degenerate into GBM, typically prognosis is better than a pure GBM.

  Anaplastic oligodendroglioma is indistinguishable from GBM on imaging and has a poor prognosis.

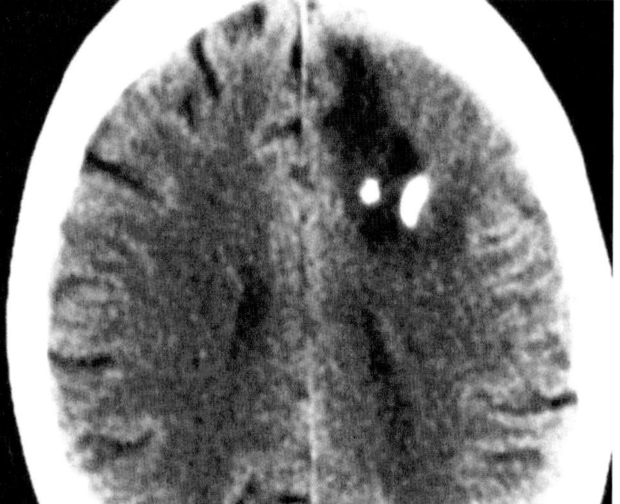

Oligodendroglioma: Noncontrast CT demonstrates a hypoattenuating mass in the left frontal lobe containing coarse calcifications. The lack of significant edema suggests a slow-growing lesion.

Image courtesy Amir Zamani, MD, Brigham and Women's Hospital.

Ependymoma

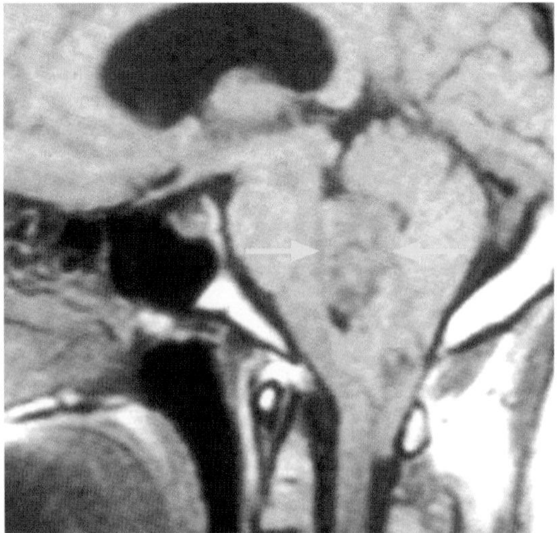
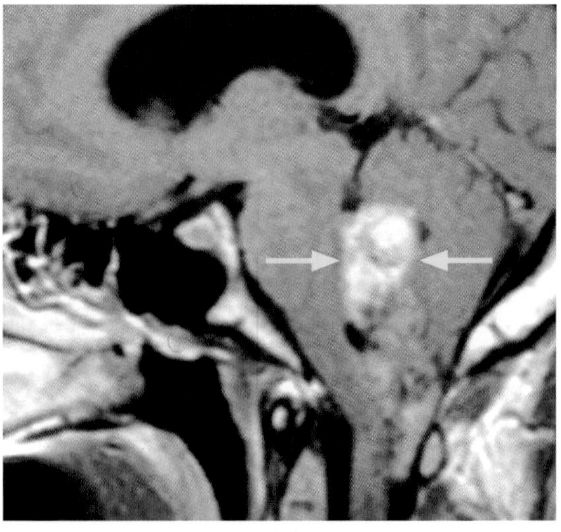

Ependymoma: Precontrast T1-weighted (left image) and post-contrast T1-weighted sagittal MRI shows a lobulated, isointense, avidly enhancing mass arising from the fourth ventricle (arrows). There is kinking of the brainstem and obstructive hydrocephalus of the third ventricle.

Case courtesy Amir Zamani, MD, Brigham and Women's Hospital.

- An ependymoma is a tumor of ependymal cells that tends to occur in the posterior fossa in children and in the spinal cord in older adults.
- The pediatric posterior fossa ependymoma has been called the *toothpaste* tumor for its propensity to fill the fourth ventricle and squeeze through the foramina of Magendie or Luschka into the adjacent basal cisterns. Medulloblastoma, the most common pediatric brain tumor, also usually arises in the posterior fossa but does not typically squeeze through the foramina.
- The adult spinal ependymoma can occur anywhere in the intramedullary spinal cord. The main differential diagnosis of an intramedullary spinal cord mass is an astrocytoma, which tends to occur in younger patients. It is not possible to reliably differentiate spinal cord ependymoma from astrocytoma on imaging.

Non-glioma primary brain tumors

Lhermitte–Duclos

- Lhermitte–Duclos, also called dysplastic cerebellar gangliocytoma, is a WHO grade I cerebellar lesion that is part hamartoma and part neoplasm.
- Lhermitte–Duclos is almost always seen in associated with Cowden syndrome (multiple hamartomas and increased risk of several cancers).
- The classical imaging finding is a *corduroy* or *tiger-striped* striated lesion in the cerebellar hemisphere. Enhancement is rare.

Embryonal tumors

- Embryonal tumors represent a spectrum of WHO grade IV, aggressive childhood malignancies that are known as primitive neuroectodermal tumors (PNET). Intracranial PNET tumors are more commonly located in the posterior fossa but may occur supratentorially.

Atypical teratoid/rhabdoid tumor (ATRT)

- Atypical teratoid/rhabdoid tumor (ATRT) is a WHO IV, aggressive tumor that may appear similar to medulloblastoma, but occurs in slightly younger patients. The majority occur in the posterior fossa. ATRT is associated with malignant rhabdoid tumor of the kidney.

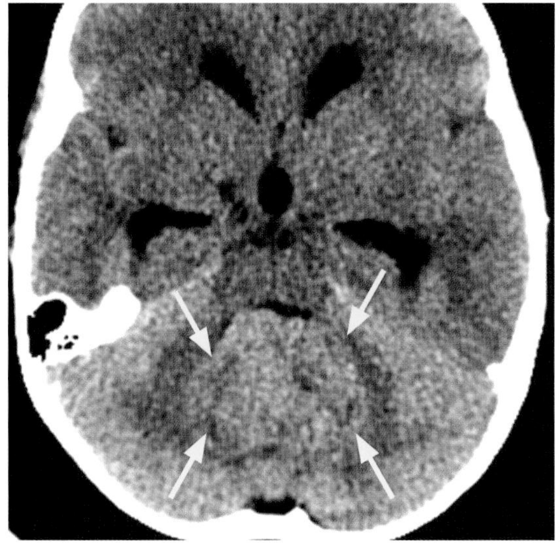

Axial unenhanced CT shows a hyperattenuating mass in the midline posterior fossa (arrows). There is near-complete effacement of the fourth ventricle, with resultant hydrocephalus.

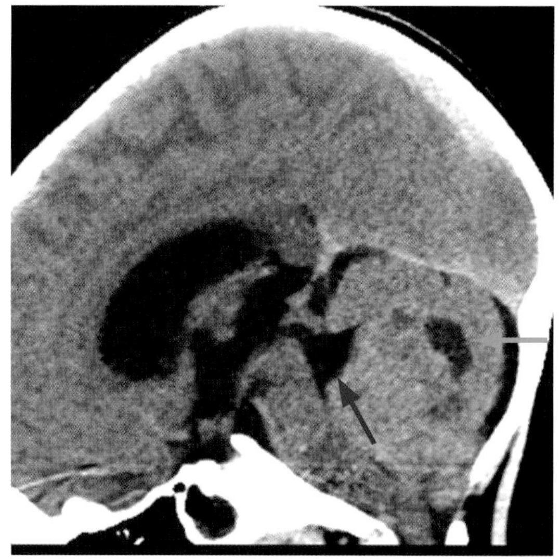

Sagittal unenhanced CT shows that the mass has displaced the fourth ventricle superiorly (red arrow) and contains a cystic component posteriorly (blue arrow).

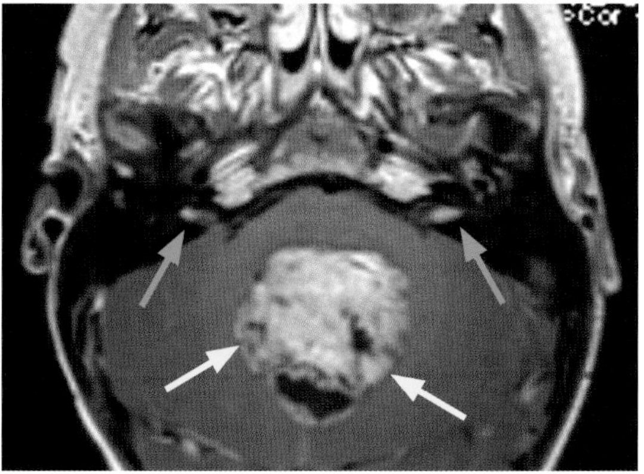

Post-contrast T1-weighted MRI shows the avidly enhancing mass (yellow arrows) completely effacing the fourth ventricle. There is enhancing leptomeningeal tumor dissemination within the internal auditory canals bilaterally (green arrows).

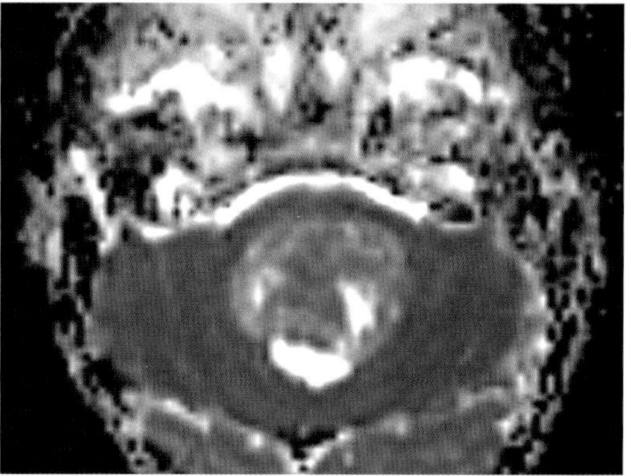

ADC map shows somewhat heterogeneous dark foci within the mass, consistent with hypercellularity.

Case courtesy Gregory Wrubel, MD, Brigham and Women's Hospital.

- Medulloblastoma is a WHO grade IV tumor of small-blue-cell origin. It is one of the most common pediatric brain tumors.
- Medulloblastoma most commonly occurs in the midline in the cerebellar vermis. It is slightly hyperattenuating on CT due to its densely packed cells and is accordingly hypointense on T2-weighted images and has low ADC values. The tumor is avidly enhancing and may appear heterogeneous due to internal hemorrhage and calcification.

  The low ADC values can be a useful finding to differentiate medulloblastoma from ependymoma and pilocytic astrocytoma, the two other most common childhood posterior fossa tumors.
- Leptomeningeal metastatic disease is present in up to 33% of patients. Sugar-coating (*Zuckerguss*) is icing-like enhancement over the brain surface. Imaging of the entire brain and spine should be performed prior to surgery.
- When medulloblastoma occurs in a young adult (as opposed to a child), the tumor tends to arise eccentrically in the posterior fossa, from the cerebellar hemisphere.

- A few low-grade, fluid-secreting tumors present as a cyst with an enhancing mural nodule.

Juvenile pilocytic astrocytoma (discussed previously in the astrocytoma section)

Hemangioblastoma

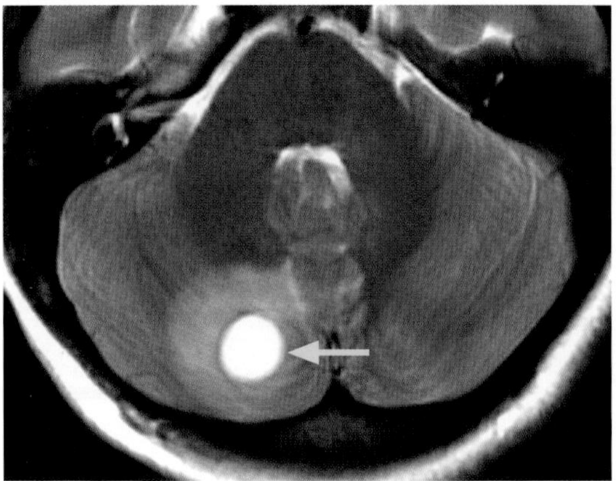
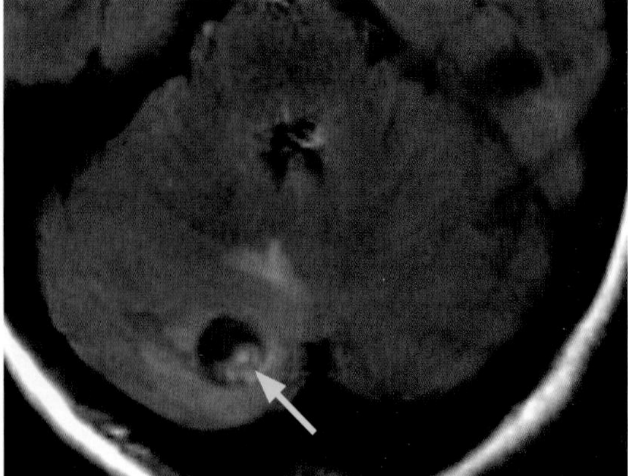

Hemangioblastoma: Axial T2-weighted MRI (left image) shows a cystic lesion (arrow) in the right cerebellar hemisphere with mild surrounding edema. The nodular component is demonstrated on FLAIR (arrow).

Case courtesy Sanjay Prabhu, MD, Boston Children's Hospital.

- Hemangioblastoma is a highly vascular WHO grade I tumor associated with von Hippel–Lindau (VHL) syndrome that occurs most commonly in the cerebellum, medulla, or spinal cord. It only rarely occurs supratentorially.
- Although associated with VHL, only 30% of patients with hemangioblastoma have VHL. Hemangioblastoma in a patient with VHL has a worse prognosis.
- The classic appearance of hemangioblastoma is a cystic mass with an enhancing mural nodule. Prominent vessels are often seen as tubular areas of flow void. Less commonly, a hemangioblastoma may be solid or hemorrhagic.
- When in the spinal cord, hemangioblastoma is often associated with a syrinx.

Pleomorphic xanthoastrocytoma (PXA)

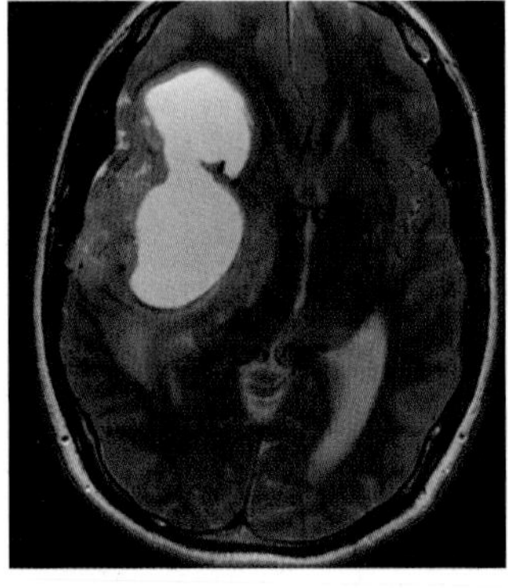
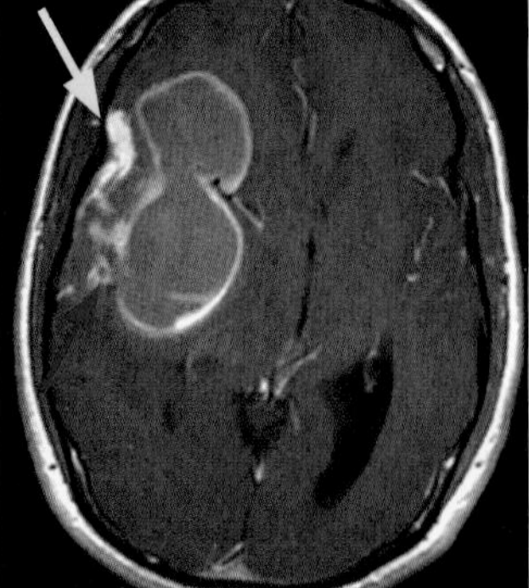

Pleomorphic xanthoastrocytoma: Axial T2-weighted (far left image) and post-contrast T1-weighted MRI shows a large right temporal, predominantly cystic mass. The mass has enhancing nodularity laterally (red arrow). The overlying dura is thickened and enhancing (yellow arrow). There is relatively little surrounding edema given the large size of the lesion. *Case courtesy Raymond Huang, MD and David Lee, MD, Brigham and Women's Hospital.*

- Pleomorphic xanthoastrocytoma (PXA) is a low-grade WHO grade II astrocytoma variant.
- PXA is a rare tumor of childhood and adolescents, typically with history of chronic epilepsy.
- The most common location of PXA is the temporal lobe, where it typically presents as a supratentorial cortical cystic mass with an enhancing mural nodule. The overlying dura may be thickened and enhancing.
- The main differential consideration, both by imaging and clinical presentation, is ganglioglioma; however, ganglioglioma does not usually cause dural thickening.

Ganglioglioma

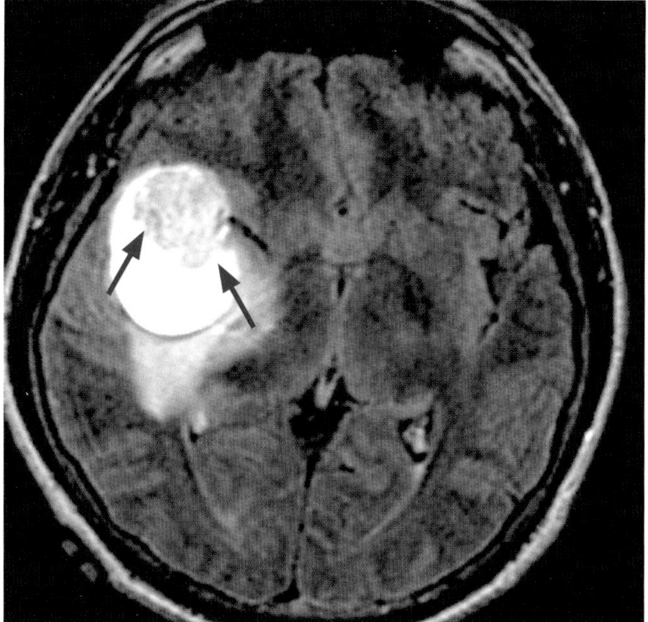

Ganglioglioma: Axial FLAIR shows a cystic lesion in the right temporal lobe with an associated large solid nodule (arrows). There is mild surrounding edema and mild mass effect with midline shift to the left.

Case courtesy Amir Zamani, MD, Brigham and Women's Hospital.

- Ganglioglioma is a rare, slow-growing neuroglial tumor that typically presents in an adolescent or young adult with medically refractory temporal lobe epilepsy.
- Ganglioglioma characteristically appears as a temporal lobe cyst and enhancing mural nodule, often with calcification. Ganglioglioma may cause calvarial remodeling and scalloping.

INTRAVENTRICULAR TUMORS

Central neurocytoma

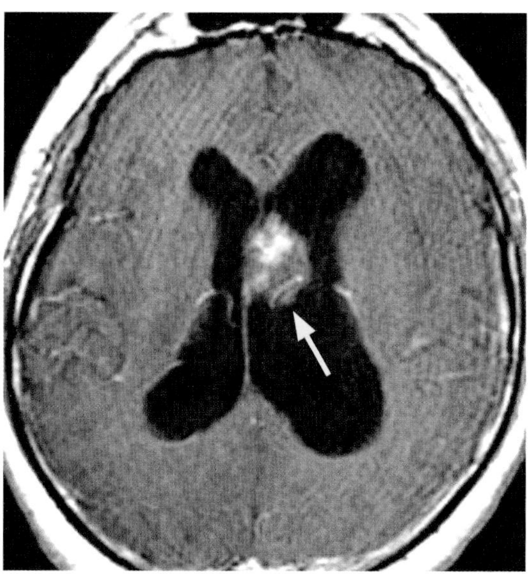

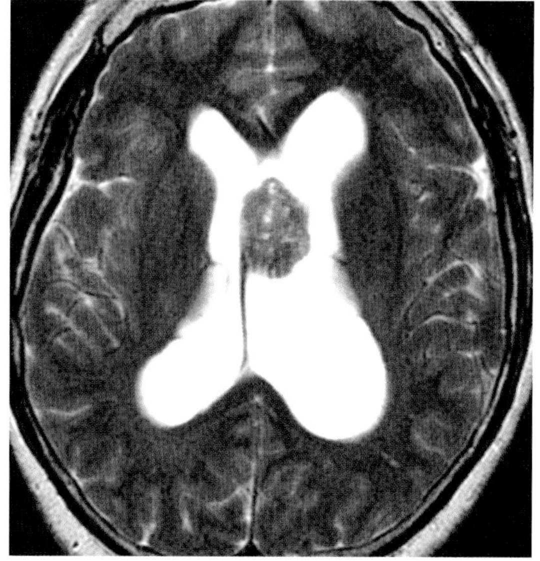

Central neurocytoma: Contrast-enhanced T1-weighted (left image) and T2-weighted MRI demonstrates a lobulated mass in the body of the left lateral ventricle (arrow) attached to the septum pellucidum. The mass enhances and contains foci of cystic change (seen as hyperintense foci on the T2-weighted image).

Case courtesy Amir Zamani, MD, Brigham and Women's Hospital.

- Central neurocytoma is a low-grade tumor likely of neuronal origin that occurs in young adults, from teenagers to young middle aged-patients. Prognosis is excellent.
- Typical imaging appearance is a lobulated mass attached to the septum pellucidum, with numerous intratumoral cystic areas. Calcification is common.

Choroid plexus papilloma/carcinoma

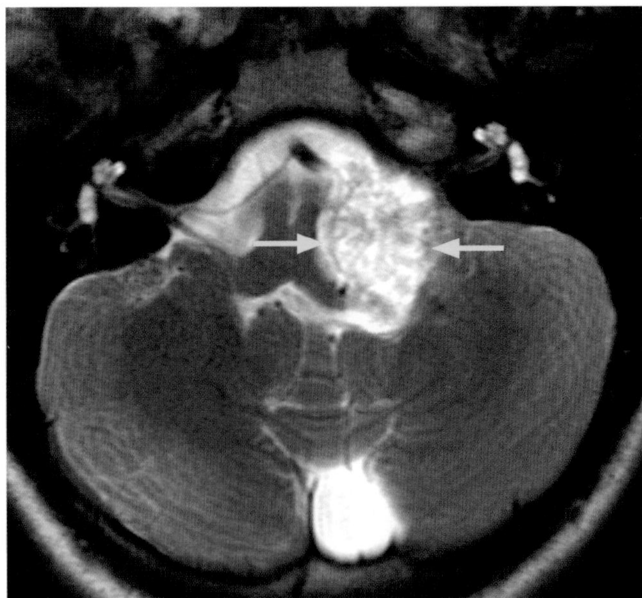

Choroid plexus papilloma: Axial T2-weighted image shows a hyperintense, cauliflower-like mass (arrows) in the left cerebellomedullary fissure deforming the medulla. The epicenter of the mass is at the foramen of Luschka, which is likely its location of origin.

Case courtesy Sanjay Prabhu, MD, Boston Children's Hospital.

- Choroid plexus papilloma is a rare intraventricular tumor. Choroid plexus papilloma is a low-grade (WHO I) neoplasm arising from choroid plexus epithelial cells. It is the most common brain tumor in babies <1 year old, but it may also occur in adults.
- T2-weighted images show a lobulated, heterogeneous or hyperintense mass that avidly enhances on T1-weighted MRI.
- In children, the atrium of the lateral ventricle is the most common location.
- In adults, the fourth ventricle is the most common location.
- Less commonly, choroid plexus papilloma may arise from the third ventricle or cerebellomedullary angle, as in the case shown.
- Choroid plexus papilloma and carcinoma (WHO grade III) are not reliably distinguishable.

Intraventricular meningioma

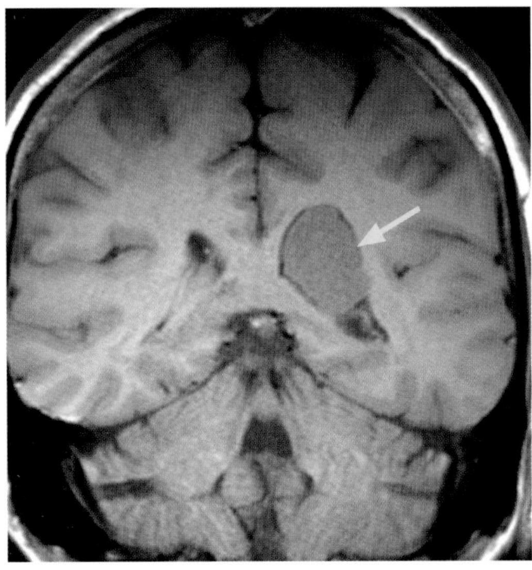

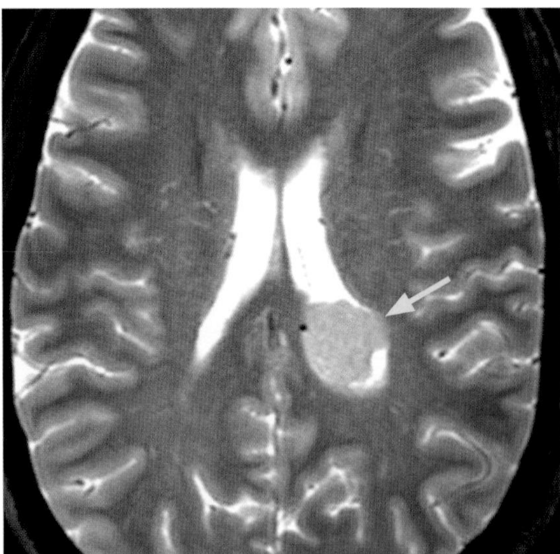

Intraventricular meningioma: Coronal T1-weighted (left image) and axial T2-weighted MRI shows a T1 hypointense, T2 slightly hyperintense mass (arrows) in the atrium of the left ventricle.

Case courtesy Mary Beth Cunnane, MD, Massachusetts Eye and Ear Infirmary.

- Intraventricular meningioma appears as a solid mass, typically in the trigone of the lateral ventricle. It tends to occur in older patients, similar to other meningiomas.
- Intraventricular meningiomas are typically hypercellular and homogeneously enhance, distinguishing them from other intraventricular neoplasms.

Subependymal giant cell astrocytoma (SEGA)

- Subependymal giant cell astrocytoma (SEGA) is a low-grade (WHO I) astrocytoma variant that is associated with tuberous sclerosis. Other findings in tuberous sclerosis include subependymal nodules and hamartomas (cortical and subcortical).
- SEGA classically is an enhancing mass in the lateral ventricle near the foramen of Monro.

Subependymoma

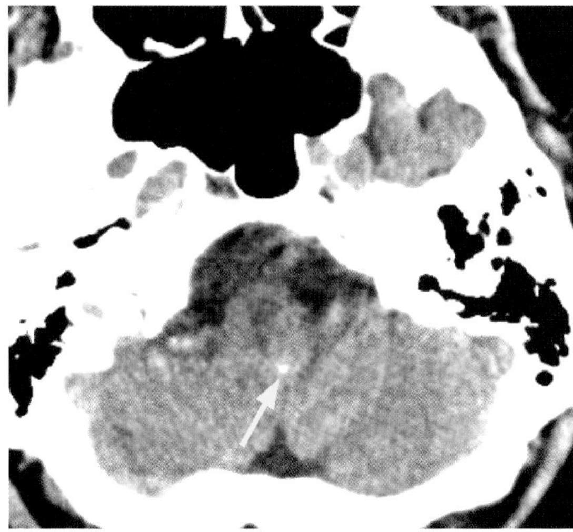

Subependymoma: Noncontrast axial CT shows a subtle focus of hyperattenuation in the region of the cerebellar vermis/fourth ventricle (arrow).

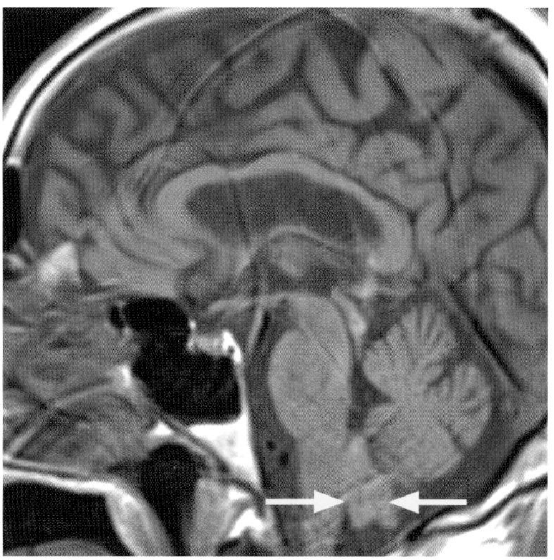

Sagittal T1-weighted MRI shows an isointense mass in the inferior fourth ventricle (arrows). The fourth ventricle is normal in size.

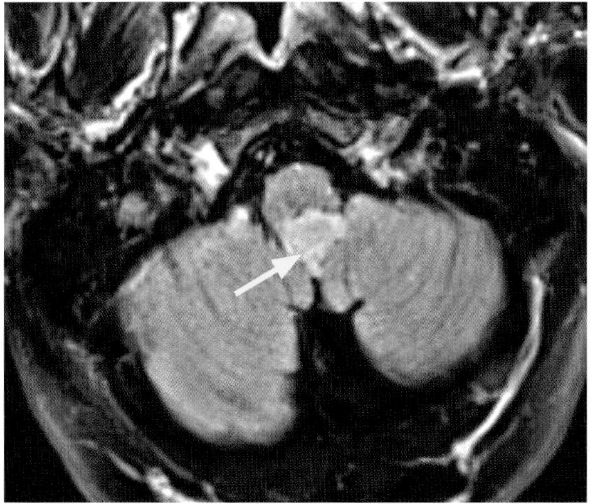

Axial FLAIR shows that the inferior fourth ventricular mass (arrow) is slightly FLAIR hyperintense.

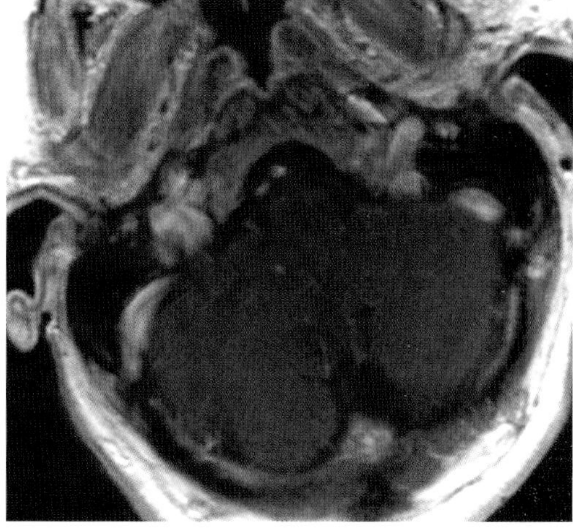

Post-contrast axial T1-weighted MRI shows absolutely no enhancement within the lesion. These lesions can be easily missed on axial T1-weighted images, with or without contrast.

- Subependymoma is a nonenhancing low-grade tumor of unclear origin thought to arise from subependymal astrocytes, ependymal cells lining the ventricles, or common precursor cells.
- Subependymoma is a tumor of middle-aged and older adults. It is often found incidentally.
- The most common locations are the obex of the 4th ventricle (inferior 4th ventricle) or at the foramen of Monro in the lateral ventricle. The tumor usually doesn't enhance.
- Despite their similar names, subependymoma is not related to subependymal giant cell astrocytoma (discussed above, associated with tuberous sclerosis) or with ependymoma.

Primary CNS lymphoma (PCNSL): Overview

- Primary CNS lymphoma is lymphoma isolated to the CNS, most commonly diffuse large B-cell lymphoma. Immature blast cells form lymphoid aggregates around small cerebral blood vessels in a periventricular location. Note that the brain does not contain native lymphoid tissue.
- PCNSL is known to "melt away" with chemoradiation but tends to recur aggressively.
- The appearance of PCNSL depends on the immune status of the patient. Regardless of immune status, however, key imaging findings are a periventricular location and high cellularity (hyperattenuating on CT, relatively hypointense on T2-weighted images, and reduced diffusivity).

Primary CNS lymphoma: Immunocompetent patient

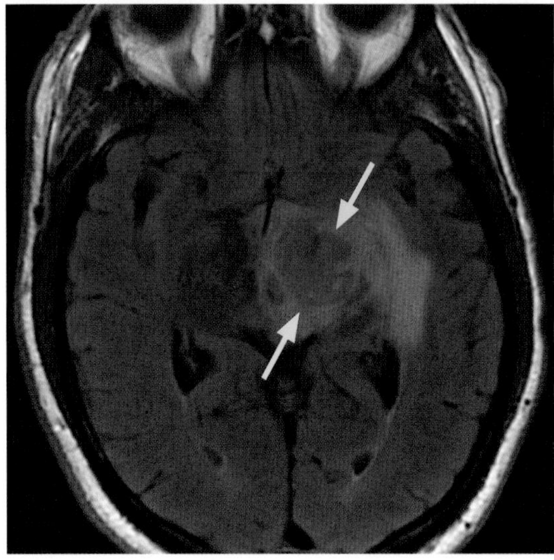

Axial FLAIR MRI demonstrates a heterogeneous mass (arrows) in the left basal ganglia with associated vasogenic edema.

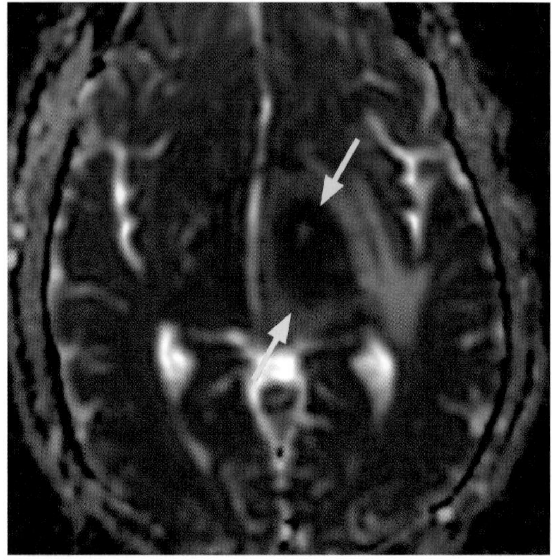

ADC map shows that the epicenter of the mass is dark (arrows), suggestive of reduced diffusivity due to hypercellularity.

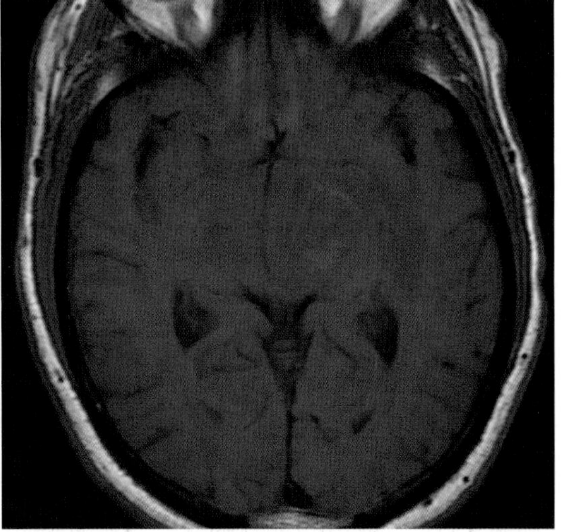

Pre-contrast T1-weighted image shows that the mass is T1 isointense.

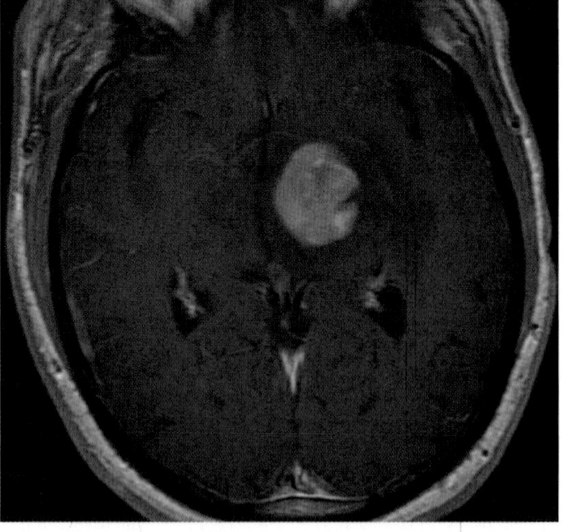

Post-contrast axial T1-weighted MRI shows intense, relatively homogeneous enhancement of the mass. There is no appreciable central necrosis.

Primary CNS lymphoma: *Case courtesy Gregory Wrubel, MD, Brigham and Women's Hospital.*

- In an immunocompetent patient, PCNSL typically presents as an **enhancing periventricular mass**, often crossing the corpus callosum to involve both hemispheres. Involvement of the frontal lobes and basal ganglia is most common.
- The differential diagnosis for a mass involving the corpus callosum includes lymphoma, glioblastoma multiforme, and demyelinating lesion.
- PCNSL in an immunocompetent individual usually enhances homogeneously, without central necrosis. This is in contrast to PCNSL in an immunocompromised patient, where central necrosis is typical.

Primary CNS lymphoma: Immunocompromised patient

- In an immunocompromised patient, PCNSL typically presents as a **periventricular ring-enhancing** lesion in the basal ganglia. The ring enhancement is caused by central necrosis. The two primary differential considerations for a ring-enhancing basal ganglial mass in an immunocompromised patient are lymphoma and toxoplasmosis.
- Several clinical and imaging options are available to differentiate between lymphoma and toxoplasmosis:

> **Empirical anti-toxoplasmosis therapy** and short-interval follow-up.
>
> **Thallium scanning**: CNS lymphoma is thallium avid and toxoplasmosis does not take up thallium.
>
> **PET**: CNS lymphoma tends to be high-grade and metabolically active. Toxoplasmosis usually does not have avid FDG uptake.
>
> **Perfusion scanning**: CNS lymphoma has increased relative cerebral blood volume while toxoplasmosis is hypovascular. Note that lymphoma and toxoplasmosis cannot be reliably differentiated by enhancement. Intra-axial enhancement is a measure of capillary leakage, not perfusion. Both will enhance.

Secondary CNS lymphoma

- Secondary CNS lymphoma represents involvement of the CNS in a patient with known extra-cerebral lymphoma. Secondary CNS lymphoma tends to involve the meninges and may cause leptomeningeal carcinomatosis or epidural cord compression.
- Less commonly, secondary CNS involvement of lymphoma may present as a parenchymal mass.

Metastatic disease to the brain

Intra-axial metastasis

- The most common primary tumors to cause parenchymal metastases are lung, breast, and melanoma.
- Most metastases are hematogenous and arise at the gray–white junction, where there is a caliber change in the small arterioles.
- Enhancement is universal, as capillaries produced by an extra-CNS primary tumor do not have a functioning blood brain barrier.
- Larger metastases often feature marked edema, while small metastases may present as tiny enhancing foci that are apparent only on the post-contrast images.

Dural neoplasms

Meningioma

- Meningioma is by far the most common extra-axial tumor. It arises from meningoepithelial cells called arachnoid "cap" cells. Meningiomas typically occur in elderly adults with a female predominance and are most often asymptomatic.
- The vast majority are benign, but 1–2% are anaplastic or malignant. Both benign and malignant meningiomas can metastasize, although this is uncommon.
- Multiple meningiomas are seen in neurofibromatosis type 2 or following radiation therapy.
- Meningiomas can occur anywhere in the neuraxis, but are most commonly supratentorial and parasagittal.
- Meningiomas may also be intraventricular (in the trigone/atrium of the lateral ventricle) or intra-osseous. Intra-osseous meningioma may mimic fibrous dysplasia.
- On noncontrast CT, meningiomas are usually hyperattenuating relative to brain and approximately 25% calcify.
- On MRI, appearance can be variable with iso- or slightly hypointense signal on T1-weighted images and variable signal intensity on T2-weighted images. There is typically a broad-based attachment to the dura.
- Meningiomas avidly enhance. An enhancing *dural tail* is thought to be due to vasoactive substances released by the meningioma rather than tumor spread to the dura.
- Despite the extra-axial location of most meningiomas, there may be extensive white matter edema, thought to be due to vasoactive factors and a pial vascular supply. There is often a discordance between the size of meningioma and degree of white matter edema, with severe edema possible even with a very small tumor.

Dural metastasis

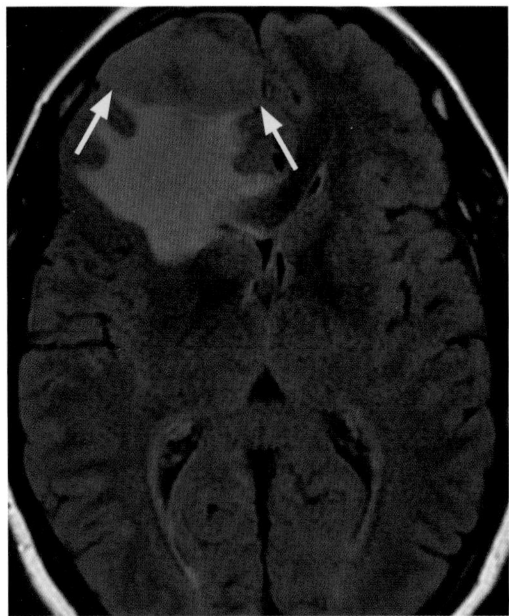

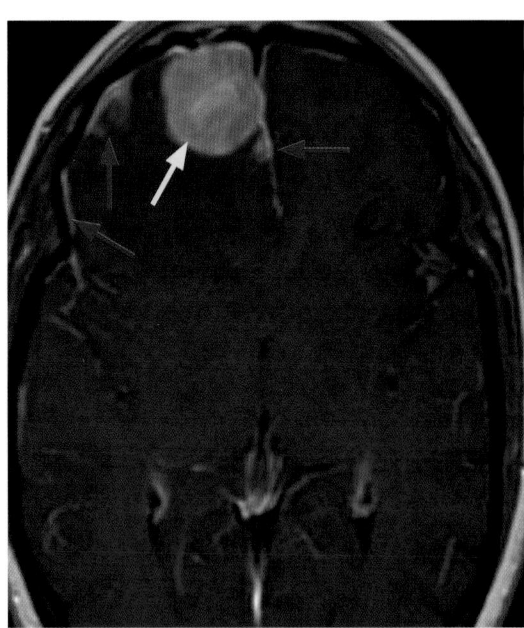

Dural metastasis: Axial FLAIR (left image) shows a right frontal mass (yellow arrows) with vasogenic edema affecting the right frontal lobe. From this image alone it is difficult to determine if the mass is intra- or extra-axial. Axial post-contrast T1-weighted (right image) MRI shows that the mass (yellow arrow) is dural based and is associated with adjacent dural enhancement (red arrows). This was a case of metastatic breast cancer.

- The most common tumors to metastasize to the dura are breast (most common), lymphoma, small cell lung cancer, and melanoma.

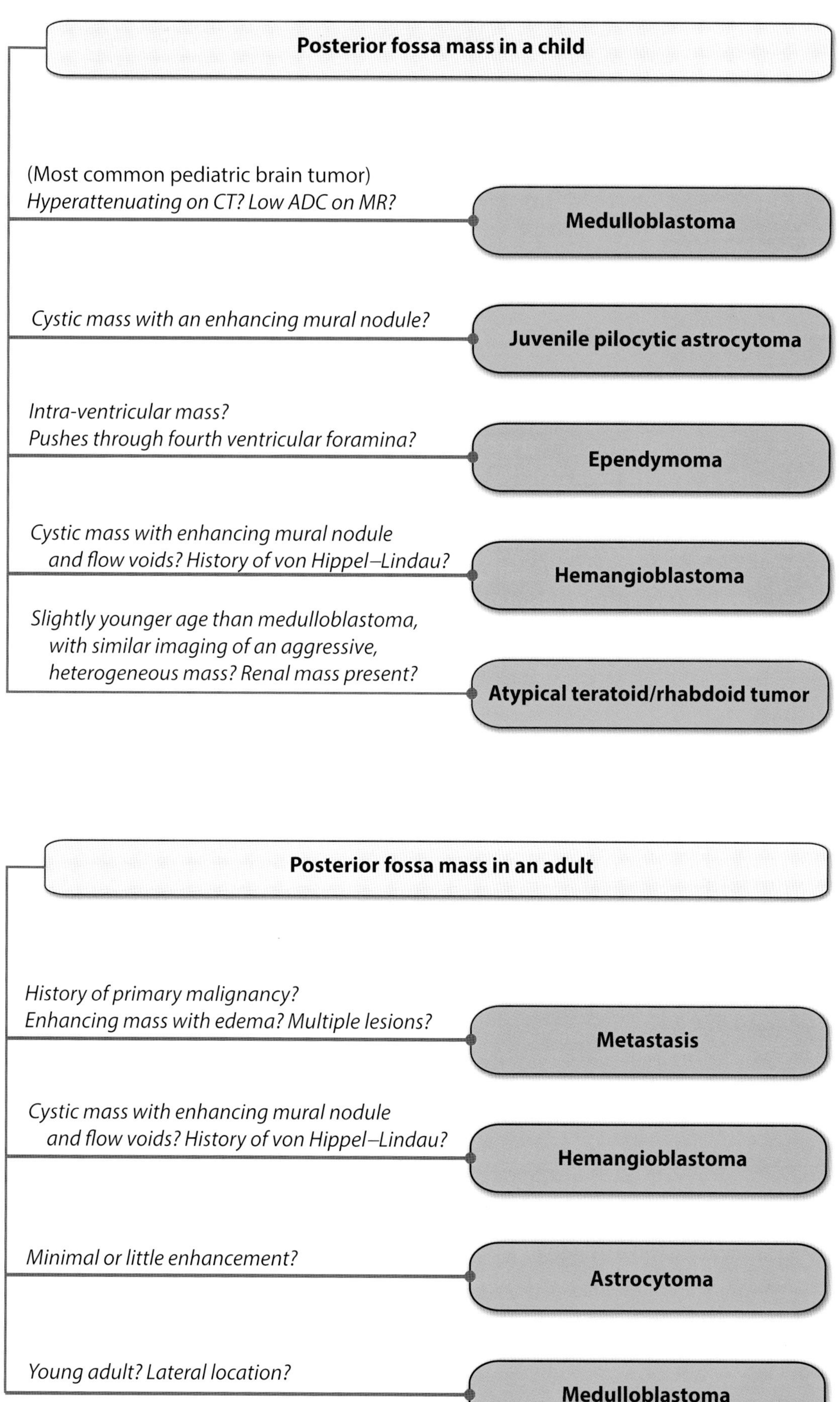
Posterior fossa mass in a child
(Most common pediatric brain tumor)
Hyperattenuating on CT? Low ADC on MR?
Medulloblastoma
Cystic mass with an enhancing mural nodule?
Juvenile pilocytic astrocytoma
Intra-ventricular mass?
Pushes through fourth ventricular foramina?
Ependymoma
Cystic mass with enhancing mural nodule
and flow voids? History of von Hippel–Lindau?
Hemangioblastoma
Slightly younger age than medulloblastoma,
with similar imaging of an aggressive,
heterogeneous mass? Renal mass present?
Atypical teratoid/rhabdoid tumor
Posterior fossa mass in an adult
History of primary malignancy?
Enhancing mass with edema? Multiple lesions?
Metastasis
Cystic mass with enhancing mural nodule
and flow voids? History of von Hippel–Lindau?
Hemangioblastoma
Minimal or little enhancement?
Astrocytoma
Young adult? Lateral location?
Medulloblastoma

Overview and anatomy of the CPA

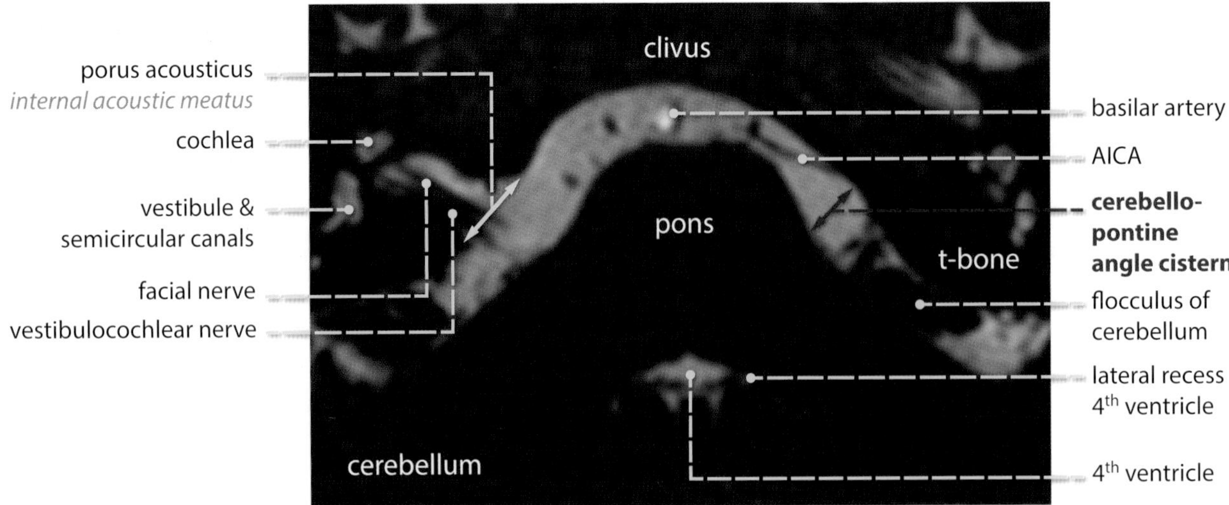

- The cerebellopontine angle (CPA) is region between the pons and cerebellum and the posterior aspect of the petrous temporal bone. Important structures of the CPA include the 5th (trigeminal), 7th (facial), and 8th (vestibulocochlear) cranial nerves, and the anterior inferior cerebellar artery (AICA).
- Most lesions of the CPA are extra-axial and located in the CPA cistern itself, although some may arise in the internal auditory canal (IAC), temporal bone, or rarely intra-axially from the pons or cerebellum. CPA masses are more common in adults.

Schwannoma

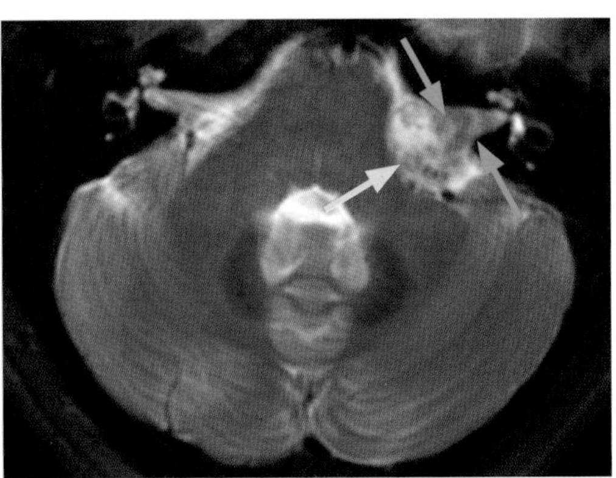
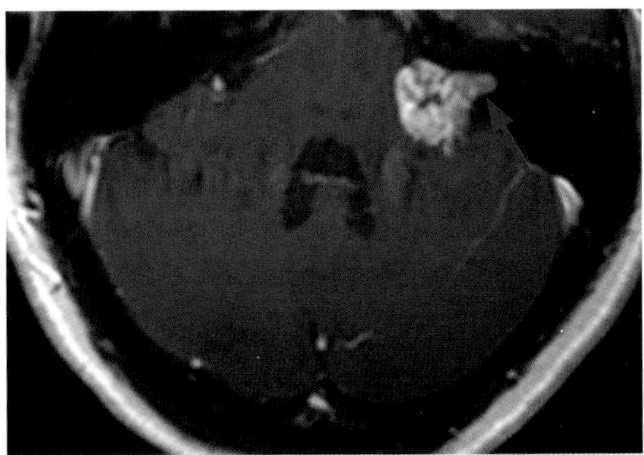

Vestibular schwannoma: Axial T2- (left image) and T1-weighted post-contrast MRI demonstrates a heterogeneously enhancing mass in the left cerebellopontine angle with an *ice cream cone* appearance that indents the cerebellar-pontine junction (yellow arrow) and protrudes into the internal acoustic meatus (red arrow). The porus acousticus is slightly widened (blue arrows).

Case courtesy Mary Beth Cunnane, MD, Massachusetts Eye and Ear Infirmary.

- Schwannoma of the vestibulocochlear nerve, also known as a vestibular schwannoma, is by far the most common cerebellopontine angle mass, representing greater than 75% of all CPA masses.
- Vestibular schwannoma is hyperintense on T2-weighted images and avidly enhances. The characteristic *ice cream cone* appearance describes the "cone" protruding through (and widening) the porus acousticus and the "ice cream" exerting mass effect on the cerebellar–pontine junction. Schwannoma may become cystic, especially when larger.
- Schwannomas of other cranial nerves in the CPA, including the facial or trigeminal nerves, are less common. Trigeminal schwannoma may extend into Meckel's cave.

Meningioma

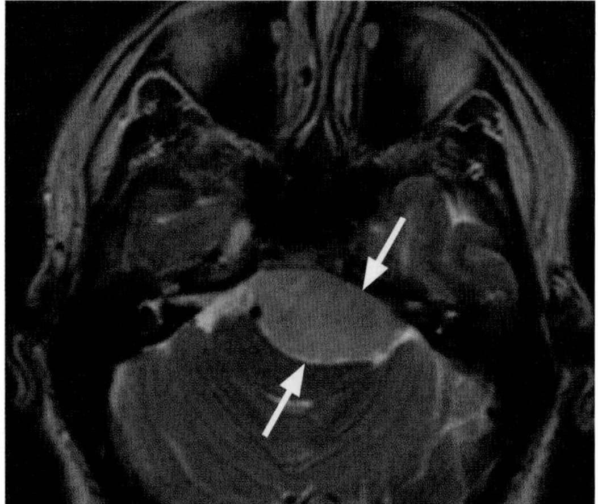

Prepontine/left CPA meningioma: Axial T2-weighted MRI (top left image) demonstrates a circumscribed, hyperintense, prepontine mass (yellow arrows).

Axial precontrast T1 (bottom left image) and postcontrast T1-weighted (bottom right image) MRI shows that the mass avidly enhances and extends from the prepontine cistern into the left CPA and left porus acousticus (red arrow). There is also extension into Dorello's canal on the left (green arrow), likely causing cranial nerve VI palsy. There is flattening of the pons. The basilar artery is nearly 180 degrees encased and mildly narrowed (blue arrow).

Case courtesy Gregory Wrubel, MD, Brigham and Women's Hospital.

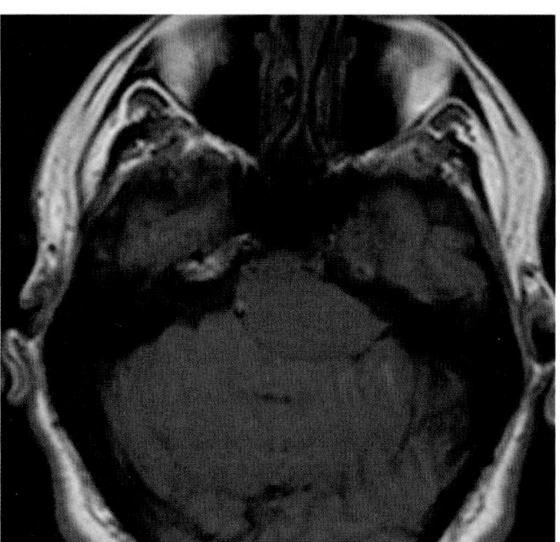

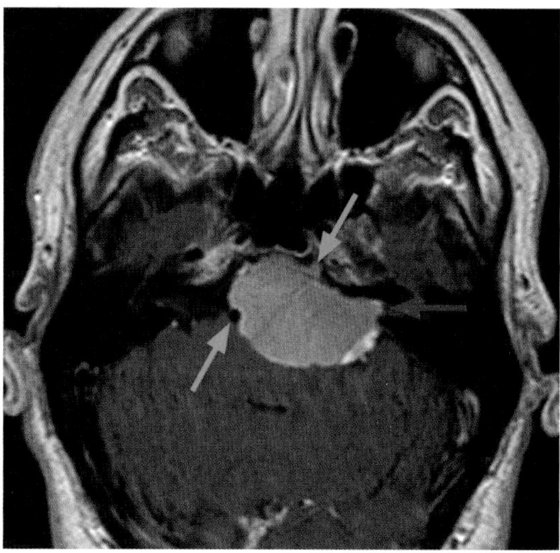

- Although meningioma is overall the most common extra-axial mass in adults, it is only the second most common mass of the CPA, representing approximately 10–15% of all CPA masses.
- Meningiomas often feature a short segment of dural enhancement and may induce adjacent bony hyperostosis. Approximately 20% calcify, in contrast to schwannomas where calcification is rare.
- In contrast to schwannoma, a CPA meningioma does not enlarge the porus acousticus.

Arachnoid cyst

- An arachnoid cyst is a benign CSF-filled lesion that is usually congenital. Although most arachnoid cysts are supratentorial, the cerebellopontine angle is the most common infratentorial location.
- An arachnoid cyst will follow CSF signal on all sequences, including complete suppression on FLAIR. Unlike an epidermoid cyst, an arachnoid cyst does not have restricted diffusion.

Aneurysm

- Vertebrobasilar aneurysm (arising from the posterior inferior cerebellar artery, anterior inferior cerebellar artery, vertebral artery, or basilar artery) may appear as a well-defined, avidly enhancing CPA lesion and may be initially mistaken for a schwannoma or meningioma on contrast-enhanced CT.
- On MRI, clues to a vascular etiology would be flow void and pulsation artifacts. MRA or CTA are diagnostic.

Epidermoid cyst

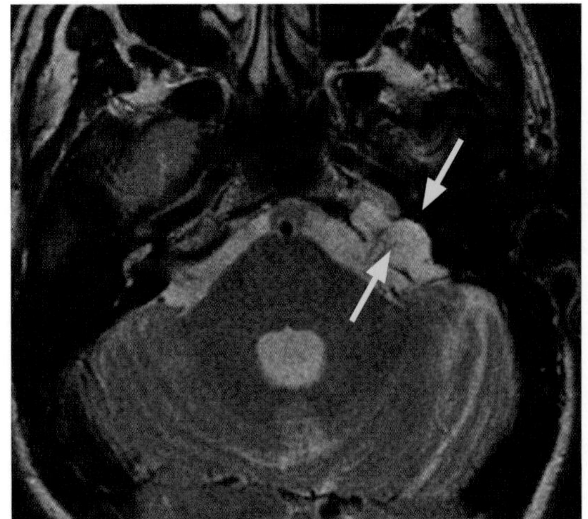

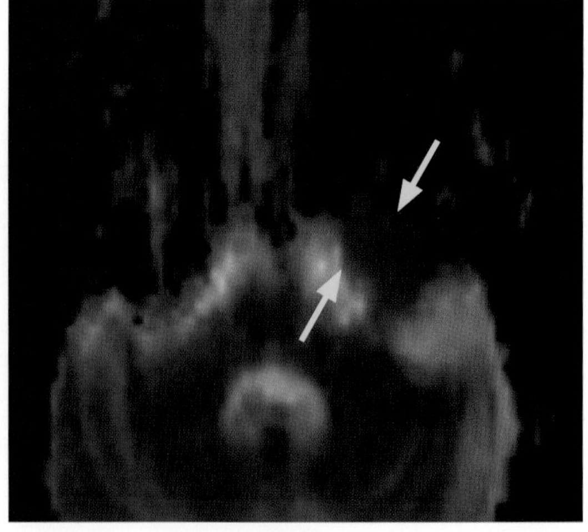

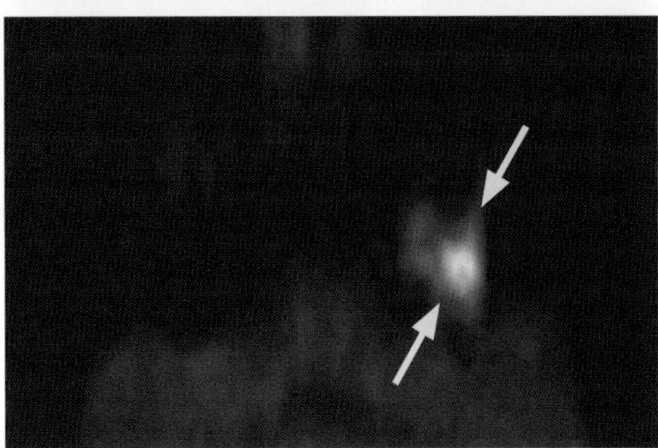

Epidermoid cyst: Axial T2-weighted MRI (top left image) shows a lobulated mass (arrows) in the left cerebellopontine angle. The mass is isointense to CSF.

ADC map (top right image) and DWI (left image) show that the mass (arrows) is dark on ADC and bright on DWI, consistent with reduced diffusivity.

Case courtesy Gregory Wrubel, MD, Brigham and Women's Hospital.

- An epidermoid cyst is a congenital lesion arising from ectopic ectodermal epithelial tissue.
- Epidermoids progressively enlarge from desquamation of keratinized epithelium lining the cyst. The mass characteristically insinuates in between structures, encasing cranial nerves and vessels. Gross pathology features a characteristic "cauliflower-like" surface.
- On CT, epidermoid cyst may mimic arachnoid cyst and appear as a water-attenuation cystic structure. On MRI, an epidermoid cyst has similar signal characteristics to CSF on T1- and T2-weighted images. Unlike arachnoid cyst, an epidermoid does not usually suppress on FLAIR.
- Diffusion sequences show very bright signal on diffusion-weighted images (a combination of restricted diffusion and T2 shine through). Postsurgical DWI follow-up is critical to detect any residual focus, which will be DWI bright.
- Rarely, epidermoids may exhibit signal hyperintensity on unenhanced T1-weighted imaging, also known as "white epidermoids."

Intra-axial neoplasm

- A posterior fossa intra-axial neoplasm may invade laterally into the CPA.
- An exophytic brainstem glioma or metastasis may invade into the CPA.
- Medulloblastoma tends to occur in the midline in children, though lateral involvement of the cerebellar hemispheres can be seen in older children or young adults.
- Ependymoma may extend into the CPA by squeezing through the lateral 4th ventricular foramina (of Luschka).
- Hemangioblastoma, associated with von Hippel–Lindau (VHL) disease, typically presents in the cerebellar hemisphere as a fluid-secreting tumor with a cyst and enhancing nodule. There are often prominent flow voids feeding the tumor.

  The other intracranial manifestation of VHL seen on imaging is an **endolymphatic sac tumor**, which occurs along the posterior petrous ridge.

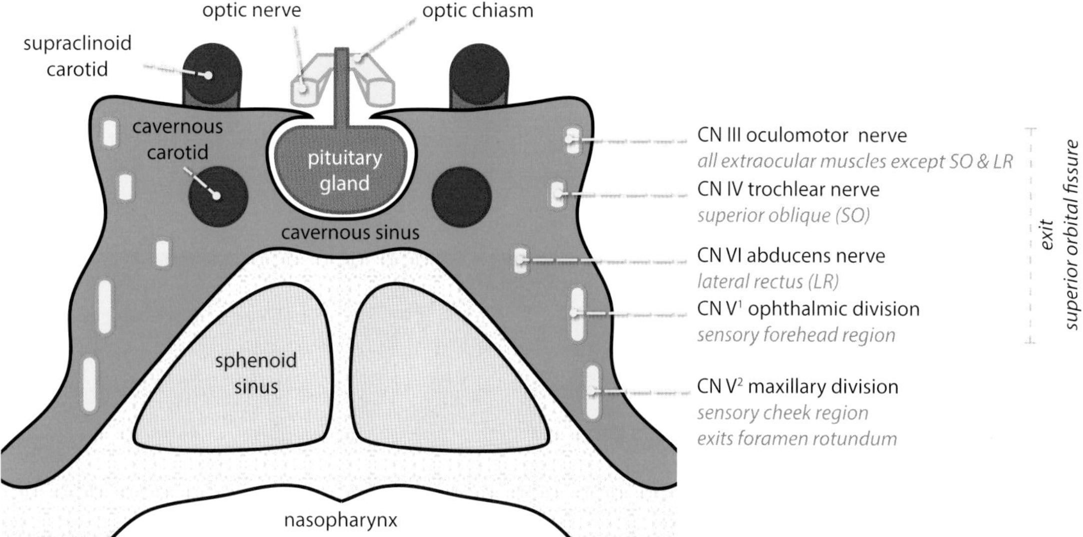

The mandibular nerve (V³) is the only segment of the trigeminal nerve that does not traverse the cavernous sinus. It exits inferiorly from Meckel's cave through the foramen ovale.

The abducens nerve (VI) enters the petrous portion of the temporal bone through Dorello's canal and is the only nerve that travels in the medial venus sinusoids.

The maxillary nerve (V²) is the only nerve of the cavernous sinus that does not exit the superior orbital fissure. Instead, it exits the foramen rotundum.

- The pituitary gland is formed from Rathke's pouch, which is a superior invagination from the primitive oral cavity. The pituitary gland sits in the sella turcica, a cup-shaped depression of the basisphenoid bone. The pituitary is composed of an anterior and a posterior lobe.

  Rathke's pouch closes off to form a vesicle that involutes. Sometimes, the involution is incomplete and a cleft can be left behind, which may give rise to craniopharyngioma or Rathke's cleft cyst.

- The anterior lobe of the pituitary produces and secretes endocrine hormones, including growth hormone, ACTH, prolactin, TSH, FSH, and LH.
- The posterior lobe of the pituitary is derived from neuroectoderm and is composed of axons from the hypothalamus, through which vasopressin and oxytocin are transported.
- The pituitary gland has a wide range of normal morphology, depending on patient age, sex, and hormonal/pregnancy status. The gland may be convex superiorly in adolescent or pregnant females. The normal posterior pituitary is hyperintense on T1-weighted MRI and is called the "posterior pituitary bright spot," best seen on sagittal images.
- The empty sella is a normal variant when seen in isolation. An empty sella is partially filled with CSF, with the gland flattened against the floor of the sella.

  Empty sella is also a component of the constellation of findings in pseudotumor cerebri. Pseudotumor cerebri, also known as idiopathic intracranial hypertension, is a syndrome associated with elevated CSF pressure, visual changes, and headaches that is typically seen in obese black females. Imaging findings include empty sella, enlargement of Meckel's cave, and optic disc protrusion into the posterior globes. The ventricles are normal in size or slightly reduced in caliber. The sigmoid or transverse sinus may be stenotic.

Approach to a sellar/parasellar mass

- The first step in evaluation of a sellar region mass is to determine if the mass is intrinsic to the pituitary or if the mass represents an adjacent extra-pituitary lesion.
- The differential for an intrinsic pituitary mass is rather limited and includes pituitary adenoma (by far the most common intrinsic pituitary mass), Rathke's cleft cyst, and hypophysitis (inflammation of the pituitary). Craniopharyngioma may rarely occur in the sella, but essentially never occurs within the pituitary gland itself.

INTRINSIC PITUITARY MASS

Pituitary microadenoma

- A pituitary microadenoma is a pituitary adenoma <10 mm in size. Patients seek medical attention due to symptoms of hormone excess, not mass effect.
- Most microadenomas are hypoenhancing relative to the pituitary, although ACTH-secreting adenomas may be hyperenhancing.

Pituitary macroadenoma

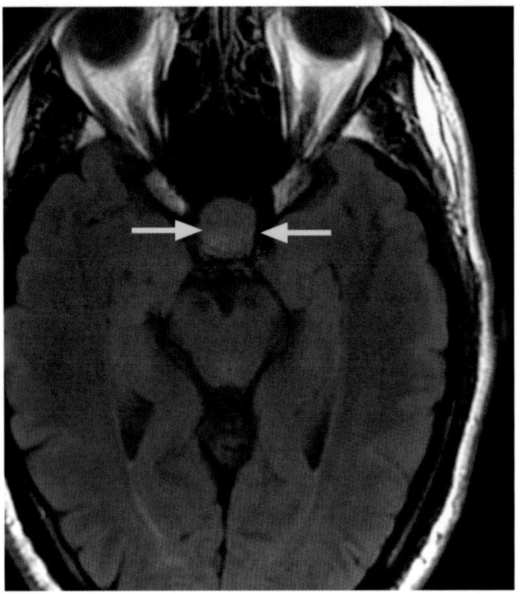

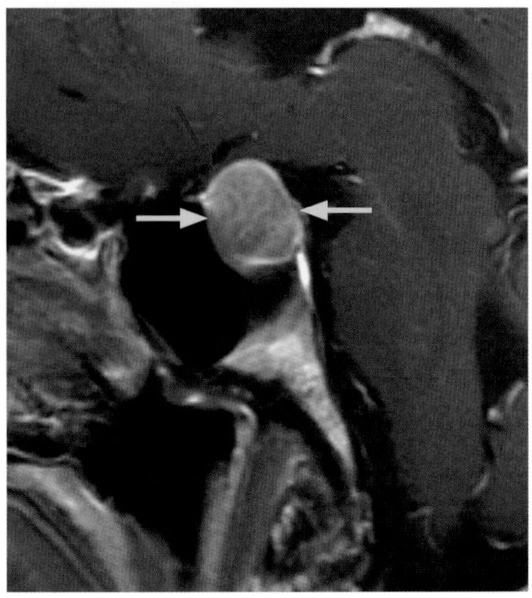

Macroadenoma: FLAIR (left image) and post-contrast sagittal T1-weighted MRI shows complete replacement of the pituitary gland by an enhancing mass (yellow arrows). The optic chiasm is displaced superiorly (red arrow).

- A macroadenoma is defined as an adenoma >10 mm in size. Patients usually present with mass effect (e.g., compression of the optic chiasm) rather than endocrine dysfunction.
- The bony sella is often enlarged. Macroadenomas may encase the carotid, but tend not to narrow it. In contrast, meningiomas or metastases can narrow the carotid. Pituitary macroadenoma may bleed after medical treatment, producing a complex MRI appearance.

  Intra-tumoral hemorrhage is distinct from pituitary apoplexy. Pituitary apoplexy is a clinical syndrome of severe headache and endocrine dysfunction caused by hemorrhage into an otherwise normal pituitary.

Lymphocytic hypophysitis

- Lymphocytic hypophysitis is an autoimmune inflammatory disorder usually seen in peripartum women that may affect the pituitary and infundibulum. It presents with diabetes insipidus, headache, visual impairment, and endocrine dysfunction.
- MRI shows thickening and intense enhancement of the pituitary stalk, usually with enlargement of the pituitary gland that may appear similar to a macroadenoma.
- Lymphocytic hypophysitis responds to steroid therapy.

Granulomatous hypophysitis

- Granulomatous inflammation of the pituitary and infundibulum can be secondary to sarcoidosis, Wegener granulomatosis, tuberculosis, and Langerhans cell histiocytosis (LCH). LCH hypophysitis is a disease of children. In all causes, imaging is identical to lymphocytic hypophysitis.

Rathke's cleft cyst

- Rathke's cleft cyst may be limited to the pituitary gland but is more commonly seen extrinsic to the pituitary.

- The differential diagnosis for an extra-pituitary lesion is broad, but the imaging findings together with clues about the patient's age and clinical presentation can usually narrow the differential diagnosis to a few entities.
- The most common suprasellar lesion in a child is craniopharyngioma, while the most common suprasellar lesion in an adult is a pituitary macroadenoma that has extended superiorly.
- The SATCHMO mnemonic may be helpful to remember the spectrum of extra-pituitary masses; however, the order of the entities is NOT based on frequency of occurrence.

  Sarcoidosis/**S**uprasellar extension of an adenoma.

  Aneurysm.

  Teratoma (dermoid cyst)/**T**olosa Hunt.

  Craniopharyngioma/**C**left cyst (Rathke's).

  Hypothalamic glioma (adults)/**H**ypothalamic hamartoma (children).

  Meningioma/**M**etastasis.

  Optic nerve glioma.

Craniopharyngioma

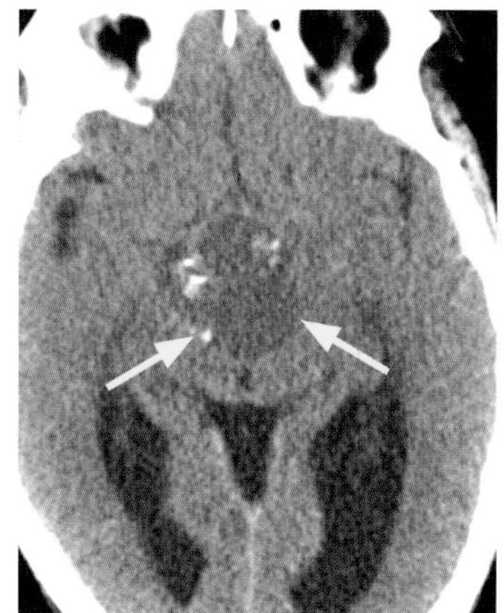 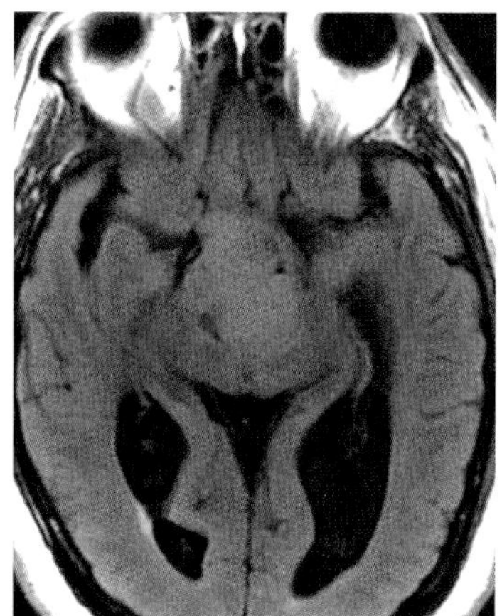 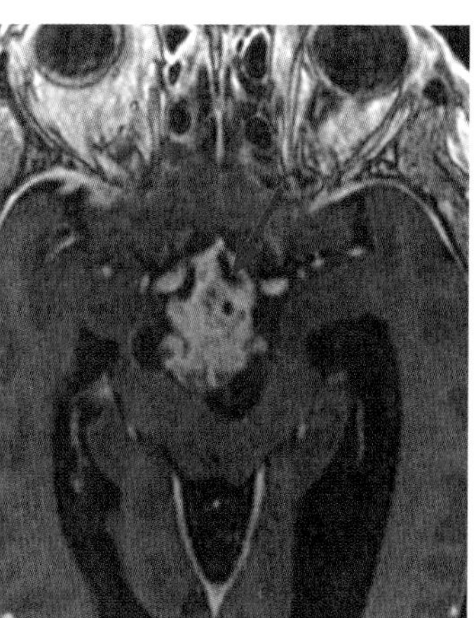

Craniopharyngioma: Noncontrast CT (left image) shows a hypoattenuating suprasellar mass (arrows) containing coarse calcifications. The suprasellar cistern is effaced. FLAIR MRI (middle image) shows an isointense, primarily solid suprasellar mass. Postcontrast T1-weighted (right image) MRI shows avid heterogeneous enhancement. There is a small cystic focus anteriorly (red arrow).

- Craniopharyngioma is the most common suprasellar lesion of childhood, arising from squamous epithelial remnants of Rathke's pouch that produce keratin.
- Craniopharyngioma occurs in a bimodal age distribution. The majority of cases are lesions of childhood, but craniopharyngioma may occur uncommonly in late middle age.
- Most involve both the sella and suprasellar regions. Although craniopharyngioma may rarely involve only the sella, it is almost always separate from the pituitary gland.
- Craniopharyngioma has potential for enamel production and almost always calcifies. The characteristic intracystic *machine-oil* seen on gross examination is composed of desquamated squamous epithelium, keratin, and cholesterol.
- MRI shows a complex cystic mass containing protein or blood products (hyperintense on T1-weighted images).
- There is avid enhancement of the solid elements and cyst walls.
- In contrast to Rathke's cleft cyst, craniopharyngioma almost always enhances, is almost always calcified, and is almost always separate from the pituitary.

Rathke's cleft cyst

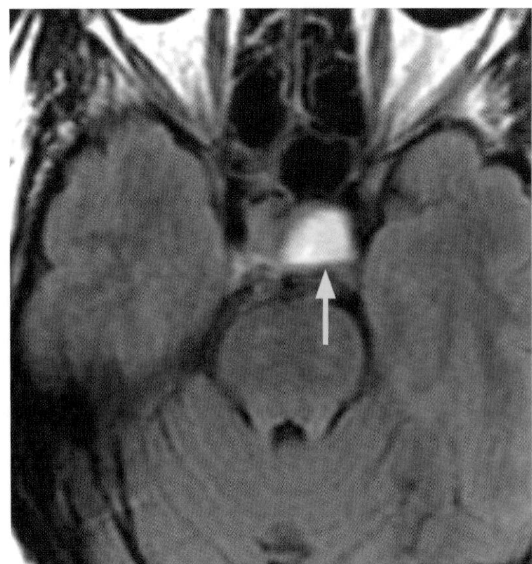

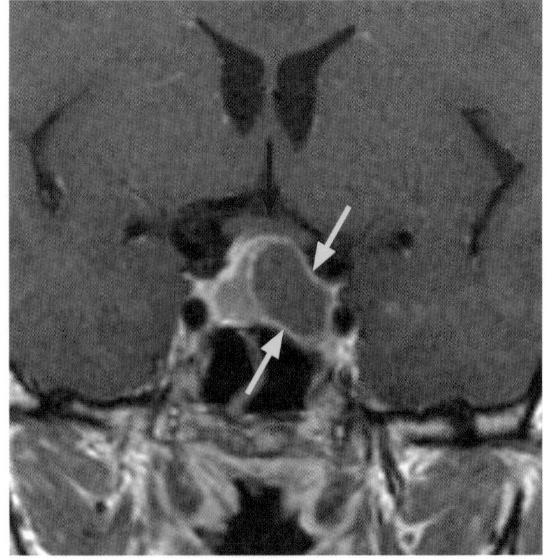

Rathke's cleft cyst: Axial FLAIR (left image) and coronal post-contrast T1-weighted MRI shows a FLAIR hyperintense, T1 hypointense parasellar mass (yellow arrows). The mass demonstrates faint peripheral rim enhancement. The pituitary is displaced to the right and the optic chiasm is displaced superiorly (red arrow).

- Similar to craniopharyngioma, Rathke's cleft cyst is also a remnant of the embryologic Rathke's pouch, the precursor of the anterior lobe of the pituitary gland. In contrast to craniopharyngioma, Rathke's cleft cyst is made of simple columnar or cuboidal epithelium.
- While craniopharyngioma is the most common suprasellar lesion of childhood, Rathke's cleft cyst is typically seen in middle-aged adults, twice as commonly in females.
- Rathke's cleft cyst is reportedly very common in autopsy studies (up to 22% incidence), but clinically is usually asymptomatic or discovered incidentally.
- Imaging appearance is dependent on the protein content of the cyst. The intra-cystic fluid may be isointense to CSF if low protein and hyperintense on T1-weighted images if high protein. High protein content may cause incomplete nulling of the intracystic fluid on FLAIR.
- The *claw* sign represents enhancing pituitary tissue completely wrapped around the cyst.
- It is usually possible to distinguish craniopharyngioma from Rathke's cleft cyst. Unlike craniopharyngioma, Rathke's cleft cyst does not enhance (although rim enhancement is often seen) and does not calcify. Rathke's cleft cyst may occasionally be inseparable from the pituitary, but craniopharyngioma is nearly always distinct.

Meningioma

- Meningioma is the second most common suprasellar tumor in adults. Most common in middle-aged females, it typically presents with visual loss due to optic pathway involvement. There are several dural reflections in the region of the sella from which a meningioma may arise, including the tuberculum sella, clinoid process, planum sphenoidale, and sphenoid wing.
- Imaging shows isointense signal on T1-weighted images, variable signal on T2-weighted images, and uniform, intense contrast enhancement. There is often an enhancing dural tail. Meningioma may cause adjacent hyperostosis due to vasoactive factors.
- An important imaging finding of a parasellar meningioma is the tendency to encase and narrow the cavernous or supraclinoid internal carotid artery.
- In contrast to pituitary adenoma, the sella is usually normal and the pituitary can be identified separately.

Astrocytoma (optic pathway glioma)

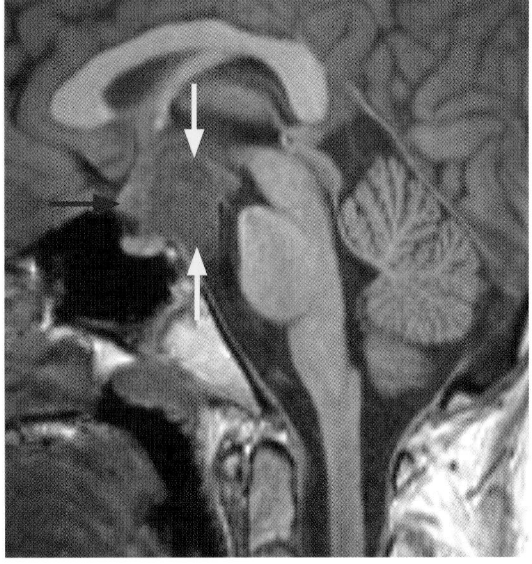

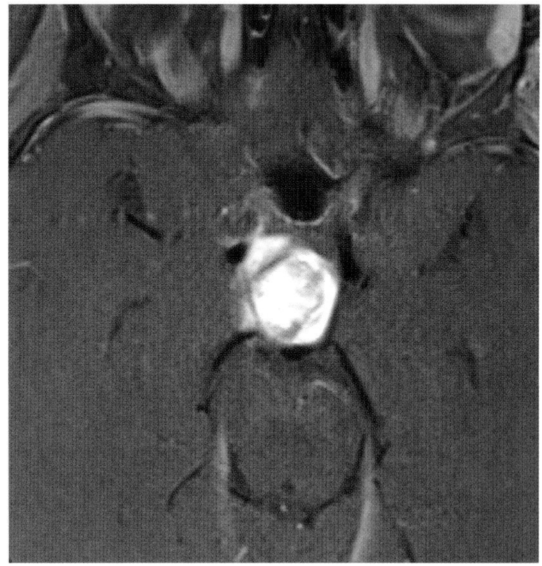

Optic pathway glioma: Sagittal T1 (left image) and post-contrast axial T1-weighted MRI shows a suprasellar mass that is slightly hypointense relative to gray matter (yellow arrows), with diffuse enlargement of the adjacent optic chiasm (red arrow). The mass demonstrates avid, slightly heterogeneous enhancement.

- An astrocytoma involving the visual pathway (optic nerve, optic chiasm, and optic tract) is the second most common suprasellar mass in children (craniopharyngioma is most common). A substantial minority of patients with optic pathway glioma have neurofibromatosis type 1. In contrast to the low-grade tumor of childhood, optic glioma is an aggressive tumor when it occurs in adults.
- Tumors are isointense on T1-weighted images, hyperintense on T2-weighted images, and usually enhance.

Germinoma

- The most common intracranial germ cell tumor is a germinoma, of which 80% arise in the pineal region and 20% arise in the parasellar region. Germinomas are primarily seen in children and adolescents.
- Imaging shows a homogeneous, intensely enhancing midline mass. The mass is hypointense on T2-weighted images and dark on ADC map due to hypercellularity.

Epidermoid and dermoid cysts

- Epidermoid and dermoid cysts are congenital benign inclusion cysts.
- Epidermoids occur most commonly in middle-aged adults in the cerebellopontine angle, but can be seen less commonly in the parasellar region. Epidermoids follow CSF signal on T1- and T2-weighted images. In contrast to a simple arachnoid cyst, epidermoid is hyperintense on FLAIR and diffusion sequences show restricted diffusion.
- Dermoids are most common in young adult males in the posterior fossa, but may occasionally occur in the parasellar region. They may contain intracystic fat which can cause chemical meningitis or ventriculitis with rupture.

Aneurysm

- A saccular supraclinoid internal carotid artery aneurysm may mimic a suprasellar tumor.
- Although parasellar aneurysms are relatively uncommon, it is essential never to biopsy a mass that may represent an aneurysm.
- Pulsation artifact may be present on conventional MRI sequences. CTA or MRA would be diagnostic.

Hypothalamic hamartoma (hamartoma of the tuber cinereum)

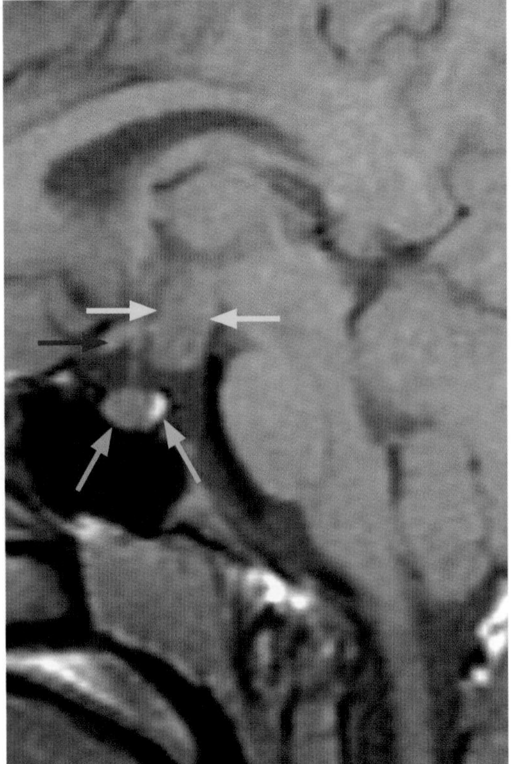

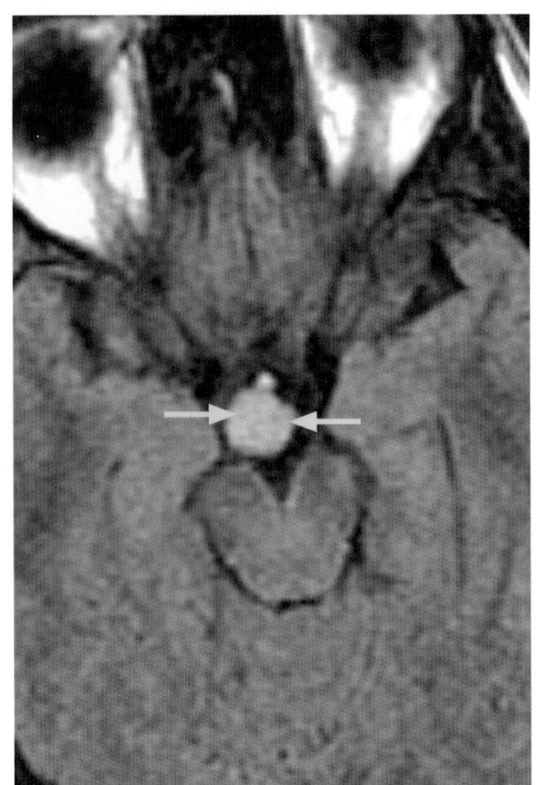

Hypothalamic hamartoma: Sagittal T1-weighted (left image) and axial FLAIR MRI shows a T1 isointense, FLAIR hyperintense suprasellar mass (yellow arrows) projecting inferiorly from the hypothalamus. The optic chiasm (red arrow), anterior pituitary (blue arrow), and posterior pituitary bright spot (green arrow), are normal.

Case courtesy Sanjay Prabhu, MD, Boston Children's Hospital.

- Hypothalamic hamartoma is not a true neoplasm, but represents ectopic hypothalamic neural tissue. It is a rare lesion of childhood that classically presents with precocious puberty and gelastic seizures (laughing spells).
- Hypothalamic hamartoma characteristically appears as a sessile mass between the pituitary stalk and the mammillary bodies.
- Hypothalamic hamartoma does *not* enhance and is isointense to gray matter.

Metastases

- Breast cancer is by far the most common lesion to metastasize to the parasellar region.

Lymphoma

- Parasellar lymphoma is rare but may occur in older adults.

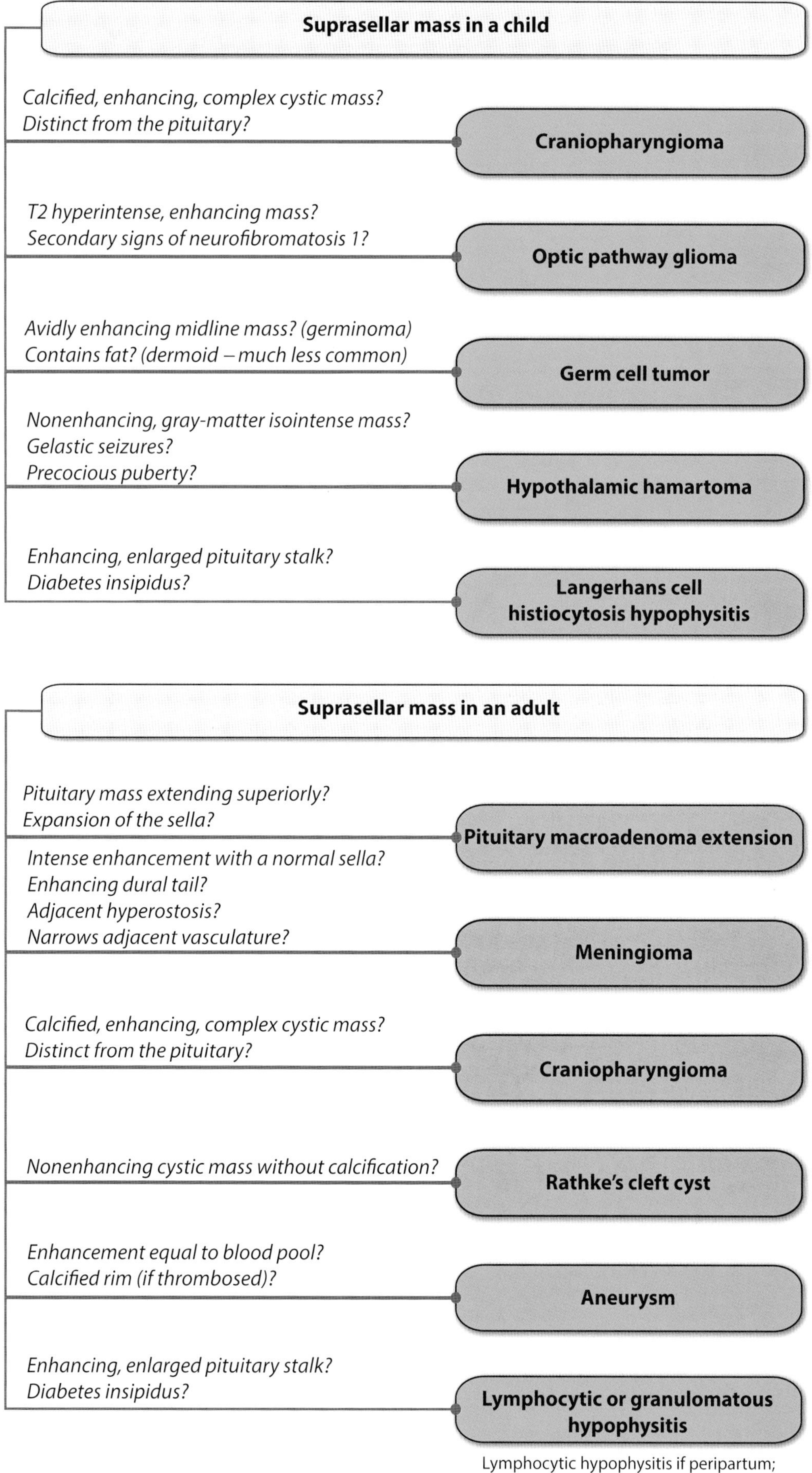
Suprasellar mass in a child
Calcified, enhancing, complex cystic mass?
Distinct from the pituitary?
Craniopharyngioma
T2 hyperintense, enhancing mass?
Secondary signs of neurofibromatosis 1?
Optic pathway glioma
Avidly enhancing midline mass? (germinoma)
Contains fat? (dermoid – much less common)
Germ cell tumor
Nonenhancing, gray-matter isointense mass?
Gelastic seizures?
Precocious puberty?
Hypothalamic hamartoma
Enhancing, enlarged pituitary stalk?
Diabetes insipidus?
Langerhans cell histiocytosis hypophysitis
Suprasellar mass in an adult
Pituitary mass extending superiorly?
Expansion of the sella?
Pituitary macroadenoma extension
Intense enhancement with a normal sella?
Enhancing dural tail?
Adjacent hyperostosis?
Narrows adjacent vasculature?
Meningioma
Calcified, enhancing, complex cystic mass?
Distinct from the pituitary?
Craniopharyngioma
Nonenhancing cystic mass without calcification?
Rathke's cleft cyst
Enhancement equal to blood pool?
Calcified rim (if thrombosed)?
Aneurysm
Enhancing, enlarged pituitary stalk?
Diabetes insipidus?
Lymphocytic or granulomatous hypophysitis
Lymphocytic hypophysitis if peripartum; granulomatous hypophysitis otherwise.

Overview and anatomy of the pineal region

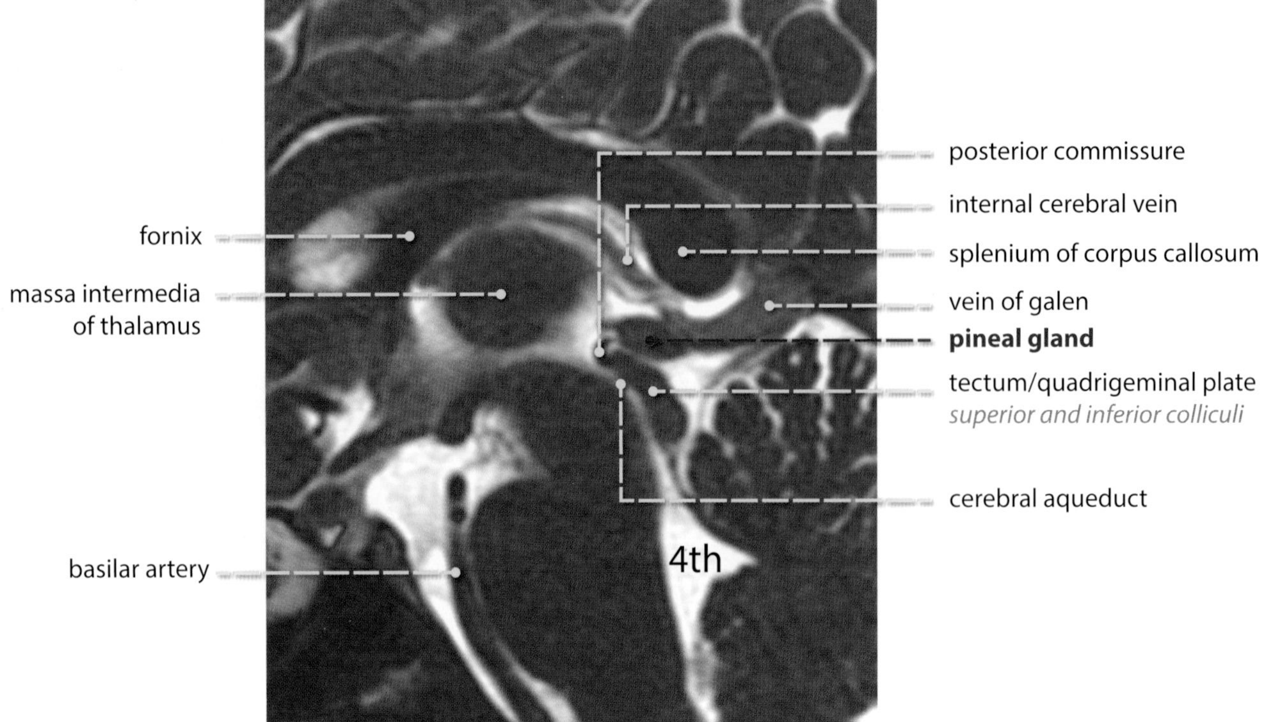

- The pineal gland is located in the midline at the level of the midbrain. It is situated between the thalami at the posterior aspect of the third ventricle. The internal cerebral veins and vein of Galen are located superior and posterior to the pineal gland, respectively.
- The principal neuronal cell of the pineal gland is the pinealocyte, which is a modified retinal neuronal cell that is innervated by the sympathetic plexus originating in the retina. The pineal gland releases melatonin, which modulates the sleep/wake cycle. The pineal gland does not have a blood brain barrier.
- A mass lesion in the pineal region may cause compression of the midbrain, compression of the cerebral aqueduct of Sylvius, or compression of the tectal plate. Compression of the tectal plate produces Parinaud syndrome, which is the inability to look up (upward gaze paralysis), pupillary light dissociation, and nystagmus.
- The first step in evaluating a pineal region mass is to determine if the lesion is arising from the pineal gland itself or from an adjacent structure.
- A mass of the pineal gland is extra-axial.
- Tumors of pineal cell origin tend to lift the internal cerebral veins, while tentorial meningiomas tend to depress the internal cerebral veins. The relationship of any pineal region mass to the internal cerebral veins is key for surgical planning and approach.

Germ cell tumor

- Extragonadal germ cell tumors can be found in the pineal gland as well as other intracranial and extracranial midline locations including the suprasellar region, mediastinum, and sacrococcygeal region. Extragonadal germ cell tumors are thought to be due to aberrant migration of totipotent germ cells during early embryogenesis.
- Germinoma and teratoma are germ cell tumors, which are the most common and second most common pineal region tumors, respectively.

- **Germinoma** (extra-gonadal seminoma) is the most common pineal region tumor and has a peak incidence in the second decade of life (age 10-19). Pineal germinoma is seen much more commonly in males, but suprasellar germinoma does not show a gender predilection.

  Germinoma is a highly cellular, avidly enhancing tumor that is slightly hyperdense on CT, isointense on T1- and T2-weighted images, and is dark on ADC map.

  Germinoma characteristically "engulfs" the pineal gland and promotes its calcification, resulting in a central area of calcification.

  Imaging of the entire neuraxis is recommended as leptomeningeal deposits can occur.

  Treatment is radiotherapy, with excellent prognosis.

  Pineal germinoma may present with a synchronous suprasellar germ cell tumor.

- **Teratoma** is the second most common pineal region tumor and confers a worse prognosis than germinoma. Teratoma has a heterogeneous imaging appearance.

  Intralesional fat is suggestive of teratoma. Teratoma is prone to hemorrhage and coarse calcification.

Pineal cyst

- Pineal cysts are seen commonly on MRI and have a prevalence as high as 40% on autopsy series. They are more common in women. Most pineal cysts are less than 1 cm and asymptomatic, but may cause symptoms due to mass effect.
- Very few pineal cysts grow and follow-up of small pineal cysts is not routinely recommended.
- Pineal cysts are usually not entirely simple. Most cysts do not fully suppress on FLAIR. Most cysts do display some peripheral enhancement, and rim calcification can be seen about 25% of the time.
- A differential consideration is a pineocytoma, which would demonstrate internal enhancement and may have cystic components. However, a truly cystic pineocytoma is considered very rare.

  A potential pitfall is that if imaging is delayed after contrast administration (by greater than 60 minutes), gadolinium may diffuse into the cyst, causing it to appear solid.

  In rare cases, it may not be possible to differentiate a hemorrhagic pineal cyst from pineocytoma.

Pineocytoma

- A pineocytoma is a low-grade (WHO grade I or II), slow-growing pinealocyte tumor.
- Any solid component should enhance. Pineocytoma may feature cystic change, however, which can make differentiation from a pineal cyst difficult.

Pineoblastoma

- Pineoblastoma is a highly malignant WHO grade IV tumor of young children, of the same primitive neuroectodermal tumor (PNET) type as medulloblastoma.
- The term trilateral retinoblastoma is used when bilateral retinoblastomas are also present (both the retina and pineal gland are light-sensing organs). The sella is additionally involved in quadrilateral retinoblastoma.
- Pineoblastoma often presents with obstructive hydrocephalus. Pineoblastoma characteristically appears as a poorly defined pineal mass that may invade into adjacent structures. High cellularity causes restricted diffusion.
- In contrast to germinoma, which "engulfs" and induces calcification of the pineal gland, pineoblastoma peripherally calcifies in a pattern that has been likened to "exploded" calcification.
- Pineoblastoma has a propensity for leptomeningeal metastasis and CSF seeding.

Metastases

- Due to the lack of a blood brain barrier, metastases to the pineal gland occur relatively commonly, but rarely in the absence of a known malignancy.
- Leptomeningeal disease is present in two-thirds of patients with pineal metastasis.

Pineal region mass (extra-pineal)

Gliomas

- Gliomas (most commonly astrocytomas) of varying grade may occur in adjacent intra-axial structures such as the tectum, midbrain, or splenium of the corpus callosum.

Vein of Galen aneurysm

- Despite the name, a vein of Galen "aneurysm" is not a true aneurysm. Instead, it represents dilation of the vein of Galen due to an arteriovenous fistula between the anterior or posterior circulation and the venous plexus leading to the vein of Galen.

Meningioma

- The tentorial apex, adjacent to the pineal gland, is a characteristic location for meningioma.
- As previously discussed, a tentorial meningioma tends to depress the internal cerebral veins, in contrast to a pineal-based mass, which typically elevates the internal cerebral veins.

Quadrigeminal plate lipoma

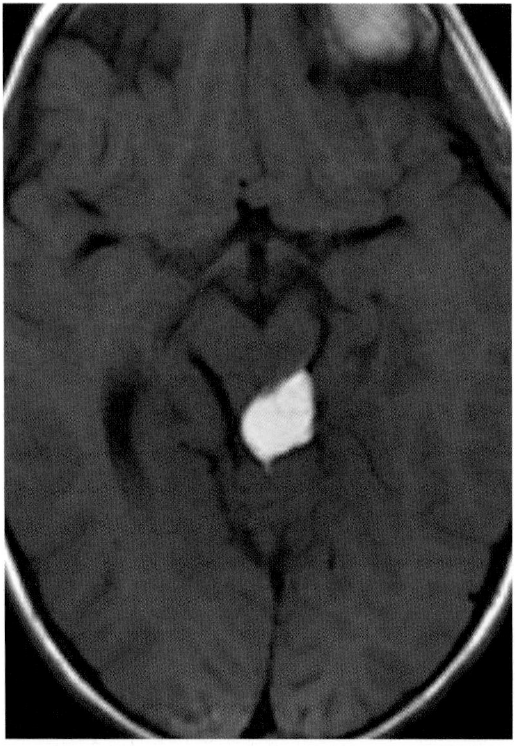
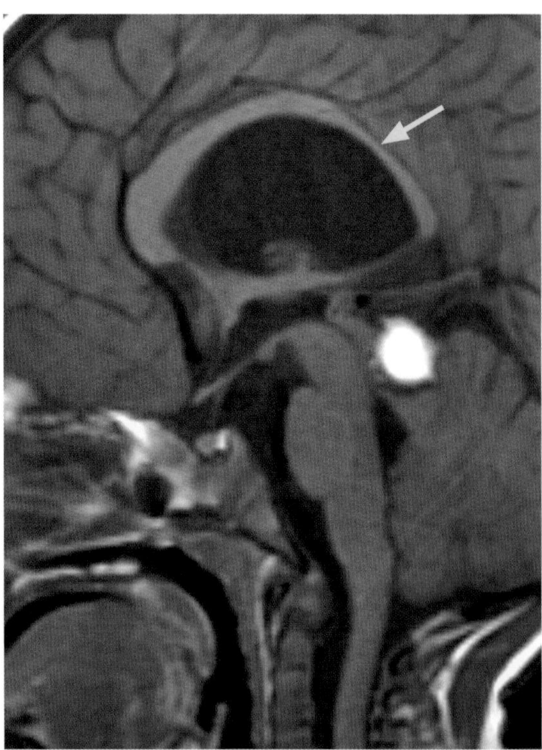

Quadrigeminal plate lipoma: Axial (left image) and sagittal (right image) T1-weighted MRI shows a lobulated, hyperintense mass of the quadrigeminal plate. Note the associated thinning of the posterior body (arrow) and splenium of the corpus callosum.

- A lipoma of the quadrigeminal plate is a rare lesion that be seen in isolation or associated with agenesis or hypoplasia of the corpus callosum.
- The quadrigeminal plate is another name for the tectum.

CEREBRAL TRAUMA

EXTRA-AXIAL HEMORRHAGE

- Acute extra-axial hemorrhage (subarachnoid, epidural, or subdural in location) is usually hyperattenuating when imaged by CT; however, blood must clot in order to be hyperattenuating. Hyperacute unclotted blood (and clotted blood in a patient with severe anemia) may be close to water attenuation on CT.

Subarachnoid hemorrhage (SAH)

- Trauma is the most common cause of subarachnoid hemorrhage (SAH), while aneurysm rupture is the most common cause of non-traumatic SAH.
- Traumatic SAH tends to occur contralateral to the side of direct impact, most often in the superficial cerebral sulci.

Epidural hematoma

- An arterial epidural hematoma is an extra-axial collection of blood external to the dura, classically caused by fracture of the squamous portion of the temporal bone and resultant tearing of the middle meningeal artery.
- An arterial epidural hematoma has a *lentiform* shape and does not cross the cranial sutures, where the dura is tightly adherent to the cranium.
- The *swirl* sign describes mixed high and low attenuation blood within the hematoma and suggests active bleeding. The low attenuation blood is hyperacute unclotted blood while the high attenuation blood is already clotted.
- A large epidural hematoma is a surgical emergency due to mass effect and risk of herniation, although small epidural hematomas can be conservatively managed with serial imaging.
- Venous epidural hematomas are far less common than arterial epidurals and are due to laceration of the dural sinuses, usually occurring in the posterior fossa in children.

Subdural hematoma

- A subdural hematoma is a crescentic extra-axial collection of blood located beneath the dura. Since it is underneath the dura, the hematoma can extend across the cranial sutures. Subdural hematomas often extend along the surfaces of the falx cerebri and tentorium cerebelli.
- Subdural hematomas typically result from tearing of cerebral veins. Patients with atrophic involutional changes are at increased risk of subdural hematoma with even minor trauma, as the cerebral veins stretch to traverse the enlarged CSF spaces.
- A particular danger is a subdural hematoma in a patient with a ventricular shunt because the shunted ventricular system does not function as a natural tamponade.

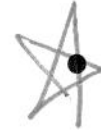

- An isodense subdural hematoma is isoattenuating to gray matter. This occurs in the subacute phase approximately 1–3 weeks after the initial injury. Three important clues alerting to the presence of an isodense subdural are increased mass effect, white matter buckling, and an apparently thickened cortex.

Intraventricular hemorrhage

- Intraventricular hemorrhage can occur due to tearing of subependymal veins or from direct extension of subarachnoid or intraparenchymal hematoma.
- Patients with intraventricular hemorrhage are at increased risk of developing noncommunicating hydrocephalus due to ependymal scarring, which may obstruct the cerebral aqueduct.

Coup/contrecoup mechanism

- The coup/contrecoup mechanism of brain trauma describes the propensity for brain to be injured both at the initial site of impact and 180° opposite the impact site, due to secondary impaction against the cranial vault.

Cortical contusion

- A cortical contusion is caused by traumatic contact of the cortical surface of the brain against the rough inner table of the skull. Contusions affect the gyral crests and can occur in a coup or a contrecoup location.
- A subacute cortical contusion may demonstrate ring enhancement and should be considered in the differential of a ring enhancing lesion if there is a history of trauma. Enhancement may continue into the chronic stage.
- A chronic contusion appears as encephalomalacia on CT. MRI is more specific, showing peripheral hemosiderin deposition as hypointense on T2-weighted images and blooming artifact on gradient echo sequences.

Intraparenchymal hematoma

- Traumatic intraparenchymal hematoma can occur in various locations, ranging from cortical contusion to basal ganglial hemorrhage (due to shearing of lenticulostriate vessels).
- Similar to a cortical contusion, a subacute intraparenchymal hematoma may show ring enhancement.

Diffuse axonal injury (DAI)/Traumatic axonal injury (TAI)

- Diffuse axonal injury (DAI) is the result of a shear-strain deformation of the brain.
- The term traumatic axonal injury (TAI) has recently been introduced as this injury pattern is thought to be multifocal rather than diffuse; however, this text will use the term DAI, as that is the more common term.
- DAI is caused by rotational deceleration and subsequent reacceleration force that exceeds the limited elastic capacity of the axons.

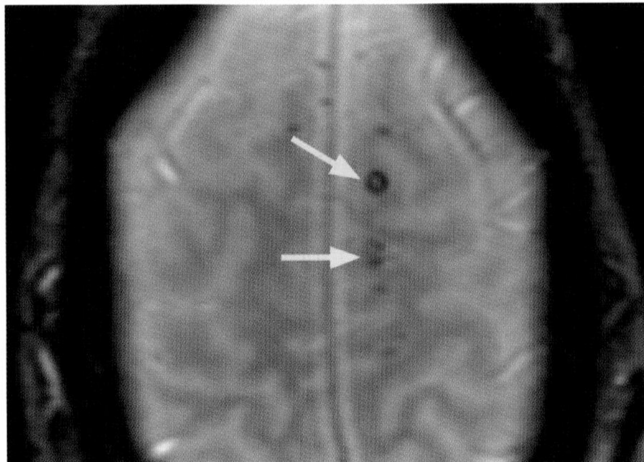

Diffuse axonal injury: Axial GRE image shows several foci of susceptibility effect along the left high convexity representing punctate hemorrhagic foci of DAI (arrows).

- The most common locations of DAI include the gray–white matter junction, the corpus callosum, and the dorsolateral midbrain. The higher the grade, the worse the prognosis.

> Grade I DAI involves only the gray–white matter junctions.
>
> Grade II DAI involves the corpus callosum.
>
> Grade III (most severe) DAI involves the dorsolateral midbrain.

- CT is relatively insensitive for detection of DAI, although hemorrhagic DAI may show tiny foci of high attenuation in the affected regions.
- MRI is much more sensitive to detect DAI, although detection relies on multiple sequences, including FLAIR, GRE, and DWI.

  GRE is extremely sensitive for hemorrhagic axonal injury; however, not all DAI is hemorrhagic.

  FLAIR is most sensitive for nonhemorrhagic DAI.

  Diffusion sequences show restricted diffusion in acute DAI due to cytotoxic edema and cell swelling.

Facial fractures

Zygomaticomaxillary complex fractures

- Commonly but incorrectly know as the *tripod* fracture, a zygomaticomaxillary complex (ZMC) fracture causes a floating zygoma by disrupting all four of the zygomatic articulations.
- The zygoma normally articulates with the frontal, maxillary, temporal, and sphenoid bones via the zygomaticofrontal, zygomaticomaxillary, zygomaticotemporal, and zygomaticosphenoid articulations.
- A ZMC fracture causes disruption of the zygomatic articulations by fractures through the following structures:

> **Lateral orbital rim** fracture: Zygomaticofrontal disruption.
>
> **Inferior orbital rim** fracture: Zygomaticomaxillary disruption.
>
> **Zygomatic arch fracture**: Zygomaticotemporal disruption.
>
> **Lateral orbital wall**: Zygomaticosphenoid disruption.

Le Fort fractures

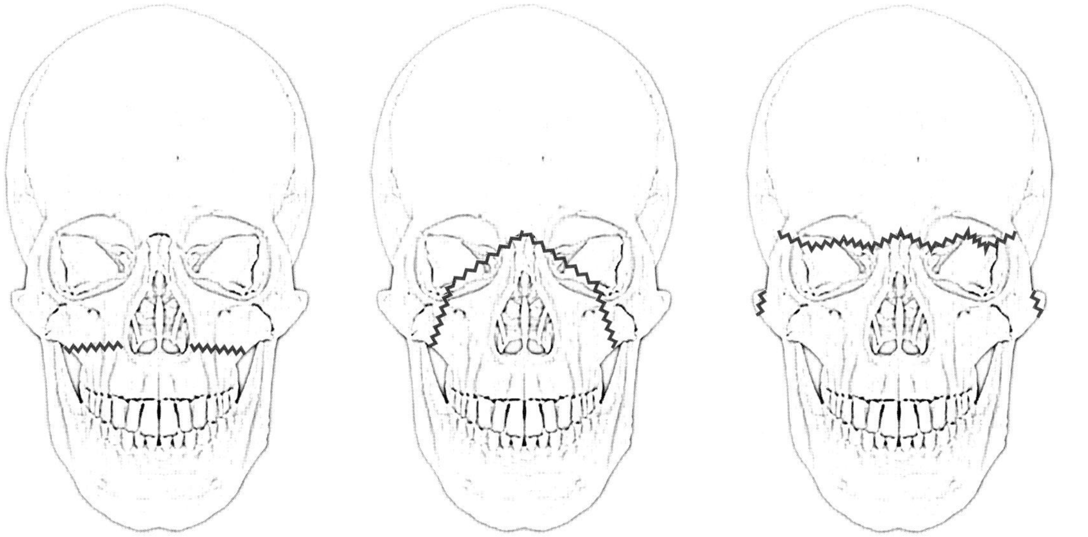

Le Fort I	*Le Fort II*	*Le Fort III*
Horizontal fracture through all walls of the maxillary sinus.	Pyramidal fracture, sparing the medial wall of the maxillary sinus.	Complete midface dissociation, with fractures through the zygomatic arch.
Allows free movement of the hard palate.	Allows free movement of the nose and hard palate (as a single unit).	Allows free movement of the entire midface.

- The Le Fort classification describes a predictable pattern of midface fractures, all of which disrupt the pterygomaxillary buttress and cause detachment of the maxilla from the skull base. All Le Fort fractures are defined by fractures through the pterygoid plates.
- Le Fort I (floating palate) detaches the maxillary alveolus from the skull base.
- Le Fort II dissociates the central midface from the skull, causing the nose and hard palate to be moved as a single unit.
- Le Fort III represents a complete midface dissociation.

Central sulcus

Find the central sulcus:

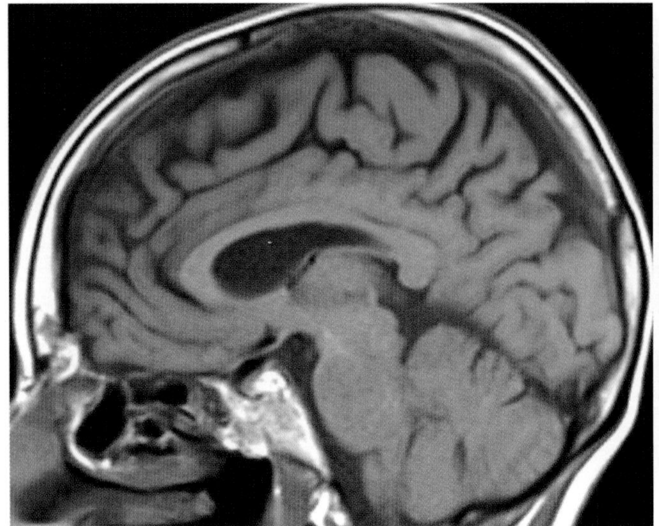

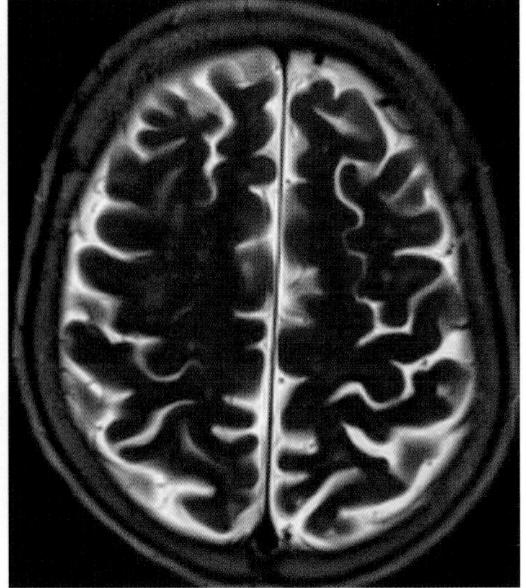

Same images, with labels:

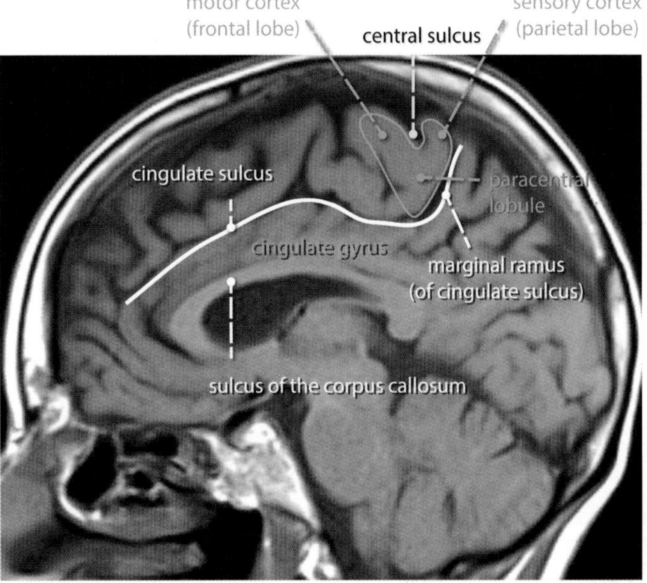

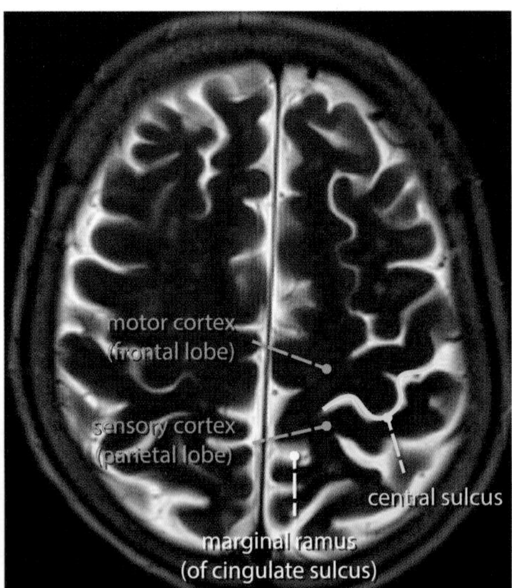

- The central sulcus separates the motor strip (frontal lobe) from the sensory cortex (parietal lobe).
- To find the central sulcus, follow the cingulate sulcus posteriorly on a slightly off-midline sagittal (left images above). The cingulate sulcus connects to the marginal ramus. Directly anterior to the marginal ramus is the paracentral lobule, which contains both the motor strip and the sensory cortex.
- On an axial image (right images above), the central sulcus forms a characteristic upside down *omega* (*Ω*). The corresponding region of motor strip, just anterior to the Ω, controls the hand.

INTERNAL CAROTID ARTERY (ICA)

Segments of the internal carotid artery

- **Cervical** (C1): Does not branch within the neck.
- **Petrous** (C2): Fixed to bone as the ICA enters the skull base, so a cervical carotid dissection is unlikely to extend intracranially.
- **Lacerum** (C3): No branches.
- **Cavernous** (C4): The **meningohypophyseal trunk** arises from the cavernous carotid to supply the pituitary, tentorium, and dura of the clivus. The **inferolateral trunk** also arises from C4 to supply the 3rd, 4th, and 6th cranial nerves, as well as the trigeminal ganglion.
- **Clinoid segment** (C5): The carotid rings are two dural rings that mark the proximal and distal portions of the clinoid segment of the ICA. The carotid rings prevent an inferiorly located aneurysm from causing intracranial subarachnoid hemorrhage with rupture.
- **Supraclinoid** (C6–C7): Gives off several key arteries:

  The **ophthalmic artery** supplies the optic nerve. It takes off just distal to the distal carotid ring in 90% of cases and can be used as a landmark for the distal ring. Aneurysms located superior to this ring can result in subarachnoid hemorrhage. Given this risk, these aneurysms are treated more aggressively than aneurysms located proximal to the distal dural ring, which are contained.

  The **posterior communicating artery** (P-comm) is an anastomosis to the posterior circulation. A fetal posterior cerebral artery (PCA) is a variant supplied entirely by the ipsilateral ICA via an enlarged P-comm.

  The **anterior choroidal artery** supplies several critical structures, despite its small size. It supplies the optic chiasm, hippocampus, and posterior limb of the internal capsule.

CIRCLE OF WILLIS

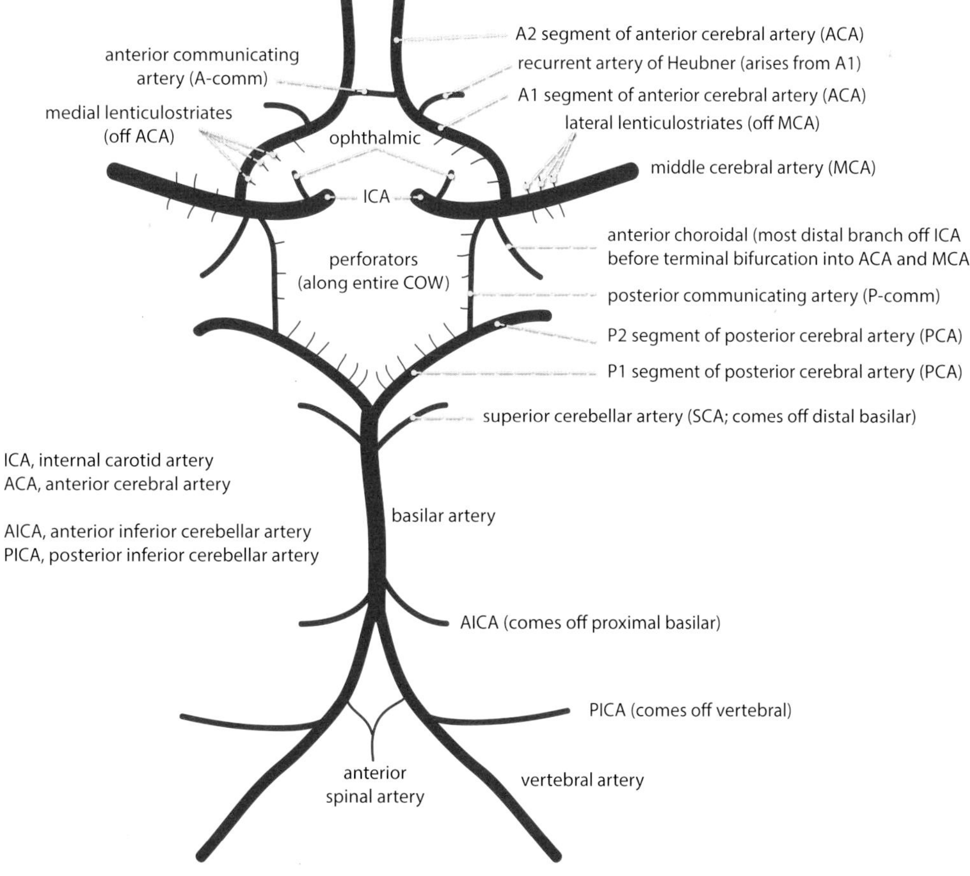

Critical small arteries arising from the circle of Willis

- The A1 segment of the anterior cerebral artery (ACA) travels above the optic nerves and give off the **recurrent artery of Heubner**, which supplies the caudate head and anterior limb of the internal capsule. The A1 segment also gives rise to the medial lenticulostriate perforator vessels, which supply the medial basal ganglia.
- Just outside the circle of Willis, the middle cerebral artery (MCA) gives rise to the lateral lenticulostriate perforator vessels to supply the lateral basal ganglia including the lateral putamen, external capsule, and the posterior limb of the internal capsule.
- The posterior communicating artery (P-comm) travels between the optic tract and the 3rd cranial nerve, giving off anterior thalamoperforator vessels. A P-comm aneurysm may cause cranial nerve III palsy due to local mass effect.
- The posterior cerebral artery (PCA) gives off thalamoperforators to supply the thalamus. **Artery of Percheron** is a variant where there is a dominant thalamic perforator supplying the ventromedial thalami bilaterally and the rostral midbrain, arising from a P1 PCA segment. An artery of Percheron infarct will result in bilateral ventromedial thalamic infarction, with or without midbrain infarction (the infarct may be V shaped if the midbrain is involved). Deep venous thrombosis may also result in bilateral thalamic infarcts.
- The anterior choroidal artery is the most distal branch of the internal carotid artery. As discussed on the previous page, it supplies the optic chiasm, hippocampus, and posterior limb of the internal capsule.

Circle of Willis normal anatomic variants

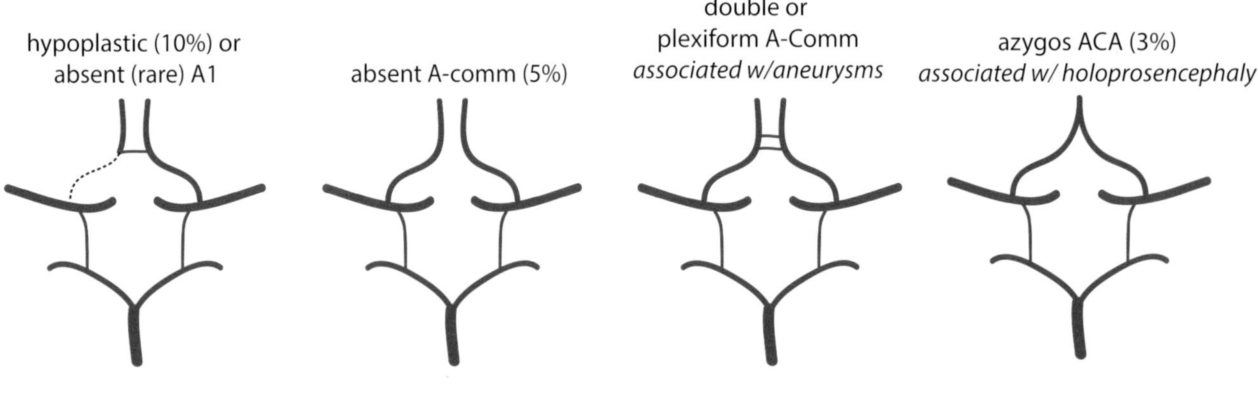

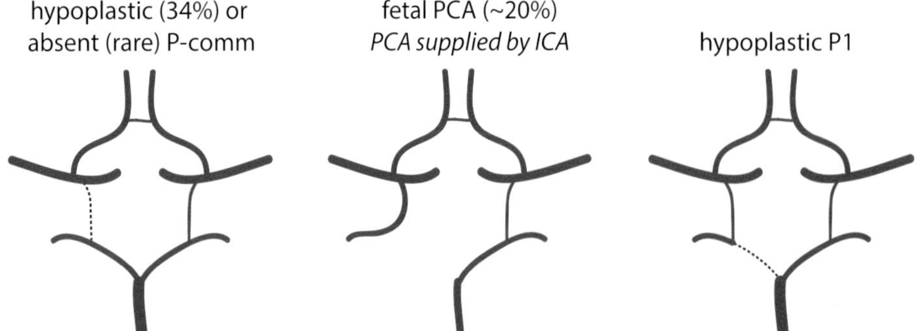

- Normal circle of Willis anatomy is only seen approximately 25% of the time.

Segmental anatomy of the middle cerebral artery

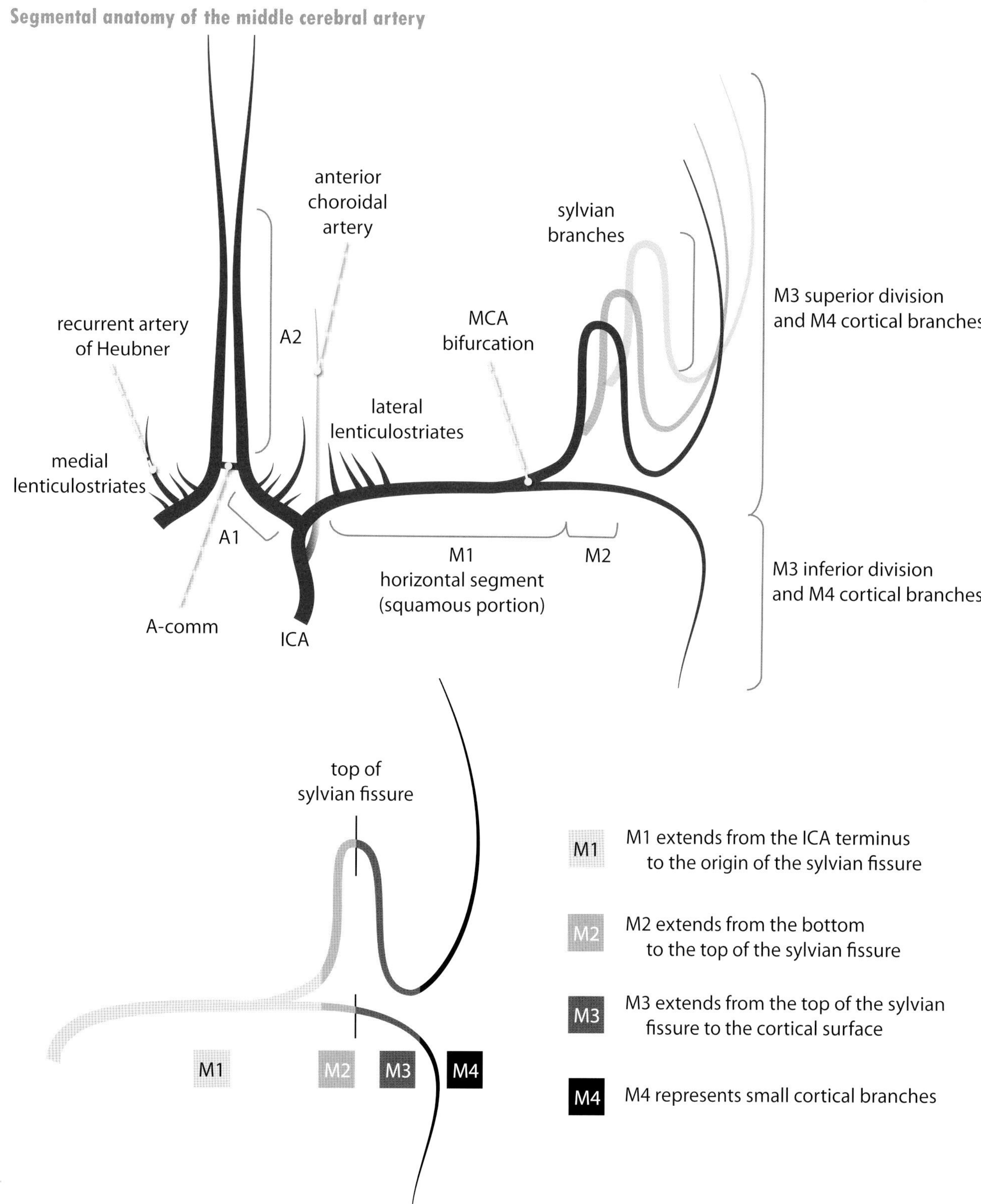

- Although the transition from M1 to M2 is technically defined as the upward point of deflection into the sylvian fissure, in practical terms, the pre-bifurcation MCA is often called M1 and the post-bifurcation MCA is called M2.

Anterior cerebral artery (ACA)

Segmental anatomy of the anterior cerebral artery

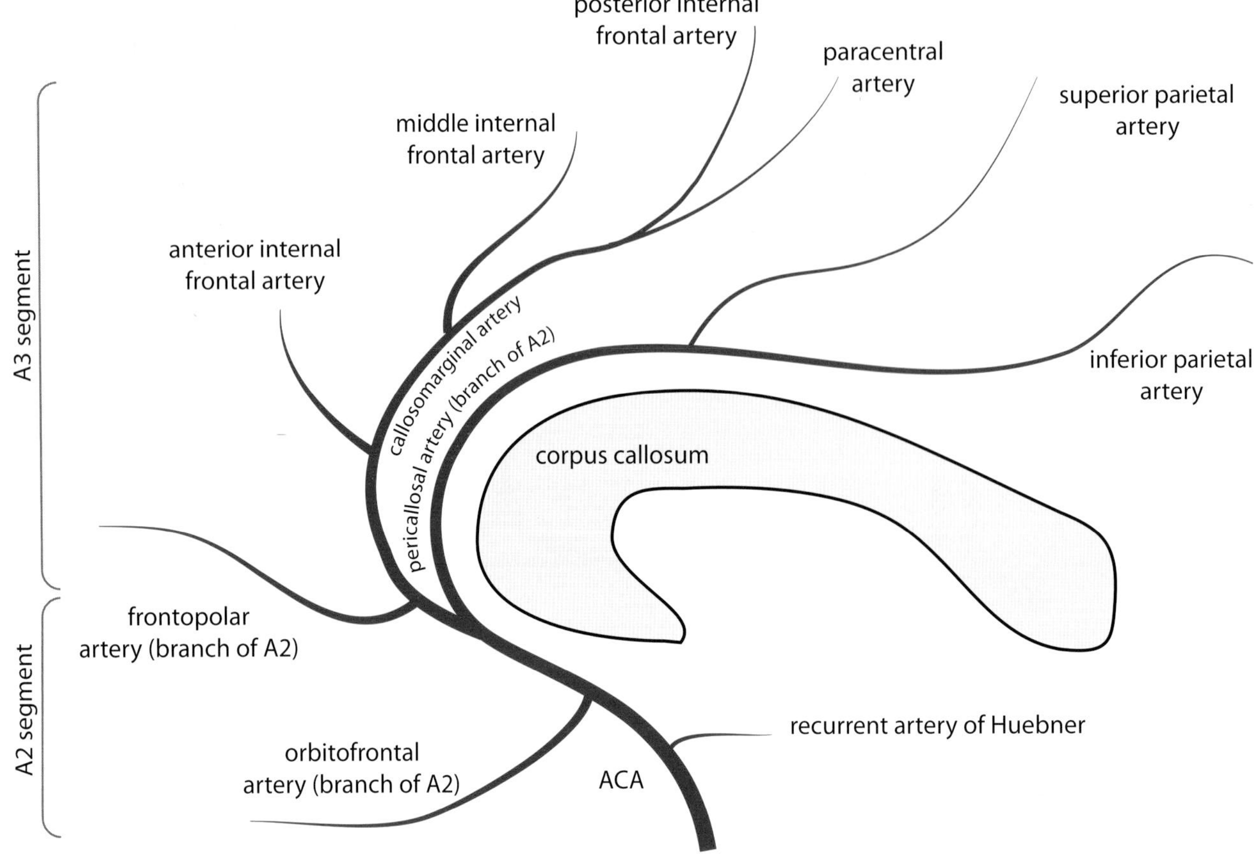

- The recurrent artery of Heubner arises most commonly from the A1 segment of the ACA, proximal to the anterior communicating artery. The recurrent artery of Heubner supplies the head of the caudate and the anterior limb of the internal capsule.

Persistent carotid–basilar connections

Overview of persistent fetal anterior–posterior connections

- A number of carotid to basilar connections are formed during embryogenesis. These fetal anterior–posterior circulation connections normally regress before birth.
- Occasionally, a fetal carotid–basilar connection may persist after birth. Each anomalous connection is named for the structures adjacent to its course in the head and neck.

Persistent trigeminal artery

- A persistent trigeminal artery is the most common persistent carotid–basilar connection and has an association with aneurysms.
- The persistent trigeminal artery courses adjacent to the trigeminal nerve. Angiography shows a characteristic *trident* or *tau* sign on the lateral view due to the artery's branching structure.
- Saltzman type I connects to the basilar artery while Saltzman type II connects to the superior cerebellar artery.

Less common carotid to basilar connections

- The otic, hypoglossal, and proatlantal intersegmental arteries are rare persistent carotid–basilar connections.

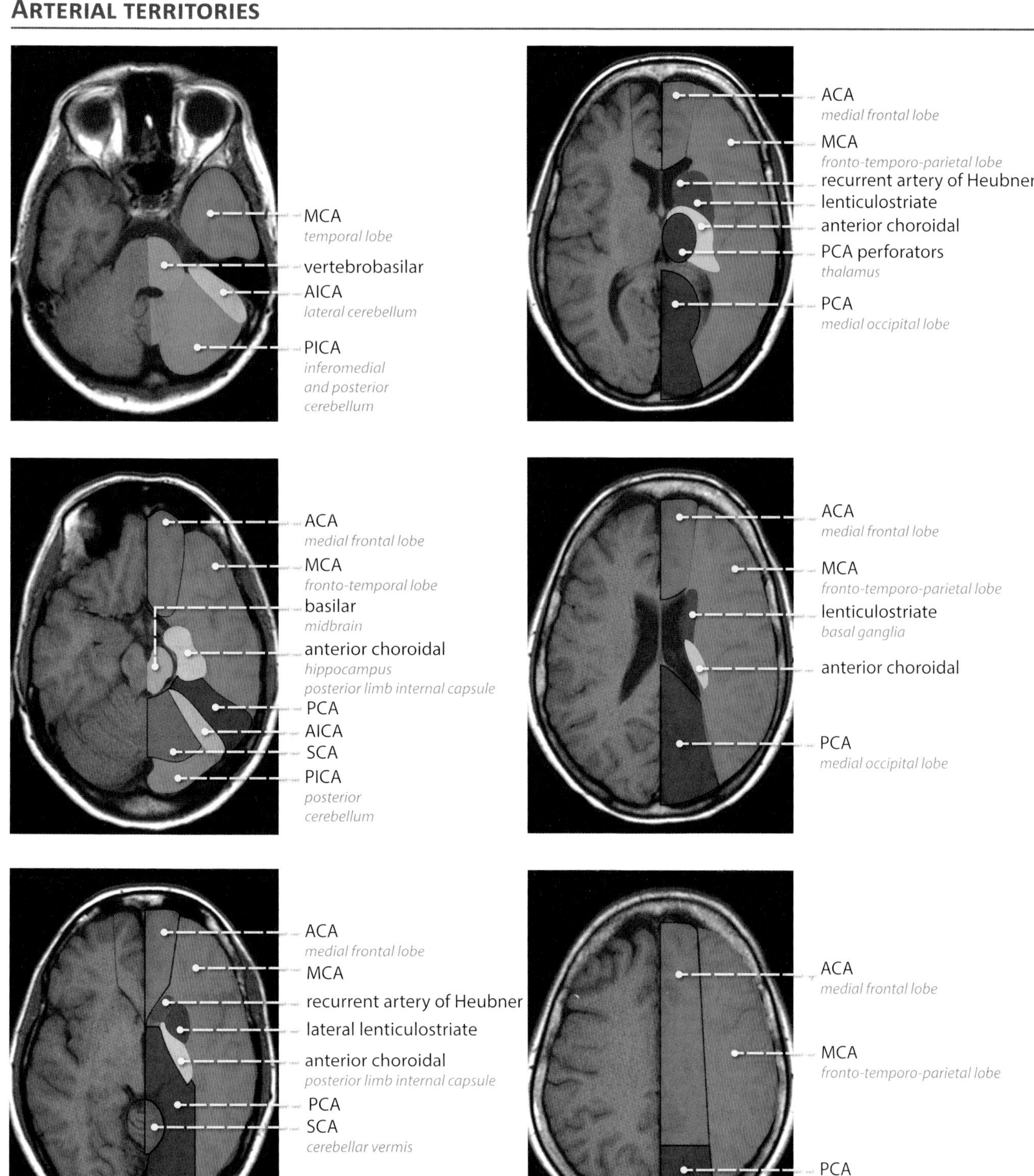
MCA
temporal lobe
vertebrobasilar
AICA
lateral cerebellum
PICA
inferomedial
and posterior
cerebellum
ACA
medial frontal lobe
MCA
fronto-temporo-parietal lobe
recurrent artery of Heubner
lenticulostriate
anterior choroidal
PCA perforators
thalamus
PCA
medial occipital lobe
ACA
medial frontal lobe
MCA
fronto-temporal lobe
basilar
midbrain
anterior choroidal
hippocampus
posterior limb internal capsule
PCA
AICA
SCA
PICA
posterior
cerebellum
ACA
medial frontal lobe
MCA
fronto-temporo-parietal lobe
lenticulostriate
basal ganglia
anterior choroidal
PCA
medial occipital lobe
ACA
medial frontal lobe
MCA
recurrent artery of Heubner
lateral lenticulostriate
anterior choroidal
posterior limb internal capsule
PCA
SCA
cerebellar vermis
ACA
medial frontal lobe
MCA
fronto-temporo-parietal lobe
PCA
medial occipital lobe

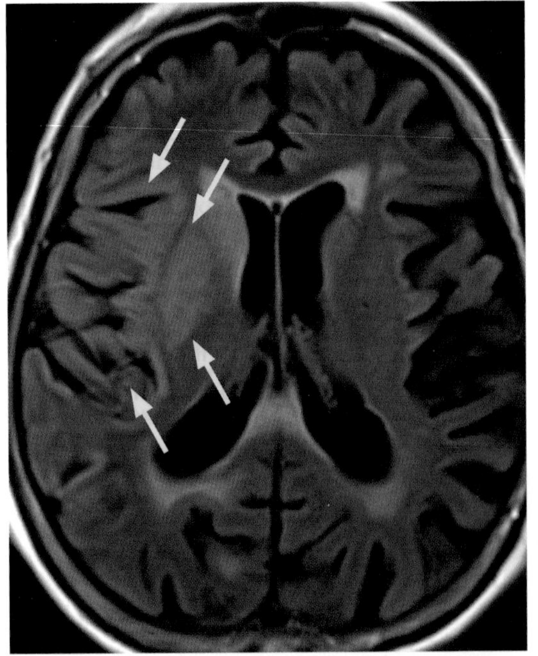

Axial FLAIR MRI shows geographic T2 prolongation in the right MCA territory (arrows) involving the right frontal and temporal lobes and right basal ganglia. The size of the T2 signal abnormality is less extensive than the infarct size apparent on DWI.

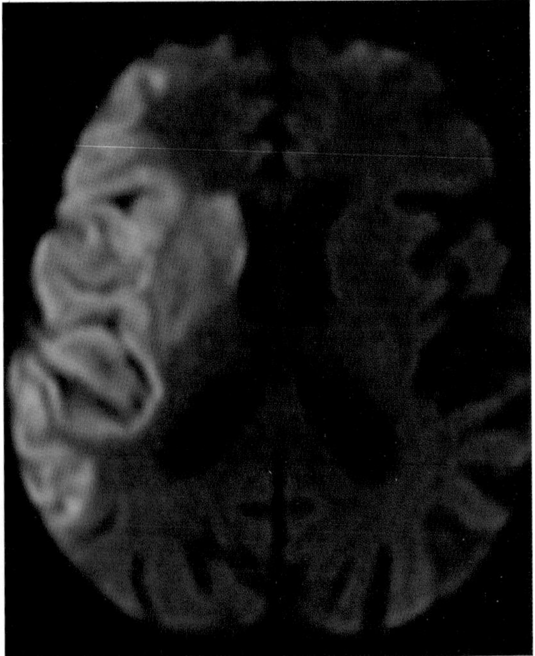

DWI shows a large region of hyperintensity in the right MCA territory involving the right frontal operculum, the right insula, the right temporal operculum, the right putamen, and the right caudate. ADC map (not shown) was dark, consistent with reduced diffusivity.

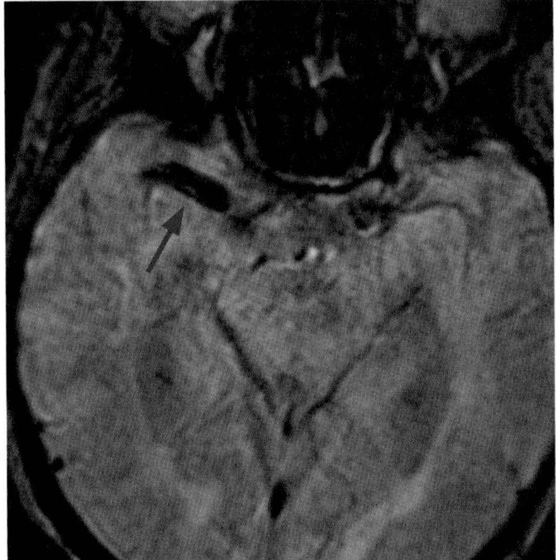

Gradient recall echo axial image shows blooming artifact (red arrow) in the right proximal MCA, which represents intraluminal thrombus and is the MRI correlate to the hyperdense artery sign that can be seen on CT.

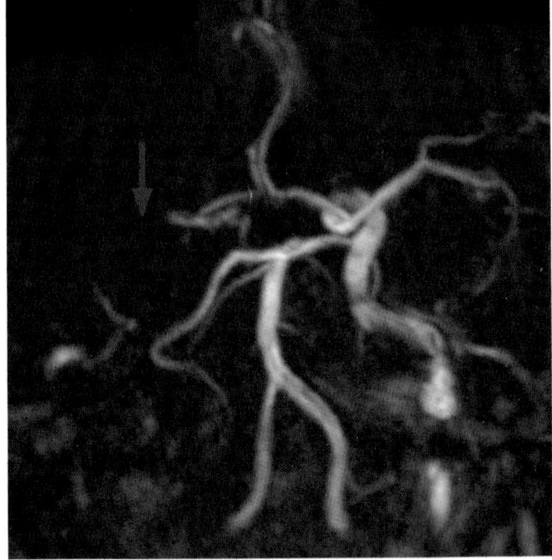

Axial oblique MIP from a time of flight MRI angiogram shows complete occlusion of the right MCA (red arrow). There is marked venous contamination on the left.

Case courtesy Gregory Wrubel, MD, Brigham and Women's Hospital, Boston

- Detailed MRI imaging of the multiple temporal stages of stroke is discussed on the following pages. For the initial evaluation, diffusion sequences can detect acute infarction with high sensitivity within minutes of symptom onset. DWI is more sensitive than FLAIR in the detection of hyperacute stroke.

EVOLUTION OF INFARCTION

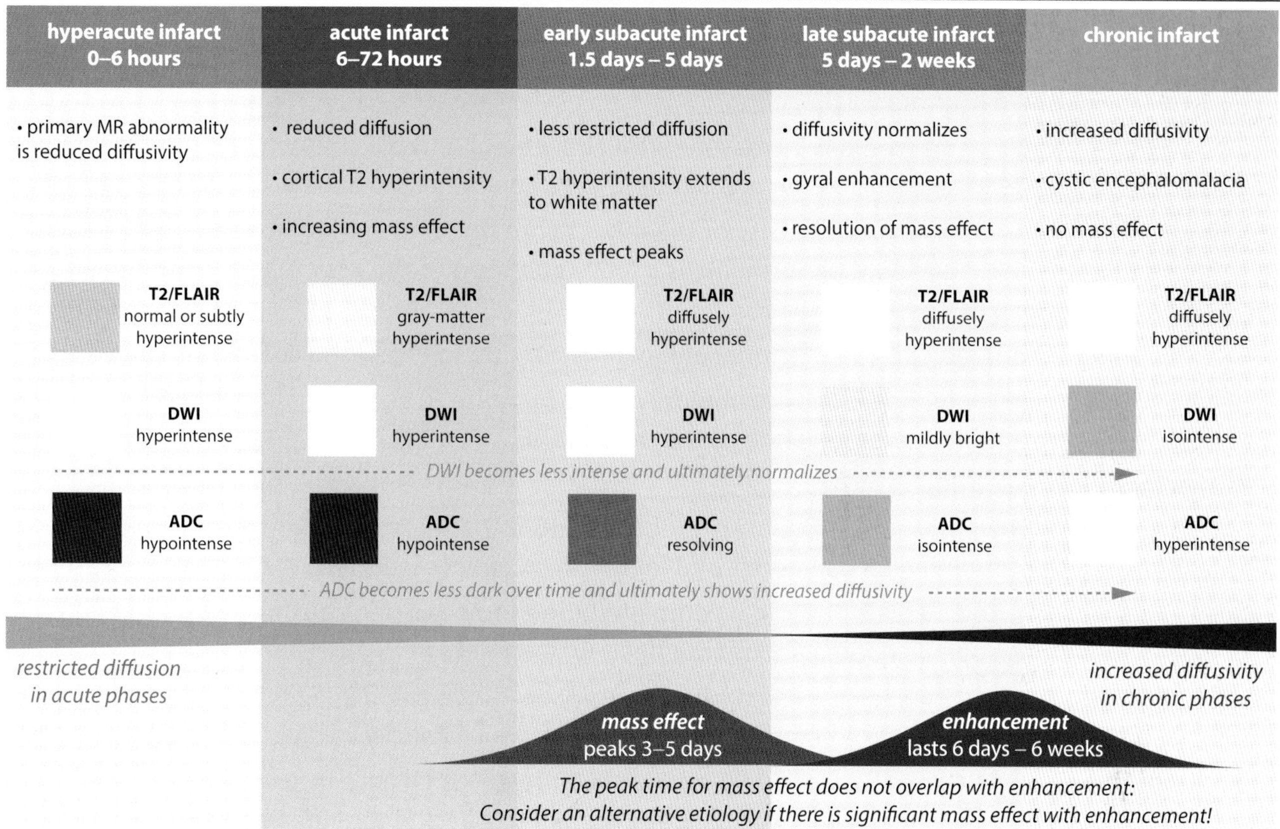

hyperacute infarct
0–6 hours
acute infarct
6–72 hours
early subacute infarct
1.5 days – 5 days
late subacute infarct
5 days – 2 weeks
chronic infarct
• primary MR abnormality is reduced diffusivity
• reduced diffusion
• cortical T2 hyperintensity
• increasing mass effect
• less restricted diffusion
• T2 hyperintensity extends to white matter
• mass effect peaks
• diffusivity normalizes
• gyral enhancement
• resolution of mass effect
• increased diffusivity
• cystic encephalomalacia
• no mass effect
T2/FLAIR normal or subtly hyperintense
T2/FLAIR gray-matter hyperintense
T2/FLAIR diffusely hyperintense
T2/FLAIR diffusely hyperintense
T2/FLAIR diffusely hyperintense
DWI hyperintense
DWI hyperintense
DWI hyperintense
DWI mildly bright
DWI isointense
DWI becomes less intense and ultimately normalizes
ADC hypointense
ADC hypointense
ADC resolving
ADC isointense
ADC hyperintense
ADC becomes less dark over time and ultimately shows increased diffusivity
restricted diffusion in acute phases
increased diffusivity in chronic phases
mass effect
peaks 3–5 days
enhancement
lasts 6 days – 6 weeks
The peak time for mass effect does not overlap with enhancement:
Consider an alternative etiology if there is significant mass effect with enhancement!

Hyperacute infarct (0–6 hours)

- Within minutes of critical ischemia, the sodium–potassium ATPase pump that maintains the normal low intracellular sodium concentration fails. Sodium and water diffuse into cells, leading to cell swelling and **cytotoxic** edema.
- Calcium also diffuses into cells, which triggers cascades that contribute to cell lysis.
- By far the most sensitive imaging modality for detection of hyperacute infarct is MRI diffusion-weighted imaging (DWI). DWI hyperintensity and ADC map hypointensity reflect reduced diffusivity, which can be seen within minutes of the ictus.
- Diffusion is reduced in an acute infarct by two factors:
  1) Shift from extracellular to intracellular water due to Na/K ATPase pump failure.
  2) Increased viscosity of infarcted brain due to cell lysis and increased extracellular protein.
- FLAIR may be normal. Subtle hyperintensity may be seen on FLAIR images in the hyperacute stage. These changes are seen less than two thirds of the time within the first six hours.
- Perfusion shows decreased cerebral blood volume of the infarct core, with or without a surrounding region of decreased cerebral blood flow, which represents the penumbra.

Acute infarct (6 hours–72 hours)

- The acute infarct phase is characterized by increase in vasogenic edema and mass effect.
- Damaged vascular endothelial cells cause leakage of extracellular fluid and increase the risk of hemorrhage.
- On imaging, there is increased sulcal effacement and mass effect. The mass effect peaks at 3–4 days, which is an overlap time between the acute and early subacute phases.
- MRI shows hyperintensity of the infarct core on T2-weighted images, best seen on FLAIR. The FLAIR abnormality is usually confined to the gray matter. DWI continues to show restricted diffusion.
- There may be some arterial enhancement, due to increased collateral flow.
- Perfusion images most commonly show increase in size of the infarct core with resultant decrease in size of the penumbra.

Early subacute infarct (1.5 days–5 days)

- In the early subacute phase, blood flow to the affected brain is re-established by leptomeningeal collaterals and ingrowth of new vessels into the region of infarction.
- The new vessels have an incomplete blood brain barrier, causing a continued increase in vasogenic edema and mass effect, which peaks at 3–4 days.
- MR imaging shows marked hyperintensity on T2-weighted images involving both gray and white matter (in contrast to the acute stage, which usually involves just the gray matter).
- The ADC map becomes less dark or even resolves if there is extensive edema; however, the DWI images typically remain bright due to underlying T2 shine through.
- Perfusion imaging shows continued expansion of the infarct core and further reduction in the ischemic penumbra.

Late subacute infarct (5 days–2 weeks)

- The subacute phase is characterized by resolution of vasogenic edema and reduction in mass effect.
- A key imaging finding is gyriform enhancement, which may occasionally be confused for a neoplasm. Unlike a tumor, however, a subacute infarction will not typically demonstrate both mass effect and enhancement simultaneously. Enhancement can be seen from approximately 6 days to 6 weeks after the initial infarct.

  The enhancement of a subacute infarct has also been described by the "2-2-2" rule, which states that enhancement begins at 2 days, peaks at 2 weeks, and disappears by 2 months.
- DWI may remain bright due to T2 shine through, although the ADC map will either return to normal or show increased diffusivity.

Chronic infarct

- In the chronic stage of infarction, cellular debris and dead brain tissue are removed by macrophages and replaced by cystic encephalomalacia and gliosis.
- Infarct involvement of the corticospinal tract may cause mass effect, mild hyperintensity on T2-weighted images, and eventual atrophy of the ipsilateral cerebral peduncle and ventral pons due to Wallerian degeneration. These changes can first be seen in the subacute phase, with atrophy being the predominant feature in the chronic stage.
- DWI has usually returned to normal in the chronic stage.
- Occasionally, cortical laminar necrosis can develop instead of encephalomalacia. Cortical laminar necrosis is a histologic finding characterized by deposition of lipid-laden macrophages after ischemia that manifests on imaging as hyperintensity on both T1- and T2-weighted images.

VASCULAR MALFORMATIONS

HIGH-FLOW LESIONS (LESIONS WITH SHUNTING)

Arteriovenous malformation (AVM)

- An arteriovenous malformation (AVM) is a congenital high-flow vascular malformation consisting of directly connecting arteries and veins without an intervening capillary bed. AVM occurs intra-axially and 85% are supratentorial. AVM usually presents with seizures or bleeding (usually parenchymal hemorrhage, rarely subarachnoid). Aneurysms of the feeding arteries or intra-nidal arteries are often seen, which predispose to bleeding.
- The **Spetzler–Martin** scale helps to evaluate surgical risk for AVM resection. A large AVM draining to a deep vein in eloquent cortex is high risk, while a small AVM draining to a superficial vein in non eloquent cortex is low risk.
- On imaging, AVM is characterized by a vascular nidus ("nest") containing numerous serpentine vessels that appear as black flow-voids on MRI. There are usually adjacent changes to the adjacent brain including gliosis (T2 prolongation), dystrophic calcification, and blood products (blooming on T2* gradient imaging). The gliosis/encephalomalacia or mineralization seen in the adjacent brain is due to alteration in vascular flow from the AVM.
- AVM replaces rather than displaces brain. It causes minimal mass effect.
- Uncommonly, a bleeding AVM may be angiographically occult if the malformed vessels are compressed by the acute hematoma.
- Factors that increase bleeding risk that are detectable by imaging include intra-nidal aneurysm, venous ectasia, venous stenosis, deep venous drainage, and posterior fossa location.
- Treatment can be with embolization, stereotactic radiation, or surgical resection.
- **Vein of Galen malformation** is a type of vascular malformation characterized by arteriovenous fistulae from thalamoperforator branches into the deep venous system. The enlarged vein is actually an enlarged median prosencephalic vein.

  In childhood, a vein of Galen malformation is the most common extracardiac cause of high output cardiac failure. Vein of Galen malformation may also be seen in adults, but clinically would be either asymptomatic or may be the cause of Parinaud syndrome due to mass effect in the pineal region.

Dural arteriovenous fistula (dAVF)

- Dural arteriovenous fistulas are a complex group of high-flow lesions characterized by arteriovenous shunts between the meningeal arterioles and dural venules.
- The primary prognostic feature is the presence and degree of *cortical venous drainage*. The **Cognard classification** I through IV describes lesions with progressively increased risk of bleeding. Type V is reserved for spinal dAVFs.

Type I: No cortical venous drainage. Lowest risk of bleeding.	**Type III**: Direct cortical venous drainage: 40% hemorrhage rate.
Type IIA: Reflux into dural sinus but not cortical veins.	**Type IV**: Direct cortical venous drainage with venous ectasia: 66% hemorrhage rate.
Type IIB: Reflux into cortical veins: 10–20% hemorrhage rate.	**Type V**: Spinal venous drainage. May cause myelopathy.

- Carotid–cavernous fistula (CCF) is a subtype of dAVF that is often caused by trauma with resultant fistula between the cavernous carotid artery and the cavernous sinus. Enlargement of the superior orbital vein and shunting within the cavernous sinus can lead to eye symptoms, such as proptosis and cranial nerve palsy.

Cavernous malformation (cavernoma)

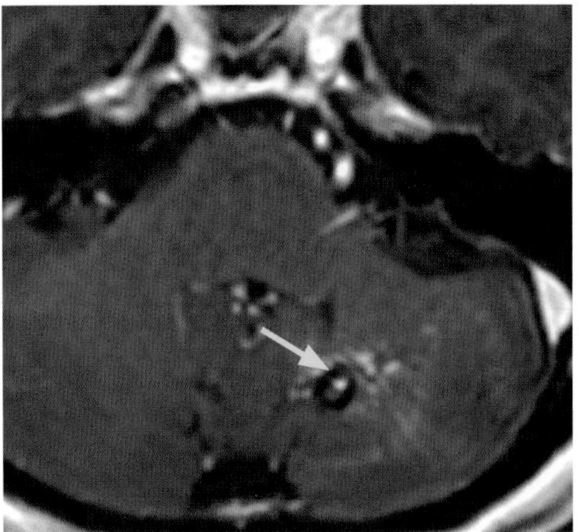

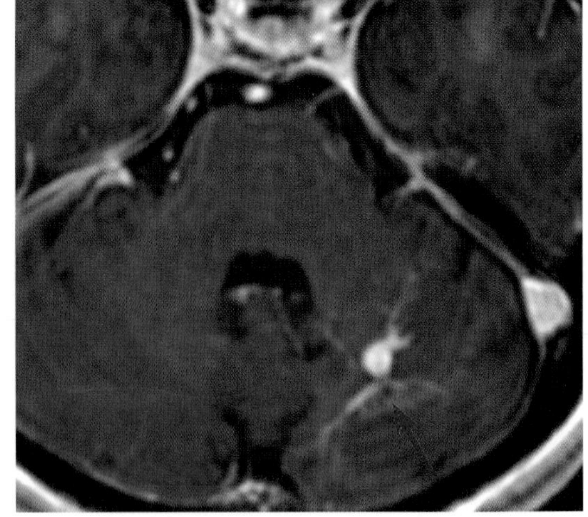

Cavernous malformation and associated DVA: Two axial contrast-enhanced T1-weighted images show a hypointense, centrally hyperintense nonenhancing cavernous malformation (yellow arrow) in the left cerebellar hemisphere. Directly superior to the cavernoma (right image) is an enhancing vascular structure with *caput medusa* morphology (red arrow), representing a developmental venous anomaly.

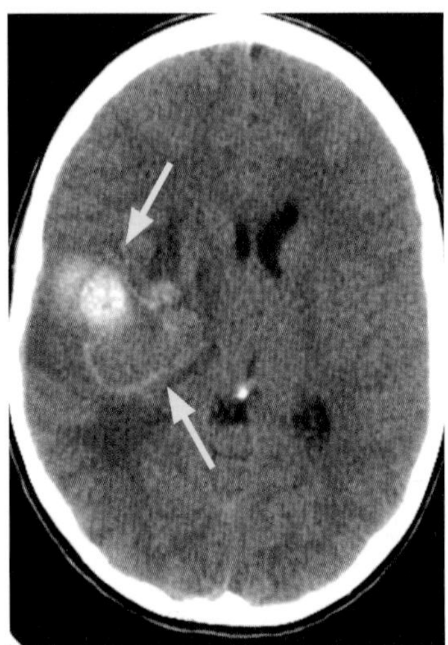

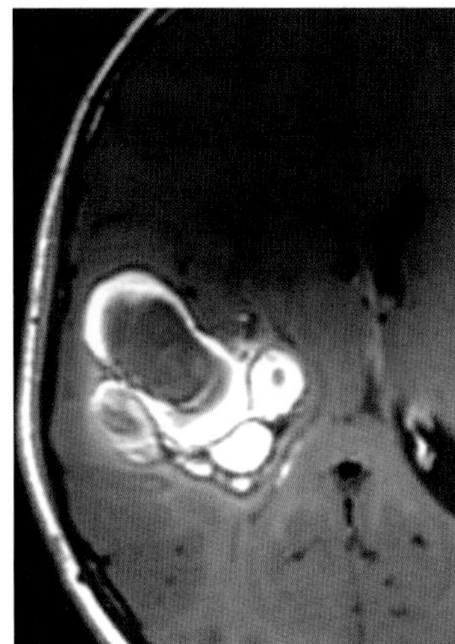

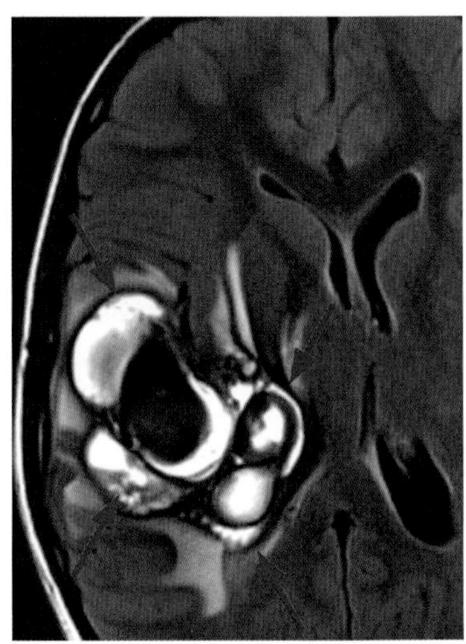

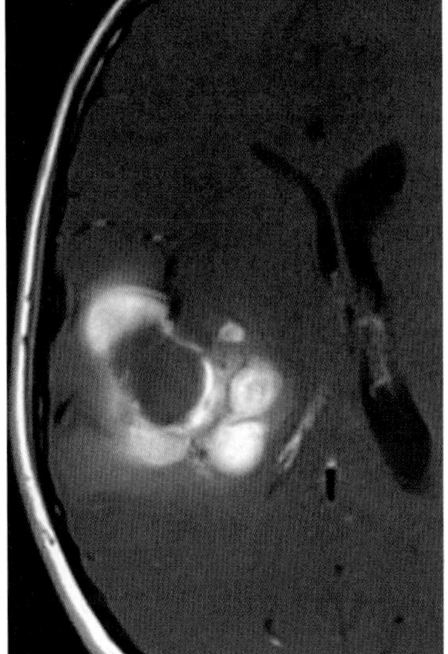

Giant cavernous malformation in a different patient:

Axial unenhanced CT (top left image) shows a hyperattenuating complex mass (arrows) in the right fronto-temporal lobe.

Unenhanced T1-weighted image (top middle image) shows the mass is predominantly cystic and hyperintense (representing blood products).

Axial FLAIR (top right image) shows that the intracystic contents are primarily hyperintense. There is a complete low signal hemosiderin ring surrounding the lesion (red arrows). There is mild surrounding edema.

Post contrast axial T1-weighted image (left image) shows no appreciable enhancement.

Case courtesy Gregory Wrubel, MD, Brigham and Women's Hospital.

- A cavernous malformation (also called a cavernoma) is a vascular hamartoma with a very small but definite bleeding risk. The clinical course of a cavernous malformation is variable and the lesion may cause seizures even in the absence of significant hemorrhage.
- Cavernous malformation is often associated with an adjacent developmental venous anomaly (DVA). There is increased risk of bleeding if a DVA is present. However, the DVA itself does not have any bleeding risk.
- When multiple, cavernous malformations represent an inherited disorder called familial cavernomatosis.
- Cavernous malformations can be induced by radiation treatment to the brain.
- Noncontrast CT shows a well-circumscribed rounded hyperattenuating lesion. The hyperattenuation is due to microcalcification within the cavernoma.
- MRI shows characteristic "popcorn-like" appearance of lobular mixed signal on T1- and T2-weighted images from blood products of various ages. There is a peripheral rim of hemosiderin which is dark on GRE and T2-weighted image. There is typically no enhancement, but intense enhancement may be seen with a long delay after contrast administration. Cavernous malformations may range in size from tiny (single focus of susceptibility artifact) to giant.
- Cavernous malformations are usually occult by vascular imaging (CTA or angiography).

Developmental venous anomaly (DVA), also called venous angioma

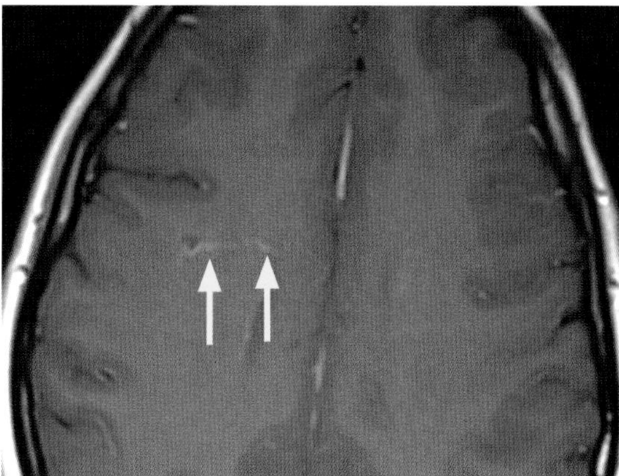

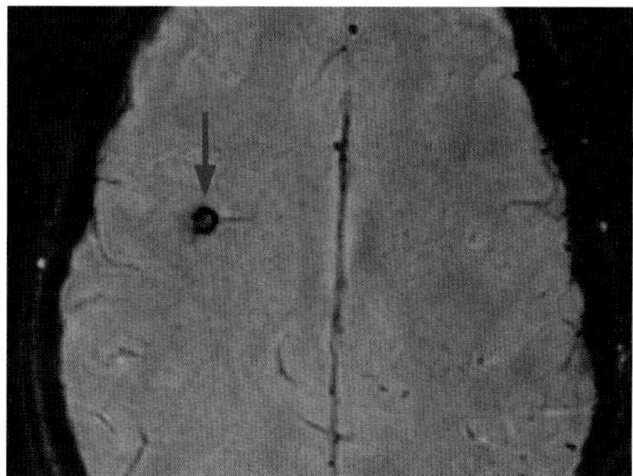

Developmental venous anomaly and a tiny cavernous malformation: Post-contrast axial T1-weighted MRI (left image) shows a subtle curvilinear enhancing structure (yellow arrow) in the right frontal white matter representing a DVA. Susceptibility weighted image (right image) shows a focus of susceptibility artifact (red arrow), suggestive of an adjacent cavernous malformation.

Case courtesy Sanjay Prabhu, MD, Boston Children's Hospital.

- A developmental venous anomaly (DVA) is an abnormal vein that provides functional venous drainage to normal brain.
- DVA can usually only be seen on contrast-enhanced images, where it appears as a radially oriented vein with a characteristic *caput medusa* appearance.
- A DVA is a Do Not Touch lesion. If resected, the patient will suffer a debilitating venous infarct. The DVA must be preserved if an adjacent cavernous malformation is resected.

Capillary telangiectasia

- A capillary telangiectasia is an asymptomatic vascular lesion composed of dilated capillaries with interspersed normal brain. A capillary telangiectasia is another Do Not Touch lesion.
- Post-contrast MRI shows a faint, brush-stroke-like enhancing lesion in the brainstem or pons, without mass effect or surrounding edema. GRE may show blooming due to susceptibility.
- Similar to cavernous malformation, capillary telangiectasia is angiographically occult.

SUBARACHNOID HEMORRHAGE (SAH)

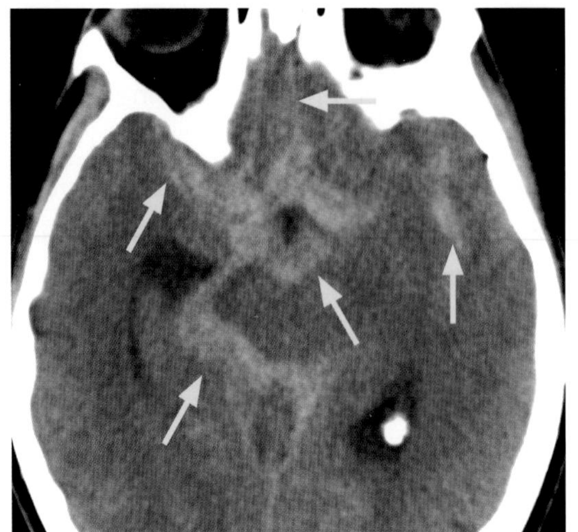

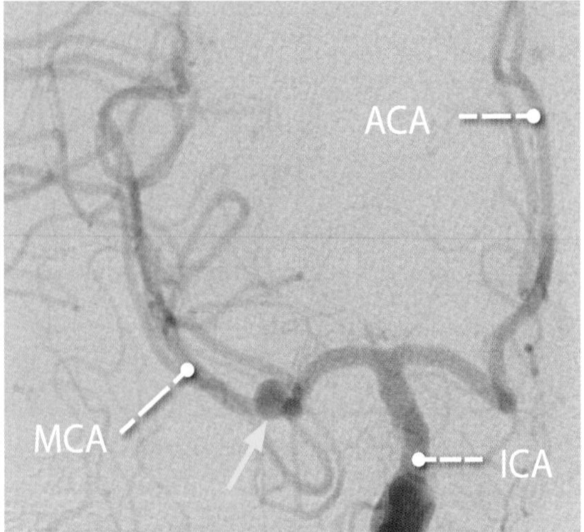

Subarachnoid hemorrhage: Noncontrast CT (left image) shows diffuse subarachnoid hemorrhage (arrows) in the basal cisterns including the suprasellar cistern, the anterior interhemispheric fissure, and the Sylvian fissure, predominantly on the right. Frontal oblique digital subtraction cerebral angiogram of the right internal carotid artery shows a small saccular aneurysm at the MCA trifurcation (yellow arrow).

- Overall, the most common cause of subarachnoid hemorrhage (SAH) is trauma. Aneurysm rupture is by far the most common cause of non-traumatic subarachnoid hemorrhage. No cause of the subarachnoid hemorrhage is identified in up to 22% of cases.
- Clinically, non-traumatic subarachnoid hemorrhage presents with thunderclap headache and meningismus.
- Noncontrast CT is the initial imaging modality in suspected subarachnoid hemorrhage. On CT, subarachnoid blood appears as high attenuation within the subarachnoid space.

> High attenuation material in the subarachnoid space may be due to SAH (by far the most common cause), meningitis, leptomeningeal carcinomatosis, or prior intrathecal contrast administration.

- Noncontrast CT is >95% sensitive for detecting subarachnoid hemorrhage within the first six hours, with sensitivity slowly decreasing to 50% by day 5. If clinical suspicion for subarachnoid hemorrhage is high with a negative CT scan, the standard of care is to perform a lumbar puncture to look for xanthochromia.
- If SAH is present on imaging or lumbar puncture shows xanthochromia, catheter angiography is the gold standard to evaluate for the presence of an aneurysm. Several recent studies have shown, however, that CT angiography is equivalent to catheter angiography in the search for a culprit aneurysm in cases of SAH.
- On MRI, acute subarachnoid hemorrhage appears hyperintense on FLAIR and demonstrates susceptibility artifact on gradient sequences.

> The differential diagnosis for increased FLAIR signal in the subarachnoid space is similar to the differential for high attenuation subarachnoid material seen on CT, including **SAH**, **meningitis**, **leptomeningeal carcinomatosis**, and **residual contrast material**. Note that meningitis and carcinomatosis will typically show leptomeningeal enhancement in addition to the abnormal FLAIR signal.
>
> Recent **oxygen** or **propofol** administration will also cause increased subarachnoid FLAIR signal.

Distribution of subarachnoid hemorrhage

- The pattern of subarachnoid hemorrhage may provide a clue to the location of the ruptured aneurysm. However, multiple aneurysms are seen in up to 20% of patients with SAH, and subarachnoid blood may redistribute if the patient was found down.
- Hemorrhage in the anterior interhemispheric fissure suggests an anterior communicating artery aneurysm (33% of intracranial aneurysms).
- Hemorrhage in the suprasellar cistern suggests a posterior communicating artery aneurysm (also 33% of intracranial aneurysms). Rarely, P-comm aneurysm rupture can result in isolated subdural hemorrhage.
- Hemorrhage in the sylvian fissure suggests a middle cerebral artery aneurysm (20% of intracranial aneurysms).
- Hemorrhage in the perimesencephalic cistern suggests either a basilar tip aneurysm (5% of intracranial aneurysms), which has a high morbidity, or the relatively benign nonaneurysmal *perimesencephalic subarachnoid hemorrhage* (subsequently discussed).

Grading of subarachnoid hemorrhage

- The **Hunt and Hess** score is the clinical grading scale for aneurysmal subarachnoid hemorrhage and is based solely on symptoms, without imaging. Grade I is the lowest grade, with only a mild headache. Grade V is the most severe, with coma or extensor posturing.
- The **Fisher grade** classifies the CT appearance of SAH. Grade 1 is negative on CT; grades 2 and 3 are <1 mm thick and >1 mm thick, respectively, and grade 4 is diffuse SAH or intraventricular or parenchymal extension.

Complications of subarachnoid hemorrhage

- **Vasospasm** is the most common cause of morbidity and mortality in patients who survive the initial episode of subarachnoid hemorrhage. The peak incidence of vasospasm occurs approximately 7 days after the initial ictus. Vasospasm may lead to stroke or hemorrhage.

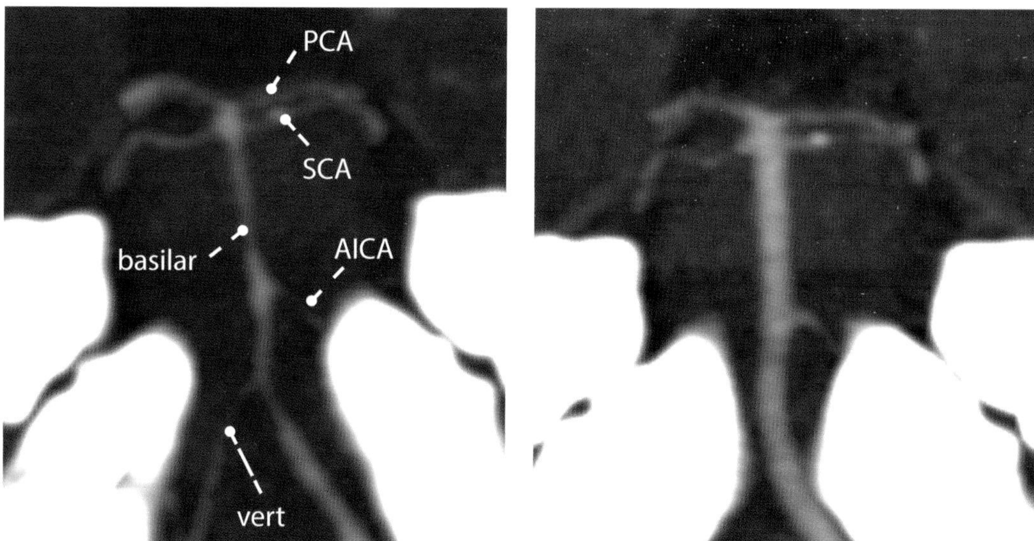

Vasospasm: Two coronal-oblique maximum-intensity projection images from subsequent CT-angiograms, in the plane of the basilar artery. The initial study (left image) shows severe narrowing of the basilar artery, left AICA (right not visible), and distal vertebral arteries. The follow-up study (right image) was performed after endovascular treatment, which shows a normal caliber of the basilar and left vertebral arteries.

The medical treatment of vasospasm is *triple-H* therapy of hypertension, hypervolemia, and hemodilution.

Endovascular treatment of vasospasm involves intra-arterial infusion of vasodilators.

- Approximately 20–30% of patients with subarachnoid hemorrhage will develop acute hydrocephalus, due to obstruction of arachnoid granulations. Treatment is ventriculostomy.

- **Superficial siderosis** is a condition caused by iron overload of pial membranes due to chronic or repeated subarachnoid bleeding. Clinically, patients with superficial siderosis present with sensorineural deafness and ataxia. On imaging, the iron causes hypointensity on T2-weighted images outlining the affected sulci.
- Imaging workup includes cranial and spinal imaging to evaluate for a source of bleeding.

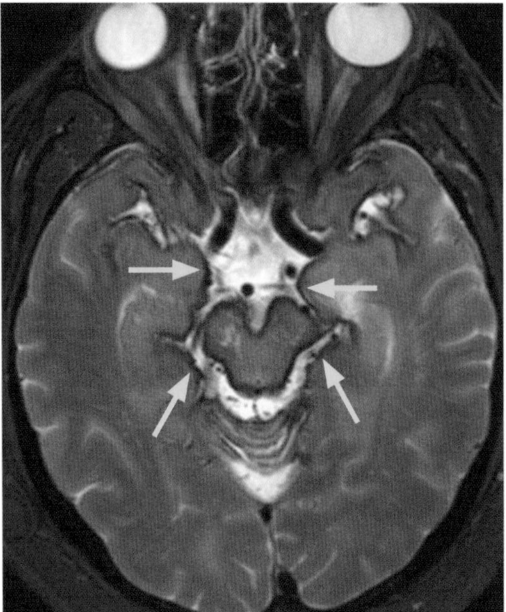

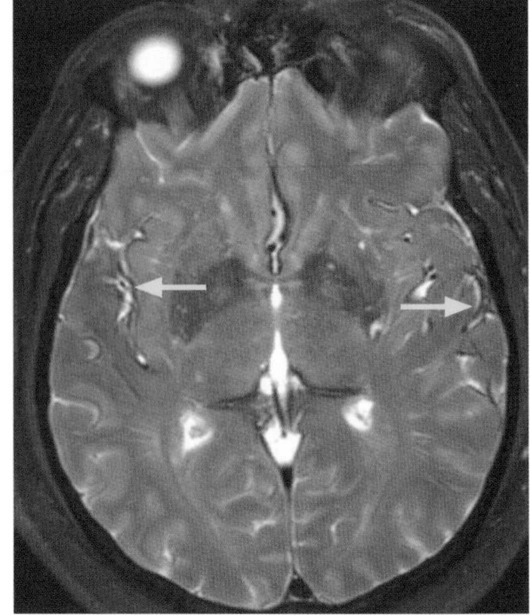

Superficial siderosis: Two axial T2-weighted images show a thin hypointense interface at the junction of the sulcal surfaces and the subarachnoid space (arrows) of the basal cisterns (left image) and the MCA territory temporal lobes (right image).

Case courtesy Mary Beth Cunnane, MD, Massachusetts Eye and Ear Infirmary.

Perimesencephalic subarachnoid hemorrhage

- Perimesencephalic subarachnoid hemorrhage is a type of nonaneurysmal subarachnoid hemorrhage that is a diagnosis of exclusion with a much better prognosis than hemorrhage due to a ruptured aneurysm.
- The hemorrhage must be limited to the cisterns directly anterior to the midbrain. The standard of care is to perform catheter angiography twice, one week apart. Both angiograms must be negative. Although the cause of the hemorrhage is unknown, it is thought to represent angiographically occult venous bleeding.
- Although the clinical presentation of perimesencephalic subarachnoid hemorrhage is similar to aneurysmal SAH (thunderclap headache), patients generally do well without residual neurological deficit. Some patients may experience mild to moderate vasospasm.

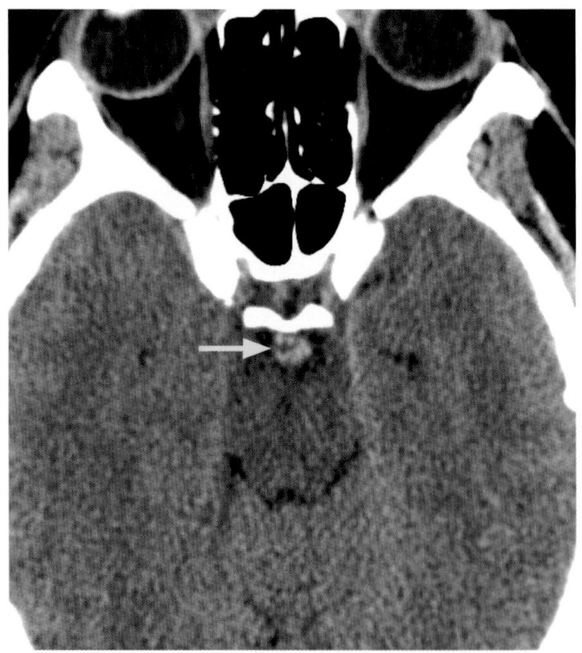

Perimesencephalic hemorrhage: Axial CT shows subarachnoid blood limited to the prepontine cistern (arrow). The membrane of Liliequist separates the prepontine cistern from the suprasellar cistern, and explains why there is no extension of blood superiorly. This patient had two negative catheter angiograms.

Reversible cerebral vasoconstriction syndrome (RCVS)

- Reversible cerebral vasoconstriction syndrome (RCVS) is a cause of nontraumatic, nonaneurysmal subarachnoid hemorrhage and ischemia. RCVS presents with thunderclap headache and is characterized by prolonged (but reversible) vasoconstriction.

Aneurysm morphology and pathology

Saccular aneurysm

- A saccular (also called *berry*) aneurysm is a focal outpouching of the arterial wall, most commonly arising at a branch point in the circle of Willis. The aneurysm points in the direction of blood flow leading into the branch point. Saccular aneurysms are seen almost exclusively in adults, with a slight female predominance. Saccular aneurysms are caused by a combination of hemodynamic stress and acquired degeneration of the vessel wall.
- Non-inherited risk factors for the development of saccular aneurysm include hypertension and inflammatory vascular disease such as Takayasu or giant cell arteritis.
- Inherited diseases that predispose to aneurysm formation include connective tissue diseases such as Marfan and Ehlers–Danlos, polycystic kidney disease, and neurofibromatosis type I.
- The aneurysm *neck* is the opening that connects the aneurysm to the parent vessel and the aneurysm *body* is the aneurysm sac. The neck:body ratio affects treatment options. Aneurysms with relatively small necks are generally easier to treat endovascularly with coils.
- Saccular aneurysms can be classified as small (<1 cm), medium (>1 cm and <2.5 cm), and giant (>2.5 cm). The larger the size, the greater the risk for rupture. Giant aneurysms often present with mass effect, causing cranial nerve palsy.

Fusiform aneurysm

- A fusiform aneurysm is segmental arterial dilation without a defined neck. Fusiform aneurysms are usually due to atherosclerosis, but may arise from chronic dissection.
- In contrast to saccular aneurysms, fusiform aneurysms do not occur at branch points.
- The vertebrobasilar system is affected more commonly than the anterior circulation.
- Fusiform aneurysms are much less common than saccular aneurysms. Since there is no aneurysm neck to exclude from the systemic circulation, fusiform aneurysms are more difficult to treat. Fusiform aneurysms of the vertebrobasilar system pose particular challenges, as critical perforating vessels may arise directly from the diseased artery.

Mycotic (infectious) aneurysm

- Mycotic aneurysms account for only 2–4% of all intracranial aneurysms and are due to septic emboli. Bacterial endocarditis is the most common embolic source.
- In contrast to saccular aneurysms, mycotic aneurysms form in the distal arterial circulation, beyond the circle of Willis. Mycotic aneurysms are fragile and have a high risk of rupture.

Oncotic aneurysm

- An oncotic aneurysm is an aneurysm caused by neoplasm.
- A benign left atrial myxoma may peripherally embolize and cause a distal oncotic aneurysm.

Traumatic pseudoaneurysm

- Aneurysms due to trauma are most commonly pseudoaneurysms, which don't contain the typical three histologic layers of the vessel wall. Usually the vessel will exhibit abnormal luminal narrowing proximal to the aneurysm. Similar to mycotic aneurysms, traumatic pseudoaneurysms tend to occur distally.
- Arteries close to bony structures (such as the basilar and vertebral artery) are prone to dissecting aneurysms.

Cerebral venous disease

Venous anatomy

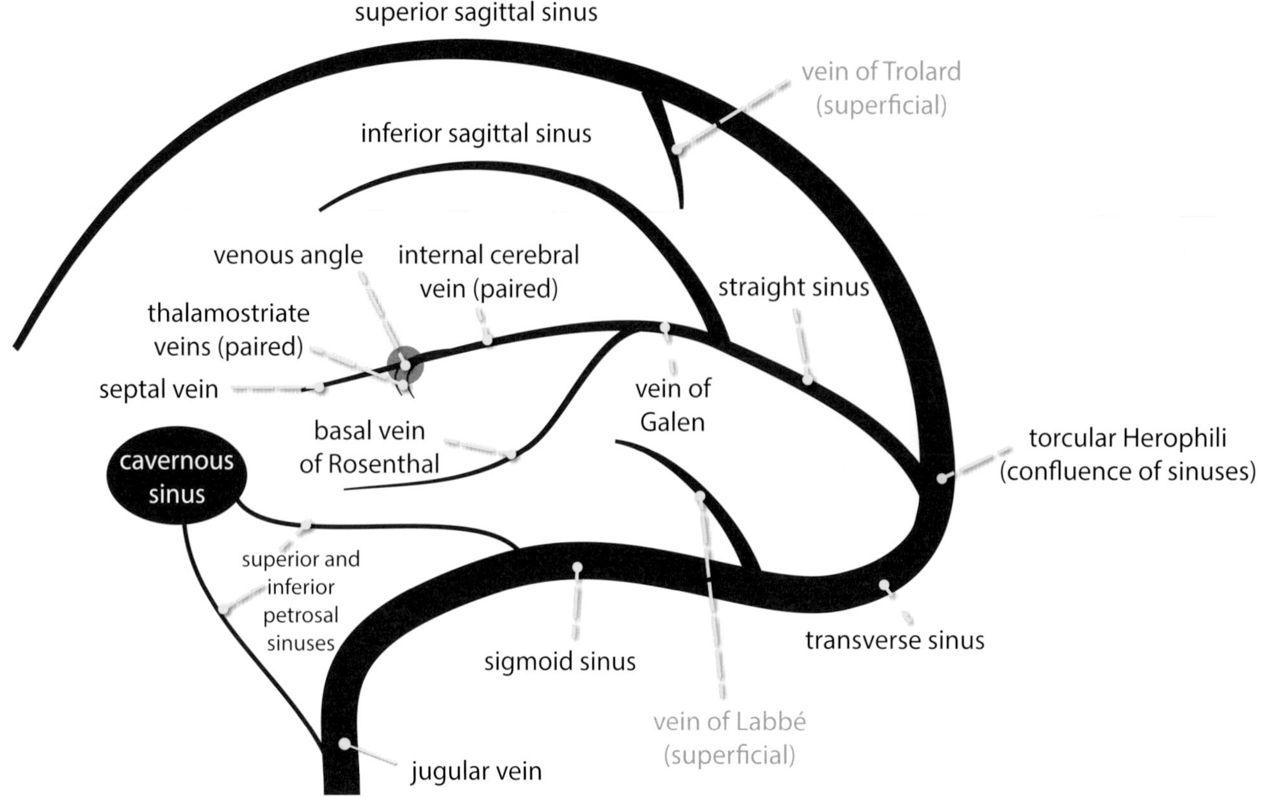

Dural sinuses

- The superior sagittal sinus (and its tributaries) drains the motor and sensory strips.
- The paired transverse sinuses are usually asymmetric, with the left transverse sinus often hypoplastic.
- The sigmoid sinus connects to the jugular bulb.
- The torcular Herophili is the confluence of the superior sagittal sinus, the transverse sinus, and the straight sinus. The word *torcular* is from the Greek word for wine press, and Herophilus was a Greek anatomist. Technically, the term *torcular Herophili* refers to the depression on the inner table of the skull produced by the confluence of sinuses, but in general use, *torcular Herophili* refers to the actual confluence of sinuses.

Deep cerebral veins

- The deep cerebral veins consist of the paired internal cerebral veins, the basal vein of Rosenthal, and the vein of Galen.
- The venous angle (red dot in the diagram above) is the intersection of the septal vein and the thalamostriate veins. The venous angle is the angiographic landmark for the foramen of Monro.

Superficial cerebral veins

- The vein of Trolard connects superficial cortical veins to the superior sagittal sinus.
- The vein of Labbé drains the temporal convexity into the transverse or sigmoid sinus. Retraction injury to the vein of Labbé during surgery may lead to venous infarction and aphasia.

Venous thrombosis

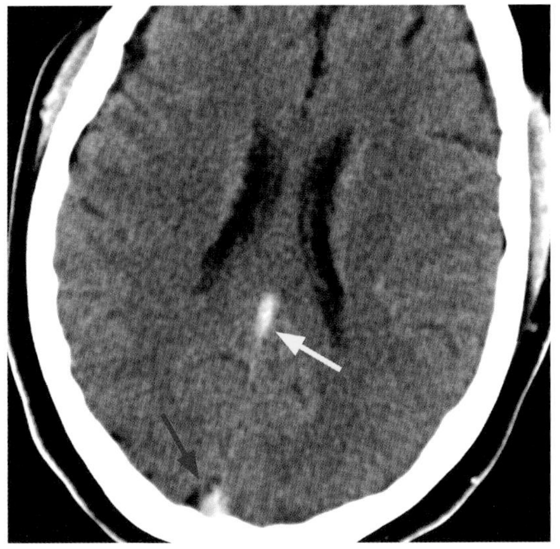

Non-contrast axial CT shows high attenuation in the vein of Galen (the *cord* sign; yellow arrow) and superior sagittal sinus near the torcular Herophili (red arrow).

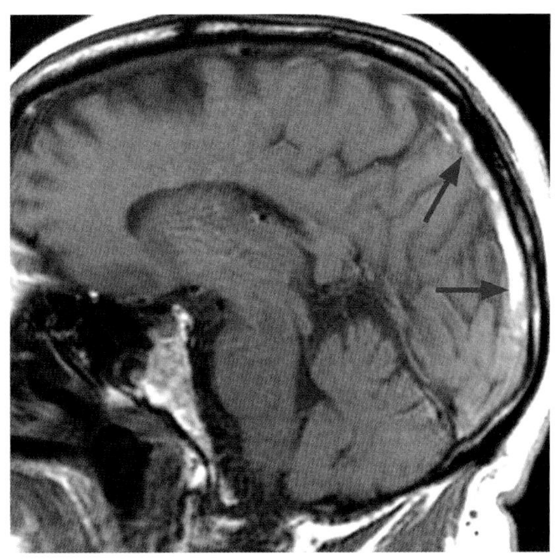

Sagittal T1-weighted MRI shows hyperintense thrombus within the superior sagittal sinus (arrows).

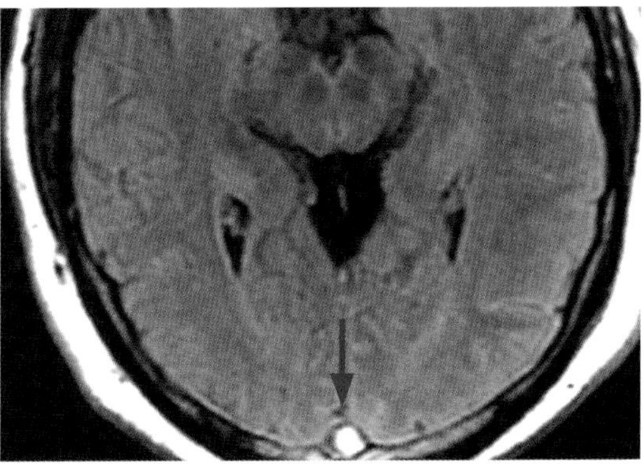

FLAIR MRI shows hyperintense thrombus within the superior sagittal sinus (arrow).

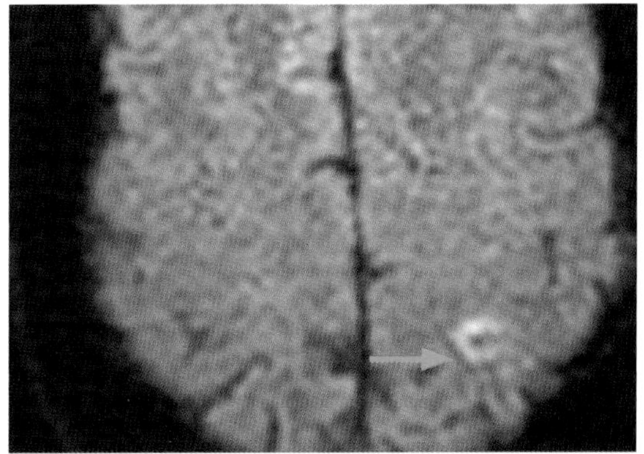

Diffusion-weighted MRI shows a subtle cortical focus of restricted diffusion (confirmed on ADC) in the left parietal lobe (arrow), a typical pattern of infarction seen with superior sagittal sinus thrombosis.

- Thrombosis of a cortical vein or a deep venous sinus is one of the more common causes of stroke in younger patients. Risk factors for venous thrombosis include pregnancy, oral contraceptives, thrombophilia, malignancy, and infection.
- A clue to the diagnosis of venous thrombosis on noncontrast CT is increased density within the thrombosed sinus or cortical vein (the *cord* sign). On contrast-enhanced CT, the *empty delta* sign signifies a filling defect in the superior sagittal sinus.
- MR venogram will show lack of flow in the thrombosed vein or dural venous sinus.
- Venous thrombosis leads to venous hypertension, which may cause infarction and parenchymal hemorrhage. There are three characteristic patterns of venous infarction, dependent on the location of the thrombosed vein:

Superior sagittal sinus thrombosis → infarction of the **parasagittal high convexity** cortex.

Deep venous system thrombosis → infarction of the **bilateral thalami.**

Transverse sinus thrombosis → infarction of the **posterior temporal lobe.**

Intraparenchymal hemorrhage

Imaging of hemorrhage

CT imaging of hemorrhage

- Noncontrast CT is usually the first imaging study performed in the emergency setting for a patient with a sudden neurologic deficit, headache, seizure, or altered level of consciousness.
- CT is highly sensitive for detection of hyperacute/acute intracranial hemorrhage, which appears hyperattenuating relative to brain parenchyma and CSF.

  Acute hemorrhage may be nearly isoattenuating to water in severe anemia (hemoglobin <8 mg/dL).

MR imaging of hemorrhage

- MR imaging of hemorrhage is complex. The characteristics of blood products change on T1- and T2-weighted sequences as the iron in hemoglobin evolves through physiologic stages:

  Intracellular oxyhemoglobin → *deoxygenation* →
  Intracellular deoxyhemoglobin → *oxidation* →
  Intracellular methemoglobin → *cell lysis* →
  Extracellular methemoglobin → *chelation* →
  Hemosiderin and ferritin

- Each stage of this evolution adheres to a reasonably constant time course in the intra-axial space and allows the radiologist to "date" the hemorrhage based on the unique signal characteristics on T1- and T2-weighted images for each stage.
- In general, all stages of hemorrhage are isointense or slightly dark on T1-weighted images, except for the methemoglobin stages, which are bright.
- Methemoglobin is bright on both T1- and T2-weighted images, except for intracellular methemoglobin, which is dark on T2-weighted images.
- In general, non hyperacute hemorrhage is dark on T2-weighted images, with the exception of extracellular methemoglobin, which is hyperintense on T2-weighted images. A hyperacute hematoma, containing primarily oxyhemoglobin, is slightly hyperintense on T2-weighted images but features a characteristic dark rim representing deoxygenation at the periphery of the clot.
- The inherent slight hyperintensity of oxygenated blood on T2-weighted images becomes apparent in slow flow states, as seen in venous hypertension and moyamoya disease. Slowly flowing blood is not susceptible to the flow-void artifact and the resultant apparently "enhancing" vasculature really represents unmasking of the normal blood signal.
- The expected evolution of blood products is highly dependent on macrophage elimination of blood breakdown products. These rules of thumb are not applicable to extra-axial blood and timing is generally not given for extra-axial blood, such as a subdural hematoma.

Treatment of hemorrhage

- In most cases, imaging is performed to evaluate for a treatable cause of hemorrhage, such as AVM or aneurysm. The mainstay of treatment of intraparenchymal hemorrhage is supportive, including blood pressure control and normalization of any coagulopathy.
- Larger hemorrhages can be evacuated surgically if there is significant mass effect or risk of herniation. In particular, a hemorrhage >3 cm in the posterior fossa would generally be treated surgically as there is increased risk of brainstem compression or hydrocephalus from fourth ventricular obstruction.

SPECIFIC STAGES OF PARENCHYMAL HEMATOMA ON MR

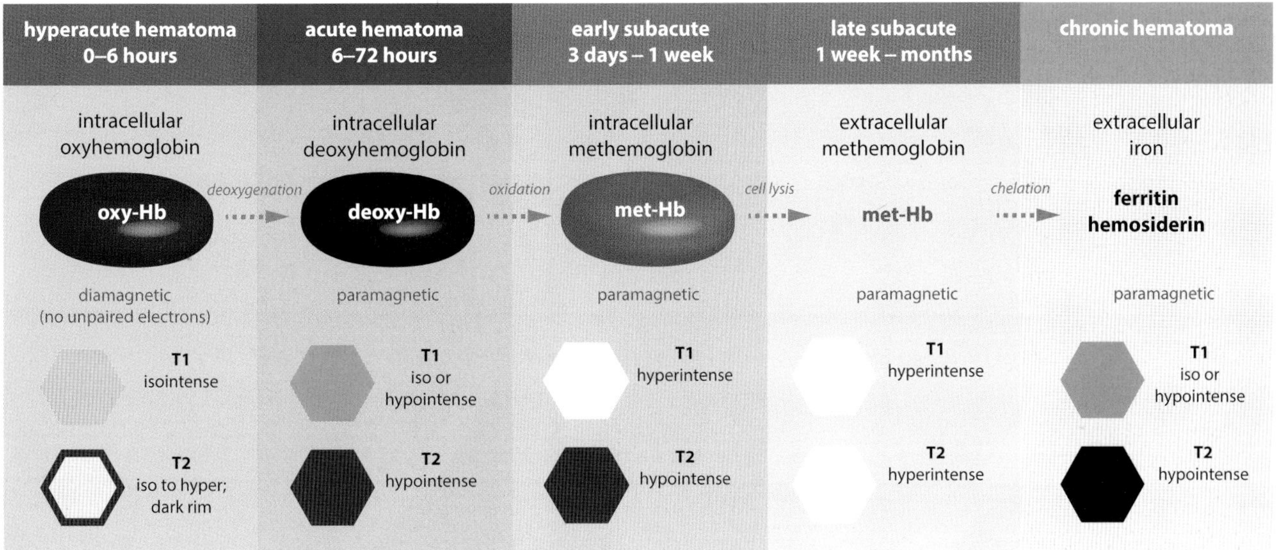

Hyperacute hematoma (<6 hours): Intracellular oxyhemoglobin

- A few hours after red cell extravasation, a hyperacute hematoma is primarily composed of intact red cells containing oxygenated hemoglobin, which is diamagnetic.
- The center of the hematoma will be isointense on T1-weighted images and iso- to slightly hyperintense on T2-weighted images.
- The key imaging finding of a hyperacute hematoma is a peripheral rim of hypointensity on T2-weighted images due to deoxygenation of the most peripheral red cells. This peripheral dark rim is most conspicuous on GRE sequences.

Acute hematoma (6–72 hours): Intracellular deoxyhemoglobin

- After the red cells desaturate (lose oxygen), the entire hematoma becomes hypointense on T2-weighted images and iso- to mildly hypointense on T1-weighted images.

Early subacute hematoma (3 days to 1 week): Intracellular methemoglobin

- The subacute phase is characterized by methemoglobin, which is paramagnetic and undergoes proton–electron dipole–dipole interactions (PEDDI) with water. PEDDI shortens T1 to cause hyperintensity on T1-weighted images. Intracellular and extracellular methemoglobin are both hyperintense on T1-weighted images.
- In the early subacute phase, blood remains hypointense on T2-weighted images due to the paramagnetic effects of methemoglobin, which remains trapped in the red cells.

Late subacute hematoma (1 week to months): Extracellular methemoglobin (after RBC lysis)

- The methemoglobin PEDDI effect persists after cell lysis, causing continued hyperintensity on T1-weighted images.
- Paramagnetic effects of methemoglobin lessens. Signal intensity on T2-weighted images increases to that of CSF, due to RBC lysis and decrease in protein concentration.
- There may be peripheral enhancement of a subacute to chronic infarct.

Chronic sequela of hemorrhage: Hemosiderin and ferritin

- Salvaged iron atoms are deposited into hemosiderin and ferritin, which become permanently trapped in the brain parenchyma after the blood brain barrier is restored.
- Susceptibility effects of the stored iron produce characteristic hypointensity on T2-weighted and GRE images.
- Chronic hemorrhage may have peripheral enhancement.

Hypertensive hemorrhage

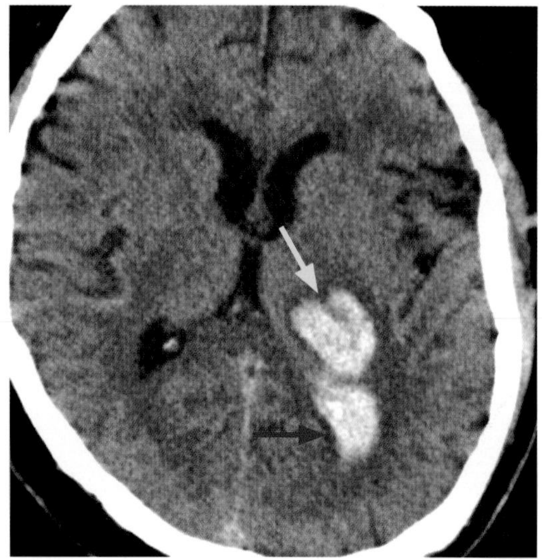
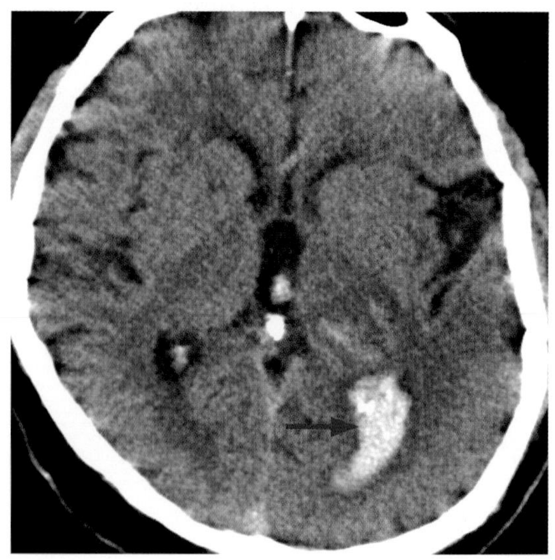

Hypertensive hemorrhage: Two contiguous noncontrast CT images show a left thalamic hemorrhage (yellow arrow) with extension into the left ventricle occipital horn (red arrows).

- Chronic hypertension is the most common cause of spontaneous adult intraparenchymal hemorrhage and is due to the secondary microangiopathic effects of chronic hypertension.
- Chronic hypertension causes arteriolar smooth muscle hyperplasia, which eventually leads to smooth muscle death and replacement with collagen. The resultant vascular ectasia predisposes to hemorrhage.
- Hypertensive hemorrhage occurs in characteristic locations in the basal ganglia, thalamus, and cerebellum.
- In addition to location, imaging (MRI or CT) findings suggestive of a hypertensive bleed include additional stigmata of hypertensive microangiopathy, such as periventricular white matter disease and prior lacunar infarcts.
- An additional MR-specific finding suggesting hypertensive hemorrhage is the presence of microhemorrhages on T2* (GRE or SWI) in the basal ganglia or brainstem.

Cerebral amyloid angiopathy (CAA)

- Cerebral amyloid angiopathy (CAA) is amyloid accumulated within the walls of small and medium arteries, ultimately causing vessel weakness and increased risk of hemorrhage.
- While the spontaneous form of CAA occurs almost exclusively in elderly adults (in which population it is the second most common cause of nontraumatic hemorrhage), a hereditary variant has an earlier age of onset.
- In addition to being a risk factor for hemorrhage, CAA can also occlude the lumens of small vessels and contribute to microangiopathy.
- The main clinical clue that a hemorrhage is secondary to CAA is that the patient is a normotensive elderly adult.
- The primary imaging feature to suggest CAA is the location of hematoma, which is almost always lobar or cortical, usually in the parietal or occipital lobes.
- An important secondary MRI finding is multiple microhemorrhages seen on T2* (GRE or SWI) within the brain parenchyma. In contrast to the microhemorrhages associated with hypertension, CAA microhemorrhages are in the cortex, not in the basal ganglia.

Aneurysmal hemorrhage

- As discussed, aneurysmal hemorrhage is by far the most common cause of nontraumatic subarachnoid hemorrhage. If an intraparenchymal hematoma is due to an aneurysm, the hematoma is usually adjacent to the ruptured aneurysm dome.
- The pattern of subarachnoid blood may help localize the aneurysm; however, if the patient was found down, then the blood will settle in the dependent portion of the brain, confounding localization.
- CT angiography is the study of choice for further evaluation of nontraumatic subarachnoid hemorrhage.

Arteriovenous malformation (AVM)

- An arteriovenous malformation is a congenital lesion consisting of abnormal high-flow arteriovenous connections without intervening normal brain.
- In case of AVM rupture, the resultant hematoma is usually parenchymal. In contrast to amyloid angiopathy, a hematoma from a bleeding AVM tends to affect younger patients.

Dural AV fistula (dAVF)

- Dural AV fistulas are a group of high-flow vascular malformations characterized by a fistulous connection between a meningeal artery and a venous sinus or cortical vein. Cavernous sinus (cavernous–carotid fistula) and posterior fossa dAVFs are the most common types.
- Imaging may show enlarged feeding arteries and enlarged or occluded dural sinuses, or enlarged cortical veins.

Venous thrombosis

- Thrombosis of cortical veins or deep venous sinuses leads to venous hypertension, which may cause infarction and parenchymal hemorrhage.

Hemorrhagic neoplasm

- Occasionally, the initial presentation of a brain tumor may be acute hemorrhage.
- The most common primary brain tumor to cause hemorrhage is glioblastoma.
- There are a relatively limited number of extracranial primary tumors known to cause hemorrhagic metastases, including:

  Choriocarcinoma.

  Melanoma.

  Thyroid carcinoma.

  Renal cell carcinoma.

  Although breast and lung cancer rarely cause hemorrhage on a per-case basis, they are such common cancers overall that they can always be considered when a hemorrhagic neoplasm is suspected.

- Patients treated with bevacizumab (trade name Avastin®, Genentech) may be at increased risk for hemorrhagic metastasis.
- Clues to the diagnosis of an underlying tumor causing hemorrhage include more-than-expected edema surrounding a hyperacute hematoma and heterogeneous blood product signal, suggesting varying breakdown stages of hemoglobin.
- The presence of multiple enhancing masses strongly suggests metastatic disease.
- In cases where the diagnosis is unclear, a follow-up MRI should be performed once the initial hemorrhage improves. If tumor is present, the MRI may show a delay in the expected evolution of blood products, persistent edema, and enhancement of the underlying tumor.

Cavernous malformation (cavernoma)

- A cavernous malformation is a vascular hamartoma that consists of low-flow endothelial-lined blood vessels without intervening normal brain.
- Although non-hemorrhagic cavernomas have a characteristic MRI appearance (with "popcorn-like" lobular mixed/high signal on T1- and T2-weighted images and a dark peripheral hemosiderin rim), once bleeding occurs, the resultant hematoma has nonspecific imaging features. The presence of a developmental venous anomaly adjacent to a hematoma may suggest the diagnosis of a recently hemorrhaged cavernoma.
- Angiography plays no role in the diagnosis. Cavernous malformations are angiographically occult.

Hemorrhagic transformation of infarct

- In most cases, the clinical or imaging diagnosis of stroke is made before hemorrhagic transformation occurs; however, hemorrhage may occasionally be the presenting feature of an infarct.
- More commonly, symptomatic hemorrhage occurs post-infarct in approximately 6–12% of patients receiving thrombolytic therapy.
- Noncontrast CT can identify risk factors for hemorrhagic transformation after thrombolytic therapy, including a relatively large region of hypoattenuation and a dense artery sign. Note that per AHA guidelines, neither of these findings is an exclusion criterion for administration of IV tPA.

Vasculitis

- Vasculitis affecting the CNS may be primary or secondary to systemic vasculitides.
- The most common presentation of vasculitis is cerebral ischemia. Less commonly, vasculitis may present with frank hemorrhage.
- Standard MRI imaging shows of vasculitis shows multiple foci of T2 prolongation in the basal ganglia and subcortical white matter.
- Noninvasive vascular imaging (CTA or MRA) is relatively insensitive to small vessel involvement, but may show irregularity of involved large or medium vessels.
- Angiography is the most sensitive test and shows multifocal areas of stenosis and dilation.

Moyamoya

- Moyamoya is a non-atherosclerotic vasculopathy characterized by progressive stenosis of the intracranial internal carotid arteries and their proximal branches, which leads to proliferation of fragile lenticulostriate collateral vessels.
- Angiography of the enlarged basal perforating arteries gives a *puff of smoke* appearance.
- The *ivy* sign on FLAIR MRI represents tubular branching hyperintense structures within the sulci, representing cortical arterial branches that appear hyperintense due to slow collateral flow.
- Patients with moyamoya disease are susceptible to aneurysm formation, especially in the posterior circulation.
- Perfusion studies show decreased flow in the affected vascular regions.

Intraparenchymal hemorrhage etiology

Elderly adult with hypertension?
*Hemorrhage in **basal ganglia**, **cerebellum**, or **thalamus**?*
*Multiple **basal ganglia** microbleeds on T2*?*
Prior lacunes and periventricular WM disease?
→ **Hypertensive hemorrhage**

***Lobar** or cortical hemorrhage?*
Elderly adult without hypertension?
*Multiple **parenchymal** microbleeds on T2*?*
→ **Amyloid angiopathy**

(Hypertensive hemorrhage and amyloid angiopathy: *older adults*)

Extensive subarachnoid blood?
Aneurysm adjacent to hematoma?
→ **Aneurysmal hemorrhage**

Parenchymal hemorrhage in a young patient?
Enlarged feeding artery?
Adjacent encephalomalacia?
→ **AVM**

Hemorrhage adjacent to cavernous sinus or in posterior fossa?
Enlarged meningeal artery or cortical vein?
→ **dAVF**

Adjacent DVA on post-contrast images?
Multiple dark spots on T2 (familial variant)?*
→ **Cavernous malformation**

(AVM, dAVF and cavernous malformation: *vascular malformations*)

Parasagittal or bilateral thalamic hemorrhage?
Young patient, especially female?
Increased density in cortical vein or dural sinus?
→ **Venous thrombosis**

More edema than expected?
More heterogeneous signal than expected?
Multiple enhancing lesions?
→ **Hemorrhagic neoplasm**

Clinical history of infarct?
History of thrombolytic therapy?
→ **Hemorrhagic infarct**

Multifocal T2 prolongation in deep WM?
History of systemic vasculitis?
Multifocal stenosis/dilation on angiography?
→ **CNS vasculitis**

Occlusion of internal carotid arteries?
Multiple collateral vessels?
→ **Moyamoya**

WHITE MATTER DISEASE

WHITE MATTER OVERVIEW

White matter imaging overview

- The typical MRI appearance of white matter injury is T2 prolongation of the affected white matter. Less commonly, *tumefactive* demyelination may be mass-like, enhance, and look very similar to a tumor.
- The key imaging finding of demyelinating disease is *minimal mass effect* relative to the lesion size.
- A frequent pattern of white matter disease consisting of scattered foci of T2 prolongation in the subcortical, deep, and periventricular white matter is seen very commonly, especially in older adults. In older patients, this pattern is most likely due to chronic microvascular ischemia. In younger patients, a similar pattern can be seen in chronic migraine headaches, as sequelae of prior infectious or inflammatory disease, and with demyelination.

Normal structures may mimic white matter disease on T2 images

- Virchow–Robin spaces are tiny perivascular spaces that follow deep penetrating vessels into the subarachnoid space. Virchow–Robin spaces follow CSF signal on all sequences, including FLAIR.

  Enlarged Virchow–Robin spaces and a J-shaped sella can be seen in the mucopolysaccharidoses.
- Ependymitis granularis represents frontal horn periventricular hyperintensity on T2-weighted images due to interstitial CSF backup. Despite the name ("-itis"), ependymitis granularis is not associated with inflammation.

IDIOPATHIC/AUTOIMMUNE/INFLAMMATORY WHITE MATTER DISEASE

Multiple sclerosis (MS)

- Multiple sclerosis (MS) is idiopathic inflammatory destruction of CNS axons in the brain and spinal cord. MS is likely autoimmune in etiology and may be associated with other autoimmune diseases such as Graves disease and myasthenia gravis.
- MS is the most common chronic demyelinating disease. It often leads to severe disability.
- MS is more common in middle-aged Caucasian females from northern latitudes.
- There are two main clinical presentations of multiple sclerosis:

  1) **Relapsing–remitting** (most common): Partial or complete resolution of each acute attack.

  2) **Progressive**: No resolution or incomplete resolution between acute attacks.

     Primary progressive: Slow onset without discrete exacerbations.

     Secondary progressive: Similar to relapsing–remitting but with less complete resolution between attacks, leading to progressive disability.
- Optic neuritis may represent the first sign of MS. The purpose of a brain MRI after optic neuritis is to look for other lesions, which may be clinically silent.
- Histopathologically, destruction of myelin is caused by lymphocytes attacking oligodendrocytes (which make CNS myelin).
- Although MRI imaging is highly sensitive, there are no pathognomonic imaging findings. The McDonald criteria, last revised in 2010, describe strict imaging findings to diagnose MS. The McDonald criteria are most useful for clinically ambiguous cases.
- In order to make the diagnosis of MS, there must be lesions separated in **space** (different areas of the CNS) and in **time** (new lesions across scans).

- Suggestive imaging findings include periventricular ovoid foci of T2 prolongation that "point" towards the ventricles, called *Dawson fingers*. The corpus callosum is often affected, best seen on sagittal FLAIR.

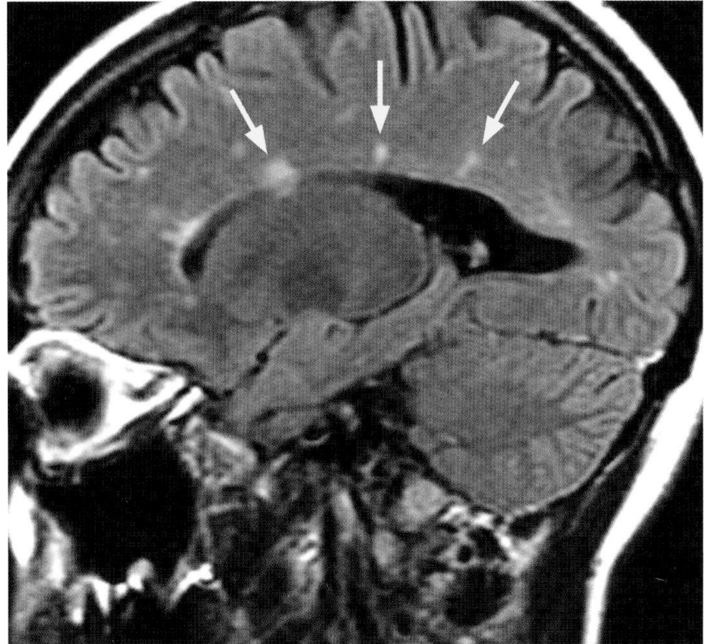

Dawson fingers in multiple sclerosis: Parasagittal FLAIR shows numerous foci of T2 prolongation (arrows) within the corpus callosum that point towards the ventricle in a patient with relapsing–remitting multiple sclerosis.

- In general, an enhancing lesion is suggestive of active demyelination, as enhancement is thought to be due to inflammatory blood brain barrier breakdown.

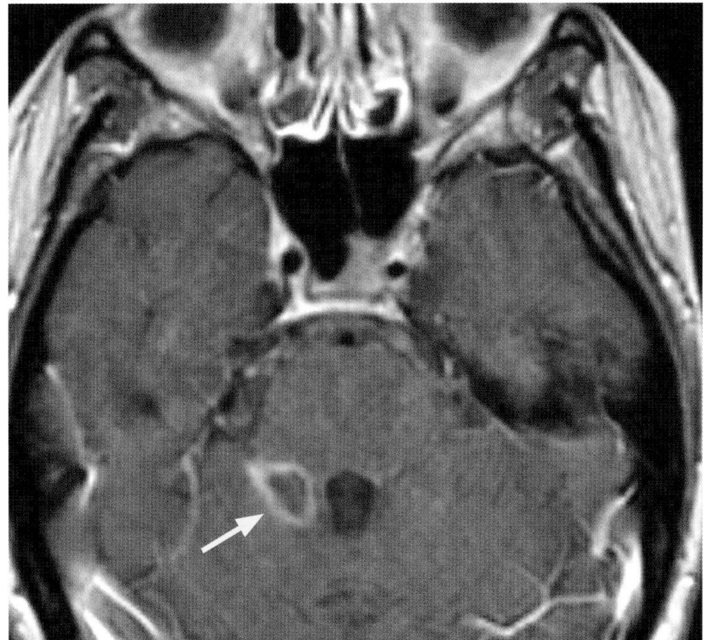

Enhancing lesion in the same patient as above, with known multiple sclerosis: Axial post-contrast T1-weighted image shows a ring-enhancing lesion in the right middle-cerebellar peduncle (arrow).

Although ring enhancement is nonspecific, the lack of any appreciable mass effect (the adjacent fourth ventricle is normal in size and shape) suggests a demyelinating lesion.

- Lesions that are dark on T1-weighted images are called "black holes" and are associated with more severe demyelination and axonal loss.
- Chronic MS leads to cortical atrophy, thinning of the corpus callosum, and changes in MRI spectroscopy, with ↓ NAA, ↑ choline, ↑ lipids, and ↑ lactate.
- *Tumefactive* MS describes the occasionally seen ring enhancement and mass-like appearance of an active MS plaque. In contrast to a brain tumor, the demyelinating lesion will *not have any significant mass effect,* and the ring of enhancement is usually incomplete.
- MS involves the spinal cord in a substantial minority of patients and the spine is routinely evaluated in patients with MS. Spinal MS involvement is usually short-segment and unilateral. Isolated spinal cord involvement is seen in up to 20% of cases of MS.

Concentric (Balo) sclerosis

- Concentric (Balo) sclerosis is a very rare variant of MS with pathognomonic alternating concentric bands of normal and abnormal myelin. It is seen more often in younger patients.

Marburg variant (acute multiple sclerosis)

- Marburg variant of MS is a fulminant manifestation of MS, leading to death within months.

Devic disease (Neuromyelitis optica)

- Devic disease is a demyelinating disease, distinct from MS, which involves both the optic nerves and spinal cord. Devic disease confers a worse prognosis compared to MS.
- NMO-IgG, an antibody to aquaporin 4, is highly specific for Devic disease. NMO-IgG activates the complement cascade and induces demyelination.
- Imaging shows MS-type lesions with involvement of the optic tracts and spinal cord. Brain lesions, if present, tend to be periventricular.

Toxic-metabolic white matter disease

Osmotic demyelination

- Osmotic demyelination is caused by a rapid change in extracellular osmolality, typically occurring after aggressive correction of hyponatremia. The quick osmotic gradient change causes endothelial damage, blood brain barrier breakdown, and release of extracellular toxins, which damage myelin.
- Patients with poor nutritional status, including alcoholics, chronic lung disease patients, and liver transplant recipients, are the most susceptible to osmotic demyelination.
- Osmotic demyelination is typically seen in the pons, but may occur elsewhere in the brainstem and deep gray nuceli. MRI features bilateral central T2 prolongation in the affected region. Signal abnormalities in the thalami and basal ganglia may also be present.

Marchiafava–Bignami

- Marchiafava–Bignami is a fulminant demyelinating disease of the corpus callosum seen in male alcoholics.

Wernicke encephalopathy

- Wernicke encephalopathy is an acute syndrome of ataxia, confusion, and oculomotor dysfunction, which may be caused either by alcoholism or generalized metabolic disturbances, such as bariatric surgery.
- On imaging, there is T2 prolongation and possible enhancement within the mammillary bodies and medial thalamus. The non-alcoholic form may also affect the cortex.

Vascular white matter disease

Posterior reversible encephalopathy syndrome (PRES)

- Posterior reversible encephalopathy syndrome (PRES) is a disorder of vasogenic edema with a posterior circulation predominance triggered by failed autoregulation and resultant hyperperfusion, most commonly caused by acute hypertension. In addition to hypertension, PRES is also associated with eclampsia, sepsis, autoimmune disorders, multidrug chemotherapy, and solid or stem cell transplantation.
- In contrast to infarction, the edema is vasogenic in etiology, not cytotoxic. Diffusion may be normal, increased, or restricted.
- Imaging shows **symmetric** regions of subcortical white matter abnormality (hypoattenuation on CT and T2 prolongation on MR), especially in the posterior circulation (occipital and parietal lobes and posterior fossa). Mild mass effect and enhancement can be seen.

Cerebral autosomal dominant arteriopathy with subcortical infarcts and leukoencephalopathy (CADASIL)

- Cerebral autosomal dominant arteriopathy with subcortical infarcts and leukoencephalopathy (CADASIL) is an inherited disease characterized by recurrent stroke, migraine, subcortical dementia, and pseudobulbar palsy, due to small vessel arteriopathy.
- The clinical hallmark of CADASIL is recurrent episodes of stroke or transient ischemic attacks, which are nearly always found to be subcortical in the white matter or basal ganglia on imaging. There is often associated migraine. It may eventually lead to dementia.
- MRI shows **symmetric** foci of T2 prolongation in the subcortical white matter, which may become confluent as the disease progresses. Anterior temporal lobe or paramedian frontal lobe foci of T2 prolongation are highly sensitive and specific for CADASIL, especially with clinical history of migraine. Although the symmetric subcortical pattern is similar to PRES, the distribution in CADASIL is anterior circulation.

Vasculitis

- CNS vasculitis is a group of vascular inflammatory disorders that primarily affects the small vessels, in particular the leptomeningeal and small parenchymal vessels.
- Etiologies include lupus, polyarteritis nodosa, giant cell arteritis, and Sjögren syndrome.
- MRI shows numerous small focal areas of T2 prolongation in subcortical and deep white matter. Although the appearance may be similar to MS, foci of hemorrhage (best seen on GRE or SWI) may be present in vasculitis, which would not be seen in multiple sclerosis.
- Vascular imaging (CT angiography and catheter angiography are more sensitive than MR angiography) shows a beaded, irregular appearance to the cerebral vessels.

Microangiopathy

- Microangiopathy describes age-related chronic axonal loss, gliosis, and ischemic changes seen in up to 80% of elderly individuals. Microangiopathy never involves the corpus callosum: If involvement of the corpus callosum is present, an alternative diagnosis should be considered, such as multiple sclerosis or neoplasm.
- Binswanger disease represents the combination of dementia and severe microangiopathy.

Infectious (viral) white matter disease

Progressive multifocal leukoencephalopathy (PML)

- Progressive multifocal leukoencephalopathy (PML) is a demyelinating disease of immunocompromised patients caused by reactivation of JC virus. There is progressive demyelination with lack of inflammatory response.
- PML occurs most commonly in AIDS patients (PML is an AIDS defining illness), but can also be seen in patients with malignancy, status post organ transplant, or with autoimmune disorders. Approximately 1 in 1,000 patients with MS treated with natalizumab (Tysabri®) may have superimposed PML and it may be difficult to distinguish between MS and PML. Diagnosis is made by PCR for JC virus DNA in CSF.
- MR imaging of PML shows **asymmetric** multifocal white matter lesions that may become confluent. There is rarely mass effect or enhancement. The arcuate (subcortical U) fibers are typically involved. Arcuate fibers are myelinated tracts at the gray–white junction that connect cortex to cortex.
- In an AIDS patient, the primary differential for white matter lesions is PML and HIV encephalitis. In contrast to PML, HIV encephalitis is usually bilateral (and symmetric), spares the subcortical white matter, and is associated with cerebral atrophy:

  Diffuse bilateral involvement, sparing of subcortical white matter, and cerebral atrophy → HIV encephalitis.

  Asymmetric involvement, involvement of subcortical white matter, and lack of atrophy → PML.

Subacute sclerosing panencephalitis (SSPE)

- Subacute sclerosing panencephalitis (SSPE) is a demyelinating disease caused by reactivation of measles virus, usually after a long latent period.
- Imaging shows periventricular white matter lesions, but in distinction to the other white matter entities, SSPE lesions tend to have surrounding edema and mass effect.

POST-VIRAL WHITE MATTER DISEASE

Acute disseminated encephalomyelitis (ADEM)

- Acute disseminated encephalomyelitis (ADEM) is a monophasic demyelinating disorder seen primarily in children that typically occurs after a viral infection or vaccination.
- The majority of patients will make a full recovery, but a minority will have permanent neurologic sequelae.
- Imaging findings can be identical to MS, and occasionally cases of presumed ADEM will be reclassified as MS due to polyphasic clinical course. Similar to MS, ADEM may involve the brain, brainstem, or spinal cord.
- Optic neuritis and spinal cord involvement can be seen in ADEM, as with MS.
- The Hurst variant (acute hemorrhagic leukoencephalitis) is a rapidly fulminant form of ADEM that leads to death within days.

  Imaging of the Hurst variant shows multifocal T2 prolongation and associated white matter hemorrhage, which may appear as confluent hematomas.

IATROGENIC WHITE MATTER DISEASE

Radiation injury

- Radiation injury causes small vessel arteritis and secondary ischemia.
- The acute phase occurs during radiation therapy, thought to reflect edema due to endothelial injury, and is of little clinical significance.
- The early delayed phase occurs between several weeks and up to six months after treatment, and is thought to be due to demyelination. MRI shows diffuse white matter T2 prolongation.
- The late delayed phase occurs months to years after radiation. It can present as white matter injury or a focal radiation necrosis.

  Mass effect, edema, and enhancement are common, and radiation necrosis should be considered in the differential of a ring enhancing mass in a patient with history of prior radiation.
- Other complications of brain radiation include the development of meningiomas, capillary telangiectasias, cavernous malformations, and/or moyamoya.

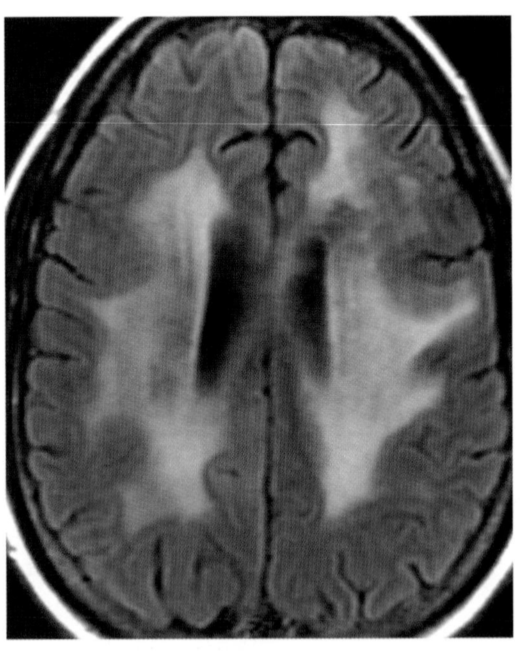

White matter radiation injury: Axial FLAIR image shows extensive confluent T2 prolongation within most of the visualized white matter. The patient had a remote history of radiation therapy for a high-grade glioma.

Chemotherapy-related white matter disease

- Chemotherapy may cause focal, multifocal, or diffuse white matter disease, especially in combination with radiation treatment.

BACTERIAL INFECTION

Pyogenic abscess

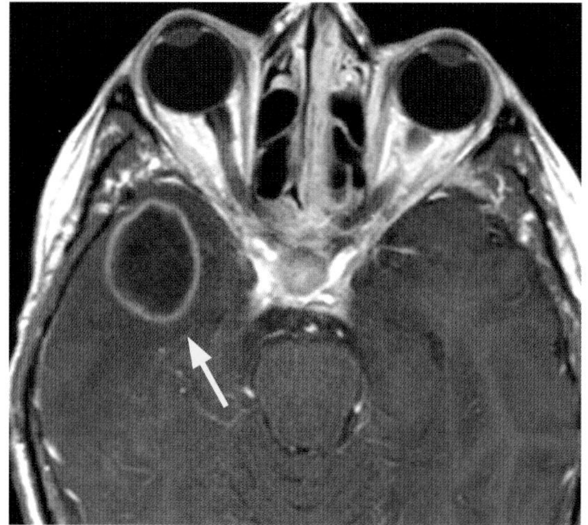

Axial contrast-enhanced T1-weighted MRI

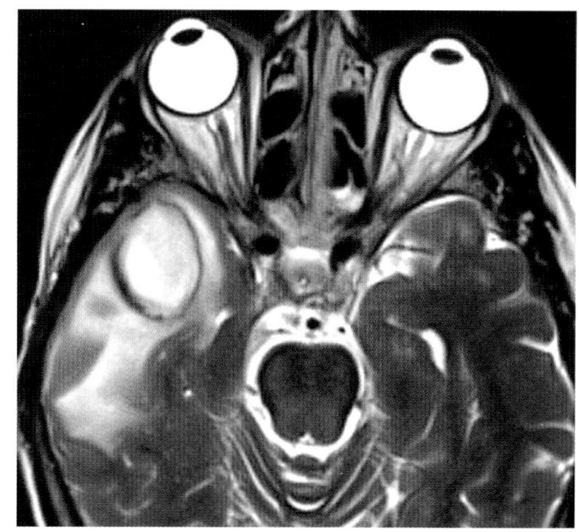

Axial T2-weighted MRI

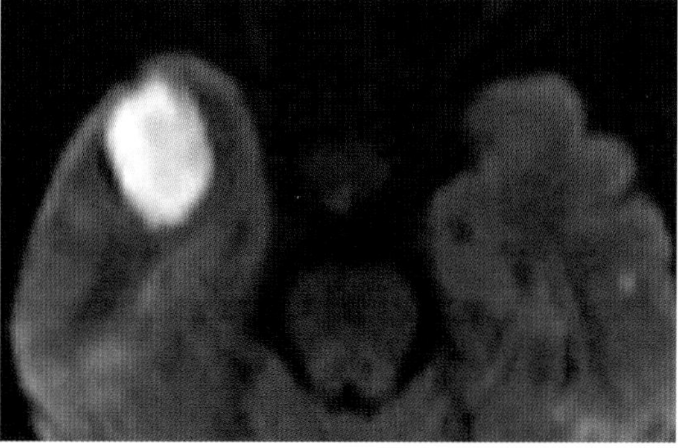

DWI

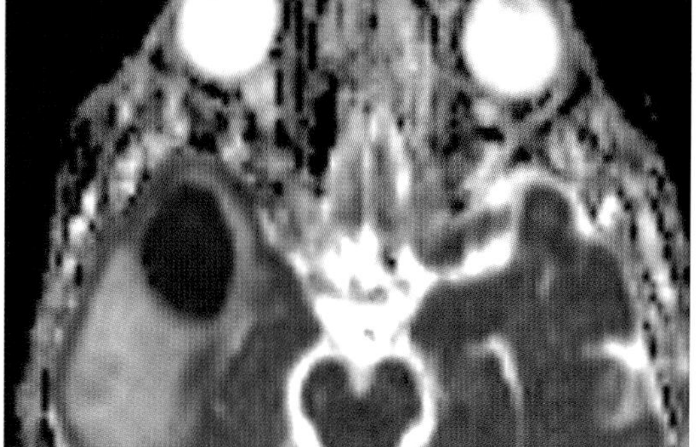

ADC map

Pyogenic abscess: A ring-enhancing lesion (arrow) in the right anterior temporal lobe features a thin, smoothly enhancing, hypointense rim on the T2-weighted image, with moderate surrounding vasogenic edema. The contents of the lesion are hyperintense on DWI and dark on ADC, consistent with restricted diffusion.

- A cerebral pyogenic abscess may be due to hematogenous dissemination, direct spread from paranasal sinusitis or mastoiditis, or a complication of bacterial meningitis.
- An abscess evolves over four stages (early cerebritis → late cerebritis → early abscess → late abscess) and takes about two weeks to fully develop. In the early stage of infection, there is nonspecific T2 prolongation in the affected region, with heterogeneous enhancement.
- After the abscess becomes discrete, the classic imaging appearance is a ring-enhancing mass. The rim is hypointense on T2-weighted images. Unlike the rim of a glioma or metastasis, an abscess rim is thin and smooth.
- When periventricular in location, an abscess classically tends to feature a thinner capsule oriented towards the ventricles. Disruption of the ventricular margin may herald impending rupture. Rupture may result in ventriculitis, with very high mortality.
- A pyogenic brain abscess almost always demonstrates restricted diffusion, appearing very bright on DWI due to restricted diffusion superimposed on inherent hyperintensity on T2-weighted images.

Tuberculoma

- A tuberculoma is a localized tuberculosis granuloma. It is not always possible to differentiate a tuberculoma from a pyogenic abscess.
- A tuberculoma tends to have central hypointensity on T2-weighted image (in contrast to a pyogenic abscess, which is hyperintense). A cystic tuberculoma, however, may mimic a pyogenic abscess. Similar to pyogenic abscess, tuberculomas tend to show restricted diffusion.

Lyme disease

- Lyme disease, caused by the spirochete *Borrelia burgdorferi*, can cause white matter disease with a nonspecific imaging appearance of T2 prolongation predominantly in the frontal subcortical white matter. Associated enhancement of multiple cranial nerves or meningeal enhancement may suggest the diagnosis.

Fungal infection

Cryptococcus

- Cryptococcosis is the most common CNS fungal infection in patients with AIDS and is caused by *Cryptococcus neoformans.* It is the third most common CNS infection in AIDS overall, after HIV encephalopathy and toxoplasmosis.
- Similar to toxoplasmosis, AIDS patients become susceptible to cryptococcus with a CD4 count less than 100 cells/μL. The most common clinical presentation is chronic basilar meningitis. The most common imaging finding is hydrocephalus, which is very nonspecific.
- *Cryptococcus* spreads along the basal ganglia perivascular spaces, leaving behind *gelatinous pseudocysts,* which appear as round water-signal lesions on T1- and T2-weighted MRI.
- *Cryptococcus* has a predilection for spread to the choroid plexus, producing ring-enhancing granulomas (called *cryptococcomas*) within the ventricles.
- Treatment is with antifungal agents including fluconazole and amphotericin B.

Parasitic infection

Neurocysticercosis

- Neurocysticercosis is the most common parasitic CNS infection of immunocompetent patients. It is caused by the tapeworm *Taenia solium* and clinically presents with seizures.
- Four stages of neurocysticercosis have been described:

> 1) **Viable/vesicular**: Imaging shows several CSF-intensity cysts, without enhancement. Many of these cystic lesions may demonstrate an eccentric "dot" representing the scolex.
>
> 2) **Colloidal**: The colloidal stage has the least specific imaging findings, presenting as ring-enhancing lesions. In contrast to a pyogenic abscess, the lesions feature *increased* diffusivity.
>
> 3) **Nodular/granular**: Edema decreases as the cyst involutes and the cyst wall thickens.
>
> 4) **Calcified**: Imaging shows small parenchymal calcifications (on CT) and small foci of susceptibility (GRE).

- Intraventricular neurocysticercosis can occur in up to 20% of cases, typically in the aqueduct of Sylvius or the fourth ventricle. Hydrocephalus may be the initial presentation, with the obstructing cyst most apparent on FLAIR images because the protein-rich intracystic fluid will not be nulled on FLAIR.
- The racemose form of neurocysticercosis is an older term describing a variant without a visible scolex, now thought to represent degeneration of the scolex.
- Treatment is with antiparasitic medications including albendazole, supplemented with steroids for edema and antiseizure medications as needed.

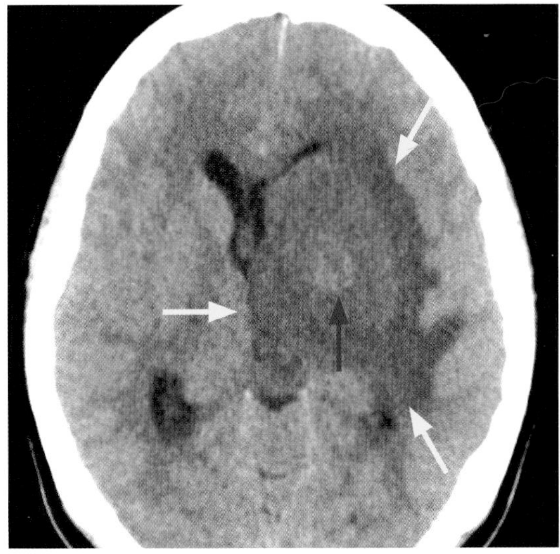

Toxoplasmosis: Axial unenhanced CT shows a large area of edema in the left basal ganglia (yellow arrows), centered on a subtle hyperattenuating mass (red arrow).

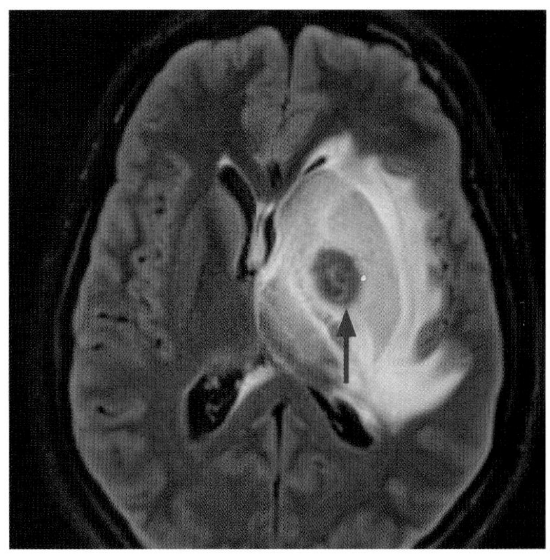

Axial FLAIR shows the extensive edema surrounding a heterogeneous rounded mass (red arrow) in the left basal ganglia.

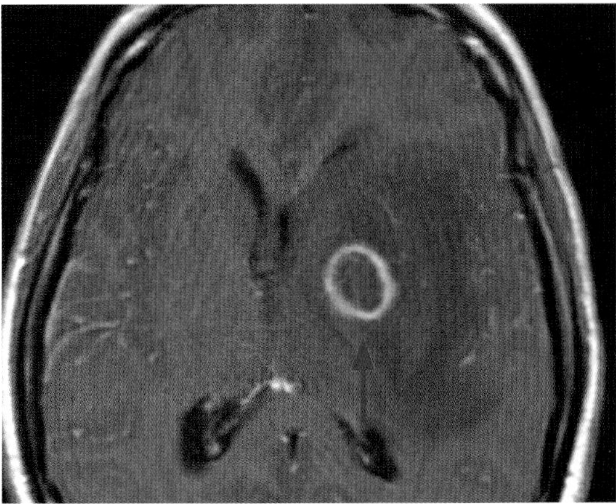

Post-contrast axial T1-weighted MRI demonstrates smooth ring-enhancement of the lesion (red arrow).

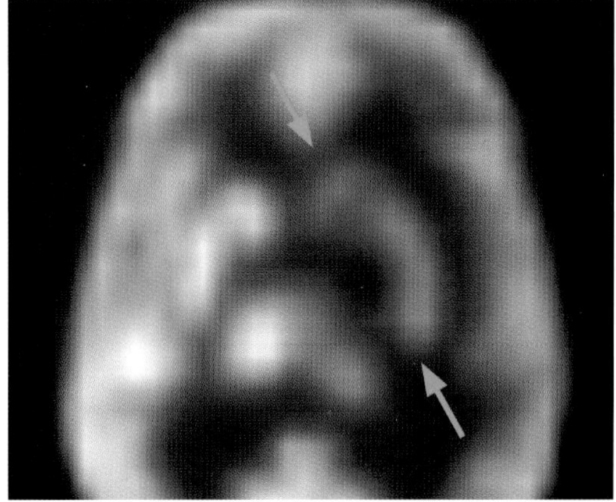

F-18-FDG PET scan shows asymmetrical, relatively decreased metabolism of the left basal ganglia (blue arrows).

- Toxoplasmosis is the most common mass lesion in AIDS patients and is caused by the parasite *Toxoplasma gondii.* AIDS patients become susceptible to the parasite with a CD4 count less than 100 cells/µL. Toxoplasmosis is the second most common CNS infection in AIDS patients, with HIV encephalitis being the most common.
- The typical appearance of toxoplasmosis is single or multiple ring-enhancing lesions in the basal ganglia.
- The *asymmetric target* sign is not frequently seen but is relatively specific and describes an eccentric nodule of enhancement along the enhancing wall of the toxoplasmosis lesion.
- The primary differential consideration of a basal ganglia mass in an immunocompromised patient is CNS lymphoma. In contrast to CNS lymphoma, toxoplasmosis does not demonstrate reduced diffusivity and does not demonstrate increased relative cerebral blood volume on perfusion imaging. Additional studies typically demonstrate toxoplasmosis to be hypometabolic on FDG–PET, and not avid on thallium scintigraphy.

Viral infection

Herpes encephalitis

- Herpes encephalitis is a devastating (if untreated), necrotizing encephalitis caused by reactivation of latent HSV-1 within the trigeminal ganglion. Clinical symptoms are nonspecific, with fever and headache often being prominent complaints. Mental status may be altered.
- *Herpes should be the first consideration in any patient with fever, mesial temporal lobe signal abnormality, and acute altered mental status.*
- Although lumbar puncture should be obtained before MRI and treatment should never be delayed for MRI, it is important to note that herpes encephalitis may be present when not clinically suspected and PCR of HSV in cerebrospinal fluid is not 100% sensitive.
- Herpes encephalitis causes edema, hemorrhage, and necrosis, typically in the medial temporal lobes and the inferior frontal lobes.
- CT is often normal but can show ill-defined hypoattenuation in the affected regions.
- MRI is much more sensitive and typically shows bilateral (but usually asymmetric) T2 prolongation in the medial temporal lobe, insular cortex, cingulate gyrus, and inferior frontal lobe. Once the infection becomes hemorrhagic, MRI will show foci of T1 shortening and gradient susceptibility. The affected areas typically demonstrate reduced diffusion.
- Enhancement may develop later in the infection, and is typically gyral in morphology.
- In an immunocompromised patient, HSV-6 infection should be considered with the above findings, although enhancement and diffusion abnormalities may be absent.
- The differential diagnosis of medial temporal lobe lesions includes MCA infarction, infiltrating glioma, limbic encephalitis, and seizure-related changes. Fever is typically absent in infarction and glioma. Herpes encephalitis should be the first consideration in any patient with fever and signal abnormality in the medial temporal lobe.
- Treatment is urgent antiviral therapy.

HIV encephalopathy

- HIV encephalopathy is the most common CNS infection in AIDS patients. It is a progressive neurodegenerative disease caused by direct infection of CNS lymphocytes and microglial cells (CNS macrophages) by the HIV virus.
- On imaging, HIV encephalitis manifests as diffuse cerebral atrophy and symmetric T2 prolongation in the periventricular and deep white matter.
- As previously discussed, in contrast to progressive multifocal leukoencephalopathy (PML), HIV encephalitis spares the subcortical U-fibers and tends to be symmetric.

Cytomegalovirus (CMV) encephalitis

- Cytomegalovirus (CMV) encephalitis only affects the immunosuppressed, typically when the CD4 cell count is less than 50 cells/μL.
- The most common CNS manifestation of CMV infection is ventriculitis or meningoencephalitis.
- The characteristic imaging features of CMV ventriculitis include subependymal FLAIR hyperintensity and enhancement throughout the ventricular system.
- In neonates, CMV is one of the most common TORCH infections and causes atrophy, encephalomalacia, ventricular enlargement, and periventricular calcification.

Creutzfeldt–Jakob disease (CJD)

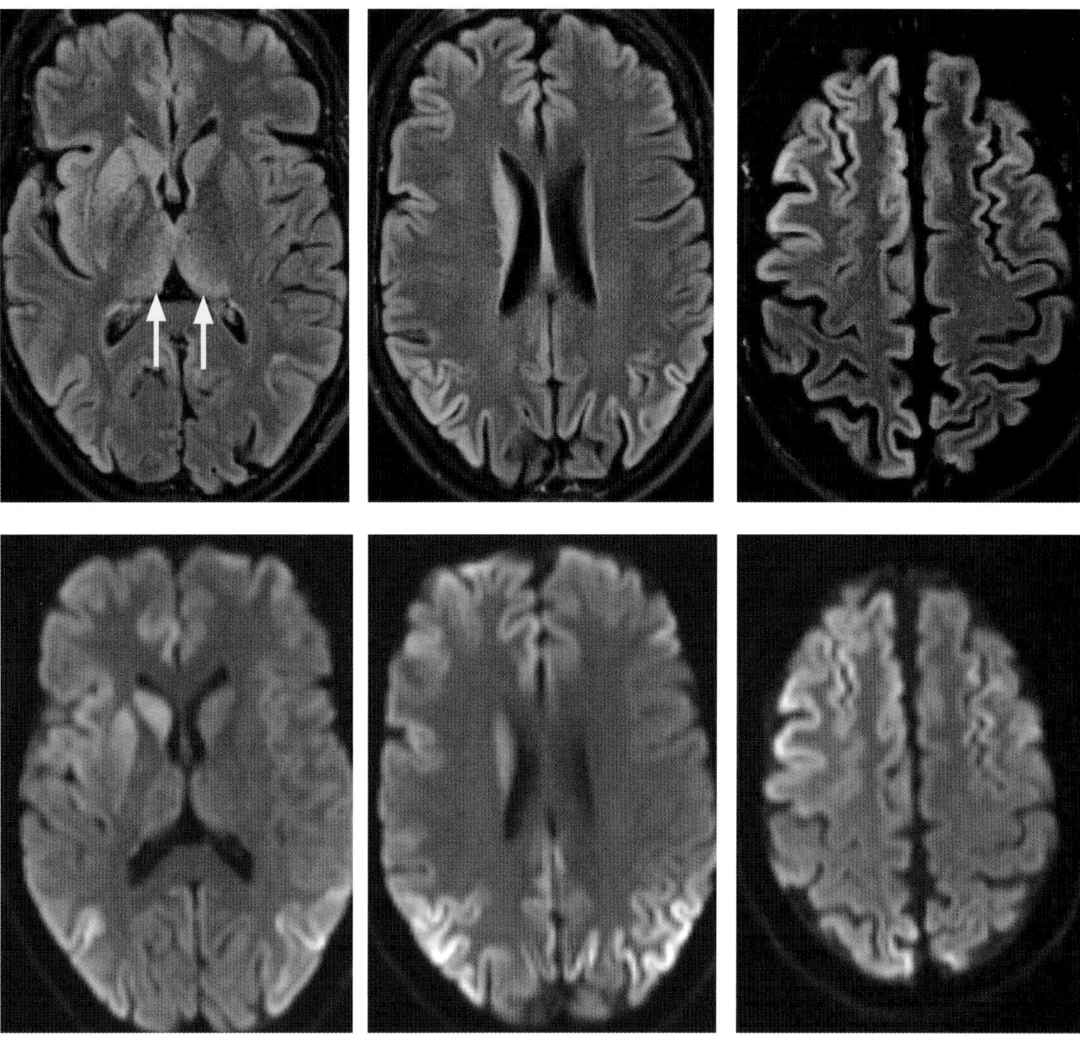

Creutzfeldt–Jakob disease: Axial FLAIR (top row), and DWI (bottom row) show diffusely increased FLAIR signal with restricted diffusion (when correlated to ADC maps, not shown) in the cerebral cortex, basal ganglia, and dorsomedial thalamus. There is relative sparing of the motor cortex (red arrows). A *hockey stick* sign is visible in the thalami on the first FLAIR image (yellow arrows).

Case courtesy Saurab Rohatgi, MD, Brigham and Women's Hospital.

- Creutzfeldt–Jakob disease (CJD) is a rare neurodegenerative disease caused by a prion.
- The typical MRI appearance of CJD is *cortical ribboning*, which describes ribbonlike FLAIR hyperintensity and restricted diffusion of the cerebral cortex. The basal ganglia and thalami are also involved. There is often sparing of the motor cortex.
- The *pulvinar* sign describes bright DWI and FLAIR signal within the pulvinar nucleus of the thalamus. The *hockey stick* sign describes bright DWI and FLAIR signal within the dorsomedial thalamus.

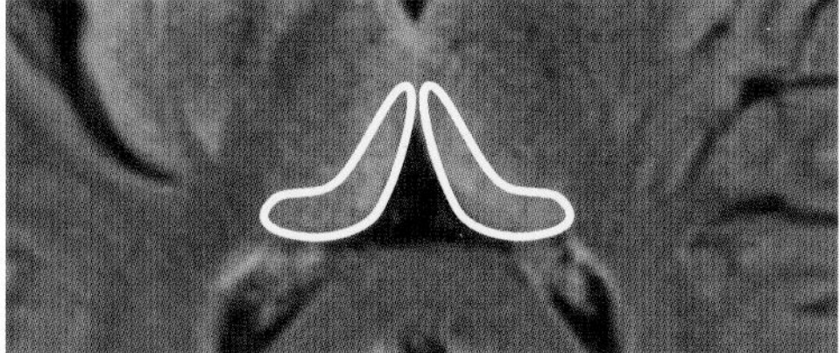

Hockey stick sign of CJD: FLAIR (close-up of top left FLAIR image above with the thalami outlined in yellow) shows hyperintensity of the dorsomedial thalami, mimicking the shape of a hockey stick.

Liver disease

- The classic brain MRI finding in liver disease is hyperintense signal on T1-weighted images in the globus pallidus and substantia nigra, thought to be due to manganese deposition.

Hypoglycemia

- Severe hypoglycemia can show bilateral T2 prolongation in the gray matter, including the cerebral cortex, hippocampi, and basal ganglia.

Hypoxic ischemic encephalopathy (HIE)

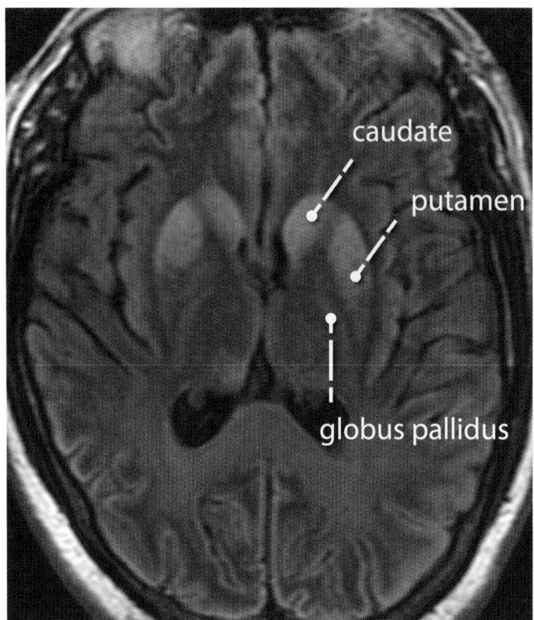

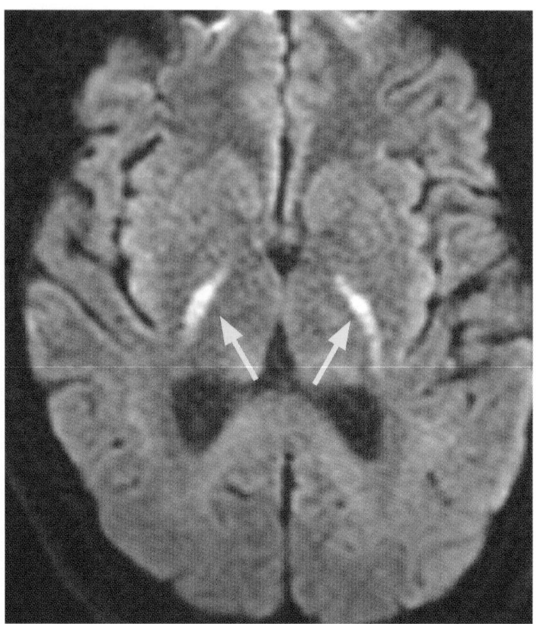

Hypoxic ischemic encephalopathy: Axial FLAIR (left image) shows symmetrical T2 prolongation in the bilateral putamina, heads of the caudate nuclei, and to a lesser extent in the globi pallidi. There is subtle FLAIR hyperintensity of the entire cortical ribbon. DWI (right image) shows marked DWI hyperintensity within the globi pallidi (arrows).

- Hypoxic ischemic encephalopathy (HIE) in adults is caused by circulatory or respiratory failure, leading to global hypoxia/anoxia.
- Severe HIE typically affects the gray matter, including the cerebral cortex, hippocampi, and basal ganglia. This distribution is similar to that of severe hypoglycemia. Involvement of the basal ganglia portends a worse prognosis.
- MR imaging shows FLAIR and/or DWI hyperintensity of the affected regions.
- On CT, there is loss of gray–white differentiation, diffuse cerebral hypoattenuation, and sulcal effacement. The *white cerebellum* sign describes the typical sparing of the cerebellum, which appears relatively hyperattenuating compared to the affected supratentorial brain.

Methanol poisoning

- Methanol poisoning can present with optic neuritis as the first symptom.
- Hemorrhagic necrosis of the putamen and white matter edema may follow.

Carbon monoxide

- Carbon monoxide poisoning typically causes symmetric T2 prolongation and restricted diffusion of the globus pallidus.

ANATOMY

Fascial anatomy of the retropharyngeal space

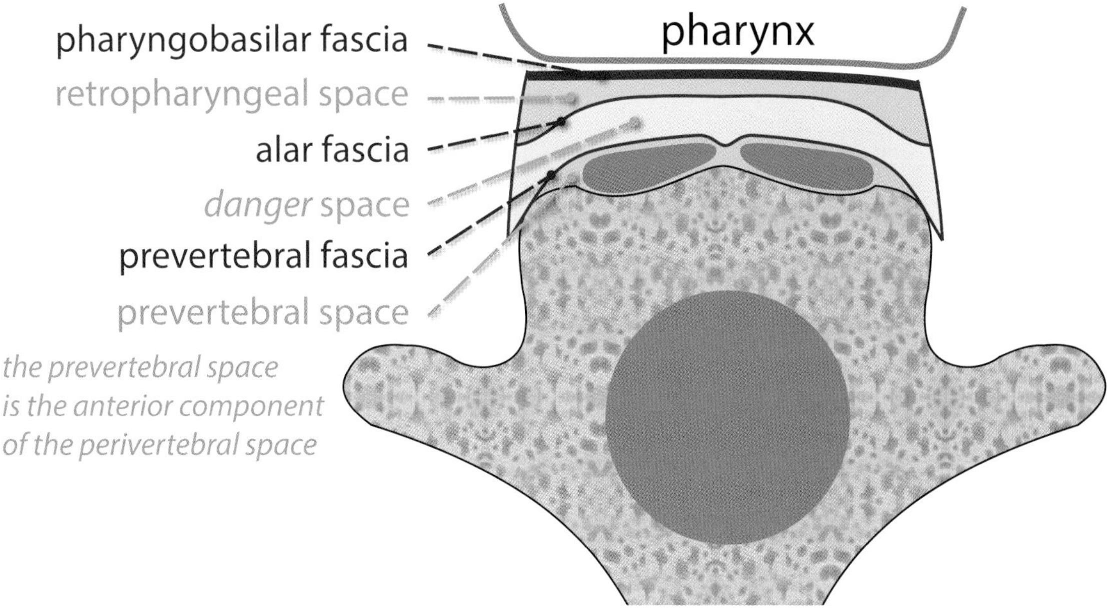

- The **retropharyngeal space** is a potential space located posterior to the pharynx, separated from the pharynx by the pharyngobasilar fascia. The retropharyngeal space extends from the base of the skull to the upper mediastinum. Directly lateral to the retropharyngeal space are the carotid and parapharyngeal spaces.
- The alar fascia is directly posterior to the retropharyngeal space. The alar fascia separates the retropharyngeal space from another potential space, the *danger* space, which acts as a trapdoor for infection to travel all the way from the neck to the diaphragm.
- The prevertebral space (the anterior component of the perivertebral space in the suprahyoid neck) is located just anterior to the vertebral body and is bounded anteriorly by the prevertebral fascia.

Fascial anatomy of the floor of the mouth

- The sublingual space is a potential space located at the base of the tongue, nestled between the genioglossus and geniohyoid muscles medially and the sling of the mylohyoid muscle inferiorly and laterally.
- Directly inferior to the sublingual space is the U-shaped submandibular space. The sublingual space is separated from the submandibular space by the mylohyoid muscle anteriorly, although the sublingual space is contiguous with the submandibular space posteriorly.

NECK INFECTIONS AND INFLAMMATION

Ludwig angina

- Ludwig angina is cellulitis of the floor of the mouth. It is an infection that can involve the submental, sublingual, and submandibular spaces.
- The tongue can rapidly become posteriorly displaced, so ensuring airway patency is a clinical priority.
- On imaging, there is stranding and swelling at the floor of the mouth.

Retropharyngeal abscess

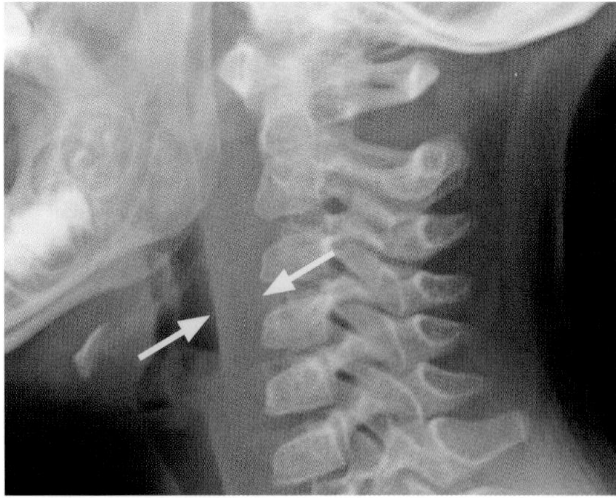

Retropharyngeal abscess: Lateral neck radiograph (top left image) demonstrates marked thickening of the prevertebral tissues (arrows).

Sagittal (bottom left image) and axial contrast-enhanced CT demonstrates a peripherally enhancing fluid collection in the retropharyngeal space (arrows), causing effacement of the right oropharynx.

Case courtesy Mary Beth Cunnane, MD, Massachusetts Eye and Ear Infirmary.

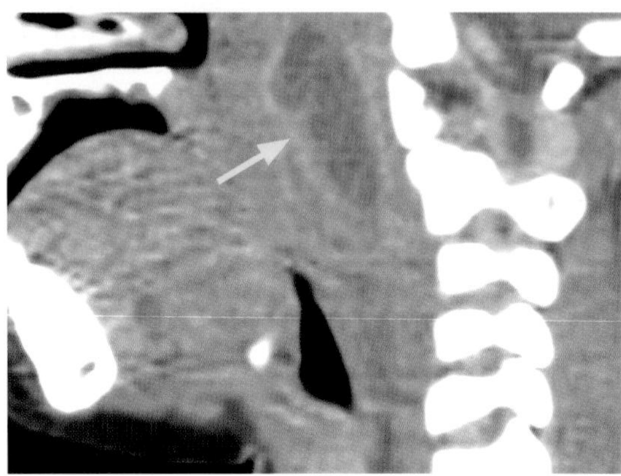

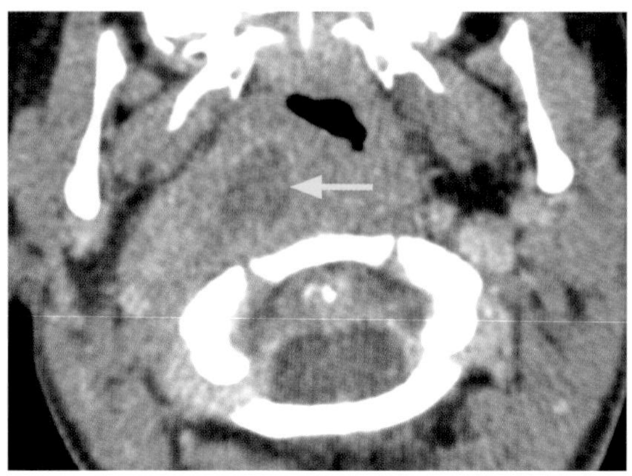

- Retropharyngeal infection may cause airway compromise.
- In children, retropharyngeal infection is most often from spread of an upper respiratory tract infection, such as pharyngitis. Enlargement of retropharyngeal lymph nodes that drain the pharynx may lead to subsequent suppuration and rupture.
- In adults, retropharyngeal infection is most often due to penetrating injury, such as fish bone ingestion or instrumentation.

Peritonsillar abscess

- Peritonsillar abscess is a complication of peritonsillar lymph node suppuration, causing the characteristic *hot-potato* voice.

Lemierre syndrome

- Lemierre syndrome is venous thrombophlebitis of the tonsillar and peritonsillar veins, often with spread to the internal jugular vein. Immunocompetent adolescents and young adults are typically affected.
- The most common infectious agent is the anaerobe *Fusobacterium necrophorum,* which is part of the normal mouth flora.
- Imaging shows enlargement, thrombosis, and mural enhancement of the affected veins.
- Metastatic pulmonary abscesses may be present.

Bezold abscess

- Bezold abscess is a complication of otomastoiditis where there is necrosis of the mastoid tip and resultant spread of infection into the adjacent soft tissue.
- On imaging, there is opacification of the middle ear and mastoid air cells, often with bony erosion of the mastoid.

FLOOR OF MOUTH CYSTIC LESIONS

Ranula

- A ranula is a mucous retention cyst that arises from the sublingual gland as a sequela of inflammation. All ranulas arise from the sublingual gland and hence begin in the sublingual space.
- A plunging ranula extends from the sublingual space into the submandibular space by protruding posteriorly over the free edge of the mylohyoid or by extending directly through a defect in the mylohyoid.
- A dermoid cyst may also present below the mandible, but is typically midline, rather than the eccentric location of a plunging ranula.

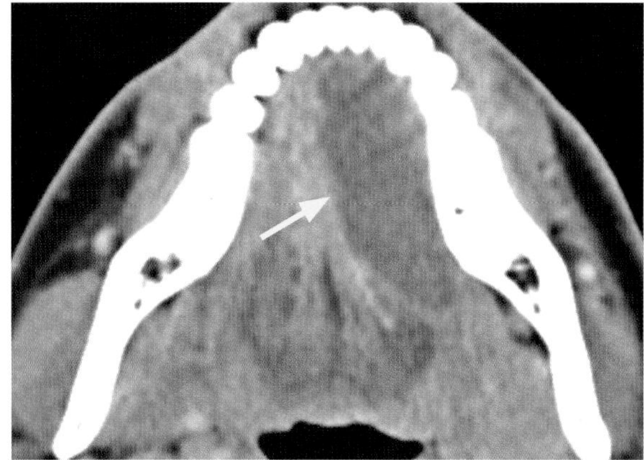

Ranula: Contrast-enhanced axial CT at the level of the mandible shows a cystic lesion (arrow) in the left sublingual space

Dermoid/epidermoid

- A dermoid is a teratomatous lesion that contains at least two germ cell layers, while an epidermoid contains only ectoderm.
- On CT, both dermoid and epidermoid will appear as a fluid-attenuation lesion, most commonly in the midline of the floor of the mouth. A pathognomonic MRI finding of dermoid is the *sack of marbles* appearance from floating fat globules. In the absence of this finding, epidermoid and dermoid can be indistinguishable in this location on MRI.

Thyroglossal duct cyst (TDC)

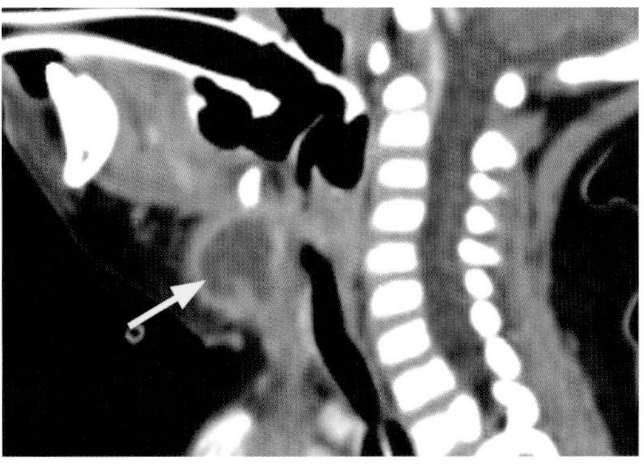

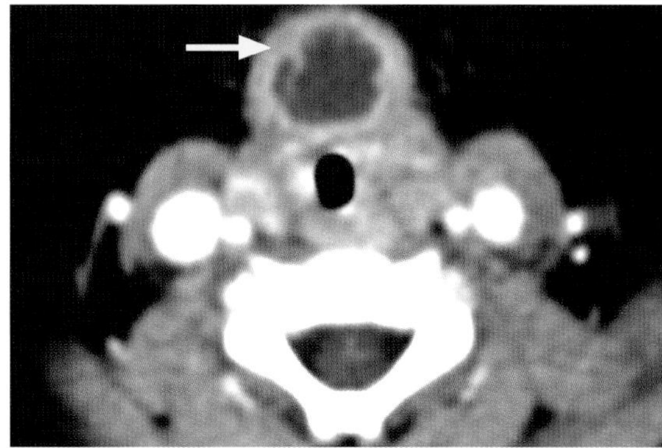

Infected thyroglossal duct cyst: Sagittal (left image) and axial enhanced CT in an intubated 13 month old shows a thick-walled, peripherally enhancing cystic structure (arrows) in the midline, inferior to the mylohyoid.

Case courtesy Mary Beth Cunnane, MD, Massachusetts Eye and Ear Infirmary.

- A thyroglossal duct cyst (TDC) is due to persistence of the thyroglossal duct. The thyroglossal duct follows the midline descent of the embryonic thyroid gland from the base of the tongue (foramen cecum) to its normal position in the neck. Most thyroglossal duct cysts present in childhood as an enlarging neck mass that elevates with tongue protrusion.
- The majority of TDCs (65%) are infrahyoid, the rest found at the level of the hyoid or above. Most TDCs are midline, but they may occur slightly off midline, especially when infrahyoid.
- Thyroid carcinoma (papillary type) is a rare complication seen in 1% of TDCs.

Cystic metastasis

- Papillary thyroid cancer and squamous cell carcinoma from the base of tongue or the tonsils may metastasize to the floor of the mouth region. These metastases tend to be cystic.

Solitary parotid region cystic lesion

First branchial cleft cyst (BCC)

- A first branchial cleft cyst (BCC) is rare and is usually located near the parotid or the external auditory canal.
- A first BCC may appear as a simple cyst; however, imaging is variable and contents may be heterogeneous, especially if superinfected.

Cystic lesions about the mandible

Second branchial cleft cyst

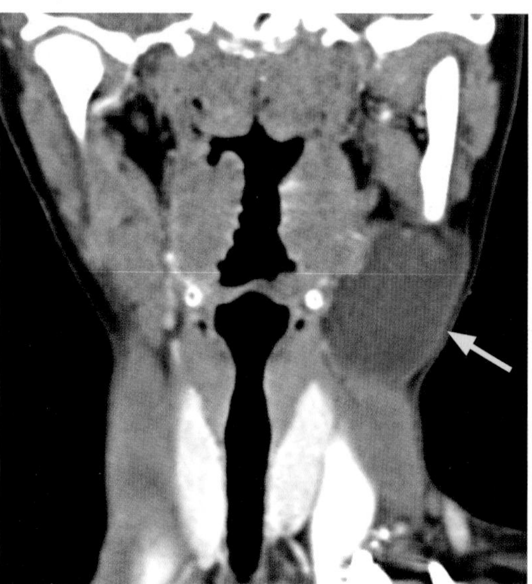
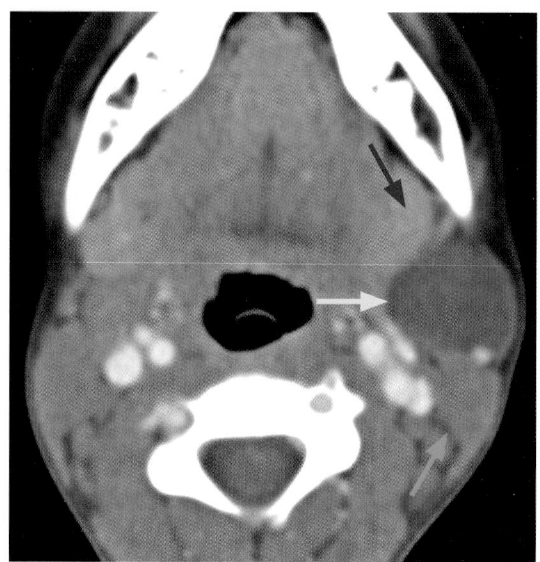

Second branchial cleft cyst: Coronal (left image) and axial contrast-enhanced CT shows a water-attenuation cystic lesion (yellow arrows) at the angle of the left mandible with minimal peripheral wall enhancement. This cyst is in the classic location of a second branchial cleft cyst: posterior to the submandibular gland (red arrow), anterior to the sternocleidomastoid muscle (blue arrow), and closely associated with the carotid sheath.

Case courtesy Mary Beth Cunnane, MD, Massachusetts Eye and Ear Infirmary.

- A branchial cleft cyst (BCC) is a congenital anomaly arising from the embryologic branchial apparatus. There are four types of congenital branchial cleft cysts, with the second type being the most common type.
- A second BCC may occur at any point along the path extending from the palatine tonsil to the supraclavicular region, but most occur near the angle of the mandible.
- The classic location of a second BCC is anterior to the sternocleidomastoid muscle, posterior to the submandibular gland, and closely associated with the carotid bifurcation.
- The cyst may become superinfected. With superinfection, the wall may enhance and there may be inflammatory changes within the surrounding soft tissues.

  Although second BCC has been described as being in the posterior submandibular space, an infected second BCC would not typically be confused with a submandibular abscess. Submandibular abscess is usually due to dental disease and is typically located immediately inferior to the mandible.

- Branchial cleft cysts are uncommon in older adults. A cystic metastasis (e.g., from papillary thyroid cancer or base of tongue/tonsillar squamous cell carcinoma) should be considered instead, especially if the cyst is irregular or has a mural nodule.

Submandibular or masticator abscess

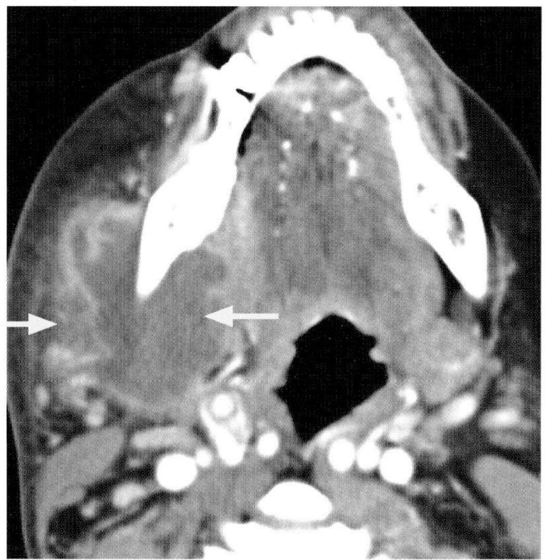

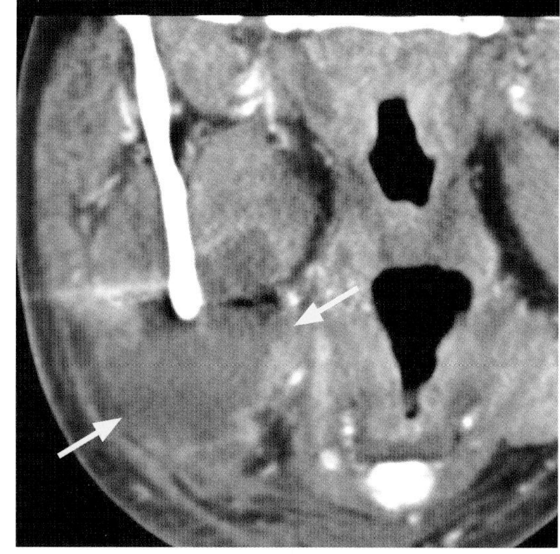

Masticator/submandibular abscess: Axial (left image) and coronal contrast-enhanced CT shows a peripherally enhancing, irregular fluid collection (arrows) abutting the angle of the right mandible, with associated stranding of the subcutaneous fat.

- A submandibular or masticator abscess may arise from dental disease (most commonly), suppurative adenopathy, or spread of adjacent salivary gland infection.
- On imaging, an abscess appears as an irregular, thick-walled, peripherally enhancing fluid collection located inferior to the mandible. Adjacent stranding of the cervical fat is usually present.
- In addition to antibiotics, aspiration is usually a key component of treatment.

Other neck cystic lesions

Lymphatic malformations

- Lymphatic malformations are congenital abnormalities that result when the embryologic lymphatics fail to connect to developing veins. There are three types of lymphatic malformations, classified by the size of the intra-lesional cystic spaces.
- **Cystic hygroma** is the most common type of lymphatic malformation, the majority being present at birth and associated with chromosomal anomalies including Turner and Down syndromes. A cystic hygroma features large lymphatic spaces. The most common location is in the posterior triangle of the neck.
- **Cavernous lymphangioma** has smaller lymphatic spaces than a cystic hygroma, while a **capillary lymphangioma** has the smallest cystic spaces.

Thornwaldt cyst

- A Thornwaldt cyst is a notochordal remnant that is usually asymptomatic, but may be a cause of halitosis. The typical location of a Thornwaldt cyst is in the midline nasopharynx.

Miscellaneous neck lesions

Lingual thyroid

- Lingual thyroid is ectopic thyroid tissue that has incompletely descended during embryologic development and remains at the floor of the mouth. Usually, the ectopic gland is the only functioning thyroid tissue, so the neck should be evaluated to confirm lack of normal gland.
- Lingual thyroid is much more common in females.
- Lingual thyroid is susceptible to standard thyroid pathology, including thyroiditis and cancer.

Larynx

Overview and anatomy

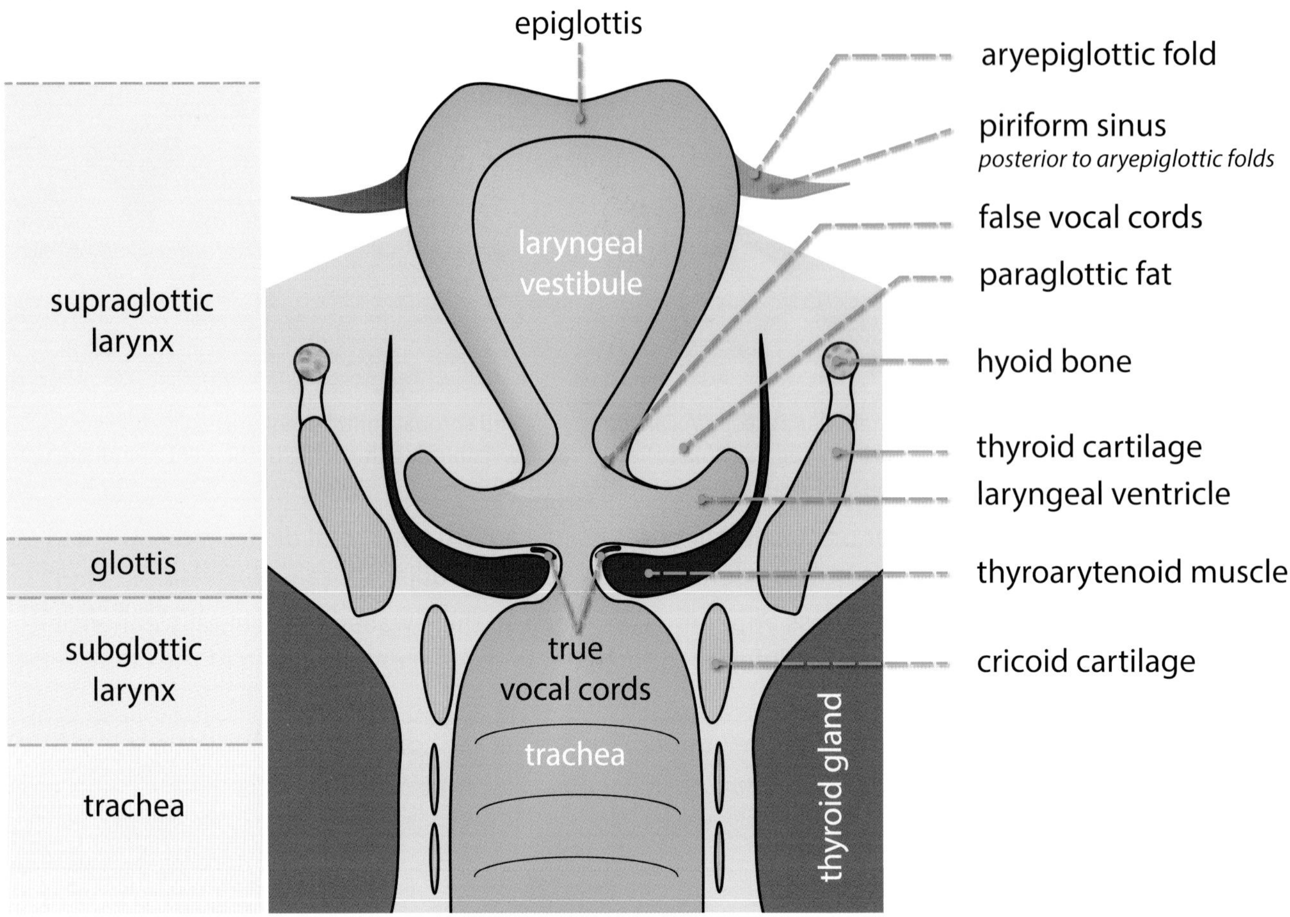

- The larynx is a fibrocartilaginous tube that extends from the skull base to the esophagus.
- The cartilaginous components of the larynx include the epiglottis, thyroid cartilage, cricoid cartilage, and arytenoids.

  The cricoid cartilage is a complete ring that provides support for the larynx.
- The entire larynx, including the epiglottis, aryepiglottic folds and false vocal cords, is lined with mucosa.

  The aryepiglottic folds are an extension of the mucosa covering the epiglottis and mark the entrance to the larynx. The aryepiglottic folds connect the epiglottis anteriorly to the arytenoids posteriorly.

  The false vocal folds are mucosal infoldings superior to the laryngeal ventricle. They can be identified on cross-sectional imaging by the presence of the paraglottic fat laterally.
- The **supraglottic larynx** extends from the epiglottis to the ventricle. The false vocal cords, the aryepiglottic folds, and the arytenoid cartilages are within the supraglottic larynx.
- The **glottis** includes the true vocal cords and the thyroarytenoid muscle. The medial fibers of the thyroarytenoid muscle comprise the vocalis muscle.

  The true vocal cords are identified in the axial plane on CT or MRI by identifying the transition of paraglottic fat to muscle (thyroarytenoid muscle) within the wall of the larynx.
- The **subglottic larynx** begins 1 cm inferior to the apex of the laryngeal ventricles and extends to the first tracheal ring.

Vocal cord paralysis

- Vocal cord paralysis is most commonly due to iatrogenic trauma from neck surgery, but may be secondary to a mass lesion along the course of the vagus or recurrent laryngeal nerves.

  The most common mass lesion to cause vocal cord paralysis is a mediastinal or thoracic mass; however, enlargement of the left atrium or pulmonary arteries may cause *cardiovocal* syndrome due to recurrent laryngeal nerve compression.

- The CT imaging of vocal cord paralysis shows a thickened, medialized aryepiglottic fold and enlargement of the piriform sinus on the affected side.
- The left recurrent laryngeal nerve is the most commonly affected nerve. Imaging for vocal cord paralysis should extend from the skull base to the level of the left pulmonary artery to cover the full course of the vagus and the left recurrent laryngeal nerves.

  The recurrent laryngeal nerve innervates all laryngeal musculature except the cricothyroid muscle, which is innervated by the superior laryngeal nerve.

Laryngocele

- A laryngocele is dilation of the laryngeal ventricle, which may be caused by high laryngeal pressures. Trumpet players, glassblowers, and patients with COPD have increased risk of developing a laryngocele. A laryngocele may be filled with air or fluid.
- An important differential consideration is ventricular obstruction by neoplasm (most commonly squamous cell carcinoma), which typically causes a fluid-filled laryngocele.

Laryngeal cancer

- The vast majority of laryngeal tumors are squamous cells of the mucosa, which are typically accessible to the otolaryngologist for direct visualization and biopsy.

  Less common tumors of the larynx (such as lymphoma and chondrosarcoma) may be submucosal and therefore not visible on laryngoscopic exam.

- The role of the radiologist in the workup of laryngeal cancer is not to offer a differential diagnosis, but to determine the extent of disease.
- The most important imaging determination is if a tumor is supraglottic, glottic, or subglottic.

  30% of tumors are supraglottic. 65% of tumors are glottic. Only 5% of tumors are subglottic.

  A transglottic tumor is usually defined as a tumor that crosses the laryngeal ventricle to involve both the false and true vocal cords, although the exact definition of a transglottic tumor varies between authors. The presence of a tranglottic tumor has important treatment implications.

- A small isolated supraglottic or glottic tumor can be treated with laser resection and preservation of laryngeal integrity. In contrast to the more superiorly located tumors, even a small subglottic or transglottic tumor requires a total laryngectomy, which is an extremely morbid surgery.

Laryngeal trauma

- Blunt trauma to the neck may compress the larynx against the cervical spine. The thyroid cartilage and cricoid cartilage are susceptible to fracture, which may be difficult to detect in young patients with incomplete ossification of these structures.
- Laryngeal trauma may also result from intubation, which can cause arytenoid dislocation.

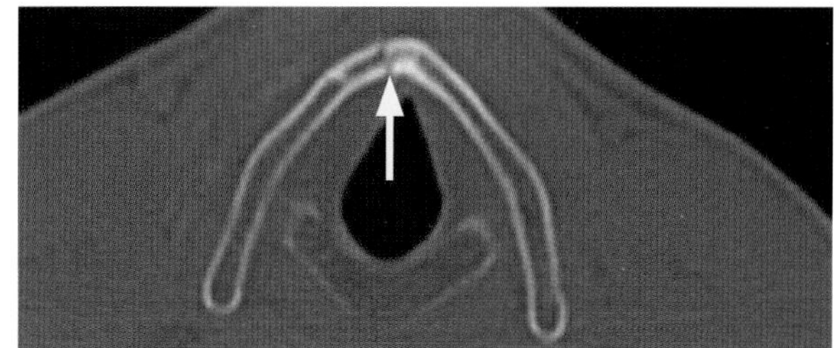

Thyroid cartilage fracture: CT in bone windows demonstrates a minimally displaced fracture of the thyroid cartilage (arrow).

Case courtesy Mary Beth Cunnane, MD, Massachusetts Eye and Ear Infirmary.

ANATOMY OF THE PARANASAL SINUSES

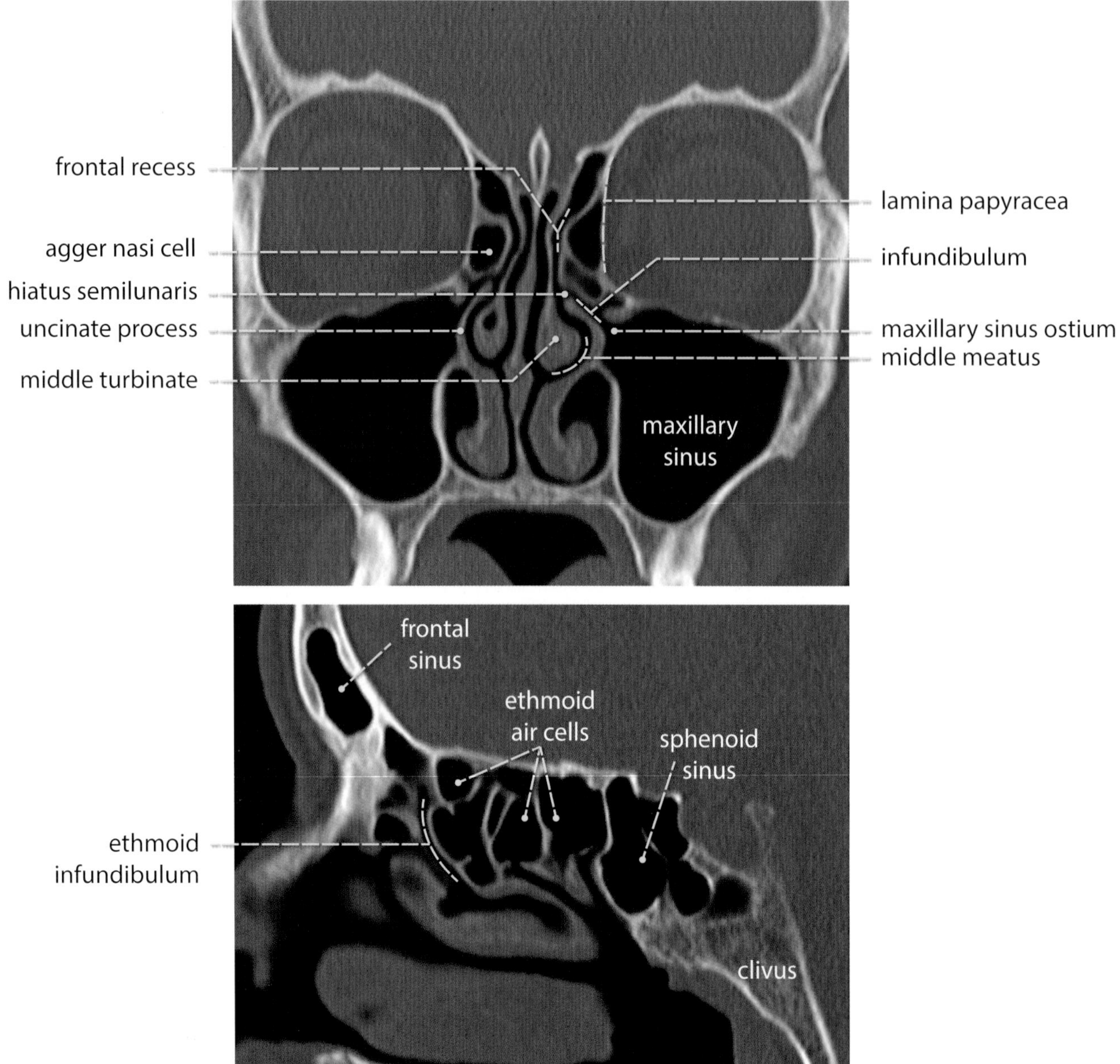

Sinus anatomy and mucosal drainage

- The sinuses are lined with ciliary mucosa that propels secretions through the drainage pathways. Each pathway should be carefully evaluated on a sinus CT.
- The ostiomeatal unit (OMU) is the common drainage pathway for the maxillary, frontal, and anterior ethmoid sinuses, which all drain into the middle meatus. Several air passages and a single bony structure (the uncinate process) make up the OMU, which is comprised of the maxillary sinus ostium, infundibulum, uncinate process, hiatus semilunaris, ethmoid bulla, and middle meatus. Some authors include the frontal recess as part of the OMU.

- Isolated sinus disease of the maxillary sinus is most likely due to obstruction of the maxillary sinus ostium or infundibulum, while sinus disease affecting the maxillary, frontal, and anterior ethmoid sinuses is most likely due to obstruction of the hiatus semilunaris.
- The maxillary sinus is the largest sinus and drains via ciliary action through the superiorly located maxillary sinus ostium.
- The ethmoid sinus is comprised of multiple small air cells, divided into anterior and posterior divisions. The basal lamella demarcates the boundary between the anterior and posterior ethmoids. The lateral wall of the ethmoid sinus is the lamina papyracea, a thin bone separating the ethmoid sinus from the orbit.

> The **anterior ethmoids** drain via the frontal recess into the **middle meatus** (via the OMU).
>
> The **posterior ethmoids** drain via tiny ostia underneath the superior turbinate into the **superior meatus**.

- The frontal sinus is absent at birth and represents an enlarged anterior ethmoid cell. The frontal sinus drains into the ethmoid infundibulum via the frontal recess.
- The sphenoid sinus drains into the ethmoid cells via the sphenoethmoidal recess. Subsequently, the posterior ethmoid cells drain into the superior meatus via individual unnamed ostia.

Turbinates and meatuses

- The turbinates are three paired bony protuberances within the nasal cavity.
- The superior meatus is adjacent to the superior turbinate. The posterior ethmoids and sphenoid sinus (via the sphenoethmoidal recess) drain into the superior meatus.
- The middle meatus is the air channel lateral to the middle turbinate and is the common drainage pathway of the maxillary, frontal, and anterior ethmoid sinuses via the OMU.
- The inferior meatus is just inferior to the inferior turbinate and is the drainage pathway of the lacrimal duct.

Presurgical evaluation of chronic sinusitis

- Chronic sinusitis is thought to be caused by obstruction of the normal drainage pathways. The goal of functional endoscopic sinus surgery (FESS) is to relieve the obstruction.
- It is essential to report certain anatomic variations that may lead to surgical complications if the surgeon is unaware of them.
- A **dehiscent lamina papyracea** appears on imaging as a medial bulging of the orbit. If the surgeon does not know about this, the orbit may be entered by accident.
- Similarly, a **dehiscent cribriform plate** may produce inferior bulging of the frontal lobe, which can be entered by mistake at endoscopic surgery.

Imaging of the sinuses

- CT is the primary modality for imaging the sinuses.
- A low mA CT technique has a similar radiation dose to a standard four-view radiographic series, and therefore, there is no role for radiography in the evaluation of sinus disease.
- MRI is not typically used in the evaluation of routine sinus disease. The MRI imaging of sinus secretions is complex, with varying signal intensities on T1- and T2-weighted images depending on the chronicity. It is possible for desiccated secretions to show low signal on T2-weighted images that could even be mistaken for normal, while CT would clearly show the fully opacified sinus. MRI does play a limited role in evaluating for suspected complications of sinusitis, such as osteomyelitis.

Named air cells

Agger nasi cell

- The agger nasi (Latin for nasal mound) cell is the most anterior ethmoid air cell. A large agger nasi cell may cause obstruction of the frontal recess.

Haller cell

- A Haller cell is an ethmoid cell located inferior to the orbit, which may compromise the maxillary ostium if the Haller cell becomes large or inflamed.

Onodi cell

- An Onodi cell is the most posterosuperior ethmoid air cell, which is located directly inferomedial to the optic nerve. An Onodi cell may be mistaken for the sphenoid sinus endoscopically, potentially placing the optic nerve at risk.

Concha bullosa

- Concha bullosa is formed when the inferior bulbous portion of the middle turbinate is pneumatized. A concha bullosa is usually incidental, but may cause septal deviation and narrowing of the infundibulum when large.

Sinonasal disease

Acute sinusitis

- Acute sinusitis is infection or inflammation of the paranasal sinuses and is a clinical diagnosis. Imaging is indicated only if a complication of sinusitis is suspected
- An air–fluid level may represent acute sinusitis, but is nonspecific. Sinus mucosal thickening most commonly represents chronic sinusitis, but can also be seen in acute sinusitis.

Chronic sinusitis

- Chronic sinusitis is inflammation of the paranasal sinus mucosa that lasts for at least 12 consecutive weeks. It is an extremely common disease, affecting more than 30 million people annually in the US.
- Similar to acute sinusitis, chronic sinusitis is a clinical diagnosis, with imaging reserved for presurgical planning or to evaluate for suspected complications.
- Chronic sinusitis is thought to be caused by obstruction of the normal drainage pathways, and the goal of functional endoscopic sinus surgery (FESS) is to relieve the obstructing lesion.

Orbital complications of sinusitis

- Direct spread of infection from the sinuses to the orbit may cause subperiosteal abscess, orbital cellulitis, or ophthalmic vein thrombosis.

Intracranial complications of sinusitis

- Direct spread of infection into the cranial cavity can cause cavernous sinus thrombosis, meningitis, or abscess. Intracranial abscesses secondary to sinusitis may be epidural, subdural, or intraparenchymal.

Bony complications of sinusitis

- Chronic inflammation of the mucoperiosteum may cause periostitis and osteomyelitis.
- Osteomyelitis of the frontal bone may cause a subgaleal abscess with associated soft-tissue edema, which is called *Pott's puffy tumor.*

Mucus retention cyst

- A mucus retention cyst is a common incidental finding representing obstruction of the small mucosal serous or mucinous glands.

Chronic allergic fungal sinusitis

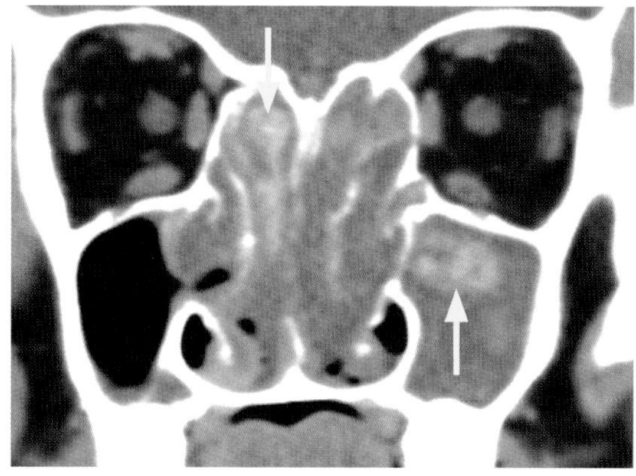
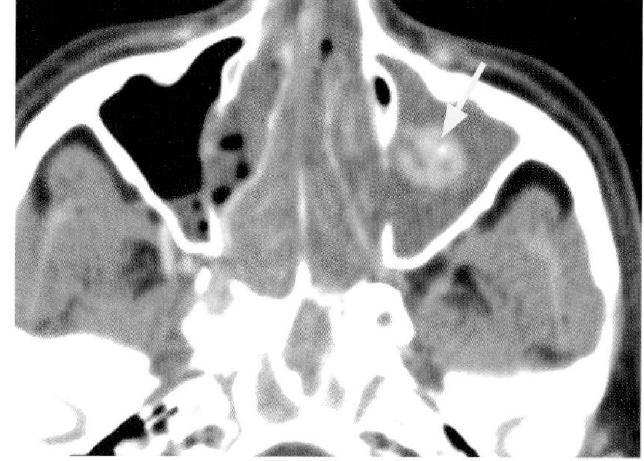

Allergic fungal sinusitis: Coronal (left image) and axial noncontrast CT shows marked pan-sinus disease with curvilinear hyperattenuation in the affected sinuses (arrows). There is erosion of the ethmoid sinus walls.

Case courtesy Mary Beth Cunnane, MD, Massachusetts Eye and Ear Infirmary.

- Chronic allergic fungal sinusitis is a noninvasive disease caused by a hypersensitivity reaction to fungi. Most patients with allergic fungal sinusitis are immunocompetent but have a history of asthma.
- On imaging, the affected sinus is expanded and airless, with thin deossified walls. The sinus contents are typically mixed attenuation with heterogeneous curvilinear high attenuation.

Acute invasive fungal sinusitis

- Acute invasive fungal sinusitis is an aggressive infection that occurs in immunosuppressed patients. *Aspergillus* and *Zygomycetes* are the most common organisms. In particular, *Aspergillus* can cause acute fulminant disease.
- The imaging of early invasive fungal sinusitis shows nonspecific sinus mucosal thickening. Later in the disease process there is often local invasion, bony destruction, and intracranial and intraorbital spread.
- Unlike chronic allergic fungal sinusitis, invasive fungal sinusitis is not hyperdense on CT.

Antrochoanal polyp

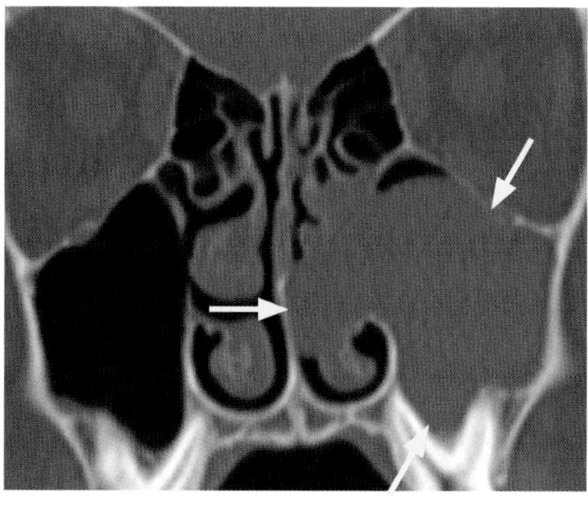
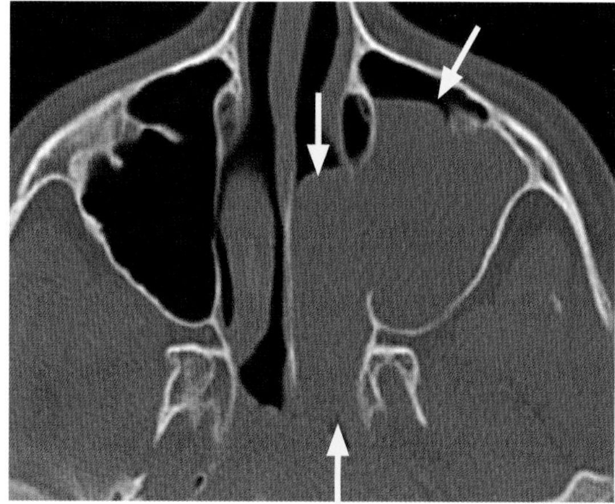

Antrochoanal polyp: Coronal (left image) and axial non-contrast CT show a polypoid lesion (arrows) involving the left maxillary sinus and nasopharynx, with erosion of the middle turbinate and medial wall of the maxillary sinus.

Case courtesy Mary Beth Cunnane, MD, Massachusetts Eye and Ear Infirmary.

- An antrochoanal polyp is a benign polyp extending from the maxillary sinus into the nasal cavity, with characteristic widening of involved ostium. It may erode bone and extend into the nasopharynx. Complete resection is necessary to prevent recurrence.

Mucocele

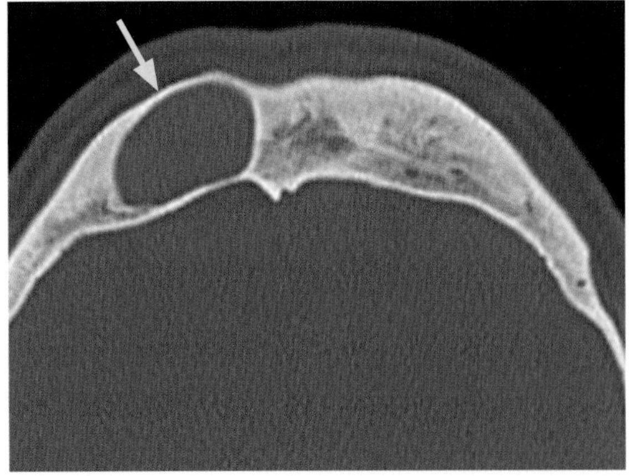

Mucocele of the frontal sinus: Axial non-contrast CT shows an expanded, fluid-filled right frontal sinus (arrow) with thinning of the sinus walls. Incidentally, the left frontal sinus is congenitally absent.

Case courtesy Mary Beth Cunnane, MD, Massachusetts Eye and Ear Infirmary.

- A mucocele is an expanded airless sinus that results from obstruction of the sinus ostia.
- Mucocele may be secondary to inflammatory sinus disease (most commonly) or tumor.
- On imaging, there is thinning of the sinus walls. The contents of the sinus tend to be homogeneous on CT and MR; however, the MRI signal intensity is variable depending on the degree of desiccation of the sinus contents. Specifically, with increasing chronicity, signal increases on T1-weighted images and decreases on T2-weighted images. In late disease, there can be markedly reduced signal on T2-weighted images that may actually simulate a normal air-filled sinus, so it's important to always look at all sequences.

Inverted papilloma

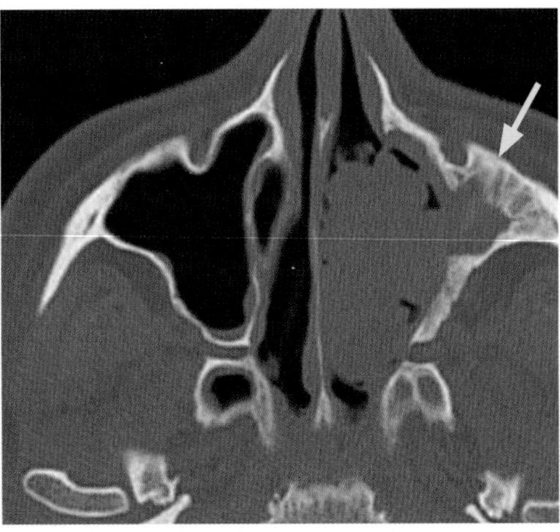

Inverted papilloma: Axial non-contrast CT shows a polypoid lesion of the left maxillary sinus with erosion of the medial wall of the maxillary sinus, the ethmoid air cells, and the turbinates. The sinus is not expanded. There is reactive bony sclerosis of the lateral wall of the maxillary sinus (arrow).

Case courtesy Mary Beth Cunnane, MD, Massachusetts Eye and Ear Infirmary.

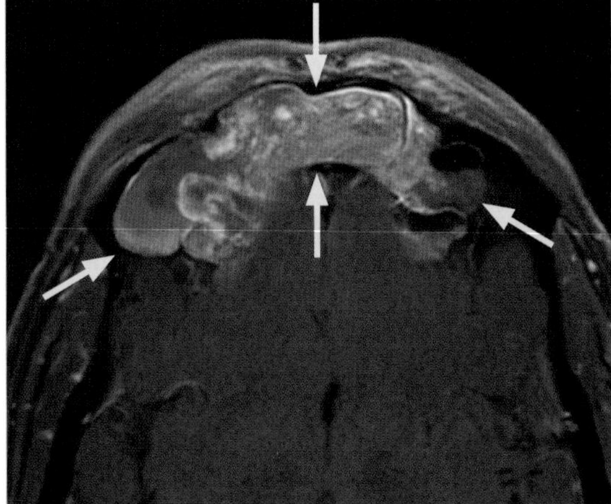

Inverted papilloma in a different patient: Axial contrast-enhanced T1-weighted MRI with fat suppression shows a lobulated extra-axial mass (arrows) arising from the frontal sinus. The mass demonstrates characteristic *cerebriform* enhancement.

Case courtesy Gregory Wrubel, MD, Brigham and Women's Hospital.

- An inverted papilloma is a benign lobulated epithelial tumor of the sinus mucosa; however, it can be associated with squamous cell carcinoma 10–20% of the time.
- The classic imaging finding on an enhanced study is a *cerebriform* pattern of enhancement, which describes curvilinear, gyriform enhancement. In contrast to a mucocele or obstructed secretions, the entire solid tumor will enhance. The tumor tends to remodel bone.
- Treatment is surgical resection and recurrences occur in approximately 15%.

Salivary glands

Anatomy of the salivary glands

- The parotid, submandibular, and sublingual glands are the major salivary glands. There are also numerous unnamed minor salivary glands in the head, neck, and trachea.

Parotid glands

- The parotid glands are the largest salivary glands. Each parotid gland is divided into superficial and deep lobes, although there is no fascial demarcation between these lobes.

  Surgeons use the facial nerve as the demarcation between the superficial and deep lobes.

  Since the facial nerve is not normally visible on imaging, radiologists use the retromandibular vein as the demarcation.
- The main parotid duct is known as Stensen's duct.
- During embryological development, the parotid gland is the last major salivary gland to become encapsulated, and is therefore the only salivary gland that contains intrinsic lymphoid tissue.
- The facial nerve exits the skull at the stylomastoid foramen and subsequently passes anterior to the posterior belly of the digastric and lateral to the styloid process before entering the parotid gland.

Submandibular gland

- The paired submandibular glands sit partly in the floor of the mouth, and partly in the neck. Each gland wraps around the free posterior margin of the mylohyoid muscle, which separates the floor of the mouth from the neck.

Sublingual gland

- The sublingual glands are the smallest major salivary glands. Each gland sits medial to the mandible at the anterior aspect of the floor of the mouth.

Minor salivary glands

- There are numerous tiny minor salivary glands spread throughout the mucosa of the paranasal sinuses, oral and nasal cavities, nasopharynx, and trachea.
- Normally, minor salivary glands are not seen on imaging; however, occasionally a neoplasm may arise from one of these normally invisible glands.
- The most common minor salivary gland tumor is the benign pleomorphic adenoma; however, a tumor of minor salivary gland origin is much more likely to be malignant than a tumor arising from the submandibular or parotid glands.

Pleomorphic adenoma

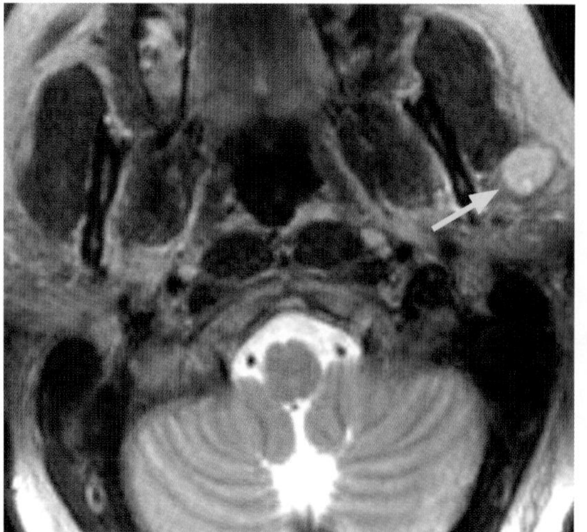

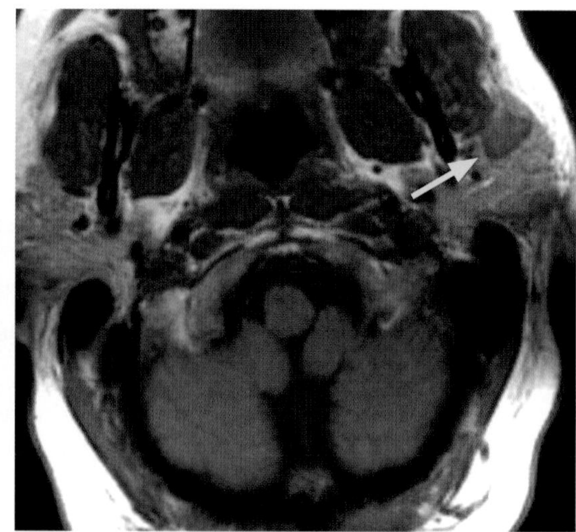

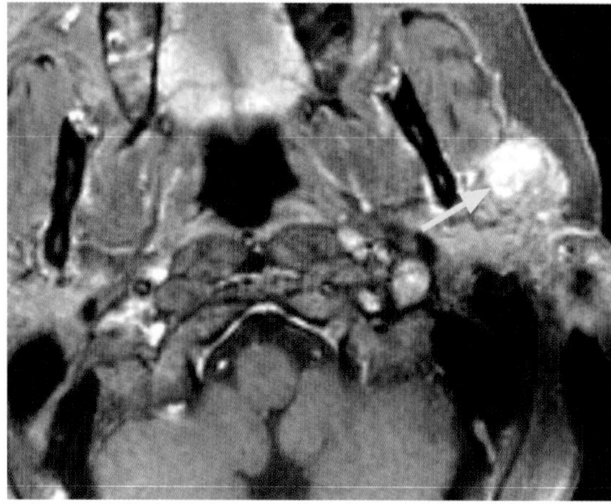

Pleomorphic adenoma: Axial T2-weighted (top left image), T1-weighted (top right image), and post-contrast fat saturated T1-weighted (bottom left image) MRI shows a T2 hyperintense, T1 hypointense, enhancing circumscribed mass (arrows) in the anterior aspect of the superficial left parotid.

Case courtesy Mary Beth Cunnane, MD, Massachusetts Eye and Ear Infirmary.

- Pleomorphic adenoma is by far the most common parotid tumor, accounting for 80% of all parotid tumors. The tumor typically presents as a small firm mass in a middle-aged patient. There is a slight female predominance.
- Although pleomorphic adenoma is benign, complete surgical resection is the standard treatment. Left unexcised, the tumors can continue to grow, and there is an increasing risk for malignant transformation to *carcinoma ex pleomorphic adenoma.* Additionally, it is not possible to distinguish between benign pleomorphic adenoma and malignant mucoepidermoid carcinoma by imaging alone.
- During surgery, the capsule of the tumor must be preserved to prevent diffuse tumor seeding.
- CT is insensitive for detecting a small parotid tumor, so MRI is preferred. The T1 and T2 characteristics of a pleomorphic adenoma are similar to water. Unlike a simple cyst, however, enhancement is typical for pleomorphic adenoma.

Warthin tumor

- Warthin tumor is the second most common benign parotid tumor, accounting for 10% of all parotid tumors. Up to 15% are bilateral and the typical patient is an elderly male. Smoking is a risk factor. Unlike pleomorphic adenoma, there is no risk of malignant transformation.
- Warthin tumor generally appears as a cystic neoplasm. Unlike pleomorphic adenoma, Warthin tumor does not enhance.

Malignant parotid neoplasm

Mucoepidermoid carcinoma

- Mucoepidermoid carcinoma is relatively uncommon (accounting for approximately 5% of all parotid tumors), but it is the most common primary parotid malignancy.
- Low-grade mucoepidermoid carcinoma typically appears as an enhancing mass that is hyperintense on T2-weighted images. This appearance is indistinguishable from benign pleomorphic adenoma on MRI.
- Treatment is surgical resection.

Adenoid cystic carcinoma

- Adenoid cystic carcinoma is the most common submandibular and sublingual gland malignancy and the second most common parotid gland malignancy.
- Adenoid cystic carcinoma has a tendency to spread along the nerves (perineural spread) and often presents with cranial nerve palsy or paresthesia.
- Adenoid cystic carcinoma has a very high risk of local recurrence.
- Metastatic disease is frequently present (in up to 50%). Even with a large metastatic burden, however, patients may survive for several years.
- The key imaging feature suggestive of adenoid cystic carcinoma is an enhancing mass with perineural spread.

Carcinoma ex pleomorphic adenoma

- A benign pleomorphic adenoma has a 1.5% risk of malignant degeneration during the first 5 years. That risk increases to 9.5% in tumors present for 15 years.
- Carcinoma ex pleomorphic adenoma tends to affect elderly patients, with the classic clinical presentation of rapid enlargement of an existing mass.
- In contrast to benign pleomorphic adenoma, malignant carcinoma ex pleomorphic adenoma is hypointense on both T1- and T2-weighted images.

Squamous cell carcinoma

- Primary squamous cell carcinoma of the parotid gland is very rare, as there are normally no squamous epithelial cells within the parotid. Chronic inflammation, however, can induce squamous metaplasia.
- Imaging demonstrates an aggressive, large mass, often with nodal metastases.

Inflammatory salivary disease

Sialolithiasis and obstructive sialadenitis

- Sialolithiasis (stone disease of the salivary ducts) can cause obstruction of the duct and resultant inflammation of the salivary gland, referred to as obstructive sialadenitis.
- The vast majority of salivary calculi (80–90%) occur in the mucus-producing submandibular gland, due to its relatively viscous and alkaline secretions. Additionally, the submandibular duct has an uphill course, which predisposes to stasis.

Sarcoidosis

- Involvement of the parotid gland is seen in up to 30% of patients with sarcoidosis, typically presenting as bilateral painless swelling.
- Uveoparotid fever, which presents with bilateral uveitis, parotid enlargement, and facial nerve palsy, is considered pathognomonic for sarcoidosis.
- Gallium-67 scintigraphy produces the classic *panda* sign from increased uptake by the lacrimal and parotid glands.

Sjögren syndrome

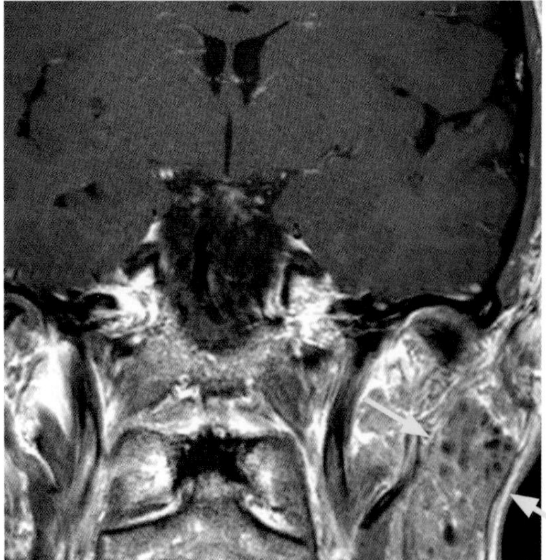

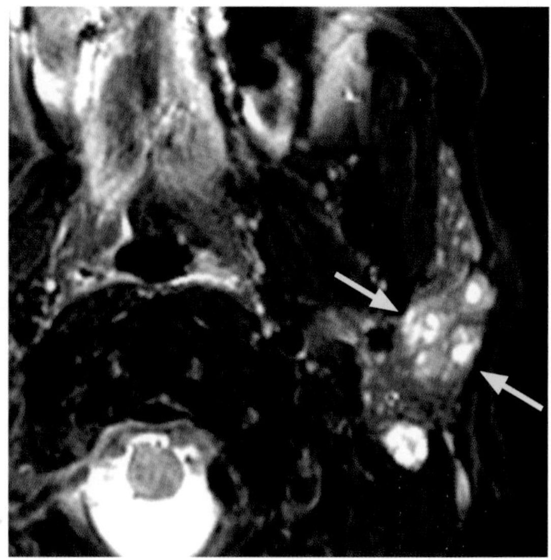

Sjögren syndrome: Coronal post-contrast T1-weighted (left image) and axial T2-weighted MRI with fat suppression shows numerous small, T2 hyperintense lesions in the left parotid (arrows), which demonstrate minimal peripheral enhancement.

Case courtesy Mary Beth Cunnane, MD, Massachusetts Eye and Ear Infirmary.

- Sjögren syndrome is an autoimmune disorder that affects the major and minor salivary glands as well as the lacrimal glands. When secondary to a systemic connective tissue disorder such as rheumatoid arthritis, the disease is referred to as secondary Sjögren syndrome. When only the salivary and lacrimal glands are affected, the disease is called primary Sjögren syndrome.
- Sjögren syndrome typically affects middle-aged females.
- On imaging, there is atrophy and fatty replacement of the salivary glandular tissue, with multiple nodules, abnormal enhancement, numerous small cystic foci, and punctate calcification.
- The risk of parotid and head and neck lymphoma is markedly increased in patients with Sjögren syndrome. Any new dominant parotid mass in the setting of Sjögren syndrome should raise concern for lymphoma.

HIV lymphoepithelial lesions

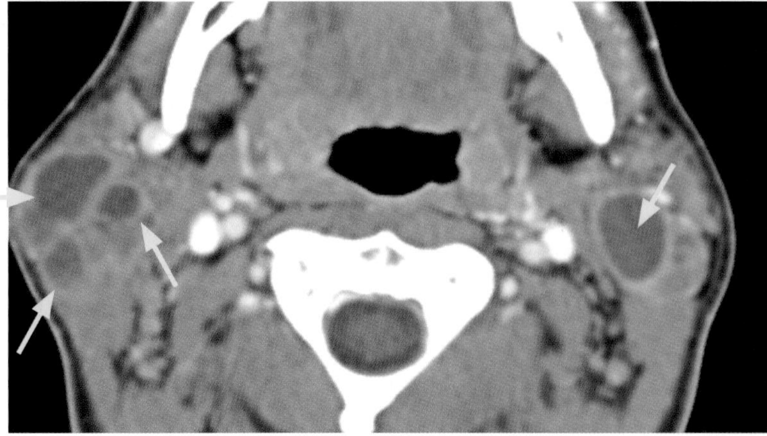

HIV lymphoepithelial lesions: Axial contrast-enhanced CT through the parotid glands shows numerous peripherally enhancing cystic lesions bilaterally (arrows).

Case courtesy Mary Beth Cunnane, MD, Massachusetts Eye and Ear Infirmary.

- Patients with HIV frequently have parotid manifestations of lymphoid dysfunction, including multiple bilateral lymphoepithelial cysts and solid masses.
- The parotid glands are the only salivary glands containing intrinsic lymphoid tissue. Therefore, only the parotid glands are affected in patients with lymphoepithelial lesions.

ANATOMY

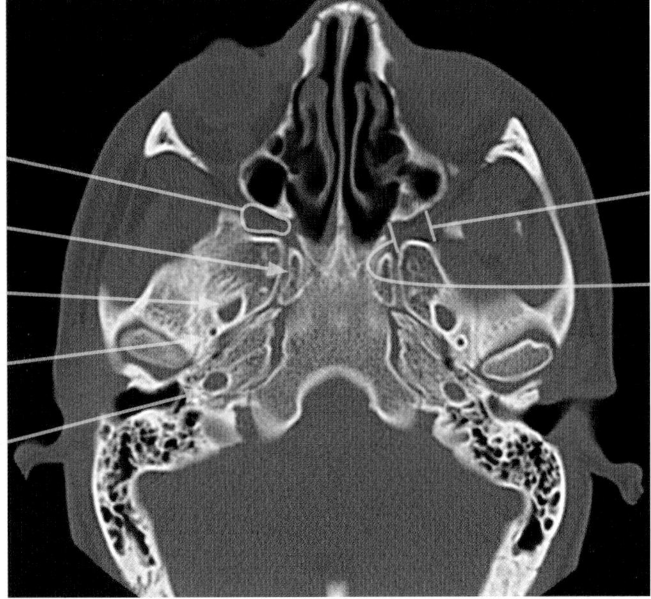

Anatomy of the pterygopalatine fossa

- The pterygopalatine fossa is the bridge between the face and the brain, and is an important potential pathway for the spread of tumor or infection.
- The pterygopalatine fossa sits directly posterior to the maxillary sinus and inferior to the inferior orbital fissure. It can be thought of as a three-dimensional box with each of the six sides leading to important structures in the face.
- The pterygopalatine fossa should contain symmetric fat and soft tissue. Asymmetry in the pterygopalatine fossa should raise concern for a mass, such as lymphoma or perineural spread of a salivary tumor (e.g., adenoid cystic carcinoma).
- The contents of the pterygopalatine fossa are the pterygopalatine ganglion and branches of the internal maxillary artery.

Foramina of the pterygopalatine fossa and central skull base

- The **pterygomaxillary fissure** is the lateral exit of the pterygopalatine fossa, which leads into the masticator space.
- The **sphenopalatine foramen** is the medial exit of the pterygopalatine fossa. It leads into the nasopharynx via the superior meatus. The nasal margin of the sphenopalatine foramen is thought to be the site of origin of juvenile nasopharyngeal angiofibroma.
- **Foramen rotundum** is the posterior opening to the middle cranial fossa. Cranial nerve V2 travels through foramen rotundum.
- The **inferior orbital fissure** is the "roof" of the pterygopalatine fossa and opens anteriorly into the orbit. The infraorbital nerve and artery travel through the inferior orbital fissure.
- The **vidian canal** is located directly below foramen rotundum. It contains the vidian nerve and vidian artery, also known as the nerve and artery of the pterygoid canal.
- The **pterygopalatine canal** is the "floor" of the pterygopalatine fossa, which leads to the oral cavity via the greater and lesser palatine foramina. The pterygopalatine canal transmits the descending palatine nerve and artery.

- The anterior skull base divides the anterior cranial fossa superiorly from the paranasal sinuses and orbits inferiorly.
- The cribriform plate of the ethmoid bone is the roof of the nasal cavity.

Benign anterior skull base neoplasms

Juvenile nasopharyngeal angiofibroma (JNA)

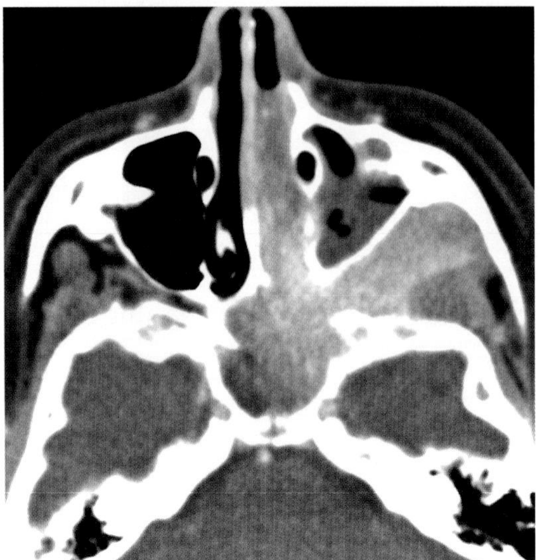

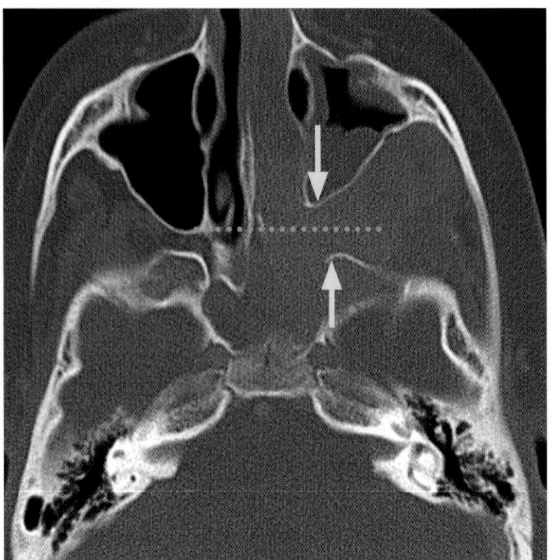

Juvenile nasopharyngeal angiofibroma: Axial contrast-enhanced CT through the pterygopalatine fossa in soft tissue (left image) and bone windows shows an avidly enhancing mass in the left nasopharynx, pterygopalatine fossa, and sphenoid sinus, with characteristic widening (arrows) of the pterygopalatine fossa. There is resultant anterior displacement of the posterior wall of the maxillary sinus relative to the left (dotted blue line).

Case courtesy Sanjay Prabhu, MD, Boston Children's Hospital.

- Juvenile nasopharyngeal angiofibroma (JNA) is a benign, highly vascular tumor seen in adolescent males. The most common clinical presentation is nasal obstruction and epistaxis.
- Despite the lack of metastatic behavior, JNA is very locally aggressive and insinuates through adjacent skull base foramina. Tumors frequently recur if incompletely resected.
- JNA arises from within the nasal aspect of the sphenopalatine foramen, which is the medial boundary of the pterygopalatine fossa.
- On imaging, JNA enhances very avidly and is centered in the nasopharynx. As the mass continues to grow, extension into the pterygopalatine fossa or the orbits is commonly seen.
- The three classic findings of JNA include:

1. Nasopharyngeal mass.
2. Expansion of the pterygopalatine fossa.
3. Anterior bowing or displacement of the posterior maxillary sinus wall.

- Pre-operative embolization is often performed to reduce the vascularity of the lesion prior to resection.

Olfactory groove meningioma

- Meningioma, a common benign neoplasm arising from arachnoid villi rests, is the most common intracranial lesion to affect the anterior skull base.
- The imaging appearance of olfactory groove meningiomas is similar to that of meningiomas elsewhere, featuring avid enhancement and an enhancing dural tail. There is often reactive bone sclerosis.

MALIGNANT ANTERIOR SKULL BASE NEOPLASMS

Overview of skull base tumors

- It is usually not possible to arrive at a single diagnosis when faced with a neoplasm involving the anterior skull base. However, the radiologist plays an important role to assist the surgeon in determining resectability and optimal surgical approach.
- Important findings to describe include the presence of bony destruction, invasion into the brain parenchyma, and extension into the orbit and cavernous sinus.

  Invasion into the brain may manifest solely as vasogenic edema, even without abnormal enhancement.

  Orbital invasion most commonly occurs through the lamina papyracea, which is the weak medial orbital wall.

Esthesioneuroblastoma

- Esthesioneuroblastoma, also known as an olfactory neuroblastoma, is a malignant neural crest tumor that arises from specialized olfactory epithelium. The histology is similar to other neural crest tumors, such as small cell lung carcinoma and neuroblastoma.
- Esthesioneuroblastoma affects patients in a bimodal age distribution, with peak incidence in the teenage years and middle age.
- On imaging, the tumor appears as an aggressive mass that is slightly hyperattenuating on CT and intermediate intensity on both T1- and T2-weighted images due to high cellularity. Calcification is often present.
- A classic finding, thought by some authors to be pathognomonic of esthesioneuroblastoma, is the presence of peripheral tumor cysts that occur at the margins of the intracranial portion of the mass.

Squamous cell carcinoma

- Squamous cell carcinoma (SCC) is by far the most common malignancy of the paranasal sinuses and the nose. The maxillary antrum is the most common primary site within the paranasal sinuses.
- On imaging, SCC of the skull base appears as an aggressive, intensely enhancing mass with bony destruction. Enhancement is the key differentiating feature from benign inflammatory processes such as sinonasal polyposis or mucocele.

Adenoid cystic carcinoma

- Adenoid cystic carcinoma may arise from minor salivary glands in the sinonasal cavity.
- Although local lymphatic spread is rare, distant metastases are seen commonly.
- Adenoid cystic carcinoma demonstrates water signal on T1- and T2-weighted images, but unlike a cyst, enhancement is characteristic.
- Adenoid cystic carcinoma arising in the region of the anterior skull base has a high rate of trigeminal nerve perineural spread. Post-contrast evaluation of the cranial nerves offers the highest sensitivity to evaluate for subtle perineural spread.

Rhabdomyosarcoma

- Rhabdomyosarcoma is the most common head and neck tumor in children. It is discussed in the pediatric imaging section.

TEMPORAL BONE

OVERVIEW OF THE TEMPORAL BONE

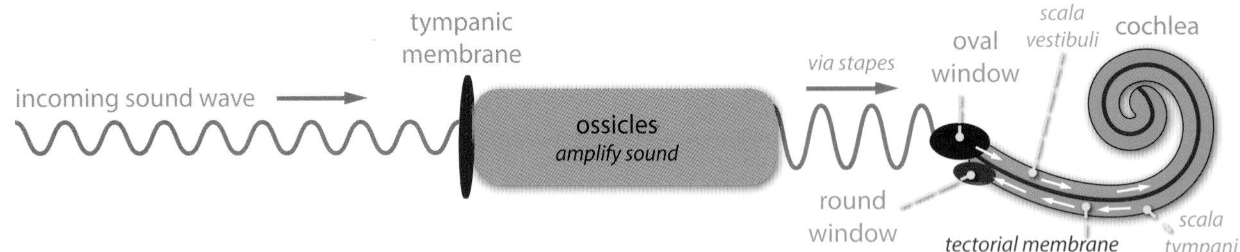

external ear

contents:

external auditory canal (EAC)

pathology:

EAC atresia
squamous cell carcinoma
swimmer's ear (acute external otitis)
surfer's ear (EAC exostosis)
malignant otitis externa
acute external otitis
first branchial cleft cyst
keratosis obturans

middle ear

contents:

tympanic membrane
ossicles:
- malleus
- incus
- stapes

stapedius muscle
facial nerve

pathology:

hypoplasia of ossicles
cholesteatoma
otitis media
mastoiditis
glomus tympanicum
aberrant internal carotid artery
dehiscent jugular bulb
oval window atresia
facial nerve schwannoma

inner ear

contents:

cochlea
semicircular canals
vestibule
utricle
saccule
vestibular aqueduct
cochlear aqueduct

pathology:

cochlear dysplasia
superior semicircular canal dehiscence
semicircular canal hypoplasia
lateral most commonly affected
enlarged vestibular aqueduct
otospongiosis/otosclerosis
Paget disease
fibrous dysplasia
labyrinthitis
petrous apicitis
cholesterol cyst

- The temporal bone can be anatomically and functionally divided into the external, middle, and inner ear. Although some pathologies can overlap, each division tends to be susceptible to unique pathologies.
- This anatomic and functional division parallels the pathway of sound waves into the brain. Sound enters the head at the external ear, is amplified by the ossicles in the middle ear, and is finally converted into electrical impulses in the inner ear.
- An additional function of the inner ear (not drawn above) is the balance and position sense provided by the vestibule and the semicircular canals. Together, the cochlea, vestibule and semicircular canals make up the *labyrinth*.

External ear and external auditory canal (EAC)

Anatomy of the external ear and external auditory canal (EAC)

- The external auditory canal (EAC) is a fibrocartilaginous tube that sound passes through before reaching the middle ear.

Congenital EAC stenosis, hypoplasia and atresia

- Congenital malformations of the external ear, including stenosis, hypoplasia, and complete atresia, are relatively common. The EAC and inner ear have different embryologic origins, so it is uncommon for both an EAC anomaly and an inner ear abnormality to be present.
- The malleus and incus are 1st branchial cleft structures and are usually abnormal in EAC atresia.

Acute external otitis

- Acute external otitis, otherwise known as *swimmer's ear*, is a bacterial infection of the external ear seen in areas of high humidity.

EAC exostosis (surfer's ear)

- EAC exostosis, also known as *surfer's ear*, is a bony exostosis of the EAC seen in those who swim/surf in cold waters.

Necrotizing external otitis (malignant otitis externa)

- Previously known as malignant otitis externa, necrotizing external otitis is a severe complication of external otitis seen in elderly diabetic or immunocompromised patients. The most common pathogens are *Pseudomonas aeruginosa* in diabetics and *Aspergillus fumigatus* in the immunocompromised.
- The infection may be fast-spreading and aggressive, with potential involvement of the middle or inner ear structures, or skull base extension.
- On imaging, there is extensive enhancement centered around the external ear, with associated bony erosion.

Keratosis obturans

- Keratosis obturans is characterized by keratin plugs within an enlarged EAC, and is typically seen in young patients with sinusitis and bronchiectasis. It is usually bilateral.

Cholesteatoma

- Acquired cholesteatomas occur more commonly in the middle ear, but should be considered in the differential of an EAC soft tissue mass, especially in the presence of bony erosion.

EAC malignancy

- The most common malignancy of the external auditory canal is squamous cell carcinoma. Risk factors are controversial but may include sun exposure or chronic inflammation.

Middle ear

Anatomy of the middle ear and adjacent facial nerve

- The middle ear begins at the tympanic membrane and includes the ossicles (malleus, incus, and stapes) and the tensor tympani and stapedius muscles.
- The handle of the malleus is attached to the tympanic membrane. Sound waves vibrate the tympanic membrane, which transmits mechanical energy directly to the malleus, and then through the malleoincudal and incudostapedial articulations to the oval window. The footplate of the stapes articulates directly with the oval window.
- The oval window is the interface between the air-filled middle ear and the fluid-filled inner ear.

Glomus tympanicum

- A glomus tympanicum is an extra-adrenal pheochromocytoma (paraganglioma) isolated to the middle ear. Glomus tympanicum is the most common primary middle ear tumor and typically presents with pulsatile tinnitus or conductive hearing loss.
- On otoscopic evaluation, a vascular red mass will be present behind the tympanic membrane.

Facial nerve schwannoma

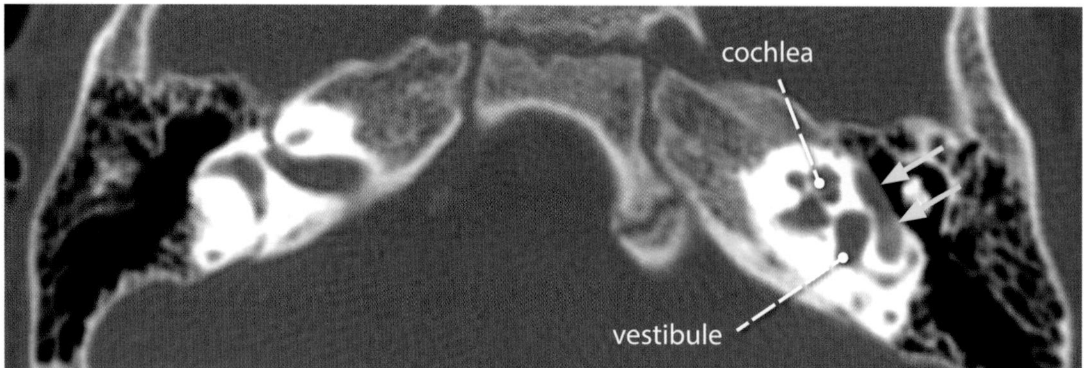

Facial nerve schwannoma: Axial CT through the temporal bone in a child shows subtle enlargement of the tympanic segment of the left facial nerve canal (arrows).

Case courtesy Sanjay Prabhu, MD, Boston Children's Hospital.

- Within the temporal bone, schwannomas of the facial nerve (CN VII) tend to be slow growing and most commonly involve the geniculate ganglion, followed by the labyrinthine and tympanic segments. The segments of the facial nerve in the temporal bone are:

> **Labyrinthine segment**. Courses from the internal auditory canal to the geniculate ganglion, which is located superior to the cochlea.
>
> → Greater superficial petrosal nerve innervates salivation.
>
> **Tympanic (horizontal) segment**. Facial nerve courses under the lateral semicircular canal.
>
> **Mastoid (descending) segment**. Facial nerve courses inferiorly, then exits the temporal bone at the stylomastoid foramen.
>
> → Nerve to stapedius.
>
> → Chorda tympani (taste to anterior 2/3 of tongue).

- The majority of patients with facial nerve schwannoma present with facial nerve palsy; however, up to 30% present without facial nerve symptoms. Larger facial nerve schwannomas can interfere with ossicular function, causing conductive hearing loss.
- On CT, the typical finding of a facial nerve schwannoma is enlargement of the bony canal through which the involved portion of the facial nerve passes. There is typically no calcification. The tumor usually demonstrates brisk contrast enhancement on MRI.

Cholesterol granuloma (cholesterol cyst)

- A cholesterol granuloma, otherwise known as a cholesterol cyst, is the most common benign petrous apex lesion, but may also occur in the middle ear. It is caused by a giant cell reaction to cholesterol crystals thought to be initially incited by an obstructed air cell.
- On otoscopic examination, a blue mass is present behind the tympanic membrane.
- Cholesterol granuloma and cholesteatoma are often considered together in the differential diagnosis of a soft tissue middle ear mass with bony erosion. In contrast to cholesterol granuloma, a cholesteatoma will show restricted diffusion and will appear as a white mass on otoscopic examination of the tympanic membrane. Cholesterol granuloma is typically hyperintense on T1-weighted images.

Cholesteatoma

- A cholesteatoma is a non-neoplastic lesion of the temporal bone which has been described as "skin in the wrong place." The name cholesteatoma is deceptive since the lesion does not contain fat and is not neoplastic. An intracranial, extra-axial "cholesteatoma" is an epidermoid cyst.
- Cholesteatomas can occur in children or adults. Cholesteatomas of the middle ear are more common in younger individuals, while cholesteatomas of the EAC are more common in middle-aged and older adults.
- A middle ear cholesteatoma is almost always acquired (accounting for 98% of all middle-ear cholesteatomas), but rarely may be congenital. There is no histopathologic difference between the congenital and acquired forms. A congenital cholesteatoma can occur anywhere within the temporal bone, while acquired cholesteatomas occur in the middle ear.
- The etiology of cholesteatoma is controversial. Acquired cholesteatoma may represent sequela of tympanic membrane perforation, inflammation, or traumatic implantation of epidermal elements. Congenital cholesteatoma may represent persistent fetal epithelial squamous cell nests.
- Clinically, congenital cholesteatomas are usually asymptomatic, but may be detectable as a white mass behind the tympanic membrane. If the cholesteatoma grows large, symptoms may mimic acquired cholesteatoma with recurrent ear disease, eustachian tube obstruction, chronic ear discharge, and mixed sensorineural and conductive hearing loss.
- In the evaluation of a suspected cholesteatoma, it is important to describe potential involvement of three key landmarks: The lateral semicircular canal, the tegmen tympani (the bony roof separating the mastoids from the brain), and the facial nerve.
- CT is very sensitive for the detection of even a small cholesteatoma, but is nonspecific and cannot differentiate between cholesteatoma and other soft tissue masses such as cholesterol granuloma or neoplasm. The typical CT appearance of cholesteatoma is a well-circumscribed soft-tissue mass with adjacent bony erosion, blunting of the scutum, and erosion of the ossicles.

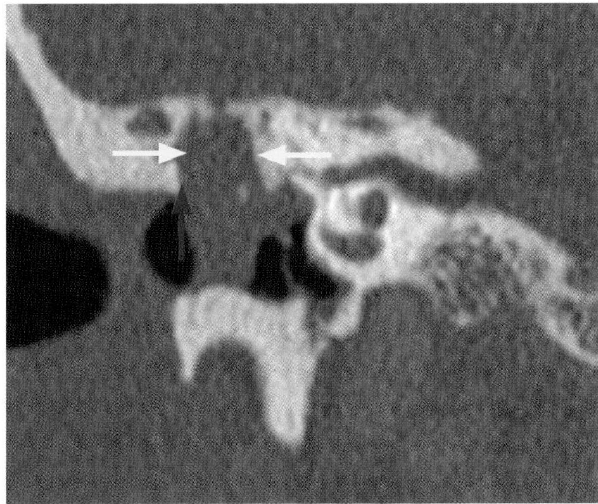

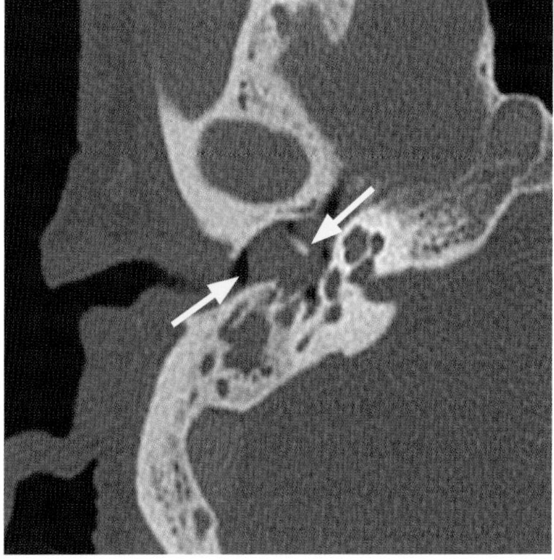

Middle ear cholesteatoma: Coronal (left image) and axial noncontrast CT through the right temporal bone demonstrates a soft tissue mass (yellow arrows) in the middle ear with near-complete erosion of the scutum (red arrow) and the ossicles, consistent with a cholesteatoma. There is opacification of the mastoid air cells.

Case courtesy Mary Beth Cunnane, MD, Massachusetts Eye and Ear Infirmary.

- The most specific MRI sequences to evaluate for cholesteatoma are post-contrast and diffusion-weighted imaging. Similar to intracranial epidermoids, cholesteatomas are hyperintense on diffusion-weighted (DWI) images and do not enhance. The DWI hyperintensity represents a combination of T2 shine through and restricted diffusion, thought to be due to the viscous contents of the cholesteatoma. Cholesteatomas are intermediate to slightly hyperintense on T2-weighted images and of variable signal intensity on T1-weighted images.

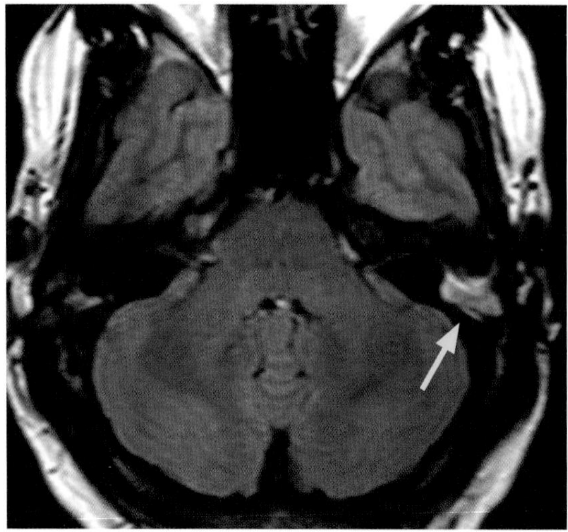

Middle ear cholesteatoma: T1-weighted axial MRI demonstrates iso- to slightly hyperintense (compared to gray matter) signal in the left middle ear (arrow).

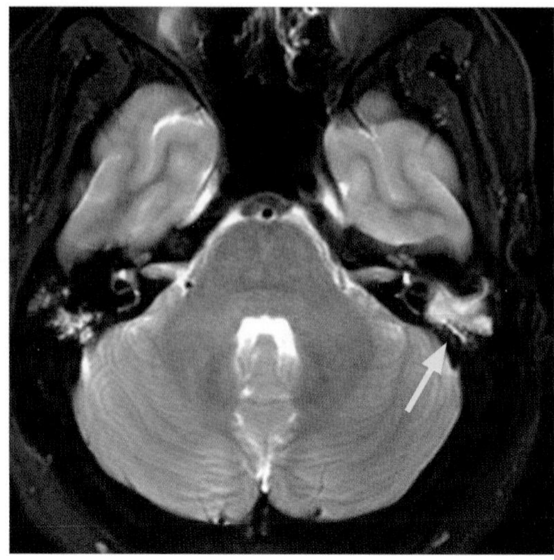

T2-weighted axial MRI with fat suppression shows that the lesion is slightly hyperintense (arrow).

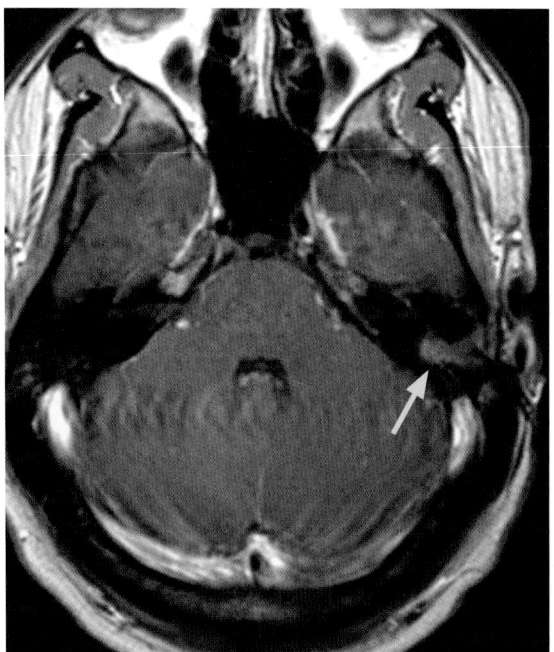

Post-contrast T1-weighted MRI shows no enhancement of the lesion (arrow).

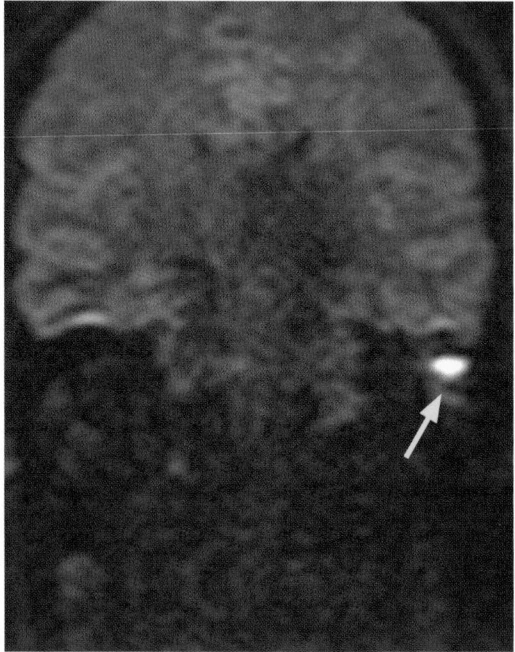

Coronal diffusion weighted image shows a focus of DWI hyperintensity in the left middle ear. Diffusion was restricted when correlated with the ADC map (not shown).

Case courtesy Mary Beth Cunnane, MD, Massachusetts Eye and Ear Infirmary.

Anatomy of the inner ear

- The inner ear consists of the otic capsule. The otic capsule is the bony superstructure containing the fluid-filled spaces of the cochlea, vestibule, and semicircular canals. The otic capsule is the densest bone in the body.
- The cochlea allows us to hear. It is a two-and-a-half turn spiral containing numerous neuroepithelial hair cells of the organ of Corti, which send electrical impulses to the spiral ganglia of the cochlea in response to mechanical bending.

  Hydraulic pressure created in the perilymph by the vibrations of the stapes against the oval window ascends to the apex of the cochlea by the scala vestibuli. Pressure waves descend back to the basal turn through the scala tympani. The vibrations from the scala tympani are transmitted through the round window, where the energy is dissipated.
- The vestibule is involved with balance. The semicircular canals are three arcs oriented in orthogonal planes that allow perception of movement in three- dimensional space.
- The vestibular aqueduct connects the crus common (the common channel of the superior and posterior semicircular canals) to the subarachnoid space at the internal auditory canal, and is thought to be involved in pressure equalization between the CSF and the inner ear.

Cochlear dysplasia (Mondini deformity)

- The most common form of congenital cochlear dysplasia is characterized by incomplete development of the normal two and a half turns of the cochlea, resulting in confluence of the apical and middle turns and preservation of a distinct basilar turn.
- The correct nomenclature for this anomaly is *incomplete partition type II,* although it is commonly referred to as the Mondini deformity. The use of the eponym *Mondini* to describe cochlear dysplasia is controversial and probably best avoided, as there is confusion amongst radiologists regarding the exact malformation originally described.
- There is a strong association between cochlear dysplasia and enlarged vestibular aqueduct.

Michel aplasia

- Michel aplasia is a very rare complete lack of development of the entire inner ear.

Enlarged vestibular aqueduct syndrome

- Although the vestibular aqueduct does not have a direct function in the physiology of hearing, there is a spectrum of congenital hearing loss associated with an enlarged vestibular aqueduct. Clinically, enlarged vestibular aqueduct syndrome may lead to progressive hearing loss while playing contact sports.
- As an internal reference, the vestibular aqueduct should not be larger than the posterior semicircular canal, which is often seen at the same level in the axial plane.

Otospongiosis (otosclerosis)

- Otospongiosis, otherwise known as otosclerosis, is a primary bone dysplasia of the otic capsule characterized by replacement of normal endochondral bone by irregular spongy bone. Otospongiosis occurs most commonly in young and middle-aged women and is bilateral 85% of the time.
- The two main types of otospongiosis are fenestral and retrofenestral types.

> The **fenestral** type of otospongiosis is more common, occurs at the fissula ante fenestrum (located directly anterior to the oval window), and usually affects the oval window.
>
> The **retrofenestral** (cochlear) type is thought to represent a more severe form with involvement of the otic capsule in addition to the lateral wall of the labyrinth. The differential diagnosis of cochlear demineralization includes retrofenestral otospongiosis, osteogenesis imperfecta in a child, fibrous dysplasia in a young adult, and Paget disease in an older adult.

- CT is the best imaging modality for evaluation of otospongiosis, which shows increased lucency of the affected bone. Findings may be extremely subtle without detailed knowledge of the normal appearance of the otic capsule.

Labyrinthitis

- Labyrinthitis is inflammation of the inner ear, which may be infectious or autoimmune.
- Labyrinthitis has been divided into three stages of chronicity based on the imaging (primarily MR) characteristics.
- **Acute labyrinthitis** is the earliest stage, presenting as pus in the inner ear. The only MRI signal abnormality of acute labyrinthitis is enhancement of the affected inner ear structures.

  The main differential consideration of acute labyrinthitis is a cochlear or intralabyrinthine schwannoma. A schwannoma tends to be focal and discrete, while labyrinthitis may produce more diffuse enhancement.
- **Fibrous labyrinthitis** represents the replacement of endolymph and perilymph with fibrous strands that cause decreased signal intensity on T2-weighted images. There may be mild (but decreased) residual post-contrast enhancement of the affected structures.
- **Labyrinthitis ossificans** is the final stage of the disease. Calcified debris replaces the normal endolymph and perilymph. CT is the best way to image labyrinthitis ossificans, as the calcification causes decreased signal intensity on T2-weighted MRI and lack of enhancement.

TEMPORAL BONE FRACTURES

- Temporal bone fractures have been historically classified by their orientation with respect to the axis of the temporal bone. A newer classification that has been the most predictive of clinical outcome divides temporal bone fractures into otic capsule-violating versus otic capsule-sparing, although the longitudinal and transverse terms remain in common use.

Longitudinal temporal bone fracture

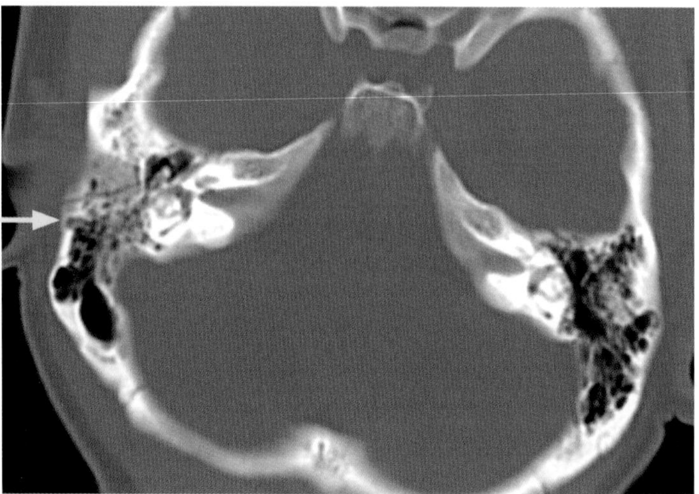

Longitudinal temporal bone fracture: Axial CT through the temporal bone shows a nondisplaced fracture (arrow) extending through the axis of the petrous portion of the temporal bone.

- A longitudinal temporal bone fracture is aligned with the long axis of the petrous portion of the temporal bone and is by far the most common type of temporal bone fracture. Longitudinal temporal bone fractures are likely to involve the ossicles and result in **conductive** hearing loss. 20% of longitudinal fractures are associated with facial nerve injury.
- If the tympanic membrane is disrupted, there is increased risk for subsequent development of an acquired cholesteatoma.

Transverse temporal bone fracture

- A transverse temporal bone fracture is perpendicular to the long axis of the petrous portion of the temporal bone. Transverse fractures are more likely to involve the bony labyrinth and result in **sensorineural** hearing loss. 50% of transverse fractures result in facial nerve injury.

Petrous apex

Anatomy of the petrous apex

- The petrous apex is the most medial portion of the temporal bone.
- The petrous apex is a bridge between the suprahyoid neck inferiorly and the intracranial compartment above, and is adjacent to several important structures such as Dorello's canal, Meckel's cave, and the petrous portion of the internal carotid artery.

  Cranial nerve VI passes through Dorello's canal.

  Meckel's cave is the site of the trigeminal ganglion.
- Normally, the petrous apex is composed of bone marrow and dense bone. The petrous apex is pneumatized in approximately 10% of the population, which increases the risk for development of a cholesterol cyst or apical petrositis.

Cholesterol cyst (cholesterol granuloma)

- A cholesterol cyst is a foreign body giant cell reaction to cholesterol crystals. It is thought to be initially instigated as a reaction to an obstructed air cell and therefore occurs more commonly in a pneumatized petrous apex.
- A cholesterol cyst is the most common primary petrous apex lesion but may also occur in the mastoid portion of the temporal bone or the middle ear.
- MR imaging of a cholesterol cyst shows an expansile mass with internal hemorrhage and fluid that does not suppress on fat suppression, unlike fatty marrow.

Apical petrositis (petrous apicitis)

- A relatively rare complication of infectious otomastoiditis, apical petrositis is also known as petrous apicitis and results when infection extends medially into a pneumatized petrous apex.
- In the early stages of apical petrositis, there is opacification of the petrous apex air cells with progressive bony demineralization and resorption, resulting in localized osteomyelitis of the skull base.
- The classic Gradenigo triad is not commonly seen, but is comprised of otomastoiditis, facial pain due to trigeminal neuropathy at Meckel's cave, and lateral rectus palsy from 6th cranial nerve palsy at Dorello's canal.
- Vascular complications of apical petrositis include internal carotid arteritis and dural venous thrombosis.

Congenital cholesteatoma

- While acquired cholesteatomas are located within the middle ear, congenital cholesteatoma can be located anywhere in the temporal bone, including the petrous apex.
- MR imaging will typically show restricted diffusion.

Schwannoma

- A petrous apex schwannoma may originate from cranial nerves V, VII, or VIII. Imaging shows a circumscribed, smoothly expansile, enhancing mass that may cause bony remodeling. Large tumors may become cystic and contain fluid levels.

Langerhans cell histiocytosis (eosinophilic granuloma)

- Langerhans cell histiocytosis (LCH) is a neoplastic proliferation of eosinophils and Langerhans cells. The temporal bone is the most common site of skull base involvement.
- CT shows a well-circumscribed destructive lesion, usually with nonsclerotic margins.
- MRI shows the LCH lesions as soft-tissue masses surrounded by bone marrow and soft tissue edema. Marked enhancement is characteristic.

Chondrosarcoma

- Chondrosarcoma is a malignant neoplasm that characteristically arises in the midline from the clivus or slightly off-midline from the petroclival synchondrosis. CT often shows a tumor with a ring-and-arc chondroid matrix, although internal matrix is not always seen. MRI shows a lobular, cauliflower-shaped, hyperintense mass on T2-weighted images.

Chordoma

- Chordoma (subsequently discussed in the section on clival lesions) most commonly arises from the clivus but may expand laterally to secondarily involve the petrous apex. In some circumstances it can be difficult to distinguish between chordoma and chondrosarcoma.

Differential diagnosis of a petrous apex lesion

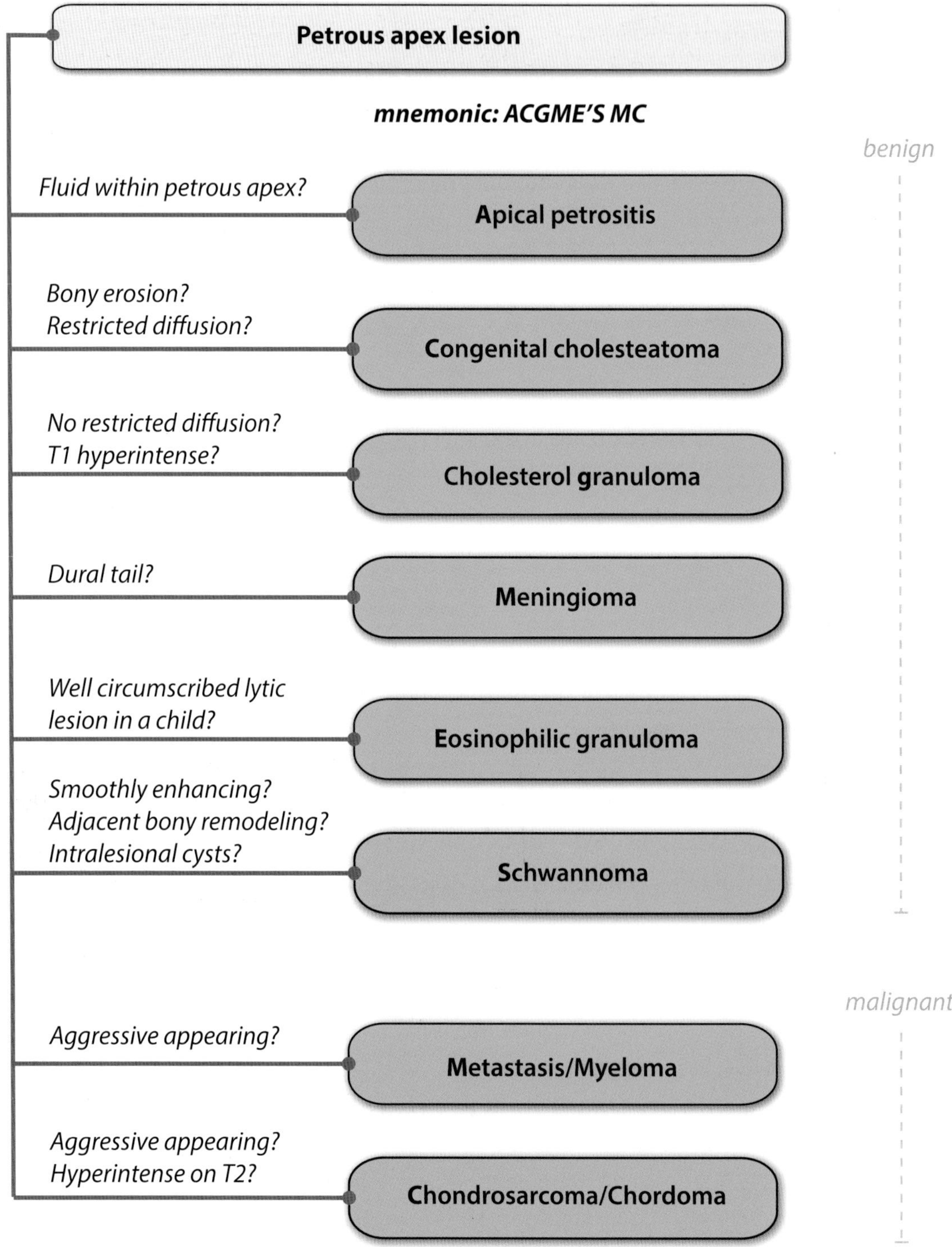

- The normal clivus in an adult should demonstrate fatty marrow signal on sagittal T1-weighted MRI. In children, the clival marrow may be low in signal due to persistent hematopoietic marrow, depending on age. While diffuse marrow replacement may represent a systemic process, focal replacement of normal marrow should raise concern for neoplastic disease.

Chordoma

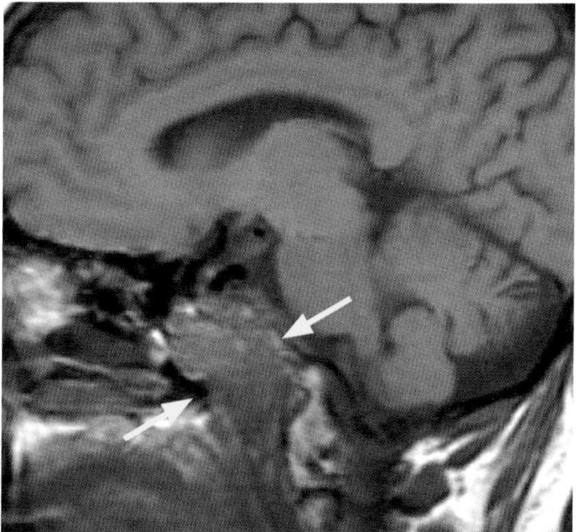

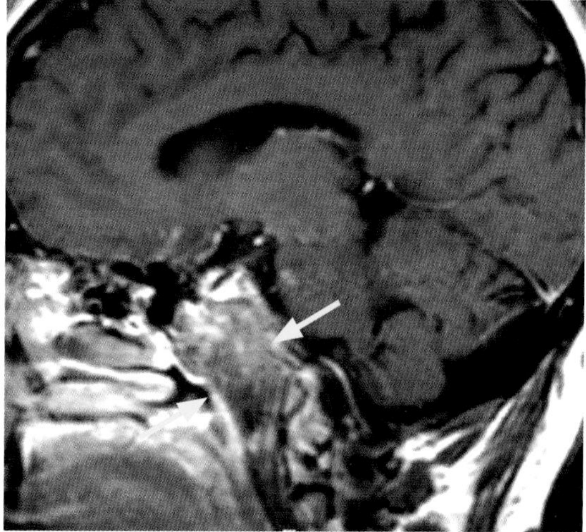

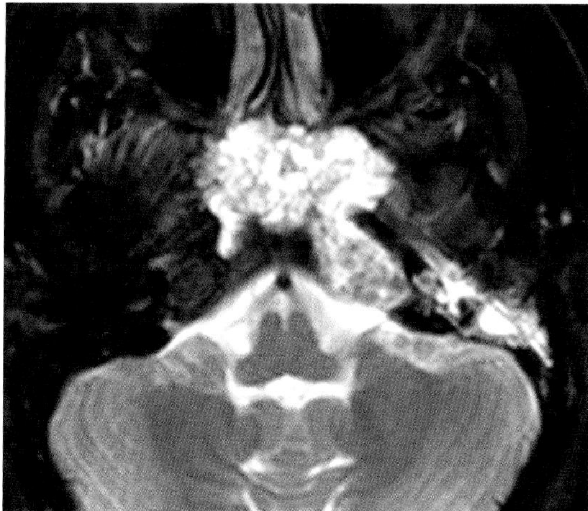

Clival chordoma:

Sagittal T1-weighted MRI (top left image) shows replacement of the normal clival marrow by an isointense mass (arrows).

Sagittal post-contrast T1-weighted MRI (top right image) shows heterogeneous enhancement of the mass (arrows).

Axial T2-weighted MRI (bottom left image) shows a microlobulated, hyperintense clival mass with extension into the left petrous apex and opacification of the left middle ear and mastoid air cells.

Case courtesy Mary Beth Cunnane, MD, Massachusetts Eye and Ear Infirmary.

- Chordoma is a locally invasive tumor arising in the midline from notochord remnants. Approximately 50% arise near the sacrum, 35% near the clivus, and the remainder in the vertebral column.
- Chordomas do not have internal matrix but calcification within the lesion may represent residual fragments of eroded bone.
- MR imaging of chordoma is similar to chondrosarcoma, appearing as a hyperintense mass on T2-weighted images with bony destruction.

Chondrosarcoma

- Chondrosarcoma may arise either centrally from the clivus or para-sagittally from the petrous apex.

Metastasis

- Breast cancer has a propensity to metastasize to the clivus.

- Paragangliomas, otherwise known as glomus tumors, are neoplasms of paraganglionic tissue that arise from sympathetic glomus bodies. These neoplasms are histologically identical to extra-adrenal pheochromocytoma. Paragangliomas occur in a few predictable locations in the head and neck. Five named glomus tumors have been described, classified by the typical locations at which they arise. Most glomus tumors are benign, but they can be locally aggressive. Less than 5% undergo malignant degeneration.
- Paragangliomas are associated with multiple endocrine neoplasia type 1 and neurofibromatosis type 1, where they are often multiple.
- Paragangliomas are highly vascular and enhance avidly.
- The classic MRI imaging pattern is the *salt and pepper* appearance due to intra-tumoral flow voids.
- Conventional angiography may be performed to provide a vascular road map and to perform pre-surgical embolization.

Glomus jugulare

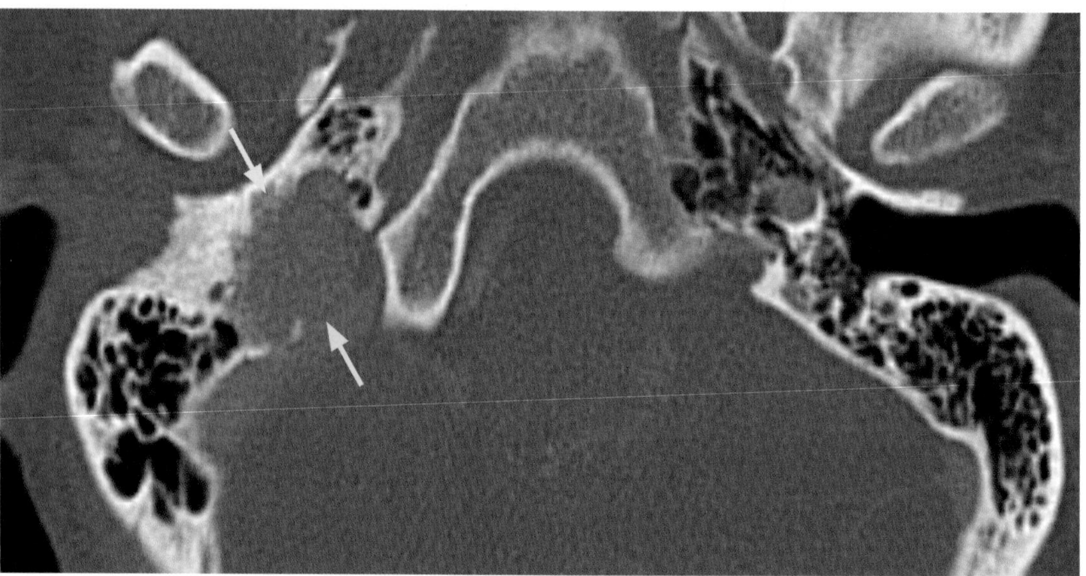

Glomus jugulare: Axial CT through the mastoid air cells shows permeative, moth-eaten bony destruction centered on the right jugular foramen (arrows).

- Glomus jugulare is the most common primary neoplasm of the jugular foramen. The typical patient is a woman in late middle age presenting with pulsatile tinnitus and conductive hearing loss.
- The *moth-eaten* bony destruction typical of paragangliomas is centered around the jugular foramen. A schwannoma or meningioma may also occur near the jugular foramen; however, schwannoma typically features smooth bony remodeling and meningioma typically causes hyperostosis.

Glomus tympanicum

- Glomus tympanicum is a paraganglioma isolated to the middle ear.
- Otoscopic evaluation shows a vascular, red, retro-tympanic mass. The differential diagnosis of a vascular, red, retro-tympanic mass includes:

Glomus tympanicum.
Aberrant carotid artery.
Tympanic membrane hemangioma.

Glomus jugulotympanicum

- Glomus jugulotympanicum is a glomus jugulare that has spread into the middle ear.

Carotid body tumor (glomus caroticum)

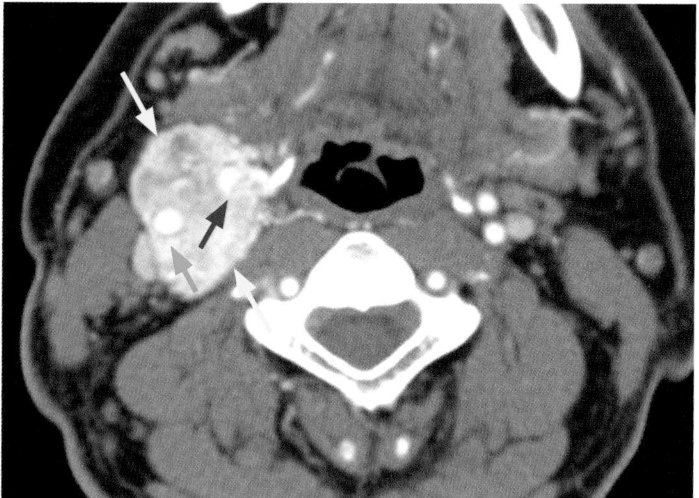

Carotid body tumor: Axial contrast-enhanced CT shows an avidly enhancing mass (yellow arrows) surrounding and splaying the right internal (red arrow) and external carotid (blue arrow) arteries.

Case courtesy Mary Beth Cunnane, MD, Massachusetts Eye and Ear Infirmary.

- Glomus caroticum, much more commonly referred to as a carotid body tumor, is a paraganglioma of the carotid body.
- It characteristically splays the internal and external carotid arteries.

Glomus vagale

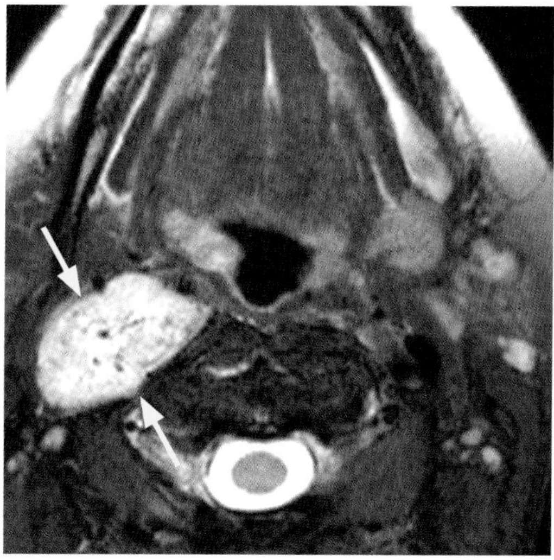

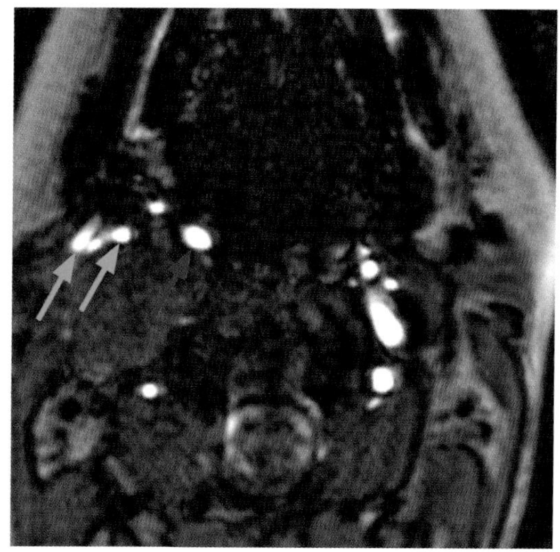

Glomus vagale: T2-weighted MRI with fat suppression (left image) shows a hyperintense mass (yellow arrows) containing punctate flow voids in the right carotid space. An axial source image from an MR angiogram (right image) shows anterior-medial displacement of the internal carotid artery (red arrow) and anterior displacement of the external carotid branches (blue arrows).

Case courtesy Mary Beth Cunnane, MD, Massachusetts Eye and Ear Infirmary.

- Glomus vagale is a paraganglioma of the vagus nerve, typically occurring at the same level of the neck as the carotid body tumor.
- Glomus vagale displaces the carotid artery (both internal and external branches) medially and anteriorly. In contrast, a carotid body tumor splays the internal and external carotids.
- A schwannoma of the vagus nerve may occur in the same location and will also displace the carotid artery medially and anteriorly. A schwannoma is generally relatively less vascular. Schwannoma may enhance avidly, but would not show the flow voids typical of a glomus vagale.

ORBITS

OVERVIEW AND ANATOMY OF THE ORBITS

Bony orbits and foramina

- The orbit is a quadrilateral, pyramidal, bony cavity made of five bones: the frontal, ethmoid, nasal, zygomatic, and the maxilla. Several of these bones are very thin and several contain pneumatized sinuses. The bony surfaces are covered with a tough periosteum, which often maintains the integrity of the orbit even in the presence of a bony fracture.
- The following structures pass through the optic foramen:

  Optic nerve.

  Ophthalmic artery.

- All of the cranial nerves (CN) of the cavernous sinus except V^2 enter the superior orbital fissure. V^2 exits the cavernous sinus via the foramen roturdum and subsequently enters the orbit via the inferior orbital fissure. The following structures pass through the superior orbital fissure:

  CN III (oculomotor nerve) innervates the superior, medial, and inferior rectus, and the inferior oblique.

  CN IV (trochlear nerve) innervates the superior oblique (mnemonic: SO_4).

  CN V^1 (ophthalmic division of trigeminal nerve) provides sensory innervation to the upper face.

  CN VI (abducens nerve) innervates the lateral rectus (mnemonic: LR_6).

  Superior ophthalmic vein, a valveless vein that can be a potential route of infection into the brain.

- The following structures pass through the inferior orbital fissure:

  CN V^2 (maxillary division of trigeminal nerve) provides sensory innervation to the inferior eyelid, upper lip, and nose.

  Infraorbital artery.

Compartments of the orbits

- The orbit can be conceptually and anatomically divided into five compartments to aid in the differential diagnosis and classification of orbital pathology, although several types of masses (e.g., orbital hemangioma and lymphoma) may not be confined to these boundaries.
- Division into **preseptal** and postseptal compartments is most useful for the evaluation of orbital infection. The orbital septum is thin connective tissue at the orbital margin that extends into the tarsus of the eyelid. The preseptal orbit is an anterior superficial potential space that does not contain any orbital structures.
- The postseptal orbit, which is essentially the entire orbit, can be further divided into four compartments: The **extraconal**, **conal**, and **intraconal** compartments, and the **globe**.
- The **extraconal** compartment contains the lacrimal gland, fat, and bony orbit.
- The **conal** compartment contains the extraocular muscles.

  All of the muscles except for the inferior oblique muscle arise from a common fibrous ring called the annulus of Zinn, located at the apex of the orbit at the optic foramen and medial superior orbital fissure.

  The inferior oblique arises from the medial orbital floor.

- The **intraconal** compartment is comprised of the structures contained within the cone of the extraocular muscles, including the optic nerve–sheath complex, sensory and motor nerves of the orbit, lymph nodes, and fat. Some authors consider the optic nervel/sheath separately.

  The optic nerve–sheath complex consists of the optic nerve, surrounding CSF, and leptomeningeal and dural coverings.

- The **globe** is considered a distinct compartment.

ORBITAL INFECTION

Overview of orbital infection

- Direct spread of infection from the paranasal sinuses is the most common etiology of orbital infection.
- Other etiologies of orbital infection are trauma, foreign body, and odontogenic infection.
- Orbital infection represents a progressive spectrum, listed below from least to most severe.

Preseptal infection

- Infection of the superficial preseptal space presents with swelling and erythema of the eyelids.

Orbital cellulitis/phlegmon

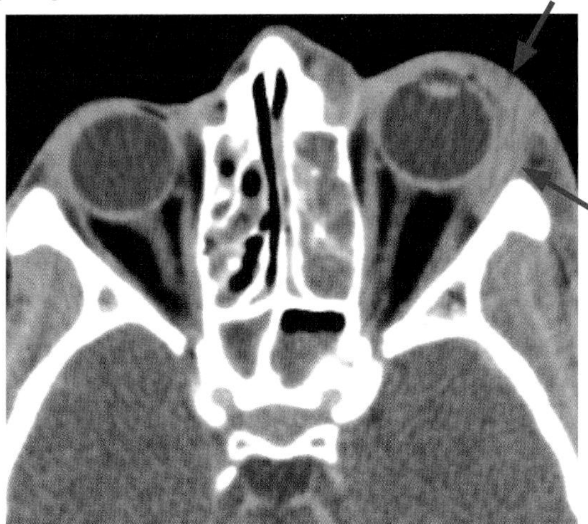
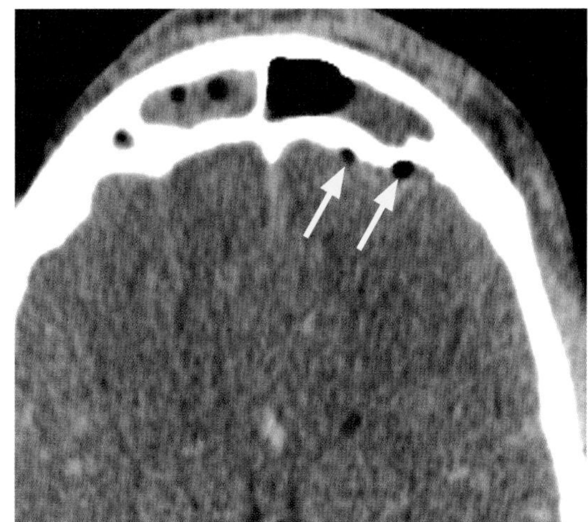

Orbital cellulitis with epidural abscess: Axial contrast-enhanced CT through the orbits (left image) shows left proptosis and both pre- and postseptal inflammatory change (red arrows), without a discrete fluid collection. There is complete opacification of the left ethmoid sinus and opacification of the sphenoid sinus. CT through the brain (right) demonstrates two locules of gas in the extra-axial space (yellow arrows) directly posterior to the left frontal sinus, representing an epidural abscess.

Case courtesy Mary Beth Cunnane, MD, Massachusetts Eye and Ear Infirmary.

- Orbital cellulitis or phlegmon is infection within the orbit that is not yet organized or peripherally ring enhancing.
- Any postseptal infection, including orbital cellulitis, may spread intracranially via the valveless ophthalmic veins and predispose to intracranial infection, as shown above.

Subperiosteal abscess

- Subperiosteal abscess is an organized infection underneath the orbital periosteum, which clinically presents with exophthalmos and visual impairment.
- Subperiosteal abscess is a surgical emergency due to the risk of permanent blindness from elevated intraocular pressure.
- Treatment is with intravenous antibiotics and surgical drainage.

Orbital abscess

- Orbital abscess is a more severe form of infection than subperiosteal abscess, clinically presenting with ophthalmoplegia in addition to the symptoms of subperiosteal abscess.

Cavernous sinus thrombosis

- Cavernous sinus thrombosis is a severe sequela of orbital infection. It may present with multiple cranial nerve palsies in addition to symptoms of orbital abscess.

Hemangioma

- There are two types of orbital hemangioma. **Cavernous hemangioma** is seen in adults and is the most common adult orbital mass, typically presenting with progressive proptosis. In contrast, orbital **capillary hemangioma** is rare and is seen only in the first year of life.
- Orbital **cavernous hemangioma** (adult hemangioma) is usually intraconal but may be extraconal. It is composed of vascular channels filled with slowly moving blood. CT shows an ovoid, enhancing intraconal or extraconal mass. Bony remodeling may be present. MRI shows a well-defined mass that is isointense on T1-weighted images and hyperintense on T2-weighted images, demonstrating early patchy enhancement that progressively fills in.

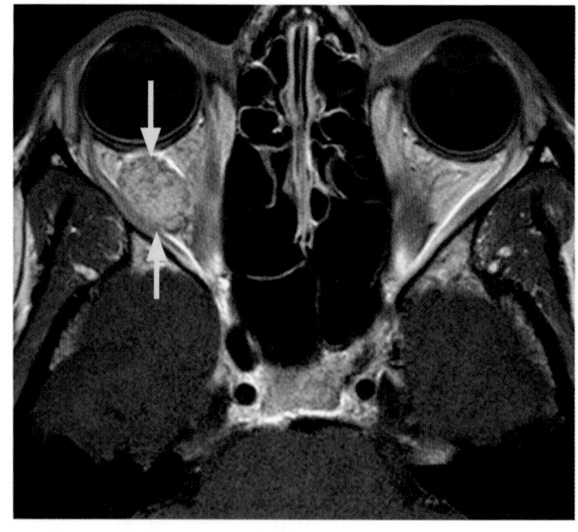

Cavernous hemangioma: Axial T1-weighted post-contrast MRI through the orbits demonstrates a well-circumscribed, intraconal ovoid mass (arrows) that demonstrates inhomogeneous, patchy enhancement.

Case courtesy Mary Beth Cunnane, MD, Massachusetts Eye and Ear Infirmary.

- **Capillary hemangioma** (pediatric hemangioma) is analogous to and often present in conjunction with associated skin lesions such as port-wine stain and strawberry hemangioma. Like these lesions, capillary hemangioma typically enlarges over the first few months of life before spontaneously involuting.

Orbital lymphoma

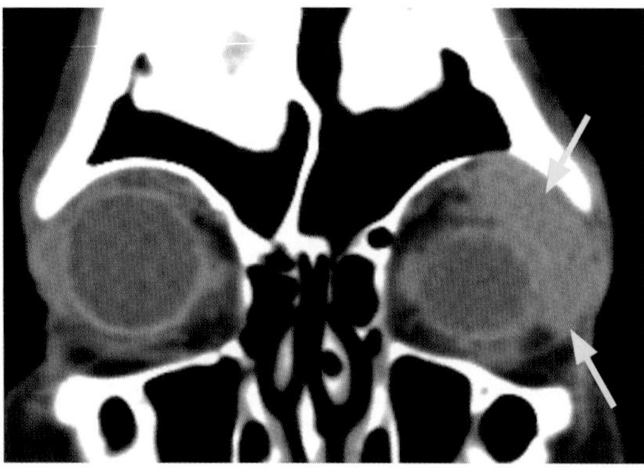

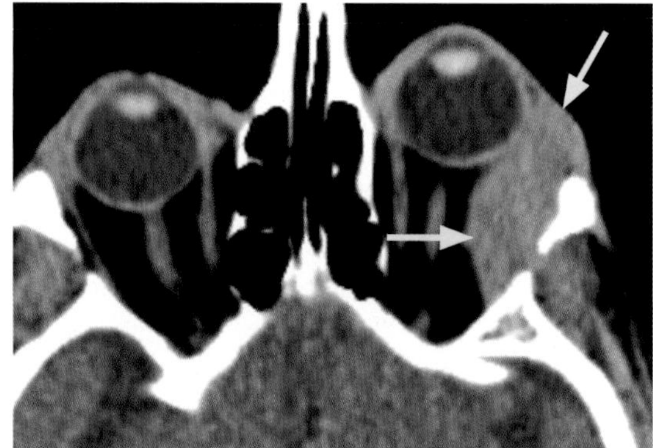

Orbital lymphoma: Coronal (left) and axial noncontrast CT through the orbits shows left-sided proptosis and an ill-defined, slightly hyperattenuating mass (arrows) in the left superior-lateral orbit. The mass conforms to the shape of the globe, rather than deforming it. The left lacrimal gland is not separately identified.

- Orbital lymphoma is usually associated with systemic disease. The lacrimal gland, located in the superolateral quadrant of the orbit, is the most common site of orbital lymphoma. When lymphoma is centered on the lacrimal gland, mass effect on the globe leads to the classic clinical presentation of painless downward proptosis.
- Orbital lymphoma is a hypercellular tumor that is hyperdense on CT and hypointense on both T1- and T2-weighted imaging.
- Orbital lymphoma and orbital pseudotumor both tend to mold to the globe, although orbital pseudotumor typically presents with pain. Other orbital masses may deform the globe.

Lymphangioma

- Lymphangioma is a benign hamartomatous lesion seen in the pediatric population. The preferred nomenclature for lymphangioma is a *low flow lymphatic malformation*.
- Lymphangiomas most commonly involve the extraconal compartment but may be found anywhere in the orbit.
- On imaging, lymphangioma appears as a multilocular cystic mass, often with complex internal contents and fluid levels from prior hemorrhage. Slight peripheral and septal enhancement is often seen.

Schwannoma/neurofibroma

- Schwannoma and neurofibroma are peripheral nerve sheath tumors with indistinguishable imaging appearances when they occur in the orbit. Schwannoma is more common.
- The most commonly affected nerves are the sensory branches of V^1, resulting in a characteristic location in the superior orbit. Involvement of other nerves, however, can produce a schwannoma anywhere in the orbit. Regardless of which nerve is involved, the location tends to be eccentric within the orbit.
- Orbital nerve-sheath tumors tend to be hypointense on T1-weighted images, hyperintense on T2-weighted images, and demonstrate enhancement.

Metastasis

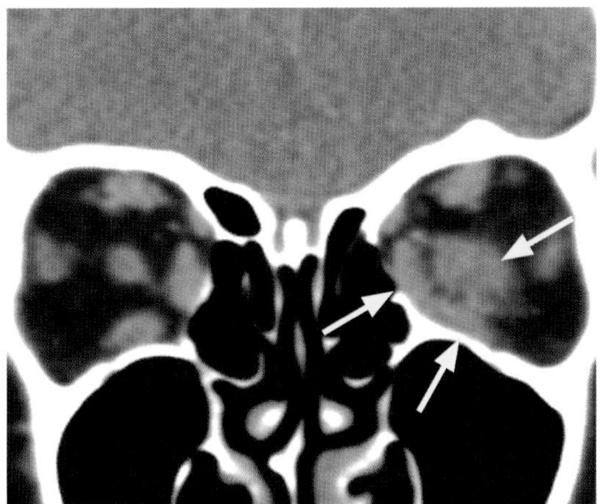
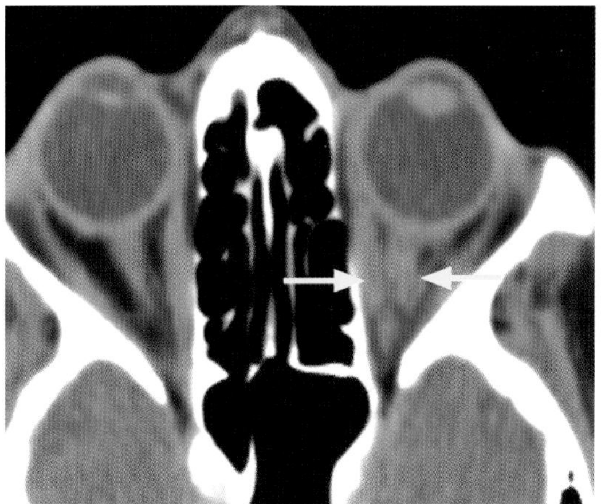

Scirrhous breast cancer metastasis: Coronal (left image) and axial CT through the orbits demonstrates ill-defined soft tissue in the left orbit (arrows), with loss of the normal definition of the optic nerve–sheath complex, medial rectus, and inferior rectus. Despite the presence of the mass, there is no significant proptosis.

Case courtesy Mary Beth Cunnane, MD, Massachusetts Eye and Ear Infirmary.

- In the adult, breast, lung, thyroid, renal cell, and melanoma are known to metastasize to the orbit. A classic imaging finding is the appearance of metastatic scirrhous breast cancer, which can prevent exophthalmos or even cause frank enophthalmos due to fibrosis.
- A special consideration in children is metastatic neuroblastoma, which classically causes an aggressive sunburst-type periosteal reaction within the involved bone.

Lacrimal gland lesion

- The lacrimal gland is composed of both epithelial salivary tissue and lymphoid tissue, and is therefore subject to diseases of these two tissue types.
- Epithelial tumors of the lacrimal gland are approximately 50% benign (e.g., pleomorphic adenoma) and 50% malignant (e.g., adenoid cystic and mucoepidermoid carcinoma).
- Diseases of lymphoid tissue, such as sarcoidosis and lymphoma, may also affect the lacrimal glands. The lacrimal gland is the most common site of orbital lymphoma.
- The lacrimal gland may also become enlarged in orbital pseudotumor.

Thyroid ophthalmopathy (thyroid eye disease)

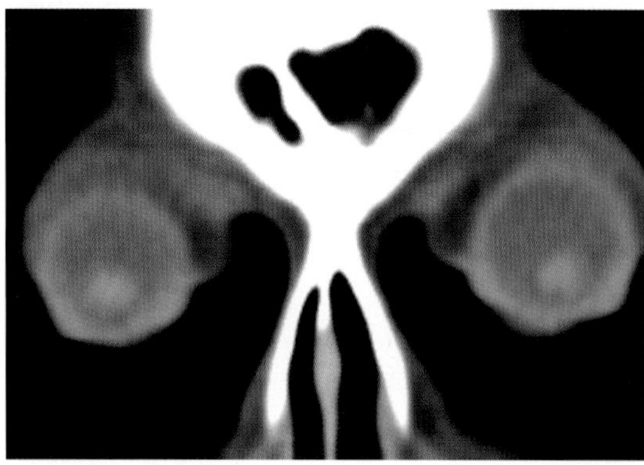
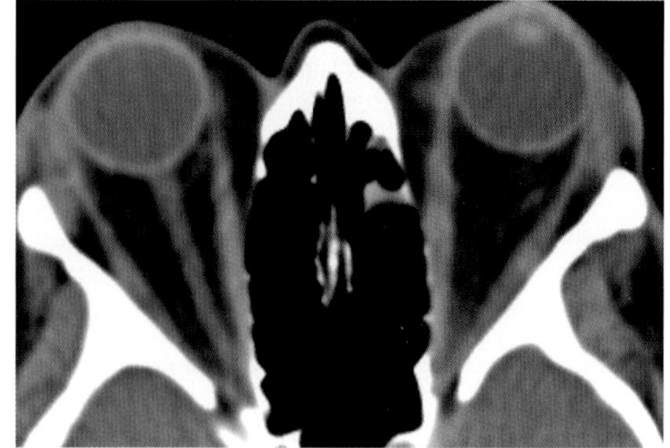

Thyroid ophthalmopathy, fatty type: Coronal (left image) and axial noncontrast CT through the orbits shows bilateral exophthalmos. The extraocular muscles do not appear abnormally thickened.

Case courtesy Mary Beth Cunnane, MD, Massachusetts Eye and Ear Infirmary.

- Thyroid ophthalmopathy (thyroid eye disease) is orbital inflammation associated with thyroid disease. It is mediated by lymphocytes that produce hyaluronic acid. Ultimately, this process leads to fibrosis of the extraocular muscles. Although thyroid ophthalmopathy is most commonly associated with Graves disease, it can occur in any thyroid disorder, even prior to the development of lab abnormalities.
- Initially, there is an increase in intra-orbital fat, which may demonstrate stranding due to inflammatory change. Subsequently, the extraocular muscles become enlarged.
- The inferior rectus muscle is most commonly affected first. The mnemonic *I'M SLow* helps remember the order of involvement of the extraocular muscles:

  Inferior rectus → **m**edial rectus → **s**uperior rectus → **l**ateral rectus
- Isolated lateral rectus enlargement is very uncommon in thyroid ophthalmopathy and should prompt a search for an alternative diagnosis, such as orbital pseudotumor.
- In contrast to pseudotumor, thyroid ophthalmopathy tends to be bilateral and spares the muscle tendons.
- Steroids are temporarily helpful, but 20% of patients will ultimately require surgery to prevent optic nerve compression at the orbital apex.

Orbital pseudotumor

- Orbital pseudotumor is idiopathic orbital inflammation mediated by an infiltrate of lymphocytes, plasma cells, and macrophages. Clinically, it presents with *painful* proptosis (in contrast to lymphoma, which is usually painless). Orbital pseudotumor is a diagnosis of exclusion that can only be made after other causes of orbital inflammation (e.g., Wegener granulomatosis, sarcoidosis, and others) have been ruled out.
- The lacrimal gland is the most commonly involved orbital structure. Several other structures in the orbit may be affected, including the anterior structures (producing uveitis) and the extraocular muscles.
- Imaging findings of orbital pseudotumor include stranding within the orbit fat, increased orbital soft tissue, and enlargement of the extraocular muscles.
- Treatment is with steroids.
- **Tolosa–Hunt syndrome** is the same pathologic process as orbital pseudotumor, but involving the cavernous sinus.

- The optic nerve is the most important structure within the intraconal orbit.

Optic nerve glioma

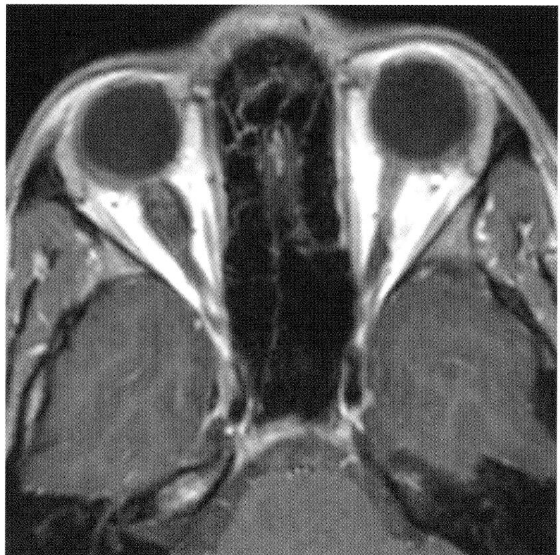

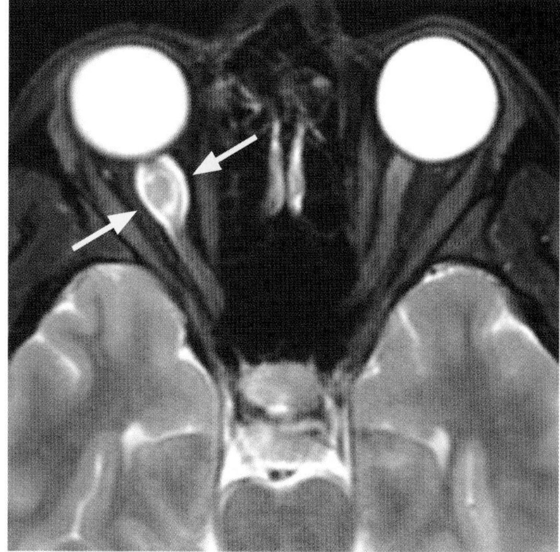

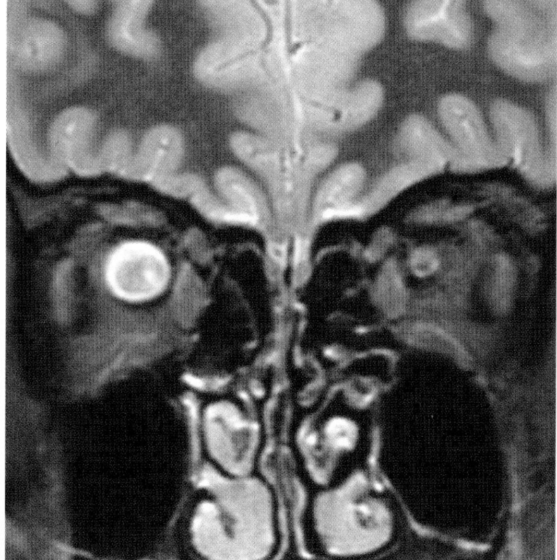

Low-grade optic nerve glioma in a young adult:

Axial T1-weighted post-contrast fat suppressed (top left image), axial T2-weighted fat suppressed (top right image), and coronal T2-weighted fat suppressed (bottom left image) MRI through the orbits demonstrates fusiform, T2 hyperintense enlargement of the distal right optic nerve (arrows) with no appreciable enhancement of the lesion.

- Optic nerve glioma is the most common tumor to arise from the optic nerve–sheath complex.
- Optic nerve glioma can affect children or adults, with differing prognosis. The tumor of childhood is typically a low-grade astrocytoma with an indolent course. Childhood tumors are associated with neurofibromatosis type 1 and are often bilateral. In contrast, optic nerve glioma of adulthood is usually an anaplastic astrocytoma or glioblastoma multiforme, with a poor prognosis.
- The MRI appearance of the low-grade childhood tumor is variable. Often there is fusiform enlargement of the optic nerve and variable enhancement. Like low-grade pilocytic astrocytomas of the posterior fossa, the tumor may have a cyst and nodule appearance.
- The aggressive adult optic glioma typically appears as an enhancing mass, which often extends intracranially to involve the optic chiasm. The tumor may involve any part of the optic tract, including the optic radiations.

Optic nerve meningioma

- Optic nerve meningioma is the second most common optic nerve-sheath tumor, arising from arachnoid cells within the leptomeninges surrounding the optic nerve.
- The typical patient is a middle-aged female with slowly progressive visual impairment, classically with preservation of the central visual field.
- On imaging, the nerve-sheath tends to be circumferentially thickened, with uniform contrast enhancement. The enhancing peripheral tumor and the nonenhancing, central optic nerve produce the *tram-track* sign on the axial image.

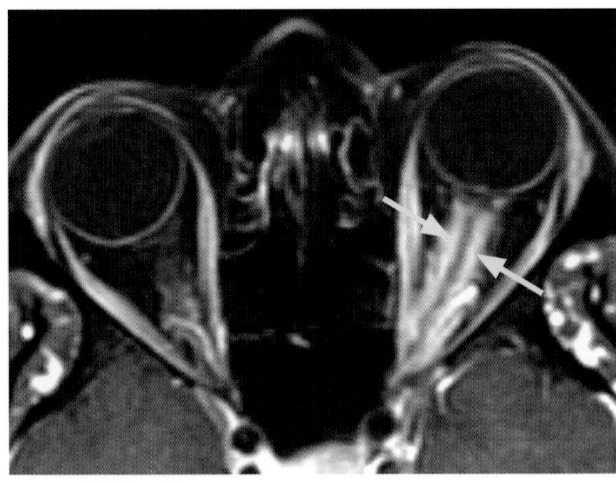

Optic nerve-sheath meningioma: Axial post-contrast fat-sat T1-weighted image demonstrates marked enhancement surrounding the left optic nerve with a *tram-track* appearance (arrows).

Optic neuritis

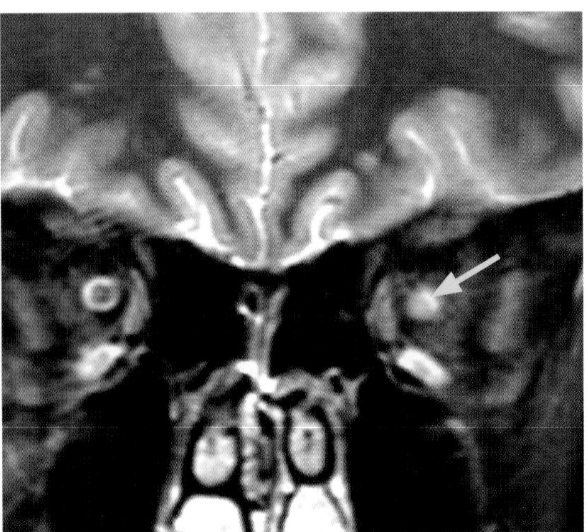

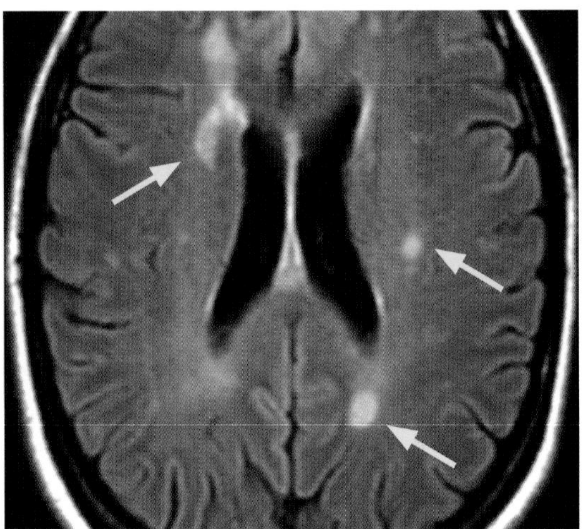

Optic neuritis due to multiple sclerosis: Coronal fat suppressed T2-weighted MRI through the orbits (left image) shows increased signal of the left optic nerve (arrow), with loss of clear distinction between the optic nerve and the surrounding normal T2 hyperintense CSF. The right optic nerve appears normal. There was no enhancement of the left optic nerve (not shown).

Axial FLAIR (right image) shows numerous foci of T2 prolongation within the periventricular white matter (arrows), in a pattern consistent with multiple sclerosis.

Case courtesy Mary Beth Cunnane, MD, Massachusetts Eye and Ear Infirmary.

- Optic neuritis is non-neoplastic inflammation of the optic nerve. It is typically painful and presents with painful subacute vision loss and reduced color perception.
- Optic neuritis is most commonly due to multiple sclerosis, but may result from other etiologies including viral infection, sarcoidosis, vasculitis, and toxin exposure.

  Optic neuritis associated with spinal demyelination (in the absence of brain lesions) is Devic syndrome, previously discussed in the section on white matter imaging.
- Acutely, there is optic nerve enlargement and T2 prolongation of the optic nerve. Enhancement suggests active disease. Chronically, the optic nerve atrophies.
- Imaging of the brain and spine should be performed to evaluate for intracranial plaques: More than 75% of patients with optic neuritis will have a brain white matter lesion.

- Lesions of the globe are seen most commonly in children.

Retinoblastoma

- Retinoblastoma is the most common primary malignant tumor of the globe.
- Retinoblastoma is almost always seen in children under 5 years old and typically presents with leukocoria (white pupillary reflex).
- Sporadic cases are often unilateral, but familial cases (associated with p53 tumor suppressor mutation) are bilateral.
- Classically, retinoblastoma appears as a hyperattenuating, enhancing retinal mass with calcification, in a normal-sized globe.
- "Trilateral" retinoblastoma describes bilateral retinoblastoma with pineal-gland pineoblastoma. "Quadrilateral" retinoblastoma is bilateral retinoblastoma, pineoblastoma, and suprasellar retinoblastoma.

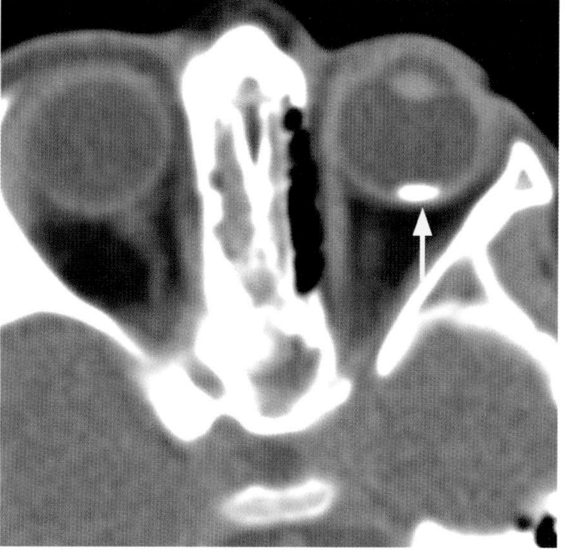

Retinoblastoma: Non-contrast axial CT through the orbits in a 20-month-old child demonstrates a normal-sized left orbit with a coarse retinal calcification (arrow).

Case courtesy Mary Beth Cunnane, MD, Massachusetts Eye and Ear Infirmary.

Coat disease

- Coat disease is a vascular disease of the retina that affects boys and features lipoproteinaceous subretinal exudates that lead to retinal detachment.

  Patients with Coat disease tend to be slightly older than those affected by retinoblastoma.
- The globe is normal in size but features subretinal soft tissue that does not enhance.

Retinopathy of prematurity (ROP)

- Retinopathy of prematurity (ROP) is seen only in premature infants and is due to prolonged oxygen therapy. Findings include abnormal vascular development, hemorrhage, and retinal detachment.
- Both eyes tend to be affected equally.
- There is bilateral microphthalmia (small globes), with increased attenuation of the globe due to prior hemorrhage.
- Though intraocular calcifications may be present (similar to retinoblastoma), ROP is distinguished from retinoblastoma by microphthalmia.
- The end-stage is phthisis bulbi, which is a shrunken, nonfunctioning globe.

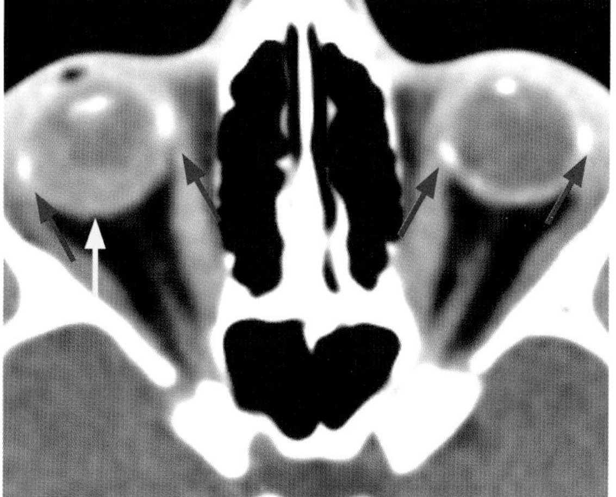

ROP: Non-contrast axial CT through the orbits shows bilateral microphthalmia with scattered orbital calcifications (red arrows). Peripheral high attenuation material in the right globe (yellow arrow) represents prior hemorrhage.

Case courtesy Mary Beth Cunnane, MD, Massachusetts Eye and Ear Infirmary.

Persistent hyperplastic primary vitreous (PHPV)

- Persistent hyperplastic primary vitreous (PHPV) is persistent embryonic vasculature within the vitreous that leads to loss of vision from hemorrhage, cataracts, and retinal detachment. Affected infants are typically full term.
- The eye is small (microphthalmia) with increased attenuation of the vitreous.
- PHPV is distinguished from retinoblastoma and ROP by the absence of calcifications.

Coloboma

- A coloboma is caused by incomplete fusion of the embryonic intraocular fissure, which can result in an elongated or malformed globe.
- Coloboma is associated with numerous syndromes including trisomies 13 and 18, and the CHARGE and VATER associations.
- Imaging shows a cone-shaped or notch-shaped deformity. Optic nerve colobomas can have outpouchings posteriorly, while iris colobomas are anterior. Colobomas that involve the uvea tend to have microphthalmos and a cyst.

Congenital orbital lesions

Sphenoid wing dysplasia

- Sphenoid wing dysplasia is seen in neurofibromatosis type 1.
- Transmission of CSF pulsation through the sphenoid wing defect may classically produce pulsatile exophthalmos.

Septo-optic dysplasia

- Septo-optic dysplasia is characterized by optic nerve hypoplasia and agenesis of the septum pellucidum.
- It is often associated with schizencephaly, a full-thickness cleft in the cerebral hemisphere that creates a communication between the ventricles and the extra-axial subarachnoid space.

Fascial spaces of the suprahyoid neck

Overview of head and neck spaces

- The complex layers of cervical fascia produce several fascially bounded spaces in the suprahyoid neck. Knowledge of these spaces is useful in creating differential diagnoses for neck masses, as specific lesions tend to arise in characteristic locations.

Pharynx

- The pharynx is a muscular tube extending from skull base to the thoracic inlet. It is the anatomic center of the head and neck, around which the other suprahyoid spaces wrap.
- The pharynx is divided into five distinct anatomic regions:

Nasopharynx: Top of pharynx behind the nasal cavity.

Oropharynx: From the level of the palate to the hyoid bone, behind the oral cavity. The posterior 1/3 of the tongue is part of the oropharynx.

Oral cavity: The space defined by the anterior 2/3 of the tongue, bounded superiorly by the palate and inferiorly by the floor of the mouth.

Hypopharynx: From the hyoid bone to the esophagus (posterior).

Larynx: From the hyoid bone to the trachea (anterior).

Masticator space

Anatomy of the masticator space

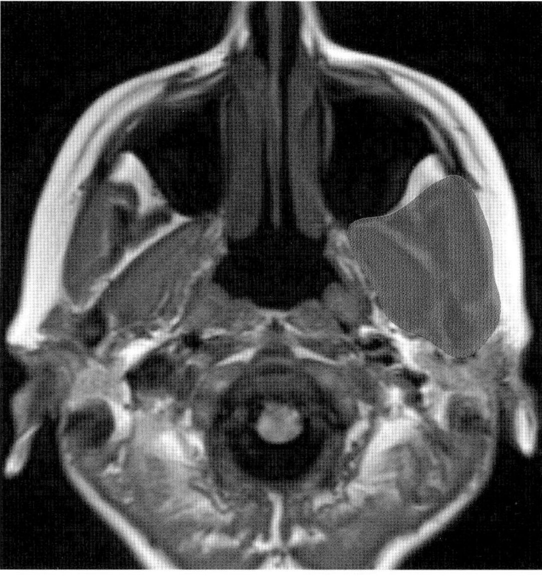

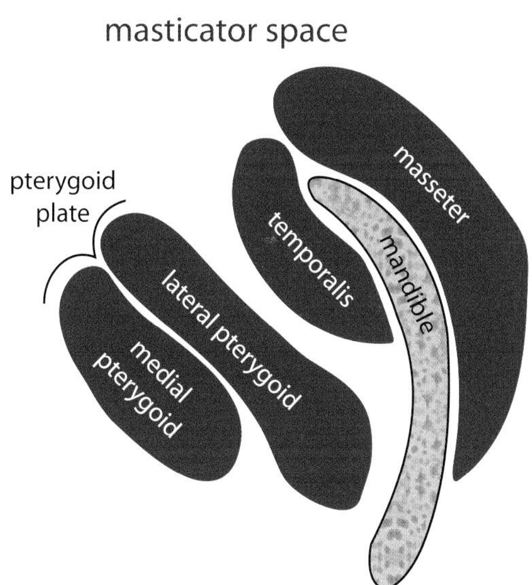

- The masticator space is located directly anterior to the parotid and contains the muscles of mastication, the mandible, and cranial nerve V3. Cranial nerve V3 (mandibular division) exits the skull through foramen ovale and innervates the muscles of mastication. If there is a lesion in the masticator space, it is important to assess for perineural spread along V3.

Differential diagnosis of a masticator space lesion

- **Odontogenic disease**

  Dental disease is the most common masticator space pathology, which can lead to abscess.
- **Mandibular lesion**

  Osteosarcoma and metastasis are the two most common malignant mandibular lesions.
- **Rhabdomyosarcoma**

  Rhabdomyosarcoma is the most common head and neck tumor of childhood.

Anatomy of the carotid space

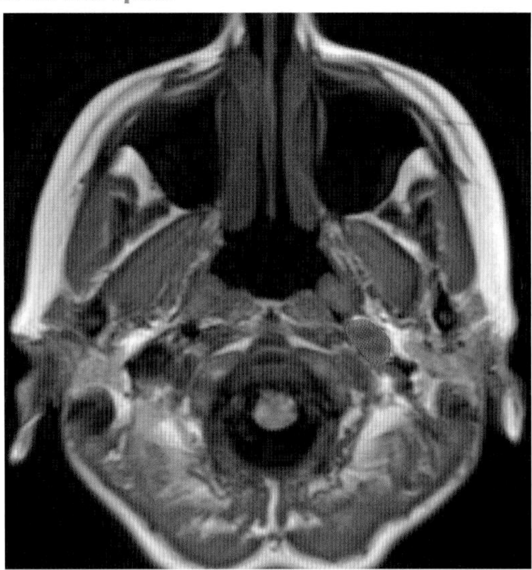

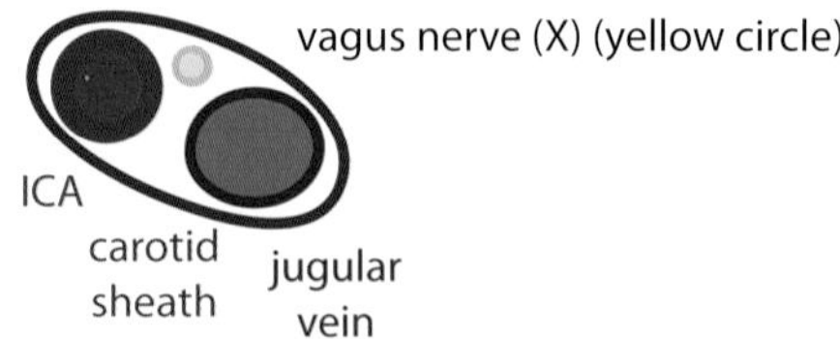

Other cranial nerves passing through the carotid space:
glossopharyngeal nerve (IX)
spinal accessory nerve (XI)
hypoglossal nerve (XII)

- The carotid space, or post-styloid parapharyngeal space, is an incomplete fascial ring surrounding the carotid artery and jugular vein. The carotid space extends from the skull base to the aortic arch. There is some controversy regarding the terminology of the carotid space, as some authors prefer the term "post-styloid parapharyngeal space" versus "carotid space." Though the former is more anatomically accurate because the fascial boundary of this space is incomplete, the latter is simpler and perhaps more helpful to generate a differential diagnosis of a mass.
- The contents of the carotid space include the carotid artery, carotid body, jugular vein, and several cranial nerves. The vagus nerve (cranial nerve X) is the only cranial nerve that remains within the carotid space the entire way into the thorax. In contrast, cranial nerves IX, XI and XII pass transiently through the carotid space. Though there are lymph nodes surrounding the carotid space, there are no lymph nodes contained within it.
- The pattern of displacement of vascular structures in the carotid space is the key to generating a differential diagnosis for a carotid space mass.

Differential diagnosis of a carotid space mass

- **Paraganglioma**

  A paraganglioma is a benign, highly vascular neoplasm of neural crest cells, featuring intense enhancement and a characteristic salt-and-pepper appearance on MRI due to intra-tumoral flow voids.

  Paraganglioma of the carotid body (carotid body tumor) splays the external and internal carotid arteries at the carotid bifurcation.

  Paraganglioma of the vagal nerve (glomus vagale) displaces the internal and external carotid arteries anteromedially.

- **Schwannoma**

  Similar to glomus vagale, schwannoma (also most commonly of the vagus nerve) also displaces the carotid arteries anteromedially. Schwannoma, however, is not nearly as vascular as paraganglioma and usually does not enhance as homogeneously.

- **Neurofibroma**

  Neurofibromas are almost always associated with neurofibromatosis type 1.

  Neurofibroma and schwannoma are indistinguishable by MRI.

Parapharyngeal space (PPS)

Anatomy of the parapharyngeal space

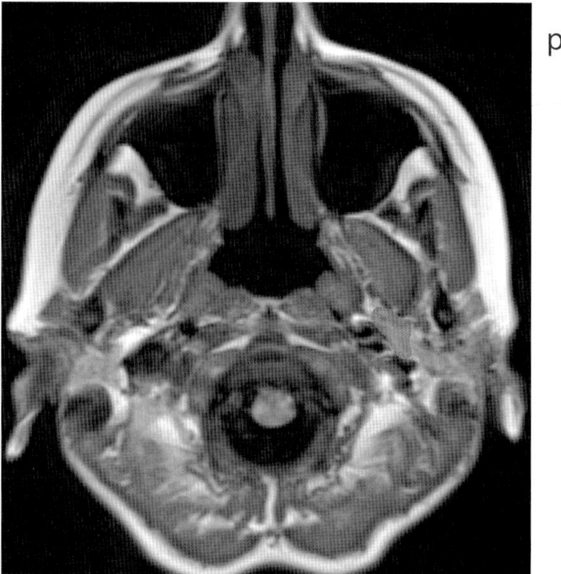

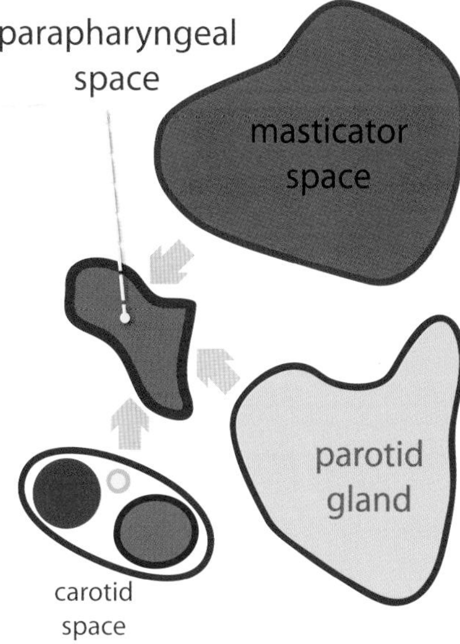

- The parapharyngeal space (PPS) is a triangular fat-filled space with no significant contents aside from occasional ectopic minor salivary gland tissue. The parapharyngeal space is relatively conspicuous on both MRI and CT due to its fat content.
- The direction of displacement of the parapharyngeal space by a mass lesion in an adjacent compartment is predictable and helpful in determining from which compartment a given mass originates.
- Masticator space lesions (e.g., masticator abscess) displace the PPS posteromedially.
- Parotid lesions (e.g., pleomorphic adenoma) displace the PPS anteromedially.
- Carotid space lesions (e.g., paraganglioma) displace the PPS anteriorly.

Perivertebral space

Anatomy of the perivertebral space

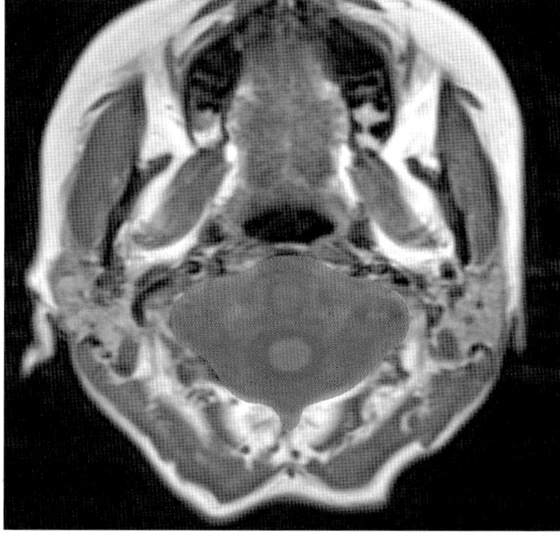

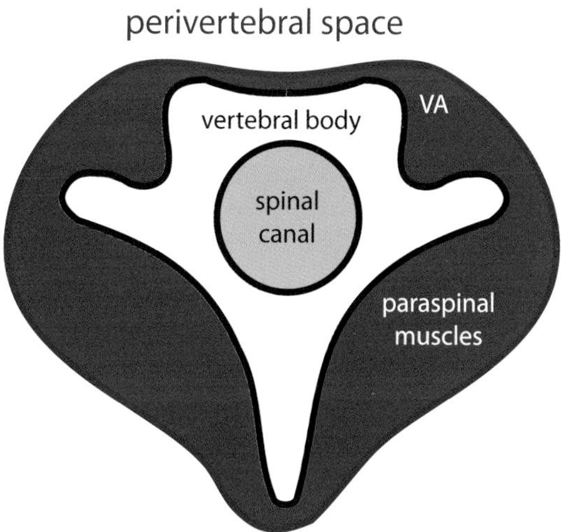

- The perivertebral space is formed by the deep layer of deep cervical fascia, which wraps entirely around the prevertebral and paraspinal muscles. The prevertebral space is the anterior component of the perivertebral space. The *peri*vertebral space is in the suprahyoid neck; the *para*vertebral space is the analogous region in the thoracolumbar spine.
- Contents include vertebral arteries, paraspinal muscles, spinal column, and exiting nerves.

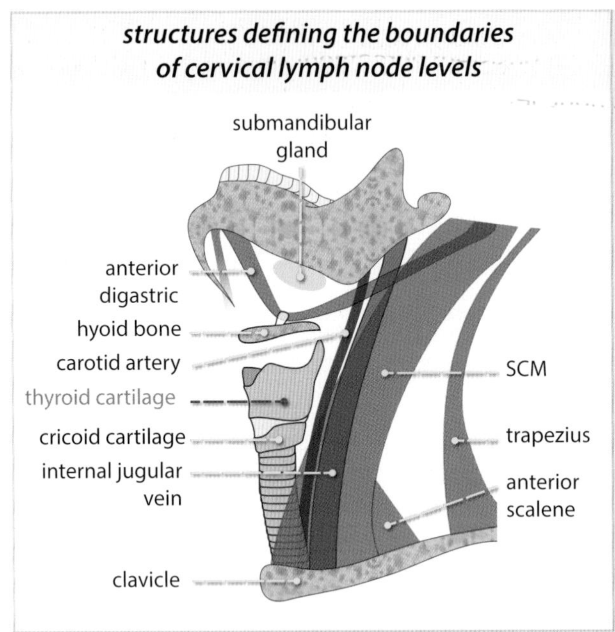
structures defining the boundaries of cervical lymph node levels
submandibular gland
anterior digastric
hyoid bone
carotid artery
thyroid cartilage
cricoid cartilage
internal jugular vein
clavicle
SCM
trapezius
anterior scalene

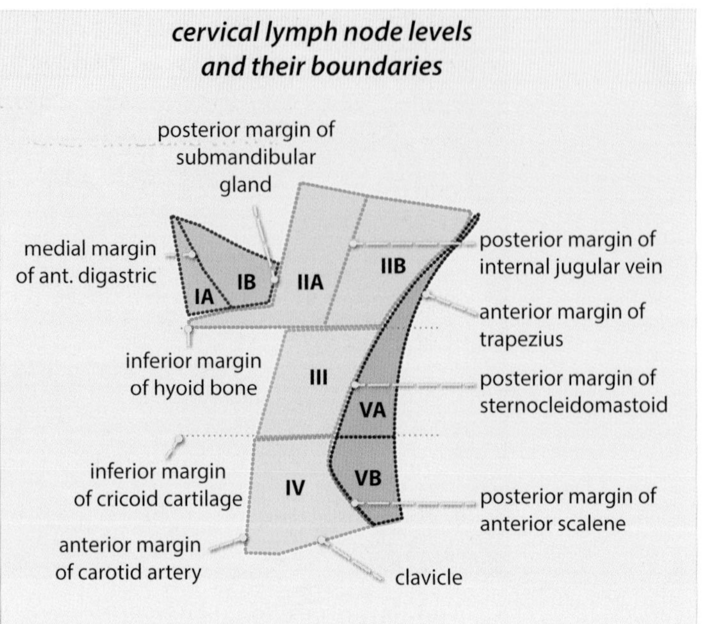
cervical lymph node levels and their boundaries
posterior margin of submandibular gland
medial margin of ant. digastric
IA
IB
IIA
IIB
III
VA
IV
VB
inferior margin of hyoid bone
inferior margin of cricoid cartilage
anterior margin of carotid artery
clavicle
posterior margin of internal jugular vein
anterior margin of trapezius
posterior margin of sternocleidomastoid
posterior margin of anterior scalene

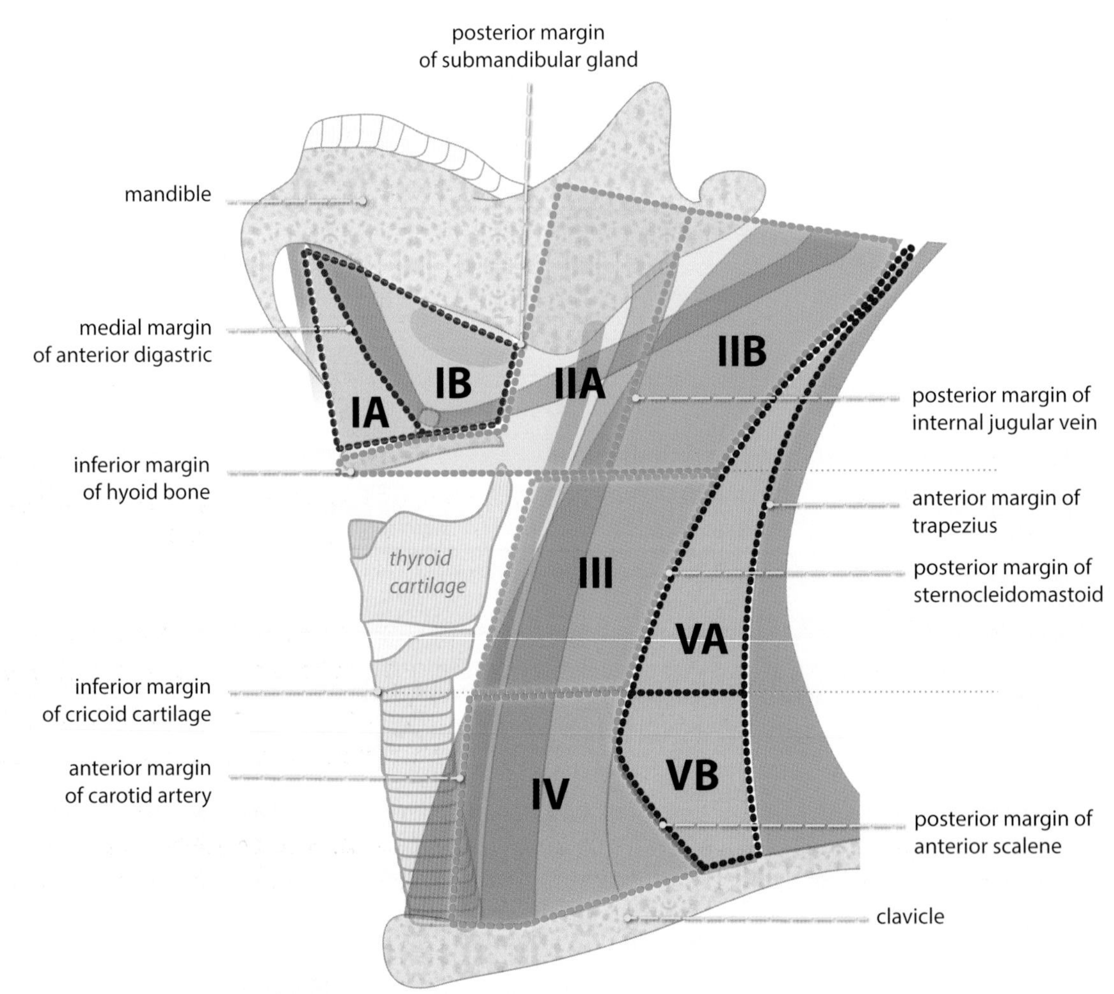
cervical lymph node levels superimposed on boundary structures
posterior margin of submandibular gland
mandible
medial margin of anterior digastric
inferior margin of hyoid bone
thyroid cartilage
inferior margin of cricoid cartilage
anterior margin of carotid artery
IA
IB
IIA
IIB
III
VA
IV
VB
posterior margin of internal jugular vein
anterior margin of trapezius
posterior margin of sternocleidomastoid
posterior margin of anterior scalene
clavicle

Cervical lymph node levels

Overview of cervical lymph nodes

- The cervical lymph nodes are divided into seven levels as recommended by the AJCC (American Joint Committee on Cancer), with consistent agreement between surgeons, oncologists, and radiologists. The lymph node levels are not defined by fascial planes, but instead are defined by anatomic landmarks and organized by patterns of lymphatic spread.
- In an adult, 90% of head and neck cancers are squamous cell carcinoma: The role of the radiologist is not to provide a differential, but to stage the disease. The degree of lymph node involvement has a substantial prognostic value. For instance, a single metastatic lymph node decreases survival from squamous cell carcinoma by 50% over an equivalent period.

Level I

- Level I lymph nodes include submental and submandibular nodes, which are superior to the hyoid bone and inferior to the mandible and mylohyoid.
- **IA** nodes are submental, lying between the medial margins of the anterior bellies of the digastrics.
- **IB** nodes are submandibular, lateral to the medial margin of the anterior belly of the digastric and extending to the posterior margin of the submandibular gland.

Level II

- Level II lymph nodes are upper internal jugular nodes, extending from the skull base to the inferior margin of the hyoid bone.
- **IIA** nodes are anterior to the posterior margin of the internal jugular vein (IJV).
- **IIB** nodes are posterior to the IJV but anterior to the posterior margin of the sternocleidomastoid muscle.

Level III

- Level III lymph nodes are middle jugular nodes, extending craniocaudally from the inferior aspect of the hyoid to the inferior aspect of the cricoid cartilage. The posterior edge of the sternocleidomastoid is the shared posterior margin for both level III and level IIB nodes.

Level IV

- Level IV nodes are inferior jugular nodes, extending from the inferior aspect of the cricoid cartilage to the clavicle. Superiorly, the posterior border is the posterior aspect of the sternocleidomastoid muscle (similar to level III and IIB nodes). Inferiorly, the posterior border is the posterior aspect of the anterior scalene muscle.

Level V

- Level V lymph nodes are posterior cervical nodes.
- **VA** nodes are superior, extending from the skull base to the inferior cricoid cartilage.
- **VB** nodes are inferior, extending from the inferior cricoid cartilage to the clavicle.

Level VI

- Level VI nodes are pretracheal nodes, which are often simply called "pretracheal." They are located anteromedially in the lower neck and bounded laterally by the carotid sheaths. Level VI extends craniocaudally from the inferior aspect of the hyoid bone to the top of the manubrium.

Level VII

- Level VII nodes are superior mediastinal nodes, which are also commonly described by their location. They are inferior to level VI and medial to the carotid sheaths, extending craniocaudally from the superior aspect of the manubrium to the brachiocephalic vein.

SPINE LESION LOCALIZATION

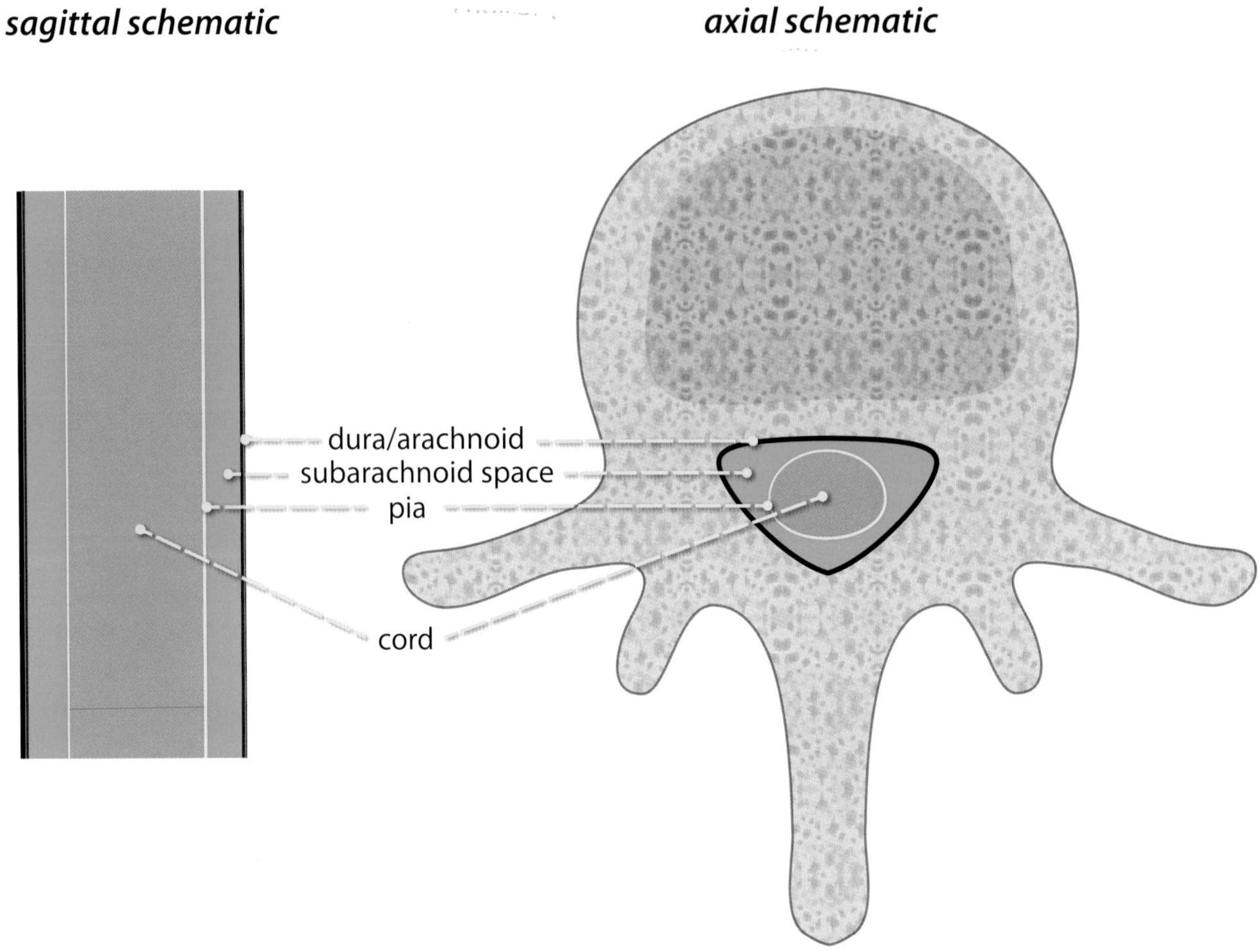

sagittal schematic

axial schematic

dura/arachnoid
subarachnoid space
pia
cord

intramedullary

ependymoma
astrocytoma
hemangioblastoma
demyelinating lesion

intradural extramedullary

schwannoma
neurofibroma
meningioma
myxopapillary ependymoma
epidermoid/dermoid
arachnoiditis

extradural

degenerative disease
vertebral neoplasm
epidural metastasis
hemangioma
epidural lipomatosis

- The first step in evaluation of any spinal lesion is to determine its compartment of origin. Each compartment has its own differential considerations.
- The three compartments are **intramedullary** (deep to the pia, usually within the substance of the cord itself), **intradural–extramedullary** (within the dura, but outside the pia), and **extradural** (external to the dura).

Overview of intramedullary lesions

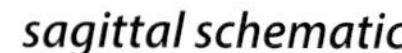

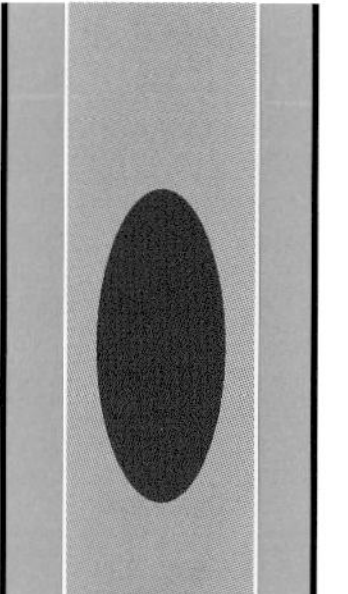

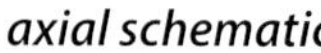

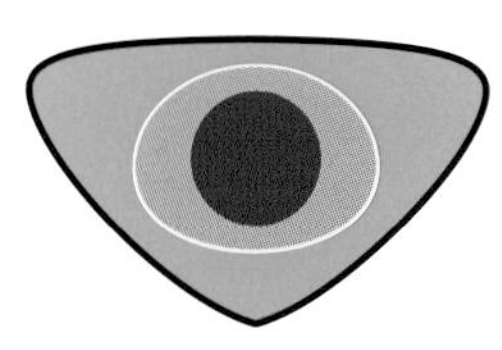

- Intramedullary lesions are located deep to the pia, typically within the substance of the cord itself. By definition, all intramedullary lesions are also intradural.
- Astrocytoma and ependymoma together make up 95% of intramedullary tumors. These two tumors have overlapping imaging features.
- Astrocytomas are more common in children and ependymomas are more common in adults.

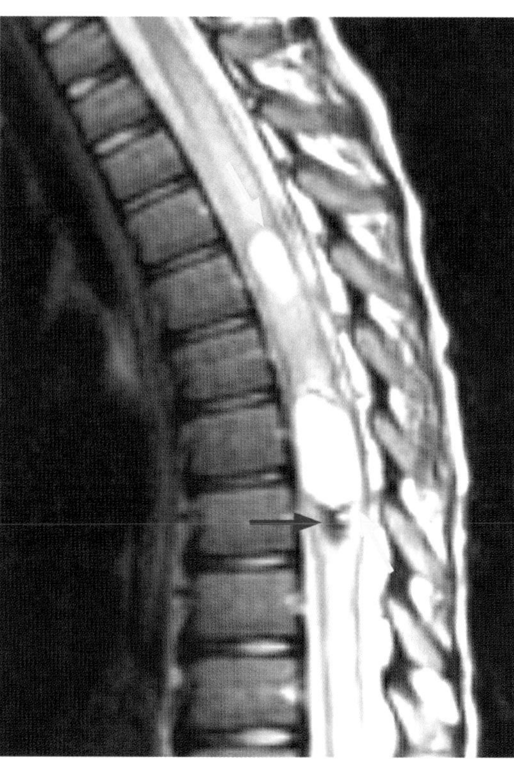

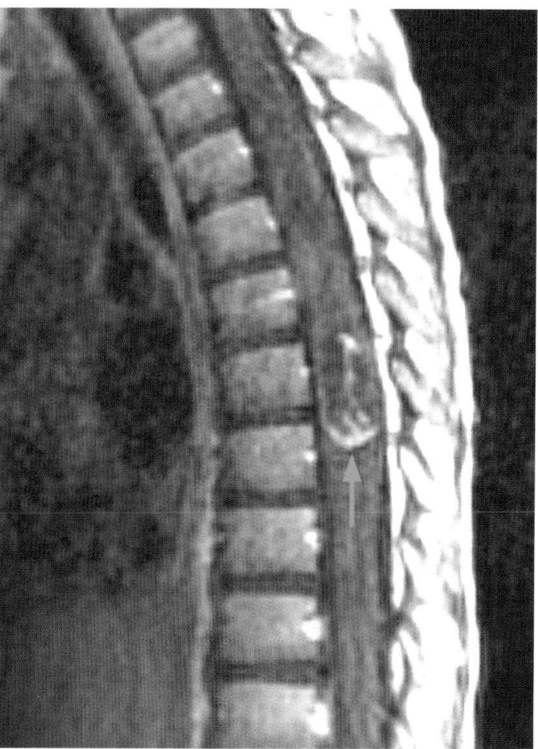

Intramedullary mass: Sagittal T2-weighted (left image) and T1-weighted postcontrast (right image) MRI shows an intramedullary mass in the thoracic spine (yellow arrows), which expands the spinal cord and causes cord signal abnormality from the mid-thoracic spine down. A focus of hypointensity on the T2-weighted image at the inferior aspect of the lesion may represent hemorrhagic material (red arrow). On the post-contrast image, the mass demonstrates wispy enhancement inferiorly (blue arrow). This was an astrocytoma.

Astrocytoma

- Astrocytoma is the most common intramedullary tumor in children. Most spinal astrocytomas are low grade. Spinal glioblastoma multiforme has been described but occurs rarely. Astrocytoma usually extends over several vertebral levels and causes fusiform dilation of the spinal cord.
- Cystic components are seen in approximately 1/3 and a syrinx may be present. Tumors almost always enhance despite being low grade. In contrast to ependymoma, hemorrhage is rare.
- Astrocytoma cannot be reliably differentiated from ependymoma based on imaging features. Hemorrhage is more commonly seen with ependymoma and may occasionally be a helpful discriminating feature.

Ependymoma

- Ependymoma is the most common intramedullary tumor in adults, arising from ependymal cells that line the central spinal canal. Ependymoma is associated with neurofibromatosis type 2, especially when seen in children.
- Ependymoma is often hemorrhagic, leading to a heterogeneous MRI appearance. Peripheral hemosiderin deposition causes a dark rim on T2-weighted images. Most ependymomas enhance. Classically, there is extensive formation of both tumoral cysts and nontumoral polar cysts. Tumoral cysts are surrounded by enhancement and must be resected with the mass. A classic radiographic finding of ependymoma is scalloping of the vertebral bodies; however, that finding is associated with advanced disease and is rarely seen today.

Hemangioblastoma

- Hemangioblastoma is a rare intramedullary tumor (distant third most common behind astrocytoma) associated with von Hippel–Lindau (VHL). One third of hemangioblastomas are associated with this syndrome.
- Characteristic imaging features are marked enhancement, cyst formation, and numerous flow voids. Up to 15% have both intramedullary and intradural–extramedullary components.

Demyelinating lesion

- An active multiple sclerosis (MS) lesion may enhance and mimic a spinal tumor, but MS is often distinguishable from a neoplasm by the absence of cord expansion (analogous to the absence of significant mass effect that is typical of intracranial tumefactive MS).

Intradural–Extramedullary Lesions

Overview of intradural–extramedullary lesions

- Intradural–extramedullary lesions are located within the dura but outside the spinal cord. Most of the time, intradural–extramedullary lesions are located in the subarachnoid space. A classic imaging appearance (not always seen) is a cleft of CSF between the lesion and the cord.
- Nerve-sheath tumors (neurofibromas and schwannomas) and meningiomas together make up about 90% of intradural–extramedullary tumors.

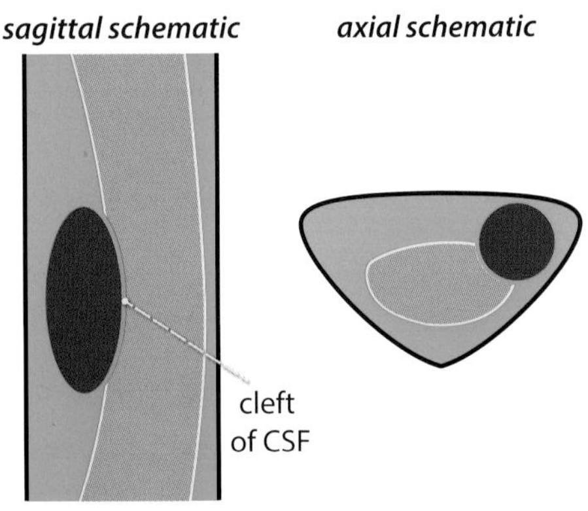

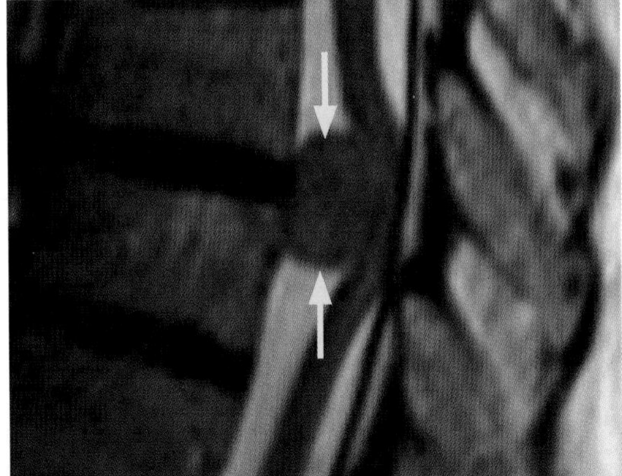

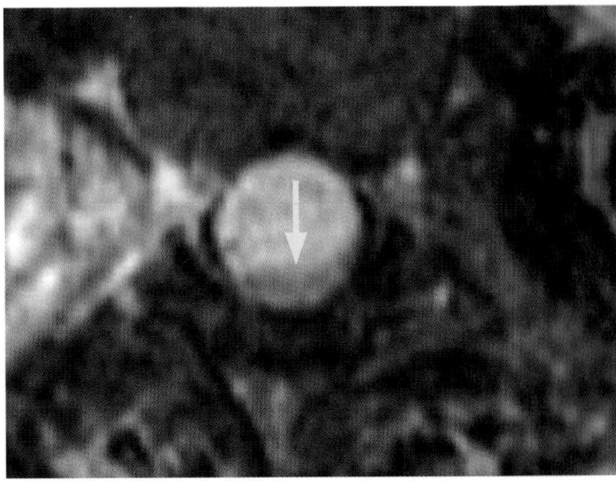

Intradural–extramedullary mass: Sagittal T2-weighted (left image) and axial T1-weighted post-contrast (right image) MRI shows an intradural thoracic mass (arrows). The mass is distinct from the spinal cord and displaces the cord posteriorly. The axial image shows severe posterior compression of the cord by the avidly enhancing mass (arrow). This was a meningioma. Usually, however, thoracic meningiomas are posterior to the spinal cord.

Nerve-sheath tumor (schwannoma, neurofibroma)

- Benign nerve-sheath tumors are the most common intradural–extramedullary tumors. Fifteen percent are both intradural–extramedullary and extradural (called "dumbbell" tumors) and 15% may be completely extradural.
- **Neurofibroma** and **schwannoma** cannot be reliably differentiated on imaging.
- Schwannoma is more common, occurs in older patients, and is encapsulated. Schwannoma can be treated by a nerve-sparing approach, which is accomplished by "shelling out" the tumor.
- Neurofibroma is associated with neurofibromatosis type 1, occurs in younger patients (early adulthood), and lacks a capsule. The complete circumference of the nerve is involved and treatment therefore necessitates nerve resection.
- Both neurofibroma and schwannoma can cause neural foraminal enlargement.
- The target sign, which is central hypointensity on T2-weighted images surrounded by a hyperintense periphery, is seen in both conditions and suggests benignity.

Meningioma

- Meningioma is a benign neoplasm arising from arachnoid cap cells. It is most commonly seen in older women.
- A classic imaging finding is a broad dural base. Meningiomas often calcify. Typical locations are anterior to the cord in the cervical spine and posterior to the cord in the thoracic spine.

Dermoid cyst

- Dermoid cyst is a congenital lesion that usually presents in childhood.
- Dermoid contains macroscopic fat, which is hyperintense on T1-weighted images.
- Rare dermoid rupture may cause potentially fatal chemical meningitis.

Epidermoid cyst

- Epidermoid cyst is a rare acquired spinal tumor. It is thought to be caused by implantation of skin elements in the subarachnoid space during neonatal spinal puncture.
- Spinal epidermoids are usually intradural–extramedullary but may rarely be intramedullary.
- Most commonly, an epidermoid cyst appears similar to a simple cyst (hypointense on T1-weighted images and hyperintense on T2-weighted images). Faint peripheral rim enhancement can be seen. Occasionally, the cyst contents may be proteinaceous, causing T1 shortening.
- As with other epidermoids, diffusivity is restricted, in contrast to an arachnoid cyst.

Myxopapillary ependymoma

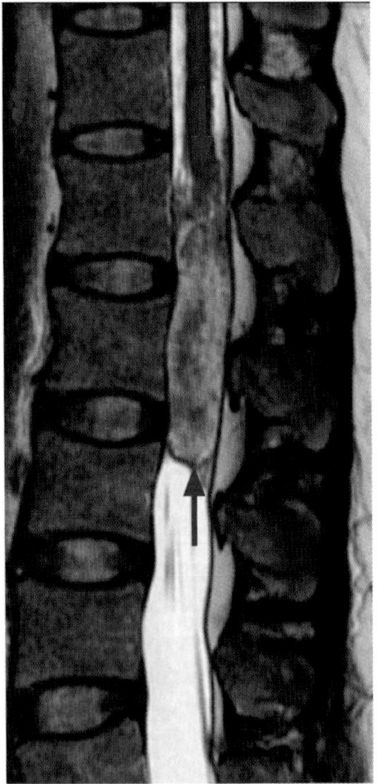
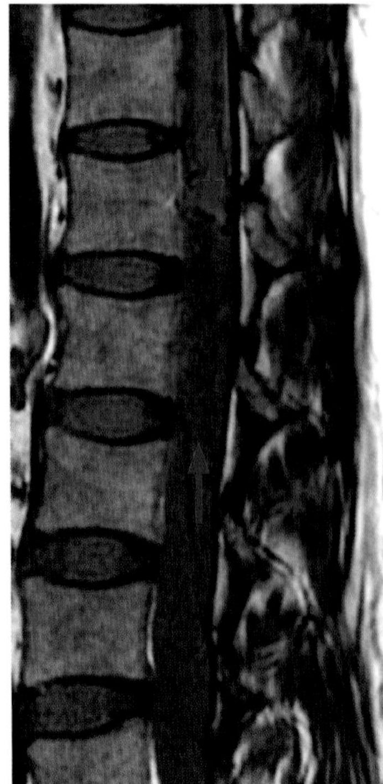
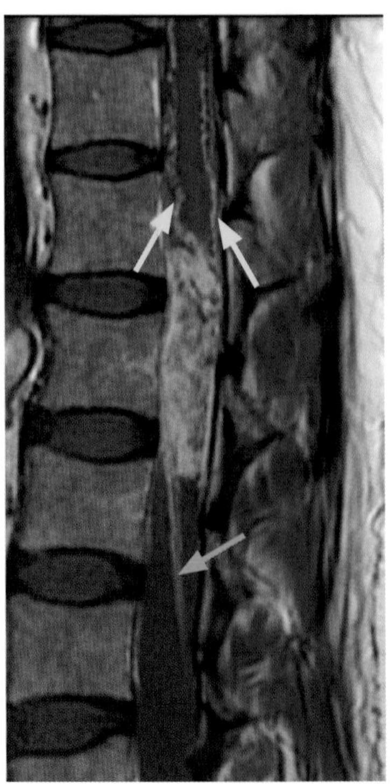

Myxopapillary ependymoma:

Sagittal T2- (left image), T1- (middle image), and post-contrast T1-weighted (right image) MRI demonstrates a heterogeneously T2 hyperintense, lobulated mass (red arrows) containing regions of hypointensity on the T2-weighted image. The mass is located at the conus medullaris and avidly enhances. There is also enhancing leptomeningeal dissemination along the surface of the more proximal cord (yellow arrows) and along the cauda equina nerve roots (blue arrow).

Case courtesy Gregory Wrubel, MD, Brigham and Women's Hospital.

- Myxopapillary ependymoma is an ependymoma variant that occurs exclusively within the conus medullaris or the filum terminale. It is the most common tumor of the conus and filum and arises from ependymal cells in the filum.
- The tumor is characterized by slow growth, classically leading to vertebral scalloping and spinal canal enlargement.
- Myxopapillary ependymoma is a highly vascular, hemorrhagic tumor, featuring a complex, lobulated MRI appearance with internal hemorrhage. Peripheral hemosiderin is often present, producing hypointensity on T2-weighted images and blooming on GRE.

Arachnoiditis

- Arachnoiditis is inflammation of the arachnoid surrounding the nerve roots, which produces a fibrinous exudate and secondary dural adhesions. In the past, tuberculosis and syphilis were common causes of arachnoiditis. Today, lumbar spine surgery is a far more common cause. Arachnoiditis may be a cause of persistent back pain after lumbar surgery.
- The primary imaging feature of arachnoiditis is displacement of the nerve roots. Three patterns have been described:

Group 1: **Central conglomerations** of nerve roots within the thecal sac.

Group 2: **Peripheral clumping** of nerve roots, causing the *empty thecal sac* sign.

Group 3: **Obliteration of the subarachnoid space**. Imaging shows increased soft tissue within the thecal sac. This is the most severe form of arachnoiditis.

EXTRADURAL LESIONS

Overview of extradural lesions

- **Extradural** lesions are located external to the dura. The epidural space is extradural.
- Degenerative lesions, such as osteophytes and herniated discs, are the most common extradural lesions.
- Other important extradural lesions include epidural metastases and infection (discitis/osteomyelitis).
- Primary extradural tumors are rare and are usually bony in origin.

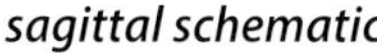

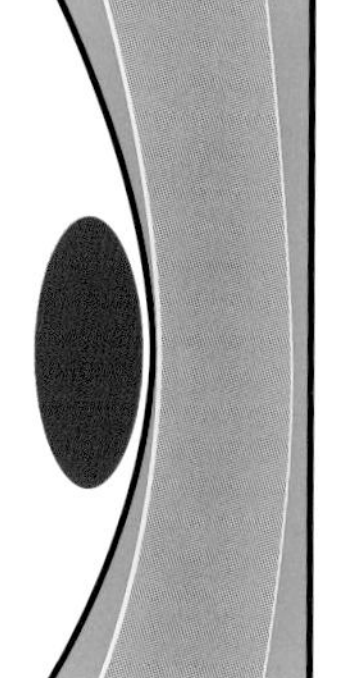

axial schematic

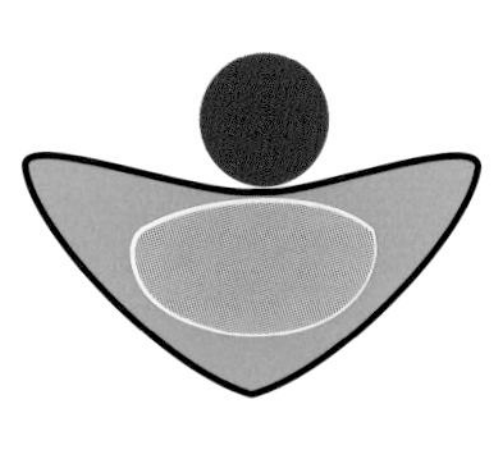

Degenerative disease

- Degenerative lesions are the most common extradural lesions, but are usually not difficult to diagnose. Degenerative spine disease is discussed in the next section.

Vertebral body/epidural metastasis

- Metastatic disease is the most common adult extradural malignancy. Breast, lung, and prostate are the most common primary tumors to metastasize to the spinal column.
- T1-weighted images are essential for evaluation of vertebral body marrow replacement. Marrow should always be more hyperintense on T1-weighted images than the intervertebral discs.
- *Focal* decrease in intensity on T1-weighted images is concerning for metastasis.
- *Diffuse* decrease in intensity on T1-weighted images is abnormal but nonspecific. The differential for diffusely decreased T1 marrow signal includes leukemia, lymphoma, myelofibrosis, HIV, and idiopathic causes.

Discitis/osteomyelitis

- It is important to consider an infectious epidural collection in the differential diagnosis for an extradural mass. This process is addressed later in this chapter.

Hemangioma

- Vertebral body hemangioma is a common, usually incidentally found, benign lesion composed of endothelium-lined vascular structures.
- Destruction of some of the bony trabeculae and thickening of the remaining trabeculae produce the characteristic striated *corduroy* appearance on plain radiographs and sagittal/coronal CT. The stippled appearance on axial CT is produced by thickened trabeculae seen on end.
- Hemangioma is typically hyperintense on both T1- and T2-weighted images.
- Although hemangioma is benign, an aggressive variant is occasionally seen in the thoracic spine. The aggressive variant may have an epidural soft tissue component that has the potential to cause cord compression.

  Although the asymptomatic variant has no sex predilection, the aggressive form of hemangioma is more common in females.

Primary osseous vertebral body tumors of middle-aged and older adults

- **Chordoma** is a malignant tumor of older adults that arises from a notochord remnant.

  Chordoma occurs most commonly in the sacrococcygeal region and second most commonly in the clivus. Up to 15% may occur in the vertebral bodies (most commonly cervical).

  Chordoma appears as a destructive, hyperintense mass on T2-weighted images. It avidly enhances.

- **Plasmacytoma** is a lytic, expansile bony lesion of late adulthood that is thought to be a precursor of multiple myeloma.

  A plasmacytoma is a solitary lesion. The presence of multiple plasmacytomas implies the diagnosis of multiple myeloma. Development of fulminant multiple myeloma, or even abnormal serum/urine protein electrophoresis, may not occur for many years after diagnosis of a plasmacytoma.

- **Chondrosarcoma** is a low-grade malignancy that appears as a hyperintense mass on T2-weighted images, similar to chordoma. Chondroid *rings-and-arcs* calcification may be seen.

Primary osseous vertebral body tumors of adolescents and young adults

- **Aneurysmal bone cyst** (ABC) is a benign, progressively destructive lesion that occurs in adolescents. Fluid levels are typically seen on MRI, though this finding is nonspecific.
- **Chondroblastoma** is a benign but aggressive neoplasm that rarely may occur in the vertebral column (vertebral body and posterior elements). Secondary ABC may be present.
- **Osteoid osteoma** is a benign, sclerotic lesion affecting the vertebral posterior elements in teenagers and young adults, with a classic clinical history of nocturnal pain relieved by NSAIDs. A central radiolucent nidus consists of vascular fibrous connecting tissue.
- **Osteosarcoma** is a malignant tumor that typically produces osteoid matrix.

Epidural lipomatosis

- Spinal epidural lipomatosis is a rare overgrowth of fat in the extradural space, which may cause compression of neural elements. In severe cases, epidural lipomatosis may cause cauda equina syndrome.
- Epidural lipomatosis may be caused by exogenous steroid administration (systemic administration much more commonly than epidural injection) or Cushing disease/syndrome. Epidural lipomatosis is a complication of morbid obesity.
- Surgery is the preferred treatment if a neurological deficit is present.

Degenerative spine

Overview of degenerative disease

Back pain

- Back pain is the second most common reason for physician visits in the US (an upper respiratory complaint is the most common reason).
- Trauma or age-related degenerative changes can cause spinal stenosis, neural foraminal stenosis, and spinal nerve impingement, all of which may cause back pain. Additionally, injury to adjacent bony, ligamentous, or muscular structures may generate pain.

Goal of imaging

- The primary goal of MRI imaging of the spine is to identify either a surgically correctable lesion or a process that could be treated by an epidural steroid injection.
- Disc bulges and herniations are commonly seen in asymptomatic people. The high prevalence of these "abnormalities" complicates correlation of clinical and imaging findings.
- Despite efforts to standardize the nomenclature with an established lexicon, there is a fair amount of inter-observer variability in the reporting of degenerative spinal lesions.

Disc bulges and herniations

- The normal intervertebral disc is composed of a central gelatinous nucleus pulposus and a fibrous peripheral annulus fibrosus. A disc bulge, or herniation, occurs when the substance of the disc (nucleus pulposus, annulus fibrosus, or both) extends beyond the disc's normal margins.

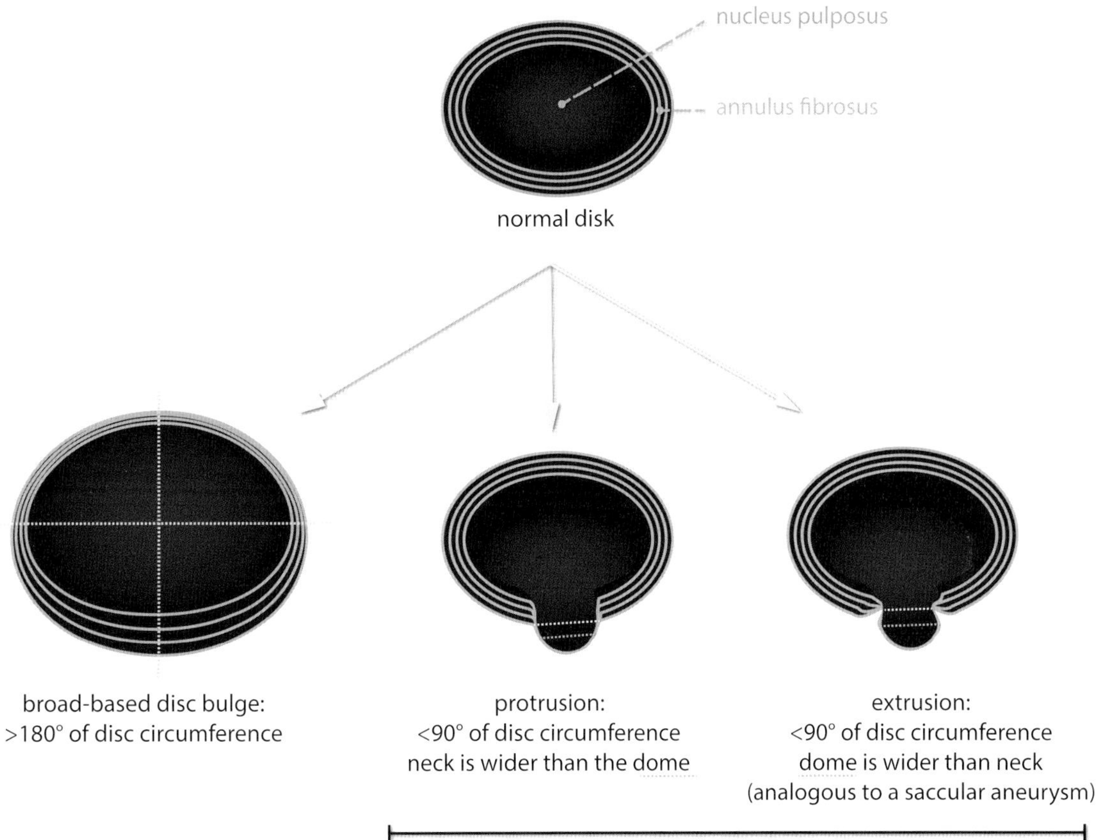

- A broad-based disc bulge is present when >180° of the disc circumference extends beyond the expected margins of the disc. Technically, the bulge must measure greater than 2 mm over greater than 180° of its circumference. In practice, the radiologist makes this diagnosis subjectively and exact measurements are typically unnecessary.
- A herniation is a focal disc bulge. Technically, a herniation must involve less than 90° of the disc circumference. In practice, measurement is rarely performed.
- The term "herniation" is a nonspecific, medicolegally charged umbrella term that is generally avoided in dictations. The preferred description for herniation is either **protrusion** or **extrusion**, depending on the morphology. In this text, "herniation" refers to both protrusions and extrusions.
- A **protrusion** is a focal herniation where the diameter of the neck is greater than the diameter of the dome.
- An **extrusion** is a focal herniation where the diameter of the neck is less than the diameter of the dome. This is analogous to a saccular aneurysm.
- Disc herniation may contribute to nerve root impingement and spinal stenosis.

- Both the medial–lateral position and the spinal level of herniation dictate which nerve root is impinged upon.
- In the thoracic and lumbar spine, each nerve root exits below its corresponding vertebral body. For instance, the L4 nerve root exits below the L4 vertebral body at L4–L5.
- In contrast, in the cervical spine, each root exits above its corresponding vertebral body. For instance, the C7 nerve root exits above the C7 vertebral body at C6–C7. At the cervicothoracic transition, the C8 nerve root exits below the C7 vertebral body and the T1 nerve root exits below the T1 vertebral body.
- Four terms describe the medial–lateral position of a herniation: **Central**, **paracentral** (adjacent to the subarticular facet joint), **foraminal**, and **far-lateral** (extra-foraminal). A medial (central or paracentral) herniation will affect the descending nerve root corresponding to the level below the disc. For instance, central or paracentral herniation of the L4–L5 disc will impinge the descending L5 root. In contrast, a lateral (foraminal or far-lateral) herniation will affect the exiting nerve root, which would be L4 at the L4–5 level.

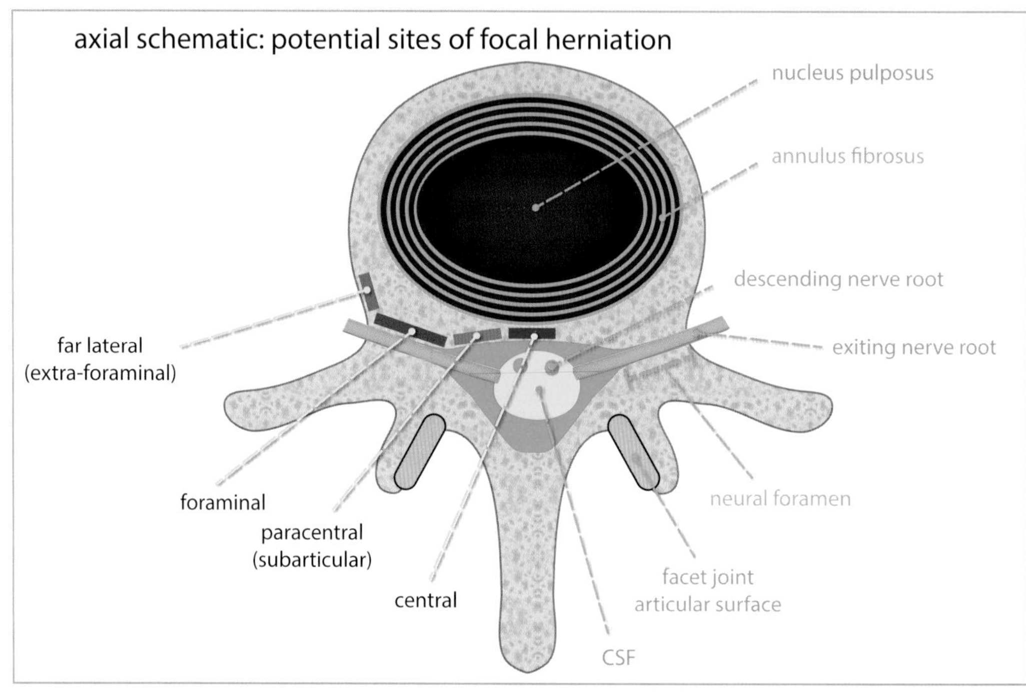

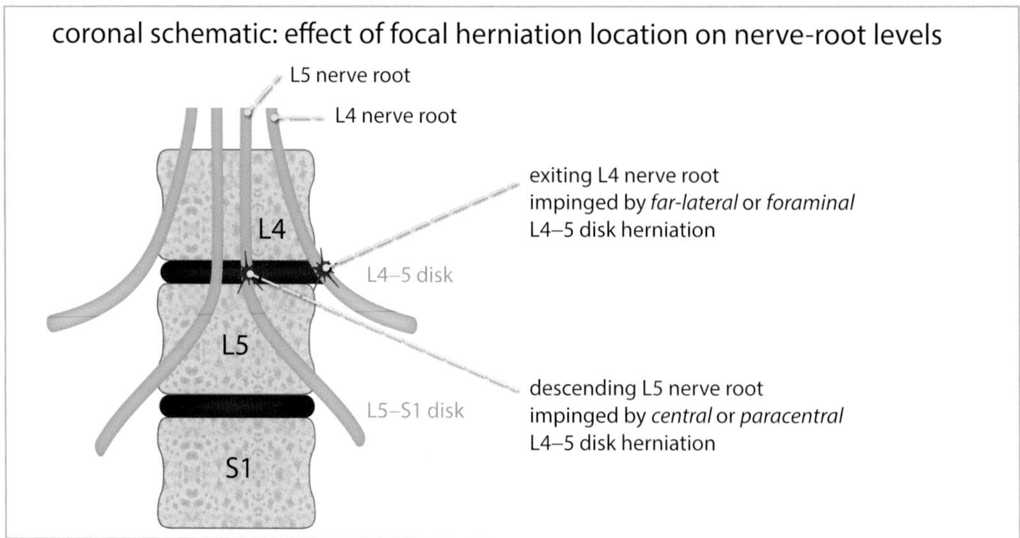

- Once protruded, disc material may separate from its parent disc to become a sequestered fragment, which may subsequently migrate inferiorly or superiorly. The surgeon needs to know about a sequestered fragment because it may preclude a minimally invasive procedure.

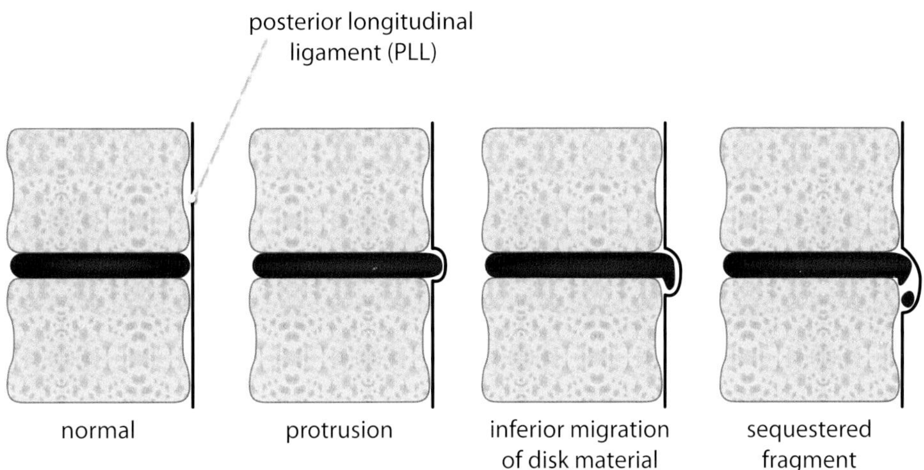

General degenerative changes

- With aging, discs tend to become desiccated, manifested as T2 shortening (hypointensity on T2-weighted images).
- Loss of disc space height may affect multiple levels.
- Osteophytes can project anteriorly or posteriorly. In the cervical spine, anterior osteophytes may cause dysphagia. Anywhere in the spine, posteriorly projecting osteophytes may contribute to spinal canal or neural foraminal stenosis.
- A **Schmorl's node** represents inferior or superior herniation of an intervertebral disc into the adjacent vertebral body endplate, which creates a rounded bony defect at the endplate. An acute Schmorl's node may be hyperintense on T2-weighted images and may contribute to back pain.

Secondary vertebral body changes – Modic changes

- Degenerative changes in the spine are associated with vertebral body endplate and subchondral marrow signal changes that were described and classified by Modic.
- **Modic type 1** changes are hyperintense on T2-weighted images and hypointense on T1-weighted images, reflecting bone marrow edema and inflammation. These changes may be associated with active back pain and their presence predicts a better outcome following lumbar spine surgery.
- **Modic type 2** changes are hyperintense on both T2- and T1-weighted images and reflect fatty proliferation within the affected marrow, thought to be secondary to chronic marrow ischemia. Modic 2 changes are less likely to be associated with active symptoms.
- **Modic type 3** changes are hypointense on both T2- and T1-weighted images and are thought to represent sclerosis. Their clinical significance is unclear.

Ligamentum flavum infolding/hypertrophy

- The ligamentum flavum lines the lamina at the posterior aspect of the spinal canal. Thickening of the ligamentum flavum can contribute to spinal canal stenosis.
- The terms "infolding," "inward buckling," and "hypertrophy" have been used to describe apparent thickening of the ligamentum flavum. The terms "infolding" or "inward buckling" are preferred by some authors as being more indicative of the actual process.

Facet arthropathy

- The intervertebral facet joints are synovial joints that can undergo the same degenerative processes as larger synovial joints, including cartilage loss, osteophytosis, sclerosis, and subchondral cystic change.
- The facet joints are located medial to the neural foramina. Degenerative changes of the facet joints (facet arthropathy) may contribute to neural foraminal narrowing.
- A synovial cyst is an epidural cyst that is associated with facet arthropathy. On MRI, a synovial cyst is hyperintense on T2-weighted images and variable signal intensity on T1-weighted images depending on the presence of internal hemorrhage. Continuity of the synovial cyst with the facet joint may not be demonstrated on MRI, but epidural injection of the facet joint will show opacification of the cyst.

  In contrast to a synovial cyst, a **Tarlov** cyst is not associated with facet arthropathy. A Tarlov cyst is a perineural cyst of the sacrum, formed within the nerve root sheath, and usually asymptomatic.

High intensity zone (annular fissure)

- *High intensity zone* is the imaging term referring to an area of hyperintense signal on T2-weighted images in the annulus fibrosus. This imaging finding is thought to correlate with fissure or tear of the annulus fibrosus and may be a cause of pain.
- The terms "annular fissure" and "annular tear" are synonymous. Annular fissure is the preferred term as *tear* implies a traumatic etiology, while this process is typically due to disc degeneration.

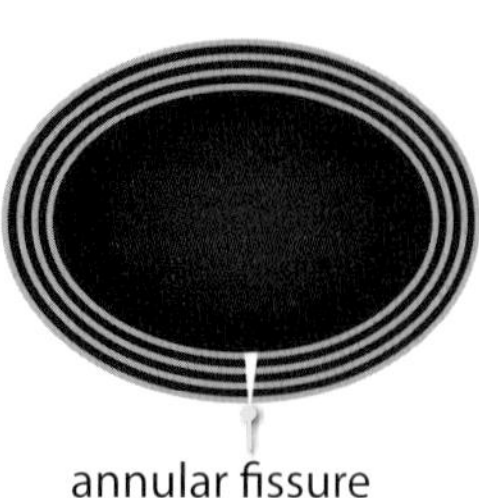

Non-degenerative hypertrophic diseases

Diffuse idiopathic skeletal hyperostosis (DISH)

- Diffuse idiopathic skeletal hyperostosis (DISH) is flowing anterior osteophytes extending at least four vertebral levels. DISH and degenerative disc disease are separate processes, though they are often seen concurrently.
- In contrast to discogenic degenerative disease, there is preservation of the disc spaces.
- Similar to ankylosing spondylitis, DISH may predispose to spinal fracture after even minor trauma due to reduced mobility of the spinal column.
- DISH is associated with ossification of the posterior longitudinal ligament.

Ossification of the posterior longitudinal ligament (OPLL)

- Ossification of the posterior longitudinal ligament (OPLL) is calcification and ossification of the posterior longitudinal ligament, which may lead to spinal canal stenosis and compression of the anterior aspect of the cord.
- OPLL is best appreciated on CT, where the abnormal ossification will be apparent in the anterior aspect of the spinal canal. MRI shows low signal in the anterior spinal canal.
- OPLL begins in the cervical spine but may extend inferiorly to the thoracic spine.

Postoperative spine

- Contrast is typically administered for postoperative MRI imaging of the spine to distinguish between recurrent disc disease and scar tissue.
- Both disc and scar appear hypointense on T2-weighted MRI. In theory, scar tissue should enhance throughout, while recurrent disc demonstrates only peripheral enhancement.
- If there is recurrent disc herniation, further surgical intervention may be indicated. In general, however, the presence of scar tissue would decrease the chance of successful relief of symptoms.

Pyogenic discitis/osteomyelitis

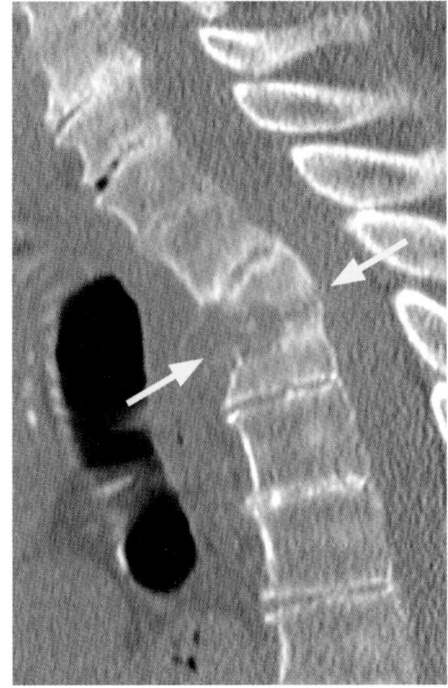

Sagittal CT

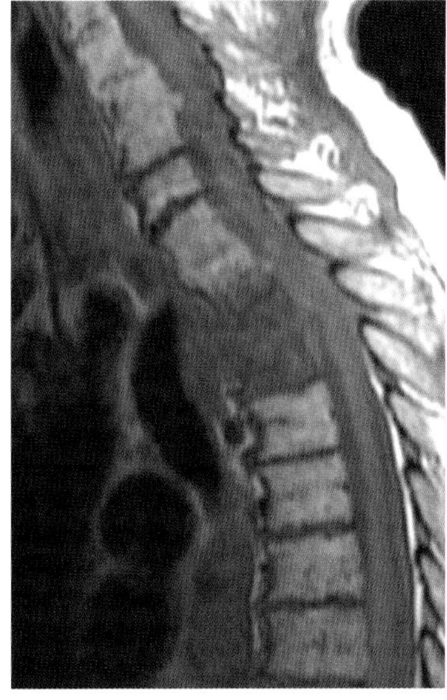

T1-weighted sagittal MRI

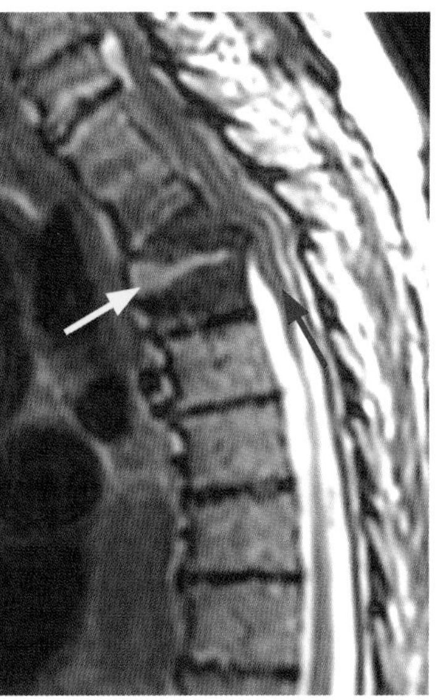

T2-weighted sagittal MRI

Pyogenic discitis/osteomyelitis: Sagittal CT (left image) shows loss of disc space height, acute kyphotic angulation, and erosion of adjacent endplates in the upper thoracic spine (arrows). There are severe degenerative changes elsewhere in the spine. T1-weighted MRI (middle image) shows diffuse marrow replacement with hypointense marrow signal in the two affected adjacent vertebral bodies and complete loss of distinction of the endplates. T2-weighted MRI (right image) shows hyperintensity in the affected disc (yellow arrow) and acute cord compression with cord signal change (red arrow).

- Pyogenic discitis/osteomyelitis is caused by bacterial infection of the intervertebral disc and the adjacent vertebrae, typically from a hematogenous source. *Staphylococcus aureus* is the most common agent.
- In adults, the vascularized subchondral bone is the initial site of infection, which spreads to the disc. In children, however, the intervertebral disc is initially infected, with subsequent spread to the vertebral endplates.
- The key imaging appearance of discitis/osteomyelitis is marrow hypointensity on T1-weighted images centered on both sides of an abnormal intervertebral disc that is hyperintense on T2-weighted images. Loss of adjacent endplate definition is usually present. On radiography, the only initial clue may be loss of disc space height. Later in the course of infection, there may be vertebral collapse.
- Adjacent soft tissue infection (paraspinal or epidural) is often present.

Tuberculous osteomyelitis

- Also called *Pott disease,* tuberculous osteomyelitis represents infection of the vertebral body with *Mycobacterium tuberculosis*. Unlike pyogenic discitis/osteomyelitis, the discs are usually spared as *M. tuberculosis* lacks the proteolytic enzymes necessary to break down the disc substance.
- Pott disease classically causes wedge-shaped compression of the anterior aspect of the vertebral body, often leading to a gibbus deformity centered at the infected vertebra.

  Gibbus deformity is an acutely angled kyphosis. Gibbus deformity may result from a vertebral compression fracture or can be seen in congenital syndromes including achondroplasia and the mucopolysaccharidoses (Hunter and Hurler syndromes).
- Approximately 10% of patients with Pott disease have active pulmonary tuberculosis.

Vascular

Dural arteriovenous fistula (dAVF)

- Dural arteriovenous fistula (dAVF) is the most common spinal vascular malformation. It typically affects older males with back pain and progressive myelopathy. Spinal dAVF is a Cognard type V dural AV fistula, as discussed in the section on CNS dAVFs.
- MRI of dAVF shows flow voids surrounding the cord. The cord is often swollen, with abnormal intramedullary T2 prolongation. CT myelography shows serpiginous filling defects in the subarachnoid space.

Infarction

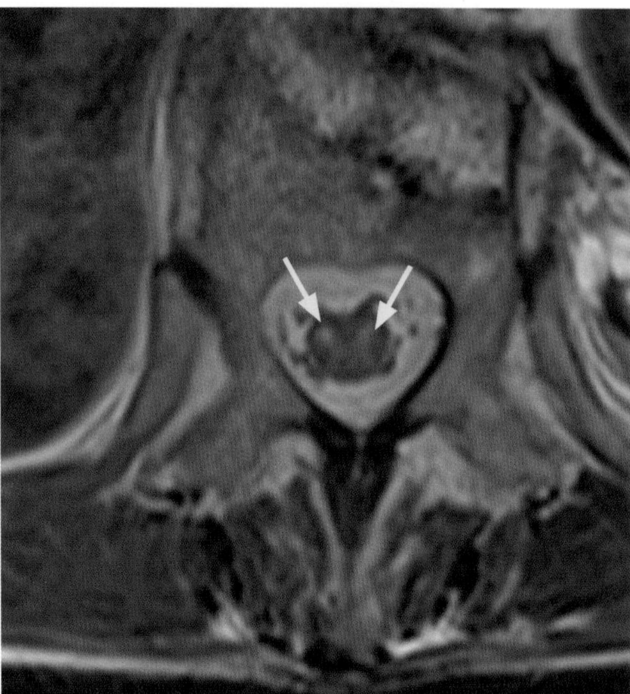

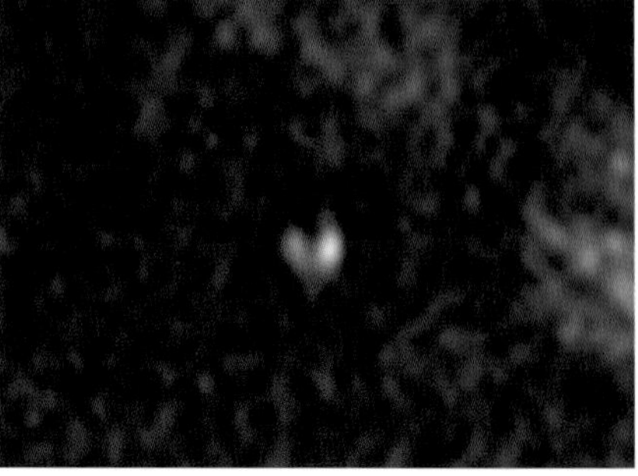

Spinal cord infarction after aortic surgery:

Axial T2-weighted MRI (left image) shows symmetric hyperintense foci involving the ventral horns of the intramedullary gray matter ("owl eye appearance").

Corresponding axial DWI (top image) shows bright spots, suggestive of restricted diffusion.

Case courtesy Gregory Wrubel, MD, Brigham and Women's Hospital.

- Spinal cord infarction is most common in the upper thoracic or thoracolumbar spine due to more precarious blood supply. The predominant blood supply to the distal cord is the artery of Adamkiewicz.
- Spinal cord infarction clinically presents with loss of bowel and bladder control, loss of perineal sensation, and impairment in both motor and sensory function of the legs.
- Risk factors for spinal cord infarction include aortic surgery (as in the case above), aortic aneurysm, arteritis, sickle cell anemia, vascular malformation, and disc herniation.
- Imaging of spinal cord infarction shows hyperintensity of the affected cord regions on T2-weighted images. The cord may be enlarged. Diffusion images typically show restricted diffusion. Concomitant vertebral body infarction may be present, which is more common in sickle cell disease and chronic steroid use.

Congenital

Tethered cord syndrome

- Tethered cord syndrome is a clinical syndrome of back and leg pain, gait spasticity, and decreased lower extremity sensation.
- Normally the conus should terminate superior to the inferior endplate of L2. If the conus terminates below this level, the cord may be tethered.
- The cord may be tethered by a thickened filum or lipoma.

Diastematomyelia

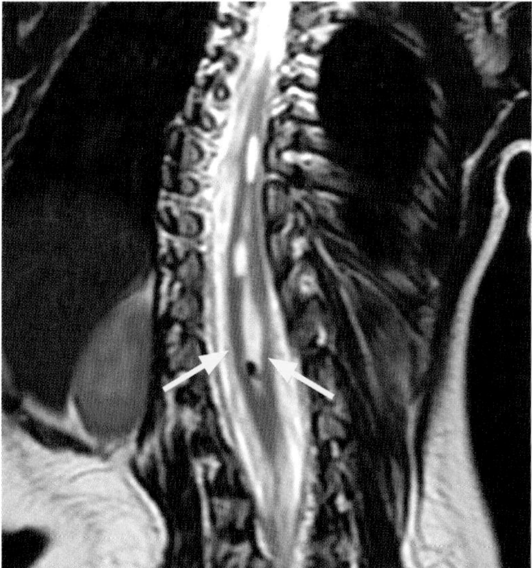

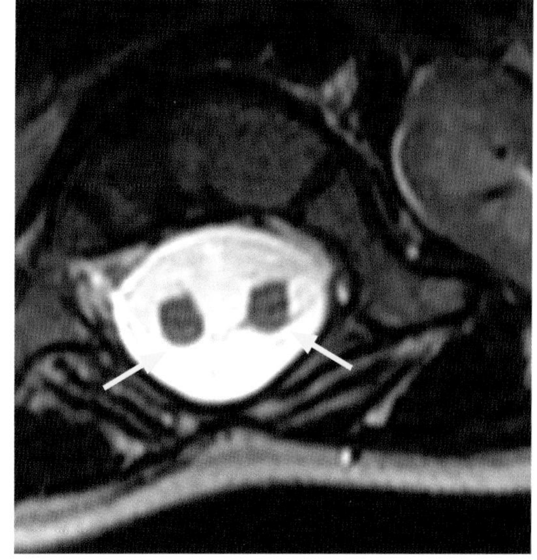

Diastematomyelia: Coronal T2-weighted MRI (left image) shows CSF between the two hemicords (arrows) and a thoracolumbar dextroscoliosis. Axial T2-weighted MRI (right image) shows two hemicords (arrows) within a single CSF space.

- Diastematomyelia is a congenitally split spinal cord, which may be a cause of scoliosis.

Fatty filum

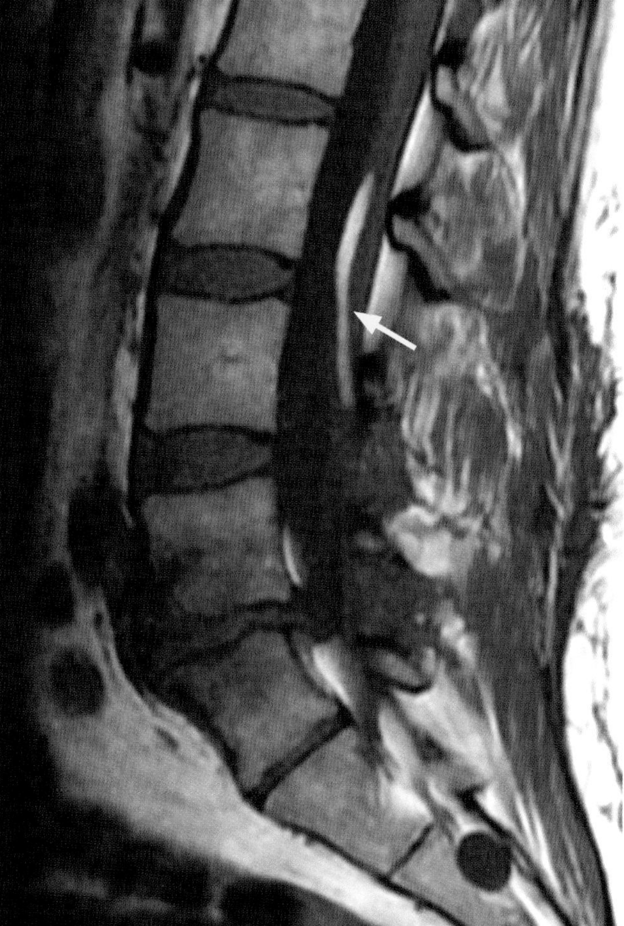

Fatty filum:

Sagittal T1-weighted MRI shows a hyperintense lesion in the filum (arrow), representing fat in the filum terminale.

- Fat within the filum terminale may be associated with diastematomyelia, tethered cord, or may be clinically insignificant.

References, resources, and further reading

General References:

Atlas, S.W. Magnetic Resonance Imaging of the Brain and Spine (4th ed.). Lippincott Williams & Wilkins. (2008).

Osborn, A. Diagnostic Neuroradiology (1st ed.). Mosby. (1994).

Yousem, D.M., Zimmerman, R.D. & Grossman, R.I. Neuroradiology The Requisites (3rd ed.). Mosby. (2010).

Fundamentals of Neuroradiology:

Smirniotopoulos, J. et al. Patterns of Contrast Enhancement in the Brain and Meninges. Radiographics, 27, 525-552(2007).

Brain Tumor Imaging and Mass Lesions:

Bonneville, F., Savatovsky, J. & Chiras, J. Imaging of cerebellopontine angle lesions: an update. Part 1: enhancing extra-axial lesions. European Radiology, 17(10), 2472-82(2007).

Bonneville, F., Savatovsky, J. & Chiras, J. Imaging of cerebellopontine angle lesions: an update. Part 2: intra-axial lesions, skull base lesions that may invade the CPA region, and non-enhancing extra-axial lesions. European Radiology, 17(11), 2908-20(2007).

Engel, U. et al. Cystic lesions of the pineal region – MRI and pathology. Neuroradiology, 42(6), 399-402(2000).

Gaillard, F. & Jones, J. Masses of the pineal region: clinical presentation and radiographic features. Postgraduate Medical Journal, 86(1020), 597-607(2010).

Rao, V.J., James, R.A & Mitra, D. Imaging characteristics of common suprasellar lesions with emphasis on MRI findings. Clinical Radiology, 63(8), 939-47(2008).

Rennert, J. & Doerfler, A. Imaging of sellar and parasellar lesions. Clinical Neurology and Neurosurgery, 109(2), 111-24(2007).

Smith, A.B., Rushing, E.J. & Smirniotopoulos, J.G. From the archives of the AFIP: lesions of the pineal region: radiologic-pathologic correlation. Radiographics, 30(7), 2001-20(2010).

Zada, G. et al. Craniopharyngioma and other cystic epithelial lesions of the sellar region: a review of clinical, imaging, and histopathological relationships. Neurosurgical Focus, 28(4), E4(2010).

Trauma:

Gean, A.D. & Fischbein, N.J. Head trauma. Neuroimaging Clinics of North America, 20(4), 527-56(2010).

Hijaz, T.A., Cento., E.A. & Walker, M.T. Imaging of head trauma. Radiologic Clinics of North America, 49(1), 81-103(2011).

Kim, J.J. & Huoh, K. Maxillofacial (midface) fractures. Neuroimaging Clinics of North America, 20(4), 581-96(2010).

Cerebrovascular and Stroke:

Adams, H.P. et al. Guidelines for the Early Management of Adults With Ischemic Stroke: A Guideline From the American Heart Association/American Stroke Association Stroke Council, Clinical Cardiology Council, Cardiovascular Radiology and Intervention C. Stroke, 38, 1655–1711(2007).

Aksoy, F.G. & Lev, M.H. Dynamic contrast-enhanced brain perfusion imaging: technique and clinical applications. Seminars in Ultrasound, CT, and MR, 21(6), 462-77(2000).

Geibprasert, S. et al. Radiologic assessment of brain arteriovenous malformations: what clinicians need to know. Radiographics, 30(2), 483-501(2010).

Leiva-Salinas, C. & Wintermark, M. Imaging of acute ischemic stroke. Neuroimaging Clinics of North America, 20(4), 455-68(2010).

Muir, K.W. et al. Imaging of acute stroke. Lancet Neurology, 5(9), 755-68(2006).

Savoiardo, M. The vascular territories of the carotid and vertebrobasilar systems. Diagrams based on CT studies of infarcts. Italian Journal of Neurological Sciences, 7(4), 405-9(1986).

Shetty, S.K. & Lev, Michael H. CT perfusion in acute stroke. Neuroimaging Clinics of North America, 15(3), 481-501, ix(2005).

Intraparenchymal Hemorrhage:

Fischbein, N.J. & Wijman, C.A. Nontraumatic intracranial hemorrhage. Neuroimaging Clinics of North America, 20(4), 469-92(2010).

White Matter Disease:

Bartynski, W.S. Posterior reversible encephalopathy syndrome, part 1: fundamental imaging and clinical features. AJNR. American Journal of Neuroradiology, 29(6), 1036-42(2008).

Bartynski, W.S. Posterior reversible encephalopathy syndrome, part 2: controversies surrounding pathophysiology of vasogenic edema. AJNR. American Journal of Neuroradiology, 29(6), 1043-9(2008).

Filippi, M. & Rocca, M.A. MRI imaging of multiple sclerosis. Radiology, 259(3), 659-81(2011).

Guidetti, D., Casali, B., Mazzei, R.L. & Dotti, M.T. Cerebral autosomal dominant arteriopathy with subcortical infarcts and leukoencephalopathy. Clinical and Experimental Hypertension, 28(3-4), 271-7(2006).

Shah, R., Bag, A.K., Chapman, P.R. & Curé, J.K. Imaging manifestations of progressive multifocal leukoencephalopathy. Clinical Radiology, 65(6), 431-9(2010).

Infection and Toxic/Metabolic:

Aiken, A.H. Central nervous system infection. Neuroimaging Clinics of North America, 20(4), 557-80(2010).

Hegde, A.N. et al. Differential diagnosis for bilateral abnormalities of the basal ganglia and thalamus. Radiographics, 31(1), 5(2011).

Neck:

Eisenkraft, B. & Som, P. The spectrum of benign and malignant etiologies of cervical node calcification. American Journal of Roentgenology, 172(5), 1433(1999).

Gor, D.M., Langer, J.E. & Loevner, L.A. Imaging of cervical lymph nodes in head and neck cancer: the basics. Radiologic Clinics of North America, 44(1), 101-10, viii(2006).

Herek, P.A., Lewis, T. & Bailitz, J.M. An unusual case of Lemierre's syndrome due to methicillin-resistant *Staphylococcus aureus*. The Journal of Emergency Medicine, 39(5), 644-6(2010).

Koeller, K., Alamo, L., Adair, C. & Smirniotopoulos, J. From the Archives of the AFIP Congenital Cystic Masses of the Neck: Radiologic-Pathologic Correlation. Radiographics, (19), 121-46(1999).

McKellop, J. A., Bou-Assaly, W. & Mukherji, S.K. Emergency head & neck imaging: infections and inflammatory processes. Neuroimaging Clinics of North America, 20(4), 651-61(2010).

Park, S.B. & Lee, J.H. Imaging Findings of Head and Neck Inflammatory Pseudotumor. Ultrasound, 193, 1180-6(2009).

Rana, R.S. & Moonis, G. Head and neck infection and inflammation. Radiologic Clinics of North America, 49(1), 165-82(2011).

Reede, D., Bergeron, R. & Som, P. CT of thyroglossal duct cysts. Radiology, 157(1), 121(1985).

Stambuk, H.E. & Patel, S.G. Imaging of the parapharyngeal space. Otolaryngologic Clinics of North America, 41(1), 77-101, vi(2008).

Wong, K.T., Lee, Y.Y.P., King, A.D. & Ahuja, A.T. Imaging of cystic or cyst-like neck masses. Clinical Radiology, 63(6), 613-22(2008).

Woo, E.K. & Connor, S.E.J. Computed tomography and magnetic resonance imaging appearances of cystic lesions in the suprahyoid neck: a pictorial review. Dento Maxillo Facial Radiology, 36(8), 451-8(2007).

Yousem, D. Suprahyoid Spaces of the Head and Neck. Seminars in Roentgenology, XXXV(1), 63-71(2000).

Paranasal Sinuses:

Beale, T.J., Madani, G. & Morley, S.J. Imaging of the Paranasal Sinuses and Nasal Cavity: Normal Anatomy and Clinically Relevant Anatomical Variants. Seminars in Ultrasound, CT, and MRI, 30(1), 2-16(2009).

Epstein, V.A. & Kern, R.C. Invasive fungal sinusitis and complications of rhinosinusitis. Otolaryngologic Clinics of North America, 41(3), 497-524, viii(2008).

Hoxworth, J.M. & Glastonbury, C.M. Orbital and intracranial complications of acute sinusitis. Neuroimaging Clinics of North America, 20(4), 511-26(2010).

Loevner, L.A. & Sonners, A.I. Imaging of neoplasms of the paranasal sinuses. Neuroimaging Clinics of North America, 14(4), 625-46(2004).

Mafee, M.F., Tran, B.H. & Chapa, A.R. Imaging of Rhinosinusitis and Its Complications. Clinical Reviews in Allergy and Immunology, 30, 165-85(2006).

Maroldi, R., Ravanelli, M., Borghesi, A. & Farina, D. Paranasal sinus imaging. European Journal of Radiology, 66(3), 372-86(2008).

Momeni, A.K., Roberts, C.C. & Chew, F.S. Imaging of chronic and exotic sinonasal disease: review. AJR. American Journal of Roentgenology, 189(6 Suppl), S35-45(2007).

Ryan, M.W. Allergic fungal rhinosinusitis. Otolaryngologic Clinics of North America, 44(3), 697-710, ix-x(2011).

Skull Base and Petrous Apex:

Borges, A. Imaging of the central skull base. Neuroimaging Clinics of North America, 19(3), 441-68(2009).

Chapman, P.R., Shah, R., Curé, J.K. & Bag, A.K. Petrous apex lesions: pictorial review. AJR. American Journal of Roentgenology, 196(3 Suppl), WS26-37 Quiz S40-3(2011).

Gore, M.R. et al. Cholesterol Granuloma of the Petrous Apex. Otolaryngologic Clinics of North America, 44(5), 1043-58(2011).

Koutourousiou, M. et al. Skull base chordomas. Otolaryngologic Clinics of North America, 44(5), 1155-71(2011).

Parmar, H., Gujar, S., Shah, G. & Mukherji, S.K. Imaging of the anterior skull base. Neuroimaging Clinics of North America, 19(3), 427-39(2009).

Schmalfuss, I.M. Petrous apex. Neuroimaging Clinics of North America, 19(3), 367-91(2009).

Temporal Bone:

Baráth, K. et al. Neuroradiology of cholesteatomas. AJNR. American Journal of Neuroradiology, 32(2), 221-9(2011).

De Foer, B. et al. Imaging of temporal bone tumors. Neuroimaging Clinics of North America, 19(3), 339-66(2009).

Lemmerling, M.M., De Foer, B., Verbist, B.M. & VandeVyver, V. Imaging of inflammatory and infectious diseases in the temporal bone. Neuroimaging Clinics of North America, 19(3), 321-37(2009).

Shah, L.M. & Wiggins, R.H. Imaging of hearing loss. Neuroimaging Clinics of North America, 19(3), 287-306(2009).

St Martin, M.B. & Hirsch, B.E. Imaging of hearing loss. Otolaryngologic Clinics of North America, 41(1), 157-78, vi-vii(2008).

Swartz, J. The otodystrophies: Diagnosis and differential diagnosis. Seminars in Ultrasound, CT, and MRI, 25(4), 305-318(2004).

Swartz, J. An overview of congenital/developmental sensorineural hearing loss with emphasis on the vestibular aqueduct syndrome. Seminars in Ultrasound, CT, and MRI, 25(4), 353-68(2004).

Yiin, R.S.Z., Tang, P.H. & Tan, T.Y. Review of congenital inner ear abnormalities on CT temporal bone. The British Journal of Radiology, 84(1005), 859-63(2011).

Orbit:

Aviv, R.I. & Casselman, J. Orbital imaging: Part 1. Normal anatomy. Clinical Radiology, 60(3), 279-87(2005).

Aviv, R.I. & Miszkiel, K. Orbital imaging: Part 2. Intraorbital pathology. Clinical Radiology, 60(3), 288-307(2005).

Chung, E.M., Specht, C. & Schroeder, J. From the Archives of the AFIP Pediatric Orbit Tumors and Tumorlike Lesions: Neuroepithelial Lesions of the Ocular Globe and Optic Nerve. Radiographics, 27, 1159-87(2007).

Goh, P.S. et al. Review of orbital imaging. European Journal of Radiology, 66(3), 387-95(2008).

Koeller, K.K. & Smirniotopoulos, J.G. Orbital masses. Seminars in Ultrasound, CT, and MR, 19(3), 272-91(1998).

Mafee, M.F., Karimi, A., Shah, J., Rapoport, M. & Ansari, S.A. Anatomy and pathology of the eye: role of MRI imaging and CT. Radiologic Clinics of North America, 44(1), 135–57(2006).

Spine:

Al-Khawaja, D., Seex, K. & Eslick, G.D. Spinal epidural lipomatosis – a brief review. Journal of Clinical Neuroscience: official journal of the Neurosurgical Society of Australasia, 15(12), 1323-6(2008).

Boo, S. & Hogg, J.P. How's your disc? Illustrative glossary of degenerative disc lesions using standardized lexicon. Current Problems in Diagnostic Radiology, 39(3), 118-24(2010).

DeSanto, J. & Ross, J.S. Spine infection/inflammation. Radiologic Clinics of North America, 49(1), 105-27(2011).

Fardon, D.F. & Milette, P.C. Nomenclature and Classification of Lumbar Disc Pathology Recommendations of the Combined Task Forces of the North American Spine Society, American Society of Spine Radiology, and American Society of Neuroradiology. Spine, 26(5), 93-113(2001).

Fayad, F. et al. Reliability of a modified Modic classification of bone marrow changes in lumbar spine MRI. Joint, Bone, Spine: revue du rhumatisme, 76(3), 286-9(2009).

Rahme, R. & Moussa, R. The modic vertebral endplate and marrow changes: pathologic significance and relation to low back pain and segmental instability of the lumbar spine. AJNR. American Journal of Neuroradiology, 29(5), 838-42(2008).

Van Goethem, J.W.M. et al. Spinal tumors. European Journal of Radiology, 50(2), 159-76(2004).

5 Musculoskeletal imaging

Contents

Basics of bones and joints

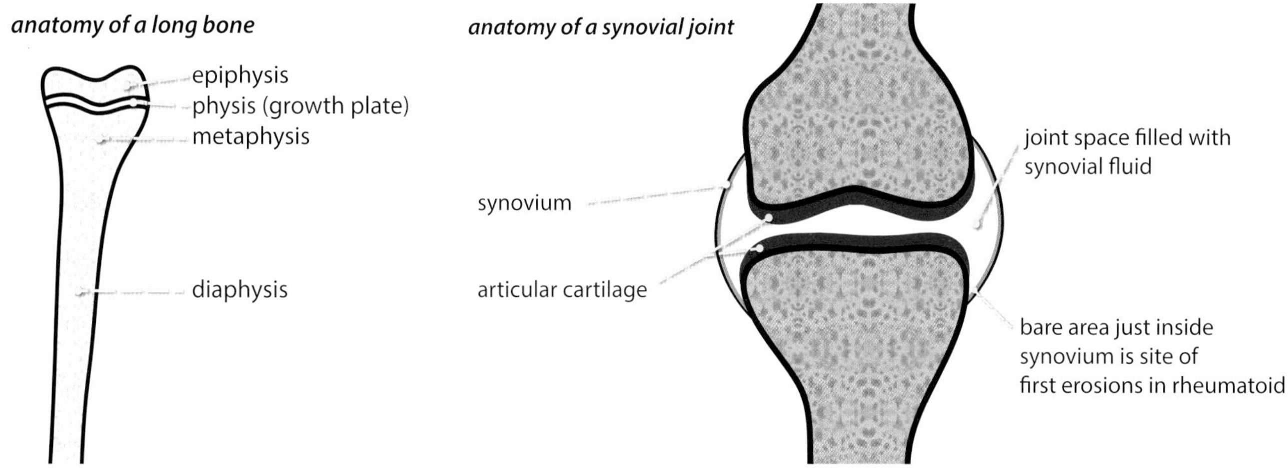

Arthritis

- The hallmark of arthritis is cartilage destruction, which may be evident on radiographs as cartilage space narrowing.
- In broad categories, arthritis can be divided into degenerative (osteoarthritis), inflammatory (rheumatoid arthritis, spondyloarthropathies, and juvenile idiopathic arthritis), crystal deposition (gout, calcium pyrophosphate dihydrate, and hydroxyapatite), hematologic (hemophilia), and metabolic categories.

Osteoarthritis (OA)

Overview of osteoarthritis

- Also called *osteoarthrosis* or *degenerative joint disease*, osteoarthritis (OA) is the result of articular cartilage breakdown from altered local mechanical factors in a susceptible individual. In addition to cartilage, OA is thought to involve the entire joint including bone, ligaments, menisci, joint capsule, synovium, and musculature.
- OA is the most common cause of cartilage loss in the middle-aged and older population.
- OA typically occurs in weight-bearing joints and the hands in a specific distribution.
- When radiographic findings of OA are seen in younger patients or in unusual locations, such as the shoulder, elbow, or ankle, then there is usually a predisposing prior trauma or other underlying arthritis.
- The radiographic hallmarks of OA, regardless of location in the body, include:

  Asymmetrical joint space narrowing.

  Sclerosis of subchondral bone, stimulated by loss of hyaline cartilage and reactive remodeling.

  Osteophytosis.

  Subchondral cystic change, due to herniation of joint fluid into bone through a cartilage defect.

  Lack of periarticular osteopenia.

- Although joint space narrowing is present in all arthritides, osteoarthritis can be diagnosed with confidence when subchondral sclerosis, osteophytosis, and subchondral cystic changes are present and inflammatory erosions are absent.

  When extensive subchondral cystic changes are present, calcium pyrophosphate dihydrate crystal deposition disease (CPPD) should be considered as well.

Osteoarthritis in the hand

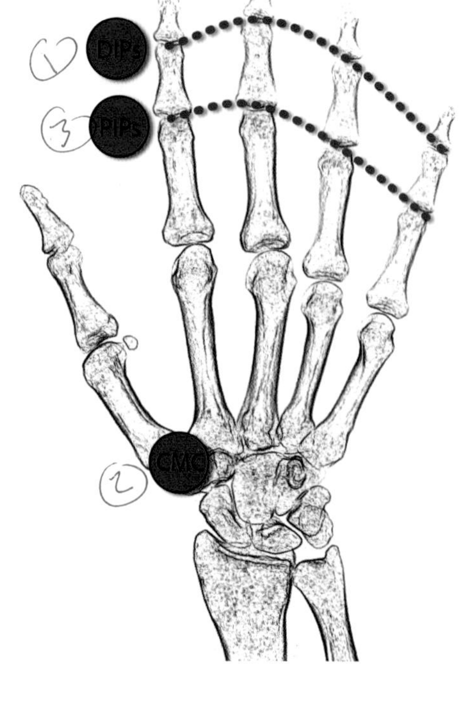

- Similar to osteoarthritis of other joints, the radiographic hallmarks of OA in the hand include cartilage space narrowing, subchondral sclerosis, and osteophytosis. Erosions are absent.
- In order of decreasing involvement, typical sites of OA in the hand include the distal interphalangeal joints (DIPs), the base of the thumb at the first carpometacarpal joint (CMC), and the proximal interphalangeal joints (PIPs).
- The most common site of osteoarthritis in the hands is the second DIP.
- Unlike rheumatoid arthritis, the metacarpophalangeal joints (MCPs) are less commonly affected.
- Large osteophytes cause characteristic soft-tissue swelling surrounding the finger joints.

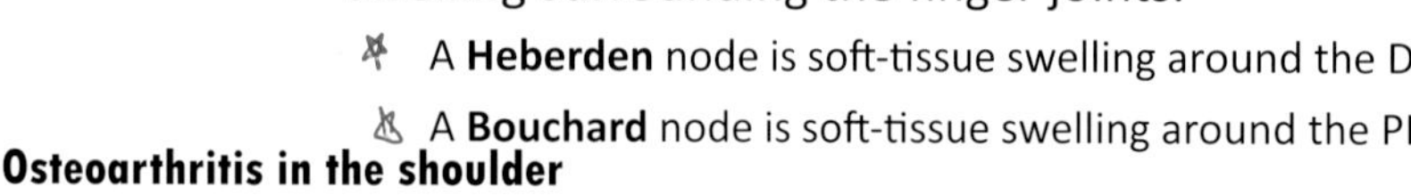

  - A **Heberden** node is soft-tissue swelling around the DIP.
  - A **Bouchard** node is soft-tissue swelling around the PIP.

Osteoarthritis in the shoulder

- The Grashey view (obtained posteriorly in 40-degree obliqued external rotation) shows the glenohumeral joint in profile and best demonstrates cartilage space narrowing.

Osteoarthritis in the foot

- The most common joint affected by OA in the foot is the metatarsophalangeal joint (MTP) of the great toe, which may lead to hallux rigidus (a stiff big toe) from dorsal osteophytes.
- Osteoarthritis also affects the talonavicular joint and is a cause of dorsal beaking.

Osteoarthritis in the knee

- There are three joint compartments in the knee: The medial and lateral tibiofemoral compartments and the patellofemoral compartment. The typical pattern for OA of the knee is asymmetrical involvement of the medial tibiofemoral compartment. Severe osteoarthritis can involve all three compartments.
- The following rule of thumb applies to OA in general, but especially in the knee: Osteophytes determine whether OA is present. The degree of joint space narrowing determines the severity of OA.
- The degree of tibiofemoral cartilage space narrowing is best determined on standing weight-bearing views, often on standing films in flexion.
- Bilateral involvement of the knees is typical.

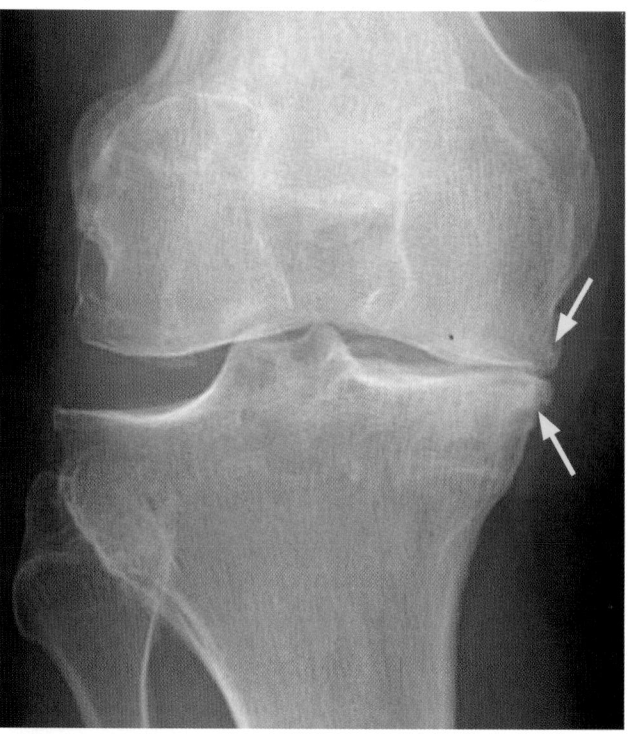

Osteoarthritis: Standing frontal radiograph of the knee shows severe cartilage space narrowing, sclerosis, and osteophytosis of the medial tibiofemoral compartment (arrows).

Osteoarthritis in the hip

- Similar to the knee, the involvement of hip osteoarthritis tends to be bilateral.
- In addition to the typical features of OA including joint space narrowing, osteophytosis, subchondral cystic change, and sclerosis, hip OA also features characteristic migration of the femoral head in a superolateral direction. Less commonly, medial migration can be seen in hip OA.
- In contrast, axial migration is seen more commonly in inflammatory arthritis.

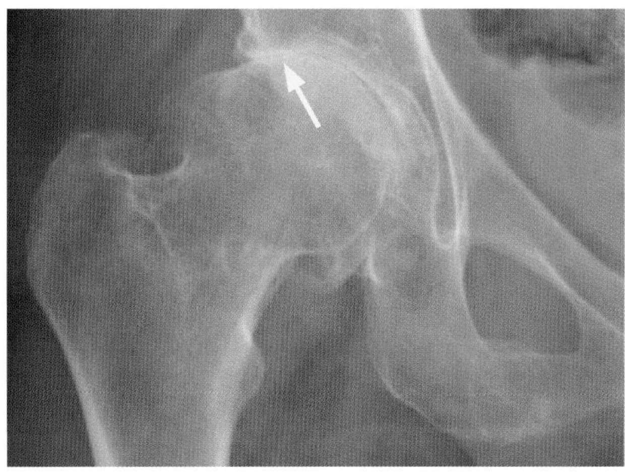

Osteoarthritis: Hip radiograph shows severe cartilage space narrowing, sclerosis, and osteophytosis of the right hip with superolateral migration (arrow) of the femoral head.

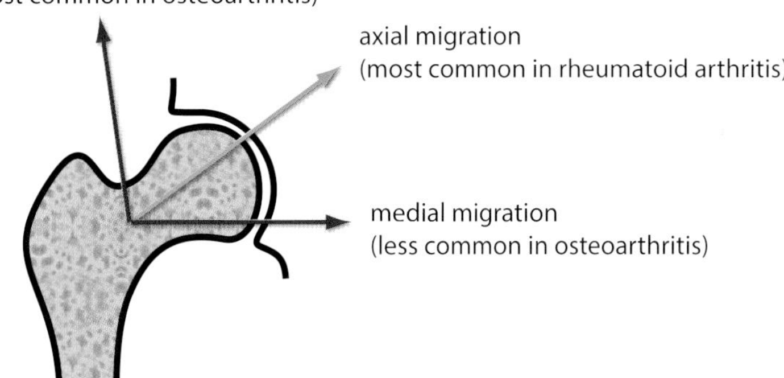

osteoarthritis

superolateral migration: superior-lateral cartilage space narrowing

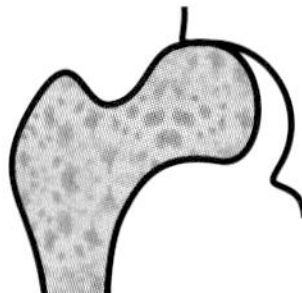

medial migration: inferomedial cartilage space narrowing

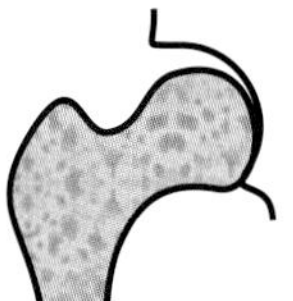

rheumatoid arthritis

axial migration: concentric cartilage space narrowing

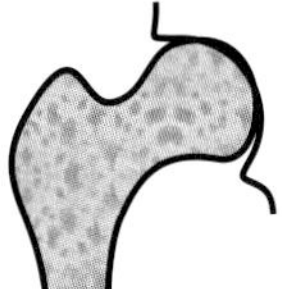

severe axial migration: protrusio deformity

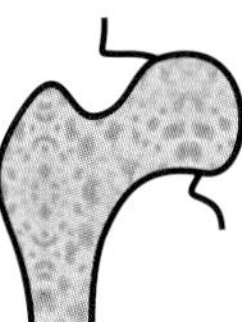

Degenerative change in the spine

- The vertebral body–disc articulations are cartilaginous joints. Vertebral body endplates are covered by hyaline cartilage that is analogous to articular cartilage in other joints. The intervertebral disk is composed of three components: The annulus fibrosus, nucleus pulposus, and the cartilaginous endplates.
- Osteoarthritis only affects synovial joints. Therefore, in the spine, osteoarthritis can occur at the facet (zygapophyseal), atlantoaxial, uncovertebral joints (in the cervical spine at C3–C7), costovertebral, and sacroiliac joints.
- The spectrum of intervertebral disk degeneration is best described as *degenerative disk disease* (DDD), which is characterized by dessication of the intervertebral discs, endplate sclerosis, and osteophytosis.
- Gas in the intervertebral disc, also called *vacuum phenomenon,* is commonly seen and is pathognomonic for degenerative disease.

  It is important not to confuse vacuum phenomenon (gas in intervertebral *disc*) with Kümmel disease, which is gas in a vertebral *body* compression fracture representing osteonecrosis.

- Complications of DDD include spinal stenosis, neural foraminal stenosis, and degenerative spondylolisthesis.
- **Diffuse idiopathic skeletal hyperostosis (DISH)** is a distinct entity from degenerative disc disease, but appears similar due to exuberant osteophytosis. DISH is defined as flowing bridging anterior osteophytes spanning at least four vertebral levels, with normal disk spaces and sacroiliac joints. The etiology of DISH is unknown. It is usually asymptomatic but may be a cause of dysphagia when it affects the cervical spine. DISH occurs in elderly patients.

  DISH is associated with **ossification of the posterior longitudinal ligament (OPLL)**, which may be a cause of spinal stenosis. OPLL may be difficult to identify on MRI and is best seen on CT.

Osteoarthritis in the sacroiliac (SI) joint

- Only the inferior portion of the sacroiliac joint is a synovial (diarthrodial) joint. The superior portion is a syndesmotic joint.
- The typical changes of OA are only seen in the inferior (synovial) portion of the SI joint.

Erosive osteoarthritis

Overview of erosive osteoarthritis

- Erosive osteoarthritis combines the clinical findings of rheumatoid arthritis (e.g., swelling) with imaging findings and distribution that are more similar to osteoarthritis.
- Erosive OA typically affects elderly females.

Erosive osteoarthritis of the hands

- The distribution of erosive osteoarthritis is limited to the hands, where the distribution is the same as degenerative OA (DIPs, CMC of the thumb, and PIPs).
- Erosive OA features a characteristic *gull-wing* appearance of the DIP joint due to central erosion and marginal osteophytes.

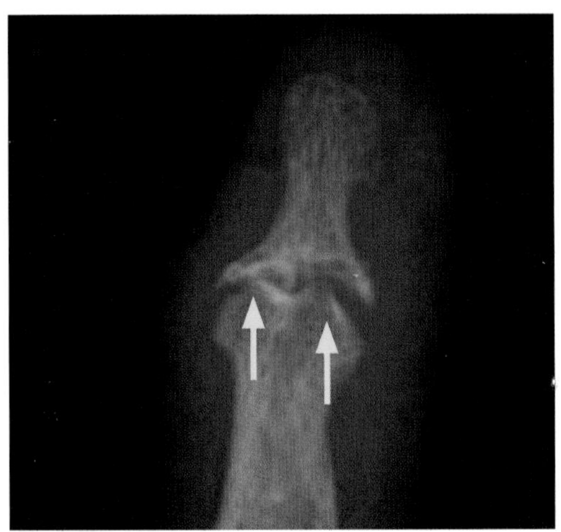

Erosive osteoarthritis: Magnified radiograph of a digit demonstrates characteristic *gull-wing* appearance of the DIP (yellow arrows).

Rheumatoid arthritis (RA)

Overview of rheumatoid arthritis

- Rheumatoid arthritis (RA) is an autoimmune disorder where the synovium is the target of a waxing and waning immune response. Rheumatoid factor (RF) is typically positive, although it is not specific. RF is an antibody directed against IgG, which activates the complement cascade. RA clinically presents with **symmetrical** joint pain, swelling, and morning stiffness.
- RA first affects the small joints in the hands and wrists. Foot involvement may occur early, so foot radiographs are routinely obtained in suspected cases of RA. In more advanced cases, RA affects the cervical spine, knees, shoulders, and hips.
- The radiographic hallmarks of RA include:

  Marginal erosions, which first occur at the intracapsular articular margins in the "bare area." The bare area is a region of exposed bone just within the joint capsule that is not covered by thick cartilage.

  Soft-tissue swelling.

  Diffuse, symmetric joint space narrowing.

  Periarticular osteopenia.

  Joint subluxations.

Rheumatoid arthritis in the hand and wrist

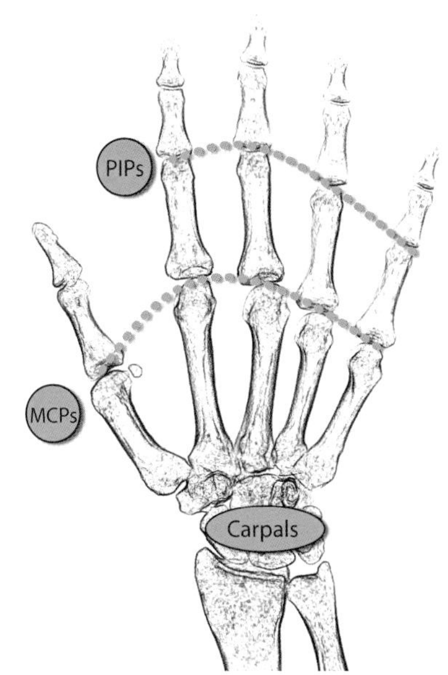

- The hands are commonly affected in patients with RA.
- Typical joints involved are the MCPs, PIPs, and the carpal articulations. The DIPs are usually spared.
- The earliest radiographic changes of RA are soft-tissue swelling and periarticular osteopenia, reflecting synovitis and hyperemia.
- Erosions occur early in disease, typically of the radial aspects of the second and third metacarpal heads, the radial and ulnar aspects of the bases of the proximal phalanges, and the ulnar styloid.
- Joint subluxations are present in more advanced disease, which typically are not reducible and lead to several common deformities, including:

  Boutonnière deformity (PIP flexion and DIP hyperextension).

  Swan neck deformity (PIP hyperextension and DIP flexion).

  Ulnar subluxation of the fingers at the MCPs.

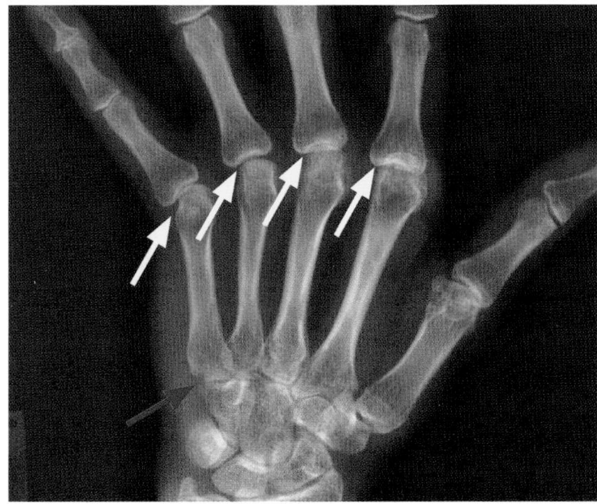

RA: PA hand radiograph shows ulnar deviation of the 2nd through 5th fingers at the MCPs (arrows). There is periarticular osteopenia. A 5th carpometacarpal joint erosion (red arrow) is better seen on the magnified image to the right.

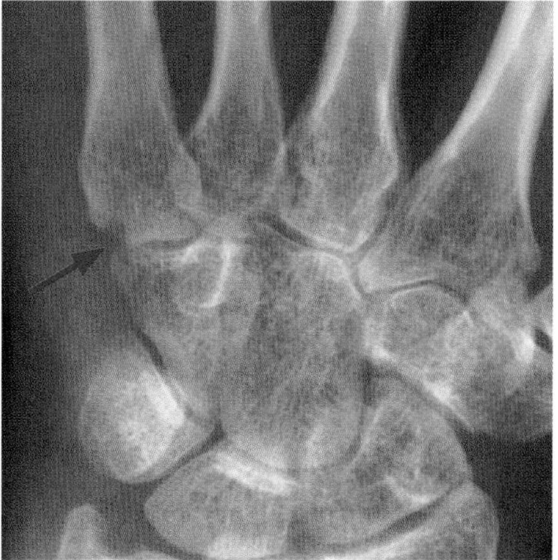

Close up of the same image better shows the erosion across the 5th carpometacarpal joint (red arrow).

- Late-stage rheumatoid arthritis may uncommonly cause ankylosis (fibro-osseous joint fusion occurring after complete cartilage loss) of the wrist. Juvenile idiopathic arthritis (discussed later), in contrast, has a higher propensity for carpal ankylosis.

Rheumatoid arthritis in the feet

- The feet are commonly involved in RA. Typically, the metatarsophalangeal (MTP) joints in the forefoot and the talocalcaneonavicular joint in the midfoot are involved. Up to 20% of patients have the MTP joint as the first site of involvement.

Rheumatoid arthritis in the hip

- RA causes concentric acetabular cartilage loss, leading to axial migration of the femoral head. In contrast, osteoarthritis more commonly causes superior acetabular cartilage space narrowing and superolateral femoral head migration.
- In severe cases, RA may cause a **protrusio deformity**, which is defined as >3 mm medial deviation of the femoral head beyond the ilioischial line in males and >6 mm in females.

Rheumatoid arthritis in the knee

- All three joint spaces (medial and lateral tibiofemoral and patellofemoral) may be affected by RA in the knee. In contrast, OA tends to first affect the medial tibiofemoral articulation. If osteophytes *and* symmetrical cartilage space narrowing are present, then secondary osteoarthritis should be considered.
- Unlike the smaller joints affected by rheumatoid arthritis, erosions are not a prominent manifestation of rheumatoid arthritis of the knee.

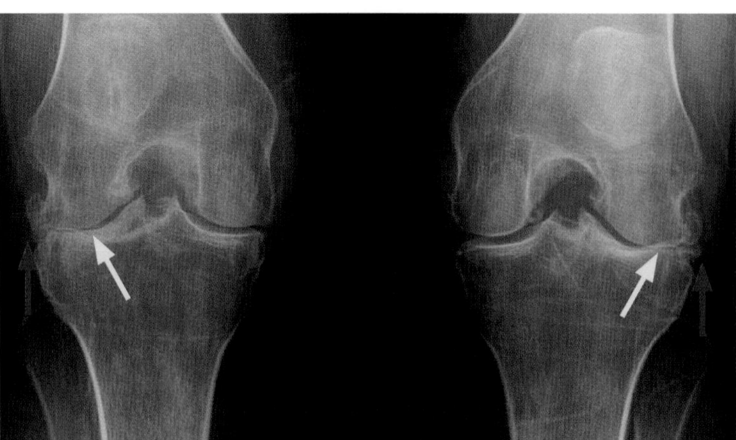

Rheumatoid arthritis with secondary osteoarthritis:

Frontal PA weight-bearing view of the knees shows cartilage space narrowing of medial and lateral tibiofemoral articulations bilaterally. The lateral tibiofemoral cartilage spaces are more markedly narrowed (yellow arrows). Prominent osteophytes laterally (red arrows) signify secondary osteoarthritis.

Rheumatoid arthritis in the spine

- The cervical spine is involved in up to 70% of patients. Involvement is increased with more severe and long-standing disease. The thoracic and lumbar spine are almost never involved.
- The general pattern of rheumatoid arthritis in the cervical spine includes subluxation at multiple levels, osteopenia, and erosions of the odontoid, facet joints, vertebral endplates, and spinous processes. Unlike osteoarthritis, there is no bone production.

Atlantoaxial subluxation in rheumatoid arthritis

- A characteristic finding of rheumatoid arthritis is **atlantoaxial (C1–C2) subluxation**. Atlantoaxial subluxation may occur in multiple directions, including anterior (most common), posterior, vertical (atlantoaxial impaction), rotatory, and lateral.
- **Anterior atlantoaxial subluxation** is caused by inflammation of adjacent bursa and resultant laxity of the transverse ligament. Anterior atlantoaxial subluxation may not be apparent if flexion radiographs are not obtained.

  Anterior atlantoaxial subluxation is present if the atlanto-dental interval (ADI) is >2.5 mm (>5 mm in children). The atlanto-dental interval is the distance between the anterior aspect of the dens and the posterior aspect of the anterior ring of C1, as measured at the inferior aspect of the C1–C2 articulation.
- **Vertical atlantoaxial subluxation** (also called atlantoaxial impaction) results from C1–C2 facet erosion and collapse, leading to protrusion of the odontoid through the foramen magnum. This may compress the midbrain.

  Direct visualization of the odontoid is usually not possible on a lateral radiograph, but impaction may cause the anterior arch of C1 (normally in line with the odontoid) to sink to the level of the body of C2.
- In the setting of RA, **posterior atlantoaxial subluxation** is usually due to odontoid erosion. It may also be caused by odontoid fracture.

Rheumatoid arthritis in the shoulder

- Rheumatoid arthritis causes chronic rotator cuff tears leading to the classic *high riding* humerus.
- Erosions tend to occur in the lateral aspect of the humeral heads. At the acromioclavicular (AC) joints, erosion may lead to "penciling" of the distal clavicle.

Rheumatoid arthritis in the elbow

- Rheumatoid arthritis involves the elbow in approximately one third of patients.

Overview of seronegative spondyloarthropathies

- The seronegative spondyloarthropathies are a group of four inflammatory arthropathies, which by definition have negative rheumatoid factor. Patients are usually HLA-B27 positive.
- The four seronegative spondyloarthropathies are ankylosing spondylitis, psoriatic arthritis, reactive arthritis (previously called Reiters arthropathy), and inflammatory bowel disease (IBD) associated arthropathy.

Sacroiliitis is a hallmark of the spondyloarthropathies

- Similar to inolvement in OA, only the inferior aspect of the sacroiliac (SI) joint is affected in seronegative spondyloarthropathies because only the inferior portion is a synovial (diarthrodial) joint. Erosions first involve the iliac aspect of the SI joint.
- Symmetric sacroiliitis is caused by IBD and ankylosing spondylitis (mnemonic: both start with vowels).

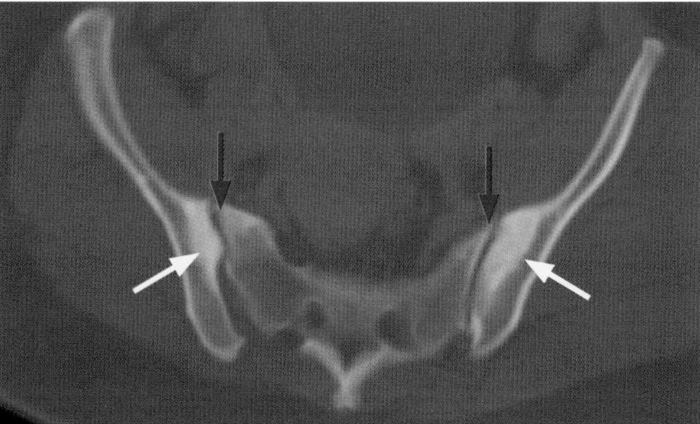

Symmetric sacroiliitis:

Axial CT through the pelvis at the level of the sacroiliac joints shows symmetric sclerosis (yellow arrows) and erosions (red arrows) at the iliac aspect of the sacroiliac joints bilaterally.

- Asymmetric sacroiliitis is caused by psoriatic arthritis and reactive arthropathy (mnemonic: both start with consonants).
- An important cause of unilateral sacroiliitis is septic arthritis, especially in an immunocompromised patient or with intravenous drug abuse. Septic arthritis usually presents with erosive changes in a patient with fever and SI joint pain.

Inflammatory bowel disease

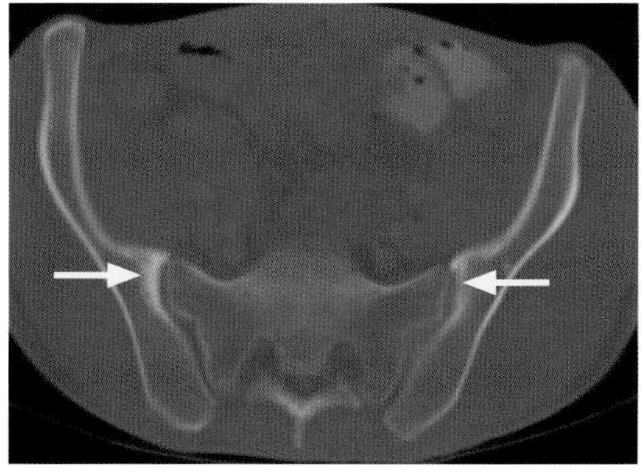

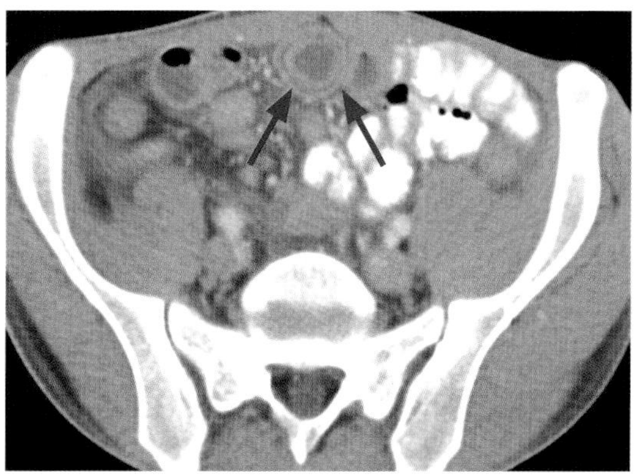

Crohn sacroiliitis: Axial CT through the pelvis in bone window (left image) shows symmetric sclerosis (yellow arrows) and erosions of the iliac aspect of the sacroiliac joints bilaterally. Soft-tissue-window CT (right image) shows bowel wall thickening, mural stratification, and hyperenhancement (red arrow), consistent with Crohn enteritis.

- Sacroiliitis associated with inflammatory bowel disease can be seen in patients with ulcerative colitis, Crohn disease, Whipple disease, and status post gastric bypass.
- IBD-associated sacroiliitis is typically symmetrical.

Ankylosing spondylitis

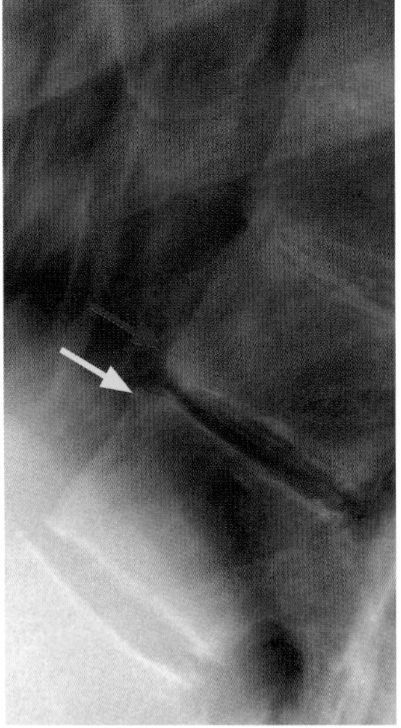

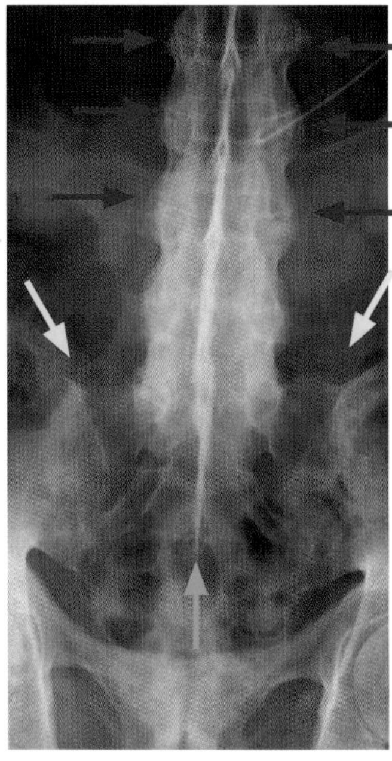

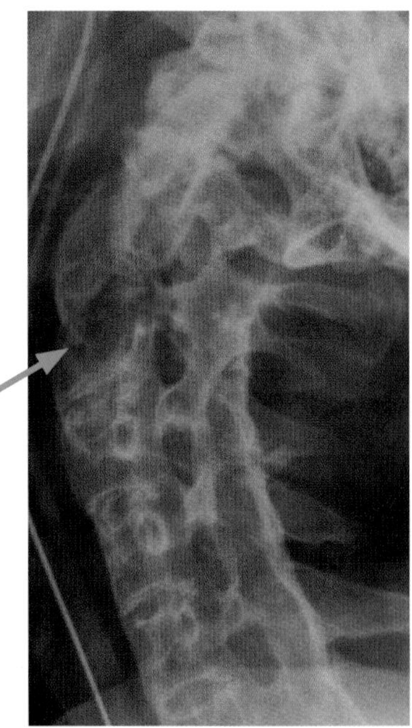

Three patients with ankylosing spondylitis:

Romanus and shiny corner lesions: Lateral radiograph of the upper lumbar spine (left image) shows an erosion of the anterior superior margin of a vertebral body at the discovertebral junction, representing a Romanus lesion (yellow arrow). The superiorly adjacent vertebral body demonstrates sclerosis of its anterior inferior margin, representing the *shiny corner* sign (red arrow). The *shiny corner* sign signifies evolution of a prior Romanus lesion.

Bamboo spine: Frontal radiograph of the sacroiliac joints and lumbar spine (middle image) demonstrates symmetrical sacroiliac joint ankylosis (yellow arrows). There are diffuse syndesmophytes, creating an undulating contour of the spinal column, representing the *bamboo spine* (red arrows). There is fusion of the spinous processes, creating the *dagger* sign (blue arrow).

Cervical fusion: Lateral radiograph of the cervical spine (right image) shows complete ankylosis of the cervical spine with fusion of the vertebral bodies and facet joints and a pseudarthrosis at C2–C3 (green arrow).

Cases courtesy Stacy Smith, MD, Brigham and Women's Hospital.

- Ankylosing spondylitis (AS) is predominantly seen in young men with HLA-B27 and presents with back pain and stiffness. AS can be associated with pulmonary fibrosis (upper lobe predominant), aortitis, and cardiac conduction defects.
- The earliest radiographic signs of AS are symmetric erosions, widening, and sclerosis of the sacroiliac joints.
- Subsequently, the spine invariably becomes involved, with radiographic findings following a specific sequence, which ascends from the lumbar to the cervical spine.

  Romanus lesions are erosions of the anterior superior or inferior edges of the vertebral body endplates caused by enthesitis (inflammation at a ligament or tendon insertion site) at attachment of the annulus fibrosus to the vertebral body.

  Shiny corners represent sclerosis of prior Romanus lesions at the corners of the vertebral bodies.

  Squaring of the vertebral body disc margins develops due to erosions and bone loss.

  Delicate syndesmophytes represents bony bridging connecting adjacent vertebral margins, which create the classic ***bamboo spine*** (spinal ankylosis) in late-stage disease.

- In advanced disease, the fully ankylosed spine is at a very high risk of fracture with even minor trauma. CT is necessary for evaluation of even minimal trauma in a patient with advanced AS and pain after trauma.
- An *Andersson lesion* is a pseudarthrosis occurring in a completely ankylosed spine.

Psoriatic arthritis

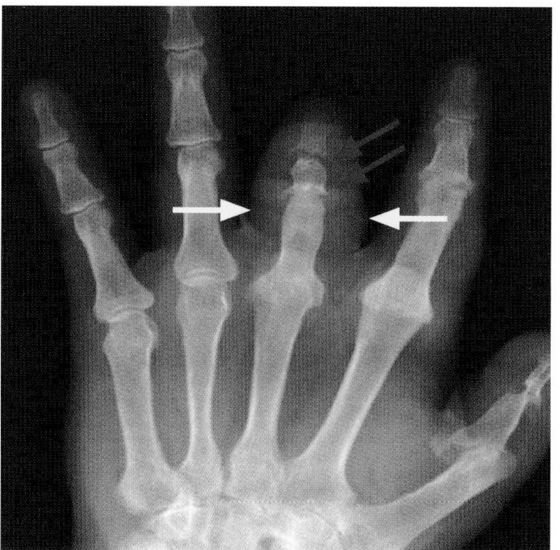

Psoriatic arthritis (arthritis mutilans form):

PA radiograph of the hand demonstrates swelling of the third digit. There are *pencil-in-cup* erosions of the DIP and PIP joints (red arrows). Multiple joint subluxations produce *telescoping* of the digits with a *main-en-lorgnette* (opera-glass hand) deformity.

Case courtesy Barbara Weissman, MD, Brigham and Women's Hospital.

- Psoriatic arthritis clinically presents as arthropathy in a patient with skin psoriasis. **Psoriatic arthritis most commonly affects the hands.** In contrast to RA, mineralization is preserved. Sacroiliitis, when present, is usually asymmetric.
- There are several patterns of psoriatic arthritis, including oligoarthritis, polyarthritis, spondyloarthropathy (producing bulky asymmetric bridging), and arthritis mutilans (a severe form usually affecting the hands, less commonly the feet).
- In the hands, the radiographic hallmark of psoriatic arthritis is diffuse soft-tissue swelling of an entire digit, producing the *sausage digit. Pencil-in-cup* erosions are also characteristic, most commonly affecting the DIPs. Although hand findings are usually bilateral, involvement tends to be asymmetric. The severe *arthritis mutilans* variant can cause marked deformity and *telescoping* digits, also known as the *main-en-lorgnette* (opera-glass hand) deformity.

  Additional findings in the hands include fluffy periostitis and ill-defined erosions of the joint margins.
- In the foot, the great toe IP and MTP joints are most commonly affected. An ivory phalanx represents osteosclerosis and is relatively specific for psoriatic arthritis. Psoriatic arthritis produces a plantar calcaneal spur with periosteal reaction. In contrast, a degenerative calcaneal spur will not feature reactive new bone.
- In the spine, psoriatic arthritis causes formation of coarse bony bridging (bulky lateral bony outgrowths), sometimes indistinguishable from reactive arthropathy (discussed below).

Reactive arthropathy (previously called Reiter disease)

- Reactive arthropathy is an inflammatory arthritis thought to be a sequela of infectious diarrhea, urethritis, or cervicitis. Sacroiliitis is usually asymmetric, as in psoriatic arthritis.
- **Reactive arthropathy predominantly affects the feet**, where it has a similar appearance to psoriatic arthritis. Initial radiographic findings include diffuse soft-tissue swelling, joint space loss, aggressive marginal erosions, and juxta-articular osteopenia. Bony mineralization is preserved in the later stage of disease.
- In particular, the calcaneus is a common site of involvement with bony proliferative changes including erosions, enthesophytes, and fluffy periosteal reaction. The posterior-superior aspect of the calcaneus is a frequent site of erosion due to adjacent bursitis. There is often secondary Achilles tendinitis and thickening of the soft tissues.
- In the hands, reactive arthropathy affects the interphalangeal joints and MTPs with erosions and diaphyseal periostitis.
- Reactive arthropathy may affect the spine with formation of coarse bony bridging, which may be difficult to distinguish from psoriatic arthritis.

Connective tissue disorders affecting the joints

Systemic lupus erythematosus (SLE)

- Joint abnormalities are seen in ~90% of patients with systemic lupus erythematosus (SLE).
- The key radiographic finding of SLE is reducible subluxations of the MCPs and PIPs. Alignment may appear normal on a PA view when the hands are compressed against the radiographic plate. Subluxations become apparent in the Norgaard ("ballcatcher's" or "you're in good hands with Allstate") or oblique views when the hand is not constrained.

Jaccoud arthropathy

- Jaccoud arthropathy was historically described as being secondary to recurrent rheumatic fever, but some authors feel that SLE and Jaccoud arthropathy are the same disease. Both entities share the same type III hypersensitivity mechanism and feature identical radiographic findings of reducible subluxations in the hand.

Scleroderma

- Scleroderma is a systemic collagen vascular disease caused by collagen deposition in the skin and soft-tissues. The fingertips are affected first, with atrophy of the distal soft tissues.
- Acroosteolysis (resorption of the distal portion of the distal phalanges) is characteristic, especially if there is accompanying calcification. The differential for acroosteolysis includes:

> **Collagen vascular disease**, including scleroderma.
>
> **Neuropathy**.
>
> **Polyvinyl chloride exposure**.
>
> **Thermal injury** (burn or frostbite). In frostbite the thumb is usually spared because it is clenched in a fist.
>
> **Hyperparathyroidism**, seen in conjunction with subperiosteal resorption.
>
> **Hajdu–Cheney**, a rare autosomal dominant syndrome characterized by short stature, craniofacial changes, and progressive acroosteolysis.

- Dystrophic soft tissue and periarticular calcifications are common in scleroderma, which causes tightening and fibrosis of the skin and often leads to joint contractures.

Polymyositis and dermatomyositis

- Polymyositis and dermatomyositis are idiopathic conditions characterized by inflammation of muscle (polymyositis) or muscle and skin (dermatomyositis). Joint abnormalities are rare, although periarticular osteopenia may be present in these conditions.
- The imaging hallmark of polymyositis and dermatomyositis is soft-tissue calcification. Intramuscular calcifications are most common, although subcutaneous calcifications may also be seen, similar to scleroderma.

Crystal deposition arthropathies

Calcium hydroxyapatite deposition disease (HADD)

- Also called calcific tendinitis, calcium hydroxyapatite deposition disease (HADD) causes crystals to be deposited in the periarticular tissues. Hydroxyapatite crystals typically do not deposit directly within the joints (the articular cartilage and synovium are spared), but instead amorphous deposition of calcium forms within tendons.
- The supraspinatus tendon in the rotator cuff is most commonly affected in the shoulder.
- Calcific tendinitis of the prevertebral longus coli muscle may cause neck pain, odynophagia, fever, and prevertebral effusion, and may clinically mimic a prevertebral abscess.
- An intra-articular variant seen in the shoulder, called **Milwaukee shoulder**, leads to rapid destruction of the rotator cuff and the glenohumeral joint.

Calcium pyrophosphate dihydrate deposition disease (CPPD)

- Calcium pyrophosphate dihydate deposition disease (CPPD) is an inflammatory arthropathy caused by intra-articular deposition of calcium pyrophosphate dihydrate crystals. Microscopically, the rhomboid crystals of CPPD are positively birefringent.
- CPPD has been called the "great mimicker" of other arthropathies. Clinical manifestations of CPPD disease include *pseudoosteoarthritis* (common), *pseudogout* (10–20%), *pseudorheumatoid* (2–6%), *pseudoneuropathic* (<2%), and asymptomatic (10–20%). CPPD is rare in a patient under 50. Crystal deposition may be idiopathic or associated with hemochromatosis, hyperparathyroidism, and hypophosphatasia.
- The hallmark radiographic finding of CPPD disease is chondrocalcinosis, which is calcification of hyaline (articular) or fibro- (meniscal) cartilage. Radiographs of the knees, wrist, and pelvis (pubic symphysis) are nearly 100% sensitive for the detection of chondrocalcinosis.
- In the wrist, chondrocalcinosis tends to affect the triangular fibrocartilage complex (TFCC). Advanced disease may lead to scapholunate advanced collapse (SLAC) wrist. SLAC wrist is proximal migration of the capitate between the dissociated scaphoid and lunate, and may also be seen in RA or trauma.

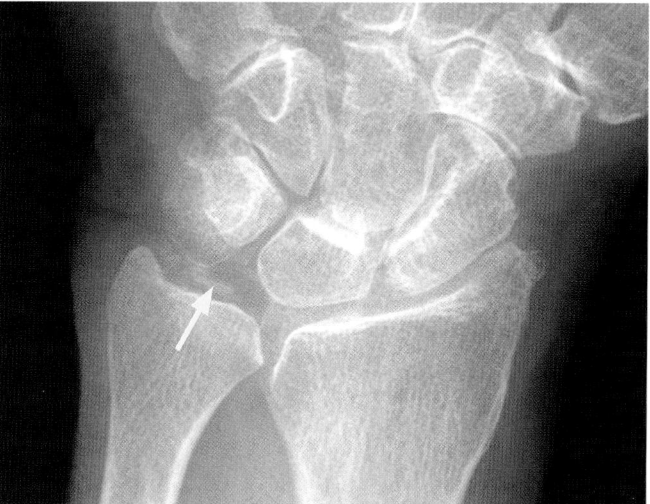

Frontal radiograph of the wrist demonstrates chondrocalcinosis of the triangular fibrocartilage complex (TFCC, arrow), a common site of chondrocalcinosis.

- In the knee, the patellofemoral compartment is affected first, but all three compartments may become involved. Isolated degenerative changes of the patellofemoral joint are highly suggestive of CPPD. Prominent subchondral cysts are also especially suggestive of CPPD.

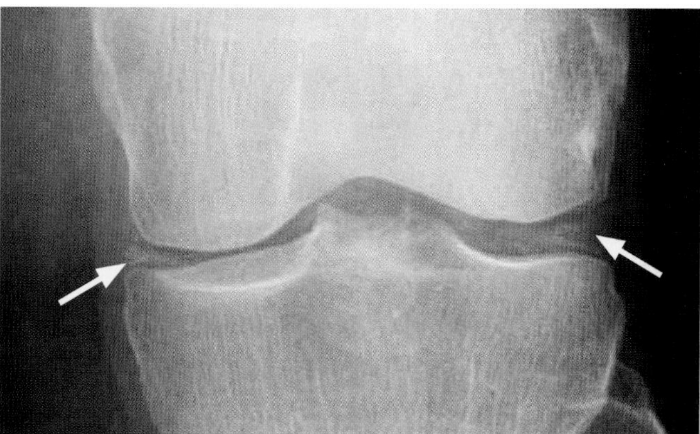

Frontal radiograph of the knee demonstrates chondrocalcinosis of the menisci in the same patient.

- In the hands, involvement of the second and third MCP joints is typical, producing characteristic *hook-like* or *drooping* osteophytes from the radial aspect of the metacarpal heads. A similar appearance can be seen in hemochromatosis, which typically features more extensive involvement of the MCPs.

Gout

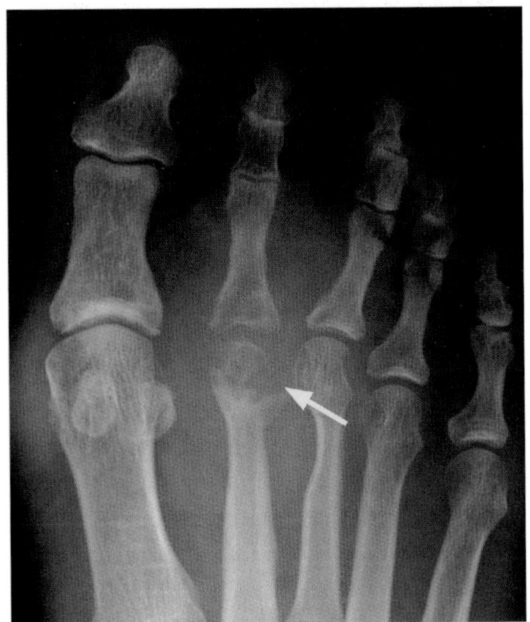

AP radiograph of the foot shows soft-tissue swelling surrounding the second MTP. An erosion of the head of the second metacarpal features a characteristic *overhanging margin* (arrow).

- Gout is a crystal-induced inflammatory arthropathy caused by sodium urate deposition in the joints. Excess uric acid may be secondary to under-excretion (more common, typically caused by renal insufficiency) or overproduction (much more rare, typically seen in younger patients).

  It takes about 10–20 years of hyperuricemia before the clinical syndrome of gout develops.

  Microscopically, gout crystals are **negatively** birefringent needle-like crystals within neutrophils.

- The great toe is most commonly involved, but gout can occur in any joint.
- Radiographic hallmarks are sharply marginated erosions with *overhanging margins*, associated with soft-tissue gouty tophi.
- Joint spaces are typically well preserved until late in the disease. Bony mineralization is preserved.

Metabolic, Hematologic, and Miscellaneous Arthropathies

Hemochromatosis

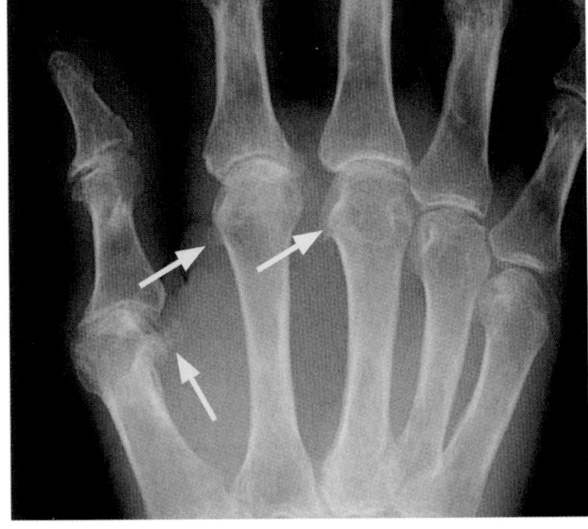

Hemochromatosis: Frontal radiograph of the hand shows cartilage loss and *beak-like* osteophytes of the 1st through 3rd MCPs (arrows).

Case courtesy Stacy Smith, MD, Brigham and Women's Hospital.

- Hemochromatosis arthropathy affects 50% of those with hemochromatosis, an autosomal recessive disease of altered iron metabolism. The arthropathy is caused by deposition of iron and calcium pyrophosphate dihydrate crystals.

  Hemochromatosis clinically presents with bronze pigmentation, diabetes, cirrhosis, congestive heart failure, and arthropathy.

- In the hand, the typical location of hemochromatosis arthropathy is the MCP joints, producing characteristic *hook-like* osteophytes at the metacarpal heads. Calcium pyrophosphate dihydrate deposition disease (CPPD) can appear identical when involvement is isolated to the 2nd and 3rd MCPs. In contrast to CPPD, hemochromatosis may involve all MCPs.

Acromegaly

- Acromegaly (excess growth hormone) causes arthropathy due to enlargement of the articular cartilage and subsequent degeneration. In contrast to all other arthropathies, joint spaces are **widened** in early disease due to cartilage hypertrophy. Later in disease, secondary osteoarthritis occurs with cartilage space narrowing.
- In the hand, beak-like osteophytes of the metacarpal heads and spade-like enlargement of the terminal tufts are characteristic.

Amyloid arthropathy

- Amyloid arthropathy is a rare noninflammatory arthropathy due to infiltration of bones, joints and soft tissues by beta-pleated sheets of amino acids. Primary systemic amyloidosis is associated with monoclonal plasma cell dyscrasia. Secondary amyloidosis is associated with chronic underlying inflammation or infection. Another form of amyloidosis is caused by β_2-microglobulin accumulation in patients on chronic hemodialysis.
- A characteristic clinical finding of amyloidosis is bulky soft-tissue nodules in the shoulder superimposed upon atrophic shoulder muscles, producing the *shoulder-pad* sign.
- Imaging findings of amyloid arthropathy are nonspecific but may resemble RA. Intra-articular deposits cause articular cartilage destruction. Soft-tissue nodules and erosions may be present.

Ochronosis (alkaptonuria)

- Ochronosis is the connective tissue manifestation of alkaptonuria. Alkaptonuria is caused by a defect in homogentisic acid oxidase, causing homogentisic acid polymers to accumulate in the visceral organs, intervertebral discs, and joints. Clinically, homogentisic acid in the urine turns black when exposed to air.
- A specific finding of ochronosis is intervertebral disc calcifications at every level with accompanying disk space narrowing.

Multicentric reticulohistiocytosis

- Multicentric reticulohistiocytosis is a rare disease where lipid-laden macrophages are deposited in soft tissues and periarticular tendons, forming skin nodules and erosions with sclerotic margins.
- The well-defined erosions of multicentric reticulohistiocytosis tend to affect the DIPs symmetrically. Other radiographic findings of multicentric reticulohistiocytosis include soft-tissue nodules and preserved bone density.
- Joint destruction may be rapid and progressive, producing an *arthritis mutilans* appearance.

Hemophilic arthropathy

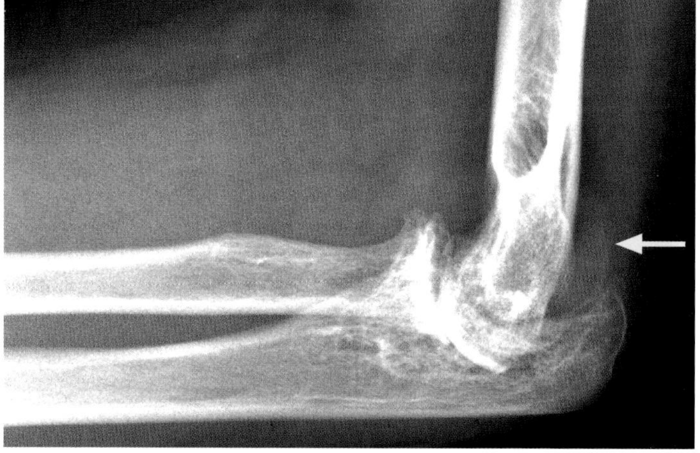

Hemophilic arthropathy: Lateral elbow radiograph shows severe joint space narrowing. Increased soft-tissue density surrounding the joint (arrow) is due to synovial hemosiderin deposition.

In this case, the radial head is not enlarged, but classically hemophilia features an enlarged radial head.

- Hemophilia is an X-linked inherited disorder of either factor VIII (hemophilia A) or IX (hemophilia B; Christmas disease) deficiency causing recurrent bleeding.
- Hemophilia most often affects the knees, elbows, and ankles. Recurrent hemarthrosis results in synovial hypertrophy and hyperemia. The hyperemia may cause epiphyseal enlargement and early fusion.

  Characteristic appearance of the elbow is an enlarged radial head and widened trochlear notch.

  Characteristic appearance of the knee is squaring of the patella and widened intercondylar notch.

- Secondary arthritis may lead to marked joint space narrowing.
- Deposition of iron in the synovium causes increased soft-tissue density around joints.
- Juvenile idiopathic arthritis (discussed below) also causes articular hyperemia and may have similar radiographic findings, especially in the knee (widened intercondylar notch) and elbow (enlarged radial head).
- **Pseudotumor of hemophilia** is a benign lesion caused by recurrent intraosseous or subperiosteal bleeding. The chronic cyclical bleeding leads to bony scalloping and pressure erosion, often with an associated soft-tissue mass.

  On radiography, pseudotumor is benign-appearing, with well-circumscribed and sclerotic margins.

  Pseudotumor may have a complex MRI appearance due to different stages of blood products.

Juvenile idiopathic arthritis (JIA), previously called juvenile rheumatoid arthritis

- Juvenile idiopathic arthritis (JIA) is a spectrum of related chronic inflammatory arthropathies affecting children under 16 years of age.
- **Monoarticular** or **pauciarticular** (most common) JIA may affect either a single joint or a few joints including the knees, ankles, elbows, or wrists.
- **Polyarticular** JIA is a systemic disease affecting multiple joints including the hands, feet, and cervical spine in addition to the joints affected by mono/pauciarticular disease.
- A variant of JIA is **Still disease**, which is a systemic disorder affecting children younger than 5, featuring acute febrile illness, rash, adenopathy, pericarditis, and mild arthralgias.
- Radiographic hallmarks of JIA are abnormal bone length or morphology due to hyperemia in a skeletally immature patient. Growth disturbances are more commonly seen in early-onset disease. Abnormal morphology results from epiphyseal overgrowth and enlargement (*ballooning*) of the ends of bone. Affected joints demonstrate premature skeletal maturation and physeal fusion.
- In the hand, premature fusion of the growth plate may cause brachydactyly.

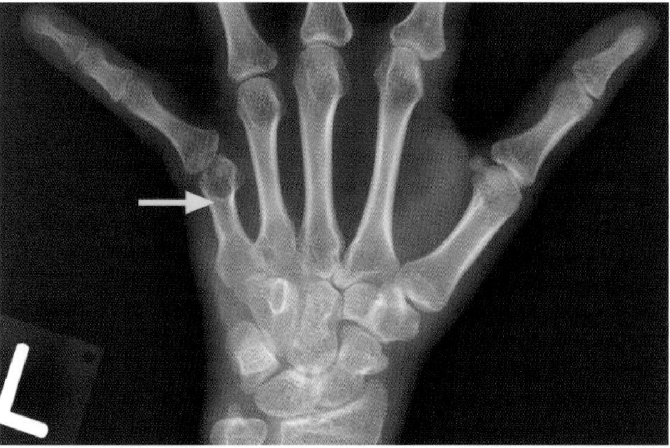

PA radiograph of the hand in a patient with juvenile idiopathic arthritis shows a shortened 5th metacarpal (arrow).

- In the knee, the characteristic appearance is a widened intercondylar notch, metaphyseal flaring, and uniform joint space narrowing. This appearance can be similar to hemophilia.
- In the elbow, there is characteristic enlargement of the radial head and trochlear notch, with uniform cartilage space narrowing. These findings can also be seen in hemophilia.
- In the hips, symmetrical cartilage space narrowing, protrusio deformity, and gracile appearance of the femoral shaft are characteristic.
- Ankylosis may occur in the wrist and zygapophyseal (facet) joints of the cervical spine. Ankylosis occurs much more commonly in juvenile idiopathic arthropathy compared to adult rheumatoid arthritis. The differential diagnosis of a child with cervical spine ankylosis is Klippel–Feil syndrome, which is failure of cervical segmentation.

Neuropathic arthropathy (Charcot joint)

- Neuropathic arthropathy, also called *Charcot joint,* is a destructive form of arthritis caused by neurosensory deficit. Lack of sensation ultimately causes severe degenerative changes with fragmentation of bone and cartilage.
- Neuropathic arthropathy clinically presents as a (usually) painless, swollen joint.
- Neuropathic arthropathy can be caused by any process that affects sensory nerves. The peripheral neuropathy of diabetes is implicated most frequently, typically affecting joints in the ankle and foot. Other causes include syringomyelia (usually affecting the upper extremity), chronic alcohol abuse, amyloid, spinal tumors, and very rarely syphilis or leprosy.
- Two forms of neuropathic arthropathy are hypertrophic (more common) and atrophic variants.
- The **hypertrophic** variant looks like *anarchy in a joint*, with destruction, dislocation (or subluxation), debris, disorganization, and *no* demineralization.

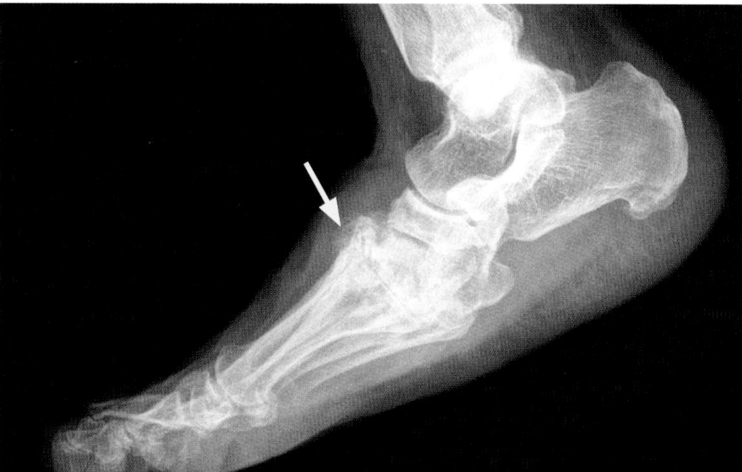

Neuropathic arthropathy:

Lateral radiograph of the foot demonstrates subluxation of the Lisfranc joint (yellow arrow). Hypertrophic degenerative changes are present at the tarsometatarsal joint There was no history of trauma.

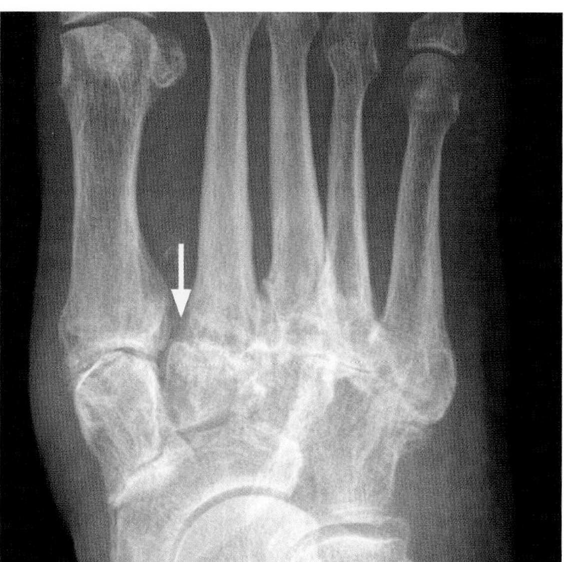

AP radiograph of the foot in the same patient shows divergent lateral subluxation of the Lisfranc joint in the same patient.

The yellow arrow points to the enlarged space between the first and second metatarsals. Offset of the second metatarsal base with the mid cuneiform may be an early finding of Lisfranc injury.

- The **atrophic** variant of neuropathic arthropathy occurs most commonly in the shoulder. It features a classic radiographic appearance of humeral head resorption with a sharp, *surgical-like* margin. Syringomyelia should be suspected in upper extremity neuropathic arthropathy and confirmed by cervical spine MRI.

Sarcoidosis

- Sarcoidosis is a multisystemic granulomatous disease. Lung findings, including adenopathy and parenchymal disease, are present in the majority of patients and are the primary manifestation of disease.
- Bony manifestations of sarcoid are rare. A characteristic finding in the hands is *lace-like* lytic lesions in the middle or distal phalanges.
- Sarcoidosis may also manifest as acute or chronic polyarthritis, although there are no distinctive radiographic patterns. Ankle involvement, especially if bilateral or associated with erythema nodosum, should raise suspicion of sarcoidosis and prompt a chest radiograph.

Putting it together: Evaluation of the hands for arthritis: ABCDEs

A: Alignment

Subluxations

- Non-reducible subluxations are seen in rheumatoid arthritis.
- Reducible subluxations are typical for systemic lupus erythematosus (SLE) or Jaccoud arthropathy. In contrast to rheumatoid, erosions are not typically seen in SLE.

Dislocations

- Joint dislocations may be present in advanced rheumatoid arthritis.

B: Bone mineral density

Evaluation of bone mineral density

- Bone mineral density is evaluated by assessing the cortical thickness of the second metacarpal shaft. The cortical thickness should be at least 1/3 of the total width of the metacarpal shaft. Evaluation of bone density helps to distinguish between inflammatory and non-inflammatory arthropathies.

Diffuse osteopenia

- Diffuse osteopenia is associated with advanced rheumatoid arthritis.
- Note that generalized osteoporosis secondary to a medical condition can be seen in any arthropathy.

Periarticular osteopenia

- Periarticular osteopenia is a nonspecific finding that can be seen in rheumatoid arthritis or the early stage of any inflammatory arthropathy.

B: Bone creation

Osteophytosis

- An osteophyte is the result of endochondral bone formation that occurs at the margins of a joint and is caused by degeneration of the adjacent articular cartilage.
- Osteophyte formation is the hallmark of osteoarthritis, but can also be seen as a secondary finding in other conditions such as CPPD and hemochromatosis.

Periosteal new bone

- Periosteal new bone formation may be triggered as a reparative response to erosive change.
- Periosteal reaction is seen in psoriatic arthritis and reactive arthropathy, but is less common in adult rheumatoid arthritis.

Bony ankylosis

- Ankylosis is the bony fusion of a joint and is seen in aggressive arthropathies that destroy articular cartilage.
- Ankylosis of the wrist and cervical spine is a typical finding in advanced juvenile idiopathic arthropathy. In advanced rheumatoid arthritis, ankylosis may uncommonly occur in the wrists.
- Ankylosis of the DIPs is a typical finding in some cases of psoriatic arthritis.

C: Calcification

- Crystal deposition diseases known to cause arthritis are calcium pyrophosphate dihydrate (CPPD) deposition disease, hydroxyapatite deposition disease (HADD), and sodium urate monohydrate arthropathy (gout).

Chondrocalcinosis

- Chondrocalcinosis is typically due to deposition of calcium pyrophosphate dihydrate crystals in cartilage, which may be idiopathic or due to hyperparathyroidism or hemochromatosis.

Calcification of tendons

- Calcification of tendons is typically caused by deposition of hydroxyapatite crystals, and is also known as calcific tendinitis. Tendon calcification can also be seen in CPPD.

Soft-tissue calcification

- The radiolucent urate crystals that make up a gouty tophus may precipitate calcium.
- Soft-tissue calcifications can also be seen in scleroderma, dermatomyositis, polymyositis, and SLE.

C: Cartilage spaces

Preserved cartilage spaces

- Gout generally features preserved cartilage spaces. Focal narrowing may be present in the region of the gouty tophi and erosion.

Asymmetrical narrowing

- Asymmetrical cartilage space narrowing is typical of osteoarthritis and gout.

Symmetrical narrowing

- Symmetrical cartilage space narrowing is seen in the inflammatory arthropathies.

Increased cartilage spaces

- Acromegaly produces cartilage space widening early in the disease, prior to the development of secondary osteoarthritis.

D: Distribution

Hand: DIP and PIP

- Osteophytes present: Osteoarthritis (no erosions); erosive osteoarthritis (erosions present).
- No osteophytes: Psoriatic arthritis (erosions present).

Hand: MCP and PIP

- Without new bone formation: Rheumatoid arthritis.

Hand: MCP only

- With erosions: Rheumatoid arthritis.
- With osteophytes: CPPD or hemochromatosis.

Wrist: CMC

- Osteophytes without erosions: Osteoarthritis.
- Osteophytes with erosions: Erosive osteoarthritis.
- Erosions without osteophytes: Gout.

Wrist: diffuse (pan-carpal)

- Inflammatory arthropathy.
- Post-traumatic osteoarthritis can occur anywhere in the wrist.

E: Erosions

- Erosions are first seen in the "bare" area of bone just inside the joint at the edge of attachment of synovium. Erosions may subsequently spread further into the joint and even destroy the entire joint in severe cases.

Variable erosions

- Rheumatoid arthritis may feature erosions in certain characteristic locations, including the radial aspect of the second and third metacarpal heads, the bases of the proximal phalanges, and the ulnar styloid.

Pencil in cup erosion

- Psoriatic arthritis.

Gullwing erosions

- Erosive osteoarthritis.

Overhanging margin of cortex

- Gout. Caused by chronic erosion from a tophus remodeling the cortex.

S: Soft-tissue swelling

Symmetrical swelling around a joint

- A characteristic finding of rheumatoid arthritis is joint distension, which radiographically appears as soft-tissue swelling, although this finding can be seen in any inflammatory arthropathy.

Asymmetrical swelling around a joint

- In osteoarthritis, characteristic locations of nodular soft-tissue swelling are due to osteophytes and capsule–ligamentous thickening.

  Heberden node: Swelling of the DIP.

  Bouchard node: Swelling of the PIP.

Swelling of an entire digit

- "Sausage digit" in the hand: Psoriatic arthritis or reactive arthropathy.
- "Sausage digit" in the foot: More commonly reactive arthropathy.

Lumpy-bumpy soft-tissue swelling

- Lumpy-bumpy soft-tissue swelling is typically caused by infiltration with a foreign substance, such as gouty tophi, sarcoidosis, amyloid, or multicentric reticulohistiocytosis.

MORPHOLOGY

Periosteal reaction

- The morphology of a bone lesion's associated periosteal reaction gives an important to clue to the rate of growth, and hence the aggressiveness, of the lesion.

Normal periosteal anatomy

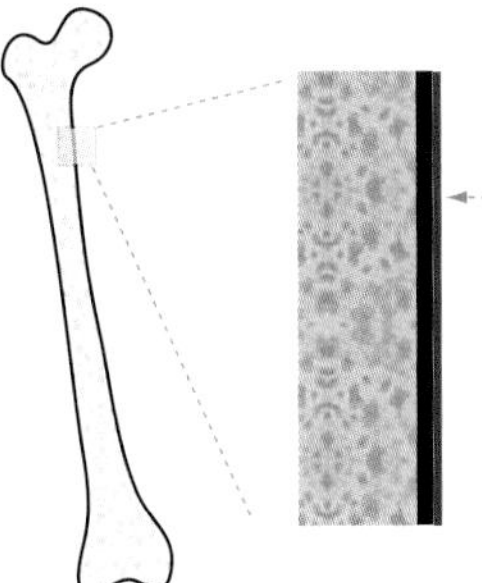

Periosteum covers essentially the entire bone excluding the joint surfaces.

Non-agressive: Solid periosteal reaction

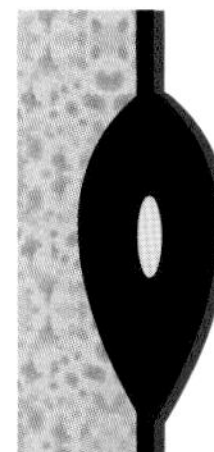

A slow-growing process, such as oseoid osteoma (radiolucent nidus), incites the periosteal cells to lay down bone in a smooth, continuous manner.

Aggressive: Lamellated periosteal reaction

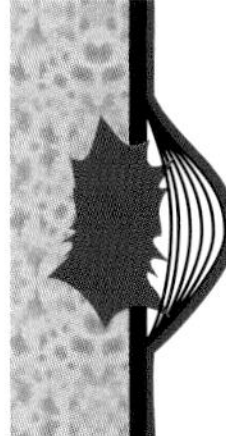

An irregularly growing process that grows in starts and stops produces a characteristic lamellated or *onion-skinned* appearance (arrows). When the lesion is growing quickly the periosteal cells don't have enough time to lay down bone.

Very aggressive: Sunburst periosteal reaction

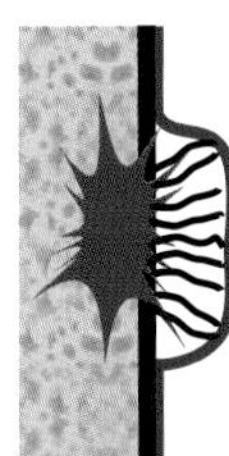

A very fast growing lesion pushes the periosteal cells outward as the lesion expands, with each periosteal cell leaving a trail of bone formation that looks like *hair on end* or *sunburst* (arrows).

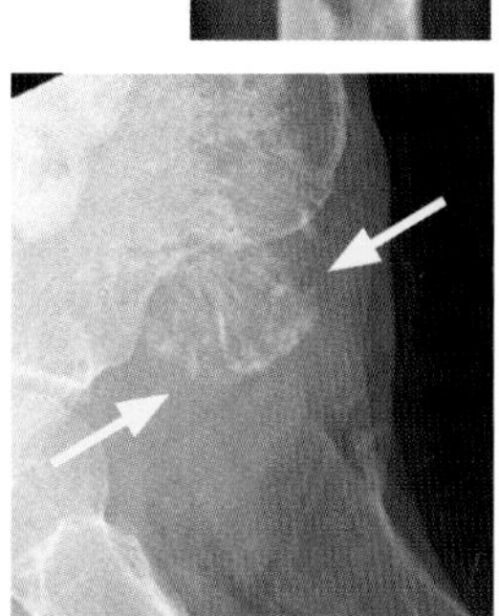

Very very aggressive: Codman triangle

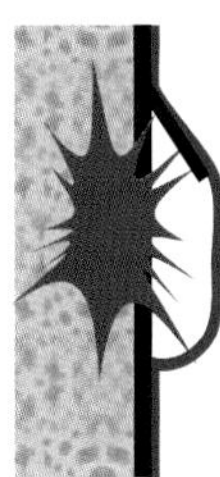

A lesion that grows so aggressively that the periosteum does not even have a chance to lay down visible calcification except at the periphery produces a characteristic *Codman triangle* (yellow arrow).

Note the associated soft tissue mass (red arrows).

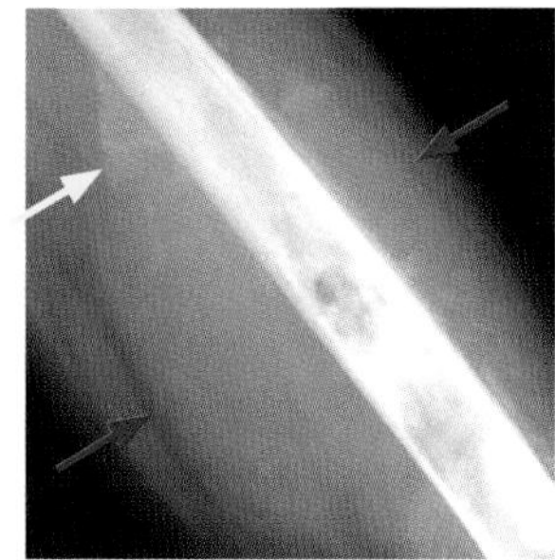

Pattern of bone destruction: Margin analysis

- Analysis of a bone lesion's margins (i.e., zone of transition from normal to abnormal bone) helps to characterize the bony destruction and stratify a lesion as aggressive or non-aggressive.
- A sharply marginated zone of transition usually denotes a less aggressive lesion with slower rate of growth. The faster the rate of growth, the more aggressive the lesion may be. A wide zone of transition suggests rapid growth and a more aggressive lesion.

Lodwick classification of bone destruction

- The Lodwick classification of bone destruction helps to stratify aggressiveness:
- Type 1: **Geographic pattern**: Margins have a thin zone of transition and may be sclerotic or well-defined.
  - IA: Thin sclerotic margins. Almost always non-aggressive.
  - 1B: Well-defined margins. Usually non-aggressive.
  - 1C: Any part of the margin is indistinct.
- Type 2: **Moth-eaten pattern**: It is difficult to define any border at all. Aggressive.
- Type 3: **Permeative**: The permeative pattern is characterized by multiple tiny holes that infiltrate the bone. This pattern is very aggressive and is seen in lymphoma, leukemia, and Ewing sarcoma.

New matrix created by tumor

- Matrix produced by an osteoid lesion, such as malignant osteosarcoma, appears as fluffy, cloud-like bone.
- Matrix produced by a chondroid lesion, such as a benign enchondroma or malignant chondrosarcoma, has a *ring and arc* or *popcorn-like* appearance.
- A *ground glass* matrix describes blurring of the trabeculae and is seen in fibrous dysplasia, a benign fibroosseous lesion involving abnormal proliferation of intraosseous fibroblasts.

Unique features

- The *fallen-fragment* sign is seen in a simple (unicameral) bone cyst with pathologic fracture.
- An *aneurysmal* or expansile appearance suggests an aneurysmal bone cyst.
- Resorption of distal clavicles or tumoral calcinosis can suggest hyperparathyroidism, which can cause brown tumors.

Patient age

- The two most likely considerations of an aggressive lytic bone lesion in a patient over age 40 are metastasis or myeloma.
- Under age 20, an aggressive lytic lesion is most likely to represent eosinophilic granuloma, infection, or Ewing sarcoma.

Location within bone

Eccentric within bone

- Giant-cell tumor, chondroblastoma, aneurysmal bone cyst, non-ossifying fibroma, and the rare chondromyxoid fibroma are located eccentrically within the bone.

Central (in the middle of a long bone)

- Simple bone cyst, enchondroma, and fibrous dysplasia are located centrally within the bone.

BONE FORMING (OSTEO-) LESIONS

Benign and incidental: Enostosis (bone island)

- Enostosis (commonly called a bone island) is an extremely common incidental finding of a small spiculated osteoblastic focus.
- A bone island is only clinically significant in that it may rarely be difficult to differentiate from an osteoblastic metastasis, osteoid osteoma, or a low-grade osteosarcoma.
- A giant variant (>2 cm) may be most difficult to differentiate from low-grade osteosarcoma.
- Bone scan of bone island is usually normal.
- Osteopoikilosis is an autosomal dominant syndrome of multiple bone islands and keloid formation.
- Osteopathia striata is a benign, asymptomatic sclerotic dysplasia characterized by linear bands of sclerosis in the long bones and fan-like sclerosis in the flat pelvic bones. Bone scan is typically normal.

Benign and incidental: Osteoma

- Osteoma is a slow-growing lesion that may arise from the cortex of the skull or the frontal/ethmoid sinuses.
- Gardner syndrome is an autosomal dominant syndrome of multiple osteomas, intestinal polyposis, and soft-tissue desmoid tumors.
- In contrast to a bone island, osteoma arises from the cortex rather than the medullary canal.

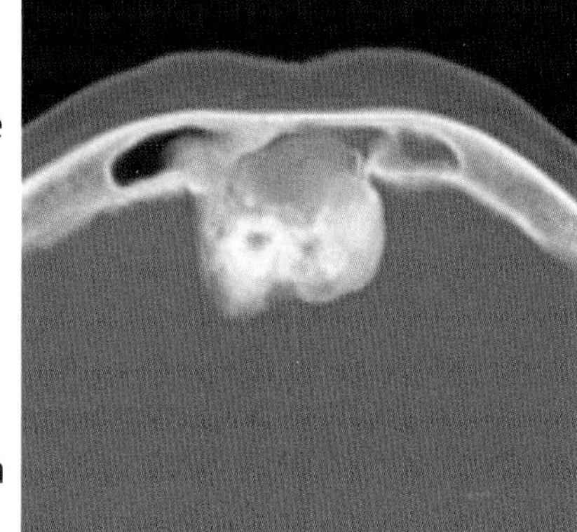

Osteoma: Axial head CT in bone window shows a densely sclerotic osteoma arising from the cortex of the frontal sinus.

Benign: Melorheostosis

- Melorheostosis (also commonly spelled melorrheostosis) is a non-neoplastic proliferation of thickened and irregular cortex with a typical *candle-wax* appearance.
- It clinically presents with pain, decreased range of motion, leg-bowing, and leg-length discrepancy.
- Melorheostosis may be associated with scleroderma-like skin lesions over the affected region.
- Melorheostosis is usually seen in a single lower limb, in the distribution of a single sclerotome. A sclerotome represents a zone supplied by a single sensory nerve.
- Melorheostosis features intense uptake on bone scan.

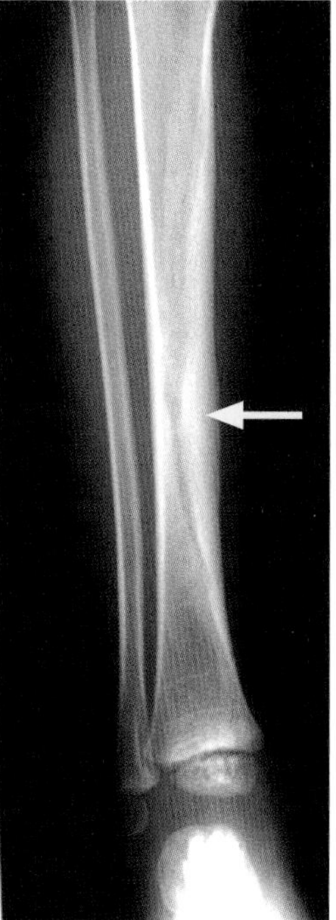

Melorheostosis: Frontal radiograph of the right tibia and fibula shows thickened, irregular wavy cortex of the medial tibia (arrow).

Case courtesy Michael Callahan, MD, Boston Children's Hospital.

Benign: Osteoid osteoma

- Osteoid osteoma is a benign osteoblastic lesion characterized by a nidus of osteoid tissue surrounded by reactive bone sclerosis. The etiology is controversial. Inflammatory, vascular, and viral causes have been proposed.
- The classic clinical presentation is night pain relieved by aspirin in a teenager or young adult.
- Osteoid osteoma tends to occur in the diaphyses of the leg long bones (femur and tibia) most commonly. About 20% occur in the posterior elements of the spine. Spinal osteoid osteoma is an important cause of painful scoliosis.
- On radiography and CT, a lucent nidus is surrounded by sclerosis. There is often central calcification within the nidus. Bone scan will be positive, with the *double density* sign representing intense uptake centrally in the region of the nidus and adjacent reactive uptake corresponding to sclerosis. Osteoid osteoma can be difficult to see on MRI alone. The nidus is usually low-signal on T1-weighted images and reactive marrow edema can obscure the lesion on T2-weighted images.

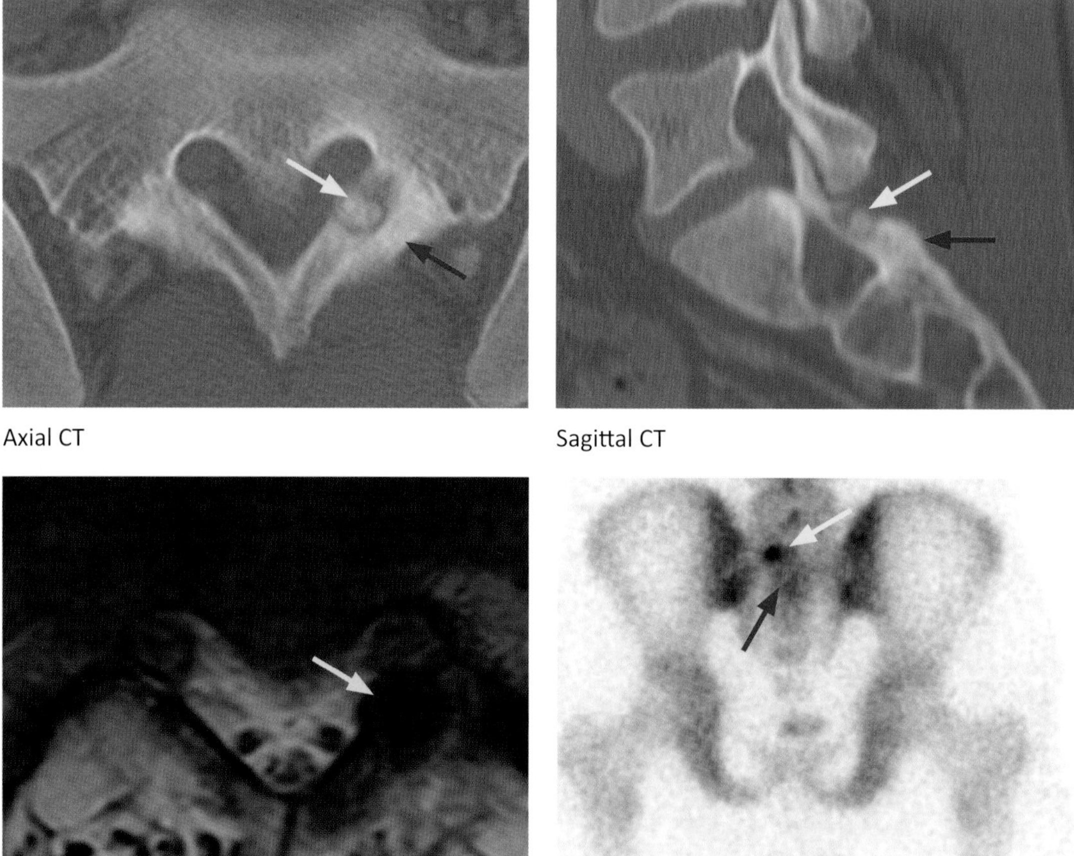

Axial CT

Sagittal CT

T1-weighted MRI

Tc-99m MDP bone scan (posterior projection)

Osteoid osteoma: CT shows a radiolucent nidus in the left sacral ala (posterior element location) with a large central calcification (yellow arrows) with adjacent sclerosis (red arrows). The lesion is less conspicuous on MRI and has very low signal on the T1-weighted image (yellow arrow). The posterior bone scan shows increased radiotracer uptake (yellow arrow) of the nidus, with a double density sign (red arrow; corresponding to reactive sclerosis).

- Treatment of osteoid osteoma is interventional radiology radiofrequency ablation, surgical curettage, or resection.

Benign: Osteoblastoma

- Osteoblastoma is a benign osteoid-producing tumor that is histologically the same as an osteoid osteoma but is greater than 2 cm in size.
- Osteoblastoma is approximately four times less common than osteoid osteoma, although it also occurs in the adolescent/young adult age range and also presents with pain. Interestingly, the pain of osteoblastoma is not typically relieved by aspirin.
- The most common location is the posterior elements of the spine, occurring anywhere from the cervical spine through the sacrum. Osteoblastoma may also occur in the femur and tibia.
- The most common radiographic appearance of osteoblastoma is a lytic lesion with mineralization. Very rarely, osteoblastoma may be aggressive with a large soft-tissue mass, but lacking metastatic potential. Secondary aneurysmal bone cyst may be seen, especially when spinal in location.
- A lytic lesion in the posterior elements of a young person may represent an osteoblastoma or aneurysmal bone cyst. If any mineralization is present within the lesion, osteoblastoma should be favored.

Malignant: Osteosarcoma

- Osteosarcoma represents a heterogeneous group of malignant tumors where the neoplastic cells are derived from osteoid lineage and most subtypes produce an osteoid matrix.
- Osteosarcoma can be primary or secondary. Secondary osteosarcoma may arise from Paget disease or after radiation. Secondary osteosarcoma in Paget disease is extremely aggressive.
- General imaging hallmarks of osteosarcoma are bony destruction, production of osteoid matrix, aggressive periosteal reaction, and an associated soft-tissue mass. Early osteosarcoma may be only evident as subtle sclerosis.
- There are more than 10 primary subtypes. The four most important subtypes are conventional (most common), telangiectatic, and the two juxtacortical subtypes including parosteal (pronounced *PAR-osteal*) and periosteal (pronounced *PERI-osteal*).
- **Conventional** (intramedullary) osteosarcoma represents 75% of osteosarcomas and occurs in adolescents/young adults usually around the knee in the metaphysis of the femur or tibia.

  Conventional osteosarcoma features an intramedullary osteoid matrix, both intramedullary and cortical bone destruction, aggressive periosteal reaction (sunburst or Codman), and a soft-tissue mass.

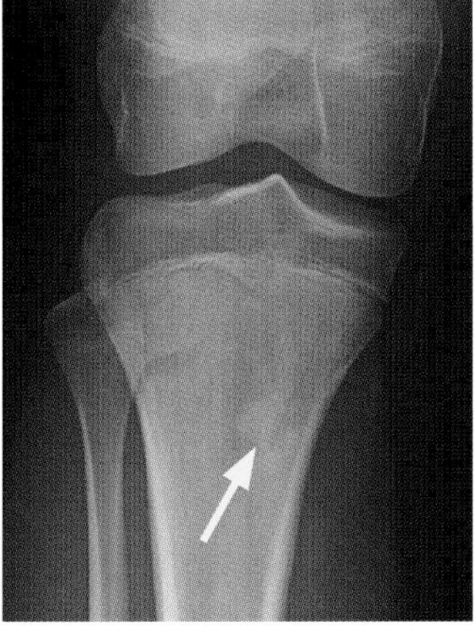

Radiograph

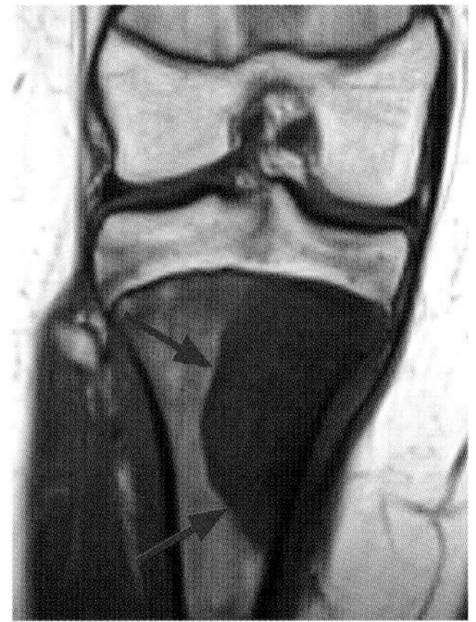

T1-weighted MRI

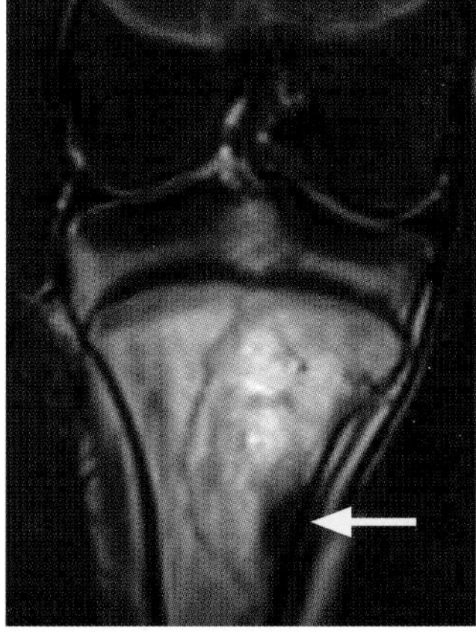

T2-weighted MRI with fat supp.

Conventional osteosarcoma: Radiograph (left image) shows a region of subtle heterogeneous sclerosis in the medial proximal tibial metaphysis (arrow). No periosteal reaction is apparent, which is unusual for osteosarcoma. T1-weighted MRI shows a well-defined region of marrow replacement by tumor (red arrows). T2-weighted MRI with fat suppression demonstrates diffuse marrow edema in the tibia, with a region of decreased T2 signal (arrow) likely corresponding to the sclerosis seen on radiography.

- **Telangiectatic** osteosarcoma is an osteolytic destructive sarcoma, which may mimic a benign aneurysmal bone cyst on imaging.

  The presence of solid nodular components on MRI helps to differentiate a telangiectatic osteosarcoma from a benign aneurysmal bone cyst.

  Unlike other osteosarcomas, telangiectatic osteosarcoma does not produce any bony matrix.

  Pathologically, telangiectatic osteosarcoma is vascular with large cystic spaces filled with blood.

  Although telangiectatic osteosarcoma is an aggressive lesion, new treatment options increase survival, which is now slightly improved compared to a conventional osteosarcoma.

- **Parosteal** (PAR-osteal) osteosarcoma is a juxtacortical osteosarcoma that arises from the outer periosteum. It most commonly occurs at the posterior aspect of distal femoral metaphysis and has a cauliflower-like exophytic morphology (mnemonic: par-boil cauliflower before eating). A lucent line may be seen separating it from the cortex.

  Patients are usually in their 3rd and 4th decades, older compared to other osteosarcoma subtypes.

  Parosteal osteosarcoma is the least malignant of all osteosarcomas, with ~90% 5-year survival.

- **Periosteal** (PERI-osteal) osteosarcoma, the other juxtacortical osteosarcoma, is a rare osteosarcoma variant arising from the inner periosteum. It features cortical thickening, aggressive periosteal reaction, and a soft-tissue mass. Histologically, periosteal osteosarcoma may show chondroid differentiation.

  The most common location of periosteal osteosarcoma is the diaphysis of the femur or tibia.

  Patients tend to be younger than 20 years old.

- Regardless of subtype, osteosarcoma may metastasize to lungs, where the metastases typically calcify.

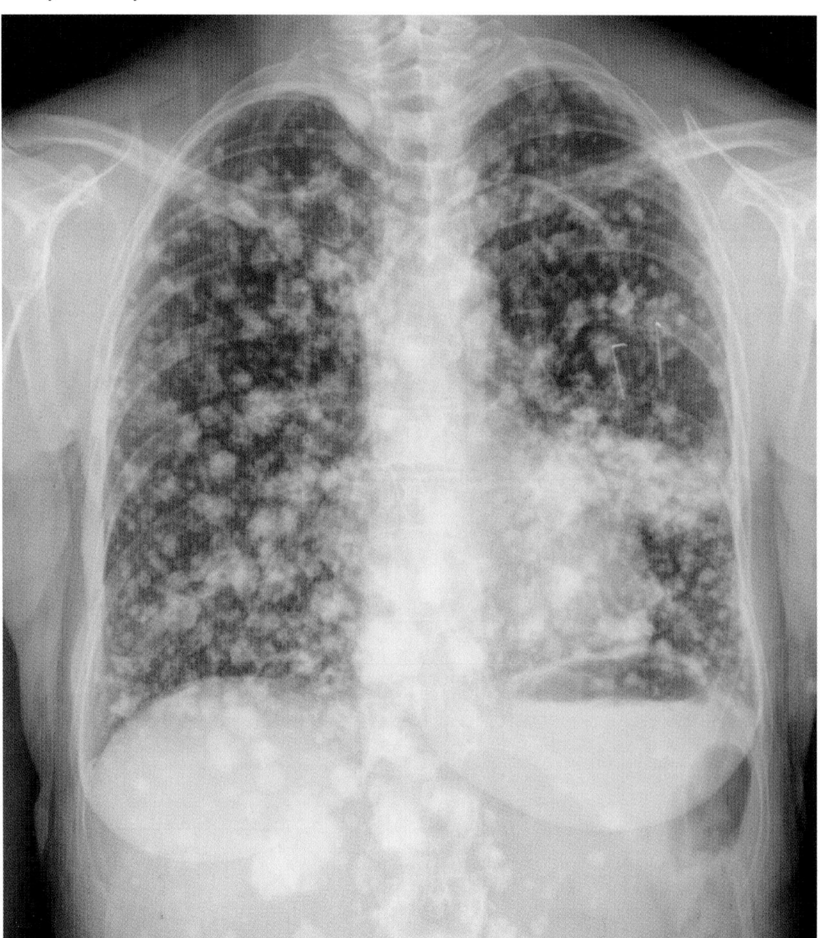

Frontal radiograph shows innumerable calcified osteosarcoma metastases in the thorax and visualized portion of the upper abdomen, demonstrating fluffy osteoid matrix.

Benign: Synovial chondromatosis/osteochondromatosis

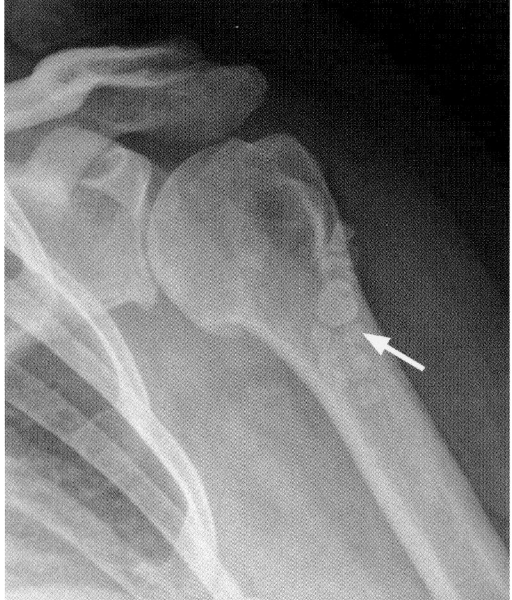

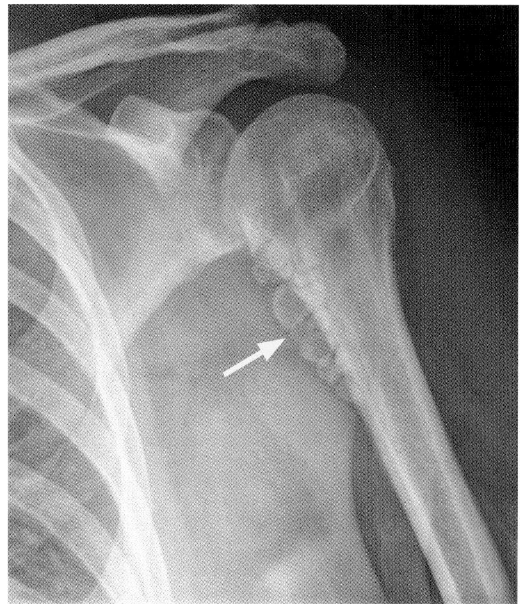

Synovial osteochondromatosis: Frontal external rotation (left image) and internal rotation (right image) radiographs of the shoulder show multiple small round calcifications tracking along the expected location of the long head of the biceps tendon sheath (arrows).

- Synovial chondromatosis is non-neoplastic synovial metaplasia characterized by the formation of intra-articular lobulated cartilaginous nodules, which may or may not ossify. It is usually a monoarticular disorder.
- The cartilaginous foci often ossify, in which case the term *osteochondromatosis* is used.
- Synovial proliferation tends not to directly cause arthropathy, although the intra-articular nodules may cause mechanical erosions and secondary osteoarthritis.
- The most common location is the knee. The shoulders, hip, and elbow may also be affected.
- Radiography shows multiple round intra-articular bodies of similar size and variable mineralization. The primary differential is intra-articular bodies from osteoarthritis; however, in osteoarthritis the bodies tend to be more varied in size and shape and fewer in number. Diagnosis can be difficult in the absence of calcification, especially if mechanical erosions are present.
- MRI appearances are variable, depending on the degree of ossification and the presence of chondroid matrix. When calcified or ossified, MRI will show multiple globular and rounded foci of low signal.
- The MRI finding of multiple intra-articular low-intensity foci is nonspecific and can also be seen in pigmented villonodular synovitis (PVNS). A radiograph will clearly show rounded calcified bodies in osteochondromatosis.
- Very rarely, malignant degenerate to chondrosarcoma may occur.

Benign: Enchondroma

- Enchondroma is a benign lesion of mature hyaline cartilage rests.
- In the long bones, enchondroma features characteristic chondroid (*popcorn* or *ring and arc)* calcifications.
- The differential diagnosis of enchondroma includes medullary bone infarct (which produces serpentine sclerosis) and chondrosarcoma.
- MRI is usually able to differentiate between infarct and enchondroma. Enchondroma has a characteristic lobulated hyperintense signal on T2-weighted images.

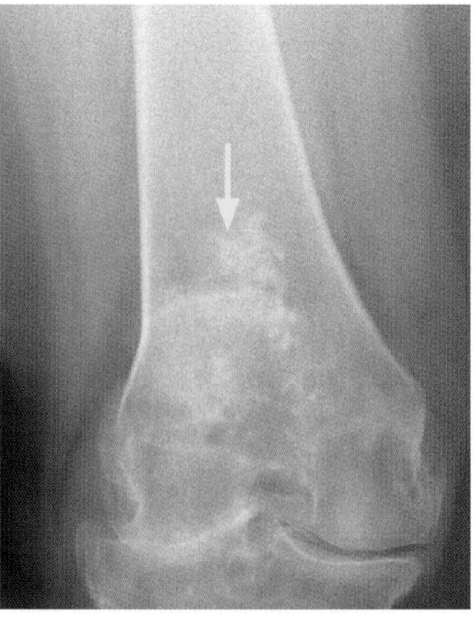

Radiograph of the distal femur shows an enchondroma with characteristic ring and arc chondroid-type calcification (arrow).

- When occurring in the hand, enchondroma typically does not produce visible matrix and appears as a geographic lytic lesion.
- Enchondroma may be complicated by pathologic fracture.

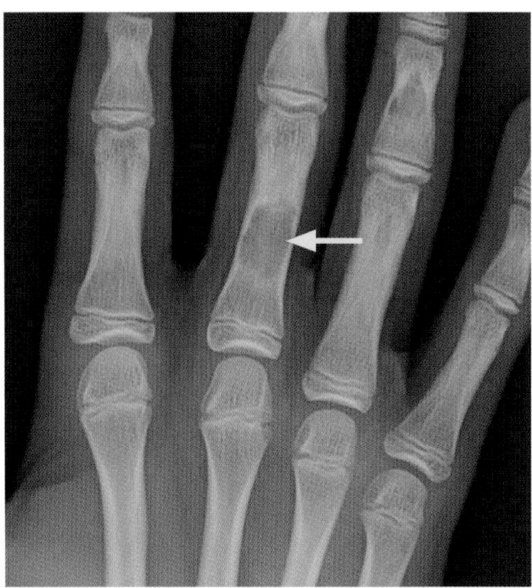

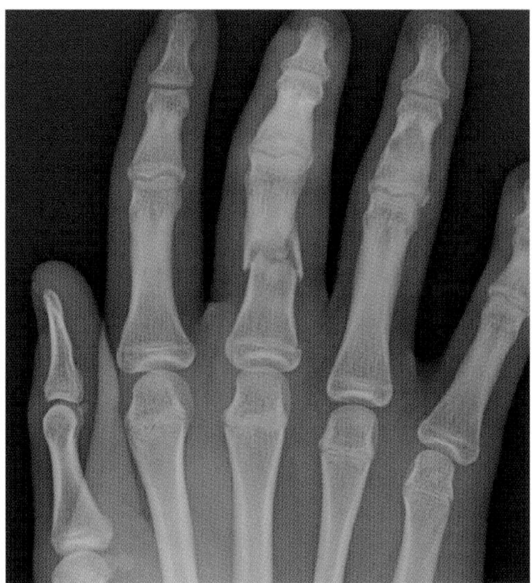

Enchondroma of the middle finger proximal phalanx (left image) complicated by pathologic fracture seen in a subsequent radiograph (right image). The enchondroma (arrow) has no perceptible chondroid matrix, which is a typical appearance of an enchondroma in the hand. Note the interval partial fusion of the physes occurring in the time interval between the two radiographs.

- Enchondroma may rarely undergo malignant transformation. Aside from Ollier and Maffucci syndrome (discussed on the following page), malignant transformation to chondrosarcoma is very rare, with the key finding being new pain in the absence of fracture. Other findings suggestive of malignant transformation include:

  Soft-tissue mass.

  Destruction of the cortex.

  Thickening of the cortex.

- Treatment of enchondroma is curettage.

- Multiple enchondromas are seen in Ollier (multiple enchondromas only) and Maffucci (multiple enchondromas and venous malformations producing phleboliths) syndromes, the two familial enchondromatoses. Both syndromes carry an increased risk of malignant transformation to chondrosarcoma, with a higher risk in Maffucci syndrome.

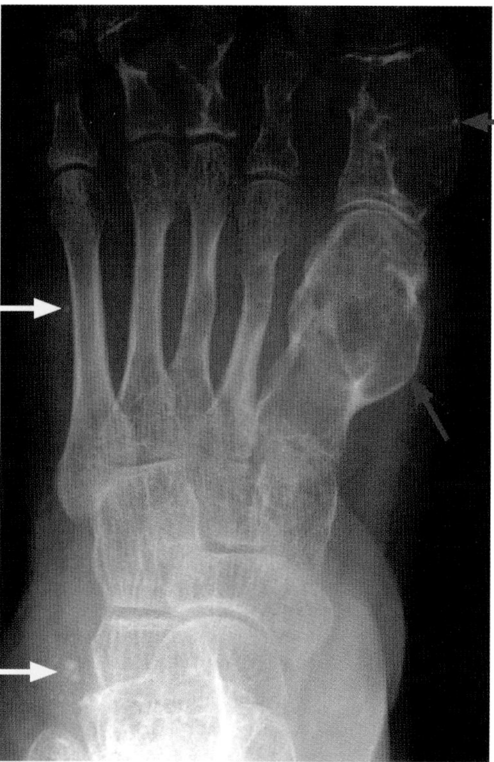

Frontal radiograph of the foot in a patient with Maffucci syndrome shows numerous expansile enchondromas most prominently in the great toe (red arrows). Multiple phleboliths (yellow arrows) represent soft-tissue venous malformations.

Note the relative paucity of chondroid calcification, which is typical of the enchondromas seen in Maffucci syndrome.

Benign: Osteochondroma

- An osteochondroma is a benign cartilage-capped bony growth projecting outward from bone, often pedunculated. It is the most common benign bone lesion.
- Osteochondroma may present clinically as a palpable mass, which usually stops growing at skeletal maturity.
- Key features are the continuity of cortex of host bone with the cortex of the osteochondroma and communication of the medullary cavities. Osteochondroma arises from the metaphysis and grows away from the epiphysis.
- An uncommon complication is malignant transformation to chondrosarcoma.

  Like enchondroma, the presence of pain in the absence of a pathologic fracture is a red flag.

  An associated soft-tissue mass is usually present with malignant transformation.

  A cartilage cap thickness >2 cm on MRI suggests malignant transformation to chondrosarcoma.

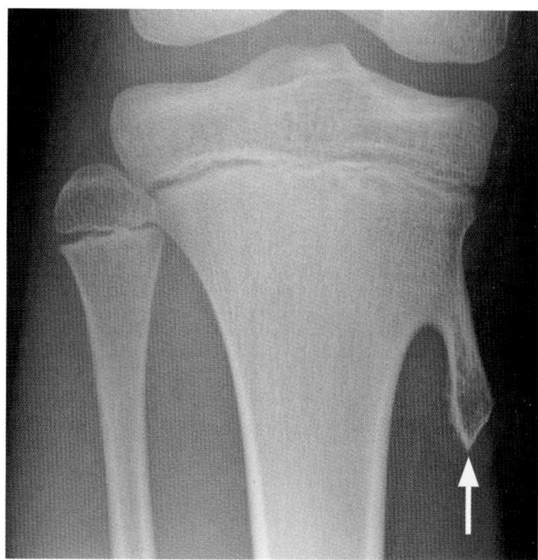

Osteochondroma: Frontal knee radiograph in a skeletally immature patient shows a pedunculated exostosis (arrow) of the tibial metaphysis, with characteristic continuity of the cortex and communication of the medullary cavities. The lesion arises from the metaphysis and projects away from the epiphysis.

- Multiple osteochondromas can be seen in familial osteochondromatosis (multiple hereditary exostoses), with increased risk for malignant transformation. Familial osteochondromatosis is an autosomal dominant skeletal dysplasia, with the knees most commonly involved.

Benign: Chondroblastoma

- Chondroblastoma is a benign lesion located eccentrically in the epiphysis of a long bone in a skeletally immature patient. It most commonly occurs about the knee or proximal humerus.
- Calcified chondroid matrix is present on almost all CT studies, but is seen only ~50% of the time on radiographs.
- Chondroblastoma is unique amongst chondroid lesions in that it typically demonstrates low or intermediate signal on T2-weighted images. Most chondroid lesions are T2 hyperintense.
- Treatment is with curettage, cryosurgery, or radiofrequency ablation. There is a low risk of local recurrence. Chondroblastoma is very rarely malignant.

Benign: Chondromyxoid fibroma

- Chondromyxoid fibroma is a very rare, benign cartilage tumor that is typically eccentric in the tibial or femoral metaphysis about the knee. It rarely demonstrates chondroid matrix.
- It usually has sclerotic margins on radiography and is high in signal on T2-weighted MRI.

Malignant: Chondrosarcoma

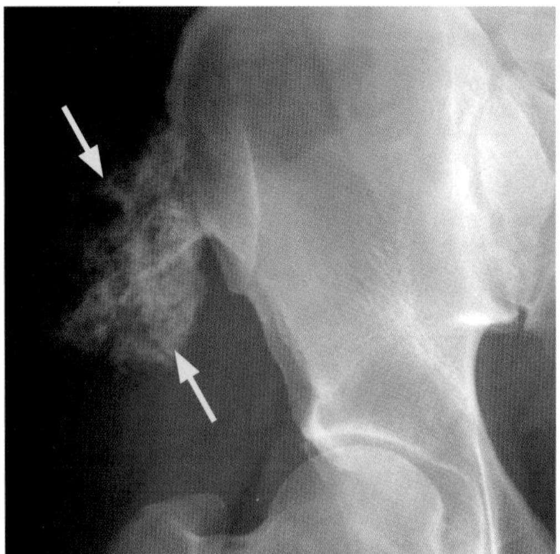

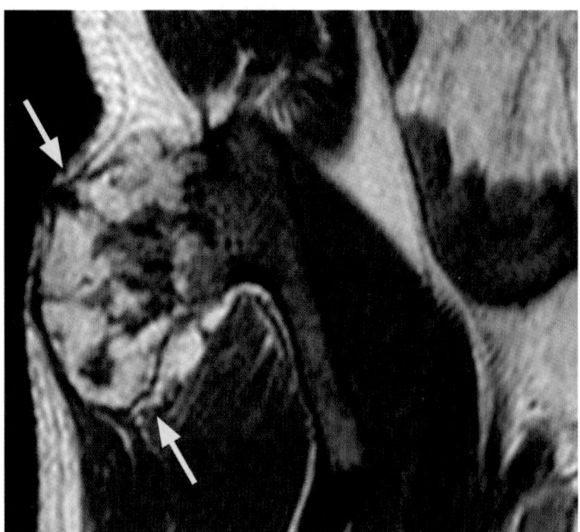

Chondrosarcoma: Frontal radiograph of the pelvis (left image) and coronal T1-weighted MRI (right image) show an exophytic lesion (arrows) arising from the right iliac crest, which is continuous with the intramedullary cavity. The lesion demonstrates ring and arc chondroid-type calcification on radiography, and is heterogeneously hyperintense with a lobulated appearance on T2-weighted MRI (arrows).

Case courtesy Roger Han, MD, Brigham and Women's Hospital.

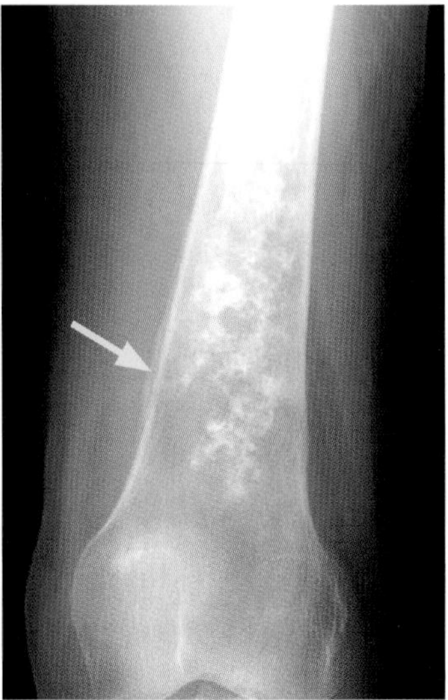

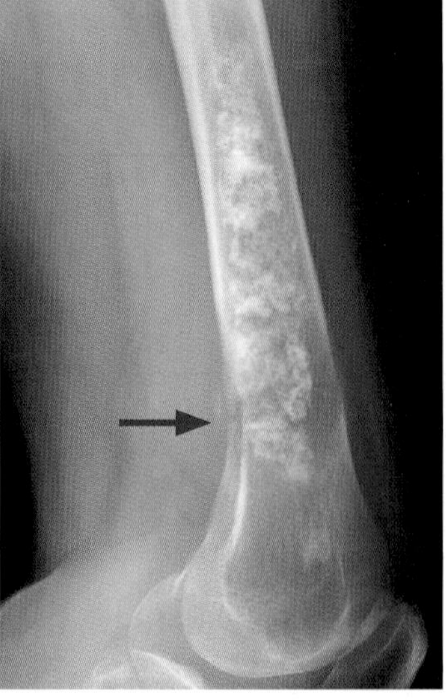

Chondrosarcoma in a different patient:

Frontal and lateral radiographs of the distal femur show an intramedullary lesion with ring and arc chondroid calcifications. Periosteal reaction (yellow arrow) and cortical disruption (red arrow) suggest aggressive behavior.

Case courtesy Stacy Smith, MD, Brigham and Women's Hospital.

- Chondrosarcoma is a malignant tumor of cartilage. Like osteosarcoma, there are multiple primary and secondary variants.
- Secondary forms arise from enchondroma (more commonly in the Maffucci and Ollier familial enchondromatoses), Paget disease, and osteochondroma (more common in familial osteochondromatosis).

    An osteochondroma with a cartilage cap thickness of >2 cm is highly suggestive of chondrosarcoma.

- The conventional (intramedullary) chondrosarcoma subtype is most common. On imaging, chondrosarcoma is typically an expansile lesion in the medullary bone, with ring and arc chondroid matrix. The tumor causes thickening and endosteal scalloping of the cortex, and there is often an associated soft-tissue mass.
- The dedifferentiated subtype of chondrosarcoma is aggressive and may contain fibrosarcoma or osteosarcoma elements.
- Other subtypes of chondrosarcoma include the rare mesenchymal and clear cell variants.

Lesions of fibrous origin

Benign: Nonossifying fibroma/fibrous cortical defect

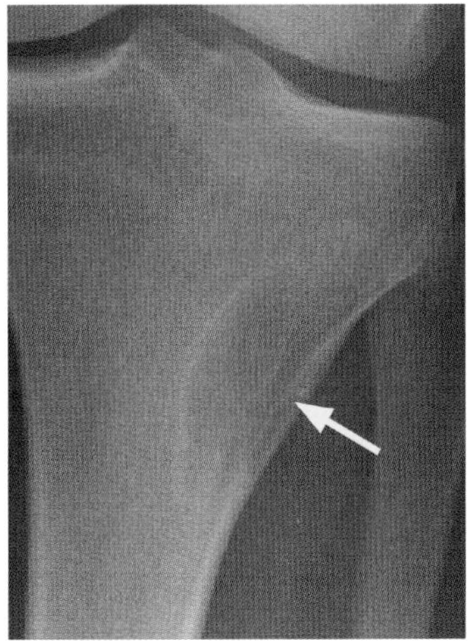
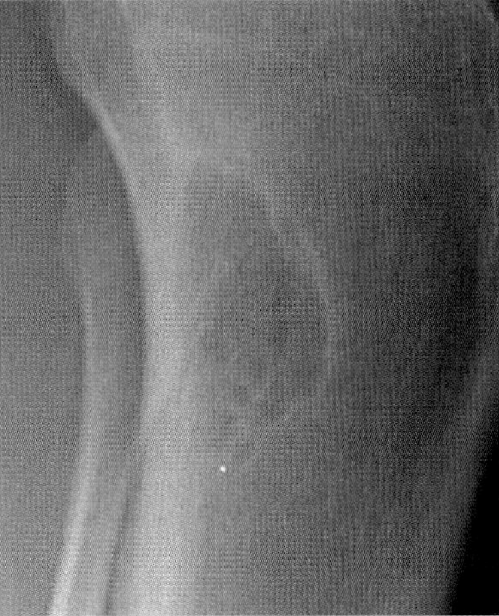

Nonossifying fibroma: Frontal (left image) and lateral (right image) radiographs of the proximal lateral tibia in a 17-year-old male show a well-defined lucent lesion in the medial tibial metaphysis. The lesion features a faint sclerotic rim in continuity with the thinned lateral cortex (arrow).

- Nonossifying fibroma (sometimes called a fibroxanthoma) is an asymptomatic and common incidental radiolucent lesion in the long bones (especially the leg) in children and adolescents. Nonossifying fibroma and fibrous cortical defect are thought to represent the same lesion; the term nonossifying fibroma is generally reserved for larger (>2 cm) or symptomatic lesions. They are the same histologically. These lesions are believed to arise from the periosteum.
- The radiographic appearance is usually diagnostic and demonstrates a lucent lesion with a narrow zone of transition, sclerotic margin, and no matrix calcification. CT or MRI may show cortical disruption or thinning, representing replacement of the cortex by fibrous tissue.
- Most lesions undergo spontaneous sclerotic involution as the patient reaches adulthood.

Malignant: Malignant fibrous histiocytoma (MFH)

- Malignant fibrous histiocytoma (MFH) is a controversial waste-basket diagnosis more recently renamed as *undifferentiated pleomorphic sarcoma not otherwise specified.* Despite the controversy and recent renaming, the term MFH is still in common use by radiologists.
- The term "fibrous" refers to the microscopy appearance of MFH, not to the cell of origin. In fact, no definite cell of origin has been determined.
- MFH is the most common adult soft-tissue sarcoma. It usually occurs in middle-aged or older adults in the thigh or the retroperitoneum, but it may occur in any extremity. Less commonly, MFH may occur in the bones, where it appears as an aggressive, lytic lesion.

Fibrous dysplasia

- Fibrous dysplasia is a benign congenital non-neoplastic condition of children and young adults characterized by replacement of normal cancellous bone by abnormal fibrous tissue.
- Fibrous dysplasia can affect one bone (monostotic) or multiple bones (polyostotic). When polyostotic, it tends to be unilateral.
- The most frequent complication is pathologic fracture, commonly at the femoral neck.
- Fibrous dysplasia of the long bones tends to be central and metadiaphyseal, often causing a bowing deformity such as the extreme varus of the *shepherd's crook.*

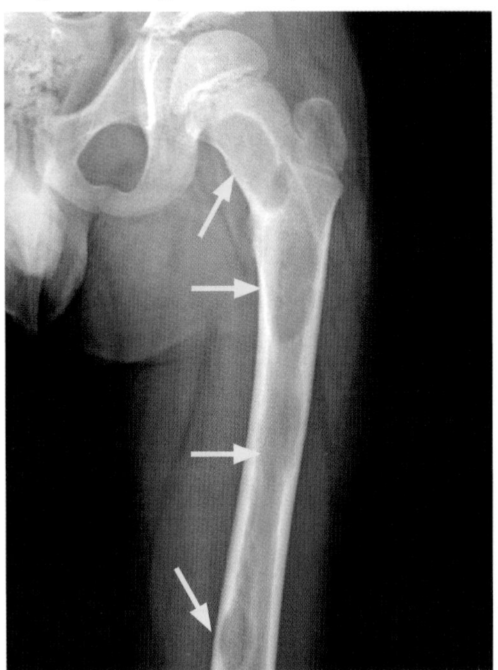

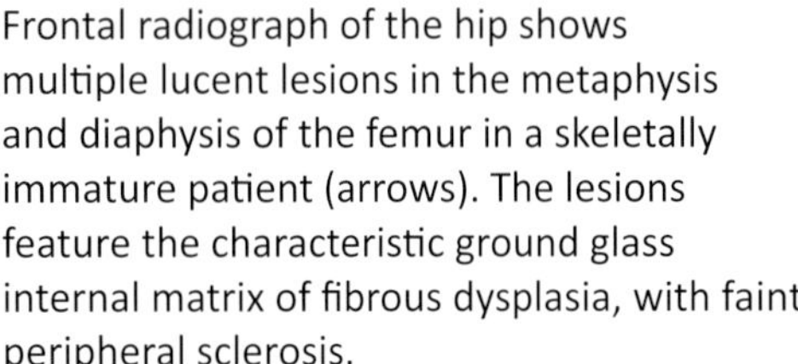

Frontal radiograph of the hip shows multiple lucent lesions in the metaphysis and diaphysis of the femur in a skeletally immature patient (arrows). The lesions feature the characteristic ground glass internal matrix of fibrous dysplasia, with faint peripheral sclerosis.

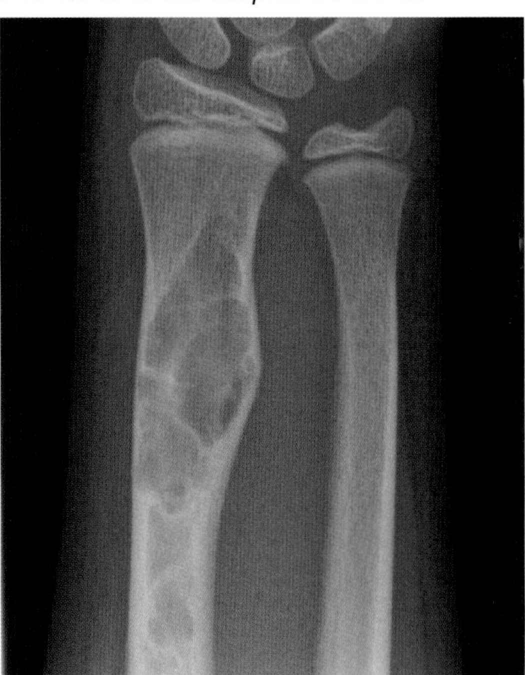

Frontal radiograph of the forearm demonstrates a multiseptated lucent lesion of the central metadiaphysis of the distal radius in a different skeletally immature patient. The differential of this appearance includes fibrous dysplasia and aneurysmal bone cyst.

- In the ribs or long bones, the matrix is typically indistinct and ground glass.
- In the pelvic bones, fibrous dysplasia is often cystic.

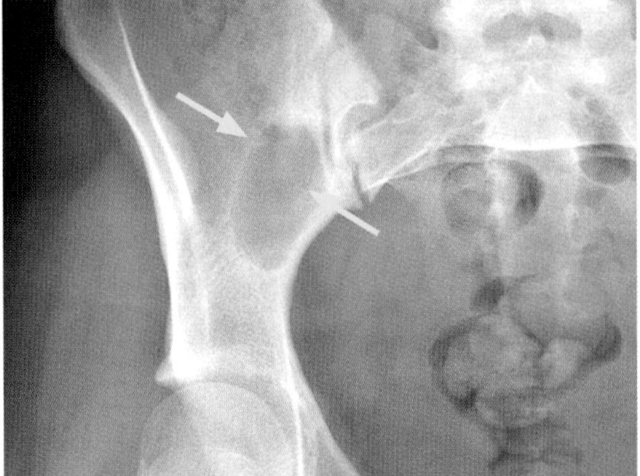

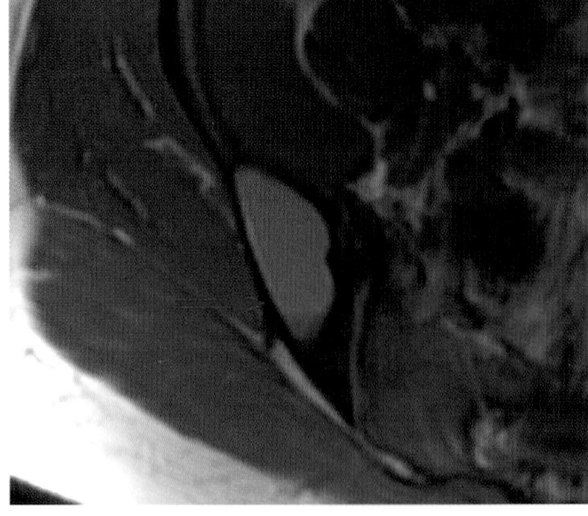

A lucent lesion of the right iliac bone (yellow arrows) shows intermediate to hyperintense signal on proton-density-weighted MRI, with a subtle fluid level (red arrow). The differential diagnosis of a cystic supra-acetabular lesion in a young adult includes cystic fibrous dysplasia and unicameral bone cyst.

- In the skull base, fibrous dysplasia is typically expansile and can look highly unusual on MRI. The primary differential of an expansile skull base lesion is Paget disease, but the age of the patient is the key: fibrous dysplasia occurs in children and young adults, while Paget occurs in older adults.

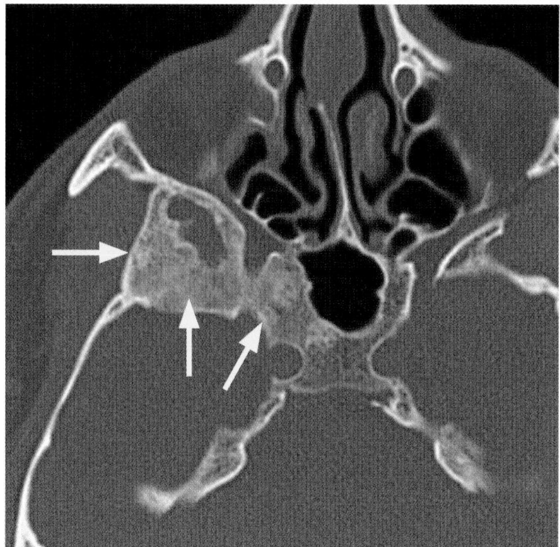

Axial CT shows the typical appearance of fibrous dysplasia of the skull base, with expansile lesions primarily of the right sphenoid bone that have a hazy, ground-glass matrix (arrows).

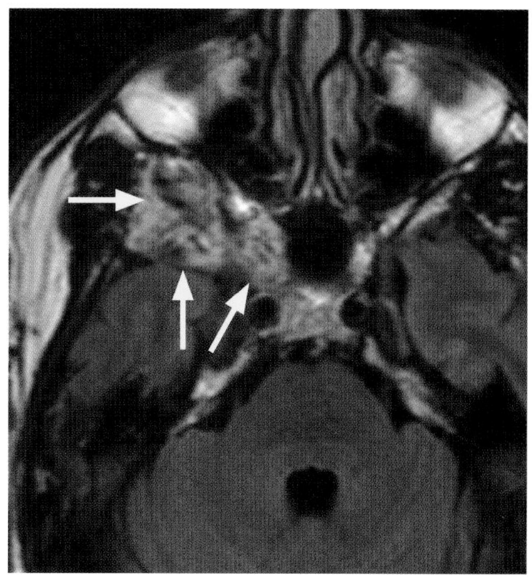

FLAIR MRI correlated to the same region as the CT to the left shows the highly heterogeneous signal of fibrous dysplasia (arrows).

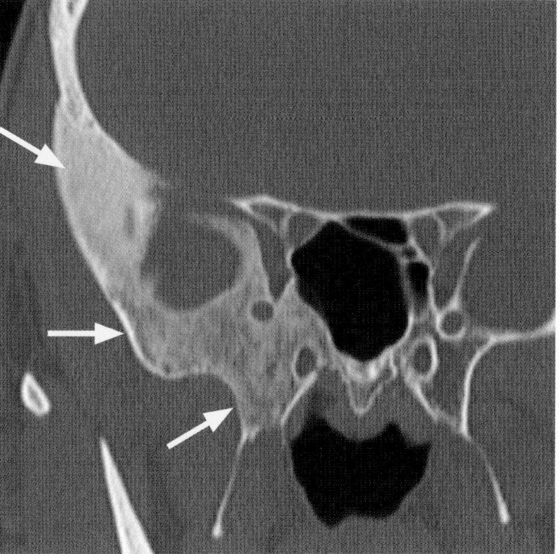

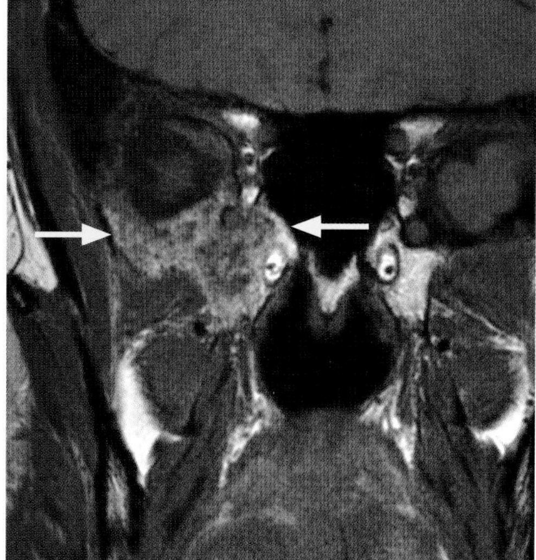

Coronal CT and T1-weighted MRI in the same patient show the true extent of the abnormality (arrows).

Case courtesy Mary Beth Cunnane, MD, Massachusetts Eye and Ear Infirmary, Boston.

- McCune–Albright syndrome is polyostotic fibrous dysplasia, precocious puberty, and cutaneous café au lait spots.
- Mazabraud syndrome is fibrous dysplasia and intramuscular myxomas, which tend to occur in the same region of the body.

Benign: Hemangioma

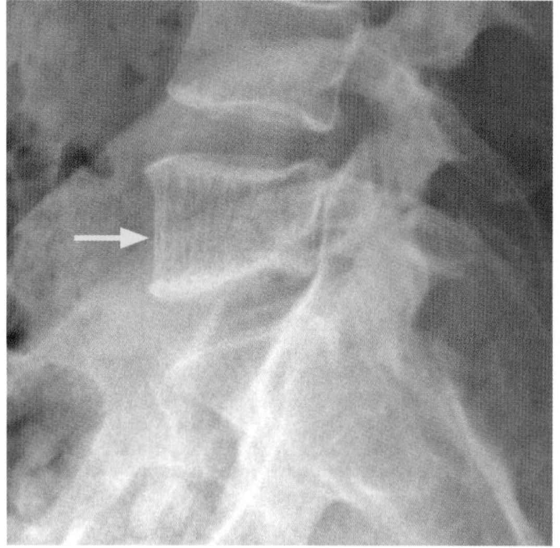

Lateral radiograph of the lumbosacral spine shows mild loss of height of the L5 vertebral body with a subtle lace-like striated trabecular appearance (arrow).

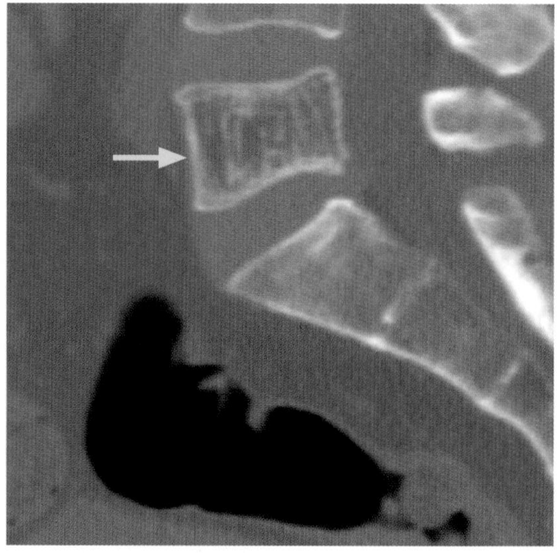

Sagittal CT shows coarsened, vertically oriented trabeculae with a typical *corduroy* appearance in L5 (arrow).

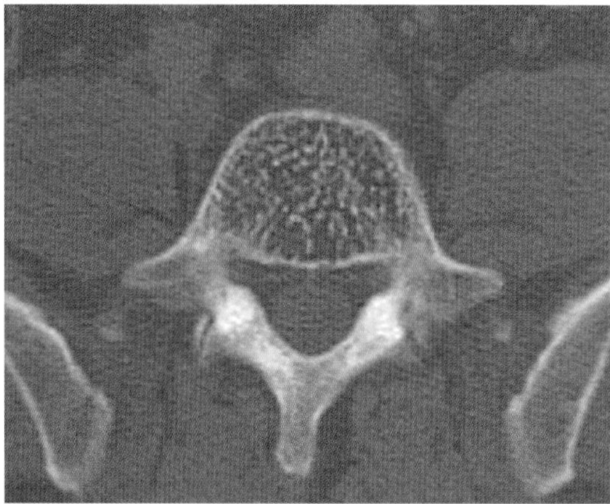

Axial CT through L5 demonstrates the typical *polka-dot* sign of the hemangioma, which involves the complete medullary cavity.

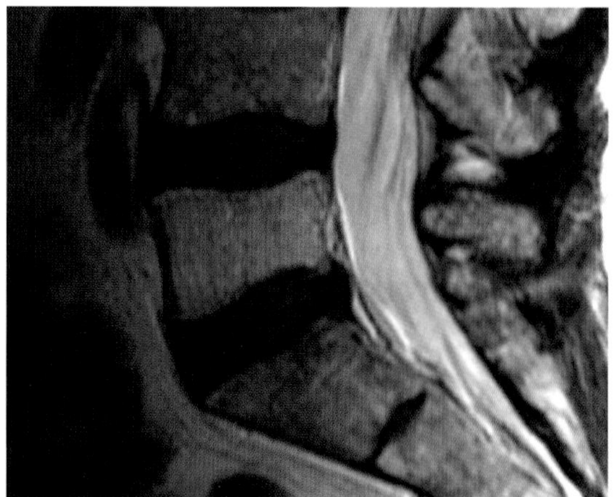

Sagittal T2-weighted MRI demonstrates high signal intensity of the L5 vertebral body.

- Hemangioma is a benign lesion that typically occurs in the vertebral body, characterized by vascular channels lined by endothelial cells.
- Although usually incidental, rarely a hemangioma may be associated with a soft-tissue mass that can cause neurologic compromise.
- Hemangioma causes reactive trabecular thickening in response to bony resorption by vascular channels.
- On MRI, high signal intensity on both T1- and T2-weighted images is from fat contained within the hemangioma. On radiography and CT, *corduroy* striations are typical. The *polka-dot* sign demonstrates thickened trabeculae imaged in cross-section.

Malignant: Angiosarcoma of bone

- Angiosarcoma looks and acts aggressively. Lung metastases are often seen.

(Usually) benign: Giant cell tumor (osteoclastoma)

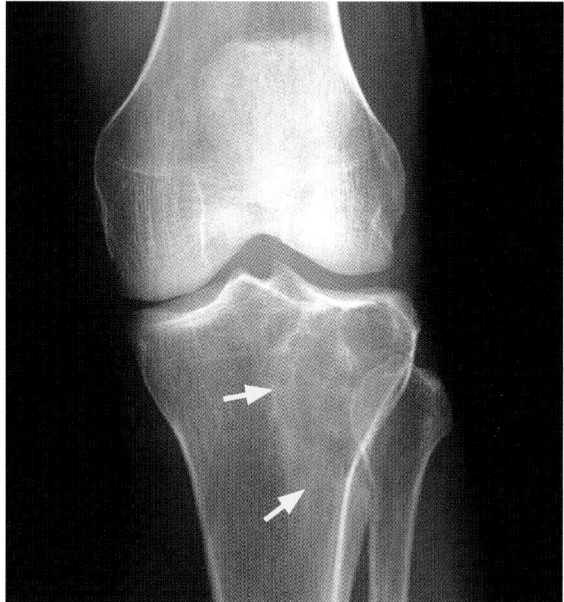

Giant cell tumor:

Frontal radiograph of the knee in a skeletally mature individual shows an eccentric lucent lesion (arrows) in the lateral tibial epiphysis and metaphysis extending to the articular surface.

Case courtesy Scott Sheehan, MD, Brigham and Women's Hospital, Boston.

- Giant cell tumor is an epiphyseal lucent lesion located eccentrically at the articular end of long bones in skeletally mature patients between ages 20 and 40. It arises from the metaphysis but crosses the closed epiphyseal plate to involve the epiphysis. The cell of origin is a multinucleated giant cell, similar in appearance to an osteoclast.
- Most giant cell tumors are benign. Approximately 5% are malignant, but it is impossible to differentiate behavior based on the appearance of the primary lesion.
- Multifocal giant cell tumors can be seen in Paget disease or hyperparathyroidism.
- Treatment is typically curettage or wide resection.

Benign: Eosinophilic granuloma (Langerhans cell histiocytosis)

- A disorder of immune regulation, Langerhans cell histiocytosis (LCH) is caused by an abnormal proliferation of histiocytes. LCH is primarily seen in children 5–10 years old and is discussed more in depth in the pediatric imaging section.
- In the skull, the classic appearance of LCH is a lytic lesion with a *beveled edge*.
- In the mandible or maxilla, LCH may cause a *floating tooth* from resorption of alveolar bone.
- In the spine, LCH may cause *vertebra plana*, which is complete collapse of the vertebral body.
- In the long bones, LCH may appear as a destructive radiolucent lesion with aggressive (often lamellated) periosteal reaction that may look like lymphoma or Ewing sarcoma.

Malignant: Ewing sarcoma

- Ewing sarcoma is a highly malignant small round cell tumor (similar to PNET) affecting children and adolescents with a male predominance. The clinical presentation is nonspecific. Ewing sarcoma usually presents with pain. Systemic symptoms including fever are often present, making the distinction between Ewing sarcoma and osteomyelitis difficult.
- Ewing sarcoma is the second most common pediatric primary bone tumor (following osteosarcoma).
- Radiographic features are of an aggressive lesion, with permeative bone destruction, aggressive periosteal reaction, and often an associated soft-tissue mass.
- In addition to Ewing sarcoma, the differential of an aggressive lytic lesion in a child includes osteomyelitis, eosinophilic granuloma, and metastatic neuroblastoma.

Malignant: Multiple myeloma (MM)/Plasmacytoma

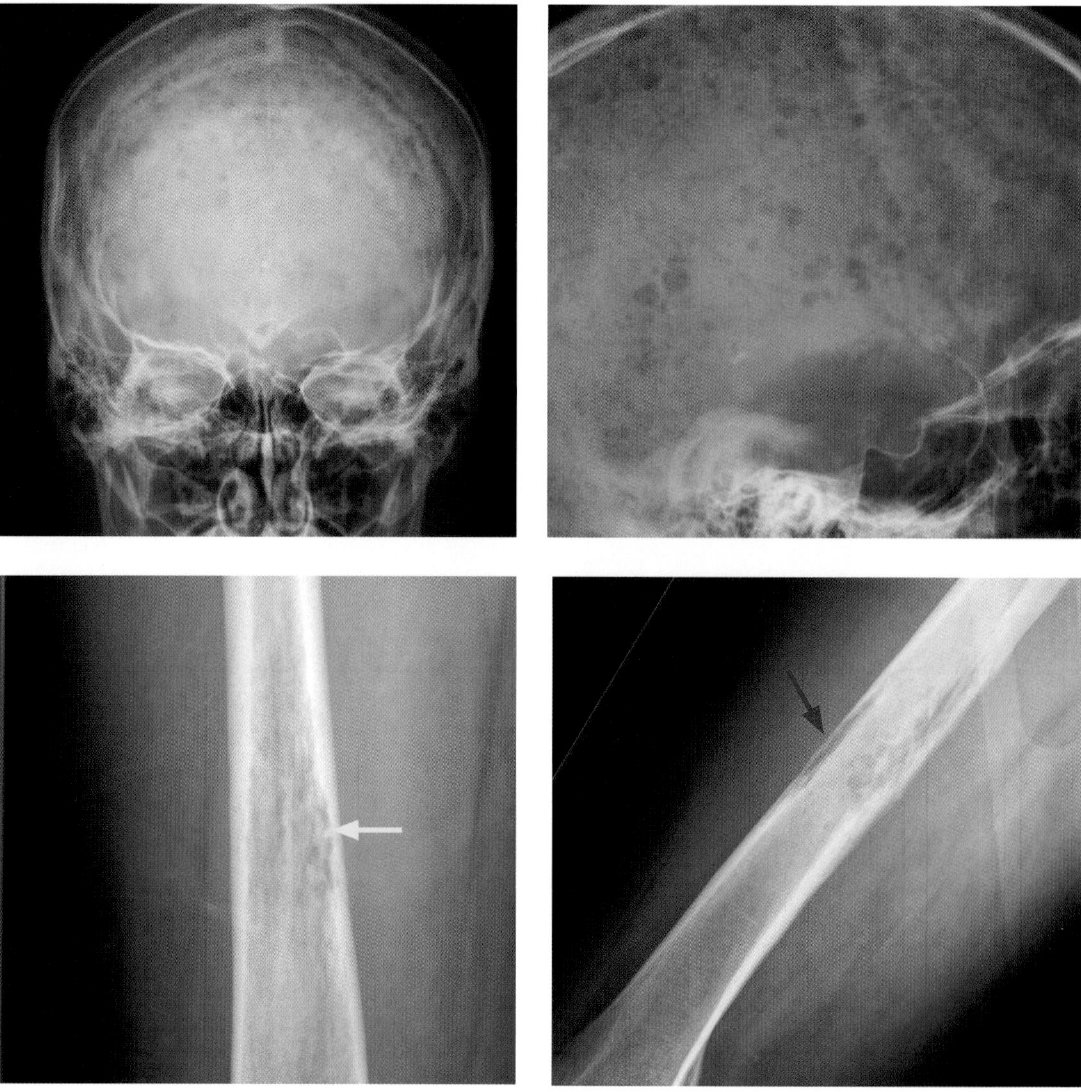

Multiple myeloma: Frontal and lateral radiographs of the skull (top images) show innumerable tiny lytic lesions. AP (bottom left image) and lateral (bottom right image) radiographs of the femur show a permeative appearance (yellow arrow), with focal cortical thinning anteriorly best seen on the lateral view (red arrow).

- Multiple myeloma is the most common primary malignant bone tumor in patients over 40.
- By far the most common presentation of myeloma is multiple lytic lesions, with the most severe form being diffuse myelomatosis with endosteal scalloping.
- Sclerosing myelomatosis is an uncommon variant, associated with POEMS syndrome:

  Polyneuropathy.

  Organomegaly (liver/spleen).

  Endocrine disturbances (amenorrhea/gynecomastia).

  Monoclonal gammopathy.

  Skin changes (hirsutism and hyperpigmentation).
- The main differential of multiple lytic lesions in an adult is metastatic disease. Multiple myeloma originates from the red marrow and usually does not involve regions where there is minimal red marrow, such as the pedicles in the spine. Multiple myeloma may be negative on bone scan, unlike most metastases.
- A solitary tumor is a plasmacytoma. Most patients with plasmacytoma will get full-blown multiple myeloma within 5 years.

Malignant: Lymphoma

- Primary bone lymphoma is very rare and tends to occur in adults over 40.
- Bone lymphoma appears as an aggressive lytic lesion, but may also be an important differential consideration for an *ivory* (diffusely sclerotic) vertebral body.
- Lymphoma is often associated with an adjacent soft-tissue mass.

Fat (lipo-) lesions

Benign: Lipoma

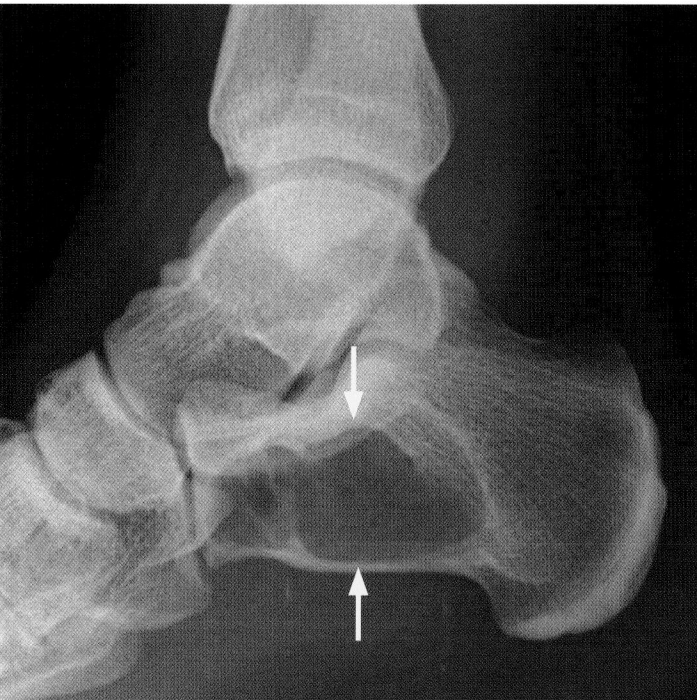

Lateral radiograph of the ankle shows a nonspecific circumscribed lucent lesion in the calcaneus (arrows) with a thin rim of peripheral sclerosis.

The differential for this lesion would include instraosseous lipoma, simple bone cyst, or aneurysmal bone cyst.

If central or ring-like calcification were present, that would more strongly favor intraosseous lipoma.

- Intraosseous lipoma is an uncommon benign neoplasm. The most common sites are the calcaneus, subtrochanteric region of the femur, distal tibia/fibula, and metatarsals. Imaging can be variable depending on the degree of fat, calcification, fibrous tissue, and peripheral sclerosis. Central or ring-like calcification is often present.
- Soft-tissue lipoma is the most common soft-tissue tumor. It is important to note that up to one third of lipomas may contain some nonadipose tissue. The presence of minimal nonadipose tissue does not suggest malignant transformation.

Malignant: Liposarcoma

- The primary differential consideration of a soft-tissue lipoma containing nonadipose tissue is a well-differentiated liposarcoma, also called an atypical lipoma.
- Features suggesting well-differentiated liposarcoma include large size (>10 cm), thick septations, globular or nodular soft tissue, or a composition consisting of <75% fat.

Notochordal lesions

Malignant: Chordoma

- Chordoma is a malignant lesion deriving from a notochord remnant. It arises in the midline of the axial skeleton, either in the spheno-occipital region, body of C2, or sacrococcygeal location.
- Chordoma is a highly destructive lesion with irregular scalloped borders.
- Calcifications may be seen within the lesion. These calcifications are due to necrosis, not bone formation.

Benign: Simple bone cyst (SBC), also called unicameral bone cyst (UBC)

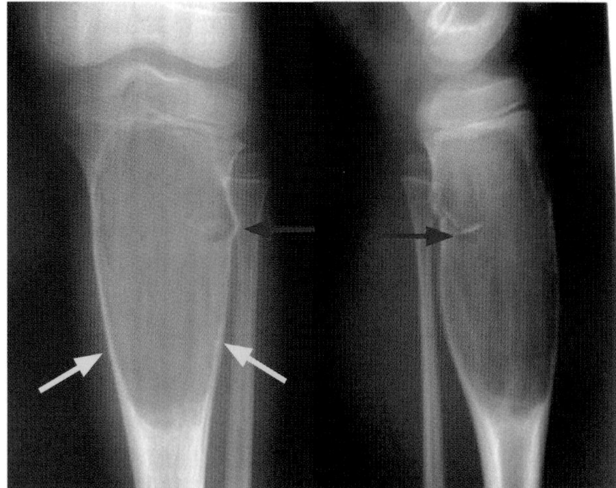

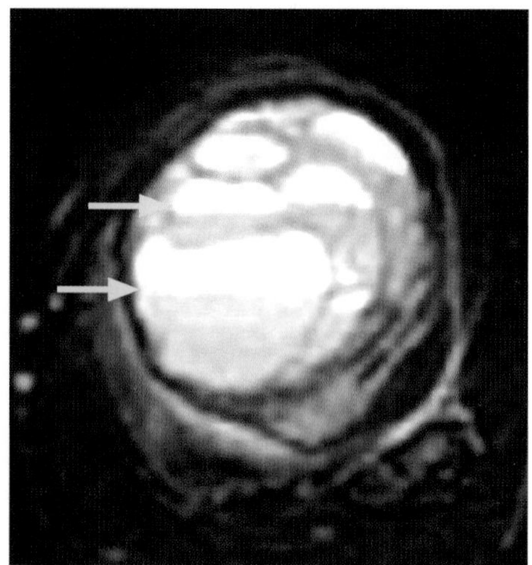

Solitary bone cyst: Frontal and lateral radiographs of the proximal tibia in a skeletally immature patient show a central, expansile lesion of the proximal tibia (yellow arrows). A pathologic fracture is present with a displaced fragment (red arrows), representing the *fallen fragment* sign. T2-weighted MRI with fat suppression (right image) shows multiple fluid levels (yellow arrows). The differential diagnosis includes an aneurysmal bone cyst.

Case courtesy Michael Callahan, MD, Boston Children's Hospital.

- Simple bone cyst/unicameral bone cyst is the result of a benign local disturbance of bone growth in children and adolescents.
- The lesion is either hollow or fluid filled and typically found in the proximal diaphysis of the humerus or femur. Other locations include the calcaneus, iliac bone, and tibia.
- SBC lacks periosteal reaction (in contrast to aneurysmal bone cyst), as long as there is no fracture.
- Up to 66% of cases are complicated by pathologic fracture. The *fallen fragment* sign represents a cortical fracture fragment that has fallen into the cyst. It is pathognomonic for SBC when seen in a young patient in a lesion in an appropriate location for SBC.
- SBC is always located centrally within a bone.
- Fluid–fluid levels are seen on MRI. Fluid levels are nonspecific and can also be seen in aneurysmal bone cyst, giant cell tumor, and telangiectatic osteosarcoma.
- One nonsurgical treatment option is the intra-lesional injection of methylprednisolone, which induces osteogenesis.

Benign: Aneurysmal bone cyst (ABC)

- Aneurysmal bone cyst (ABC) is an expansile or "aneurysmal" multicystic lesion seen in children and adolescents.
- Histologically, ABC is made of blood-filled sinusoids and solid fibrous elements. ABC may arise secondarily within a pre-existing tumor. This is important to consider if an aggressive lesion is biopsied and the pathology returns ABC, as this may imply that the true lesion was not sampled.
- Unlike SBC, ABC can be located anywhere in bone (central or eccentric). It may occur in the posterior elements of the spine. Unlike SBC, ABC often features a "buttressing" smooth periosteal reaction at the proximal and distal aspects. Like SBC, fluid levels are present.

Malignant: Adamantinoma

- Adamantinoma is a very rare, low-grade malignant tumor occurring in the tibia with a *soap-bubble* appearance. It may be difficult to differentiate from fibrous dysplasia.

Osseous metastasis

- Osseous metastases are over ten times more common than primary bone tumors.
- Most metastases occur in the red bone marrow, most commonly in the axial skeleton.
- It can be difficult to differentiate a pathologic vertebral body fracture (associated with an underlying tumor) from an osteoporotic fracture, but involvement of the pedicle or posterior vertebral body suggests metastasis.
- A fracture of the lesser trochanter should raise concern for pathologic fracture.
- A solitary sternal lesion is highly predictive of metastasis in a patient with breast cancer.

Lytic osseous metastases

- Lung (most common purely lytic).
- Breast (lytic or blastic).
- Thyroid.
- Kidney.
- Stomach, colon (lytic or blastic).

Blastic (sclerotic) osseous metastases

- Breast (lytic or blastic).
- Prostate, seminoma.
- Transitional cell carcinoma.
- Mucinous tumors.
- Carcinoid.

Benign tumor mimics

Myositis ossificans

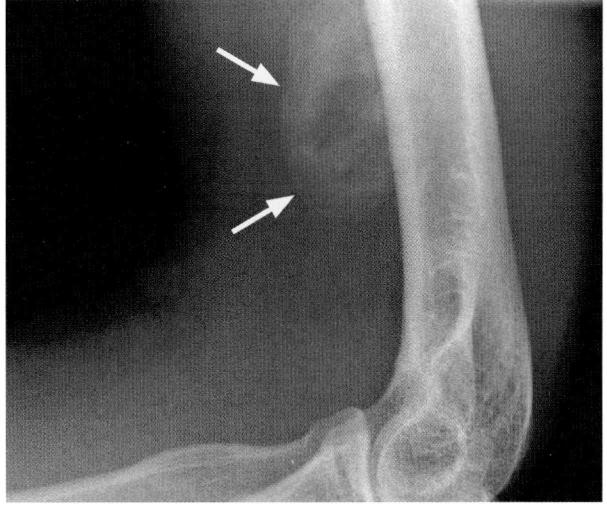

Myositis ossificans:

Lateral radiograph of the elbow shows peripheral osteoid within a mass abutting the anterior humeral cortex. The peripheral ossification (arrows) suggests myositis ossificans, at least 5 weeks old.

The main differential diagnosis is parosteal osteosarcoma; however, the peripheral ossification more strongly suggests myositis ossificans. This case was followed and confirmed by close-interval follow-up imaging.

- Myositis ossificans (MO) is heterotopic bone formation in the skeletal muscle secondary to trauma, although the history of trauma may not be remembered and the trauma may be minor. MO most commonly occurs around the elbow and thigh, which are prone to trauma.
- Myositis ossificans may mimic parosteal osteosarcoma. Parosteal osteosarcoma is usually more heavily calcified centrally, while myositis ossificans is typically more calcified peripherally.
- If myositis ossificans is suspected, a biopsy should not be performed. A biopsy can lead to unnecessary surgery, as the histology may resemble sarcoma.
- The appearance of myositis ossificans evolves over a period of weeks to months:

Weeks 1–2: Soft-tissue mass only.

Weeks 3–4: Formation of amorphous osteoid matrix. May cause periosteal reaction of adjacent bone. This stage is most suggestive of an early osteosarcoma.

Weeks 5–8: The periphery of the lesion matures into compact bone.

Up to 6 months: Ossification continues to mature.

>6 months: Typically decreases in size.

Brown tumor

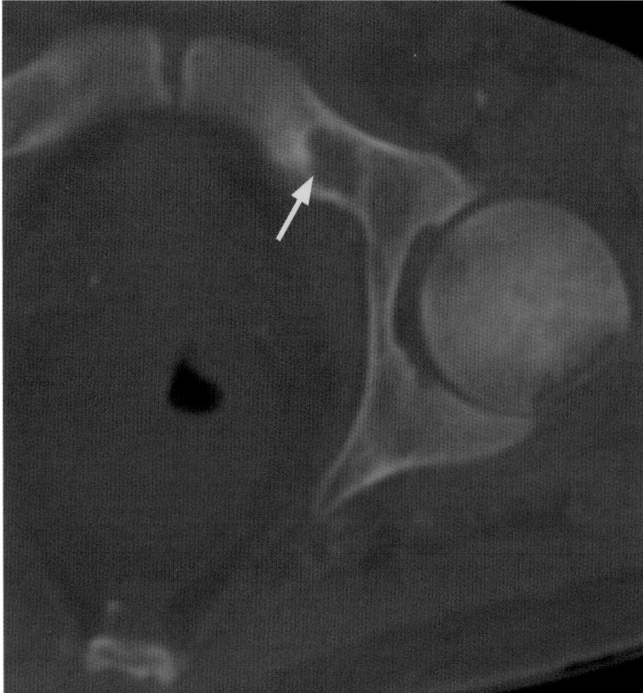

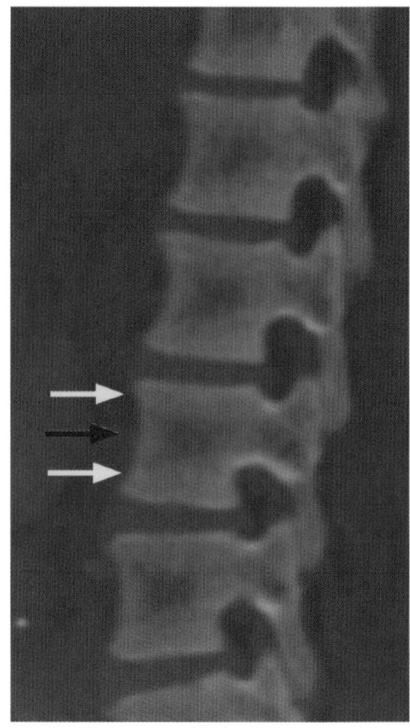

Brown tumor: Axial CT (left image) shows a nonspecific lytic lesion with a faint sclerotic margin in the left superior pubic ramus (arrow) in a patient with renal osteodystrophy and secondary hyperparathyroidism. Note the *rugger jersey* spine on the sagittal CT with alternating bands of sclerosis (yellow arrows) and relative central lucency (red arrow).

- A brown tumor is a benign lytic lesion seen in patients with hyperparathyroidism, caused by increased osteoclast activation.
- Brown tumor does not have any specific imaging features and may be difficult to differentiate from a giant cell tumor both radiologically and pathologically.
- Associated features of hyperparathyroidism are usually present, including:

> Osteopenia.
>
> Subperiosteal bone resorption (especially of the radial aspect of the 2nd and 3rd middle phalanges and the acromial ends of clavicles).
>
> Soft-tissue calcifications.

- Lab abnormalities associated with hyperparathyroidism (in addition to elevated PTH level) include elevated calcium and decreased phosphorous.
- If hyperparathyroidism is secondary to renal failure, secondary findings of renal osteodystrophy may be seen as well, such as rugger jersey spine.

Osteomyelitis

- Osteomyelitis, discussed on the following page, may cause a permeative or lytic bony lesion that can be indistinguishable from an aggressive malignancy.

OSTEOMYELITIS

Overview of osteomyelitis

- Literally meaning "inflammation (-itis) of the bone (osteo-) marrow (-myelo-)," osteomyelitis is infection in bone. Osteomyelitis has protean clinical and imaging manifestations, with an end pathway of chronic progressive bony destruction if untreated.
- Osteomyelitis can be classified by route of spread (hematogenous, contiguous spread, or direct inoculation) or by chronicity (acute or chronic), although any route of spread can lead to either acute or chronic disease.
- The anatomic distribution and clinical presentation of osteomyelitis are highly dependent on the age of the patient, the specific organism, and the presence of any underlying disorders, such as vascular insufficiency or compromised immunity.

  In adults, osteomyelitis typically arises from either contiguous spread or direct inoculation, such as in diabetic foot infections, open fractures, or as a complication of surgery. Infection is usually polymicrobial.

  In children, hematogenous spread of infection is more common, usually from *Staphylococcus aureus*.

Terminology of osteomyelitis

- *Osteitis* is inflammation/infection of the cortex.
- *Periostitis* is inflammation/infection of the periosteum.
- A *sequestrum* is a piece of necrotic bone that is separated (sequestered) from viable bone by granulation tissue. A sequestrum is a surgical lesion that can chronically harbor living organisms and function as a nidus for recurrent infection if not resected.
- An *involucrum* is living bone surrounding necrotic bone.
- A *cloaca* is an opening on the involucrum.
- A *sinus tract* is an opening from the infection to the skin surface.
- A *Brodie* abscess is a form of subacute osteomyelitis characterized by central lucency and peripheral sclerosis. The radiographic differential diagnosis of a Brodie abscess is an osteoid osteoma.

Hematogenous osteomyelitis

- Acute hematogenous osteomyelitis is usually seen in infants and children. The highly vascularized metaphyses of long bones are most commonly affected. Metaphyseal venules have sluggish flow, which facilitate bacterial invasion.
- In infants up to 12 months old, infections can involve the metaphysis, epiphysis, and joint due to the presence of bridging vessels that cross the physis. In older children, infection tends to be isolated to the metaphysis. In adults, the physes are closed but hematogenous metaphyseal infection is uncommon.

infant

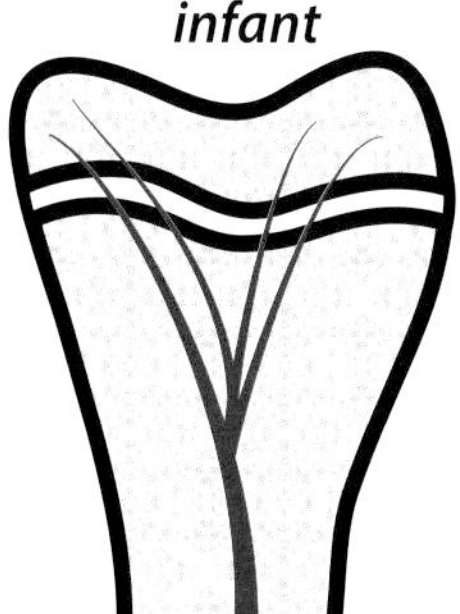

child

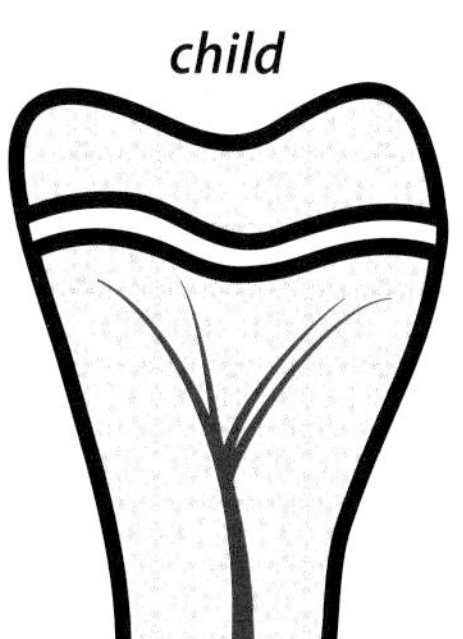

adult

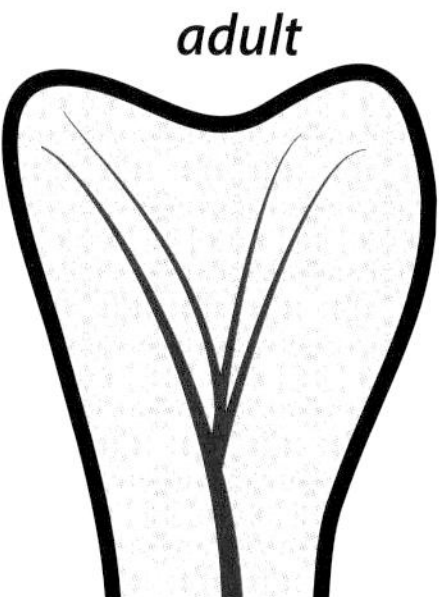

- Hematogenous infection is typically caused by a single organism. If blood cultures are positive then that specific organism can be targeted and biopsy is generally not needed.
- Hematogenous osteomyelitis occurs from the inside out, beginning with infection of the medullary cavity. Secondary involvement of the cortex occurs as bacteria spread through Haversian and Volkmann canals into the periosteum and subsequently the soft tissues. In infants and children, the periosteum is loosely adherent to the bone, causing prominent lifting of the periosteum by infection. This manifests radiographically as exuberant periostitis. In contrast, in adults the periosteum is more tightly adherent to bone and periostitis is less prominent.

hematogenous osteomyelitis

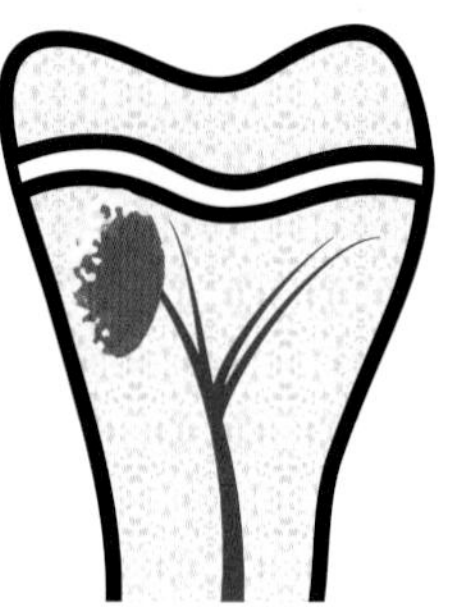

initial infection is intramedullary

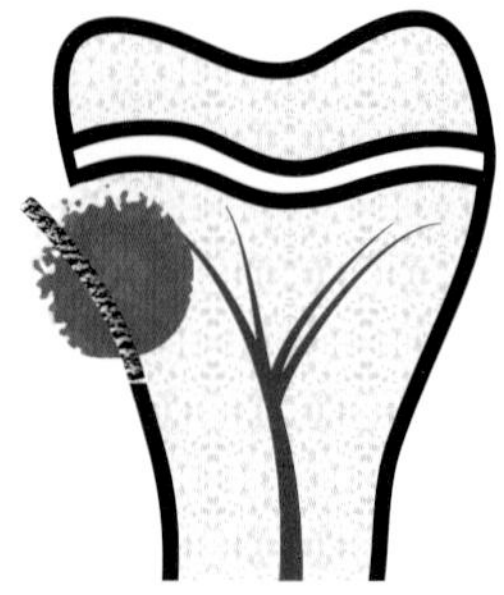

infection spreads through the cortex and uplifts the periosteum

- In adults, hematogenous osteomyelitis most commonly affects the spine.
- Chronic osteomyelitis may produce infected nonviable tissue (sequestrum). An involucrum is living bone that surrounds the sequestrum. The involucrum may be perforated by cloacae, which can open to the skin to form a sinus tract. *Chronic drainage of a sinus tract predisposes to squamous cell carcinoma.*
- Initial subtle radiographic changes in hematogenous osteomyelitis include focal soft-tissue swelling, regional osteopenia, and obliteration of the soft-tissue fat planes.
- The radiographic appearance of medullary infection is a focal, ill-defined lucent metaphyseal lesion. The lucency may cross the epiphysis in young children, where epiphyseal bridging vessels may be still patent. Periosteal reaction may appear aggressive and lamellated, mimicking Ewing sarcoma.

Contiguous focus osteomyelitis

- Osteomyelitis in adults is most commonly from contiguous spread of infection, characterized by penetration of the periosteum and cortex and subsequent medullary invasion.

contiguous focus osteomyelitis

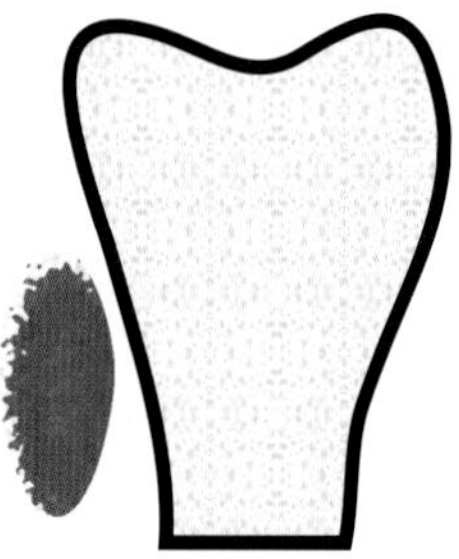

soft-tissue infection

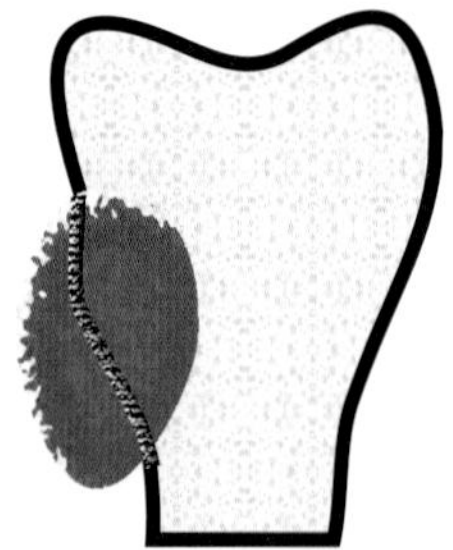

periosteal and cortical penetration

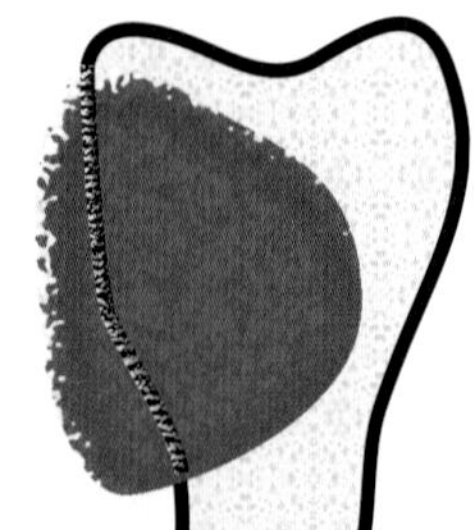

medullary invasion

- One of the most common causes of adult osteomyelitis is contiguous spread of a diabetic foot ulcer to the bones. Diabetic neuropathy leads to development of foot ulcers due to unrecognized trauma and impaired vascular reserve.

- The primary differential diagnosis of diabetic foot osteomyelitis is a neuropathic joint, a common sequela of diabetic neuropathy.

  Neuropathic arthropathy usually affects the midfoot and features polyarticular involvement, absence of contiguous soft-tissue infection, and absence of an associated ulcer/sinus tract. The bony cortex is intact.

  In contrast, diabetic foot osteomyelitis is almost always associated with a cutaneous ulcer and a sinus tract to the bone. The cortex of the involved bone is often disrupted.

  Abnormal marrow signal is seen in both neuropathic arthropathy and diabetic foot osteomyelitis.

- In contrast to hematogenous osteomyelitis, contiguous focus osteomyelitis is typically polymicrobial and biopsy is generally warranted to ensure proper treatment.

Subacute osteomyelitis

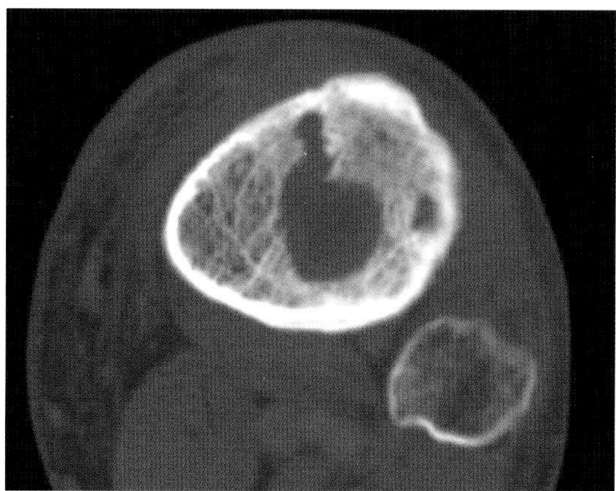
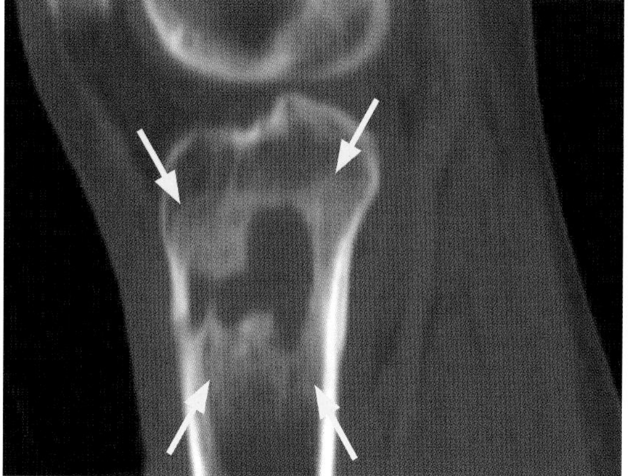

Brodie abscess: Axial (left image) and sagittal unenhanced CT of the proximal tibia demonstrates a central, intramedullary circumscribed lucent lesion. Peripheral sclerosis (arrows) is better demonstrated on the sagittal image. *Case courtesy Stacy Smith, MD, Brigham and Women's Hospital.*

- Brodie abscess is a characteristic lesion of subacute osteomyelitis, consisting of a walled-off intraosseous infection surrounded by granulation tissue and sclerotic bone. A Brodie abscess is essentially an intraosseous bone abscess.

Chronic osteomyelitis

- Chronic osteomyelitis is an indolent infection lasting greater than 6 weeks. Devascularized, necrotic bone leads to a sequestrum surrounded by granulation tissue and involucrum.
- Chronic osteomyelitis can cause a mixed lytic and sclerotic appearance, with a thickened cortex.
- It can be difficult to differentiate between active and inactive chronic osteomyelitis. Serial radiographs in active chronic osteomyelitis may show development of periosteal reaction.
- Sclerosing osteomyelitis, also known as osteomyelitis of *Garré,* is an uncommon form of chronic osteomyelitis characterized by sclerosis and thickening of bone. The differential diagnosis of sclerosing osteomyelitis includes lymphoma, sclerotic metastasis, and osteoid osteoma.

Specific organisms causing osteomyelitis

- **Staphylococcus**: *Staph. aureus* is the most common cause of hematogenous osteomyelitis.
- **Salmonella**: Osteomyelitis from *Salmonella* is typically seen in patients with sickle cell disease, with a propensity to affect the diaphysis. It may be difficult to distinguish between diaphyseal bone infarct and osteomyelitis in sickle cell patients.
- **Pseudomonas**: Osteomyelitis from *Pseudomonas aeruginosa* is classically caused by a puncture wound of the foot through a sneaker.
- **Tuberculosis**: The most common musculoskeletal infection with *Mycobacterium tuberculosis* is infection of the spine, also known as Pott disease.

Specific locations

- Hand and finger: The metacarpals and phalanges may become infected after a bite wound.
- Toe: A stubbed great toe with nail-bed injury is at risk for osteomyelitis of the distal phalanx, due to the location of periosteum immediately adjacent to the nail bed.
- Spine: Vertebral osteomyelitis/discitis in an adult may be caused by hematogenous arterial spread, spinal surgery, or spread of a genitourinary infection through the epidural venous Batson plexus. Infection begins in the subendplate region of the vertebral body and subsequently spreads to the endplate, intervertebral disc, and adjacent vertebral body.

  In contrast, in children discitis is thought to represent direct hematogenous seeding of the persistently-vascularized disc.

Imaging osteomyelitis

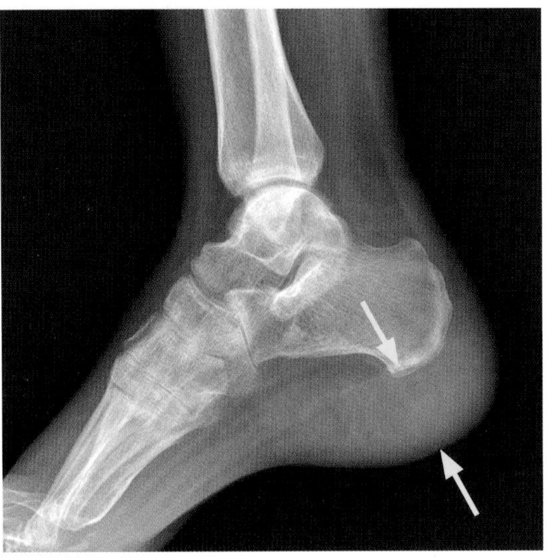

Calcaneal osteomyelitis due to foreign body: Radiograph shows marked thickening of the heel pad (arrows). No bony changes are evident.

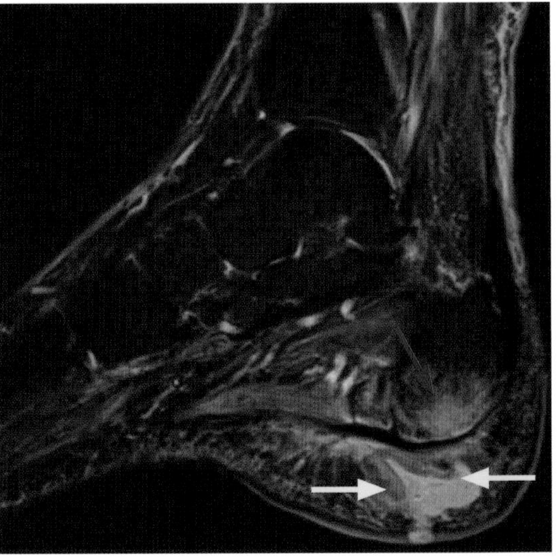

Sagittal STIR MRI shows calcaneal bone marrow edema (red arrow) and a fluid collection (yellow arrows) within the heel pad, contiguous with the skin.

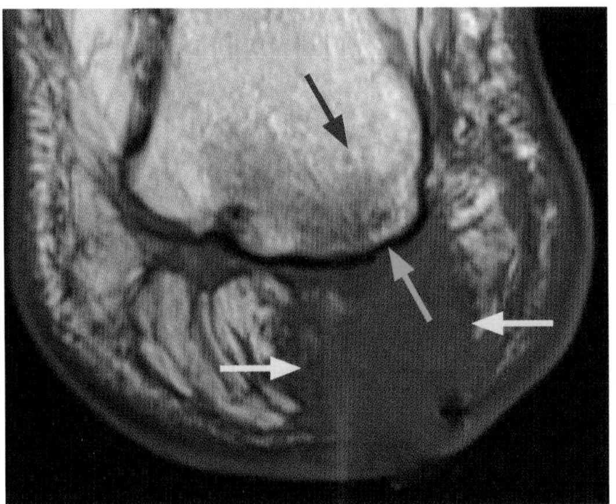

Coronal T1-weighted MRI shows the low-signal fluid collection in the heel pad (yellow arrows), regional decreased T1 marrow signal (red arrow), and irregularity of the calcaneal cortex (blue arrow).

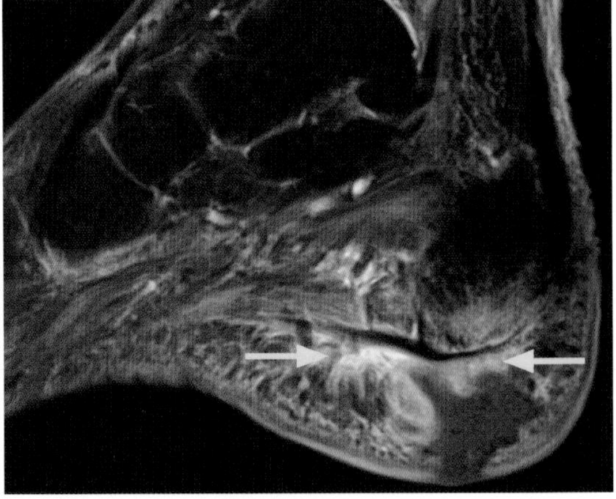

Sagittal T1-weighted post-contrast MRI with fat suppression shows marked enhancement (yellow arrows) surrounding the abscess and enhancement of the surrounding soft tissues.

Case courtesy Marie Koch, MD, Brigham and Women's Hospital, Boston.

- Radiographs are typically the first modality to evaluate suspected osteomyelitis, although it typically takes between 10 and 14 days for radiographic changes to be evident.

- Radiographic findings depend on the route of spread. Early radiographic changes of hematogenous osteomyelitis include focal osteopenia due to reactive hyperemia, followed by a lucent medullary lesion. In contiguous focus osteomyelitis, the first radiographic sign may be soft-tissue swelling and periosteal reaction, followed by erosion of the cortex.
- Scintigraphy and MRI imaging are more sensitive to detect early osteomyelitis.
- Three-phase Tc-99m MDP bone scan becomes positive within 24–48 hours after the onset of symptoms. Acute osteomyelitis is positive on all three phases (flow, blood pool, and delayed).

  In contrast, cellulitis is positive on flow and blood pool phases, and negative on delayed.

  Although highly sensitive, Tc-99m bone scan is less specific than leukocyte scintigraphy and MRI.
- Combining WBC and sulfur colloid scintigraphy adds specificity in the evaluation of osteomyelitis because bone marrow is replaced by infection and white cells. Actively infected bone marrow will show discordantly increased uptake on the WBC scan and reduced activity on sulfur colloid.

  Note that WBC scan imaging is not sensitive for spinal osteomyelitis, thought to be due to the inability of leukocytes to migrate into an encapsulated infection.

  WBC scan can be performed with either Indium-111-WBC or Tc-99m-HMPAO-WBC. Indium WBC scan has higher radiation dose, takes 24 hours to perform, and the image has more noise. The disadvantage of Tc-99m-HMPAO is its tendency to dissociate, leading to genitourinary excretion of radiotracer.
- MRI is highly sensitive to detect early osteomyelitis within 3–5 days. MRI has similar sensitivity to radionuclide studies, but greater specificity. MRI can better delineate the extent of infection, any fluid collections that must be treated surgically, sinus tracts, and skin ulcers.
- The hallmark of MRI imaging of osteomyelitis is replacement of the normal fatty marrow signal. Edema and exudates cause high marrow signal on T2-weighted images and low signal on T1-weighted images. Increased signal of the cortical bone, normally low signal on all sequences, signifies infectious involvement. MRI has very high negative predictive value: A negative MRI essentially excludes osteomyelitis. Gadolinium is helpful to delineate any fluid collections and to evaluate for the presence of nonenhancing necrotic bone (sequestrum).

Soft-tissue infections

Septic arthritis

- Septic arthritis is infection of a joint. The gold standard for diagnosis of septic arthritis is joint aspiration.
- The imaging and clinical hallmark of septic arthritis is a joint effusion.
- In children, the hip is a common site of septic arthritis caused by contiguous extension of proximal femoral metaphyseal osteomyelitis. The proximal femoral metaphysis is within the hip joint capsule.
- If untreated, septic arthritis can lead to rapid joint destruction and eventual ankylosis.
- Intravenous drug abusers are susceptible to infection of the sacroiliac and acromioclavicular joints.

Necrotizing fasciitis

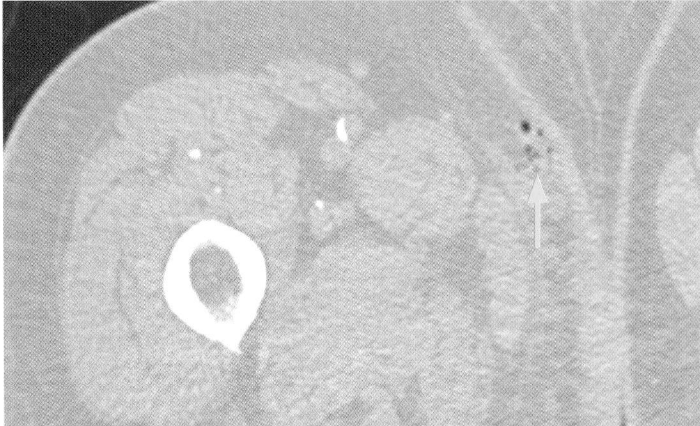

Necrotizing fasciitis:

Unenhanced CT through the proximal thigh shows several tiny locules of gas (arrow) in the medial subcutaneous tissues.

- Necrotizing fasciitis is an extremely aggressive soft tissue infection caused by *Clostridium* or other gram-positive rods. It is a surgical emergency, requiring immediate debridement.
- The characteristic radiographic and CT finding of necrotizing fasciitis is gas bubbles in the soft tissues.

DIFFUSE BONE DISEASE

MULTIFACTORIAL BONE DISEASE

Osteoporosis

- Osteoporosis is the most common metabolic bone disease and is defined as a T score of <–2.5, where a T score of –1 is a bone density one standard deviation below the mean for healthy young women.

  The Z score is the standard deviations from *age-matched* women. It is not used to determine osteoporosis.
- Osteopenia may be secondary to numerous nutritional, endocrine, and other etiologies.
- Vitamin or nutritional deficiencies can cause osteoporosis, including:

  Osteomalacia (Looser zone).

  Alcoholism.

  Hypophosphatemia.

  Scurvy (Wimberger sign).
- Endocrine disturbances can impact calcium metabolism, causing osteoporosis, including:

  Hyperparathyroidism (subperiosteal resorption).

  Cushing disease or any increase in endogenous/exogenous steroids.
- Diffuse malignancy, such as myelomatosis, can cause diffuse bony demineralization.
- Genetic causes of osteoporosis include:

  Osteogenesis imperfecta.

  Gaucher disease.

  Anemia, including sickle cell and thalassemia.
- Focal osteopenia has a more limited list of causes, including:

  Immobility/disuse.

  Reflex sympathetic dystrophy.

  Transient regional osteoporosis of the hip.

Vitamin-deficiency bone disease

Scurvy

- Scurvy (hypovitaminosis C) causes generalized osteopenia because osteoblasts require vitamin C to form mature osteoid tissue.
- Other signs of scurvy include the *Wimberger ring* sign, which is increased epiphyseal sclerosis due to disorganized epiphyseal ossification, and a *Pelkin's fracture*, which is a metaphyseal corner fracture. A dense metaphyseal line may be present.

Osteomalacia

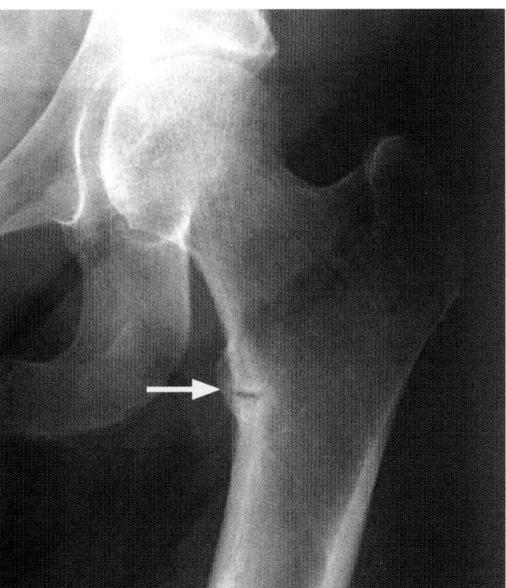

Osteomalacia: Frontal radiograph of the hip demonstrates an incomplete linear lucency (arrow) through the medial (weight-bearing) proximal femur, representing a Looser zone.

Case courtesy Stacy Smith, MD, Brigham and Women's Hospital.

- Osteomalacia is faulty mineralization of bone matrix caused by vitamin D deficiency. The same process is called osteomalacia in adults and rickets in children. Rickets is discussed in the pediatric imaging section.
- Osteomalacia manifests as diffuse osteopenia; however, a *Looser zone* (pseudofracture) is highly specific. A *Looser zone* is a cortical stress fracture that is filled with abnormal, poorly mineralized osteoid and appears as a radiolucency through the cortex. Common sites for *Looser zones* are the medial proximal femurs, distal scapulae, and pubic bones.
- Osteomalacia may be complicated by insufficiency fracture.

Endocrine bone disease

Acromegaly

- Acromegaly is the clinical syndrome caused by excess growth hormone. When the growth hormone excess occurs when the physes are open, the bones will grow longitudinally, leading to gigantism. However, when the hormone excess occurs once the physes have closed then the bones cannot lengthen and instead obtain a characteristic appearance of acral (distal) growth and widening.
- In the head there is enlargement of frontal sinuses, thickening of cranial bones, and an enlarged jaw.
- In the hands, *beak-like* osteophytes of the metacarpal heads and *spade-like* overgrowths of the distal phalanges are characteristic. Initially, joint spaces are widened, but may become narrowed later in the disease due to secondary osteoarthritis.
- In the feet, a characteristic finding is increased heel-pad thickness greater than 24 mm.

  24 mm is a normal heel-pad thickness for a 150 lb. person, with approximately 1 mm allowed for each additional 25 lb. in body weight. For instance, a 250 lb. person may have a heel-pad of 28 mm.

Hyperparathyroidism (Recklinghausen disease of bone)

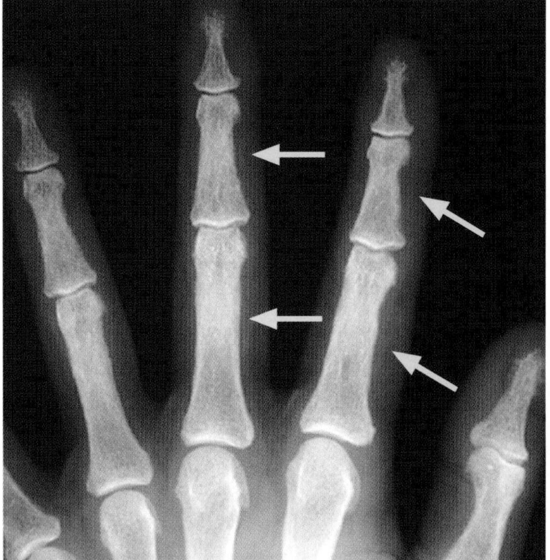

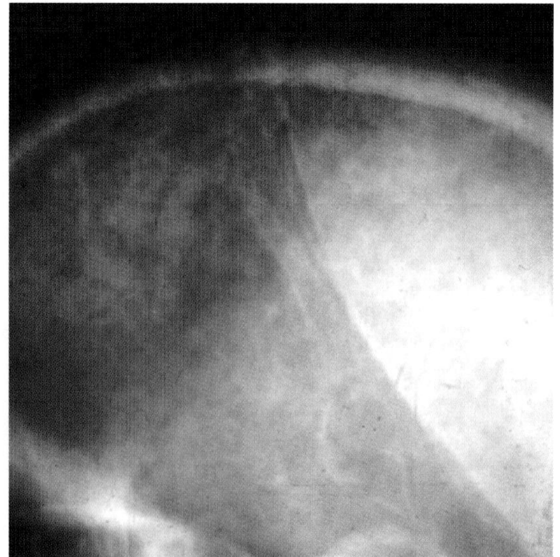

Hyperparathyroidism: Radiograph of the hand (left image) shows subperiosteal resorption and scalloping of the radial margins of the 2rd and 3rd proximal and middle phalanges (arrows). Lateral skull radiograph in a different patient shows the classic *salt-and-pepper* appearance due to trabecular resorption.

Cases courtesy Stacy Smith, MD, Brigham and Women's Hospital.

- Hyperparathyroidism is excess parathyroid hormone (PTH). PTH is normally secreted in response to hypocalcemia and maintains serum calcium levels by stimulating osteoclasts.
- Primary hyperparathyroidism is autonomously increased secretion from an overactive parathyroid gland, typically due to a parathyroid adenoma. Serum calcium is high and phosphate is low.
- Secondary hyperparathyroidism is increased secretion of PTH by a normal gland in response to hypocalcemia secondary to renal failure. Serum calcium is usually normal.
- Tertiary hyperparathyroidism is seen after prolonged secondary hyperparathyroidism, where the parathyroid glands escape regulatory control and oversecrete PTH.
- The radiological hallmarks of hyperparathyroidism are diffuse bony demineralization and subperiosteal and subligamentous bone resorption.

Skull: The classic *salt-and-pepper* skull is due to trabecular resorption.

Hands: Subperiosteal resorption of the radial aspects of the 2rd and 3rd middle phalanges is specific for hyperparathyroidism.

Clavicle: Subperiosteal resorption of the clavicle tends affect the acromial (distal) aspect.

Knee: Subperiosteal bone resorption can be seen in the medial proximal tibial metaphysis.

Teeth: Loss of lamina dura surrounding the tooth socket can occasionally be seen.

Anywhere: Brown tumors are more common in primary hyperparathyroidism.

Everywhere: Diffuse osteopenia results from continued osteoclast activation.

- Calcium pyrophosphate dihydrate deposition (CPPD) may occur, which is more common in primary hyperparathyroidism.
- Soft-tissue calcification, periosteal reaction, and sclerosis are seen more commonly in secondary hyperparathyroidism.
- Complications of hyperparathyroidism include insufficiency fracture and increased propensity for ligaments and tendons to rupture.

Renal osteodystrophy

- Renal osteodystrophy is due to the combined effects of abnormal vitamin D metabolism (osteomalacia) and secondary hyperparathyroidism from prolonged renal failure.
- In addition to renal osteodystrophy, patients with renal failure have an increased risk of additional bone disorders including osteomyelitis, avascular necrosis (if on steroids), and amyloidosis (from chronic dialysis).
- Unlike osteomalacia, *Looser zones* are uncommon in renal osteodystrophy.
- The characteristic *rugger jersey spine* describes sclerosis of the vertebral body endplates.
- Soft-tissue and vascular calcifications are often present.

Hypothyroidism

- In children, hypothyroidism causes a delay in skeletal and dental maturity.
- Hypothyroidism may cause bullet-shaped vertebral bodies and Wormian bones in the skull.
- Hypothyroidism is associated with slipped capital femoral epiphysis.

Hypoparathyroidism

- Hypoparathyroidism is most commonly a consequence of parathyroid gland resection for hyperparathyroidism.
- Hypoparathyroidism causes metastatic deposition of calcium. In particular, calcium is deposited in the subcutaneous tissues and in the basal ganglia.

Pseudohypoparathyroidism and pseudo-pseudohypoparathyroidism

- Pseudohypoparathyroidism is due to a defect of the parathyroid hormone (PTH) receptor.
- In pseudo-pseudohypoparathyroidism, the PTH level is normal and PTH receptor is normal, but the patient's phenotype is indistinguishable from that of pseudohypoparathyroidism.
- Both entities clinically present with obesity, round facies, short stature, and brachydactyly (short fingers).
- The classic radiographic finding is a short metacarpal of either the 4th or 5th digit or the thumb.

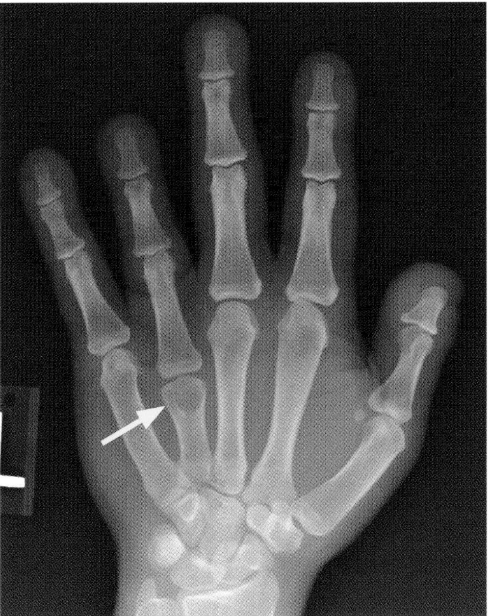

Pseudohypoparathyroidism: Radiograph of the hand shows a markedly shortened 4th metacarpal (arrow).

In addition to pseudohypoparathyroidism and pseudo-pseudohypoparathyroidism, an additional differential consideration for a short 4th metacarpal includes Turner syndrome.

Hyperthyroidism

- Hyperthyroidism causes accelerated bony maturation in children. Thyroid acropachy is a rare cause of diaphyseal periosteal reaction of multiple bones including the metacarpals, metatarsals, and phalanges, seen in the setting of treated hyperthyroidism.

Paget disease

- Paget disease is a progressive disturbance of osteoclastic and osteoblastic regulation seen in older adults. It may be seen in up to 10% of patients over 80 years old, but it is rare in patients under age 40. The cause of Paget disease is unknown, but paramyxovirus may be involved.
- Symptoms of Paget disease include bone pain, osseous enlargement or bowing, compression of cranial nerves, and high output cardiac failure. Weakened subchondral bone commonly leads to osteoarthritis.
- Paget disease affects the skull, spine, and pelvis most commonly, followed by the articular ends of the femur, proximal tibia, and proximal humerus. Involvement of the ribs and scapula can occur but is uncommon.
- Three sequential phases are described, although there is often overlap between the phases and the disease may not always progress through the three stages in order.

> **Phase I: Osteolytic** phase is due to hyperactivated osteoclasts and resultant active bone resorption.
>
> **Phase II: Mixed lytic and sclerotic** phase is continued bony resorption and new bone formation.
>
> **Phase III: Sclerotic** phase is dominated by increased bone density and sclerosis.

- Chronic Paget disease shows thickening of cortex, coarse irregular trabecular pattern, and expansion of bone. This appearance has been called a *caricature* of normal bone.
- **Paget of the skull**: In the osteolytic phase (phase I), the typical appearance is a sharply marginated geographic lytic region called *osteoporosis circumscripta*. In the mixed phase (phase II), the classic appearance is the *cotton wool* skull, which looks as though an artist dabbed paint on the skull with a piece of cotton.
- **Paget of the vertebral bodies**: The mixed phase (phase II) can produce either the classic *picture frame* vertebral body (with increased density of the periphery of the vertebral body, as opposed to the *rugger jersey spine* of renal osteodystrophy, which features sclerosis of just the superior and inferior endplates) or an ivory (diffusely sclerotic) vertebral body.
- **Paget of the pelvis:** When Paget disease involves the pelvis, the typical appearance is asymmetric coarsened trabecular thickening, with thickening of the iliopectineal and ilioischial lines. Acetabular protrusio may result.

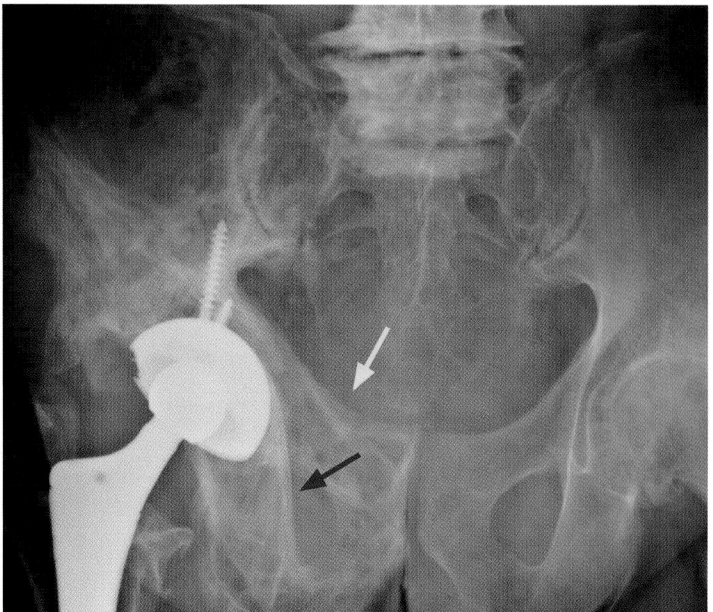

Paget disease of the right hemipelvis: Frontal radiograph of the pelvis shows expansion of the inferior and superior pubic rami with coarsened trabecular pattern and cortical thickening. There is thickening of both the iliopectineal (yellow arrow) and ilioischial (red arrow) lines.

A right total hip replacement is present, secondary to pathologic fracture of the proximal femur. Acetabular protrusio is present on the right.

- **Paget of the long bones**: The lytic phase (phase I) progresses from the proximal articular end of bone into the diaphysis with a sharply marginated border. This border has been called the *blade of grass* or *flame-shaped margin* and allows differentiation from a neoplasm. As Paget disease progresses through its phases, it may cause bowing of the long bones and coxa vara deformity of the proximal femur.
- Complications of Paget disease include pathologic fracture, malignant degeneration (most commonly osteosarcoma), secondary giant cell tumor, and secondary osteoarthritis.

Hereditary hyperphosphatasia (juvenile Paget)

- Hereditary hyperphosphatasia, also called juvenile Paget disease, is an autosomal recessive disease of infants and young children. There is cortical thickening, trabecular thickening, osteopenia, and bowing of all bones in the body, resulting in severe deformity.
- Aside from the young age of the patients and diffuse involvement, the radiography of juvenile Paget otherwise appears very similar to adult Paget disease. There may be sparing of the articular ends of bones (epiphyseal sparing) in juvenile Paget disease.

Osteopetrosis

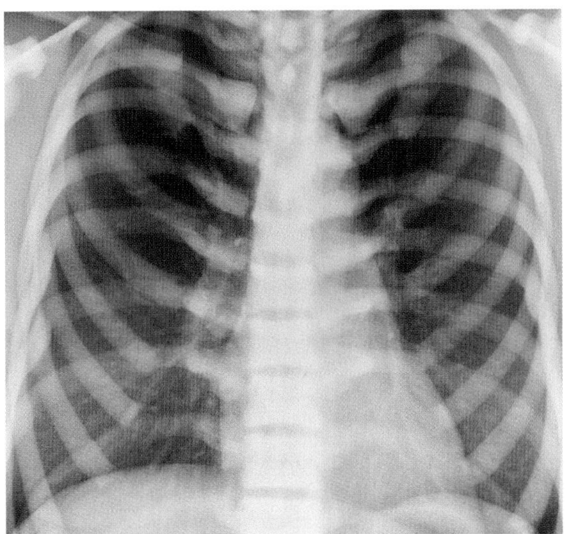

Osteopetrosis: Chest radiograph shows dramatic sclerosis of all the visualized bones in the thorax.

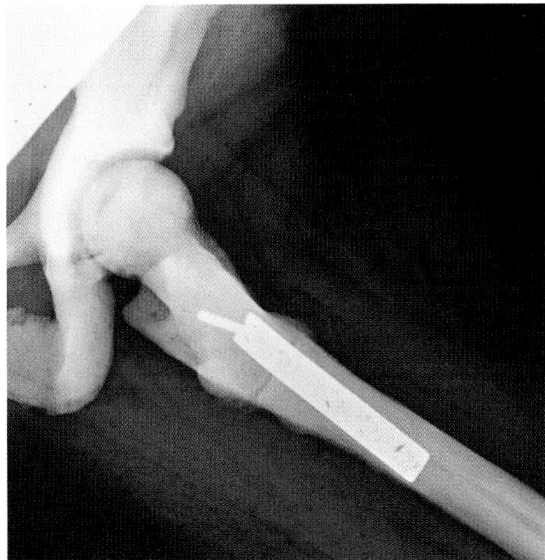

Radiograph of the femur in the same patient shows a fracture of the proximal femur, status post ORIF.

- Osteopetrosis is an extremely rare deficiency of osteoclastic carbonic anhydrase, which leads to inability of osteoclasts to resorb bone.
- Osteopetrosis is characterized by diffuse, marked sclerosis of the entire skeleton. The bones are extremely brittle, which typically leads to multiple fractures.
- The vertebral bodies may have a *sandwich* or *rugger jersey* appearance similar to renal osteodystrophy, but diffuse bony sclerosis is more marked in osteopetrosis.

Gaucher disease

- Gaucher disease is caused by an autosomal recessive defect in glucocerebrosidase, leading to abnormal cerebroside deposition in altered macrophages called Gaucher cells. Gaucher cells cause bone infarctions, medullary expansion, and hepatosplenomegaly.
- The classic *Erlenmeyer flask* deformity of long bones is a result of abnormal modeling.
- Characteristic *H-shaped* vertebral bodies are due to endplate avascular necrosis.

  H-shaped vertebral bodies are not specific to Gaucher disease, and are in fact seen more commonly in sickle cell disease. The size of the spleen can differentiate between sickle cell and Gaucher disease: Sickle cell causes splenic auto-infarction, while patients with Gaucher disease have splenomegaly.

Sickle cell disease

- Sickle cell disease is an autosomal recessive defect in the beta-chain of hemoglobin. Red cells are sickle-shaped and cause microvascular occlusion. The three osseous manifestations of sickle cell disease are bone infarcts, dramatically increased risk of osteomyelitis, and marrow expansion/hyperplasia.
- **Sickle cell bone infarcts**: Infarcts and avascular necrosis are caused by microvascular occlusion from the sickled red cells. Avascular necrosis of vertebral body endplates causes the characteristic *H-shaped* or *Lincoln-log* vertebral bodies. Other common locations for infarction include the femoral heads and the diaphyses and metaphyses of long bones.

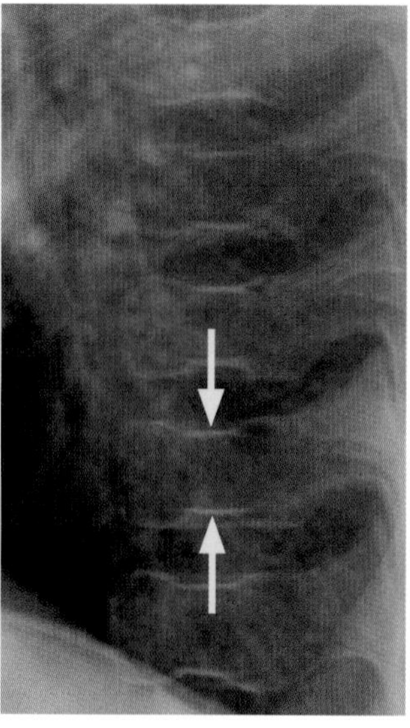

H-shaped vertebral bodies: Lateral thoracic spine radiograph shows characteristic central endplate depressions of the vertebral bodies (arrows) representing vertebral body avascular necrosis.

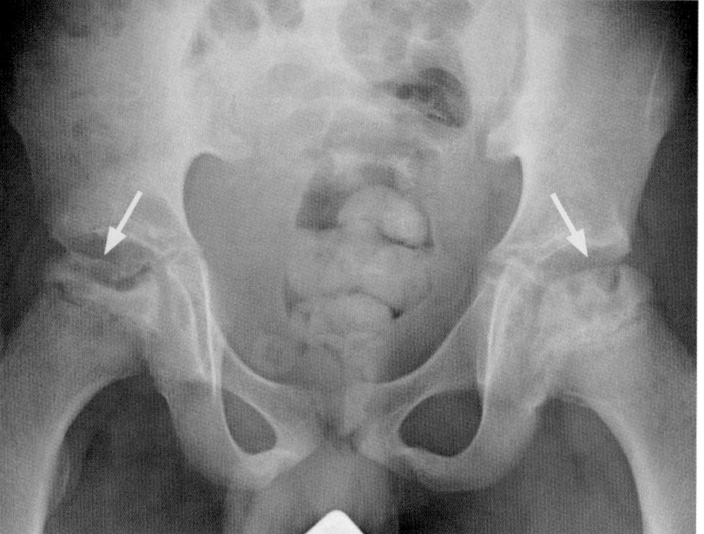

Bilateral femoral head avascular necrosis: Frontal pelvic radiograph in a skeletally immature patient with sickle cell anemia shows marked flattening and sclerosis of both femoral heads (arrows), representing advanced (Ficat stage IV) avascular necrosis.

The Ficat staging of avascular necrosis is subsequently discussed.

In advanced sickle cell, patchy sclerosis from multiple bone infarctions may become nearly confluent, producing diffusely sclerotic bones.

Sickle cell dactylitis (also called hand–foot syndrome) is a special consideration in very young children who have persistent hematopoietic marrow in the digits of the hands and feet. Microvascular occlusion exacerbated by cold temperature causes dactylitis, which is evident on radiographs as soft-tissue swelling and periosteal reaction.

- **Sickle cell osteomyelitis**: Patients with sickle cell have an approximately 100x increased risk of osteomyelitis, most frequently with *Salmonella* species.
- **Sickle cell marrow expansion**: The radiographic findings of marrow expansion are more pronounced in thalassemia, but similar findings can be seen in sickle cell.

MRI of the bone marrow shows diffusely low signal on T1-weighted images, reflecting diffuse red (cellular) marrow.

In the long bones, chronic stimulation of red cell production causes widening of the medullary spaces and coarsening of the trabeculae, which results in osteopenia and increased risk of insufficiency fracture.

In the skull, marrow expansion can cause *hair-on-end* striations and widening of the medullary cavity.

Involvement of the facial bones and extramedullary hematopoiesis are seen more commonly in thalassemia.

Thalassemia

- Thalassemia is an autosomal recessive congenital anemia that is caused by a defect in the alpha or beta hemoglobin subunits.
- Similar to sickle cell disease, the osseous hallmarks of thalassemia are bone infarcts, marrow hyperplasia, and infection. However, in contrast to sickle cell, the marrow expansion is much more prominent as the anemia can be more severe.
- In the hand, marrow expansion can cause widening and squaring of the phalanges and metacarpals.
- In the skull, the hair-on-end striations are a classic manifestation of marrow expansion.
- In the facial bones, marrow expansion may obliterate the paranasal sinuses, causing the typical rodent-like facies.
- In the long bones, the marrow expansion may cause an Erlenmeyer flask deformity.

Myelofibrosis

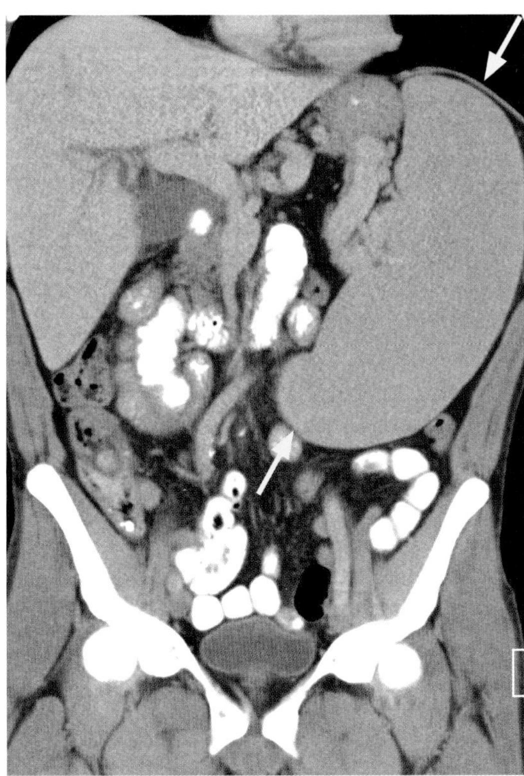
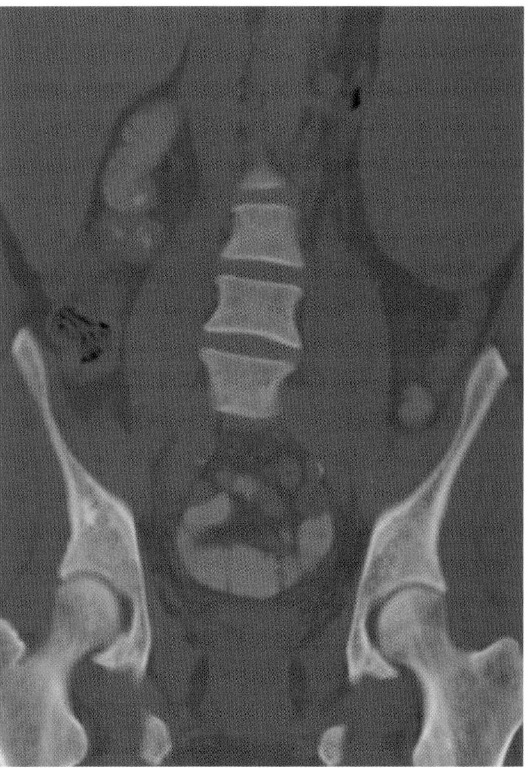

Myelofibrosis: Coronal CT in soft-tissue (left image) and bone windows show splenomegaly (arrows) and diffusely dense bones.

- Myelofibrosis is progressive fibrosis of bone marrow in older patients, leading to anemia and splenomegaly. Bone marrow fibrosis leads to diffusely sclerotic bones.

Mastocytosis

- Mastocytosis is abnormal proliferation of mast cells. It may result in either diffuse osteoporosis or sclerosis from the reaction of the marrow to the infiltrating mast cells.

DIFFERENTIAL DIAGNOSIS OF COMMON BONE LESIONS

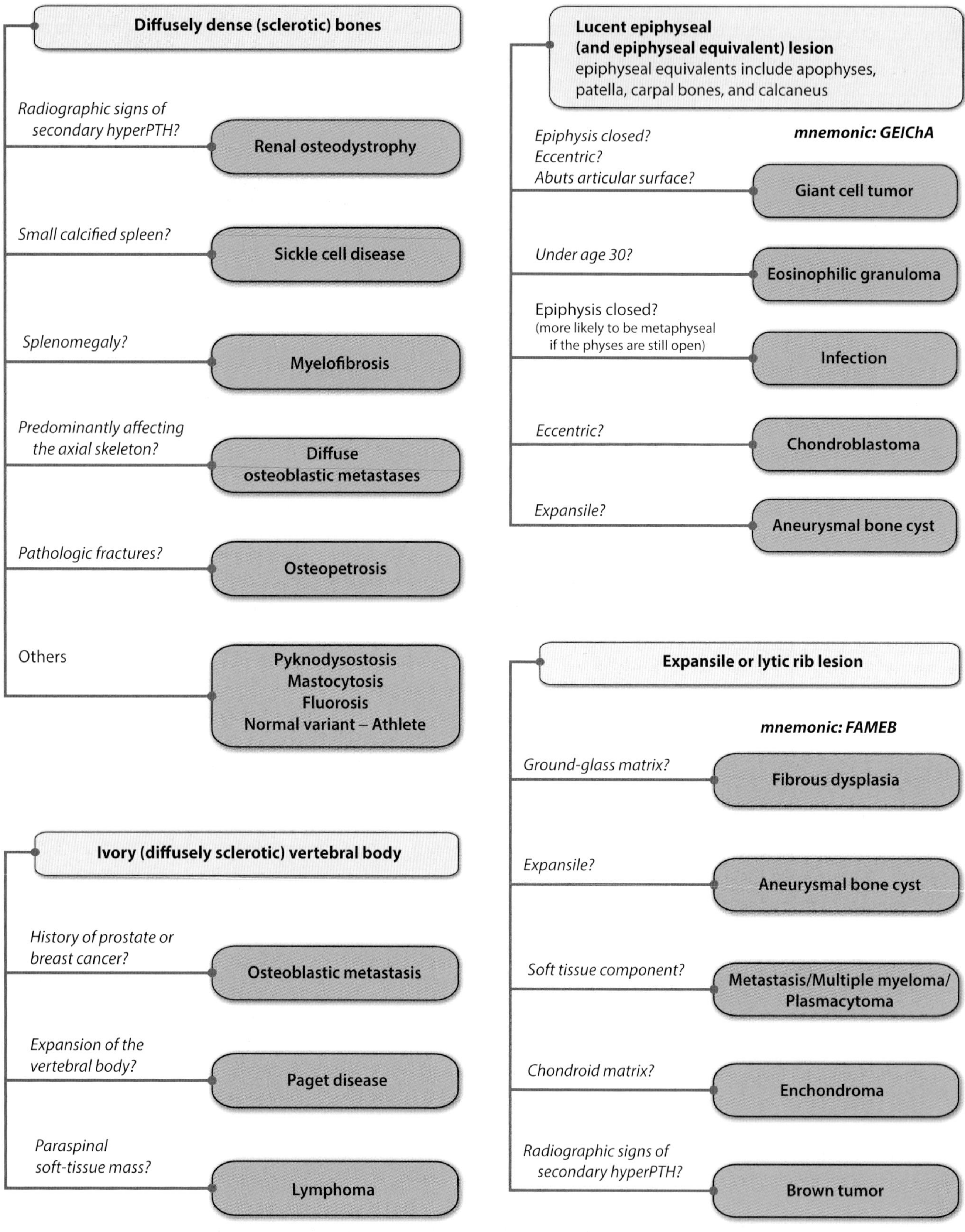

Diffusely dense (sclerotic) bones
Radiographic signs of secondary hyperPTH?
Renal osteodystrophy
Small calcified spleen?
Sickle cell disease
Splenomegaly?
Myelofibrosis
Predominantly affecting the axial skeleton?
Diffuse osteoblastic metastases
Pathologic fractures?
Osteopetrosis
Others
Pyknodysostosis
Mastocytosis
Fluorosis
Normal variant – Athlete
Ivory (diffusely sclerotic) vertebral body
History of prostate or breast cancer?
Osteoblastic metastasis
Expansion of the vertebral body?
Paget disease
Paraspinal soft-tissue mass?
Lymphoma
Lucent epiphyseal (and epiphyseal equivalent) lesion
epiphyseal equivalents include apophyses, patella, carpal bones, and calcaneus
mnemonic: GEIChA
Epiphysis closed? Eccentric? Abuts articular surface?
Giant cell tumor
Under age 30?
Eosinophilic granuloma
Epiphysis closed? (more likely to be metaphyseal if the physes are still open)
Infection
Eccentric?
Chondroblastoma
Expansile?
Aneurysmal bone cyst
Expansile or lytic rib lesion
mnemonic: FAMEB
Ground-glass matrix?
Fibrous dysplasia
Expansile?
Aneurysmal bone cyst
Soft tissue component?
Metastasis/Multiple myeloma/Plasmacytoma
Chondroid matrix?
Enchondroma
Radiographic signs of secondary hyperPTH?
Brown tumor

FRACTURES

Terminology

fracture direction

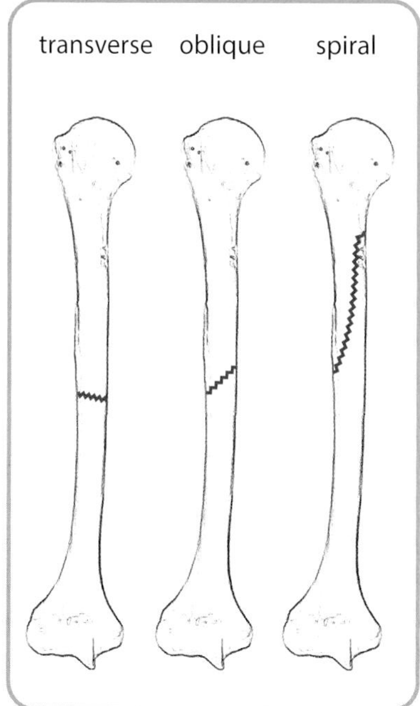

position of distal fragment

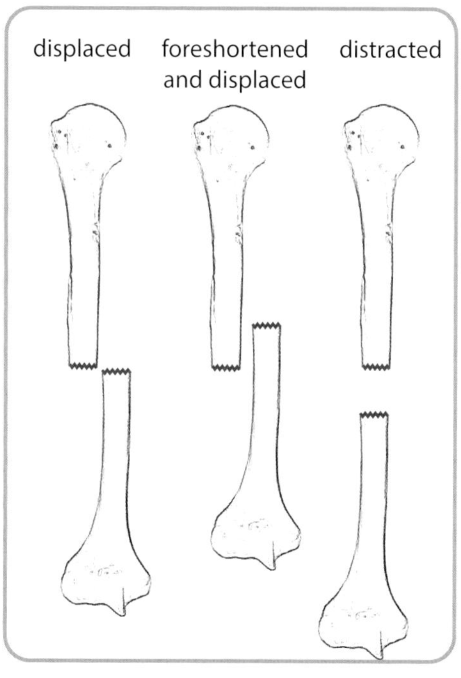

special types of comminuted fractures

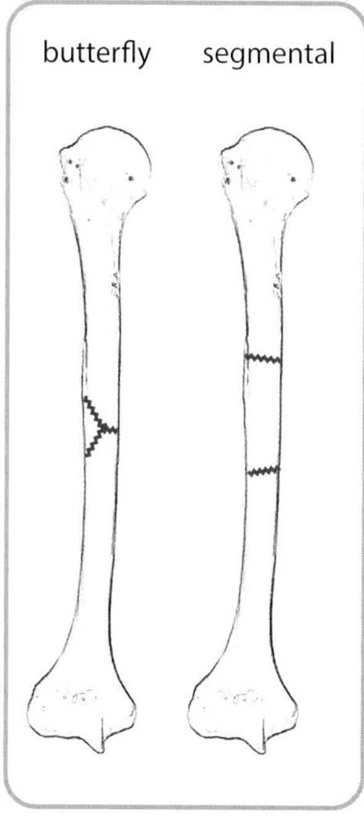

angulation of distal fragment

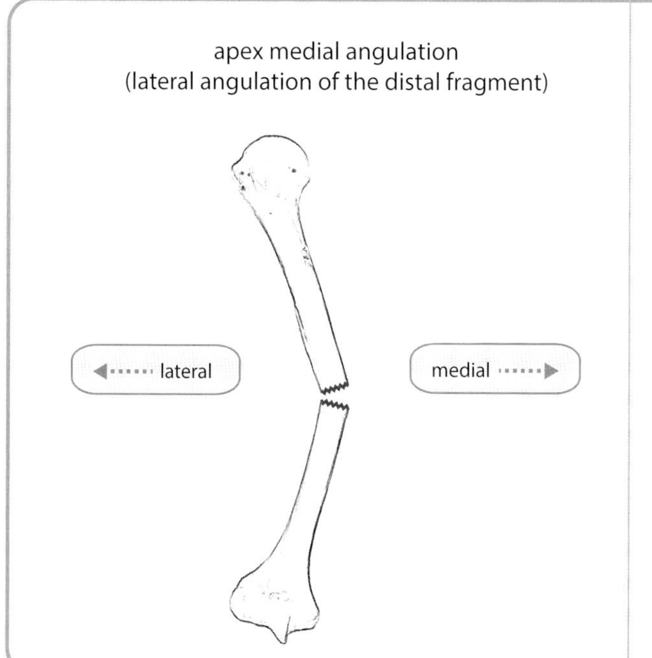

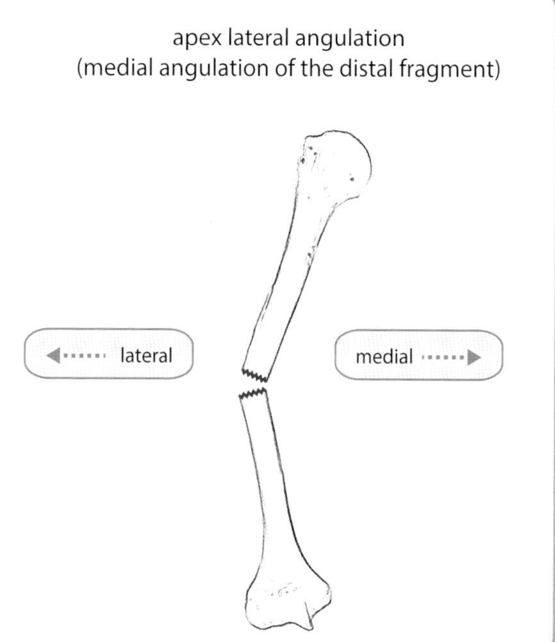

- When describing a long-bone fracture, the fracture location (proximal, mid-shaft, distal), direction of fracture, angulation, and position of the distal segment should be described.
- A comminuted fracture is defined as >2 fracture fragments.
- It is essential to mention if a fracture extends to the articular surface of a joint.

- A stress fracture may be a *fatigue* fracture (abnormal repetitive stress on a normal bone) or an *insufficiency* fracture (normal stress on an abnormal bone; e.g., in the setting of demineralization due to osteoporosis or metabolic bone disease). The term *stress* fracture is often used interchangeably with *fatigue* fracture, although these terms are not synonyms.
- A pathologic fracture is caused by normal stress on a bone weakened by an underlying lesion (typically tumor, but also including infection, fibrous dysplasia, and Paget disease).

Basics of MR

Tendons

- A normal tendon is dark on all MRI sequences.
- A normal tendon may have artifactually increased signal due to the magic angle phenomenon. Because tendons have fibers coursing along a single direction (demonstrating anisotropy), tendons may demonstrate artifactually increased signal on short TE sequences when oriented 55 degrees relative to the bore of the magnet. This phenomenon is called the magic angle artifact.

  Short TE sequences include T1-weighted images, proton density, and GRE.

  T2-weighted sequences are generally not susceptible to the magic angle artifact.

  Unlike true tendon pathology, the magic angle artifact disappears with a long TE and the tendon will otherwise have a normal morphology.

Tenosynovitis

- Tenosynovitis is inflammation surrounding a tendon. Tenosynovitis may be secondary to repetitive motion, inflammatory arthritis, or infection.
- On MRI, fluid completely surrounds the tendon circumferentially.
- A potential pitfall is that fluid can track along tendon sheaths that communicate directly with an adjacent joint (such as the long head of the biceps tendon in the shoulder). This should not be confused with tenosynovitis. Similarly, a small amount of fluid in the synovial sheath of the posterior tibialis tendon in the foot is also normal.
- A variant form, called stenosing tenosynovitis, features several loculated collections of fluid in the tendon sheath.

  Stenosing tenosynovitis can be seen surrounding the flexor hallucis longus tendon at the medial ankle in os trigonum syndrome and about the wrist in de Quervain's stenosing tenosynovitis.

Myxoid degeneration (tendinosis)

- Aging or overuse often leads to myxoid degeneration, which is synonymous with tendinosis.

  The word *tendinitis* should not be used as myxoid degeneration is not due to inflammation.

- MRI of myxoid degeneration/tendinosis will show intermediate intra-substance (within the tendon) signal. The tendon may be either normal in size or enlarged. If fluid-intensity signal is seen within a tendon, concern should be raised for a partial tear, although MR cannot always reliably differentiate between tendinosis and partial tear.

Partial tear

- A partial tendon tear represents incomplete disruption of the fibers and can have a varied MRI appearance. The tendon may be thickened, thinned, or contain intra-substance fluid.

Complete tear

- A complete disruption of the tendon will appear as complete discontinuity of the tendon. There is often retraction of the tendon remnants.

Foot and Ankle

Forefoot

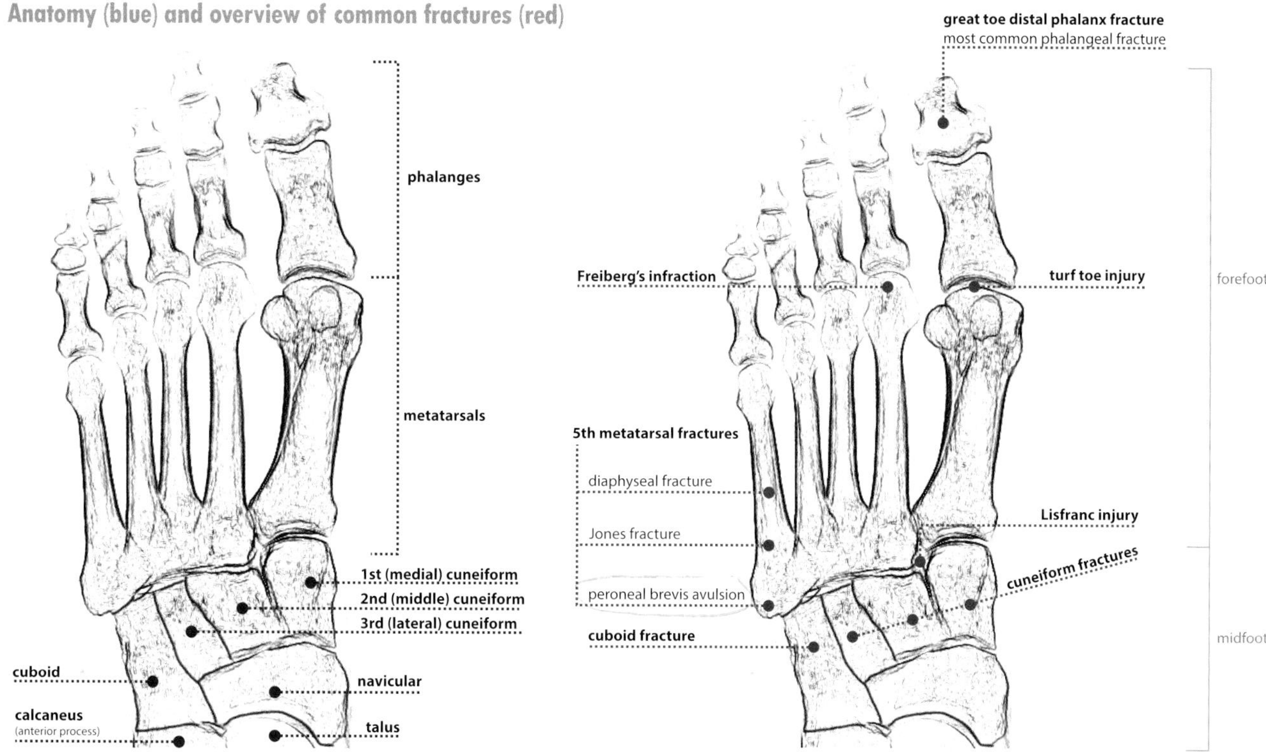

Fifth metatarsal fractures

- Metatarsal base avulsion (zone 1) is a fracture at the most proximal base of the 5th metatarsal.

  Treatment is conservative, with a boot.

  The peroneus brevis and lateral aspect of the plantar aponeurosis attach at the 5th metatarsal base.

- Jones fracture (zone 2) is a fracture of the metaphyseal–diaphyseal junction.

  A Jones fracture carries a worse prognosis compared to an avulsion fracture due to reduced blood supply at the metaphyseal–diaphyseal junction. Treatment is variable and may require surgery.

- The metatarsal shaft (zone 3) is a common location for stress fracture.

  Treatment may be surgical.

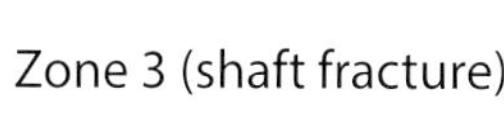

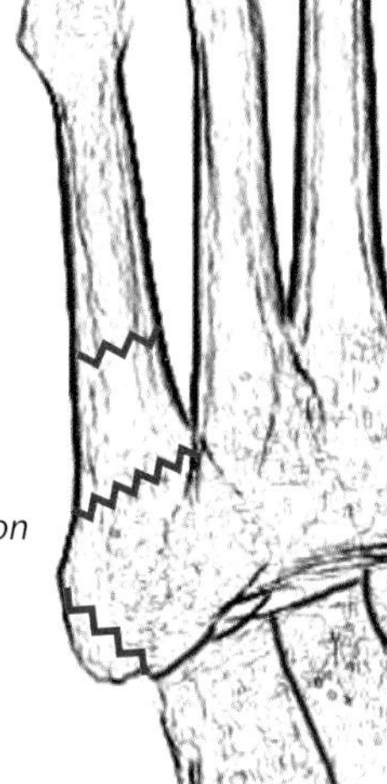

Freiberg's infraction

- Freiberg's infraction is avascular necrosis of the second metatarsal head. It is caused by repetitive stress or poorly fitting shoes (such as high-heels) and usually occurs in young women.

Metatarsal stress fracture

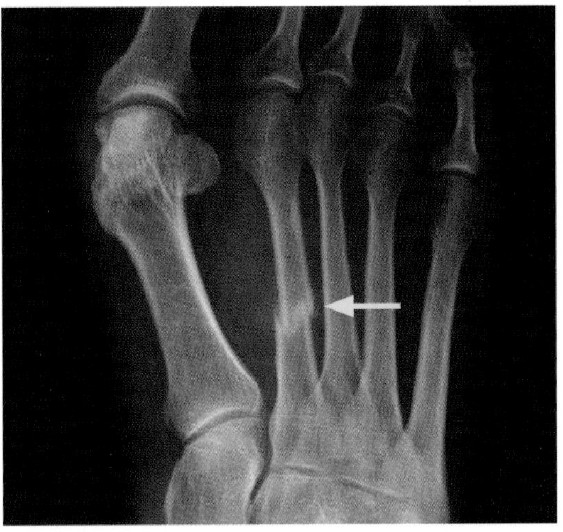

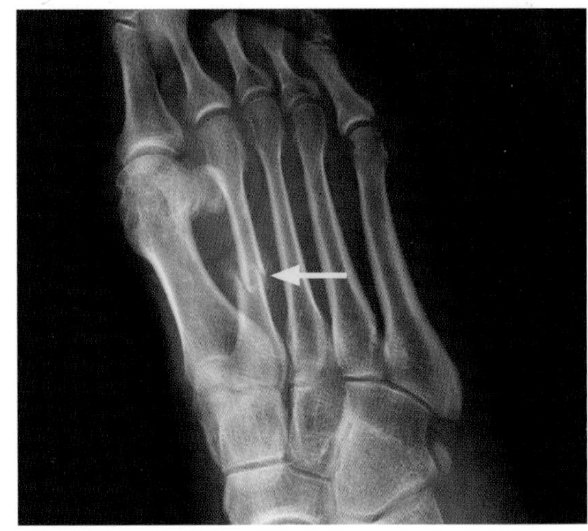

Second metatarsal stress fracture: Frontal (left image) and oblique (right image) radiographs of the foot show a minimally displaced mid-diaphyseal fracture (arrows) of the second metatarsal. There is minimal associated callus formation.

Case courtesy Barbara N. Weissman, MD, Brigham and Women's Hospital.

- The first radiographic sign of a metatarsal stress fracture is a barely perceptible linear cortical lucency. Usually, stress fractures are not apparent on radiographs until periostitis and callus have begun to form.

Sesamoid fracture

- Fracture of the great toe sesamoid bones is typically caused by extreme hyperextension or dorsal dislocation (which may be transient) of the first metatarsophalangeal joint.

  The flexor hallucis brevis attaches to the sesamoids; the medial head attaches to the tibial (medial) sesamoid and the lateral head attaches to the fibular (lateral) sesamoid.

- A bipartite sesamoid is a normal variant that may simulate a sesamoid fracture; however, a bipartite sesamoid will be round in shape and its margins will be completely corticated. Additionally, the sum of the parts of the bipartite sesamoid will be larger in size than the other sesamoid.
- The term *turf toe* has been used to describe a wide range of injuries at the first MTP joint including sesamoid fracture.

Lisfranc fracture-dislocation

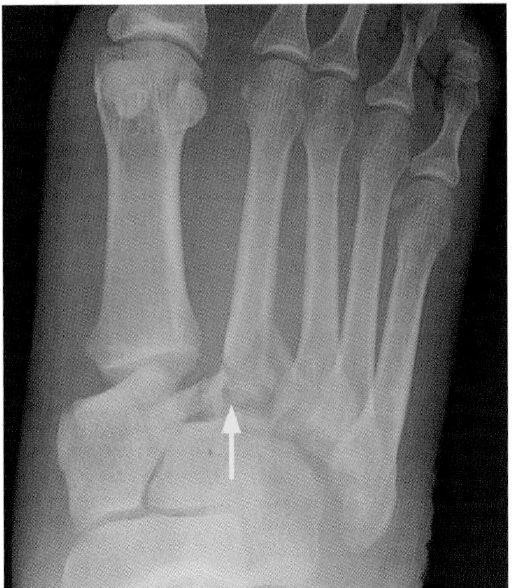

Frontal radiograph of the foot shows a homolateral dislocation at the Lisfranc joint, with fracture of the base of the second metatarsal (arrow).

- The tarsometatarsal joint is the Lisfranc joint, named after the French surgeon in the Napoleonic wars who performed amputations at this joint. The stability of the joint depends on multiple ligaments, with the Lisfranc ligament being the most important. The Lisfranc ligament is an interosseous ligamentous complex attaching the medial cuneiform to the second metatarsal base.

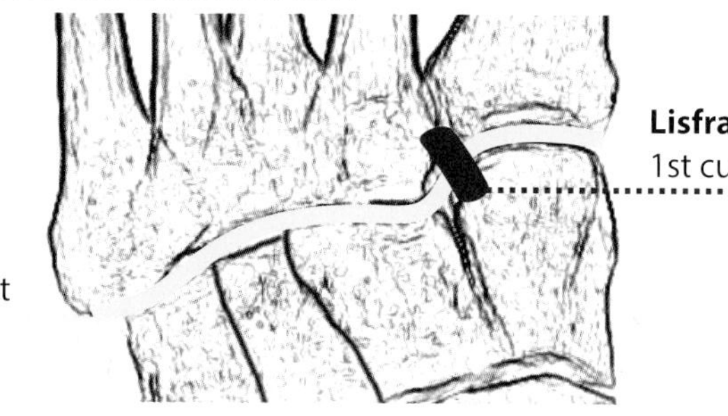

- A Lisfranc fracture-dislocation is a fracture-dislocation of the tarsometatarsal joint. The treatment of a Lisfranc injury is surgical. A missed or untreated Lisfranc injury can lead to debilitating osteoarthritis and flattening of the longitudinal arch.
- Subtle malalignment of the tarsometatarsal joint may signal serious ligamentous injury. Weight-bearing radiographs are the most sensitive. Careful evaluation of the alignment of the Lisfranc joint must always be performed, as in this normal example below.

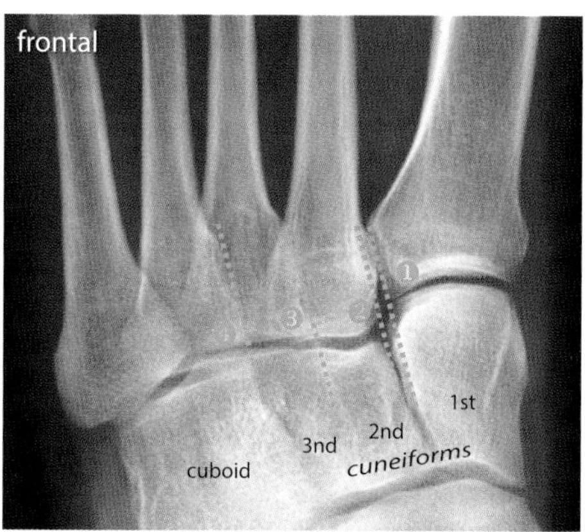

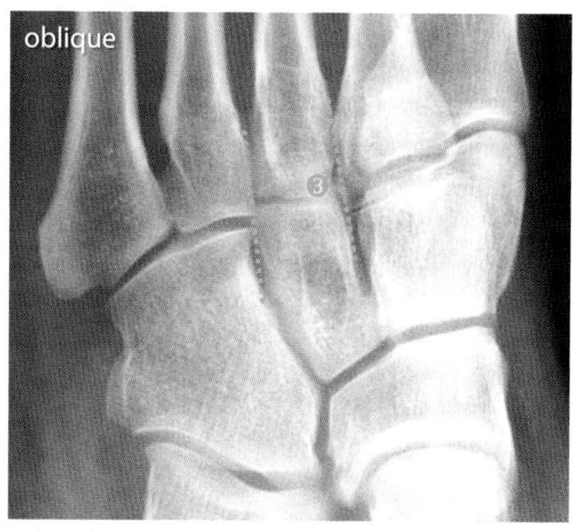

1. lateral base of 1st metatarsal should be aligned with lateral aspect of 1st cuneiform
2. medial base of 2nd metatarsal should be aligned with medial aspect of 2nd cuneiform
3. medial base of 3rd metatarsal should be aligned with medial aspect of 3rd cuneiform
4. medial base of 4th metatarsal should be aligned with medial aspect of cuboid

easier to see on oblique (3, 4)

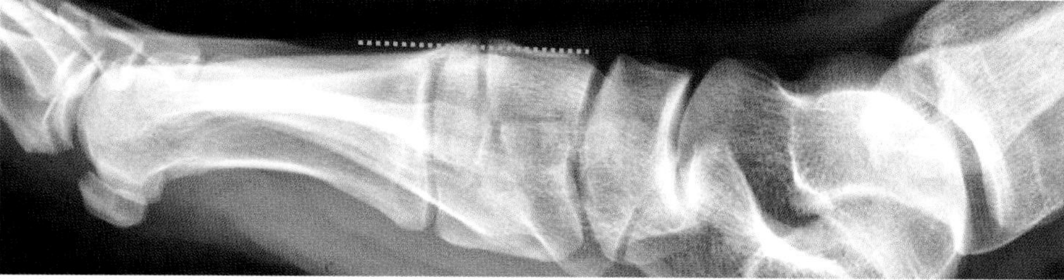

the dorsal profile of the tarsometatarsal (Lisfranc) joint should be uninterrupted

- Lisfranc injuries are classified into homolateral and divergent based on the direction of dislocation of the first metatarsal. In a divergent Lisfranc injury, the first metatarsal is medially dislocated and the 2nd through 5th metatarsals are laterally dislocated. In homolateral injury, all metatarsals will dislocate laterally.

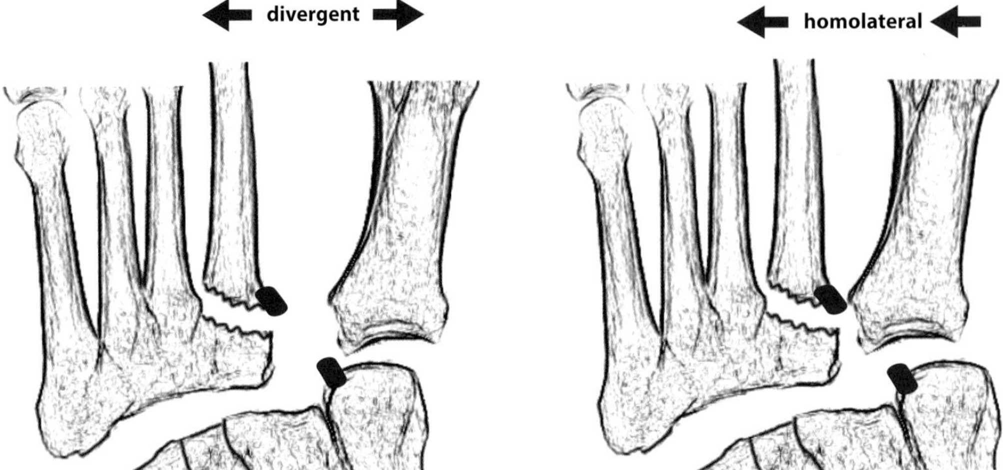

Navicular osteonecrosis

- Osteonecrosis of the navicular is called Kohler disease in childhood and Müeller–Weiss disease in adults. Kohler disease is typically self limited and occurs more commonly in boys, while Mueller–Weiss disease is more severe in course and occurs more commonly in adult women.

MIDFOOT AND HINDFOOT TRAUMA

Overview of common fractures

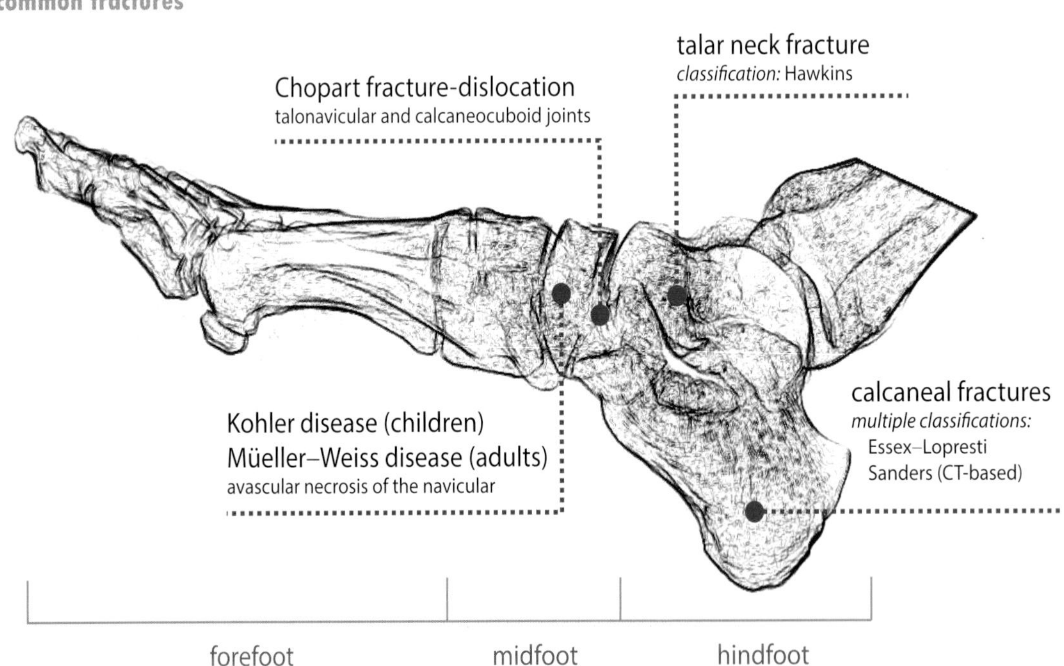

Chopart fracture-dislocation

- The Chopart joint is formed by the talonavicular and calcaneocuboid joints.
- Chopart fracture-dislocation is typically caused by high-impact trauma. Associated fractures of the calcaneus, cuboid, and navicular bones are often present.

Calcaneal fracture

- The calcaneus is the most commonly fractured tarsal bone.
- Traumatic fractures of the calcaneus are typically the result of a high-impact injury, such as a fall from height, in which case the fracture is known as the *lover's fracture.* In such cases, there is a high association with other serious injuries including lumbar spine fractures, traumatic aortic rupture, and renal vascular pedicle avulsion. If a traumatic calcaneal fracture is identified, further imaging of the lumbar spine and/or abdomen is recommended.
- Subtle fractures may not be directly visible; however, a decrease in the **Boehler angle** to less than 20 degrees is diagnostic of a calcaneal fracture.

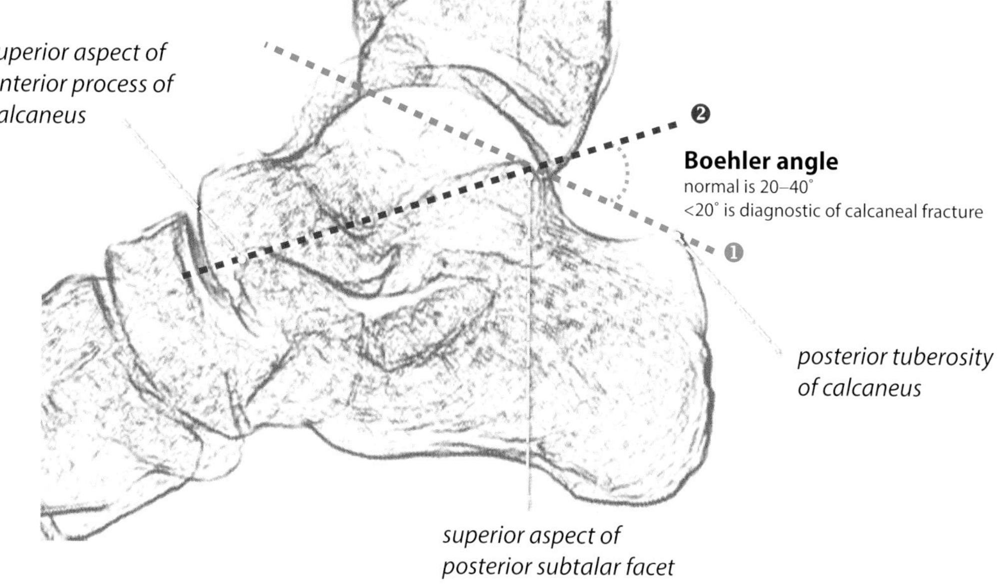

The Boehler angle is formed by drawing two lines:
❶ superior aspect of posterior tuberosity of calcaneus to the superior aspect of posterior subtalar facet
❷ superior aspect of anterior process of calcaneus to superior aspect of posterior subtalar articular surface

A Boehler angle <20° is diagnostic of a calcaneal fracture.
A normal Boehler angle (20–40°) does not exclude a calcaneal fracture.

- The Essex–Lopresti classification divides calcaneal fractures into those sparing the subtalar joint (25%) and fractures extending into the subtalar joint (75%).
- The Sanders classification is based on the number of comminuted fragments as seen on coronal CT.

Calcaneal stress fracture

- A stress fracture of the calcaneus typically appears as a fluffy band of sclerosis within the calcaneus, with an intact cortex. Boehler's angle is normal.

Talar fracture

- Fractures of the talus can be divided anatomically into lateral process, posterior process, head, body, and neck fractures.
- Fractures of the talar neck are classified by the Hawkins classification. A talar neck fracture may disrupt the blood supply to the talus and predispose to osteonecrosis.
- The Hawkins sign describes a subchondral lucent band seen on the frontal ankle radiograph 6–8 weeks after ankle immobilization. The lucent band represents increased bone reabsorption from active hyperemia. The presence of the Hawkins sign implies an intact blood supply to the talar dome and is a good prognostic indicator in talar neck fractures. Absence of the Hawkins sign suggests avascular necrosis.

Osteochondral lesion of the talus

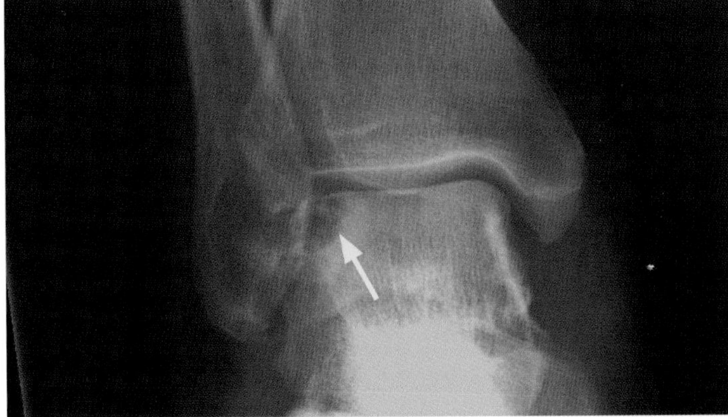

Talar osteochondral lesion:

Frontal radiograph of the ankle shows crescentic lucency (arrow) of the lateral talar dome with underlying sclerotic change.

- Osteochondral lesion of the talus is an umbrella term including osteochondrosis dissecans from chronic repetitive microtrauma and acute traumatic osteochondral fracture.

  Osteochondrosis dissecans is preferred over the older terminology of osteochondritis dissecans. The suffix *-itis* is misleading as this entity is not inflammatory.

- Osteochondral lesions and their staging are discussed in the knee section.
- In the talus, an osteochondral lesion appears on radiography as a crescentic lucency of the talar dome. MRI imaging is similar to MRI imaging of knee osteochondral lesions.

Hindfoot (tarsal) coalition

- Abnormal fusion of two tarsal bones may be a cause of hindfoot pain. Hindfoot coalitions often present in adolescence as the coalition begins to ossify. A coalition may be fibrous, cartilagineous, or osseous.
- The vast majority of hindfoot coalitions are either talocalcaneal (fusion of the talus and calcaneus) or calcaneonavicular (fusion of the calcaneus and navicular).
- **Talocalcaneal coalition** occurs most commonly at the middle subtalar facet.

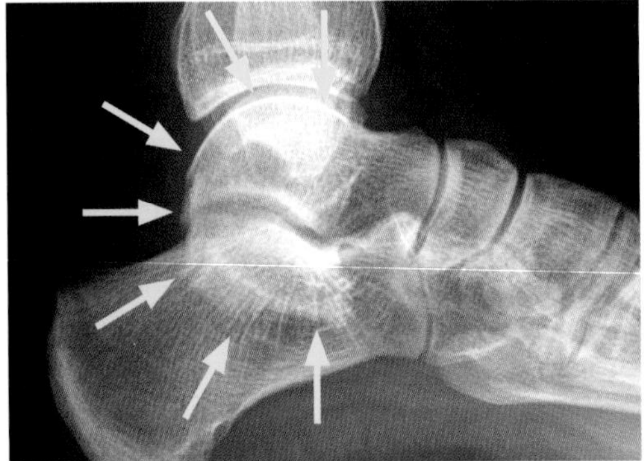

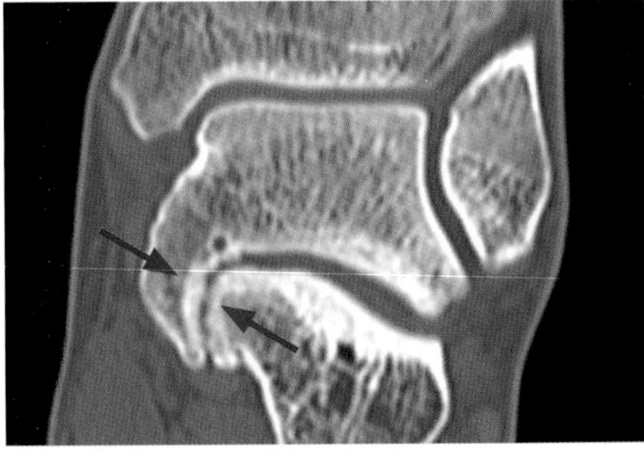

Talocalcaneal coalition: Lateral radiograph of the ankle (left image) shows the classic *C* sign (yellow arrows) representing the fused medial talus and sustentaculum tali. A fibrous coalition (red arrows) is confirmed on the coronal CT (right image), with sclerosis and subchondral cysts of the middle subtalar facet.

The C sign on the lateral radiograph describes a continuous C-shaped contour of the fused middle subtalar facet (medial talus fused with the sustentaculum tali). The C sign is not sensitive for the detection of talocalcaneal coalition, but may be helpful when seen.

The *talar beak* sign on the lateral radiograph describes a triangular-shaped beaking at the anterior-superior aspect of the talus.

- **Calcaneonavicular coalition** is fusion between the anterior process of the calcaneus and the navicular.

  The *anteater* sign represents the elongated anterior process of the calcaneus, which looks like an anteater's nose on the lateral view.

Ankle tendon anatomy

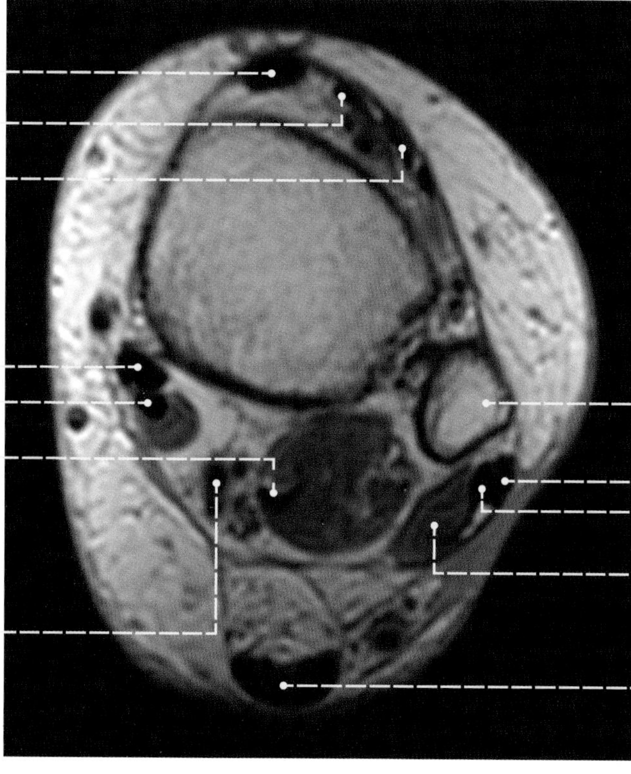

tibialis anterior tendon
extensor hallucis longus
extensor digitorum longus
anterior extensor tendons (Tom, Harry, and Dick from medial to lateral)
tibialis posterior
flexor digitorum longus
flexor hallucis longus tendon (and adjacent muscle)
posterior flexor tendons (Tom, Dick, and Harry from medial to lateral)
posterior tibial artery
fibula
peroneus longus tendon
peroneus brevis tendon
peroneus brevis muscle
Achilles tendon

Lateral ankle tendons and ligaments

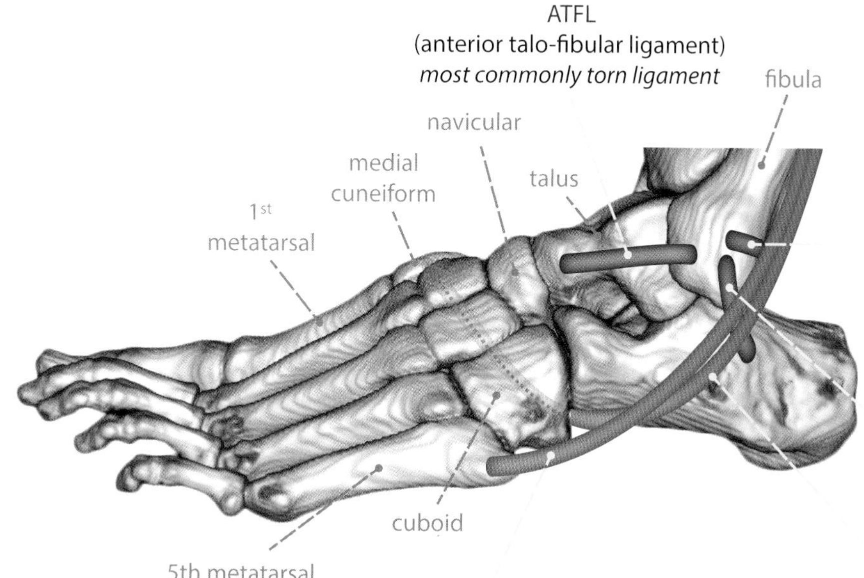

ATFL
(anterior talo-fibular ligament)
most commonly torn ligament
fibula
navicular
medial cuneiform
talus
1st metatarsal
PTFL
(posterior talo-fibular ligament)
very strong, rarely torn
calcaneofibular ligament
next most commonly torn
cuboid
5th metatarsal
peroneus brevis tendon
attaches to base of 5th metatarsal
peroneus longus tendon
runs under foot, attaches to medial cuneiform and first metatarsal
(only medial cuneiform attachment shown)

Medial ankle ligaments

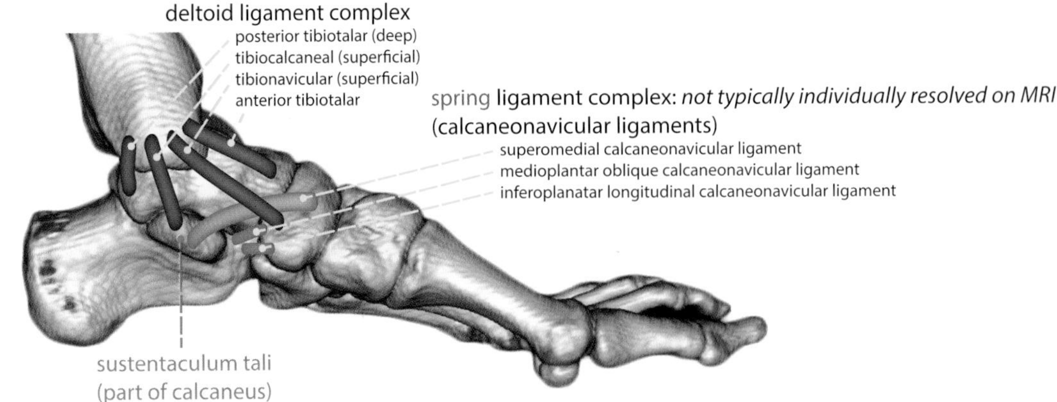

along with the posterior tibial tendon (not drawn), the spring ligament complex functions to maintain the arch of the foot*

**most common cause of acquired flat foot is posterior tibial tendon tear (especially in diabetic patients)*

Medial ankle tendons

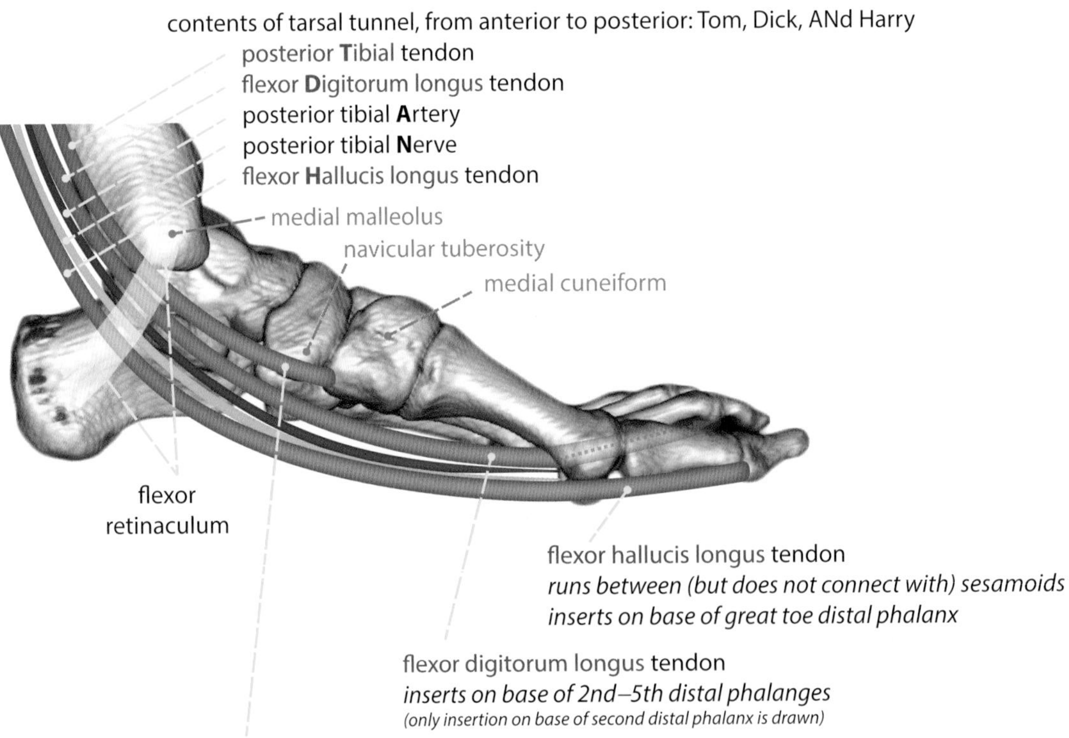

Anterior extensor tendons

- Arranged from medial to lateral, the anterior extensor tendons can be remembered with the mnemonic "Tom, Harry, and Dick":

  Tibialis anterior.

  Extensor **H**allucis longus.

  Extensor **D**igitorum longus.

- The anterior tibial artery runs anteriorly with the extensor tendons.

Ankle fractures

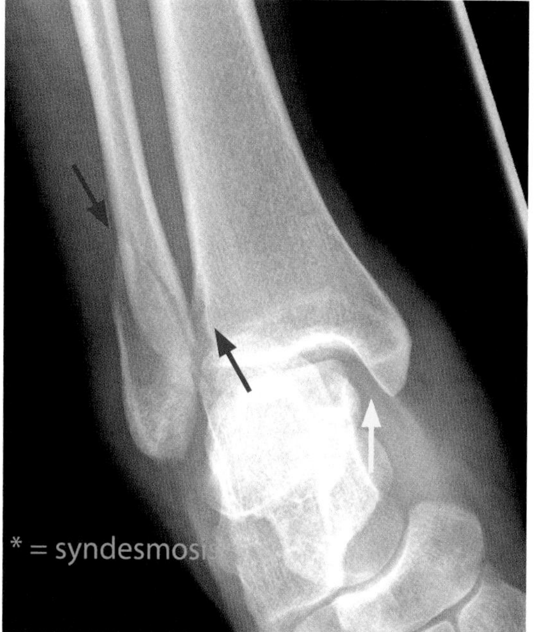

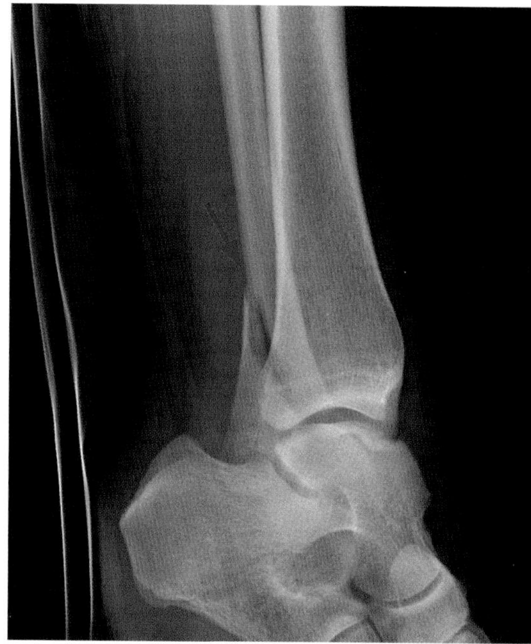

Weber B (Lauge–Hansen supination–external rotation) ankle fracture:

Oblique (left image) and lateral ankle radiographs show an oblique fracture (red arrows) through the distal fibula at the level of the syndesmosis (blue star). There is widening of the medial clear space (yellow arrow).

- Ankle sprains and fractures are the most common of all joint injuries.
- The Danis–Weber classification is the simplest classification of ankle fractures and divides ankle fractures based on the level of the fibular fracture and resultant syndesmotic injury.

  The syndesmosis is a fibrous ligamentous complex that connects the distal tibia and fibula, where the distal fibula fits into a groove in the distal tibia. It is formed by the anterior and posterior tibiofibular ligaments. The interosseous membrane connects the lengths of the tibia and fibula, superior to the syndesmosis.
- Danis–Weber A is a distal fibular fracture with an intact syndesmosis.
- Danis–Weber B is a more proximal transsyndesmotic fracture, usually associated with partial syndesmotic rupture.
- Danis–Weber C is a high fibular fracture above the level of the syndesmosis, usually associated with total syndesmotic rupture and subsequent ankle mortise instability.
- The Lauge–Hansen classification divides ankle fractures based on the directional mechanism of trauma. A supination–adduction injury correlates to Weber A; supination–external rotation correlates to Weber B; and pronation–external rotation correlates to Weber C.

Named ankle fractures

- **Tillaux** fracture is a Salter Harris III fracture of the lateral tibial epiphyses, typically seen in adolescents.
- **Triplane** fracture (also known as a Marmor–Lynn fracture) represents three distinct fractures through the distal tibia: A vertical epiphyseal fracture, horizontal physeal fracture, and oblique metaphyseal fracture.
- **Wagstaffe–LeFort** fracture is an avulsion of the anterior distal fibula at site of insertion of the anterior tibiofibular ligament.

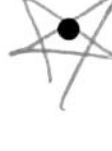

- **Maisonneuve** fracture is a high (proximal) fibular fracture associated with an interosseous membrane tear or medial malleolar fracture. Isolated imaging of the ankle may only detect subtle widening of the ankle mortise, which should prompt a more proximal radiograph.

- **Pilon** fracture is a comminuted vertically oriented fracture of the distal tibia, with resultant disruption of the tibial plafond. A pilon fracture is caused by axial loading.

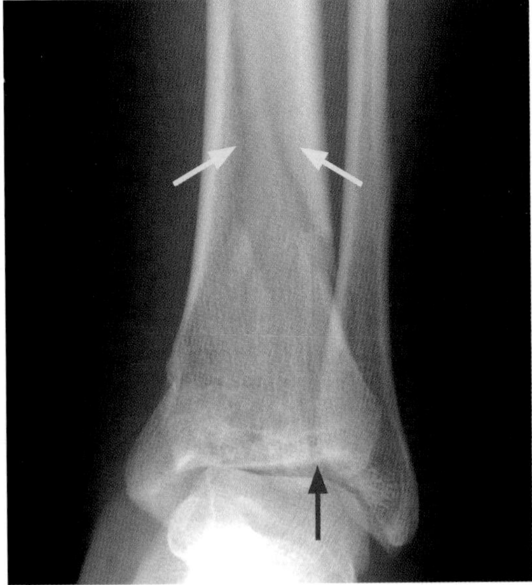

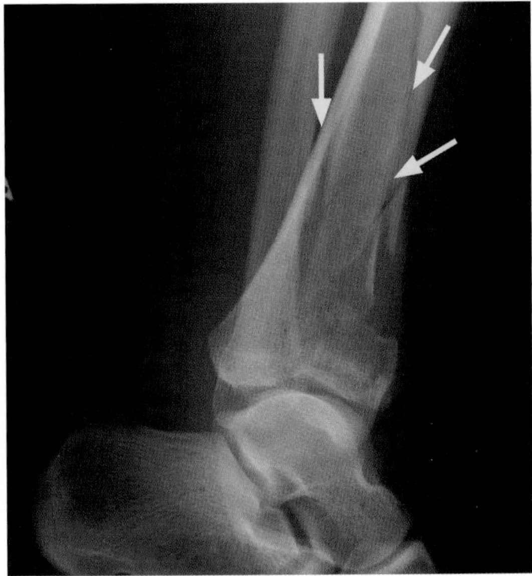

Pilon fracture: Frontal (left image) and lateral (right image) radiographs of the ankle show comminuted oblique and vertically oriented fractures (yellow arrows) of the distal tibia with disruption of the ankle mortise and tibial plafond (red arrow).

Achilles tendon injury

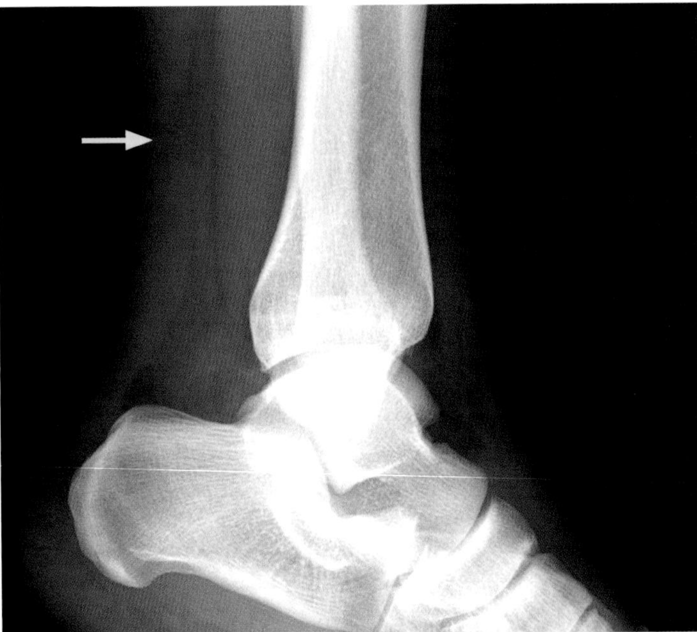

Achilles tendon rupture:

Lateral radiograph shows a subtle disruption of the contour of the Achilles tendon (arrow).

There is also increased soft tissue and fluid in Kager's fat pad. Kager's fat pad is a radiolucent triangle bounded by the flexor hallucis longus anteriorly, the calcaneus inferiorly, and the Achilles tendon posteriorly.

- The Achilles tendon is the most commonly injured ankle tendon.
- Achilles tendinosis can sometimes be evident on radiography as thickening of the tendon.

  Achilles thickening is not specific for tendinosis. Thickening of the Achilles tendon can also be caused by xanthomas in patients with a hyperlipidemia syndrome.
- Compete Achilles rupture is usually evident on clinical exam. Radiography shows discontinuity of the tendon contour, with increased soft tissue in Keger's fat pad.
- The differential diagnosis of increased soft tissue in Kager's fat pad includes:

  Achilles tendon injury.

  Accessory soleus muscle (most common soft-tissue mass seen in Kager's fat pad).

  Haglund disease, which is retrocalcaneal bursitis associated with thickening of the distal Achilles tendon. Poorly fitting shoes may be a cause, leading to the nickname *pump bumps*.

Knee and knee MRI

Knee trauma

Knee dislocation

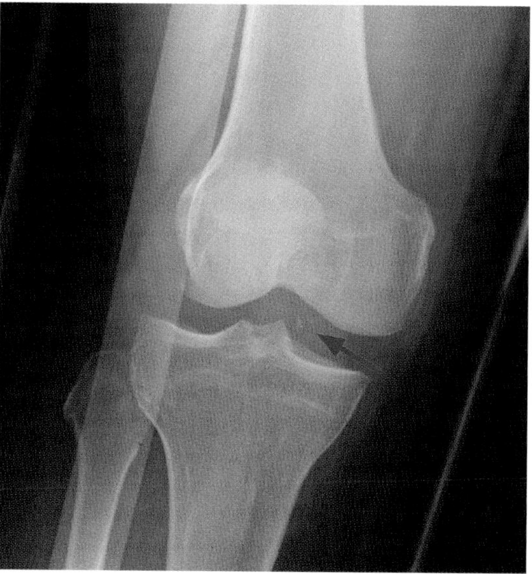

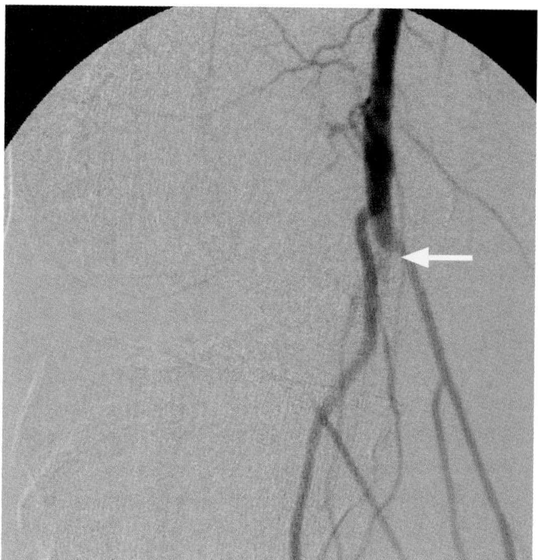

Posterior dislocation with vascular injury: Frontal radiograph of the knee (left image) shows marked widening of the joint space with slight lateral displacement of the tibia. The widened joint space suggests a dislocation. An ossific fragment projects over the joint space (red arrow). Intraoperative digital subtraction angiogram (right image) demonstrates a complete traumatic occlusion of the popliteal artery (arrow) just above the knee.

- The knee may dislocate in any direction, although anteriorly is the most common.
- There is a high risk for vascular injury to the popliteal artery, and a vascular injury may be present even if the distal pulses are still intact. CT angiography is therefore typically recommended for all knee dislocations.

Patellar fracture

- Patellar fracture may be caused by a direct blow (usually causing a comminuted fracture) or extreme sudden tension of the extensor mechanism (usually causing a distracted fracture).
- It is important to distinguish a fracture from a bipartite or multipartite patella, which are normal variants and will have well corticated margins. A dorsal defect of the patella is another normal variant, appearing as a round lucency at the superior articular (dorsal) aspect of the patella.

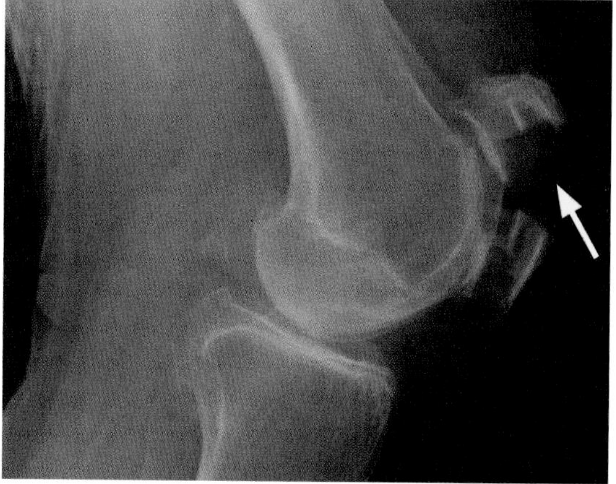

Lateral radiograph of the knee shows a distracted patellar fracture (arrow), suggestive of an injury caused by extreme tension of the extensor mechanism.

Tibial plateau fracture

- Tibial plateau fractures are classified by the Schatzker classification.
- Lateral tibial plateau fractures are more stable than medial tibial plateau fractures.

Menisci

Normal anatomy

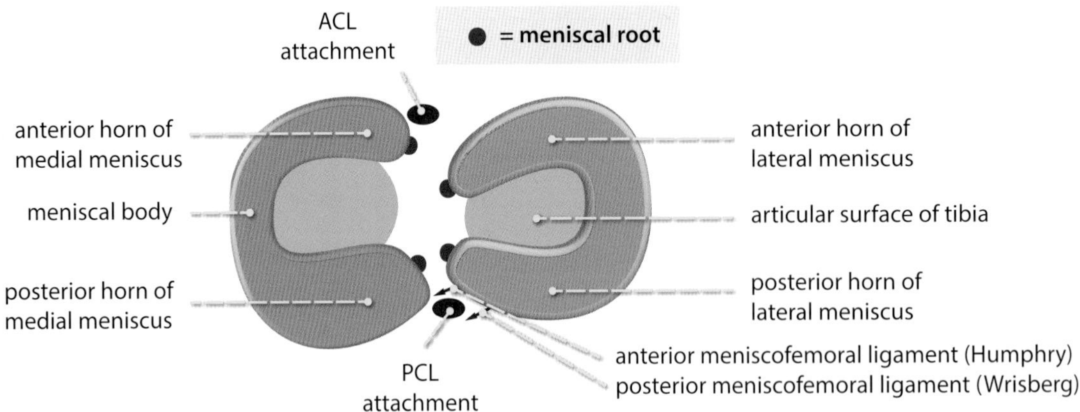

- The medial and lateral menisci are crescent-shaped fibrocartilaginous structures that form a discontinuous figure-eight to stabilize the knee and disperse the axial loading.
- Each meniscus consists of an anterior and a posterior horn.

  The posterior horn of the medial meniscus is larger than its anterior horn.

  Both horns of the lateral meniscus are the same size.
- Each meniscus is attached to the tibial plateau by an anterior and posterior meniscal root. Trauma to the meniscal root may cause meniscal extrusion.
- There are two meniscofemoral ligaments, which extend from the posterior horn of the lateral meniscus to the medial femoral condyle. It is important not to mistake a meniscofemoral ligament (which are variably present) for a meniscal tear.

  The ligament of Humphry is anterior to PCL; the ligament of Wrisberg is posterior to the PCL.
- The peripheral third of each meniscus is relatively vascular and is called the *red zone.* The central portion of the meniscus is considered avascular.
- Meniscal injuries confined to the red zone may heal spontaneously or after surgical repair, while more central meniscal injuries generally do not heal.

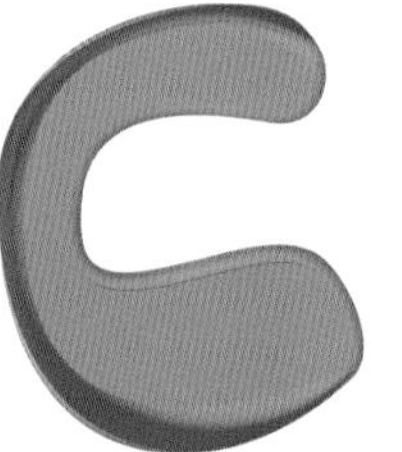

The peripheral 10–30% of the meniscus is the red zone, which is more highly vascularized than the central portion.

Normal appearance of menisci on MR

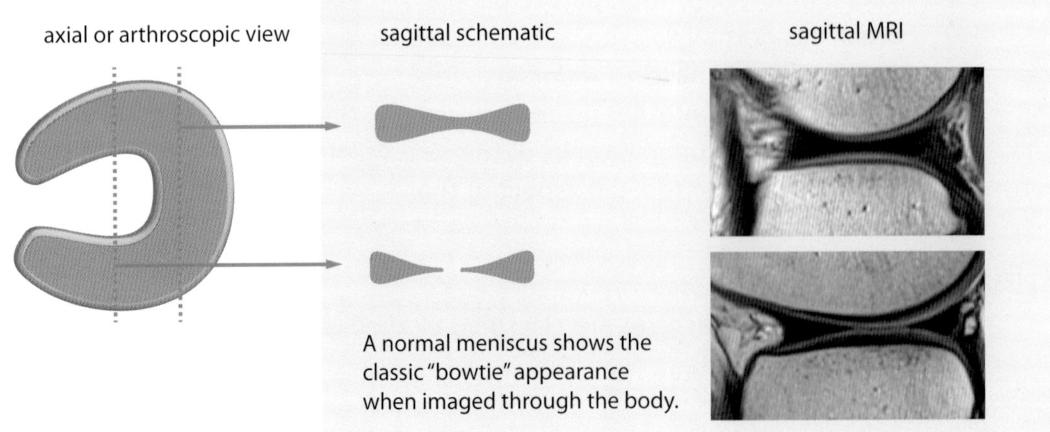

A normal meniscus shows the classic "bowtie" appearance when imaged through the body.

Case courtesy Nehal Shah, MD, Brigham and Women's Hospital.

Myxoid degeneration versus tear

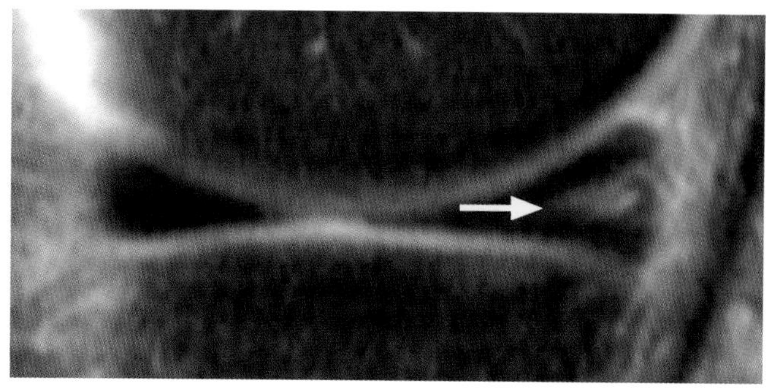

Meniscus myxoid degeneration: Sagittal fluid-sensitive MRI demonstrates increased globular signal (arrow) in the peripheral meniscus that does not extend to the articular surface.

Case courtesy Nehal Shah, MD, Brigham and Women's Hospital.

- Myxoid degeneration is increased signal within the meniscus that does not extend to the meniscal surface. It is not thought to cause symptoms and is not treated.
- In contrast, a meniscal tear is seen as a linear band of increased signal that *does* extend to the articular surface. The morphology of the meniscus is commonly abnormal. MRI is >90% sensitive and specific for the diagnosis of meniscal tears.

Oblique/horizontal tear

oblique meniscal tear

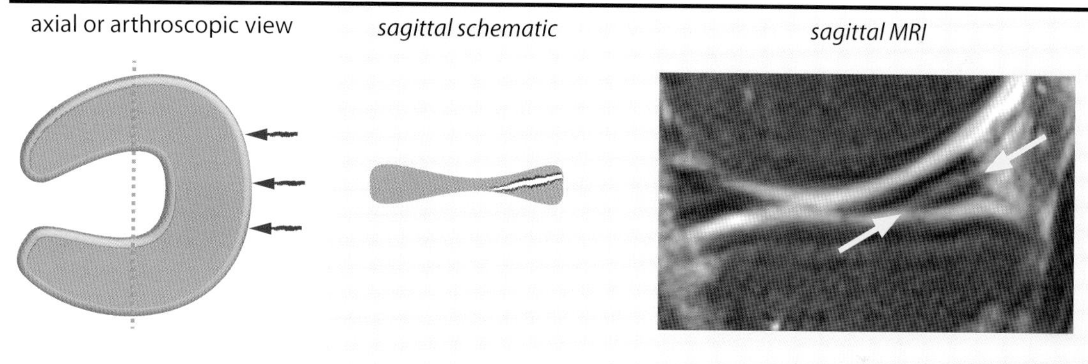

horizontal meniscal tear

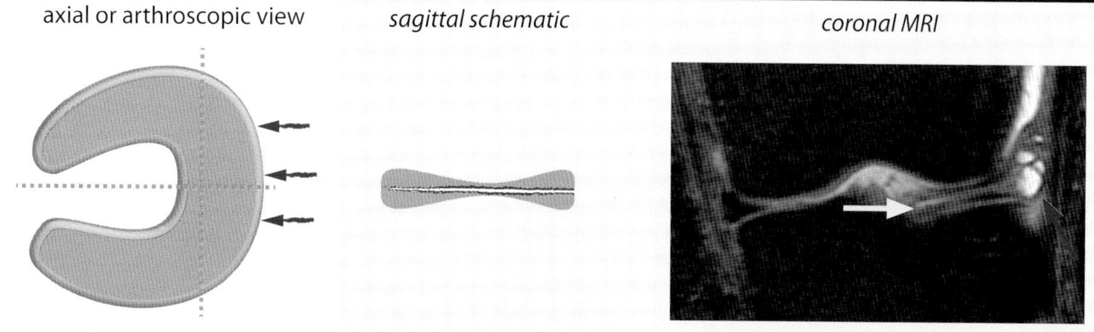

Since the cleavage plane is parallel to the tibial plateau, the surface of the meniscus will appear normal.

A true horizontal tear cleaves the meniscus in a plane parallel to the tibial plateau. The plane of cleavage appears similar in both the sagittal (as in the schematic) and coronal views. Note the associated parameniscal cysts (red arrow).

Case courtesy Nehal Shah, MD, Brigham and Women's Hospital.

- The terms *oblique* and *horizontal* are sometimes used interchangeably when referring to meniscal tears. Strictly speaking, however, a horizontal tear remains parallel to the tibial plateau, while an oblique tear may be at a slight angle to the tibial plateau.
- An oblique/horizontal tear is the most common meniscal tear, typically occurring in the posterior horn of the medial meniscus.
- Oblique and horizontal tears are more often degenerative, rather than due to trauma.

Vertical/longitudinal tear

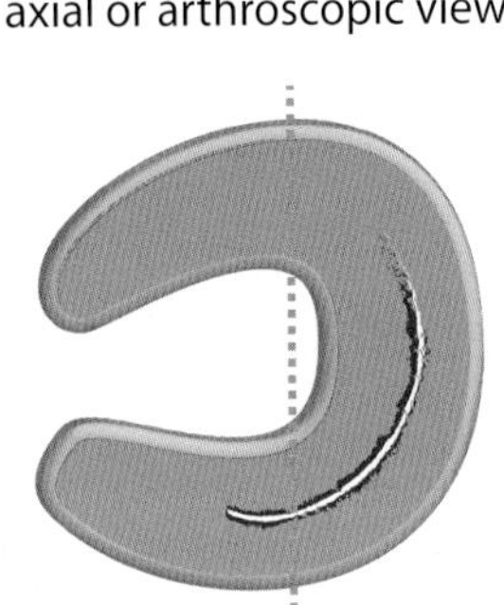

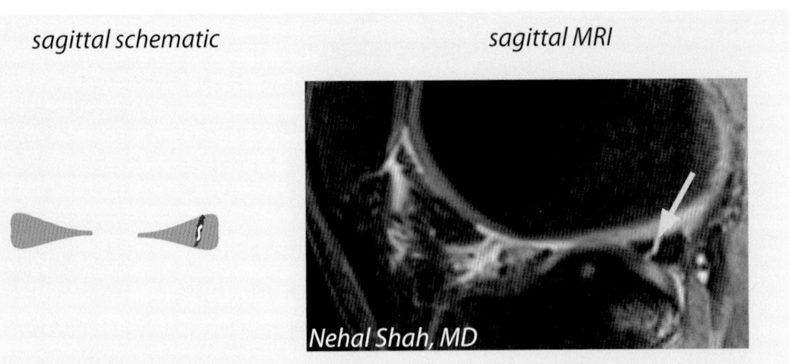

A vertical (longitudinal) tear is present (arrow) demonstrating complete superior-to-inferior surface extension.

- The vertical (synonymous with longitudinal) tear is a curved tear that follows the contour of the meniscus. On serial sagittal images, the tear will be in a vertical orientation and will remain a fixed distance from the edge of the meniscus.

Bucket-handle tear

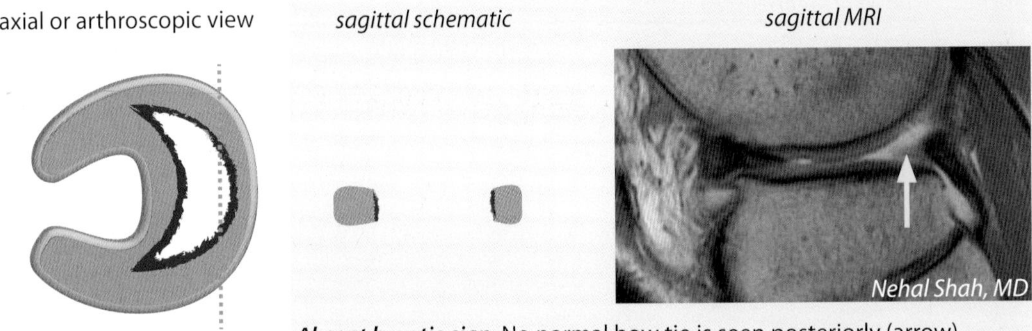

Absent bow tie sign: No normal bow tie is seen posteriorly (arrow).

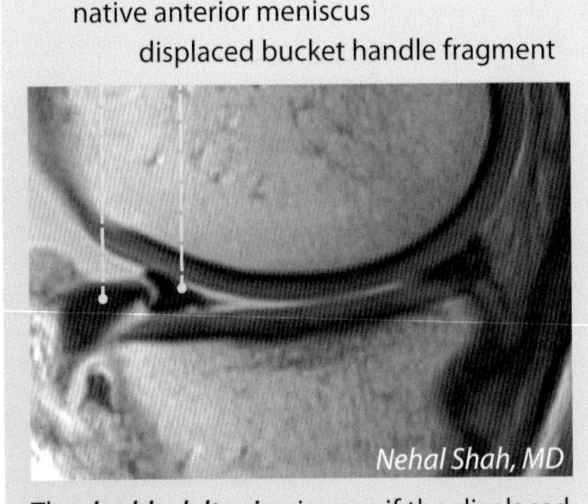

The ***double delta sign*** is seen if the displaced fragment flips anteriorly.

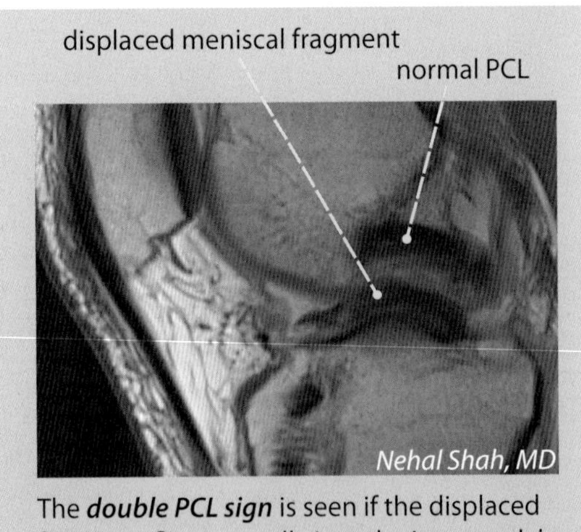

The ***double PCL sign*** is seen if the displaced fragment flips centrally into the intercondylar notch.

- A bucket-handle tear is the result of an extensive vertical tear, occurring when the free inner edge of the meniscus (medial meniscus most commonly) gets displaced or flipped over.
- The most sensitive imaging finding of a bucket-handle tear is the *absent bow tie* sign, seen when there are fewer than two "bow ties" on adjacent 4 mm-thick sagittal slices.
- The most common location of the displaced meniscal fragment is the intercondylar notch, but the meniscal fragment may also displace anteriorly or posteriorly.
- Anterior displacement produces the *double delta* sign on sagittal MRI (either meniscus).
- Posterior displacement produces the *double PCL* sign on sagittal MRI (medial meniscus only).

Radial/transverse tear

radial tear of meniscal body

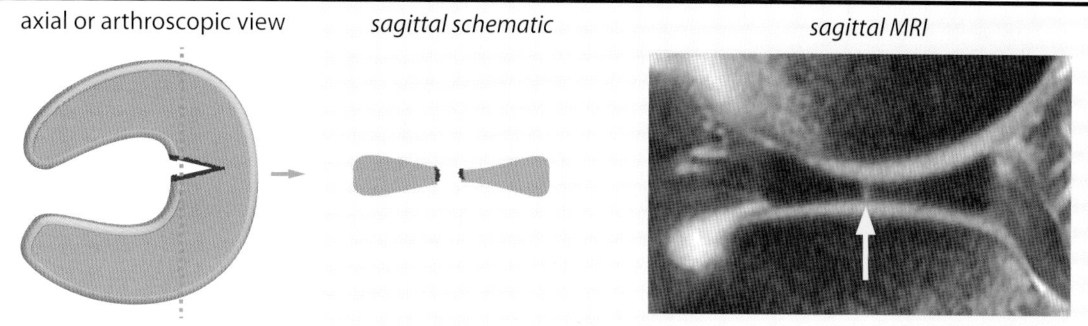

Radial tear is a vertically oriented tear extending from the free edge of the meniscus to the periphery.

radial tear of meniscal horn

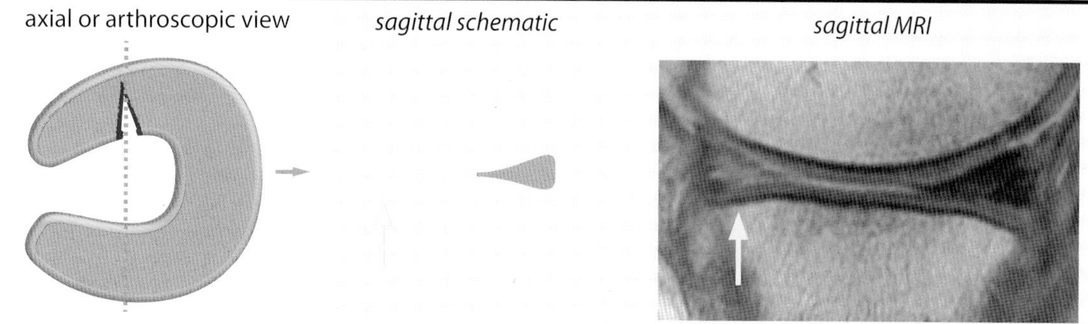

Ghost meniscus sign: No meniscal tissue is seen when the plane of imaging is directly through the radial tear (arrows).

Cases courtesy Nehal Shah, MD, Brigham and Women's Hospital.

- A radial tear (also known as a transverse tear) is a vertically oriented tear that is perpendicular to the arc of the meniscus. In contrast, the previously discussed vertical/longitudinal tear follows the curve of the meniscus.
- On a single image, a radial tear may be indistinguishable from a vertical/longitudinal tear. On serial sagittal images, however, the radial tear will change position relative to the edge of the meniscus. This phenomenon is the *marching cleft* sign.
- Depending on the orientation of the tear in relation to the scan plane, a radial tear may also show the *ghost meniscus* sign. The ghost meniscus is typically described as absence of the posterior horn of the meniscus on sagittal images (although it may also occur with absence of the anterior horn, as seen above). It occurs in tears adjacent to the intercondylar notch.
- Radial tears are associated with a high rate of meniscal extrusion, which may lead to osteoarthritis if not treated.

Meniscal cyst

- A meniscal cyst is loculated fluid adjacent to the meniscus, thought to result from extension of joint fluid through a meniscal tear.
- Meniscal cysts are most commonly associated with horizontal cleavage tears.
- It is important to mention the presence of a meniscal cyst because the meniscal cyst may continue to cause symptoms even if the meniscus is resected. Not all cysts are able to be visualized by arthroscopy.

Discoid meniscus

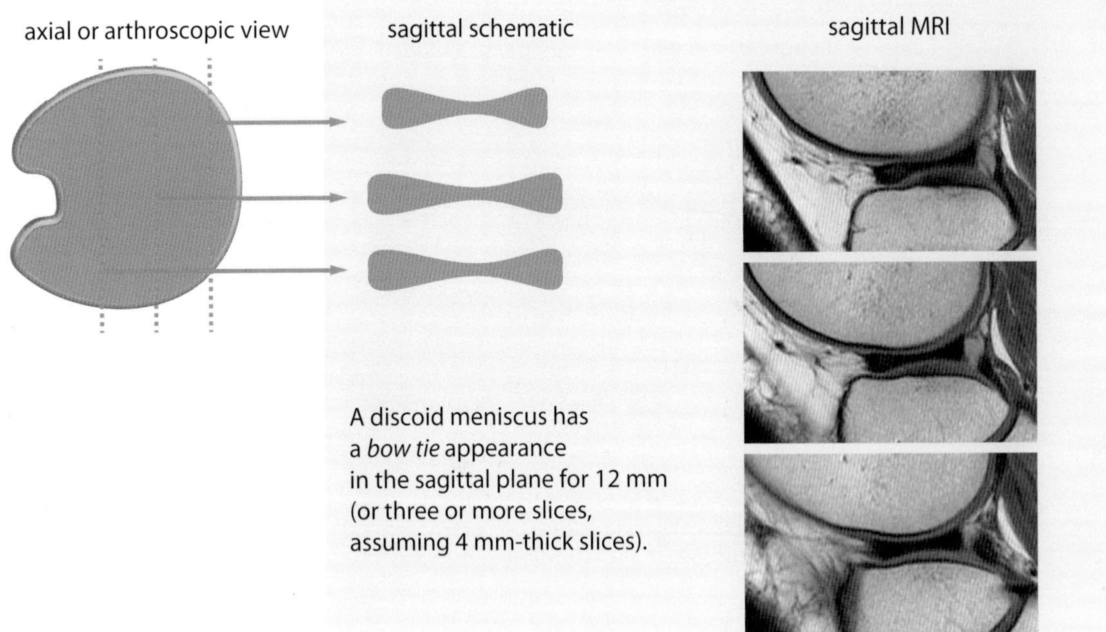
axial or arthroscopic view
sagittal schematic
sagittal MRI
A discoid meniscus has a *bow tie* appearance in the sagittal plane for 12 mm (or three or more slices, assuming 4 mm-thick slices).

Case courtesy Nehal Shah, MD, Brigham and Women's Hospital.

- Discoid meniscus is a spectrum of congenital malformations of the meniscus that ranges from increased thickness of the meniscus to a complete disc-like shape. Discoid meniscus is defined by having a portion of the meniscus extending to the central tibial plateau.
- Discoid meniscus typically affects children and is a common cause of joint-line pain, clicking, or locking in a child or adolescent. Discoid meniscus is prone to undergo cystic degeneration and tear. Even in the absence of a tear, a discoid meniscus may be symptomatic.
- The lateral meniscus is more commonly affected.
- On MRI, a meniscus is discoid if an oval or *bow tie-shaped* meniscus is seen on three or more contiguous sagittal slices with standard 4 mm-thick sagittal slices (representing 12 mm in medial–lateral thickness).

Anterior cruciate ligament (ACL)

- The anterior cruciate ligament (ACL) arises from the femoral intercondylar notch and attaches on the anterior tibial plateau, directly lateral to the tibial spine. The tibial attachment of the ACL is stronger than its femoral origin. The ACL is composed of two fiber bundles, a small anteromedial band and larger posterolateral band.

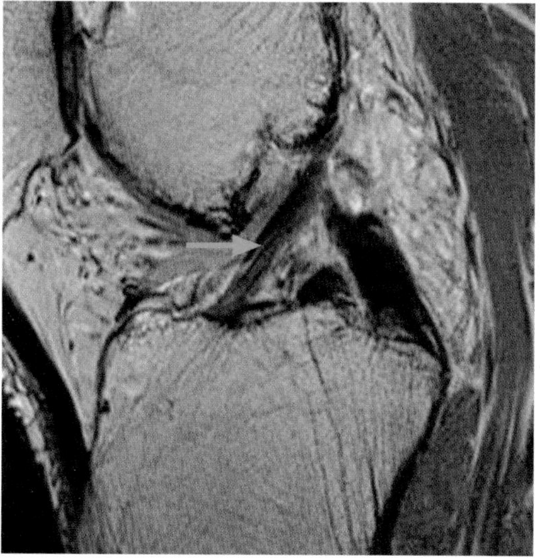

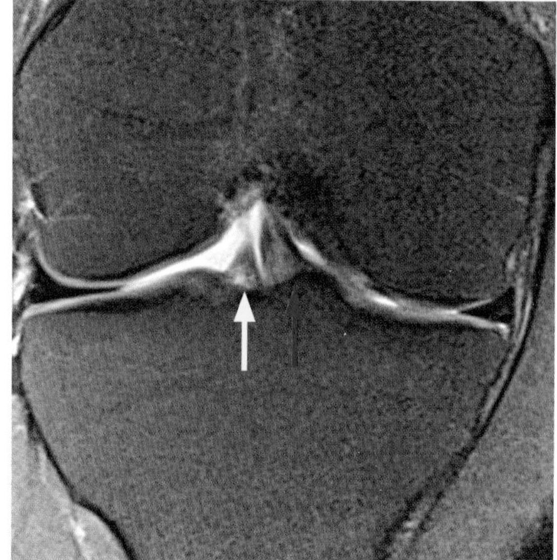

Normal ACL: Sagittal proton-density (left image) and coronal proton-density fat-sat (right image) MRI shows the normal course of the ACL fibers with the typical striated appearance (blue arrow) on the sagittal image. The coronal image demonstrates the smaller anteromedial (yellow arrow) and larger posterolateral (red arrow) fiber bundles in the intercondylar notch.

Case courtesy Nehal Shah, MD, Brigham and Women's Hospital.

ACL tear

- ACL tear is typically caused by an acute injury.
- MRI of ACL tear may show either frank discontinuity of the ligament fibers or abnormal course and signal of the ligament.

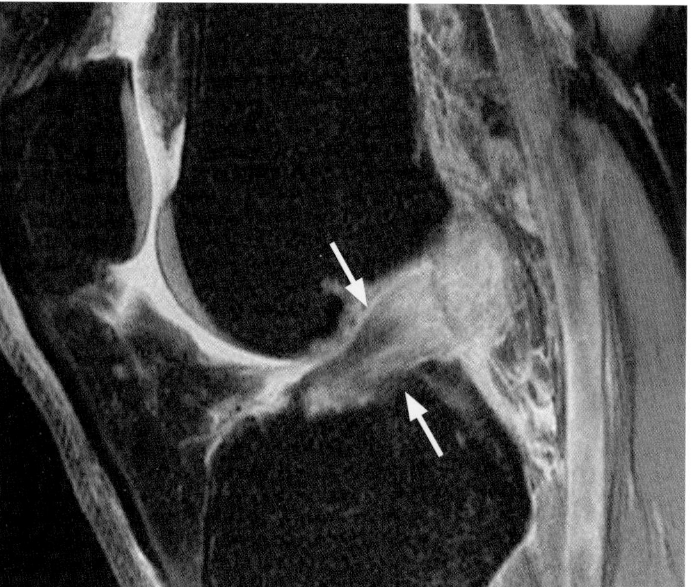

ACL tear: Sagittal fluid-sensitive MRI demonstrates frank rupture of the ACL (arrows), with discontinuity of the fibers and increased signal.

Case courtesy Nehal Shah, MD, Brigham and Women's Hospital.

- ACL injury is often associated with meniscal and MCL tears (O'Donoghue's triad). Posterolateral corner knee injuries are also frequently seen in association with ACL injury.

- There are multiple secondary findings of ACL injury. A characteristic bone contusion pattern with bone marrow edema in the lateral femoral condyle and the posterolateral tibial plateau is highly suggestive of ACL injury. Secondary buckling of the posterior collateral ligament (PCL) may also be seen due to anterior displacement of the tibia (positive *drawer* sign).

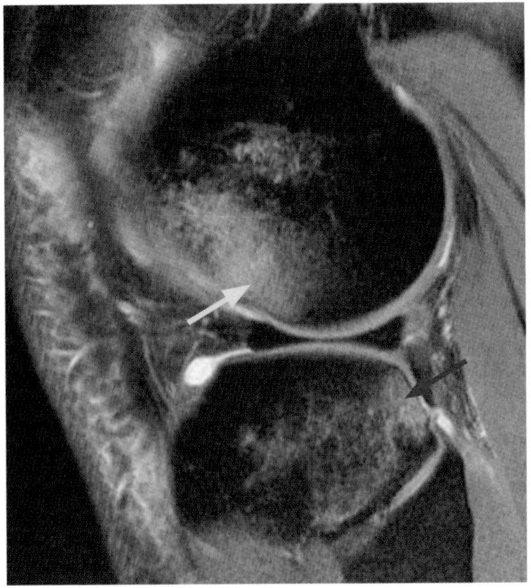

Secondary findings of ACL tear: Sagittal fluid-sensitive MRI image shows bone marrow edema in the lateral femoral condyle (yellow arrow) and posterolateral tibial plateau (red arrow), a pattern characteristic of ACL injury.

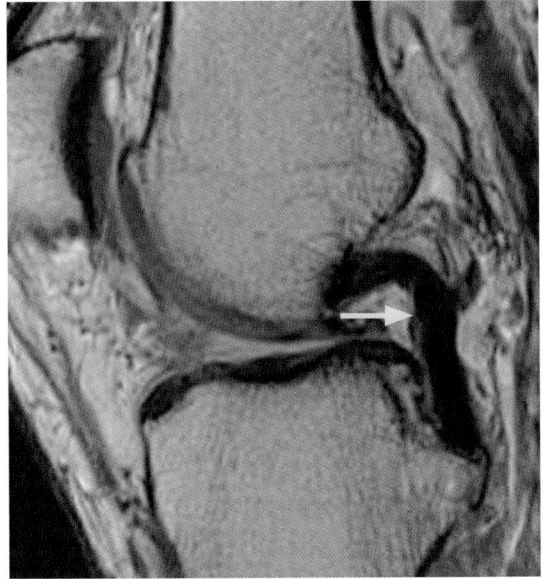

Secondary findings of ACL tear in a different patient: Sagittal proton-density MRI shows buckling of the PCL (arrow), suggestive of an ACL injury.

Cases courtesy Nehal Shah, MD, Brigham and Women's Hospital.

- A clue to ACL injury on radiography is a *Segond* fracture, which is an avulsion fracture of the lateral tibia plateau. Segond fracture is associated with both ACL injury and iliotibial (IT) band injury. The IT band inserts on Gerdy's tubercle of the tibia.

  The Segond fracture is thought to represent detachment of the lateral capsular ligament.

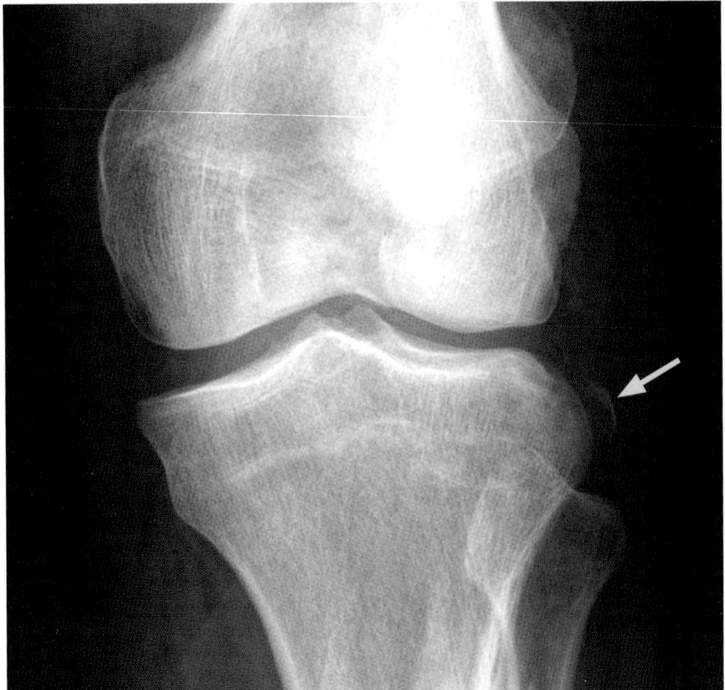

Segond fracture: Frontal knee radiograph shows an avulsion fracture of the lateral tibial plateau (arrow).

These fractures can be easily missed on radiography, but are important to diagnose.

MRI should be recommended if a Segond fracture is seen.

- After ACL reconstruction, the ACL graft should run parallel to the intercondylar notch, behind Blumensaat's line (a line drawn on radiography along the intercondylar roof).

  If the reconstructed ACL is too steep → graft can be impinged by the femur with leg extension.

  If the reconstructed ACL is too lax → graft may not provide enough stability.

  A complication of ACL reconstruction is the ***cyclops*** lesion, which is nodular scarring in Hoffa's fat pad.

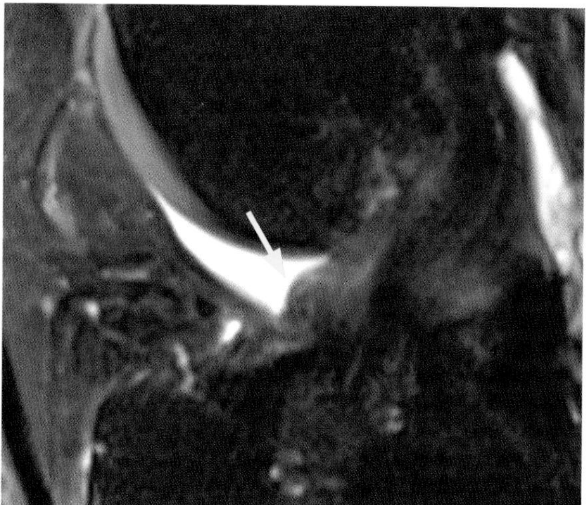

Cyclops lesion post ACL reconstruction: Fluid-sensitive sagittal MRI shows nodular soft-tissue (arrow) anterior to the reconstructed ACL.

Case courtesy Nehal Shah, MD, Brigham and Women's Hospital.

Posterior cruciate ligament (PCL)

- The posterior cruciate ligament (PCL) is a stronger, thicker ligament than the ACL. It also arises from the femoral intercondylar notch (more anteriorly than the ACL), but inserts on the posterior tibial plateau.

  The PCL is normally low signal on all sequences.

  The PCL is much less commonly injured than the ACL.

PCL tear

- In contrast to an ACL tear, a complete disruption of the PCL fibers is uncommon.
- The typical MRI appearance of PCL injury is increased laxity of the PCL, with or without abnormal high signal on T2-weighted images.

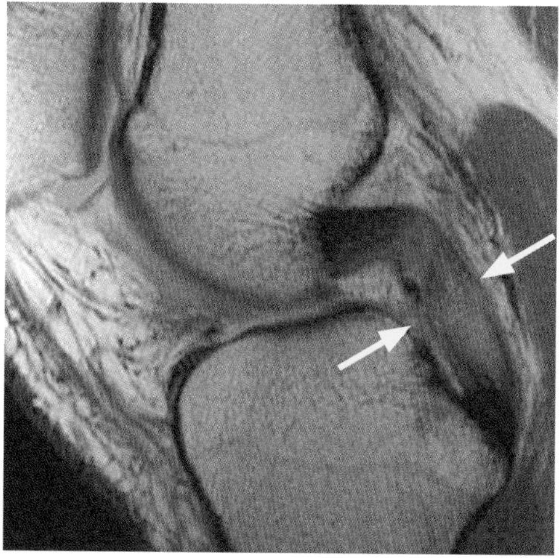

PCL interstitial tear: Sagittal proton-density MRI shows a PCL interstitial tear (arrows) with increased thickness, abnormal signal, and increased laxity of the PCL.

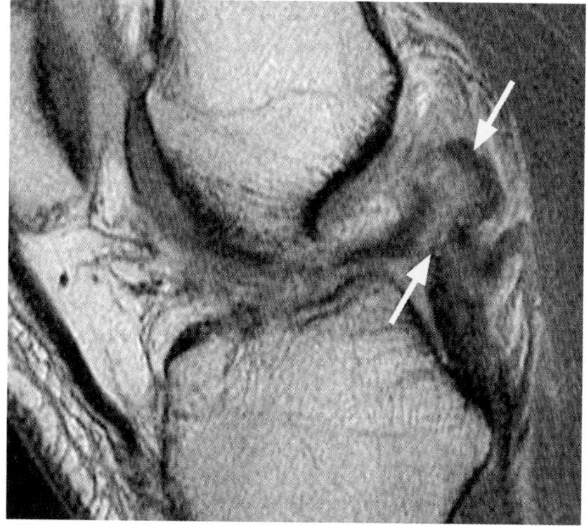

PCL complete tear (in a different patient): Sagittal proton-density MRI shows complete rupture of the PCL with frank discontinuity of the fibers (arrows).

Cases courtesy Nehal Shah, MD, Brigham and Women's Hospital.

- PCL tears tend to be less frequently repaired compared to ACL tears.

Medial collateral ligament (MCL)

- The medial collateral ligament (MCL) arises from the posterior aspect of the medial femoral condyle and attaches to the medial tibial metaphysis, deep to the pes anserinus.
  - The MCL fibers are interlaced with the joint capsule and the medial meniscus.
  - The MCL is an extrasynovial structure and is not visualized by arthroscopy.

MCL injury

- MCL injuries are commonly divided into three grades:

Grade 1 (MCL sprain): High signal in the medial soft tissues with normal signal of the ligament.
Grade 2 (severe sprain/partial tear): High signal or partial disruption within the MCL fibers.
Grade 3 (complete tear): Complete disruption of the MCL.

- The Pellegrini–Stieda lesion is post-traumatic calcification medial to the medial femoral condyle, which may be secondary to MCL avulsion injury.

Lateral collateral ligament (LCL) complex

- The lateral collateral ligament (LCL) complex is composed of many structures, three of which are routinely evaluated by MRI. From posterior to anterior, these structures are: Biceps femoris tendon (most posterior), LCL, and iliotibial band (most anterior).

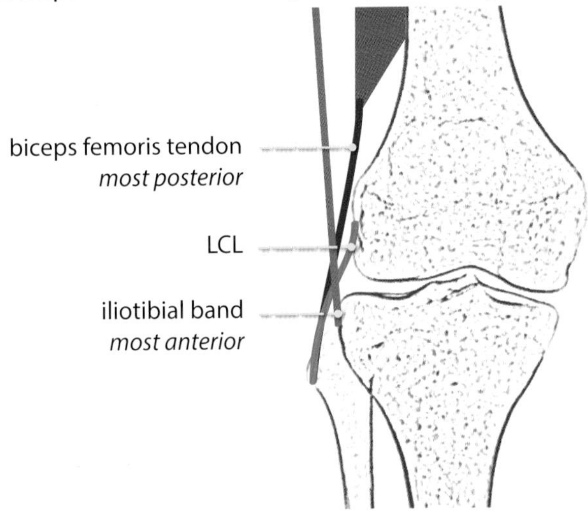

The biceps femoris tendon and the LCL both attach on the lateral fibular head, where they often have a conjoined tendon.

The iliotibial band attaches to Gerdy's tubercle on the proximal lateral tibia.

LCL injury

- LCL injury is less common than MCL injury and is usually associated with injury to other structures in the posterolateral corner. Injury to the posterolateral corner is a surgical near-emergency as there is poor outcome without prompt intervention.
- The posterolateral corner of the knee is a complex region consisting of:
  - LCL complex, consisting of the biceps femoris tendon, LCL, and the iliotibial band.
  - Arcuate ligament, a Y-shaped ligament connecting the fibula to the lateral femur.
  - Popliteofibular ligaments, which are important lateral stabilizers.
  - Popliteus tendon, which inserts on the lateral femur.

Iliotibial band syndrome

- Fluid surrounding (both superficial and deep to) the iliotibial band may represent iliotibial (IT) band syndrome, which is caused by friction between the anterolateral femur and the tendon of the iliotibial band.
- Clinically, IT band syndrome may be a cause of anterolateral knee pain and is seen commonly in runners.
- It is important to distinguish IT band syndrome from a lateral meniscus tear. Both may present with lateral knee pain, but treatment of iliotibial band syndrome is nonsurgical.

Normal anatomy of the extensor mechanism

- The **extensor mechanism** is composed of the conjoined quadriceps tendon (attaches to the patella), the patella, and the patellar tendon (attaches to the tibial tuberosity).

  The patella is a sesamoid bone and is enclosed within the quadriceps tendon.
- Three of the quadriceps muscles (vastus intermedius, medialis, and lateralis) originate from the femur. The rectus femoris arises from the anterior inferior iliac spine (AIIS).

Patella alta and patella baja

- *Patella alta* is an abnormally high patella and *patella baja* is an abnormally low patella.
- The Insall-Salvati ratio can help determine the craniocaudal alignment of the patella, based on a sagittal MRI or lateral radiograph (ideally with 30 degrees of flexion). The Insall-Salvati ratio is defined as the ratio of the patellar tendon length to the patellar length. An Insall-Salvati ratio >1.2 is suggestive of patella alta, and a ratio <0.8 is suggestive of patella baja.

Quadriceps tendon tear

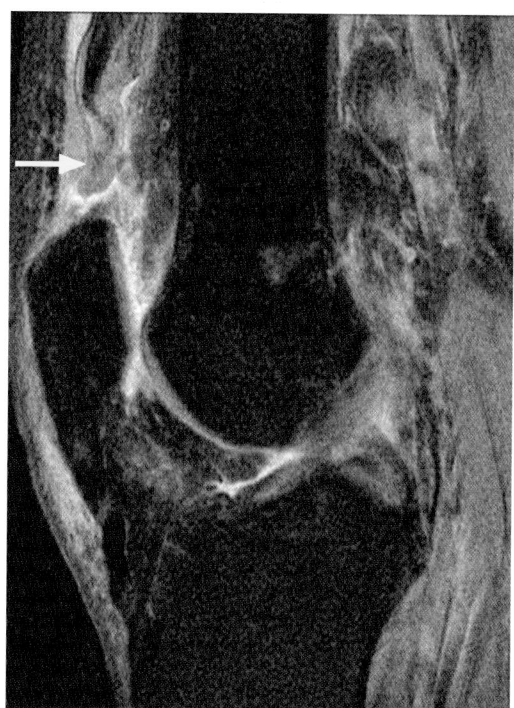
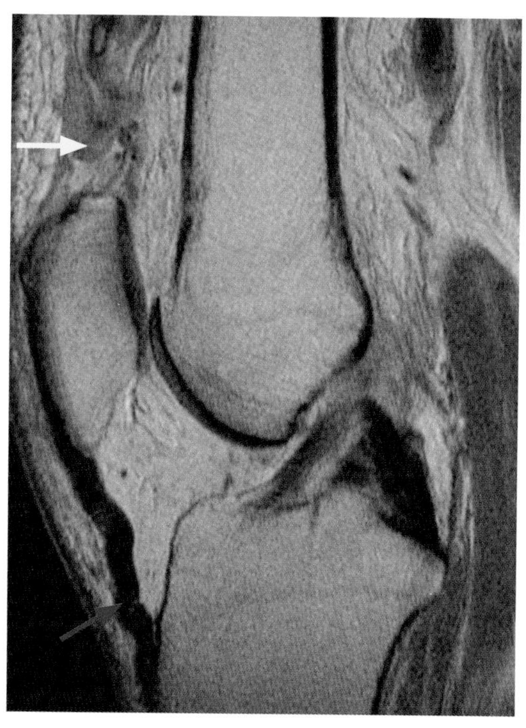

Quadriceps tendon tear: Sagittal proton density fat-saturated (left image) and proton density (right image) MRI shows complete disruption of the distal quadriceps tendon (yellow arrows) with surrounding marked edema. There is secondary buckling of the patellar tendon (red arrow).

Case courtesy Nehal Shah, MD, Brigham and Women's Hospital.

- Tear of the quadriceps tendon clinically presents with loss of knee extension.
- Quadriceps tendon tear most commonly occurs within 2 cm of the patella and may be evident on radiography due to the resultant *patella baja* (patella too low).

Patellar tendon injury

- Similar to quadriceps tendon tear, patellar tendon tear clinically presents with loss of knee extension. In contrast to quadriceps tendon tear, tear of the patella tendon causes superior displacement of the patella (*patella alta*).
- Patellar tendinosis is seen on MRI as thickening of the patellar tendon. This is known as *jumper's knee.*

Lateral patellar dislocation

- Traumatic lateral patellar dislocation leaves behind a distinctive pattern of injury, even if the patella reduces back to the normal position. Bone marrow contusions of the lateral femoral condyle and the medial patellar facet are typical, with tearing of the medial retinaculum.

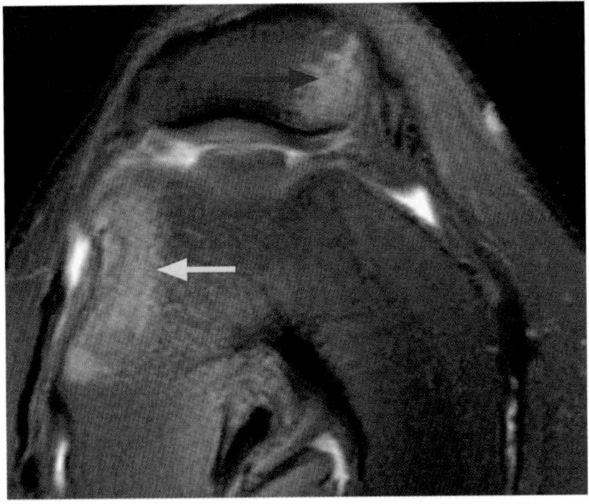

Lateral patellar dislocation: Axial fluid-sensitive MRI demonstrates the typical bone marrow edema pattern, with contusions of the lateral femoral condyle (yellow arrow) and medial patellar facet (red arrow).

The patella has relocated to its anatomic position.

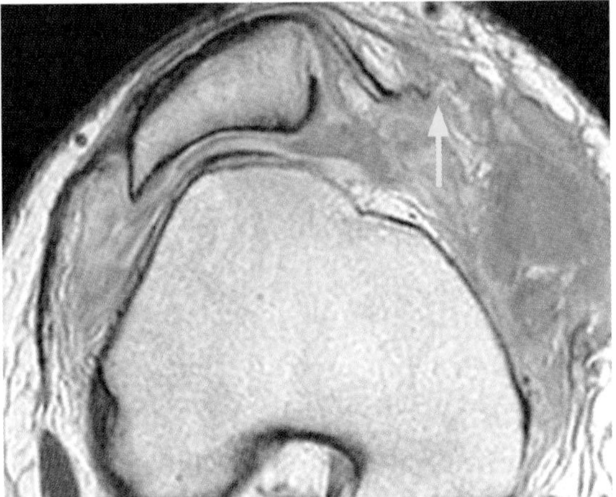

Lateral patellar dislocation in a different patient: Axial proton-density MRI shows persistent lateral subluxation of the patella, with complete tearing of the medial retinaculum (yellow arrow).

Cases courtesy Nehal Shah, MD, Brigham and Women's Hospital.

Osgood–Schlatter disease

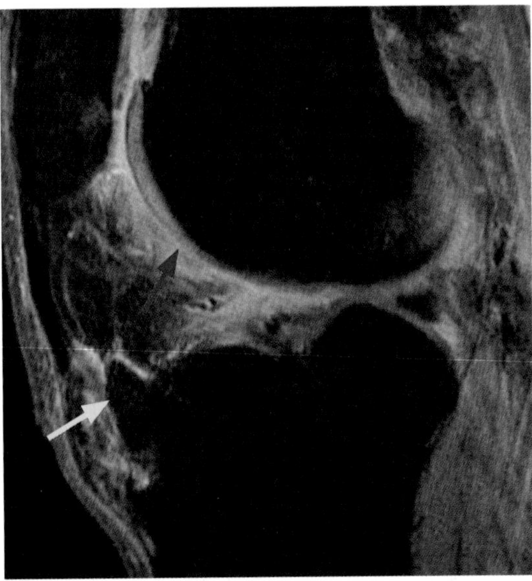

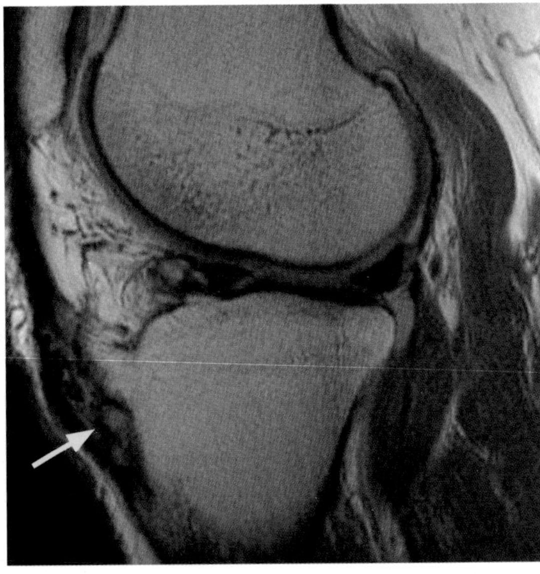

Osgood–Schlatter disease: Sagittal fluid-sensitive (left image) and proton density (right image) MRI shows an enlarged, fragmented tibial tubercle (yellow arrows). There is associated edema anterior to the tibial tubercle and within Hoffa's fat pad (red arrow).

Case courtesy Nehal Shah, MD, Brigham and Women's Hospital.

- Osgood–Schlatter disease is an osteochondrosis of the tibial tubercle, thought to be caused by repetitive microtrauma. It occurs in adolescents.
- Radiographs show an enlarged tibial tuberosity with fragmentation and adjacent edema.
- MRI shows increased signal of the distal patellar tendon, marrow edema within the tibial tubercle, and edema within Hoffa's fat pad.

KNEE CARTILAGE

Overview and anatomy

- The cartilage of each of the three major compartments (patellofemoral, medial tibiofemoral, and lateral tibiofemoral) should be routinely evaluated on every knee MRI.
- Further subdividing the patellofemoral cartilage, there are three facets of patellar cartilage (medial, lateral, and odd facets; the medial and lateral facets are divided by the median ridge) and three segments of trochlear cartilage (medial, central, and lateral). The trochlea is the femoral groove where the patella lies.

Cartilage thinning or injury

- Cartilage thinning is reported as <50%, 50%, or >50% thinning.
- Cartilage injury may manifest as surface irregularity, fissuring, or delamination. Delamination is a dissecting-type detachment of the cartilage undersurface from bone.

Osteochondrosis dissecans (OCD)

- Osteochondrosis dissecans (OCD) is an osteochondral (affecting both articular cartilage and bone) injury thought to be caused by repetitive trauma, which tends to occur in adolescents.

  The term osteochondr*itis* dissecans should be avoided as there is no inflammation involved.
- The etiology of OCD is thought to be due to cartilage dehydration and subsequent stiffening, which transmits greater force to the subchondral bone each time the joint is loaded.
- The most common joints affected are the knee, ankle, and elbow, in typical locations:

  Knee (most common): Lateral aspect of medial femoral condyle.

  Ankle (second most common): Posteromedial or anterolateral talar dome.

  Elbow (in gymnasts or throwing athletes): Anterolateral capitellum.
- An "unstable" osteochondral fragment means the lesion is unattached to bone. An unstable lesion may develop secondary osteoarthritis if not treated. The most important goal of MRI is to determine stability of an osteochondral fragment. A curvilinear region of high signal on a fluid-sensitive sequence interposed between the fragment and the underlying bone suggests that the fragment is unstable.
- MRI staging of OCD:

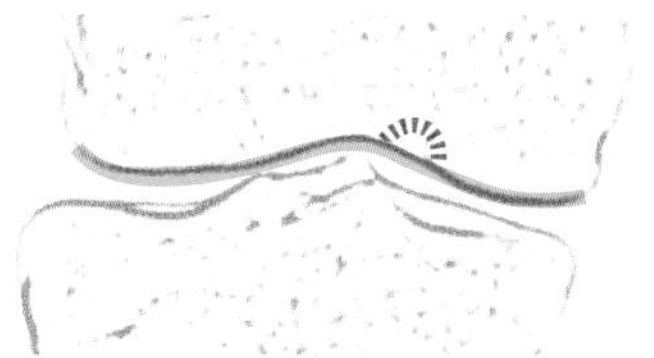

stage 1 OCD: intact articular cartilage
radiograph: normal
T2-weighted image (T2WI): bone marrow edema

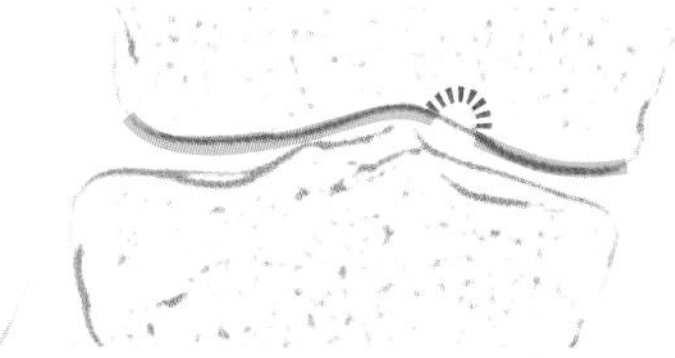

stage 2 OCD: articular cartilage defect
radiograph: semicircular fragment
T2WI: cartilage defect; low-signal line surrounding lesion

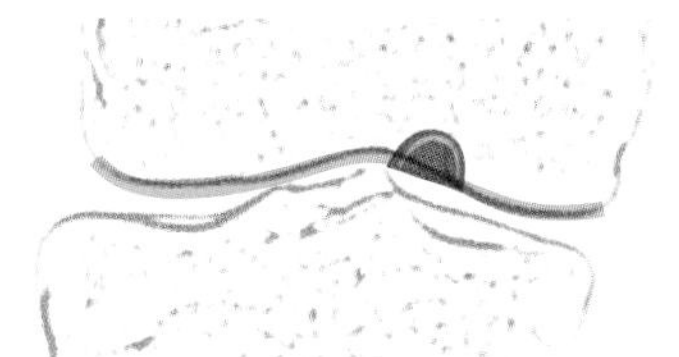

stage 3 OCD: displaceable fragment
radiograph: semicircular fragment
T2WI: high-signal line surrounding fragment

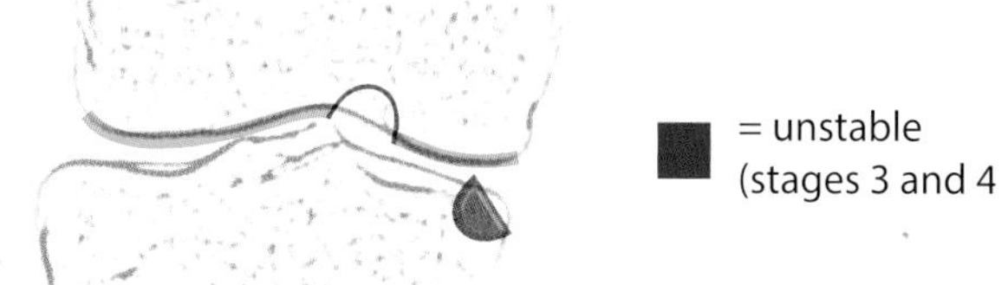

stage 4 OCD: displaced fragment
radiograph: defect or loose body
T2WI: defect and/or loose body

- *Osteochondral injury* is an acute (not repetitive) traumatic injury of cartilage and bone.

Pigmented villonodular synovitis (PVNS)

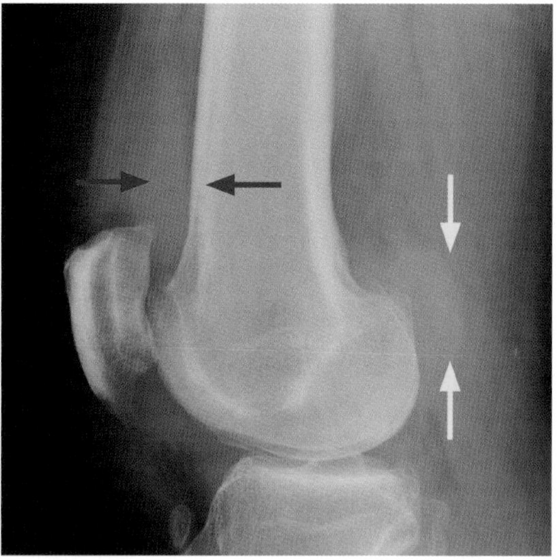

PVNS: Lateral knee radiograph shows a dense knee effusion (red arrows) and a soft-tissue mass posterior to the knee (yellow arrows).

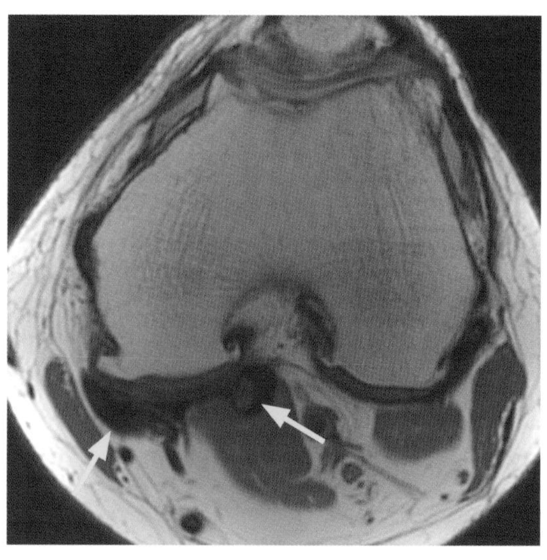

Axial proton-density MRI in the same patient shows low signal masses (arrows) posterior to the knee.

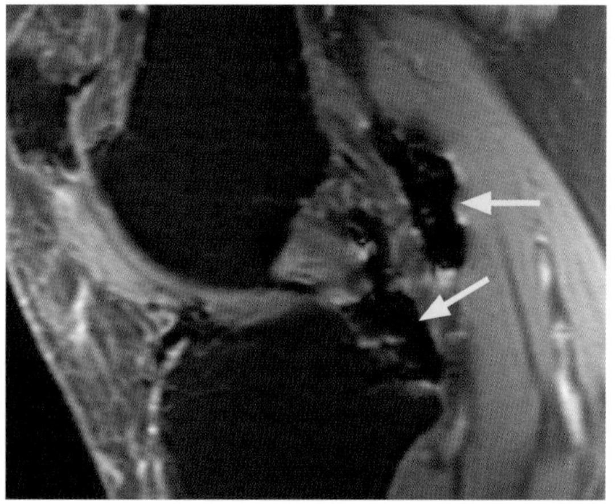

Sagittal gradient echo MRI shows the extremely dark masses accentuated by susceptibility artifact (arrows).

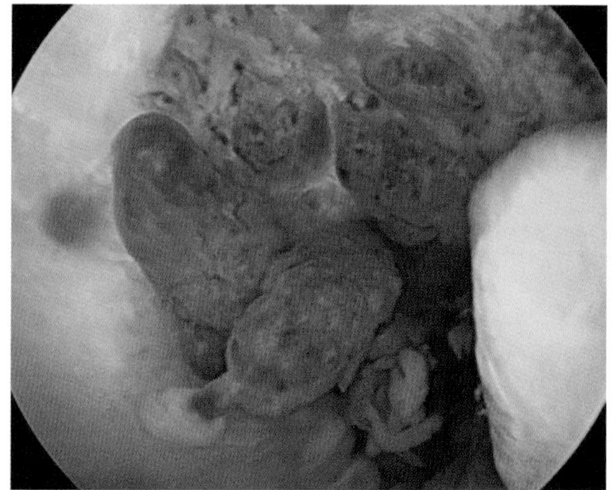

At arthroscopy, multiple synovial-based masses are evident.

- Pigmented villonodular synovitis (PVNS) is a benign hyperplastic proliferation of the synovium within the joint, now thought to represent a tumor. The same process outside of the joint is called giant cell tumor of the tendon sheath.
- The knee is by far the most common location for PVNS.
- PVNS presents as knee pain and swelling, with recurrent dark brown effusions from prior hemorrhage.
- PVNS most commonly diffusely affects a joint, but it may also be focal. Focal PVNS can clinically mimic internal derangement.
- Recurrent hemorrhage leads to residual intra-articular hemosiderin, which is paramagnetic. The paramagnetic effects of hemosiderin cause T1 prolongation and T2 shortening, resulting in dark signal on both T1- and T2-weighted images, with blooming on gradient-echo sequences.

Lipoma arborescens

- Lipoma arborescens is overgrowth of intracapsular synovial fatty tissue, causing lobulated and globular intra-articular fatty masses.
- Lipoma arborescens is treated with synovectomy to prevent premature osteoarthritis.

KNEE SOFT TISSUES

Baker's cyst

- Baker's cyst is a popliteal cyst caused from a ball-valve type communication with the knee joint.
- The typical location is between the semi**m**embranosus tendon and **m**edial head of the gastrocnemius muscle (mnemonic: Baker's **M&M**).
- An important differential consideration is a popliteal aneurysm.

Tennis leg

- Tears of either the plantaris tendon or the medial head of the gastrocnemius have both been called tennis leg.

HIP AND HIP MRI

HIP ANATOMY

Bony acetabulum

- The acetabulum is formed by the fusion of three bones: The ilium superiorly, the pubis anteriorly, and ischium posteriorly.
- Pediatric radiographs of the hip clearly show the separation of these three bones, which meet at the triradiate cartilage to form the acetabulum.

Cartilage, labrum, and ligaments

- The articular surface of the acetabulum is lined by a horseshoe-shaped thin articular cartilage. The center of the acetabulum, called the pulvinar, is not covered by cartilage.
- The labrum forms a fibrocartilaginous ring approximately 270 degrees around the periphery of the acetabulum. The labrum blends with the transverse ligament anterior/inferiorly. Note that there is no labrum at the anterior/inferior aspect of the acetabulum where the transverse ligament lies.

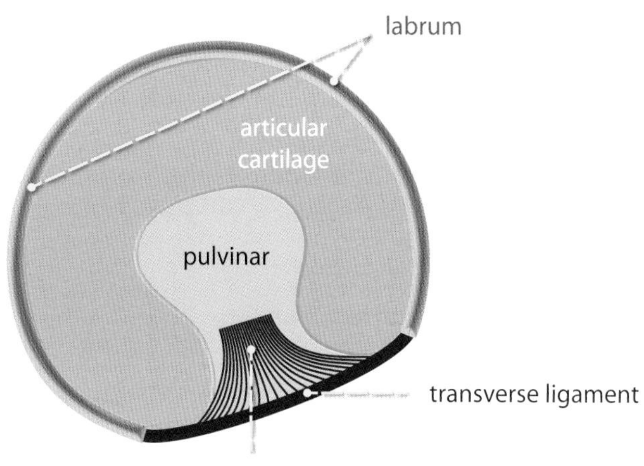

- The transverse ligament gives off fibers that form the ligamentum teres, which connects to the femoral head at its central fovea.

Cross-sectional anatomy of the hip musculature

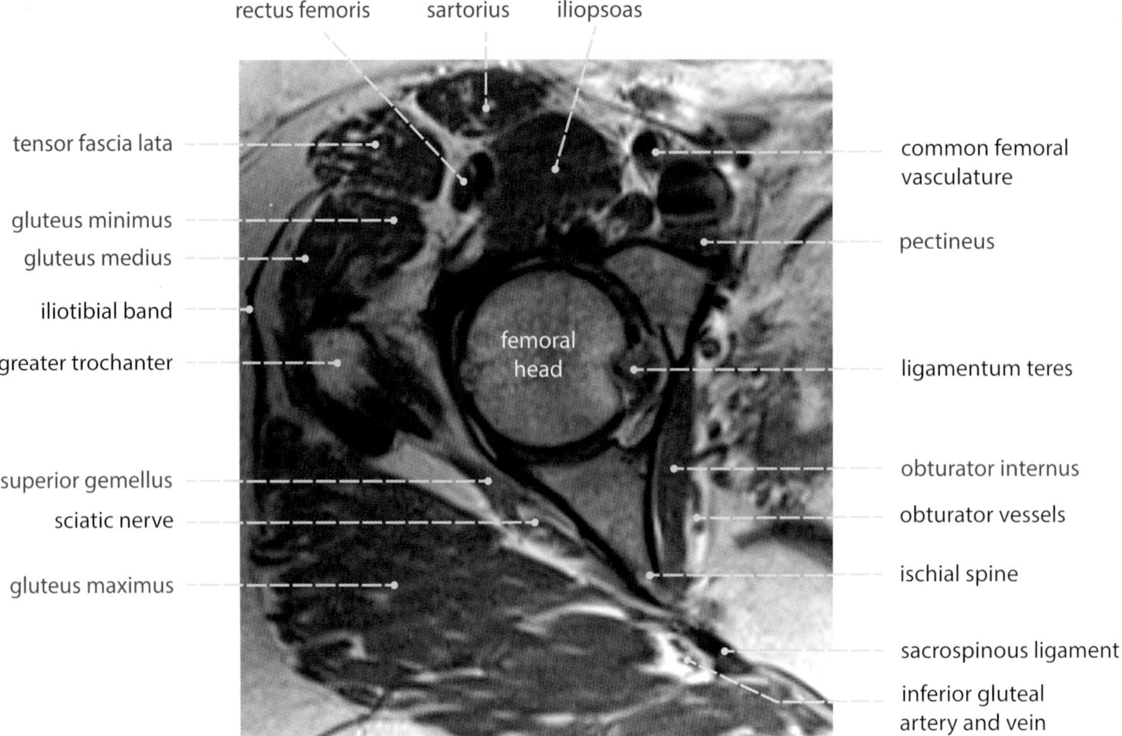

Normal radiographic anatomy of the hip

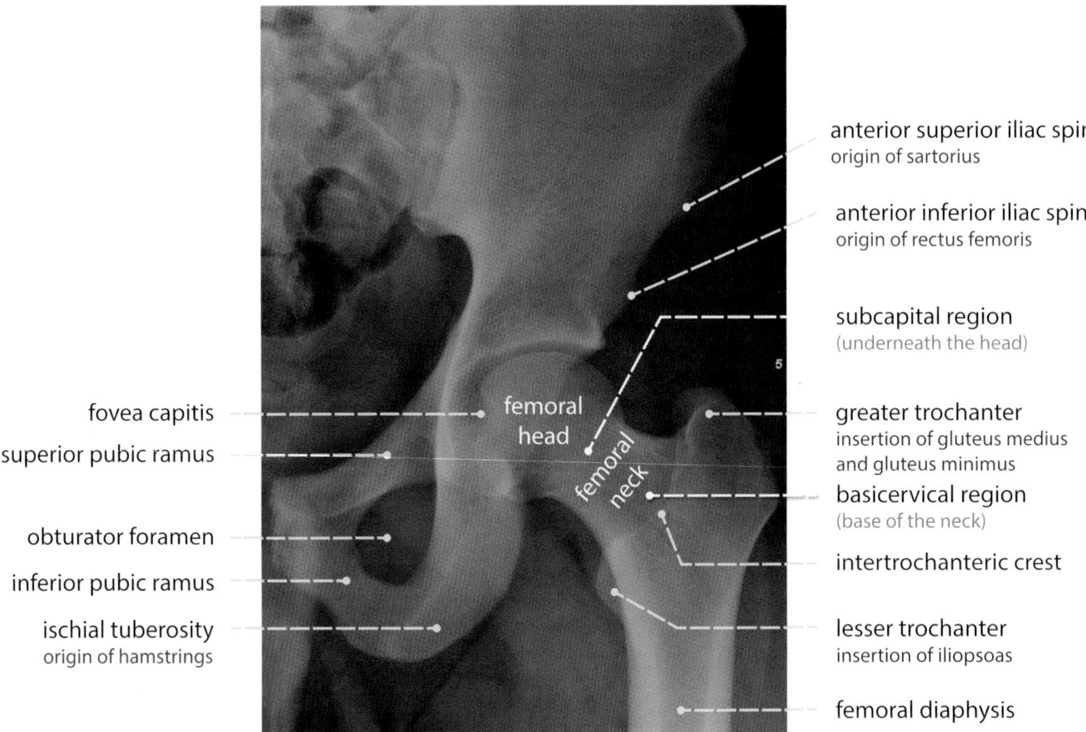

- The femoral head is mostly covered by articular cartilage except at the fovea capitis (central fovea), which is a central depression and attachment site to the ligamentum teres.
- The greater and lesser trochanters are apophyses. The greater trochanter is the insertion site for the gluteus medius, gluteus minimus, obturator internus and externus, and the piriformis. The lesser trochanter is the insertion site for the iliopsoas.

  A lesser trochanteric fracture in an adult is considered pathologic until proven otherwise.

Acetabular fracture

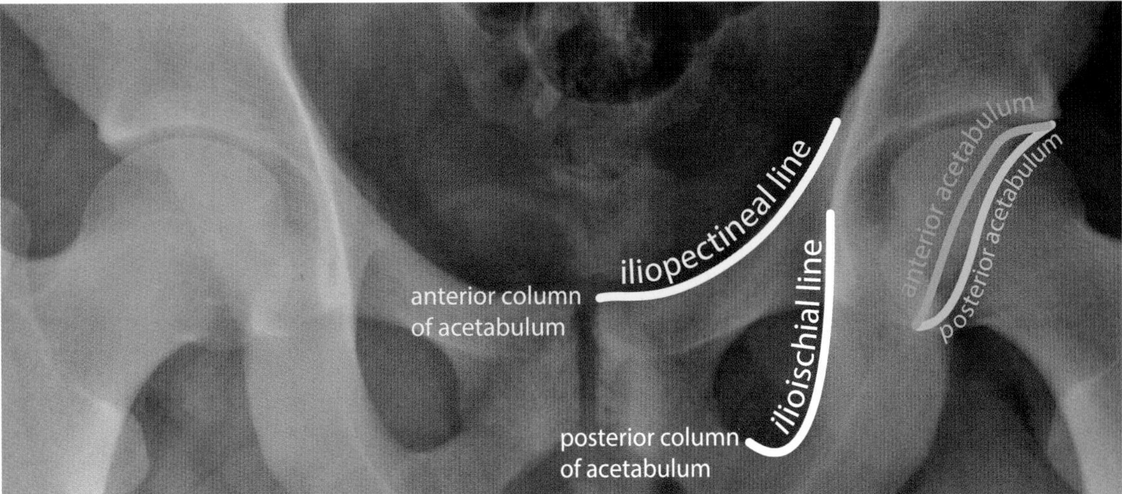

- Discontinuity of either the iliopectineal or ilioischial lines may represent a fracture of the anterior or posterior column of the acetabulum.

  The **iliopectineal line** (also called iliopubic line) represents the border of the anterior column of the acetabulum. The **ilioischial line** represents the border of the posterior column of the acetabulum.

- The anterior and posterior walls of the acetabulum can usually be directly seen projecting over the femoral head. The posterior wall is more lateral.
- Classification of acetabular fractures is complex and multiple classifications have been introduced. The most widely used classification scheme is the Judet–Letournel classification, which describes 10 types of acetabular fractures.
- The Judet–Letournel classification describes five elementary patterns: fractures of the posterior wall, posterior column, anterior wall, anterior column, and transverse fractures. Five combination patterns are also described. The Judet-Letournel types are not related to fracture complexity or prognosis.
- The posterior wall of the acetabulum is the most commonly fractured element, alone or in combination with other injuries.

Overview of proximal femur fractures

- A "hip fracture" is a nonspecific term encompassing a range of fractures of the proximal femur, including femoral head, neck, intertrochanteric, and subtrochanteric fractures.
- Femoral head and neck fractures are intracapsular. In contrast, intertrochanteric and subtrochanteric fractures are extracapsular. Extracapsular fractures are usually caused by direct injury, such as a fall, and tend to affect older individuals.
- An important complication of an intracapsular (head or neck) fracture is osteonecrosis. The majority of the blood supply to the femoral head is from the circumflex femoral arteries, which create a ring at the base of the femoral neck and send off ascending branches to the femoral head. This blood supply may be disrupted in an intracapsular fracture.

  Only minimal blood supply to the femoral head arises from small arteries in the ligamentum teres.

- In contrast to intracapsular fractures, extracapsular (intertrochanteric and subtrochanteric) fractures rarely lead to osteonecrosis. The medial femoral circumflex artery and its branches are usually not disrupted with an extracapsular fracture. Additionally, there is robust blood supply from the muscles that attach at the trochanters (gluteus medius and minimus → greater trochanter; iliopsoas → lesser trochanter).

Femoral head fracture-dislocation (intracapsular)

- Femoral head fractures are associated with posterior hip dislocations. Complications of femoral head fracture include avascular necrosis and post-traumatic arthritis.
- Orthopedists use the Pipkin classification to characterize femoral head fracture-dislocations.

  Type I: Fracture inferior to the central fovea. There is disruption of the ligamentum teres.

  Type II: Fracture superior to the central fovea. The ligamentum teres remains attached to the fracture fragment.

  Type III: Type I or II with associated femoral neck fracture.

  Type IV: Type I or II with associated superoposterior acetabular rim fracture.

Femoral neck fracture (intracapsular)

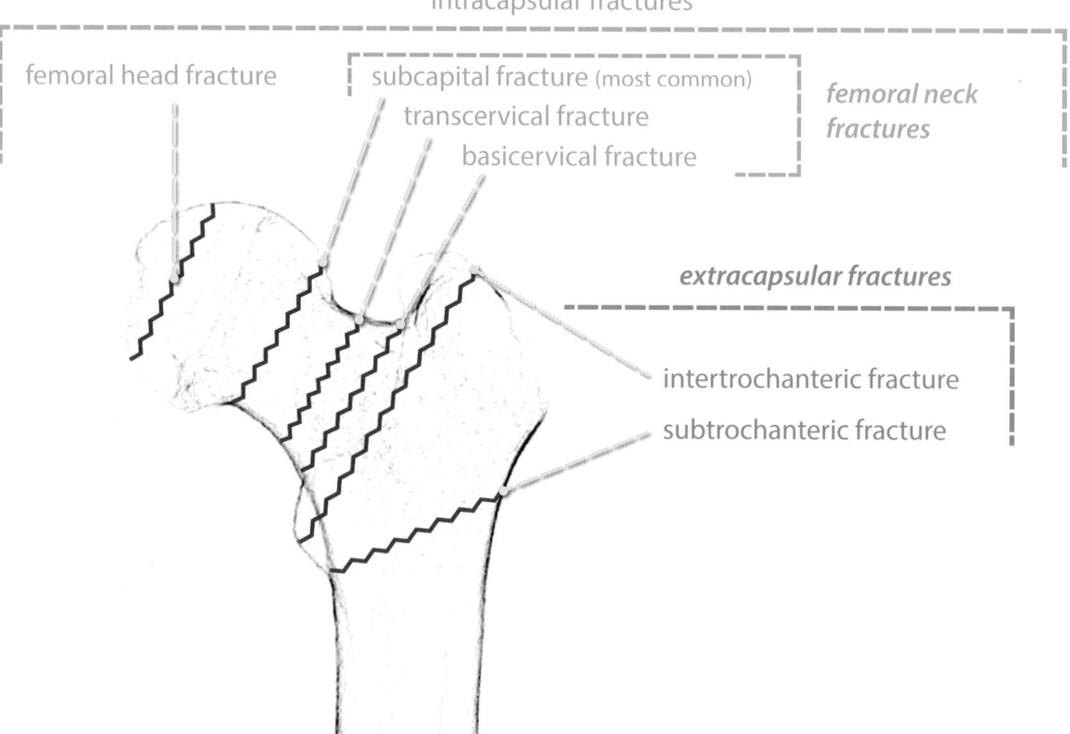

- Femoral neck fractures can be divided into three categories based on location: Subcapital (directly below the femoral head), transcervical (through the neck), and basicervical (at the base of the femoral neck). Subcapital fractures are the most common.
- The Garden classification of subcapital femoral neck fractures (diagrammed on the following page) is based on the degree of valgus displacement and is commonly used by radiologists. Note that **varus** is defined as an angle with apex pointed laterally and **valgus** is defined as an angle with apex pointed medially (mnemonic: "fair" **L**ady and "vulgar" **M**outh).

> **Stage I**: Impacted or incomplete femoral neck fracture, with valgus orientation of the femoral head/neck trabeculae and varus orientation of the femoral head and acetabulum. The femoral shaft is externally rotated. The medial trabeculae of the femoral head and neck form an angle >180°. This fracture is stable and has a good prognosis.
>
> **Stage II**: Complete, nondisplaced fracture. The trabeculae of the femoral head and neck are in mild varus and form an angle of approximately 160°. This fracture also has a good prognosis.
>
> **Stage III**: Complete, partially displaced fracture. There is more marked varus alignment of the trabecular pattern of the femoral head and neck, usually forming an angle <160°.
>
> **Stage IV**: Complete, displaced fracture. The trabecular pattern of the femoral head is aligned with that of the acetabulum, which is the normal anatomic alignment.

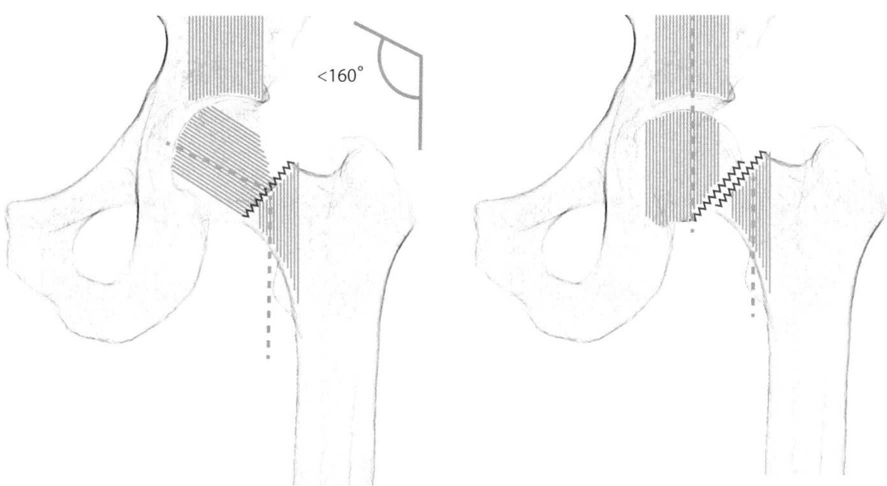

Garden stage I:
impacted or incomplete fracture
trabeculae of femoral head and neck are in valgus (>180°)
>180°
Garden stage II:
complete, nondisplaced fracture
trabeculae of femoral head and neck are in varus, usually forming an angle of approximately 160°
~160°
Garden stage III:
complete, partially displaced fracture
trabeculae of femoral head and neck are in more marked varus, usually forming an angle <160°
<160°
Garden stage IV:
complete, fully displaced fracture
trabeculae of femoral head , neck, and acetabulum are aligned

Intertrochanteric fracture (extracapsular)

- The Boyd–Griffin and Evans classifications are used to describe intertrochanteric fractures by orthopedists. These classifications are rarely used by radiologists.

Subtrochanteric fracture (extracapsular)

- Fractures at or inferior to the lesser trochanter are subtrochanteric fractures. Subtrochanteric fractures are classified using the Fielding or Seinsheimer classifications by orthopedists.

Hip MRI technique

Imaging of metallic hip arthroplasties

- It is possible to image metallic hip arthroplasties by optimizing MRI technique. In general, field strength should be as low as reasonable and fast spin echo sequences should be used instead of GRE.
- The receiver bandwidth should be increased as much as possible. This will increase the amount of noise, so the number of acquisitions (NEX) will need to be proportionally increased.
- Artifacts can be directed in the superior–inferior plane so the region directly medial and lateral to the implant (where loosening would be seen) is not obscured.
- Voxel size should be decreased by decreasing slice thickness and increasing the matrix size.

Indications for hip MRI

Occult traumatic fracture

- Radiographs are relatively insensitive for the detection of a nondisplaced femoral neck fracture.
- The MRI appearance of a fracture is a hypointense fracture line on T1- and T2-weighted images, associated with hyperintense edema signal on T2-weighted images.
- MRI may be able to suggest an alternative etiology for the patient's pain. For instance, a sacral fracture may clinically present as hip pain.

Occult stress fracture

- Stress fractures can be categorized as **fatigue** fractures (due to abnormal stress on normal bone) and **insufficiency** fractures (due to normal stress on demineralized bone).
- Radiographs are relatively insensitive for detection of hip stress fractures. When visible on a radiograph, a stress fracture typically appears as a band of sclerosis.
- MRI appearance of a stress fracture is similar to an acute traumatic fracture with a hypointense fracture line associated with hyperintense edema signal on T2-weighted MRI.
- A classic location of a stress fracture is the inferomedial femoral neck.
- Less commonly, a stress fracture may occur in the superior femoral head.

  Superior femoral head stress fractures may be difficult to differentiate from avascular necrosis (AVN), especially if large field of view imaging of both hips is acquired.

  Both AVN and fracture are characterized by a subchondral hypointense line on T1-weighted images; however, it has been suggested that the shape of the hypointense line in the coronal plane may be able to differentiate between AVN and subchondral insufficiency fracture. The hypointense line of AVN is typically smooth and concave to the articular surface, while subchondral insufficiency fracture usually produces an irregular low-intensity fracture line convex to the articular surface. Additionally, a history of corticosteroid use or alcohol abuse is typically present with AVN.

- Atypical locations of femoral stress fractures, such as lateral femoral diaphyseal and transverse diaphyseal fractures, may be secondary to bisphosphonate use.
- Treatment of stress fractures is typically conservative and a follow-up MRI in 8 weeks should show resolution of the edema. Persistent edema on the follow-up study suggests treatment failure.
- In addition to the proximal femur, stress fractures may occur at several sites in the pelvis, including the superior and inferior pubic rami, sacrum, and acetabular roof.

Avascular necrosis (AVN)

- Avascular necrosis (AVN) is focal ischemia of the epiphyseal region or subchondral bone. AVN leads to trabecular necrosis, which increases susceptibility to stress fracture, eventual collapse, and secondary osteoarthritis if untreated. The more general term *osteonecrosis* indicates necrosis of bone and marrow elements.
- The femoral head is especially susceptible to AVN because of precarious blood supply. The blood supply to the femoral head is primarily through the medial femoral circumflex artery, which enters the femoral neck and gives off posterosuperior epiphyseal branches that course along the femoral neck to supply the femoral head.
- As previously discussed, intracapsular proximal femur fractures have a high risk of AVN, including femoral neck fractures in the elderly and transient subluxation in athletes.
- Nontraumatic causes of AVN are usually systemic, including red-cell abnormalities (e.g., sickle cell disease), abnormalities of marrow packing (e.g., Gaucher disease), or secondary effects of medications including steroids, alcohol, or immunosuppression from transplant. Systemic causes of AVN tend to be bilateral.

  A clue to the presence of Gaucher disease is splenomegaly with AVN.

  A clue to the presence of sickle cell is a small calcified spleen with AVN.
- The most common site of AVN is the proximal femur. The second most common site is the proximal humerus.
- The **Ficat** staging system is based on *radiographic* appearance.

  Stage 1: Normal radiograph, with signs of AVN visible on MRI (discussed below) or bone scan (reduced tracer uptake in the femoral head). Treatment is core femoral head drilling.

  Stage 2: Cystic and sclerotic changes. Treatment is same as stage I.

  Stage 3: There is loss of the normal spherical shape of the femoral had due to collapse of subchondral bone. A subchondral lucent line representing the *crescent* sign may be visible on radiographs. Treatment is variable.

  Stage 4: Flattening of the femoral head and secondary osteoarthritis. Treatment is joint replacement.
- Several systems have been proposed for the MRI classification of AVN, including a modified Ficat system and the Mitchell system. The Mitchell system characterizes the changes in MRI signal only. It has been suggested that the modified Ficat system is more clinically useful as it accounts for the progression in ischemia that results in collapse of the femoral head.
- The most common appearance of AVN on MRI is a geographic subchondral lesion outlined by a serpentine low signal rim on T1-weighted images. The subchondral anterior-superior portions of the femoral head, at 10 o'clock and 2 o'clock on coronal images, are typical locations.
- The *double line* sign is seen on T2-weighted MRI and is comprised of a peripheral low-intensity rim and an inner high-intensity band. The double line sign is thought to be pathognomonic for AVN.
- Bone marrow edema is present in 50% and clinically correlates with pain.
- The complete description of AVN should include the presence of collapse (CT is most sensitive, followed by radiographs), the size of the T1 signal abnormality (as percentage of involved areas of the femoral head), and presence of secondary involvement of the acetabulum.

Transient bone marrow edema (TBME)

- Transient bone marrow edema (TBME), also called transient osteoporosis of the hip, is a controversial entity that is a diagnosis of exclusion and may actually reflect a combination of disorders including sympathetic nervous system overactivity, stress fracture, or transient ischemia.
- The traditional teaching is that TBME is a self-limited clinical entity lasting a few months. It is characterized by severe hip pain in young to middle-aged adults (more commonly men, although it was first described in women in the third trimester of pregnancy).
- Radiographs show regional osteopenia in the femoral head without any secondary signs of arthritis. The cartilage space is preserved and there are no erosions or morphologic abnormalities of the acetabulum.
- T1-weighted MRI shows diffuse low signal corresponding to diffusely high signal on T2-weighted images. The signal abnormality may extend from the femoral head into the femoral neck.
- As TBME may be a wastebasket diagnosis, it is essential to always evaluate for subtle lesions to explain these findings. For instance, a subchondral hypointense line on T1-weighted images may represent a fracture, or a small focus of AVN may be apparent.

Labral injury

- The acetabular labrum is analogous to the glenoid labrum in the shoulder. The acetabular labrum is a ring of fibrocartilage that functionally deepens the acetabulum. Unlike the shoulder, however, the femoroacetabular joint is a ball-in-socket joint that is inherently stable and does not rely on the extensive ligamentous and muscular support that maintains active and passive stability in the shoulder.
- Some authors advocate that hip labral injuries be called detachments rather than tears, but the use of this suggested terminology is inconsistent.
- Although labral detachment may be due to acute trauma, labral injuries are more commonly due to chronic repetitive microtrauma. Femoroacetabular morphologic abnormalities, such as developmental dysplasia of the hip (discussed in the pediatric imaging section) and femoral acetabular impingement may predispose to labral injury.
- Labral injuries are best diagnosed with MR arthrography, which shows focal contrast undermining a portion of the labrum.
- The most common location for labral injury is anterosuperior. There is no labrum at the inferior aspect of the hip joint.

Femoroacetabular impingement (FAI)

Overview and controversy of femoroacetabular impingement (FAI)

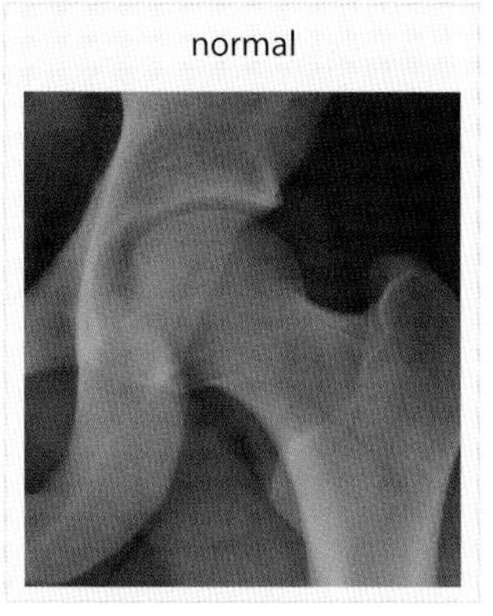

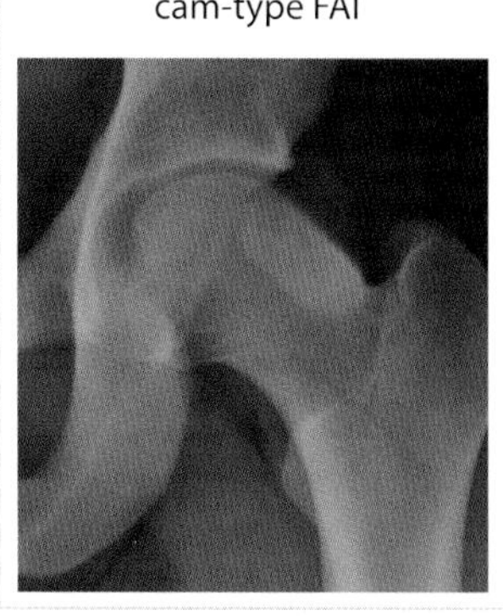

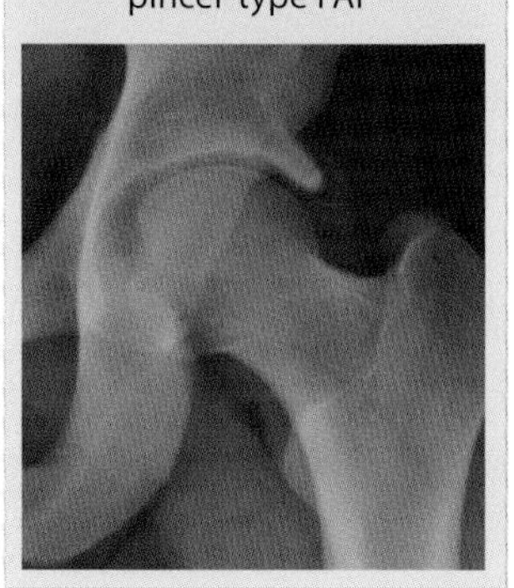

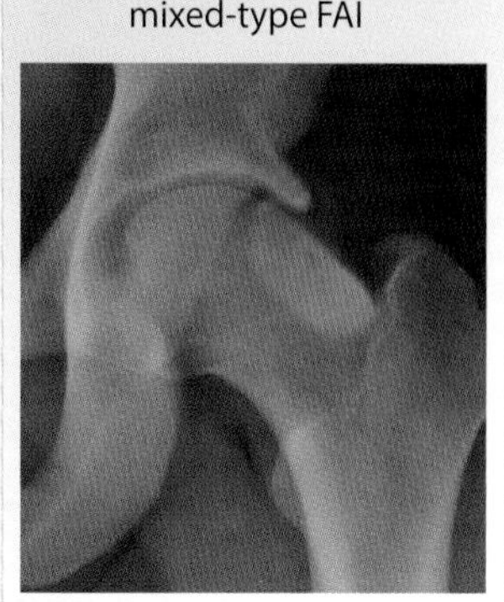

- Femoroacetabular impingement (FAI) is abnormal abutment of the femur with the acetabulum at extremes of range of motion.
- Two types of impingement have been described, depending on whether the femoral head/neck junction (cam-type) or the acetabulum (pincer-type) is abnormal.
- Chronic microtrauma of the femoral head abutting against the acetabulum may cause acetabular labral tears in young athletic individuals and may accelerate the development of hip osteoarthritis.
- While FAI may be an important cause of hip osteoarthritis in young patients, there is controversy as to whether a diagnosis of impingement can be made based on the imaging findings in the absence of the clinical syndrome.
- Impingement is primarily a clinical diagnosis and there is a significant subset of patients with abnormal morphology of the acetabulum or femoral head/neck junction who are asymptomatic.
- Labral injury secondary to FAI (typically occurring in the anterosuperior labrum) is often associated with underlying chondral injury as well.
- Regardless of the controversy, FAI is an important concept to be aware of in the young adult. A general consensus is that imaging findings suggestive of FAI should be described with the disclaimer that these findings may predispose to impingement in the presence of pain.

Cam-type impingement

- An abnormal bump at the femoral head–neck junction may be due to a variety of causes, such as childhood slipped capital femoral epiphysis, Legg–Calve–Perthes disease, sequela of developmental hip dysplasia (which ironically is characterized by acetabular *undercoverage)*, and malunited fracture.
- Cam-type impingement is most common in young athletic males.
- The *pistol-grip deformity* describes the abnormal morphology of the femoral head–neck junction that resembles an old-time pistol, with the femoral head/neck representing the handle and the femoral diaphysis the barrel.
- The alpha angle defines the degree of abnormal femoral bump. An alpha angle is measured on oblique axial MRI or CT. An alpha angle of >55 degrees is abnormal.

  To measure the alpha angle, a line through the femoral neck bisecting the center of the femoral head is interfaced with a second line connecting the center of the femoral head to the most proximal abnormal contour of the femoral head/neck.
- Cam-type impingement is treated with femoral osteoplasty.

Pincer-type impingement

- Pincer-type FAI is caused by overcoverage of the acetabulum.
- Pincer-type impingement is most common in middle-aged females.
- The *crossover* sign (also called cranial acetabular retroversion) is seen in pincer-type FAI and represents the superior aspect of the anterior acetabular wall crossing over the posterior acetabular wall on a frontal radiograph.

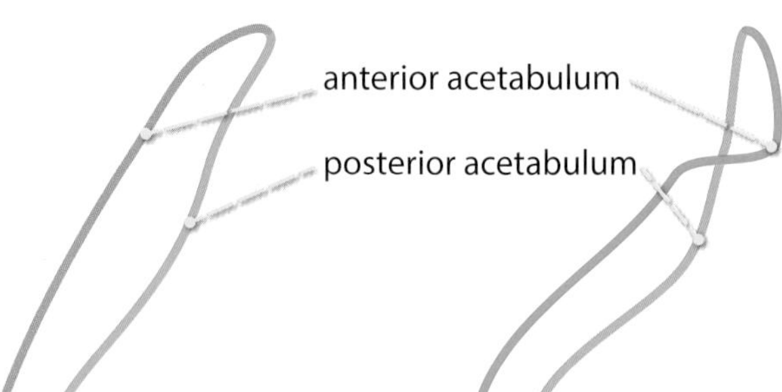

- Treatment of pincer-type FAI is surgical trimming of the acetabular rim.

Mixed-type impingement

- Mixed-type impingement is the most common form of FAI. It features abnormalities of both the femoral head/neck junction and the acetabulum.

Lumbar/Thoracic Spine

Lumbar/Thoracic Spine Trauma

Three column concept

- The three column concept of functional spinal anatomy helps to evaluate the stability of thoracolumbar spinal trauma. A spinal injury where the integrity of two of the three columns is preserved is generally considered stable, while a severe injury to all three columns is most likely to be unstable. Two column injuries may be stable or unstable.
- The *anterior column* is comprised of the anterior two thirds of the vertebral body, including the anterior longitudinal ligament.
- The *middle column* consists of the posterior third of the vertebral body and the posterior longitudinal ligament.
- The *posterior column* represents the posterior elements and the posterior ligaments (consisting of the supraspinous and infraspinous ligaments, and the ligamentum flavum).

Chance fracture

- A Chance fracture, also known as a *seat belt* fracture, is a flexion distraction injury caused by acute forward flexion of the spine during sudden deceleration.
- There is horizontal splitting of the vertebra, beginning posteriorly in the spinous process or lamina and extending anteriorly through the vertebral body.

Spondylolysis

- Spondylolysis is a fracture of the pars interarticularis, which may be secondary to chronic stress or an acute fracture.
- On oblique radiographs, spondylolysis is seen as a defect in the neck of the "scotty dog."
- Spondylolysis leads to spondylolisthesis, which is anterior–posterior subluxation of one vertebral body relative to another.

CERVICAL SPINE TRAUMA

- Intervals: The **basion-dental interval** and **atlanto-dental interval** (also known as the atlanto-axial interval) should be evaluated in every lateral cervical spine radiograph. An increased basion-dental interval >12 mm suggests craniocervical dissociation. An increased atlanto-dental interval >2.5 mm (some authors suggest 3 mm as a cutoff) can be seen in ligamentous laxity and resultant subluxation.

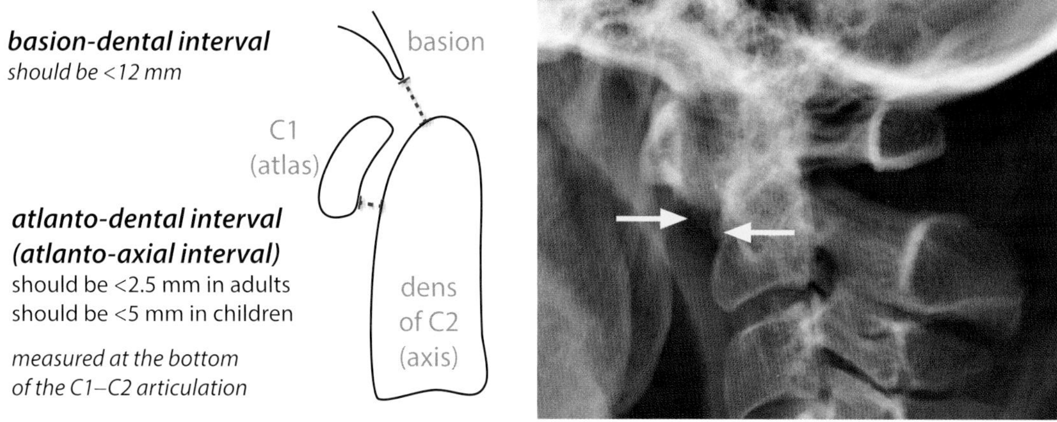

The atlanto-dental interval (ADI), also known as the atlanto-axial interval, should <2.5 mm in adults. Lateral cervical spine radiograph shows widening of the ADI (arrows) to >1 cm, indicative of anterior subluxation.

The C1 vertebral body is known as the *atlas* (who carried the globe on his shoulders) and does not have a body; instead it provides structural support via its lateral masses. C2 is known as the *axis* (allows rotation).

- Lines: Every lateral cervical spine radiograph should be evaluated for continuity and smoothness of the four primary osseous contours.

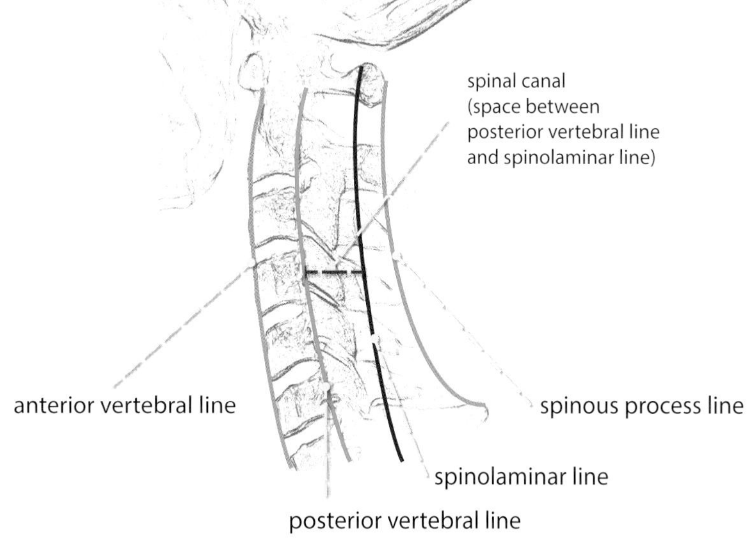

Anterior vertebral line: Traces the anterior margin of the vertebral bodies. The prevertebral soft tissues are located anterior to the anterior vertebral line.

Posterior vertebral line: Traces the posterior margin of the vertebral bodies and the anterior margin of the spinal canal. The spinal canal is the space between the posterior vertebral and spinolaminar lines.

Spinolaminar line: Traces the posterior margin of the spinal canal.

Spinous process line: Traces the posterior tips of the spinous processes.

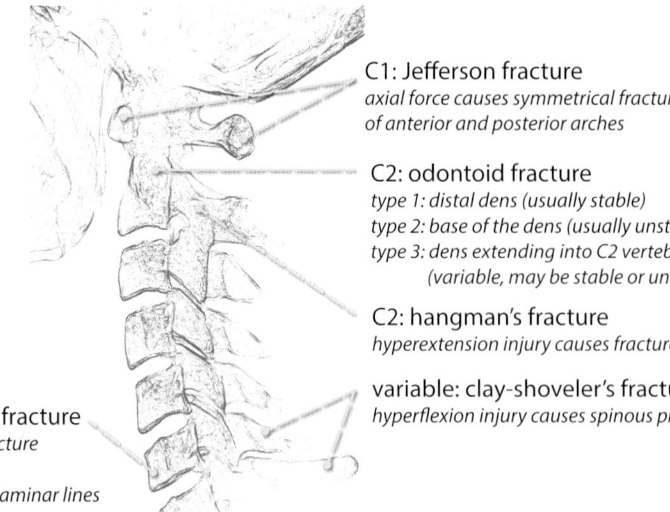
C1: Jefferson fracture
axial force causes symmetrical fractures of anterior and posterior arches
C2: odontoid fracture
type 1: distal dens (usually stable)
type 2: base of the dens (usually unstable)
type 3: dens extending into C2 vertebral body (variable, may be stable or unstable)
C2: hangman's fracture
hyperextension injury causes fracture of the arches of C2
variable: clay-shoveler's fracture
hyperflexion injury causes spinous process fracture
variable: flexion teardrop fracture
most unstable cervical spine fracture associated with disruption of posterior vertebral and spinolaminar lines

Jefferson fracture

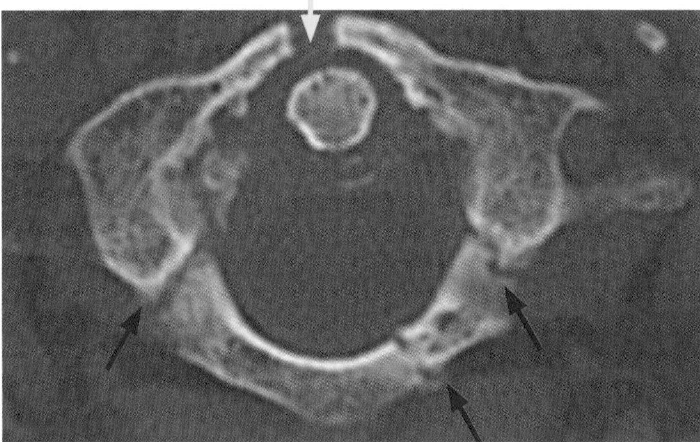

Jefferson fracture: Axial CT demonstrates a fracture of the anterior arch of C1 near the midline (yellow arrow) and bilateral posterior arch fractures (red arrows).

- A Jefferson fracture results from acute axial blow to the vertex of the head, causing symmetrical fractures of the anterior and posterior arches of C1.
- On an open-mouth odontoid radiograph, the lateral masses of C1 are displaced laterally. Jefferson fracture is best seen on axial CT, however.

Odontoid fracture

- Fractures of the odontoid process of C2 are usually caused by flexion injuries.
- **Type I** odontoid fracture is a fracture of the distal tip of the dens. Type I odontoid fractures are considered stable and treatment is generally conservative. The differential diagnosis of a Type I odontoid fracture is an os odontoideum, a normal variant secondary ossification center located at the tip of the dens.
- **Type II** odontoid fracture is a fracture of the base of the dens. It is considered an unstable injury and treatment is typically surgical fusion.
- **Type III** odontoid fracture is a fracture of the base of the dens extending into the C2 vertebral body. Type III fractures have been described as stable and unstable, depending on the reference.

Hangman's fracture

- Hangman's fracture is traumatic spondylolysis of C2. It results from hyperextension and distraction, causing bilateral fractures through the pedicles of C2.
- The characteristic radiographic finding is disruption of the spinolaminar line.
- A hangman's fracture with >3 mm displacement of C2 on C3 is likely unstable.

Burst fracture

- A burst fracture is similar in mechanism (axial loading) and appearance to a Jefferson fracture, but occurs lower in the cervical spine, at C2–C7.

Flexion teardrop fracture

- Flexion teardrop fracture is the most severe cervical spinal injury that is potentially compatible with life. It is caused by a hyperflexion and compression injury and results in posterior displacement of the affected vertebral body into the spinal canal.
- The key radiographic finding is an avulsed bony fragment from the anterior-inferior aspect of the vertebral body, caused by anterior longitudinal ligament avulsion. There is retropulsion of the affected vertebral body, which is often rotated and appears shorter in anterior–posterior dimension than the adjacent vertebrae.
- Flexion teardrop fracture can cause anterior cord syndrome due to compression of the pyramidal tracts and anterior spinothalamic tracts. This clinically presents as complete paralysis and loss of pain and temperature sensation. The dorsal column usually remains intact, preserving touch and vibration sense.

Extension teardrop fracture

- In contrast to a flexion teardrop fracture, an extension teardrop fracture is a stable fracture that usually occurs higher in the cervical spine, at C2 or C3.
- On the lateral radiograph, an anterior/inferior avulsion fragment is seen, similar to flexion teardrop. Unlike a flexion teardrop fracture, there is no subluxation and the spinolaminar line is not disrupted.

Clay-shoveler's fracture

- A clay-shoveler's fracture is a displaced avulsion fracture of a spinous process. It is caused by forced flexion.
- Clay-shoveler's fracture occurs in the lower cervical/upper thoracic spine, from C6–T1.

Bilateral interfacetal dislocation (locked facets)

- Bilateral interfacetal dislocation, also called bilateral locked facets, is a hyperflexion injury caused by complete disruption of all spinal ligaments and resultant anterior dislocation of the affected vertebra by >50%.
- Bilateral interfacetal dislocation is unstable with a high risk of cord damage.
- Bilateral interfacetal dislocation typically occurs in the lower cervical spine.
- The *naked facet* sign is seen when the superior articular facets are not covered by the adjacent inferior articular facets.
- *Perched facets* are a less severe variation of locked facets. The inferior articular facets of the superior vertebral body are subluxated (but not displaced) and *perched* upon the superior articular process of the inferior vertebra. Perched facets feature anterior subluxation of >3 mm but less than the 50% seen in a complete dislocation.

Unilateral interfacetal dislocation

- Unilateral interfacetal dislocation is dislocation of a single facet joint, caused by hyperflexion with rotation opposite the site of the dislocation.
- Unilateral interfacetal dislocation is considered a stable fracture.

Grisel syndrome

- Grisel syndrome is nontraumatic rotatory subluxation of the atlantoaxial joint (C1–C2) secondary to an inflammatory mass, most commonly occurring as a sequela of pharyngitis or retropharyngeal abscess.

Bony anatomy of the shoulder

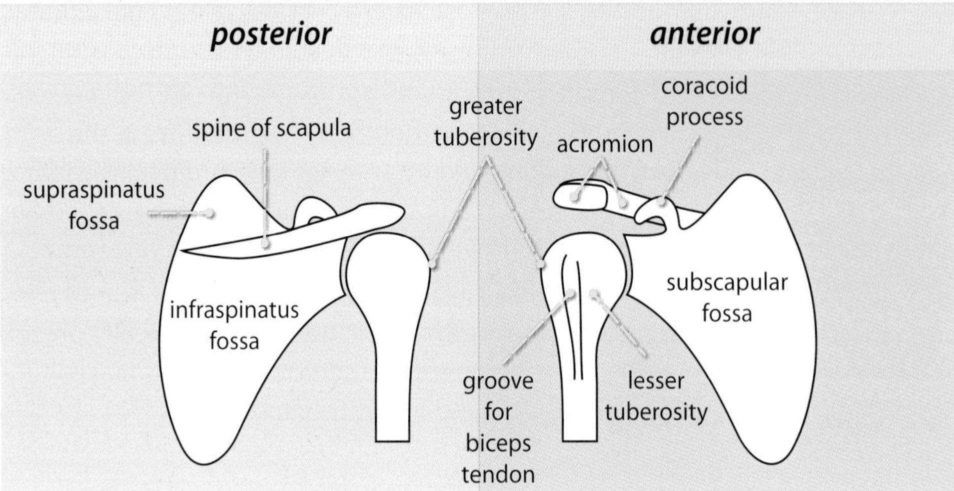

Acromioclavicular joint

Acromioclavicular (AC) joint separation

- Injuries to the acromioclavicular (AC) joint typically occur in young athletic adults, most commonly from a downward blow to the lateral shoulder. AC joint injuries range from an AC ligament sprain (grade I) to complete disruption of the AC joint capsule and associated coracoclavicular (CC) ligaments (grades III–VI).
- The normal AC joint space should be <5 mm and the normal CC distance is <11–13 mm, with a wide range of normal variation. An asymmetry of >50% side-to-side is abnormal. Passive traction, with the patient holding a weight, may be necessary to unmask an injury.
- Displacement of the acromion and clavicle determines AC ligament integrity, while the coracoclavicular interspace is assessed to evaluate the CC ligaments.
- Grade I: AC ligament sprain. Radiographs are normal.
- Grade II: Disruption of the AC ligament with intact CC ligaments.
- Grade III: AC joint and CC ligamentous disruption. CC interspace is widened 25–100% relative to the contralateral side.
- Grade IV: Distal clavicle displaced posteriorly into trapezius (seen on CT or axillary view).
- Grade V: Severe grade III injury, with >100% displacement relative to the other side.
- Grade VI: Inferior dislocation of the distal clavicle.

Glenohumeral dislocation

Anterior glenohumeral dislocation

- Anterior dislocation of the humerus with respect to the glenoid is by far the most common type of shoulder dislocation. Anterior dislocation is usually caused by direct force on the arm. The humeral head usually dislocates in an antero-inferior direction.
- Diagnosis of anterior dislocation is best made on an axillary view.
- As the humeral head recoils from the dislocation force, the posterolateral humeral head strikes the anterior-inferior glenoid. This impaction may fracture the humeral head, the glenoid, or both.

- The **Hill–Sachs** lesion is a compression fracture of the posterolateral aspect of the humeral head (**H**ill–Sachs and **h**umerus both start with **H**). On radiography, the Hill-Sachs lesion is best demonstrated on an AP radiograph with the arm in internal rotation.
- The **Bankart** lesion is an injury of the anterior-inferior rim of the glenoid. It usually involves the cartilaginous labrum only. A bony Bankart is a fracture of the bony glenoid.

Posterior glenohumeral dislocation

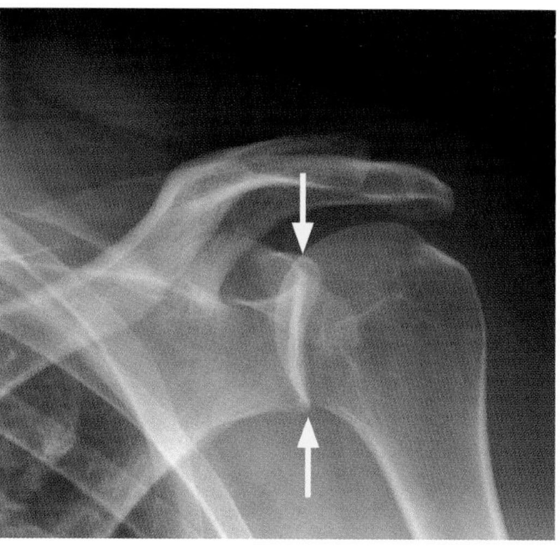
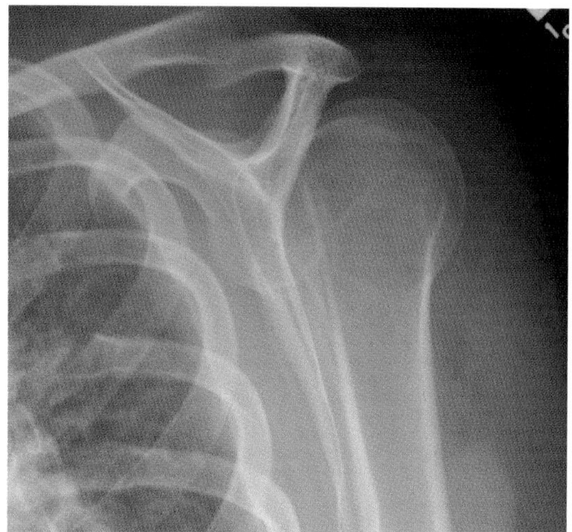

Posterior shoulder dislocation: Grashey (40 degree oblique; left image) radiograph shows overlap of the humeral head and the glenoid (arrows); normally, the glenohumeral joint space should be clear on this view. Posterior displacement of the humerus with respect to the glenoid is confirmed on the transscapular Y view (right image).

- Posterior dislocation represents only 2–3% of dislocations and is usually due to severe muscle spasm, such as from seizure or electrocution. The humeral head is dislocated posteriorly in these situations since the posterior pulling muscles of the back are generally stronger than the anterior pushing muscles.
- Diagnosis of a posterior dislocation is much more challenging compared to an anterior dislocation, as the standard frontal radiograph of the shoulder may look close to normal.
- Transscapular Y view or axillary view will best show the posterior dislocation.

  When possible, diagnosis is usually straightforward on an axillary view; however, many patients with posterior shoulder dislocation will not be able to abduct the arm.
- In a normal shoulder, a Grashey (40 degree oblique) view should show clear space between the glenoid and the humeral head; however, in case of posterior dislocation there will be overlap of the medially displaced humeral head with the glenoid.
- The *lightbulb* sign describes the appearance of the humeral head due to the fixed internal rotation of the arm often seen in posterior dislocation.
- The *trough* sign describes a compression fracture of the anteromedial aspect of the humeral head, also known as a reverse Hill–Sachs, from impaction of the humeral head on the posterior glenoid rim upon recoil.

Inferior glenohumeral dislocation (luxatio erecta)

- Inferior dislocation, also called *luxatio erecta,* is rare (occurring in approximately 1% of dislocations) and is usually caused by direct force to a fully abducted arm.
- Inferior dislocation is often associated with rotator cuff tear and greater tuberosity fracture.
- Inferior dislocation may cause injury to the axillary nerve or artery.

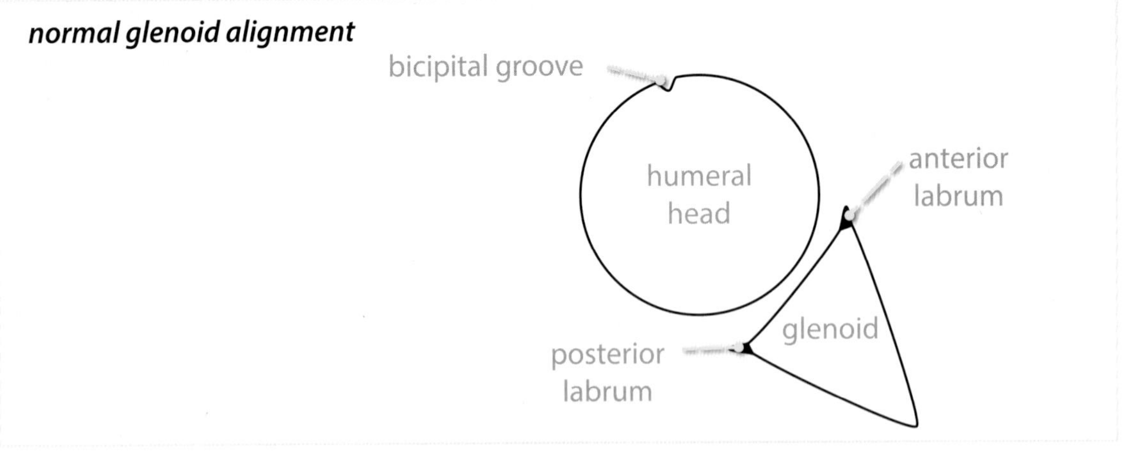

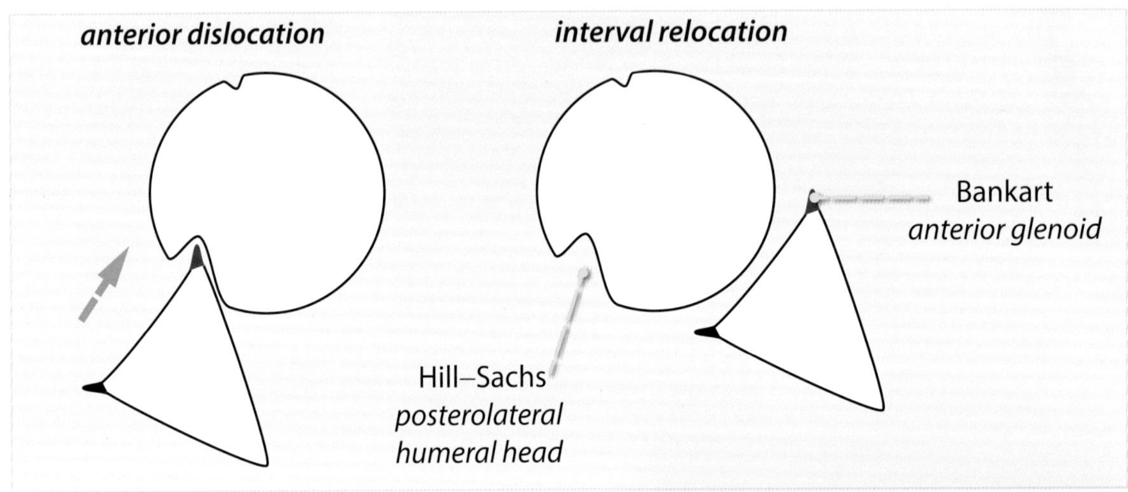

Hill–Sachs: Axial T1-weighted MR arthrogram with fat suppression shows a wedge-shaped compression fracture of the posterolateral humeral head (arrow).

Case courtesy Kirstin Small, MD, Brigham and Women's Hospital.

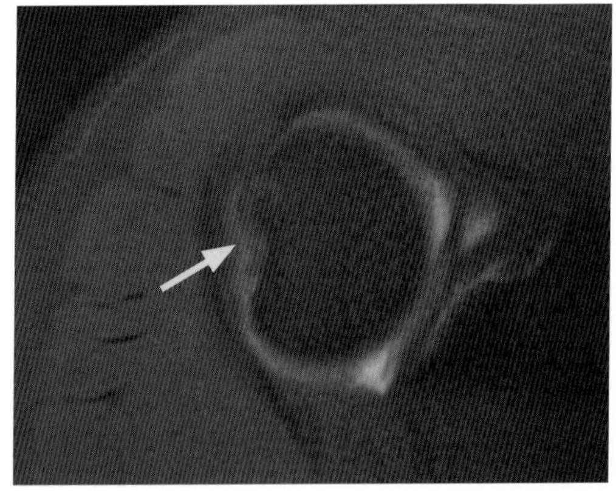

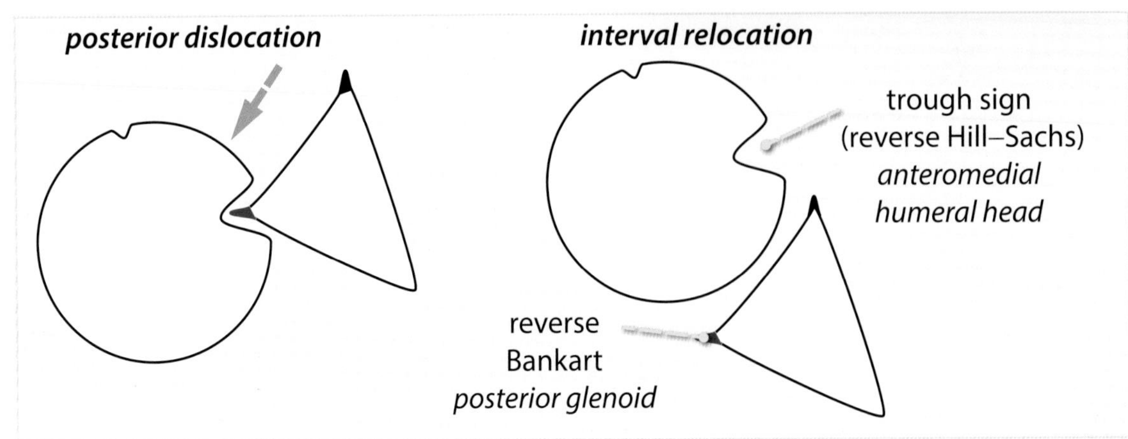

SHOULDER BURSAE

- The subacromial and subdeltoid bursae normally communicate with each other. This combined subacromial/subdeltoid bursa is not normally in communication with the glenohumeral joint.
- Fluid injected into the glenohumeral joint that extends into the subacromial/subdeltoid bursa is seen with a complete rotator cuff tear. A gap in the rotator cuff will almost always be evident.

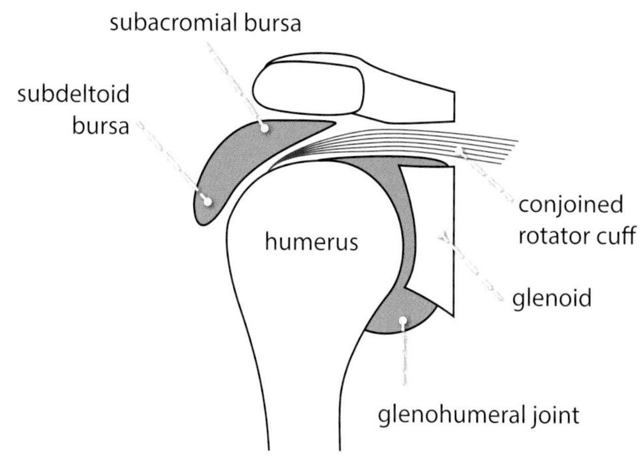

CORACOACROMIAL ARCH AND IMPINGEMENT SYNDROME

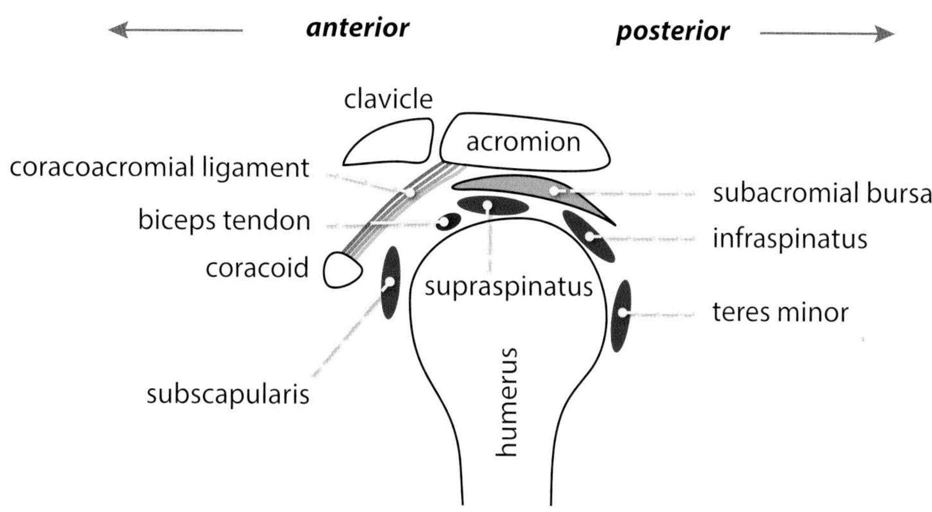

- Impingement syndrome is a clinical diagnosis that can have a variety of causes and MRI findings. Shoulder impingement was originally described as chronic compression/irritation of the structures that pass through the coracoacromial arch, including the supraspinatus tendon, biceps tendon, and subacromial bursa.
- Rotator cuff tears are often associated with chronic impingement, although there is controversy whether the cuff tears are a result of chronic mechanical impingement or whether degeneration leads to cuff tears, resulting in impingement syndrome.
- **Extrinsic impingement** is caused by structural abnormalities external to the joint and is divided into primary and subcoracoid impingement.

  Primary external impingement is common and is due to a variation in the anatomy of the coracoacromial arch (e.g., subacromial enthesophyte, hooked acromion, AC joint osteophytes, os acromiale, or thickened coracoacromial ligament). Primary external impingement is typically seen in young athletes involved with throwing or repetitive overhead movement. Chronic primary external impingement may cause the supraspinatus tendon and/or the proximal aspect of the long head of the biceps tendon to become degenerated, partially torn, or even completely torn. The subacromial bursa, immediately inferior to the acromion, may become inflamed, leading to subacromial/subdeltoid bursitis.

  Subcoracoid impingement is less common and occurs when the coracohumeral distance narrows.
- **Intrinsic impingement** is related to glenohumeral instability and is caused by abnormalities of the rotator cuff and joint capsule, without abnormality of the coracoacromial arch.

Acromial shape and orientation

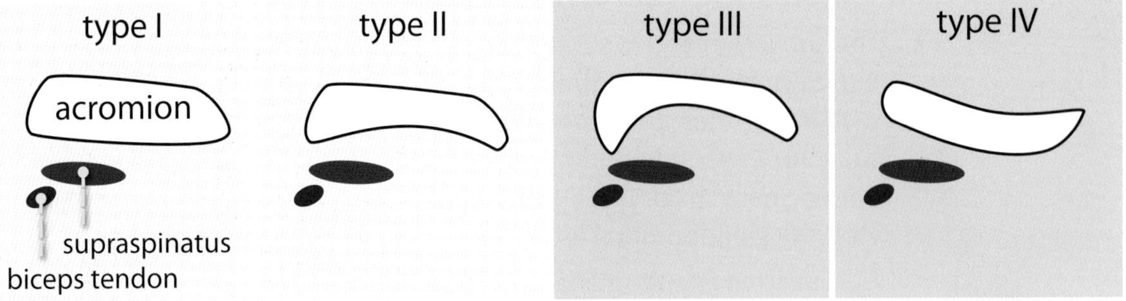

- The impact of acromial shape on impingement syndrome is controversial. An acromion with a hooked undersurface (type III) or convex undersurface (type IV) may contribute to impingement (primary external type) and lead to subsequent rotator cuff tears.
- Friction of the acromion against the immediately underlying supraspinatus and biceps tendons may predispose to injury from impingement.

Os acromiale

- An os acromiale is a persistent accessory ossification center of the acromion seen in up to 15% of patients. It is best evaluated on the axial images.
- Although the presence of an os acromiale may be an asymptomatic normal variant, the presence of marrow edema suggests that the os may be a cause of pain.
- Treatment is resection or fusion.

ROTATOR CUFF

Anatomy of the rotator cuff

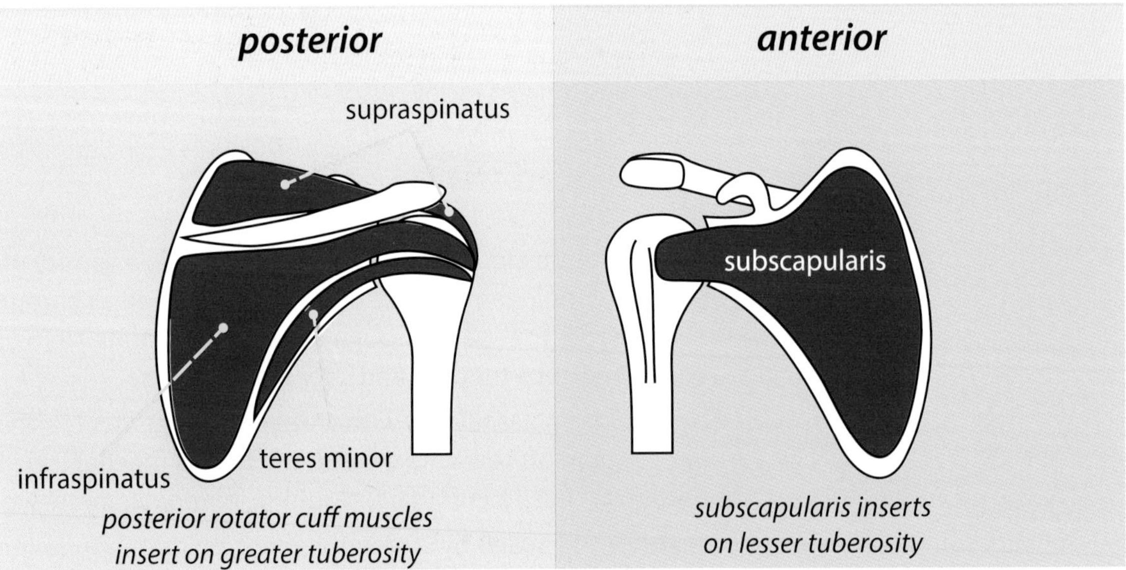

- The rotator cuff is an essential active stabilizer of the glenohumeral joint and is formed by the four rotator cuff muscles (supraspinatus, infraspinatus, teres minor, and subscapularis) and their tendons.
- The supraspinatus, infraspinatus, and teres minor are located posterior to the body of the scapula and insert on the greater tuberosity. The subscapularis is anterior to the scapula and inserts on the lesser tuberosity.

coronal

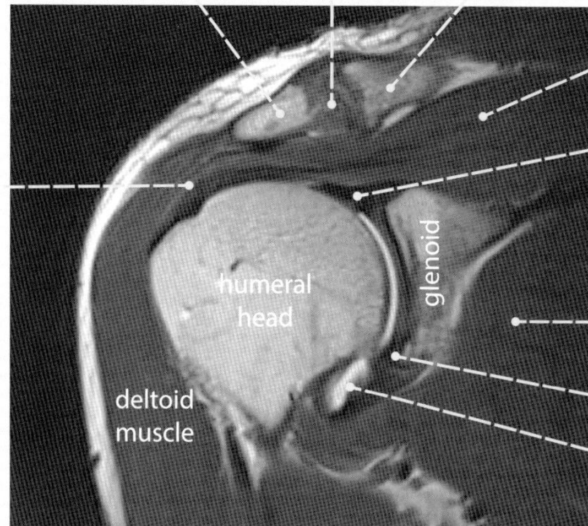

axial

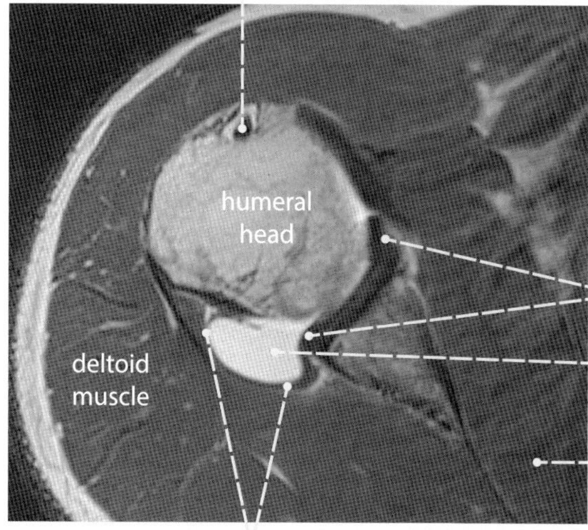

sagittal

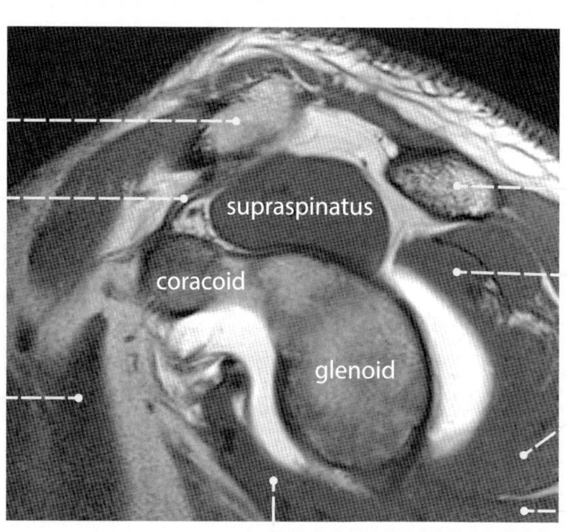

Images courtesy Kirstin Small, MD, Brigham and Women's Hospital.

Tendinosis/tendinopathy

- Tendinosis (also called tendinopathy) is mucoid degeneration of the tendon, without active inflammation. Tendinosis manifests on imaging as diffuse or focal thickening and intermediate signal intensity on T1- and T2-weighted images. On T2-weighted images, the tendinosis does not appear as hyperintense as fluid.
- The *magic-angle* phenomenon may simulate tendinosis or even a partial tear. The *magic-angle* effect is due to the anisotropy of the tendon's collagen fibers and occurs when the collagen fibers are oriented at 55 degrees relative to the magnetic field (B0) with short TE times (for instance T1-weighted images, proton density, and GRE).

Overview of rotator cuff tears

- Tears of the rotator cuff can be partial or complete.
- Complete rotator cuff tears allow communication between the subacromial/ subdeltoid bursa and the glenohumeral joint.
- The *footprint* is the attachment of the tendons at the greater tuberosity. The critical zone is a potentially undervascularized portion of the distal supraspinatus tendon approximately 1 cm proximal to the insertion on the footprint. Relatively decreased vascular supply may predispose to rupture in this location.

Partial-thickness rotator cuff tear

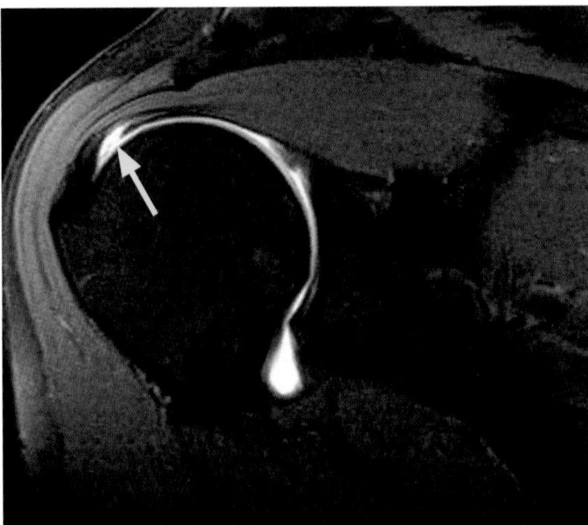

Partial articular surface supraspinatus tear:

Coronal T1-weighted MR arthrogram with fat suppression demonstrates discontinuity of the articular surface of the distal fibers of the supraspinatus tendon (arrow).

Case courtesy Kirstin M. Small, MD, Brigham and Women's Hospital.

- The most commonly injured rotator cuff muscle is the supraspinatus, followed by the infraspinatus. The teres minor is the least commonly injured rotator cuff muscle.
- A partial-thickness tear features abnormal signal in a portion of the muscle or tendon but not extending through its entire thickness. MR arthrography will *not* show communication between the injected glenohumeral joint and the subacromial/ subdeltoid bursa.

  Partial-thickness tears can be challenging to diagnose without MR arthrography. Reparative granulation tissue can obscure the abnormal signal that would otherwise indicate a tear.
- Partial tears can be divided into bursal-surface, articular surface, or intrasubstance tears. Articular-surface tears are by far the most common type of partial tear.
- A *rim rent* tear is the most common type of partial tear. Also called the PASTA lesion (partial thickness articular supraspinatus tendon avulsion), the rim rent tear is an avulsion-type partial tear of the articular surface of the supraspinatus as it inserts on the greater tuberosity.

  Less commonly, an analogous lesion can be seen in the infraspinatus.
- The PAINT (partial articular tear with intratendinous extension) lesion is a partial rotator cuff tear at the articular surface that also extends into the tendon.

Full-thickness rotator cuff tear

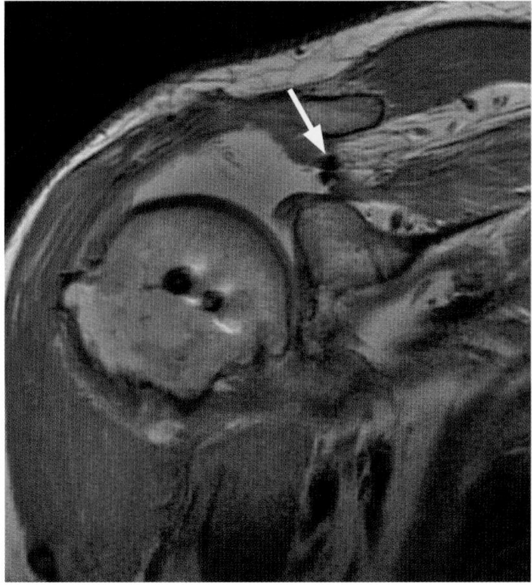
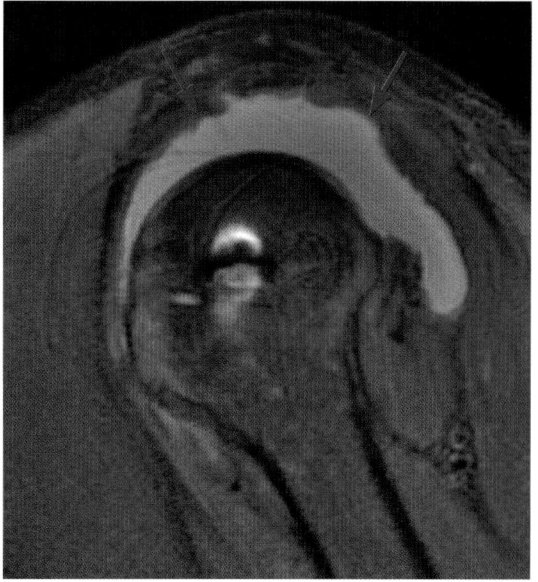

Full-thickness rotator cuff tear: Coronal proton-density (left image) and sagittal fat-saturated proton-density (right image) conventional MRI demonstrates complete discontinuity of the supraspinatus tendon with the tendon retracted proximally (yellow arrow). There is a large effusion, demonstrating continuity of the glenohumeral joint and the subacromial/subdeltoid bursa (red arrows). Susceptibility artifact is present in the humeral head, consistent with prior rotator cuff repair.

Case courtesy Kirstin M. Small, MD, Brigham and Women's Hospital.

- A full-thickness rotator cuff tear is seen on MR arthrography when fluid injected into the glenohumeral joint extends into the subacromial/subdeltoid bursa. In the absence of injected gadolinium, a full-thickness tear can be diagnosed if abnormal signal extends through the fibers of the tendon. A gap in the tendon is almost always present.
- Similar to partial tears, the supraspinatus is most commonly torn.
- Approximately 30–40% of supraspinatus tears are also associated with a tear of the infraspinatus.

  The infraspinatus is rarely torn in isolation; however, isolated infraspinatus tears can be seen in the setting of posterior instability. The posterior capsule and labrum should be carefully evaluated in such cases.

- A chronic full-thickness rotator cuff tear due to rheumatoid arthritis has a classic imaging appearance. The humeral head migrates superiorly and may articulate with the acromion in severe cases.
- Full-thickness rotator cuff tears are classified by the length of the affected tendon/muscle, ranging from small (<1 cm) to massive (>5 cm).

Rotator cuff atrophy

- Atrophy of the rotator cuff is most commonly due to chronic rotator cuff tear. Fatty degeneration may occur within 4 weeks of injury and is usually irreversible. The extent of muscle degeneration correlates with outcome following surgical repair. The degree of fatty infiltration of the rotator cuff muscles should be routinely assessed in the sagittal plane. The degree of fatty replacement can be graded with the Goutallier classification:

Grade 0: Normal muscle, no fat.	**Grade 3**: Fatty infiltration, equal muscle and fat.
Grade 1: Muscle contains a few fatty streaks.	**Grade 4**: Fatty infiltration, more fat than muscle.
Grade 2: Fatty infiltration, more muscle than fat.	

- Less commonly, rotator cuff atrophy may be secondary to denervation atrophy, subsequently discussed. Denervation atrophy is usually associated with a paralabral cyst.

Adhesive capsulitis

- Adhesive capsulitis, clinically known as *frozen shoulder*, is thickening and contraction of the glenohumeral joint capsule due to inflammation of the joint capsule and synovium.
- Adhesive capsulitis is primarily a clinical diagnosis, but MRI findings include thickening of the joint capsule and synovium >4 mm, assessed at the level of the axillary pouch.

SHOULDER LIGAMENTS AND ROTATOR INTERVAL

Anatomy of the shoulder ligaments

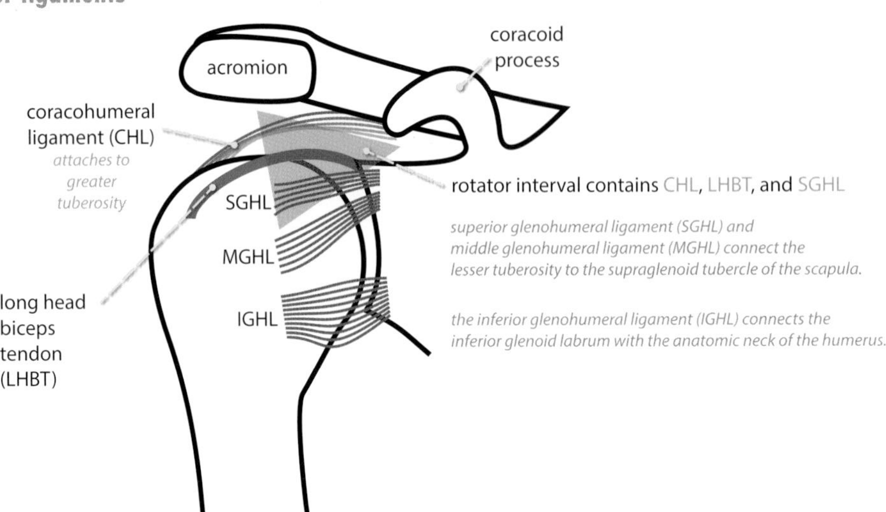

- The *rotator interval* is a triangular region that allows rotational motion around the coracoid process. It is located between the supraspinatus and subscapularis tendons. The rotator interval contains the coracohumeral ligament (CHL), the long head of the biceps tendon (LHBT), and the superior glenohumeral ligament (SGHL).
- The CHL connects the lateral aspect of the coracoid process to the greater tubercle of the humerus, where the CHL blends with the supraspinatus tendon. The CHL helps to stabilize the intraarticular biceps tendon together with the superior glenohumeral ligament as the *biceps pulley*. The CHL is located external to the joint capsule.
- The three glenohumeral ligaments are derived from the labrum and form a portion of the joint capsule.
- The superior glenohumeral ligament (SGHL) connects the lesser tuberosity to the supraglenoid tubercle of the scapula.
- The middle glenohumeral ligament (MGHL) also connects the lesser tuberosity to the supraglenoid tubercle of the scapula. The MGHL is congenitally absent in up to one third of patients. Tears of the MGHL are associated with superior labral tears.
- The inferior glenohumeral ligament (IGHL) connects the anatomic neck of the humerus to the inferior glenoid labrum. The IGHL is by far the most important component of the capsulolabral complex for maintaining stability in abduction and external rotation. The IGHL contains three components (the anterior band, the axillary pouch, and the posterior band), all of which are all well-seen on sagittal MR:

  The **anterior band** of the IGHL provides anterior stability. There are several lesions of the anterior band of the IGHL that are associated with anterior instability, discussed on the following page.

  The IGHL forms the **axillary pouch** of the glenohumeral joint capsule.

  The **posterior band** contributes to posterior stability. The IGHL is the only glenohumeral ligament to have a posterior component.
- The long head of the biceps tendon (LHBT) attaches to the anterosuperior glenoid rim along with the SGHL and MGHL.

Anatomy of the biceps tendon

- The long head of the biceps tendon originates at the superior labrum and courses in the intertubercular groove. The biceps tendon sheath communicates with the glenohumeral joint. Fluid in the tendon sheath may be normal.
- The biceps pulley is a capsuloligamentous complex that stabilizes the biceps tendon in a sling within the bicipital groove. The biceps pulley is formed by the superior glenohumeral ligament, coracohumeral ligament, and the distal fibers of the subscapularis tendon.

Biceps tendon tear

- Approximately 33% of supraspinatus tendon tears are associated with biceps tendon injury (complete tear, partial tear, or degeneration).
- The biceps tendon is at risk for impingement due to its location partially underneath the supraspinatus tendon in the coracoacromial arch.
- In cases of an acute tear, the biceps muscle may retract distally. An empty intertubercular groove may signify a complete tear with retraction or a biceps tendon dislocation.

Biceps tendon subluxation

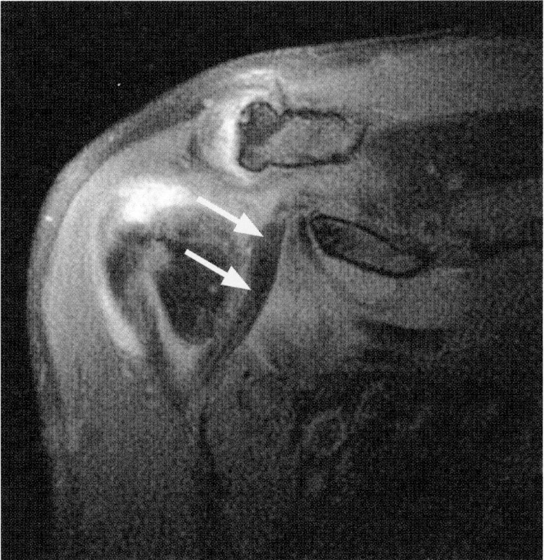

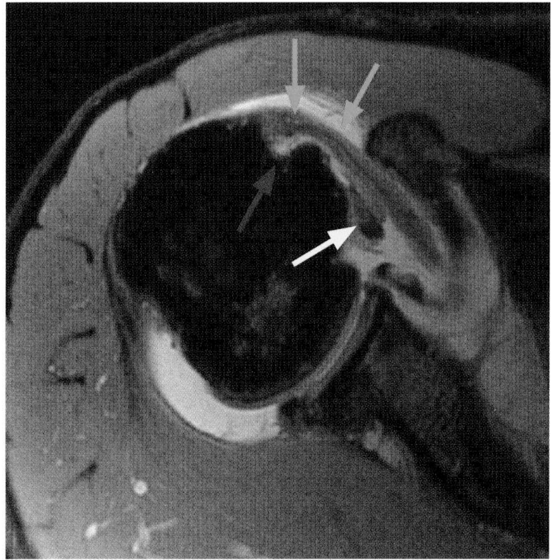

Biceps tendon subluxation: Coronal (left image) and axial T1-weighted MR arthrogram with fat suppression shows medial intra-articular subluxation of the biceps tendon (yellow arrows). The bicipital groove is empty, best seen on the axial image (red arrow). The blue arrows denote the subscapularis tendon, seen on the axial image.

Case courtesy Kirstin M. Small, MD, Brigham and Women's Hospital.

- Biceps tendon subluxation is defined as a tendon displaced from, but remaining in contact with, the bicipital groove.
- Biceps tendon subluxation and dislocation are associated with injury to the transverse ligament. The transverse humeral ligament attaches to the greater and lesser tuberosities and normally holds the biceps tendon in place.

Biceps tendon dislocation

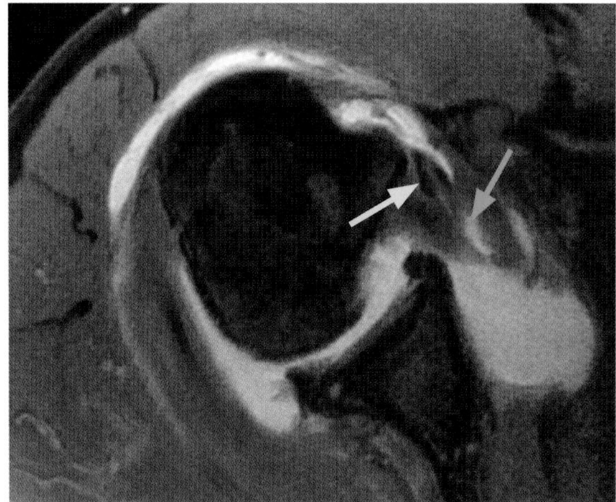

Biceps tendon dislocation:

Axial T1-weighted image with fat suppression from an MR arthrogram shows medial dislocation of the biceps tendon (yellow arrow) into the subscapularis. An interstitial tear of the subscapularis tendon is present (blue arrow).

Case courtesy Kirstin M. Small, MD, Brigham and Women's Hospital.

- Biceps tendon dislocation is often seen in conjunction with injury of both the transverse ligament and the biceps pulley.
- Medial dislocation of the biceps tendon is associated with tear of the subscapularis tendon (in contrast to biceps tears, which are more frequently associated with supraspinatus injury).
- Axial MRI best demonstrates biceps tendon dislocation. The bicipital groove is empty and the tendon can usually be seen medial to the bicipital groove.

Instability: Overview and anatomy

Overview of instability

- Shoulder instability is abnormal motion of the humeral head with respect to the glenoid during movement, producing pain, clicking, or the feeling of an unstable joint.
- Instability can manifest as dislocation, subluxation, or microinstability (repetitive motion).
- The stability of the glenohumeral joint is mostly provided by dynamic and static soft-tissue stabilizers, as there is minimal inherent osseous stability.
- The dynamic stabilizers of the joint include the rotator cuff and biceps tendons.
- The static stabilizer of the joint is the capsulo-labro-ligamentous complex, which is composed of the bony glenoid fossa, labrum, coracohumeral ligament, and superior, middle, and inferior glenohumeral ligaments.
- There are several labral, ligamentous, and osseous injuries associated with instability, but it is unclear whether the structural abnormalities are secondary to instability or a cause of it.
- There are various classifications of instability incorporating clinical, etiological, and imaging findings.
- Instability can also be classified as traumatic or atraumatic.

  Traumatic instability usually causes instability in one direction only, is associated with a Bankart lesion, and is treated surgically. Traumatic instability is referred to as **TUBS** (traumatic, unidirectional, Bankart, surgical).

  Atraumatic instability can be divided into two types. The **AIOS** (acquired, instability, overstress, surgery) pattern is usually seen in athletes with repetitive movements causing microinstability. **AMBRI** (atraumatic, multidirectional, bilateral, rehabilitation, inferior capsule shift) lesions are due to congenital joint laxity.
- Radiologists usually classify instability based on the direction of joint subluxation (anterior, posterior, multidirectional, or superior). Similar to traumatic shoulder dislocations, anterior instability accounts for the vast majority (95%) of cases.

Anatomy of the glenoid labrum

- The glenoid labrum is a fibrocartilaginous ring-like structure that rests on the glenoid hyaline cartilage and surrounds the glenoid. The labrum increases the surface area and depth of the glenoid cavity. It also provides a suction effect, adhering the humeral head to the glenoid with motion.

sagittal schematic of the glenoid fossa, glenoid labrum, and glenohumeral ligaments

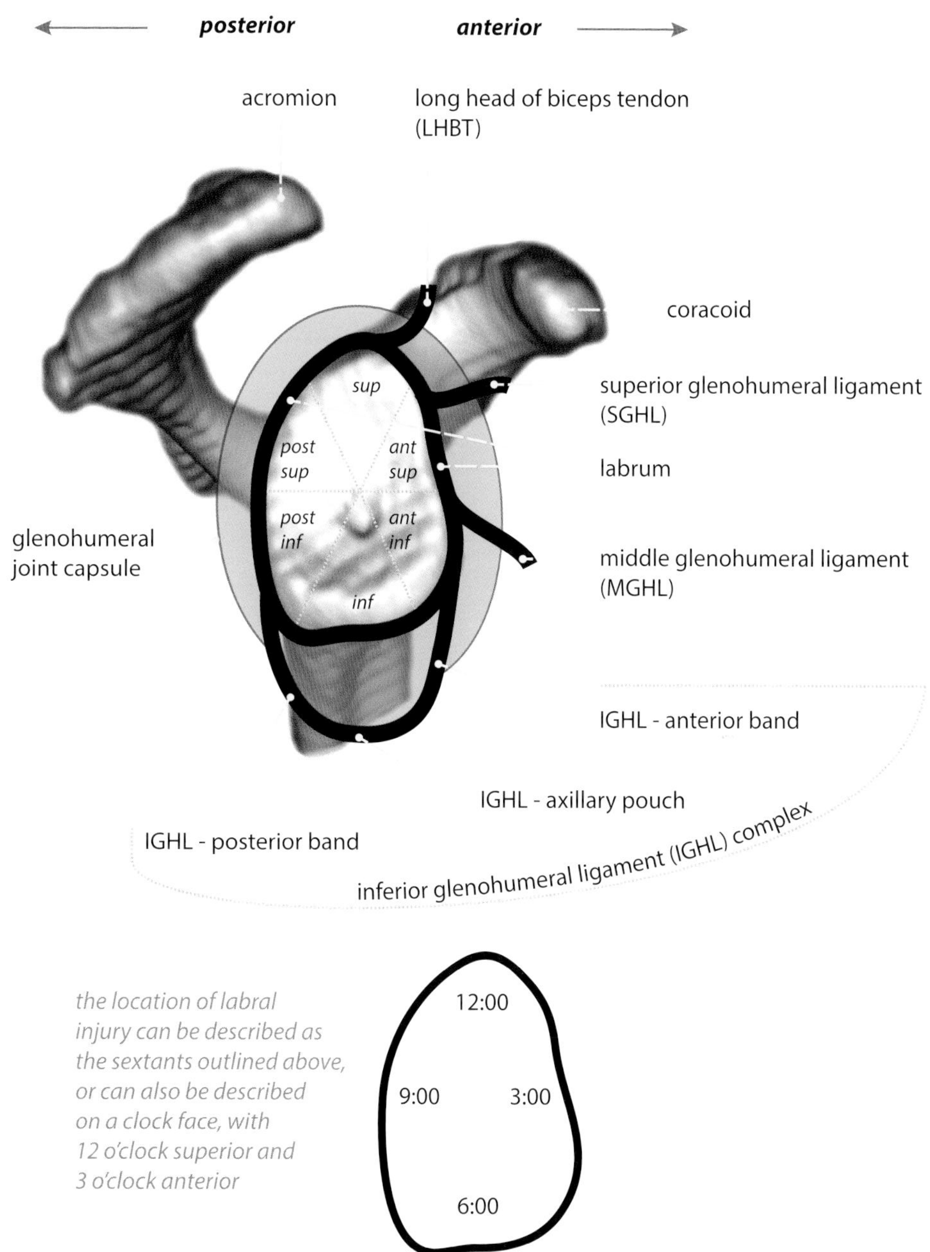

- Other important stabilizers of the joint attach directly to the labrum, including the glenohumeral ligaments, the biceps tendon, and the joint capsule

Labral normal variants

- A **sublabral foramen** (seen in 10% of patients) is a normal variant where the anterosuperior segment is not attached to the bony glenoid.
- A **Buford complex** is a less common (seen in up to 6.5%) normal variant where a cord-like middle glenohumeral ligament is seen in combination with an absent anterosuperior labrum.

- Most of the alphabet-soup instability lesions are located at the anterior-inferior aspect of the glenohumeral joint and are associated with the anterior band of the inferior glenohumeral ligament.

Bankart lesion

- The Bankart lesion is an injury of the anteroinferior labrum due to anterior glenohumeral dislocation. Specifically, a Bankart is detachment of the anteroinferior labrum from the glenoid, with stripping of the scapular periosteum.
- The labrum may migrate superiorly and appear as a balled-up mass-like object, producing the glenoid labrum ovoid mass (GLOM) sign. The differential diagnosis for a black intra-articular mass on MRI includes:

  GLOM sign (if a Bankart lesion is present inferiorly).

  Dislocated biceps tendon.

  Air bubble (if an MR arthrogram was performed).

- An osseous Bankart (or "bony Bankart") is a fracture of the anterior-inferior glenoid rim, which predisposes to recurrent dislocation due to glenoid insufficiency.

Hill–Sachs

- Hill–Sachs is an impaction fracture of the posterolateral humeral head caused by anterior dislocation. The Hill–Sachs lesion can be diagnosed by scrolling through sequential axial images: With standard 5 mm slices, the normal humeral head should appear round in three consecutive slices starting superiorly. If a Hill–Sachs lesion is present, there will be a posterolateral notch in the humeral head.
- Subtle Hill–Sachs can also be detected as bone marrow edema in this location, without fracture.

Anterior labro-ligamentous periosteal sleeve avulsion (ALPSA)

- An anterior labro-ligamentous periosteal sleeve avulsion (ALPSA) is a variant of the Bankart lesion and also represents an anterior-inferior labral injury. In contrast to the Bankart lesion, the scapular periosteum is intact with an ALPSA.
- Similar to the GLOM sign discussed above, the avulsed anterior-inferior labrum is balled up. However, since the labrum remains attached to the periosteum in an ALPSA lesion, the labrum is displaced inferomedially relative to the glenoid (as opposed to superiorly with the GLOM sign).

Perthes lesion

- The Perthes lesion is an avulsion of the anterior-inferior labrum, where the labrum remains attached to the scapular periosteum.
- Because the labrum remains attached to periosteum and may remain in its anatomic position, the Perthes lesion can be very difficult to visualize. MR arthrography with ABER (abduction–external rotation) positioning is often necessary for diagnosis.

Humeral avulsion of the inferior glenohumeral ligament (HAGL)

- Humeral avulsion of the inferior glenohumeral ligament (HAGL) is avulsion of the humeral attachment of the IGHL. This lesion occurs on the opposite (humeral) site of the IGHL compared to the Bankart/ALPSA/Perthes lesions.
- HAGL is associated with subscapularis tendon tears.

Bony HAGL (BHAGL)

- A BHAGL is a HAGL lesion with an additional bony avulsion of the anatomic neck of the humerus, caused by avulsion of the IGHL.

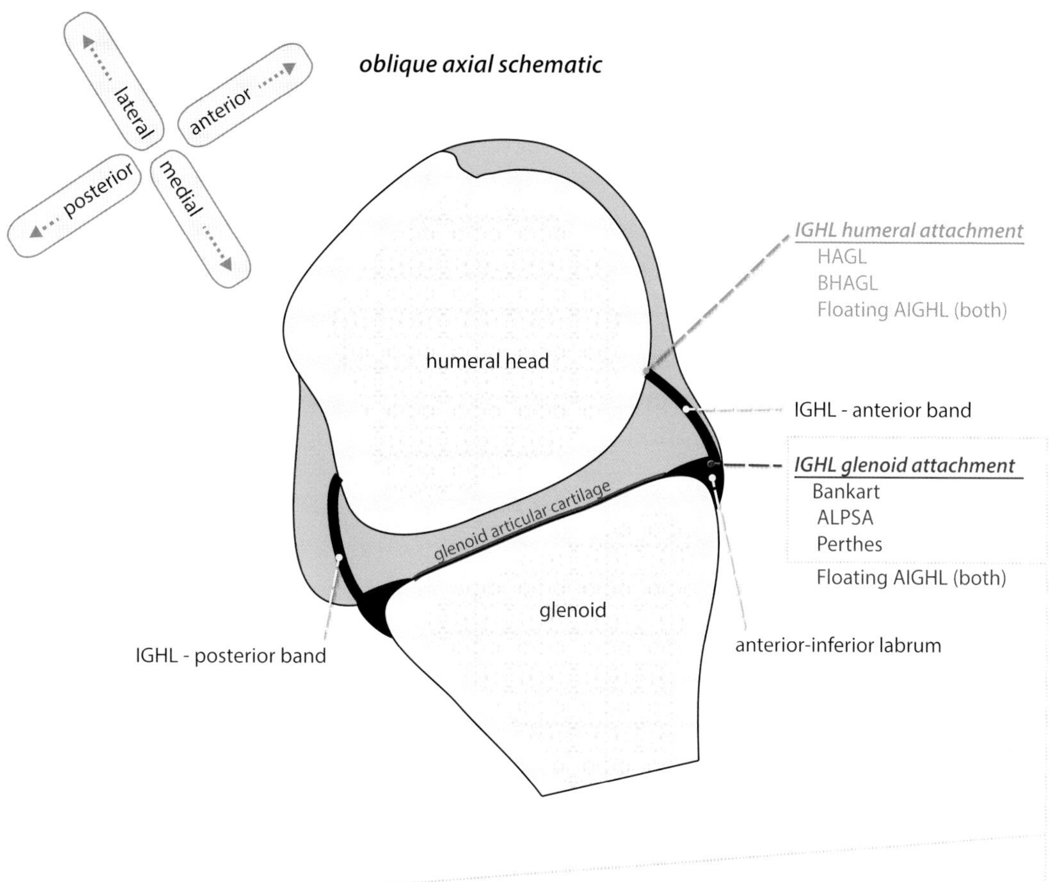

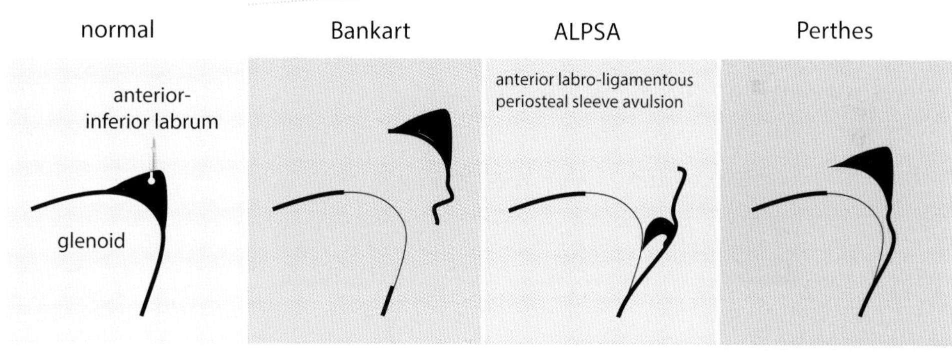

labrum detached from glenoid with stripping of the scapular periosteum

Bankart variant with balled-up labrum and intact scapular periosteum

avulsion of labrum, which remains attached to scapular periosteum

Posterior instability

- Posterior instability is uncommon, accounting for less than 5% of instability.
- The injuries associated with posterior instability are highly variable and include several posterior variations of anterior lesions such as posterior HAGL (PHAGL), reverse Bankart (posterior glenoid fracture), and reverse Hill–Sachs/*trough* sign.
- Tears of the infraspinatus and teres minor are associated with posterior instability, as these rotator cuff muscles insert on the posterior aspect of the greater tuberosity.
- Hypoplastic posterior glenoid may be a congenital cause of posterior instability.
- The Bennett lesion, also known as *thrower's exostosis*, is extra-articular posterior ossification associated with posterior labral injury. The Bennett lesion is often seen in baseball pitchers and is thought to be the result of avulsion of the posterior band of the IGHL. Ossification can be confirmed with an axillary shoulder radiograph.

Miscellaneous lesions not associated with instability

Superior labrum anterior posterior (SLAP) tear

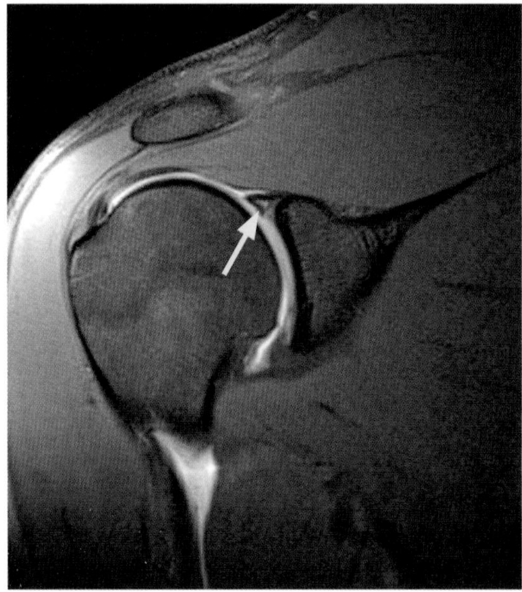
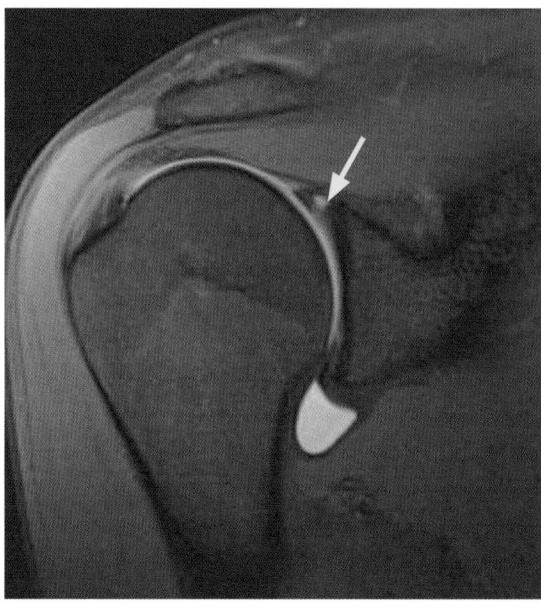

SLAP tear (type II): Coronal T1-weighted MR arthrogram with fat suppression shows high signal within the superior labrum (yellow arrows) extending from anterior to posterior.

Case courtesy Kirstin M. Small, MD, Brigham and Women's Hospital.

- A superior labrum anterior posterior (SLAP) tear is an anterior–posterior oriented tear of the superior labrum centered at the attachment of the biceps tendon. The biceps tendon inserts onto the anterior-superior labrum. There were originally four types of SLAP lesions described; however, now there are up to 10 different subcategories of SLAP lesions.
- Type I SLAP is isolated fraying of the superior portion of the labrum without a frank tear. The biceps tendon is intact.
- Type II SLAP is the most frequent type of SLAP and features labral fraying in conjunction with stripping of the superior labrum. Type II SLAP lesions are most commonly associated with repetitive microtrauma.
- Type III SLAP is a bucket-handle tear of the superior labrum, analogous to a bucket-handle tear of the knee meniscus.
- Type IV SLAP is also a bucket-handle tear of the superior labrum, with additional extension into the biceps tendon.

Glenoid labral articular disruption (GLAD)

- Glenoid labral articular disruption (GLAD) is a superficial tear of the anterior-inferior labrum, with adjacent glenoid articular cartilage injury.
- Although the GLAD lesion occurs at the anterior-inferior labrum, the same site as the Bankart, ALPSA, and Perthes lesions, GLAD is usually not caused by or associated with instability.
- GLAD lesions may lead to post-traumatic arthritis and intra-articular bodies.

Paralabral cysts

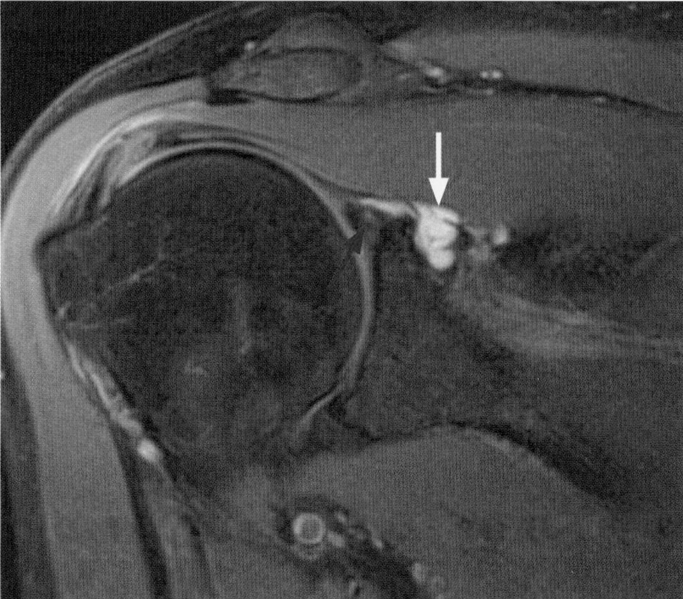

Paralabral cyst and labral tear:

Coronal T2-weighted MRI with fat suppression shows a lobulated paralabral cyst (yellow arrow) medial to the glenoid.

There is globular intermediate signal within the labrum (red arrow), highly suggestive of labral tear especially in the presence of an adjacent paralabral cyst.

Case courtesy Kirstin M. Small, MD, Brigham and Women's Hospital.

- Similar to the formation of parameniscal cysts adjacent to meniscal tears, paralabral cysts form adjacent to labral tears. Paralabral cysts are usually seen in the soft tissues adjacent to the labrum but may extend into bone.
- The presence of a paralabral cyst is a very specific finding for a labral tear even when abnormal labral signal is not seen.
- A paralabral cyst may compress a nerve and cause an entrapment neuropathy.

Entrapment neuropathies

Quadrilateral space syndrome

- The quadrilateral space is located at the posterior aspect of the axilla. It is formed by the humerus (laterally), the long head of the triceps muscle (medially), teres minor (superiorly), and teres major (inferiorly).
- The axillary nerve and posterior humeral circumflex artery travel through the quadrilateral space. The axillary nerve provides motor fibers to the teres minor and deltoid.
- Entrapment of the axillary nerve in the quadrilateral space may cause teres minor paresthesias and eventual atrophy, with or without deltoid involvement.

Suprascapular nerve entrapment at the suprascapular notch

- The proximal suprascapular nerve provides motor innervation to the supraspinatus and infraspinatus muscles. Entrapment of the suprascapular nerve at the suprascapular notch, most commonly from a paralabral cyst associated with a superior labral tear, causes atrophy of both the supraspinatus and infraspinatus.

Suprascapular nerve entrapment at the spinoglenoid notch

- The distal suprascapular nerve provides motor innervation to the infraspinatus muscle only. Entrapment of the distal suprascapular nerve at the spinoglenoid notch will cause isolated atrophy of the infraspinatus.

Summary of entrapment neuropathies

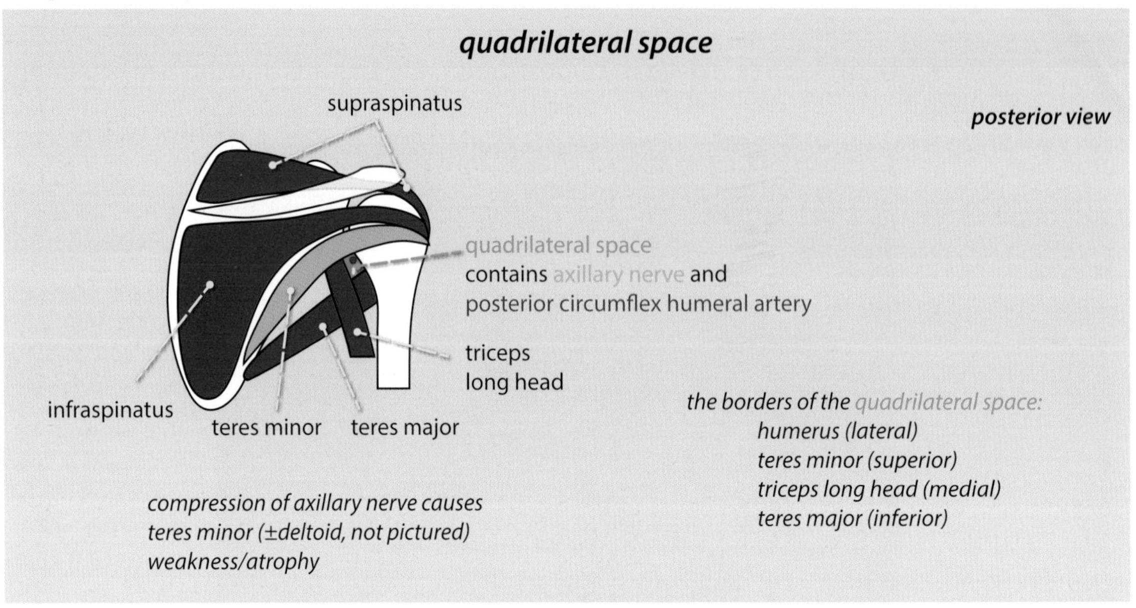

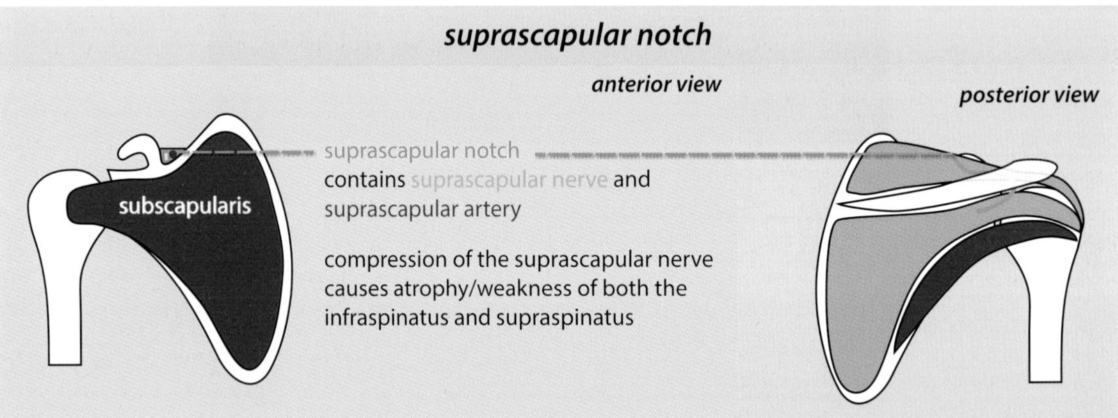

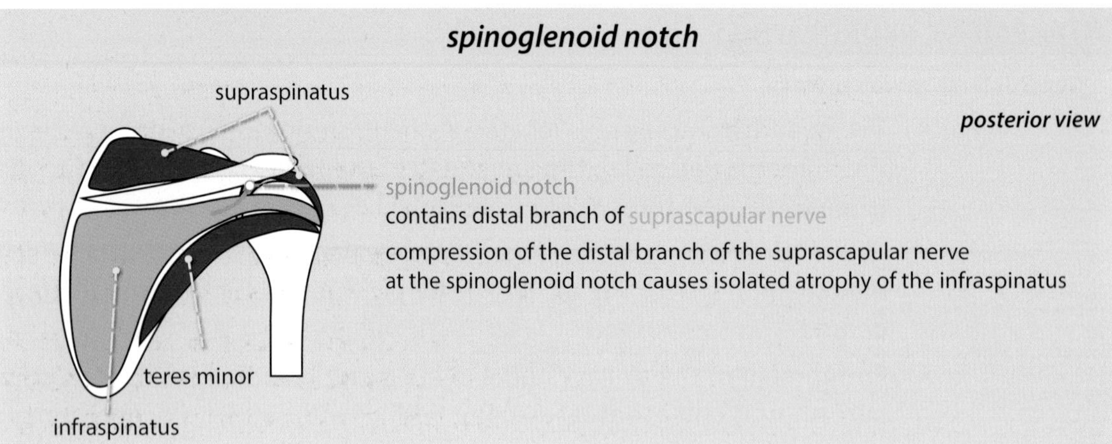

Parsonage–Turner

- Parsonage–Turner syndrome is idiopathic brachial neuropathy, which may cause rotator cuff atrophy. It is a diagnosis of exclusion and a structural cause for atrophy (e.g., a mass or cyst compressing a nerve) must be ruled out.

ELBOW AND FOREARM TRAUMA

Elbow dislocation

- The most common elbow dislocation is posterior dislocation of both the radius and ulna with respect to the humerus.
- Elbow dislocations are frequently associated with ulnar fractures. These fractures may be more distal than imaged in a typical elbow radiograph, so forearm radiographs should be obtained in the setting of an elbow dislocation.

Radial head fracture

- A radial head fracture is the most common elbow fracture in adults.
- The *fat pad* sign is elevation of the anterior and/or posterior fat pads due to an elbow effusion. Elevation of the posterior fat pad is considered nearly diagnostic for fracture (most commonly radial head fracture in adults). The *sail* sign represents elevation of the anterior fat pad only and is less specific for fracture.
- If a fat pad sign is present and no fracture is seen, additional views (typically of the radial head) or CT should be obtained.

Supracondylar fracture

- Supracondylar fracture is the most common elbow fracture in children.

Essex–Lopresti fracture-dislocation

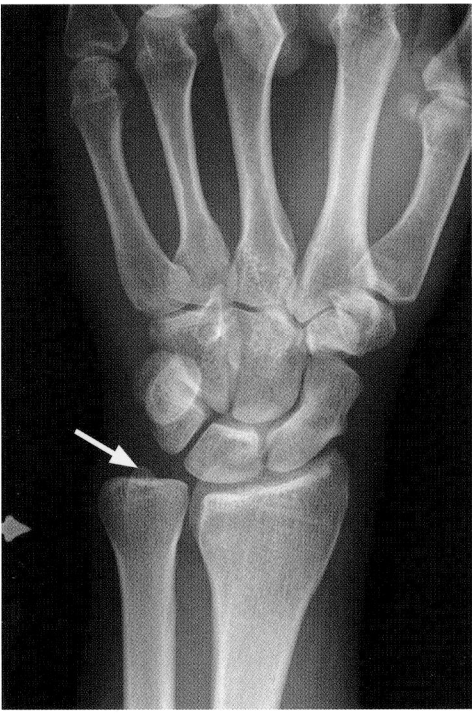

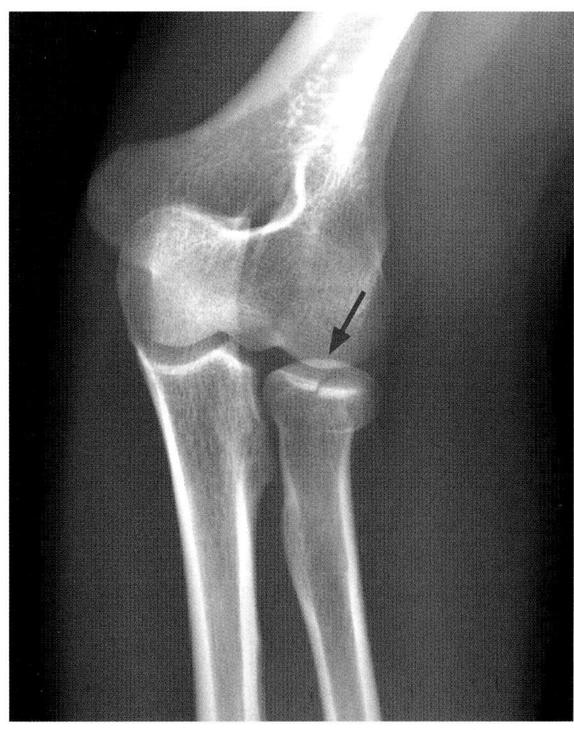

Essex–Lopresti fracture dislocation: Frontal radiograph of the wrist (left image) shows a probable ulnar (medial) dislocation of the ulna at the distal radioulnar joint. Although the dislocation is subtle, the ulna is abnormally rotated as evidenced by the radial displacement of the radial styloid (yellow arrow).

Frontal elbow radiograph shows a nondisplaced radial head fracture (red arrow).

- Essex–Lopresti fracture-dislocation is radial head fracture and tearing of the interosseous membrane with ulnar dislocation at the distal radioulnar joint.

Monteggia fracture-dislocation

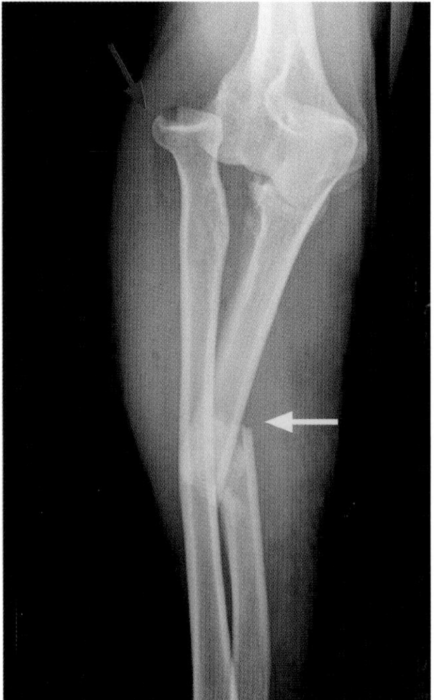

Monteggia fracture-dislocation:

Frontal radiograph of the proximal forearm shows a mid-diaphyseal ulnar fracture (yellow arrow) and radial head dislocation (red arrow).

Case courtesy Stacy Smith, MD, Brigham and Women's Hospital.

- Monteggia fracture-dislocation is an ulnar fracture and radial dislocation at the elbow.

Galeazzi fracture-dislocation

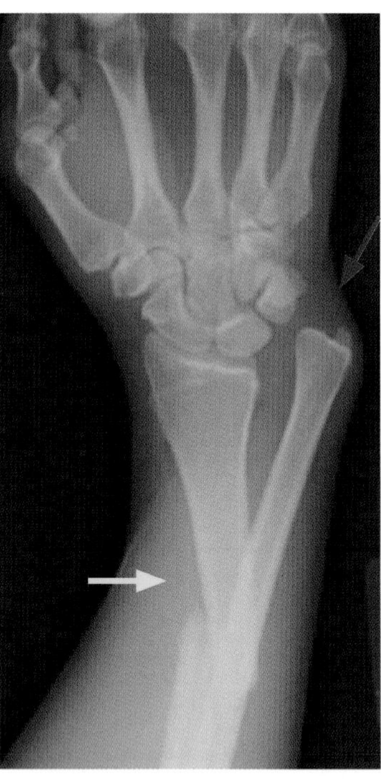

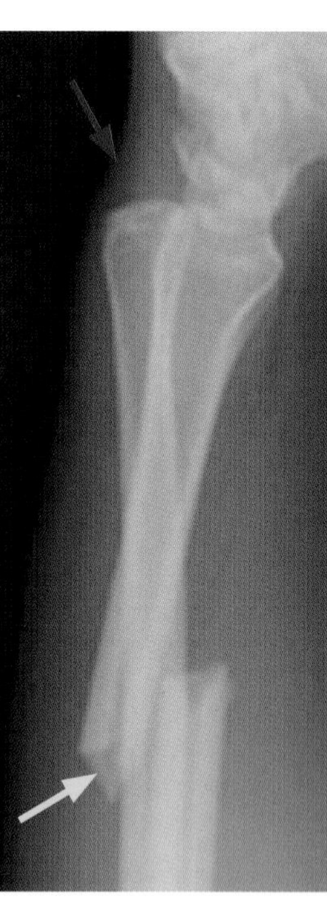

Galeazzi fracture-dislocation:

Frontal and lateral radiographs of the forearm show a radial diaphyseal fracture of the distal third of the radial diaphysis (yellow arrows) and distal ulnar dislocation (red arrows). The radial shaft fracture has radial and volar angulation and foreshortening.

Case courtesy Stacy Smith, MD, Brigham and Women's Hospital.

- Galeazzi fracture-dislocation is fracture of the distal third of the radius with ulnar dislocation at the distal radioulnar joint.

Colles fracture

- Colles fracture is a distal radius fracture with dorsal angulation. The fracture is usually intra-articular. Colles fracture is the most common injury to the distal forearm.
- Colles fracture typically results from a fall on an outstretched hand (FOOSH).

Hutchinson (chauffeur's) fracture

- Hutchinson (chauffeur's) fracture is a fracture of the radial (lateral) aspect of the distal radius extending into the radial styloid and the radiocarpal joint.

COMMON HAND AND WRIST FRACTURES

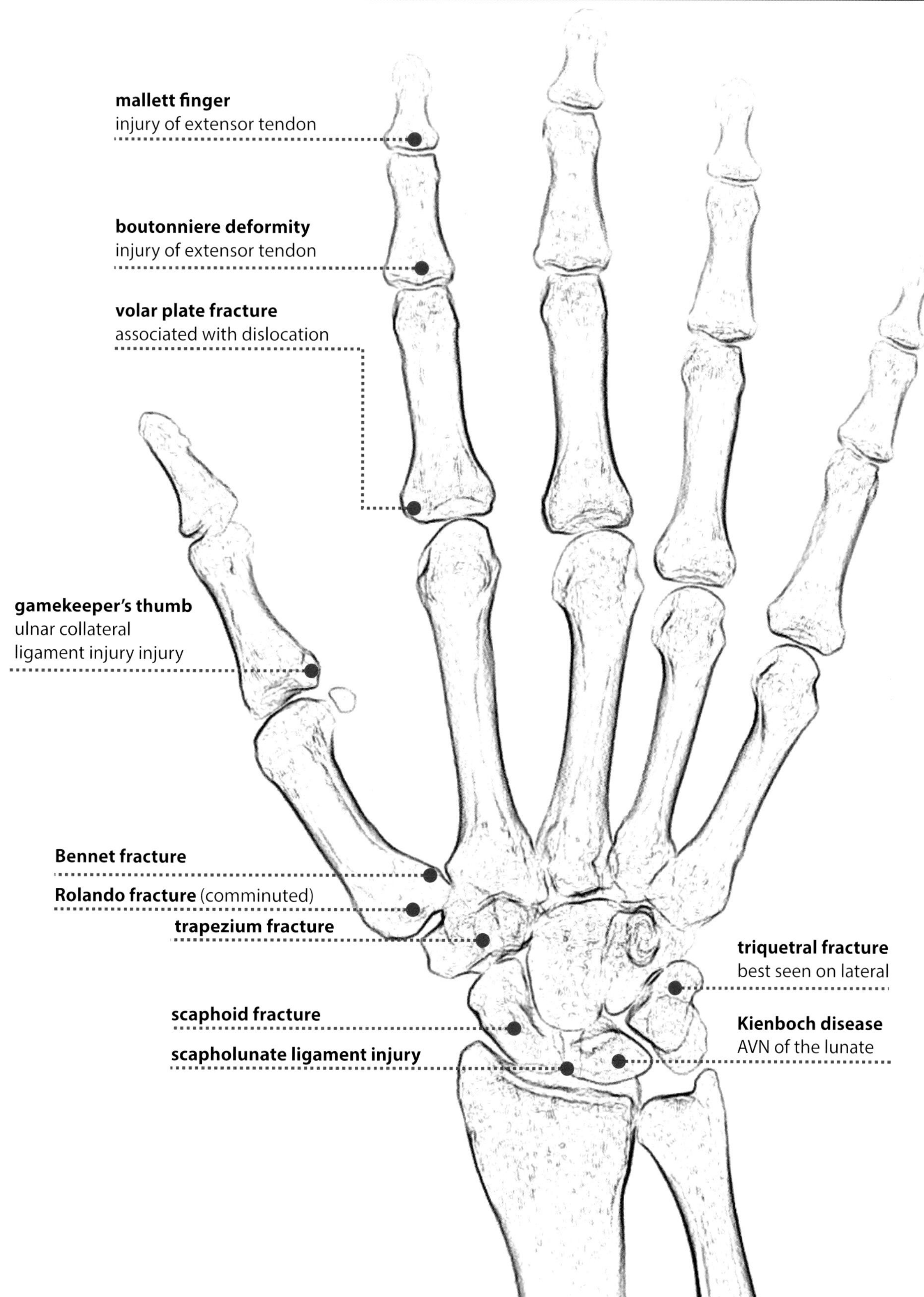
mallett finger
injury of extensor tendon
boutonniere deformity
injury of extensor tendon
volar plate fracture
associated with dislocation
gamekeeper's thumb
ulnar collateral
ligament injury injury
Bennet fracture
Rolando fracture (comminuted)
trapezium fracture
scaphoid fracture
scapholunate ligament injury
triquetral fracture
best seen on lateral
Kienboch disease
AVN of the lunate

Carpal anatomy and alignment

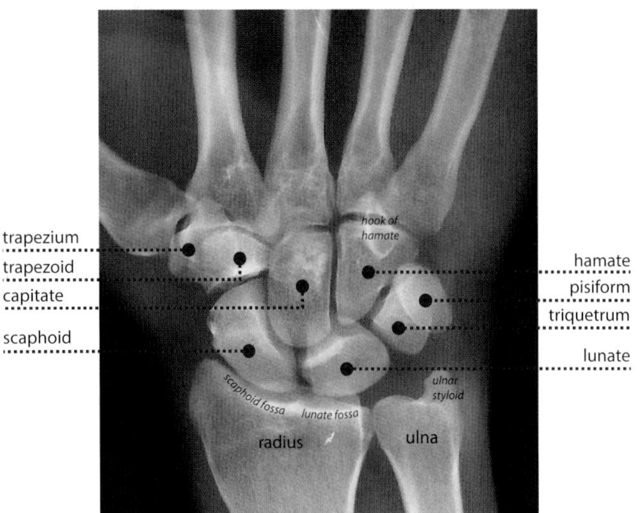

Arcs of Gilula should be smooth and continuous. Disruption may be a sign of ligamentous injury or fracture.

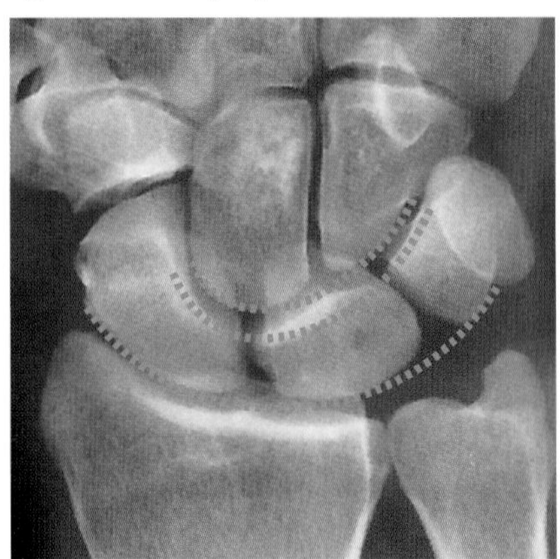

Lunate and perilunate dislocation

normal alignment	perilunate dislocation	lunate dislocation
capitate / lunate / radius	capitate / lunate / radius	capitate / lunate / radius

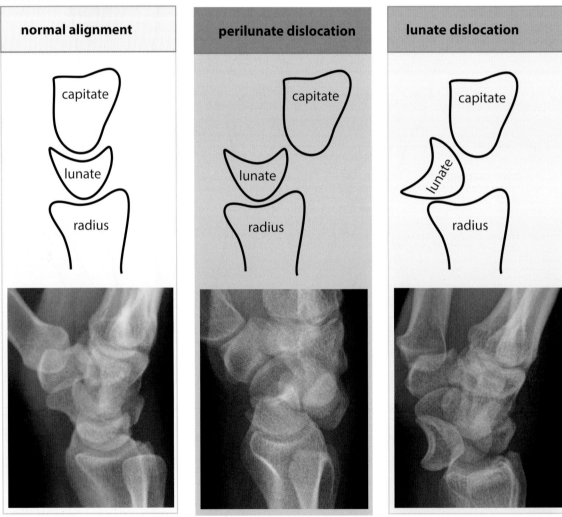

- In a **perilunate dislocation**, the lunate is aligned with the radius, but capitate is not aligned with the lunate. Dislocation is *next to* the lunate (*peri*-lunate).
- In a **lunate dislocation**, the lunate is dislocated volarly, but the capitate is still relatively aligned with the radius. The lunate itself is dislocated *(lunate dislocation).*

Scapholunate ligament injury

- Scapholunate ligament injury is one of the many patterns of injury caused by a fall on an outstretched arm.
- The *Terry Thomas* sign represents increased distance of scapholunate interval, thought to resemble the gap between the front teeth of the famous British actor from the 60s.
- Scapholunate advanced collapse (SLAC) wrist is a sequela of chronic scapholunate ligament injury, which may be secondary to osteoarthritis, CPPD arthropathy, or chronic untreated scapholunate dissociation.
- The capitate migrates proximally to fill the abnormal gap between the scaphoid and lunate.

Scaphoid fracture

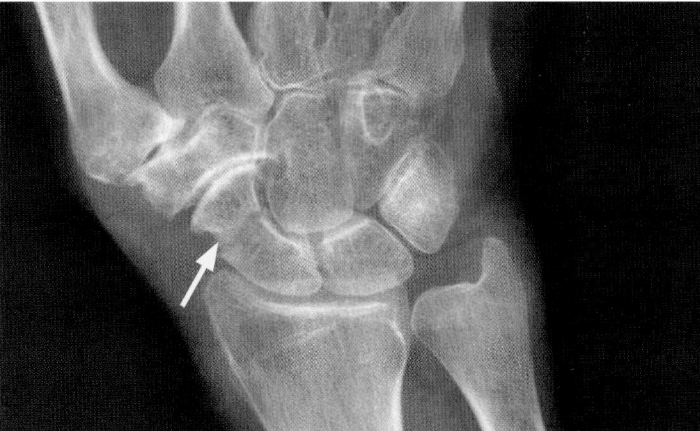

Scaphoid fracture: Radiograph of the wrist shows a minimally displaced fracture of the scaphoid (arrow).

- Blood supply to the scaphoid is interosseous, from distal to proximal. The proximal pole of the scaphoid has a tenuous blood supply and proximal fractures have the highest risk of avascular necrosis.

Triquetral fracture

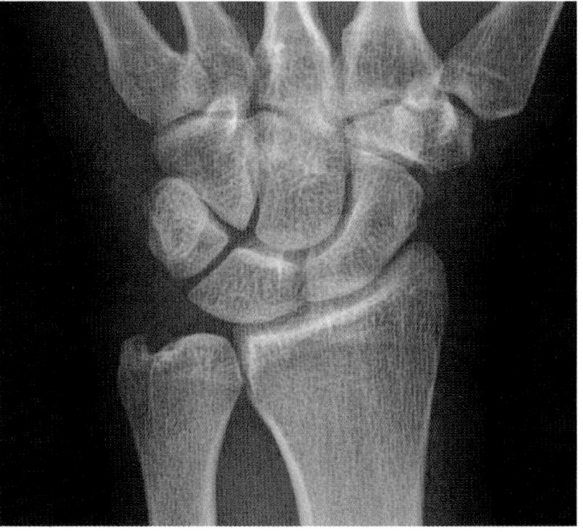

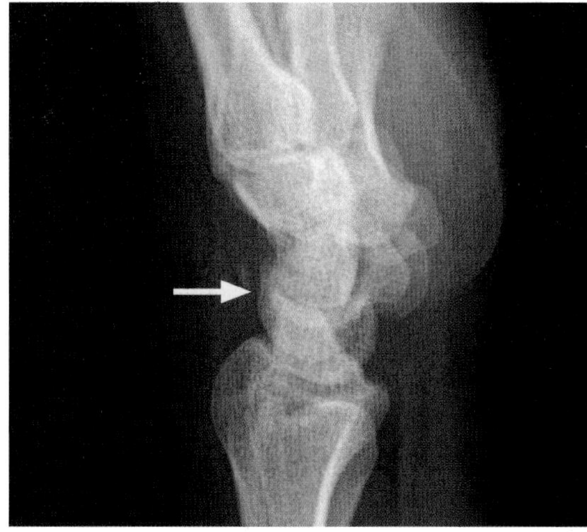

Triquetral fracture: Frontal radiograph (left image) of the wrist is normal. Lateral radiograph shows an avulsion fragment dorsal to the triquetrum (arrow).

- Fracture of the triquetrum can be subtle to detect on the frontal radiograph. Triquetral fractures are best seen on the lateral view of the wrist as an avulsion fragment dorsal to the triquetrum.

Kienbock disease

- Kienbock disease is avascular necrosis of the lunate. It is associated with negative ulnar variance (i.e., ulna shorter than the radius), and thought to be caused by increased load on the lunate.

Fingers and Hand Trauma

Extension tendon injuries

normal anatomy **mallet finger** **boutonniere deformity**

distal phalanx
lateral extensor slips
converge on base of distal phalanx
middle phalanx
central band of extensor tendon
inserts on base of middle phalanx

mallet finger
disruption of extensor tendon
at distal phalanx

boutonniere deformity
disruption of extensor tendon
at middle phalanx

- **Mallet finger**: Mallet finger is disruption of the extensor tendon at the distal phalanx. It is caused by direct impact on the tip of the finger. Mallet finger may be associated with an avulsion fragment of the distal phalanx, which is clinically an important distinction.
- On physical exam, the distal interphalangeal (DIP) joint cannot be straightened.
- **Boutonniere deformity** is injury to the medial slip of the extensor tendon. It is seen most commonly in the setting of rheumatoid arthritis, but it may be post-traumatic.
- The proximal interphalangeal (PIP) joint herniates through the lateral slips of the common extensor tendon and becomes entrapped, causing fixed flexion of the PIP and extension of the DIP.

Gamekeeper's thumb (skier's thumb)

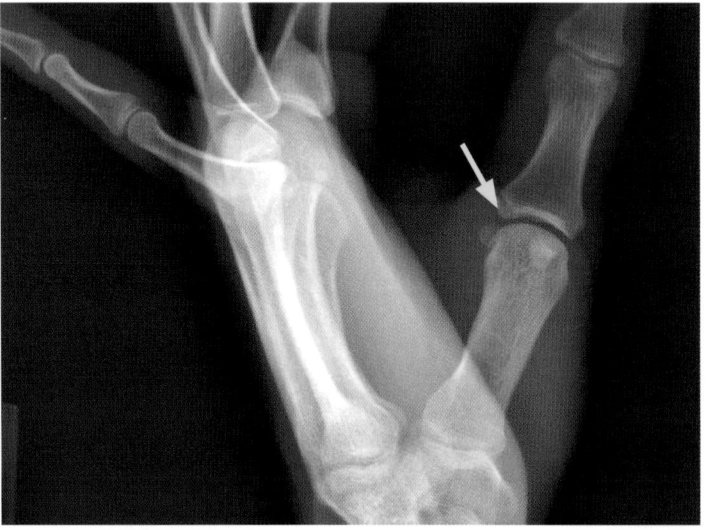

Gamekeeper's thumb with associated nondisplaced avulsion fragment:

Radiograph of the thumb demonstrates a nondisplaced avulsion fragment at the base of the thumb proximal phalanx (arrow).

- Gamekeeper's (also known as skier's) thumb is injury to the ulnar collateral ligament (UCL) at the base of the thumb proximal phalanx. It is caused by forced abduction of the thumb. Gamekeeper's thumb may be associated with an avulsion fragment of the base of the proximal phalanx.
- Incomplete UCL tears can be treated conservatively; however, complete UCL tears must be treated surgically.
- The *Stener lesion* is a complication of UCL injury and represents complete UCL disruption with interposition of the adductor aponeurosis. The Stener lesion must be treated surgically.

Bennett fracture

- A Bennett fracture is an intra-articular fracture of the base of the thumb metacarpal.

Rolando fracture

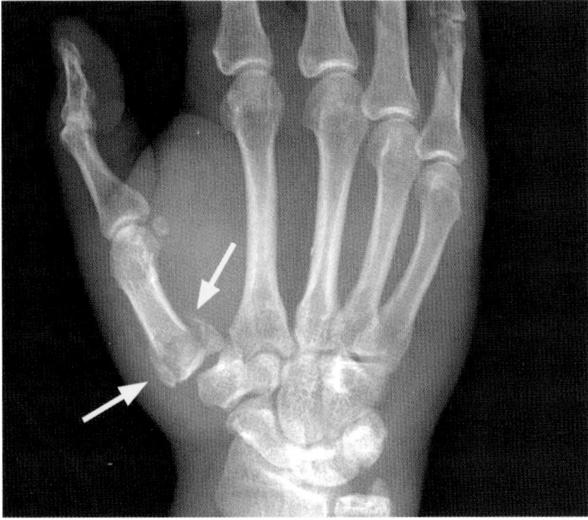

Rolando fracture: PA radiograph of the hand demonstrates a comminuted intra-articular fracture at the base of the thumb metacarpal (arrows).

- A Rolando fracture is a comminuted Bennett fracture.

Boxer's fracture

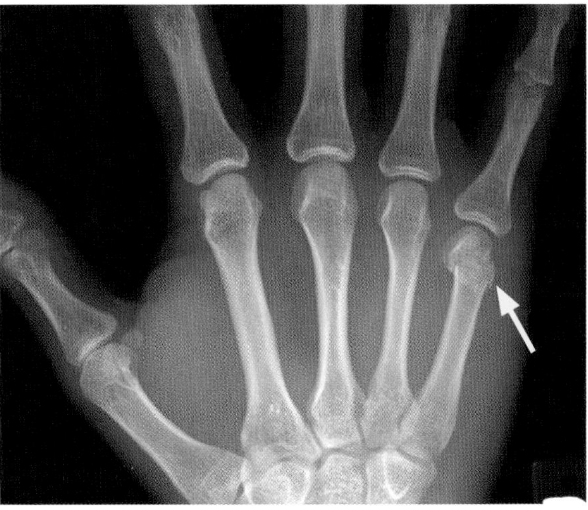

Boxer's fracture: PA radiograph of the hand shows a fracture of the 5th metacarpal neck (arrow).

- A Boxer's fracture is a metacarpal neck fracture, most commonly occurring in the 5th metacarpal.

Volar plate fracture

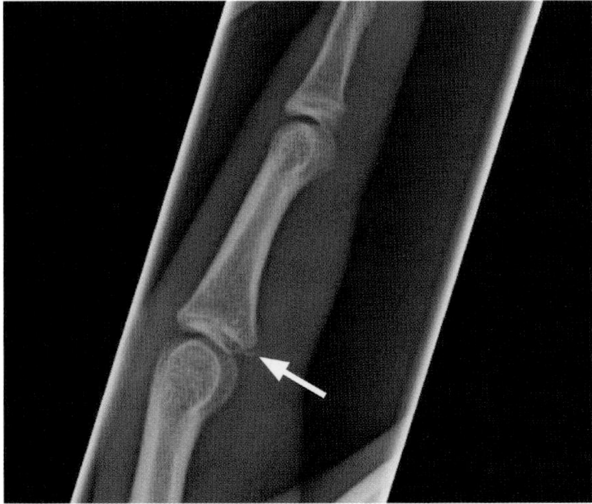

Volar plate fracture: Lateral radiograph shows a subtle tiny avulsion fragment (arrow) of the volar aspect of the middle phalanx at the PIP joint.

- A volar plate fracture is an avulsion fracture of the volar aspect of the proximal middle phalanx, caused by hyperextension.

References, resources, and further reading

General References:

Brower A.C. Arthritis in Black and White. (2nd ed.). Saunders. (1997).

Chew, F.S. & Roberts, C.C. Musculoskeletal Imaging: A Teaching File (2nd ed.). Lippincott Williams & Wilkins. (2005).

Greenspan, A. Orthopedic Imaging: A Practical Approach (5th ed.). Lippincott Williams & Wilkins. (2010).

Helms, C.A. et al. Musculoskeletal MRI (2nd ed.). Saunders. (2008).

Manaster, B., May, D. & Disler, D.G. Musculoskeletal Imaging: The Requisites (3rd ed.). Mosby. (2006).

Weissman, B. Imaging of Arthritis and Metabolic Bone Disease (1st ed.). Mosby. (2009).

Arthritis:

Bennett D., Ohashi K., Elkhoury G. Spondyloarthropathies: ankylosing spondylitis and psoriatic arthritis. Radiologic Clinics of North America, 42(1), 121-34(2004).

Jacobson J.A. et al. Radiographic Evaluation of Arthritis: Inflammatory Conditions. Radiology, 248(2), 378-89(2008).

Jacobson J.A. et al. Radiographic Evaluation of Arthritis : Degenerative Joint Disease and Variations. Radiology, 248(3), 737-47(2008).

Steinbach L.S. Calcium pyrophosphate dihydrate and calcium hydroxyapatite crystal deposition diseases: imaging perspectives. Radiologic Clinics of North America, 42(1), 185-205, vii(2004).

Neoplasms:

Miller T.T. Bone tumors and tumorlike conditions: analysis with conventional radiography. Radiology, 246(3), 662-74(2008).

Nomikos G.C. et al. Primary bone tumors of the lower extremities. Radiologic Clinics of North America, 40, 971-90(2002).

Infection:

Bancroft, L.W. MRI imaging of infectious processes of the knee. Radiologic Clinics of North America, 45(6), 931–41, v(2007).

Donovan, A. & Schweitzer, M.E. Current concepts in imaging diabetic pedal osteomyelitis. Radiologic Clinics of North America, 46(6), 1105–24, vii(2008).

Pineda, C., Vargas, A. & Rodríguez, A.V. Imaging of osteomyelitis: current concepts. Infectious Disease Clinics of North America, 20(4), 789–825(2006).

Foot and Ankle:

Choplin, R.H. et al. CT with 3D rendering of the tendons of the foot and ankle: technique, normal anatomy, and disease. Radiographics, 24(2), 343-56(2004).

Kong, A., Cassumbhoy, R. & Subramaniam, R.M. Magnetic resonance imaging of ankle tendons and ligaments: part I - anatomy. Australasian Radiology, 51(4), 315-23(2007).

Leffler, S. & Disler, D.G. MRI imaging of tendon, ligament , and osseous abnormalities of the ankle and hindfoot. Radiologic Clinics of North America, 40, 1147-70(2002).

Rosenberg, Z.S., Beltran, J. & Bencardino, J.T. From the RSNA Refresher Courses MRI Imaging of the Ankle and Foot. Radiographics, (20), 153-79(2000).

Knee:

Barr, M.S. & Anderson, M.W. The knee: bone marrow abnormalities. Radiologic Clinics of North America, 40, 1109-20(2002).

Fox, M.G. MRI imaging of the meniscus: review, current trends, and clinical implications. Radiologic Clinics of North America, 45(6), 1033-53, vii(2007).

Frick, M.A., Wenger, D.E. & Adkins, M. MRI imaging of synovial disorders of the knee: an update. Radiologic Clinics of North America, 45(6), 1017-31, vii(2007).

Mccauley, T.R. MRI imaging of chondral and osteochondral injuries of the knee. Radiologic Clinics of North America, 40, 1095-107(2002).

Phillips, M. & Pomeranz, S. Imaging of Osteochondritis Dissecans of the Knee. Operative Techniques in Sports Medicine, 16(2), 52-64(2008).

Hip:

Anderson, S.E., Siebenrock, K.A. & Tannast, M. Femoroacetabular impingement: evidence of an established hip abnormality. Radiology, 257(1), 8-13(2010).

Hong, R.J., Hughes, T.H., Gentili, A. & Chung, C.B. Magnetic resonance imaging of the hip. Journal of Magnetic Resonance Imaging: JMRI, 27(3), 435-45(2008).

Ikemura, S. et al. MRI evaluation of collapsed femoral heads in patients 60 years old or older: Differentiation of subchondral insufficiency fracture from osteonecrosis of the femoral head. AJR. American Journal of Roentgenology, 195(1), W63–8(2010).

Kwek, E.B.K. et al. An emerging pattern of subtrochanteric stress fractures: a long-term complication of alendronate therapy? Injury, 39(2), 224-31(2008).

Palmer, W.E. Femoroacetabular impingement: caution is warranted in making imaging-based assumptions and diagnoses. Radiology, 257(1), 4-7(2010).

Ragab, Y., Emad, Y. & Abou-Zeid, A. Bone marrow edema syndromes of the hip: MRI features in different hip disorders. Clinical Rheumatology, 27(4), 475-82(2008).

Sweeney, J.P., Helms, C.A., Minagi, H. & Louie, K. The Widened Teardrop Distance: A Plain Film indicator of Hip Joint Effusion in Adults. Radiology, 149, 117-19(1987).

Spine:

Bagley, L.J. Imaging of spinal trauma. Radiologic Clinics of North America, 44(1), 1-12, vii(2006).

Greenbaum, J., Walters, N. & Levy, P.D. An evidenced-based approach to radiographic assessment of cervical spine injuries in the emergency department. The Journal of Emergency Medicine, 36(1), 64-71.(2009).

Phal, P.M. & Anderson, J.C. Imaging in spinal trauma. Seminars in Roentgenology, 41(3), 190-5(2006).

Shoulder:

Chang, D., Mohana-Borges, A., Borso, M. & Chung, C.B. SLAP lesions: anatomy, clinical presentation, MRI imaging diagnosis and characterization. European Journal of Radiology, 68(1), 72-87(2008).

Morag, Y. et al. MRI Imaging of Rotator Cuff Injury: What the Clinician Needs to Know. Radiographics, 26, 1045-66(2006).

Omoumi, P., Teixeira, P., Lecouvet, F. & Chung, C.B. Glenohumeral joint instability. Journal of Magnetic Resonance Imaging: JMRI, 33(1), 2-16(2011).

Opsha, O. et al. MRI of the rotator cuff and internal derangement. European Journal of Radiology, 68(1), 36-56(2008).

Elbow, Forearm, Wrist, and Hand:

Chen, C. et al. Scapholunate advanced collapse: a common wrist abnormality in calcium pyrophosphate dihydrate crystal deposition disease. Radiology, 177(2), 459(1990).

Hauger, O. et al. Pulley system in the fingers: normal anatomy and simulated lesions in cadavers at MRI imaging, CT, and US with and without contrast material distention of the tendon sheath. Radiology, 217(1), 201-12(2000).

Sof, C.M. & Potter, H.G. Imaging of elbow injuries in the child and adult athlete. Radiologic Clinics of North America, 40, 251-65(2002).

Staebler, A., Heuck, A. & Reiser, M. Imaging of the hand: degeneration, impingement and overuse. European Journal of Radiology, 25(2), 118-28(1997).

6 Ultrasound

Contents

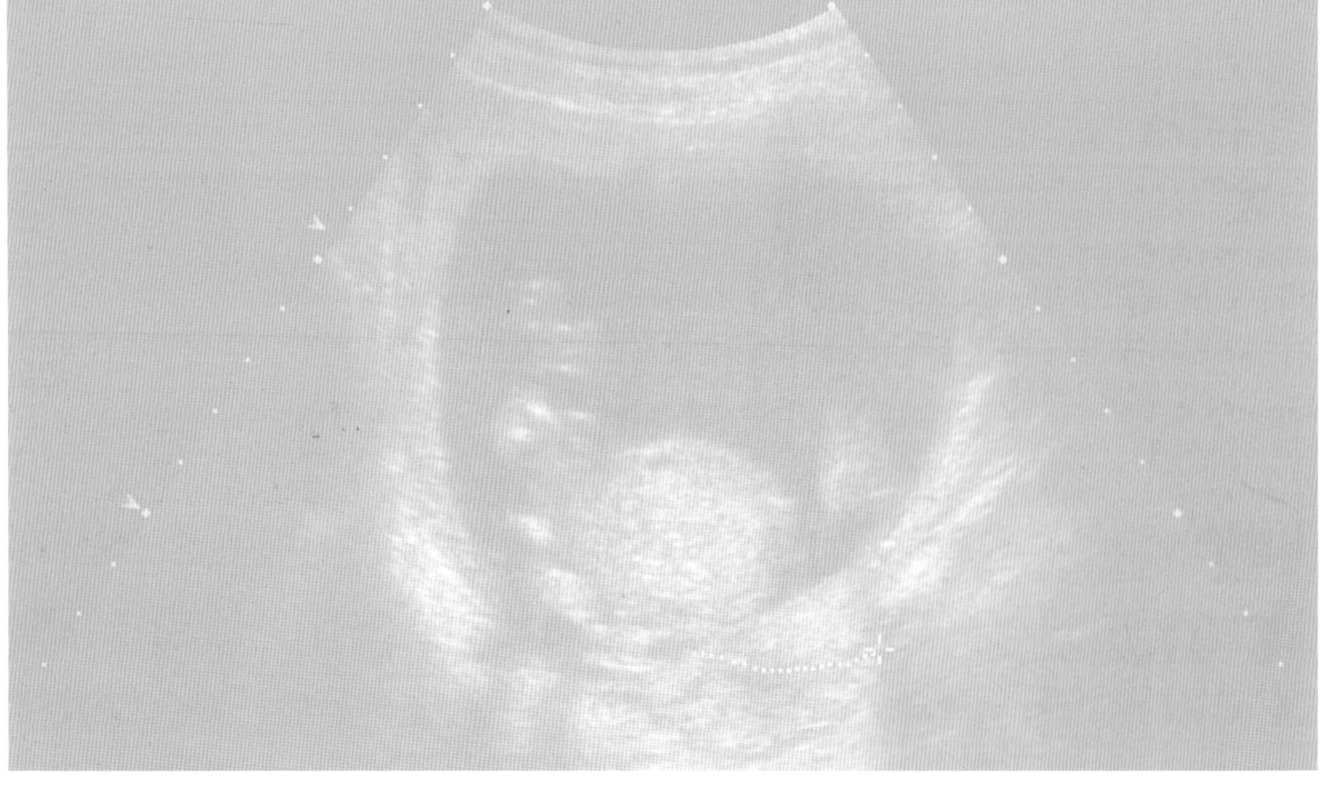

GALLSTONES AND CHOLECYSTITIS

Cholelithiasis

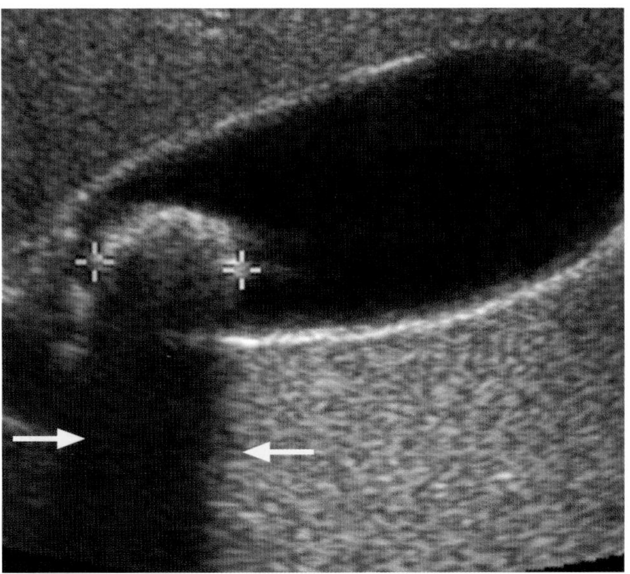

Single gallstone: Sagittal ultrasound of the gallbladder shows an echogenic gallstone (calipers) in the gallbladder neck, with posterior acoustic shadowing (arrows).

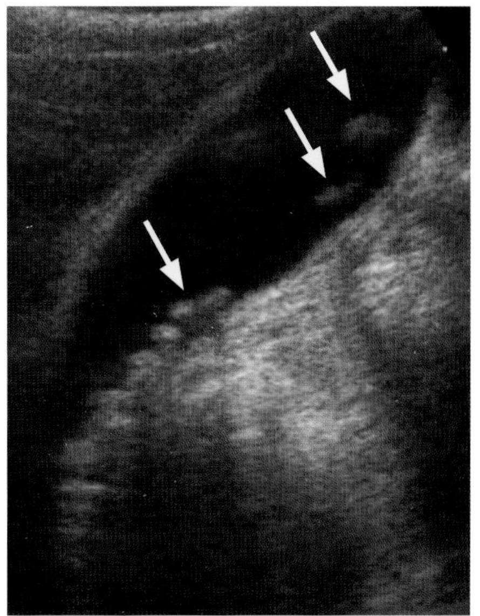

Multiple small gallstones: Sagittal ultrasound of the gallbladder in a different patient shows multiple small shadowing gallstones (arrows).

- Cholelithiasis is the presence of a gallbladder stone or stones, without associated inflammation.
- The classic clinical presentation of symptomatic cholelithiasis is colicky pain after eating a fatty meal, but it is common to see gallstones incidentally in asymptomatic patients.
- Risk factors for developing gallstones include female sex, obesity, pregnancy, middle age, and diabetes.
- The ultrasound diagnosis of gallstones is usually straightforward. Stones are echogenic with posterior acoustic shadowing and are often mobile. It is often helpful to reposition the patient (typically in the left lateral decubitus position) while scanning to assess whether the stones layer dependently to differentiate stones from polyps or other masses.
- A gallbladder completely filled with stones can be more challenging to identify. The *wall-echo-shadow* (WES) sign describes the appearance of a gallbladder full of multiple stones (or one giant stone).

  Two parallel echogenic arcs represent the gallbladder wall and leading edge of the stone, with an intervening thin layer of hypoechoic bile. The gallstone typically casts a prominent shadow.
- The differential diagnosis of echogenic material within the gallbladder includes:

Gallstone(s) (mobile, shadowing).

Gallbladder sludge (mobile, non-shadowing).

Gallbladder polyp (non-mobile, non-shadowing, often attached to the gallbladder wall via a stalk, may be vascular).

Hyperplastic cholecystoses (non-mobile, multiple polyps).

Acute calculous cholecystitis

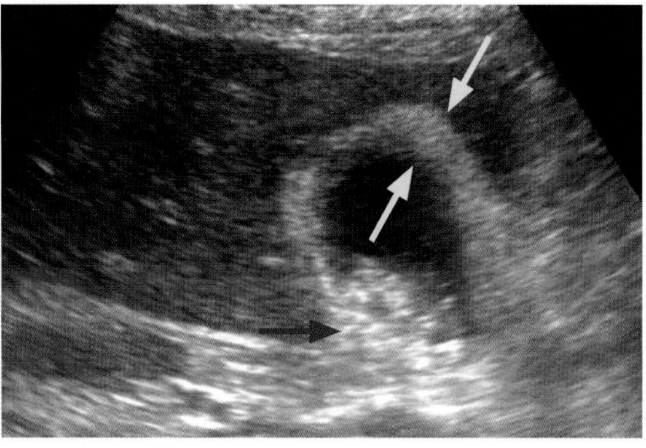

Acute cholecystitis: Oblique sagittal ultrasound through the gallbladder demonstrates a thickened, echogenic gallbladder wall (arrows). The gallbladder contains numerous echogenic gallstones (red arrow).

- Acute cholecystitis is inflammation of the gallbladder, usually due to a gallstone impacting the cystic duct. Ultrasound is the first-line evaluation of suspected acute cholecystitis.
- Acute cholecystitis clinically presents with right upper quadrant (RUQ) pain and fever.
- There is no 100% specific ultrasound finding for acute cholecystitis. However, gallstones are seen >90% of the time and a positive sonographic Murphy's sign (RUQ pain with pressure from the transducer) also has a high positive predictive value. Other findings include:

> Gallbladder wall thickening >3 mm.
>
> Distended gallbladder >4 cm in diameter.
>
> Pericholecystic fluid.
>
> Color Doppler showing hyperemic gallbladder wall.
>
> Hyperechoic fat in the gallbladder fossa (ultrasound correlate to CT finding of fat stranding).

- Complications of acute cholecystitis are rare but serious.

> **Emphysematous cholecystitis** is gas in the gallbladder wall and has a high risk of gallbladder perforation.
>
> **Gangrenous cholecystitis** is necrosis of the gallbladder wall. Sonographic findings include layering echogenic material in the gallbladder lumen representing hemorrhage and sloughed membranes.
>
> **Gallbladder perforation** appears as focal discontinuity of the gallbladder wall. Perihepatic ascites containing dirty echoes is often present.

- Surgical treatment of uncomplicated acute calculous cholecystitis is cholecystectomy. In patients who are not good surgical candidates, a temporizing percutaneous cholecystostomy tube can be placed prior to definitive surgical cholecystectomy.

Acalculous cholecystitis

- Acalculous cholecystitis is cholecystitis without gallstones, typically seen in very sick patients. Risk factors include sepsis, prolonged total parenteral nutrition, and trauma.
- The ultrasound appearance is similar to acute cholecystitis but without stones. Since many patients are ventilated or obtunded, it's often not possible to evaluate for sonographic Murphy's sign.
- Treatment of acalculous cholecystitis is typically interventional radiology percutaneous cholecystostomy. Unlike the treatment of calculous cholecystitis, cholecystostomy is often the definitive therapy.

Emphysematous cholecystitis

- Emphysematous cholecystitis is a rapidly progressive form of acute cholecystitis characterized by gas in the gallbladder wall. Emphysematous cholecystitis is associated with gallbladder ischemia causing bacterial translocation. Treatment is urgent surgery.
- On ultrasound, gas is usually present in both the gallbladder lumen and wall, which appears as echogenic lines and foci with posterior dirty shadowing.

Porcelain gallbladder

- A porcelain gallbladder is a calcified gallbladder wall due to either chronic irritation from supersaturated bile or repeated bouts of gallbladder obstruction.
- Porcelain gallbladder is associated with an increased risk of gallbladder cancer, but the incidence is controversial. In general, prophylactic cholecystectomy is the standard of care.
- On ultrasound, the wall of the gallbladder is echogenic, and there are almost always associated gallstones.
- The differential diagnosis of an echogenic gallbladder wall includes a porcelain gallbladder, a gallbladder packed full of stones (which will feature the *wall-echo-shadow* sign), or emphysematous cholecystitis (intramural gas will have dirty shadowing).

Courvoisier gallbladder

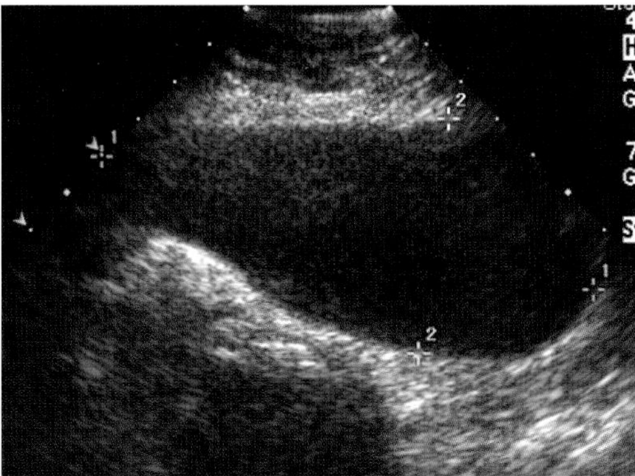

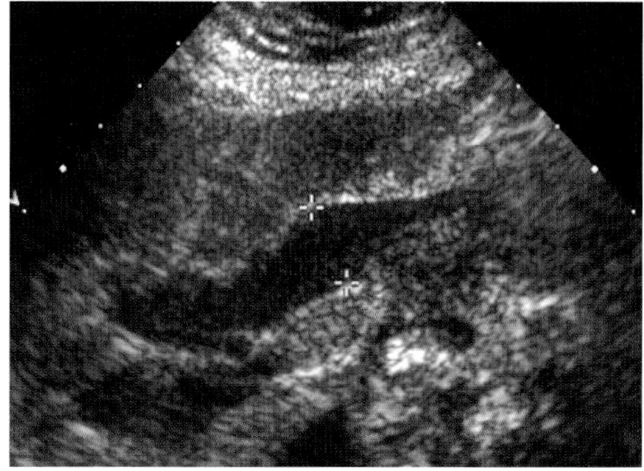

Courvoisier gallbladder: Sagittal ultrasound of the gallbladder (left image, marked with calipers) demonstrates a massively distended gallbladder. The common bile duct (right image, indicated by calipers) is also distended due to chronic malignant obstruction.

Case courtesy Julie Ritner, MD, Brigham and Women's Hospital.

- The Courvoisier gallbladder refers to a markedly dilated gallbladder (originally described as being so large as to be directly palpable) from malignant obstruction of the common bile duct.
- A markedly distended gallbladder implies chronic obstruction of either the cystic duct (when seen in isolation) or the common bile duct (when seen in combination with dilation of the common bile duct and intrahepatic biliary dilation).

Hyperplastic cholecystoses

Overview of hyperplastic cholecystoses

- The hyperplastic cholecystoses are a spectrum of non-neoplastic proliferative disorders caused by deposition of cholesterol-laden macrophages within the wall of the gallbladder. The cholecystoses range from abnormalities of the gallbladder wall (adenomyomatosis and strawberry gallbladder) to gallbladder polyps extending into the lumen.

Adenomyomatosis

- Adenomyomatosis is cholesterol deposition in mural Rokitansky–Aschoff sinuses.

  It is important not to confuse with adenomyosis of the uterus: It may be helpful to remember that there are three **L**'s in gallbladder, and adenomyomatosis is a **l**onger word than adenomyosis.
- The ultrasound hallmark of adenomyomatosis is the *comet-tail* artifact due to reflections off of tiny crystals seen in a focally thickened and echogenic gallbladder wall.

Strawberry gallbladder (cholesterolosis of the gallbladder)

- Strawberry gallbladder is a pathologic diagnosis that is not apparent by imaging. It is characterized by tiny mural cholesterol deposits likened to strawberry seeds.

Gallbladder polyps

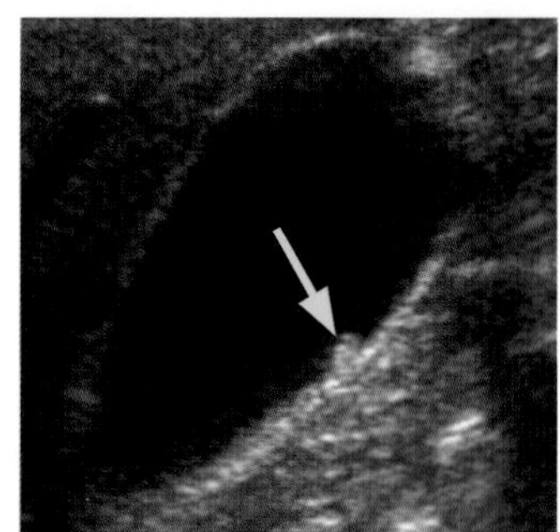

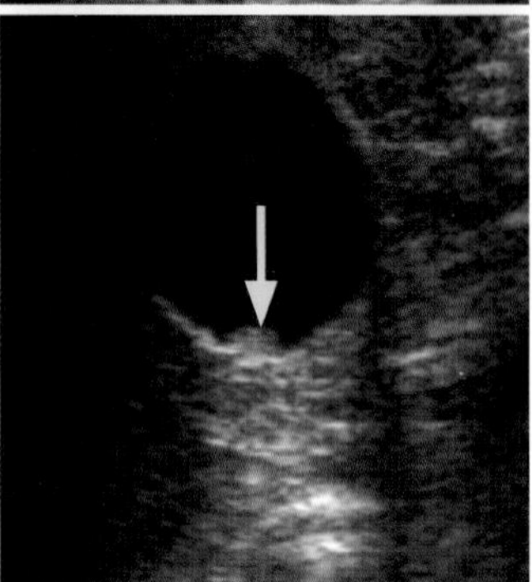

Gallbladder polyp:
Sagittal and transverse views of the gallbladder show a small non-shadowing echogenic lesion (arrows). After repositioning the patient, this was shown to be non-mobile.

- Most gallbladder polyps are benign cholesterol polyps that are part of the hyperplastic cholecystosis spectrum. Rarely (<5%), polyps may be premalignant adenomas.
- Clinically, gallbladder polyps may cause right upper quadrant pain or even cholecystitis if the cystic duct is obstructed.
- The following characteristics, known as the *six S's,* increase the risk for a polyp being malignant:

> **S**ize >10 mm or rapid growth. As a caveat, ultrasound has limited sensitivity and specificity in detecting small polyps (<10 mm), especially in the presence of gallstones.
>
> **S**ingle: A solitary polyp is more suspicious for malignancy. In contrast, benign cholesterol polyps tend to be multiple.
>
> **S**essile (broad-based): Sessile morphology is suspicious. A polyp is more likely benign if pedunculated.
>
> **S**tones: The presence of stones may induce chronic inflammation, which can predispose towards malignancy.
>
> Primary **S**clerosing cholangitis increases risk of malignancy.
>
> **S**ixty (age) or greater.

- In patients with several of these high-risk features, cholecystectomy should be considered in the presence of a polyp greater than 6 mm in size.
- The typical ultrasound appearance of a polyp is a non-mobile, non-shadowing polypoid lesion extending from the wall into the lumen of the gallbladder. There may be vascular flow in the stalk.
- The main differential consideration is adherent sludge, which will not have any vascular flow.

GALLBLADDER CANCER

Primary gallbladder carcinoma

- Gallbladder cancer is a rare malignancy with a poor prognosis. A typical clinical presentation may include right upper quadrant pain, weight loss, and jaundice.
- Risk factors for development of gallbladder cancer include:

> Gallstones and chronic cholecystitis.
>
> Porcelain gallbladder (somewhat controversial).
>
> Primary sclerosing cholangitis.
>
> Inflammatory bowel disease (ulcerative colitis more frequently than Crohn disease).
>
> Adenomatous polyp >10 mm or >6 mm with multiple risk factors, as described above.

- Ultrasound shows a polypoid mass with increased vascularity in the gallbladder. There is often direct invasion into the liver.
  - Regional adenopathy occurs early.
  - Bile duct obstruction may be present.

Gallbladder metastases

- Metastases to the gallbladder are uncommon.
- Hepatocellular carcinoma can spread directly to the gallbladder through the bile ducts.
- Melanoma can spread hematogenously to the gallbladder mucosa.

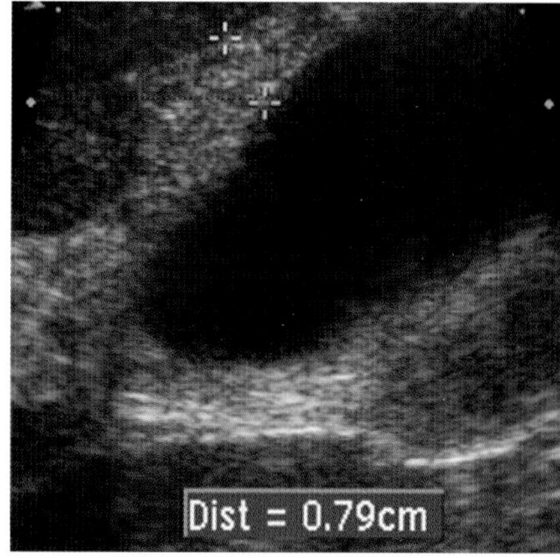

Sagittal ultrasound of the gallbladder shows diffuse wall thickening to 8 mm (calipers). In this case, the wall thickening was due to cirrhosis and resultant hypoproteinemia.

Diffuse gallbladder wall thickening >3 mm (common causes in bold)

- Fluid-overload/edematous states:
  - **Cirrhosis:** Hypoalbuminemia leads to diffuse gallbladder wall thickening.
  - **Congestive heart failure.**
  - Protein-wasting nephropathy.
- Inflammatory/infectious:
  - **Cholecystitis**, usually with associated cholelithiasis.
  - **Hepatitis.**
  - Pancreatitis.
  - Diverticulitis.
- Infiltrative neoplastic disease:
  - Gallbladder carcinoma.
  - Metastases to gallbladder (rare).
- Post-prandial state.

Focal gallbladder wall thickening (common causes in bold)

- Hyperplastic cholecystoses: **Adenomyomatosis and cholesterol polyp.**
- Vascular: **Varices.**

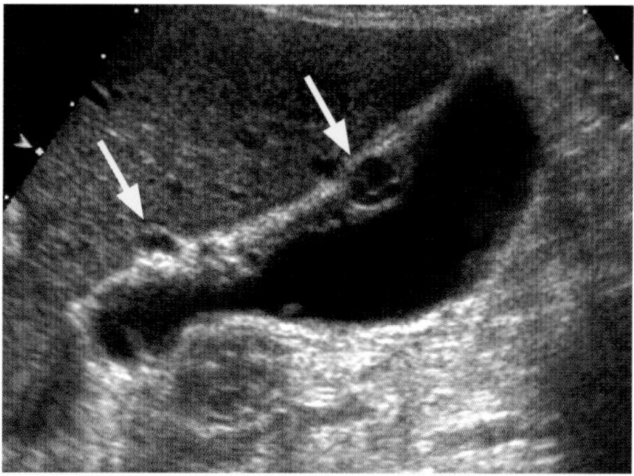

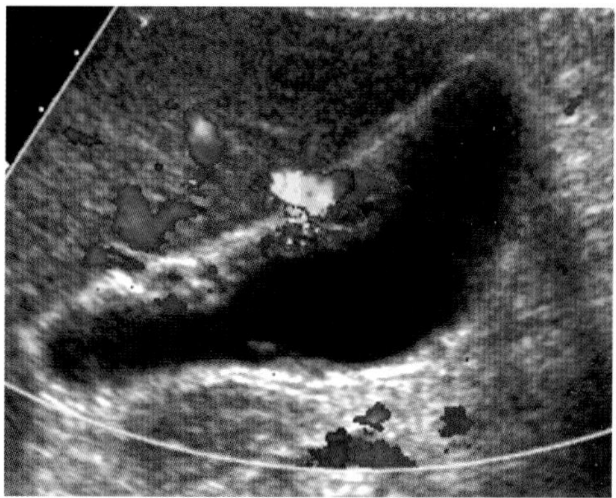

Gallbladder varices due to portal hypertension: Sagittal grayscale ultrasound of the gallbladder (left image) demonstrates several hypoechoic, cystic-appearing structures within the gallbladder wall (arrows). Color Doppler (right image) confirms the vascular etiology.

Case courtesy Julie Ritner, MD, Brigham and Women's Hospital.

- Neoplastic disease:
  - Adenomatous polyp.
  - Gallbladder carcinoma.
  - Adjacent hepatic tumor.

Non-shadowing "mass" in the gallbladder lumen

- Tumefactive sludge (mobile).
- Blood/pus (mobile).
- Gallbladder polyp (immobile).
- Gallbladder carcinoma (immobile).

Echogenic gallbladder wall

- Porcelain gallbladder.
- Gallbladder full of stones (signified by the wall-echo-shadow sign).
- Emphysematous cholecystitis.

Bile duct anatomy

- Sagittal view of the normal porta hepatis on CT and ultrasound:

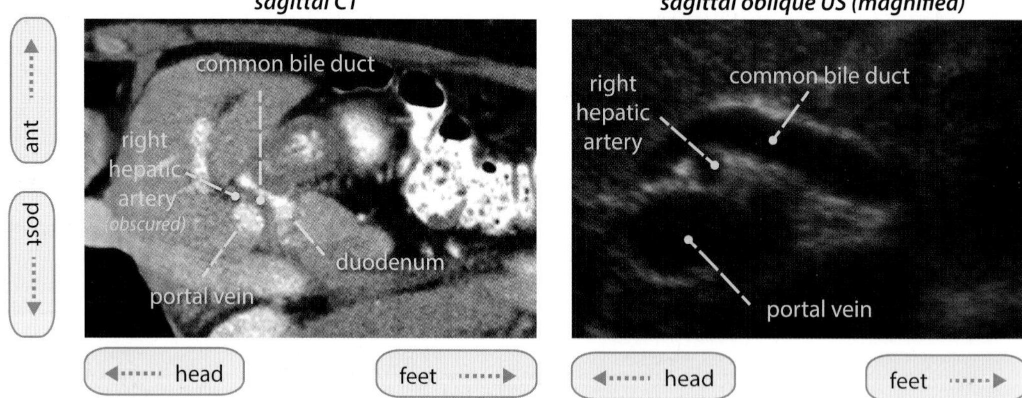

Choledocholithiasis

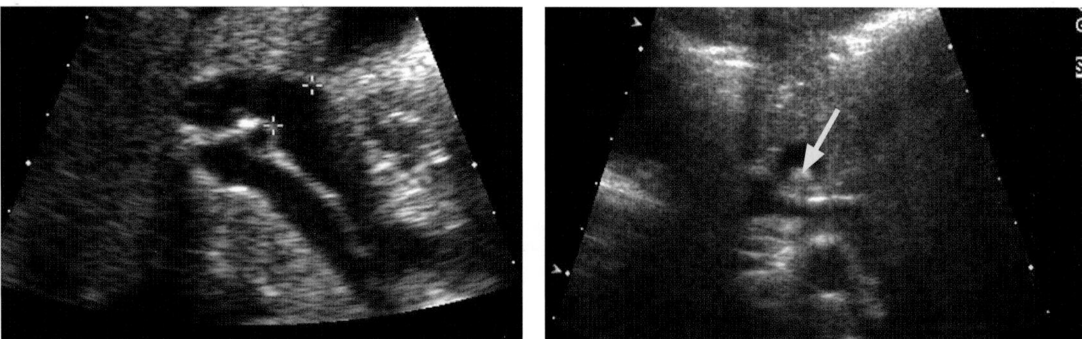

Choledocholithiasis: Sagittal ultrasound (left image) of the porta hepatis (in the same orientation as the reference anatomic image above) demonstrates common bile duct dilation (calipers) to 1.1 cm. Transverse scan (right image) through the region of the head of the pancreas shows an echogenic gallstone within the distal common bile duct (arrow).

Case courtesy Julie Ritner, MD, Brigham and Women's Hospital.

- Choledocholithiasis is a stone in the common bile duct, generally treated with ERCP.

Mirizzi syndrome

- Mirizzi syndrome is seen when a stone in the cystic duct causes inflammation and external compression of the adjacent common hepatic duct (CHD).
- Essential for the surgeon to know about preoperatively because the CHD may be mistakenly ligated instead of the cystic duct. Additionally, inflammation can cause the gallstone to erode into the CHD and cause a cysto-choledochal fistula and biliary obstruction.
- On ultrasound, a stone is typically impacted in the distal cystic duct, and the CHD is dilated. The cystic duct tends to run in parallel with the CHD.

Pneumobilia

- Pneumobilia is air in the biliary tree. It is commonly seen after biliary interventions, but may be due to cholecystoenteric fistula or rarely emphysematous cholecystitis.
- On ultrasound, small echogenic gas bubbles are seen **centrally** in the liver with posterior dirty shadowing.
- In contrast to pneumobilia, portal venous gas (which implies bowel ischemia until proven otherwise) is peripheral and causes a spiky appearance of the portal vein spectral Doppler waveform.

Cholangiocarcinoma

- Cholangiocarcinoma is cancer of the bile ducts. It classically presents with painless jaundice. Most cases of cholangiocarcinoma are sporadic, although key risk factors include chronic biliary disease (in the US) and liver fluke infection (in the Far East).
- The hilum is the most common location of cholangiocarcinoma. A hilar cholangiocarcinoma is known as a Klatskin tumor. Intrahepatic cholangiocarcinoma occurs uncommonly (10%).
- Ultrasound plays a role in the initial evaluation of adjacent adenopathy and vascular structures. Local nodes include porta hepatis and hepatoduodenal ligament nodes. If more distal nodal disease is present, then the tumor is generally considered unresectable.

Biliary ductal dilation

- A rule of thumb for assessing the common bile duct diameter (CBD) is to assume that the CBD ought to be 6 mm or less before age 60, but may still be normal if 1 mm larger per decade after that age. For example, an 8 mm duct in an 80-year-old patient may be considered normal.

  Some sources, however, suggest very small differences with age (mean duct diameter of 3.6 mm for 60-year-old patients and 4.0 mm for 85-year-old patients).

  For the hepatic ducts, >2 mm in size or >40% of the adjacent portal vein diameter is abnormal.
- The common bile duct is approximately 1.6 mm wider (on average) in patients who have undergone cholecystectomy, compared to patients who have not had a cholecystectomy.
- In general, malignancy causes more prominent ductal dilation than benign disease.

LIVER

DIFFUSE METABOLIC PARENCHYMAL LIVER DISEASE

Hepatic steatosis

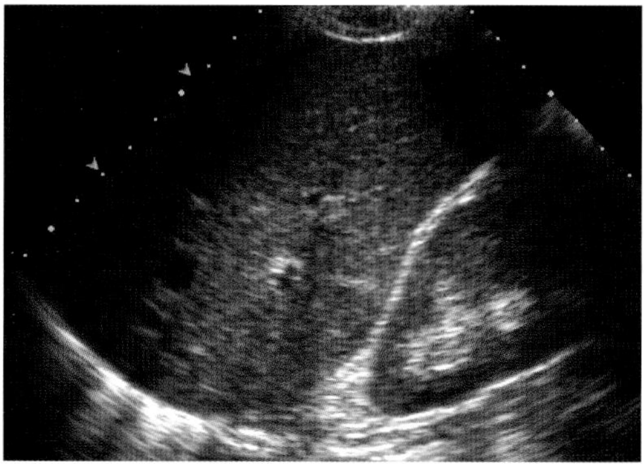

Normal liver: Ultrasound of the liver and kidney shows the normal isoechoic appearance of liver relative to renal cortex.

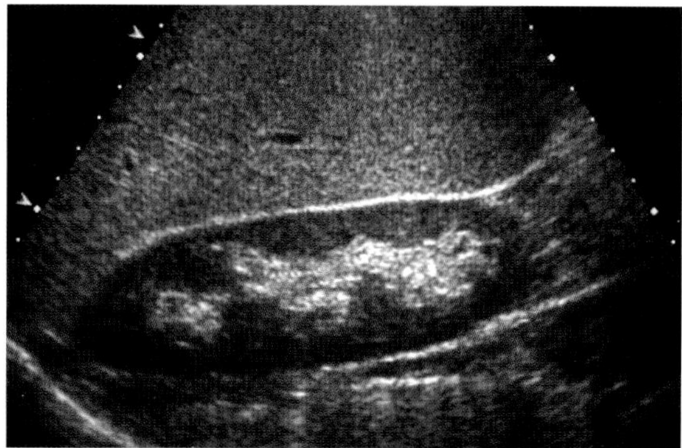

Hepatic steatosis: Ultrasound in a different patient shows diffusely increased echogenicity of the liver when compared to the renal cortex.

- Hepatic steatosis is the accumulation of excess fat within hepatocytes due to a metabolic derangement (obesity or diabetes), hepatotoxins (EtOH), or prolonged fasting.
- Ultrasound shows a diffuse increase in hepatic echogenicity. Normally, the liver and kidney should have the same echogenicity. With fatty infiltration, the liver appears more echogenic than the kidney. Hepatic steatosis also causes increased sound attenuation, leading to poor visualization of deeper structures.
- Focal fat sparing is a geographic area of hypoechogenicity in an otherwise fatty liver.

  A characteristic location of focal fat sparing is the gallbladder fossa.

Cirrhosis

- Cirrhosis is the replacement of functioning hepatocytes with dysfunctional fibrotic tissue, due to long-standing repeated cycles of hepatocyte injury and repair.
- Micronodular cirrhosis causes cirrhotic nodules less than 3 mm in size and is most commonly associated with alcoholism.
- Macronodular cirrhosis features larger nodules (>3 mm) separated by wide scars and fibrous septae. Macronodular cirrhosis is caused by fulminant viral hepatitis which does not uniformly affect the liver.
- The typical ultrasound appearance of cirrhosis is a coarse, heterogeneously increased liver echotexture with a nodular external contour. In early cirrhosis, the superficial nodularity is best appreciated with a high-frequency linear probe. The caudate lobe is often spared and hypertrophies in response to increased demand (the caudate has direct venous drainage into the IVC and therefore can bypass the hypertensive portal system). End-stage cirrhosis is characterized by a shrunken, nodular liver.
- Signs of portal hypertension are often present, including an enlarged portal vein, splenomegaly, varices, portosystemic shunts, and a patent umbilical vein. Imaging of portal hypertension is discussed in detail in the liver Doppler section.

LIVER INFECTIONS

Viral hepatitis

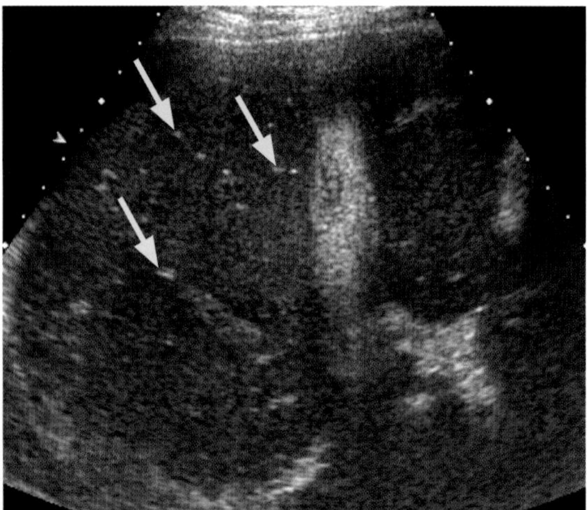

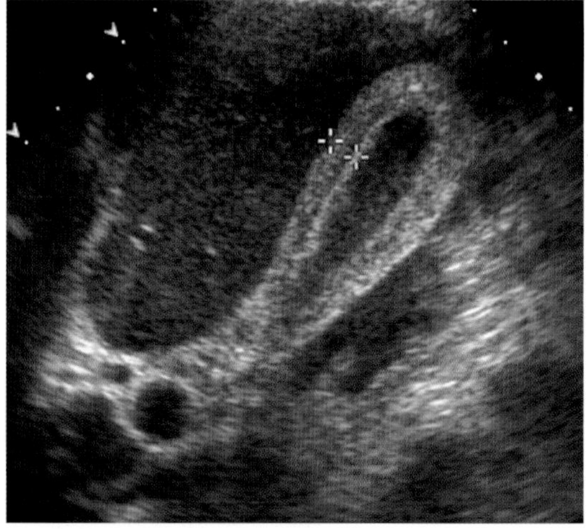

Viral hepatitis: Sagittal image of the liver (left image) demonstrates increased echogenicity of the portal triads appearing as numerous echogenic dots (arrows) that produce a *starry sky* appearance. Sagittal view of the gallbladder in the same patient (right image) shows marked diffuse gallbladder wall thickening (calipers), which is commonly seen in acute hepatitis.

Case courtesy Julie Ritner, MD, Brigham and Women's Hospital.

- Viral hepatitis is infection of the liver by a hepatotropic virus. Hepatitis B and C cause chronic disease.
- The most common ultrasound finding is a normal liver. Occasionally periportal edema produces the characteristic *starry sky* pattern of increased portal triad echogenicity.
- Acute hepatitis is often associated with diffuse severe gallbladder wall thickening.

Pyogenic abscess

- Pyogenic abscess is caused by pus-forming organisms and is usually due to spread from intestinal or biliary infection (most commonly *E. coli*).
- Infection starts as an ill-defined area of altered echogenicity (phlegmon stage) that evolves into a well-defined hypoechoic structure with internal echoes (mature abscess).

Amebic abscess

- Amebic abscess is caused by *Entamoeba histolytica*. A near-universal presenting symptom is pain, seen in 99% of patients. The most common location is near the dome of the right lobe.
- On ultrasound, an amebic abscess is indistinguishable from a pyogenic abscess and appears as a hypoechoic structure with low-level internal echoes.
- Antimicrobial therapy is usually sufficient treatment, and drainage is rarely necessary.

Echinococcal cyst (hydatid disease)

- Echinococcal cyst is caused by larvae of *Echinococcus granulosus*, most commonly found in endemic areas in the Middle East, Mediterranean, and South America.
- There is a risk of anaphylaxis with peritoneal spillage of cyst fluid, although these are often biopsied and drained uneventfully. Medical treatment is albendazole or mebendazole.
- Classic ultrasound appearance is a large liver cyst with numerous peripheral daughter cysts.

  A highly suggestive finding is the change in position of daughter cysts as the patient is repositioned.

  The *water-lily* sign is an undulating membrane within the hydatid cyst.

  Hydatid sand is a fine sediment caused by separation of the membranes from the endocyst.

Candidiasis

- Hepatic candidiasis is a rare infection in the immunocompromised due to *Candida albicans* or *Candida glabrata.*
- On imaging, there are multiple tiny targetoid lesions. The presence of concurrent similar-appearing lesions in the spleen is highly suggestive of hepatosplenic candidiasis.

Hepatic *Pneumocystis jiroveci*

- Hepatic *Pneumocystis jiroveci* is seen in disseminated disease in the severely immunocompromised. Hepatic infection is classically secondary to the use of inhaled pentamidine to treat *Pneumocystis* pneumonia, as pentamidine is not absorbed systemically and thus would not prevent hepatic infection.
- Ultrasound shows multiple punctate echogenic calcifications in the liver and often spleen.

Benign hepatic neoplasms (in order of frequency)

Cavernous hemangioma

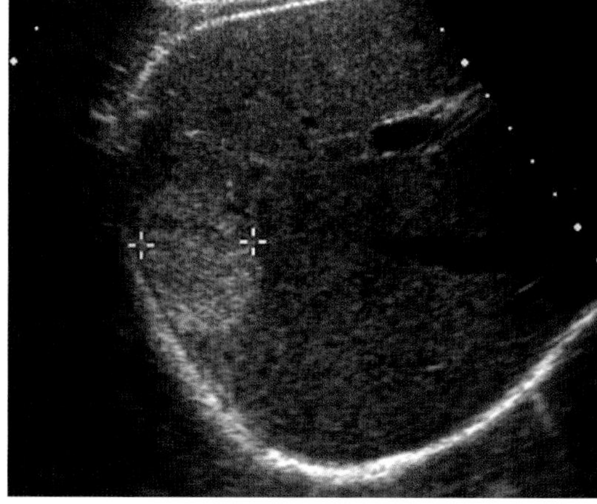

Cavernous hemangioma: Transverse ultrasound through the right lobe of the liver demonstrates a circumscribed slightly heterogeneous echogenic mass (calipers) with mild posterior acoustic enhancement.

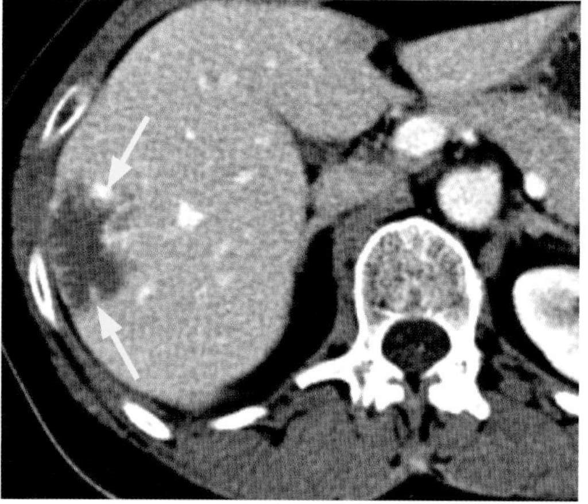

Portal venous phase axial contrast-enhanced CT demonstrates a hypoattenuating lesion with discontinuous peripheral nodular enhancement (arrows), typical of a hemangioma.

Case courtesy Julie Ritner, MD, Brigham and Women's Hospital.

- Hepatic cavernous hemangioma is the most common benign hepatic neoplasm.
- The classic ultrasound appearance of hemangioma is a solitary, circumscribed, homogeneously **echogenic** mass with no flow on color Doppler. Posterior acoustic enhancement is nonspecific but may be present. When seen, posterior acoustic enhancement is thought to correlate with hypervascularity. A hypoechoic halo should *never* be seen – this finding suggests malignancy.
- Hepatic hemangioma can rarely have an atypical hypoechoic appearance when seen in a fatty liver.
- If a solitary, classic-appearing hemangioma is seen and the patient has an otherwise normal-appearing liver, normal LFTs, no known malignancy, and is asymptomatic, then no further workup is required.
- Any heterogeneity or atypical ultrasound findings should prompt consideration of an alternative diagnosis. The differential of a hyperechoic hepatic mass includes hyperechoic hepatocellular carcinoma or metastatic disease (even in the absence of a halo). In a patient with cirrhosis or any known primary malignancy, further workup (MRI or CT) is usually warranted if the mass is new, even if classic appearing.

Focal nodular hyperplasia (FNH)

- Focal nodular hyperplasia (FNH) is a benign hyperplastic hepatic mass with a central non-fibrotic stellate scar consisting of biliary ductules and venules.
- Ultrasound findings are nonspecific. The central scar is rarely seen on ultrasound, and even when it is, this finding can be seen in other lesions, including hepatocellular carcinoma, giant hemangioma, or adenoma.
- FNH is often difficult to detect on sonography. It may be nearly isoechoic to normal liver and manifest on imaging as a subtle displacement of the hepatic contour.
- Doppler findings of FNH include a *spoke-wheel* configuration of arterial vessels.
- MRI or Tc-99m sulfur colloid scintigraphy can confirm (classically, FNH has increased uptake of sulfur colloid). MRI is by far the more useful test.

Hepatic adenoma

- Hepatic adenoma is a benign liver tumor associated with oral contraceptives, anabolic steroids, and type I glycogen storage disease (von Gierke's disease - in which case adenomas will be multiple).
- Due to high incidence of hemorrhage, adenomas are usually resected.
- There are no specific ultrasound features to distinguish an adenoma from other hepatic masses. An adenoma may be hyperechoic, isoechoic, or hypoechoic relative to normal liver.
- Adenoma is usually photopenic on Tc-99m sulfur colloid scintigraphy (in contrast to FNH).

Hepatic lipoma

- Hepatic lipoma is a benign neoplasm composed of fat that appears as a well-defined hyperechoic mass. It may appear identical to hemangioma or hyperechoic hepatocellular carcinoma.
- When multiple, may be associated with tuberous sclerosis and renal angiomyolipomas.

Biliary cystadenoma

- Biliary cystadenoma is a benign cystic mass lined with biliary-type epithelium.
- Although benign, most are surgically resected since malignant transformation may occur.
- Biliary cystadenoma appears as a multiseptated cystic mass on all imaging modalities. Mural nodules should be regarded with suspicion. The presence of mural nodularity suggests malignant transformation to cystadenocarcinoma.

Hepatic metastases

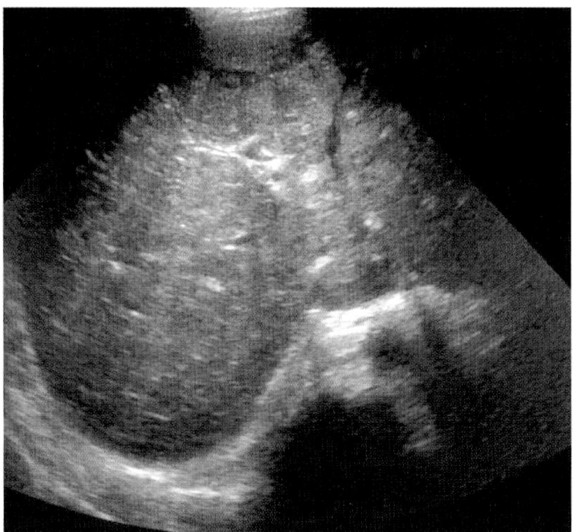

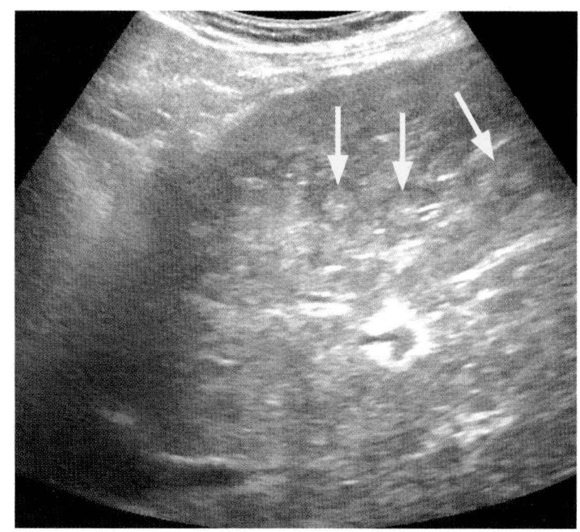

Innumerable liver metastases, initially difficult to see due to technique: Initial scanning with a low-frequency vector probe (left image) demonstrates a coarsened hepatic echotexture without definite mass. This appearance may mimic cirrhosis. When a higher frequency curved probe is used (right image), innumerable target lesions (arrows) become apparent, consistent with innumerable hepatic metastases.

Case courtesy Julie Ritner, MD, Brigham and Women's Hospital.

- Metastatic disease to the liver is far more common than primary hepatocellular carcinoma.
- Metastases can have a variable ultrasound appearance, although the classic finding is a hypoechoic rim producing a *target* sign.
- Hypoechoic hepatic metastases include:

  Breast (can be either hypoechoic or hyperechoic).

  Pancreas.

  Lung.

  Lymphoma.
- Hyperechoic hepatic metastases include:

  Colon cancer is hyperechoic in greater than 50% of cases. A hyperechoic appearance may suggest a better prognosis.

  Renal cell carcinoma.

  Breast (can be either hyperechoic or hypoechoic).

  Carcinoid.

  Choriocarcinoma.
- Calcified hepatic metastases (hyperechoic with acoustic shadowing) include:

  Colon cancer (especially mucinous type).

  Gastric adenocarcinoma.

  Osteosarcoma (very rare).
- Cystic hepatic metastases include:

  Ovarian cystadenocarcinoma.

  Gastrointestinal sarcoma.
- Infiltrative metastases include:

  Lung.

  Breast. In particular, treated breast cancer may cause a *pseudo-cirrhosis* appearance.

  Prostate.

Hepatocellular carcinoma (HCC)

- Hepatocellular carcinoma (HCC) is a hepatic malignancy arising in the setting of chronic inflammation.
- Patients with cirrhosis or chronic viral hepatitis are regularly screened for HCC with serum alpha-fetoprotein levels and ultrasound.

  Ultrasound is not very sensitive to detect small HCC in end-stage cirrhotic livers.
- HCC has a variety of ultrasound appearances — therefore, a mass in a cirrhotic liver is considered HCC until proven otherwise. High Doppler flow may be present, especially at the periphery of the mass, due to arteriovenous shunting.
- HCC has a propensity for venous invasion. The portal veins should always be carefully evaluated in the presence of a hepatic mass. Internal Doppler flow within a venous clot suggests a tumor thrombus.

Fibrolamellar carcinoma

- Fibrolamellar carcinoma is a variant of HCC seen in young adults without cirrhosis and is not associated with elevated alpha-fetoprotein.
- Fibrolamellar carcinoma has a much better prognosis compared to typical HCC.

Hepatic lymphoma

- Primary hepatic lymphoma may present as a single mass or multiple masses.
- Lymphoma tends to be hypoechoic and may demonstate the *target* sign typical of metastases.

Post-transplant lymphoproliferative disorder (PTLD)

- Post-transplant lymphoproliferative disorder (PTLD) is a type of lymphoma caused by Epstein–Barr virus that arises after solid organ or bone marrow transplant. Patients with renal transplants are at particular risk for development of PTLD. PTLD may occur anywhere, regardless of which organ was transplanted.
- Treatment is reduction/withdrawal of immunosuppression.
- PTLD appears as a mass with a variable and nonspecific ultrasound appearance. Therefore, it is important to mention PTLD if a liver mass is seen in a transplant patient.

LIVER: COMMON IMAGING PATTERNS

Multicystic liver

- Multiple simple cysts.
- Caroli disease (saccular dilation of the intrahepatic bile ducts).
- Autosomal dominant polycystic kidney disease (ADPKD): Liver cysts seen in >50% of patients.

Liver cyst with internal echoes

- Simple cyst with internal hemorrhage.
- Liver abscess.
- Hematoma.
- Necrotic or cystic metastasis (ovarian cystadenocarcinoma or gastrointestinal sarcoma).

Multiple echogenic liver lesions

- Prior granulomatous disease exposure.
- Disseminated pneumocystis in AIDS. Classic history is treatment with inhaled pentamidine, which does not have systemic absorption.

PORTAL VEINS

Anatomy

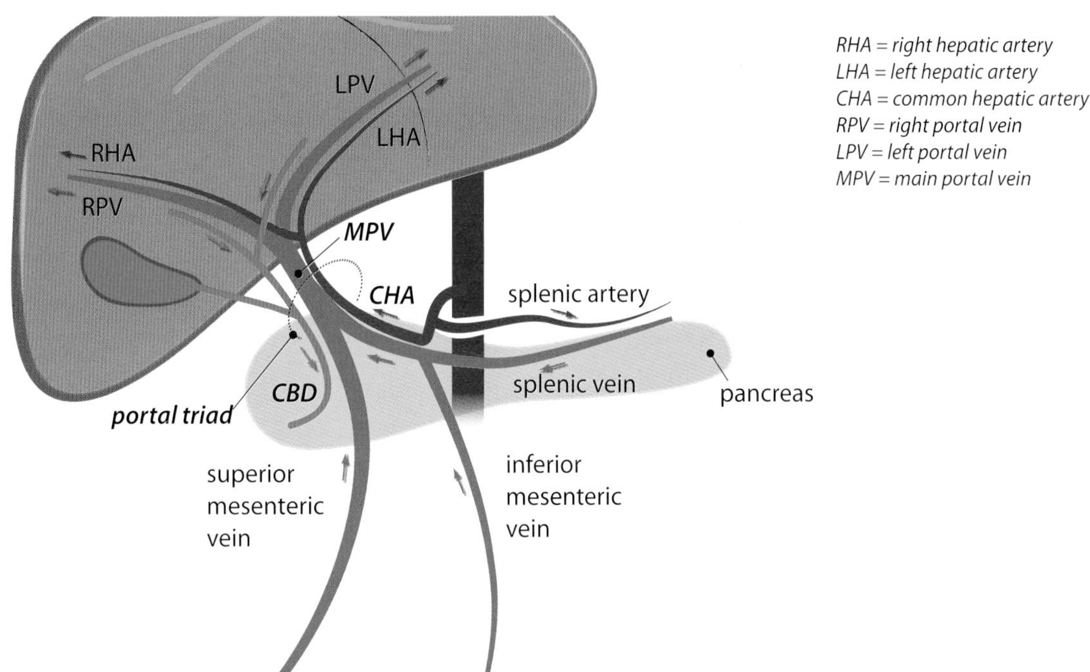

Portal hypertension

- Portal hypertension is increased pressure of the portal venous system. It can be classified in relation to the hepatic capillary bed as pre-sinusoidal, sinusoidal, or post-sinusoidal:

  Pre-sinusoidal: Insult is proximal to the hepatic parenchyma, such as portal vein thrombosis.

  Sinusoidal: Insult is hepatic in origin, such as cirrhosis.

  Post-sinusoidal: Insult is beyond the liver, such as Budd–Chiari (hepatic vein thrombosis) or IVC thrombosis.

- Normally, the portal veins and hepatic arteries flow in the same direction, toward the liver. This direction is called *hepatopetal* flow (*-petal* = toward). The normal portal venous waveform is above the baseline (hepatopetal) and gently undulating.

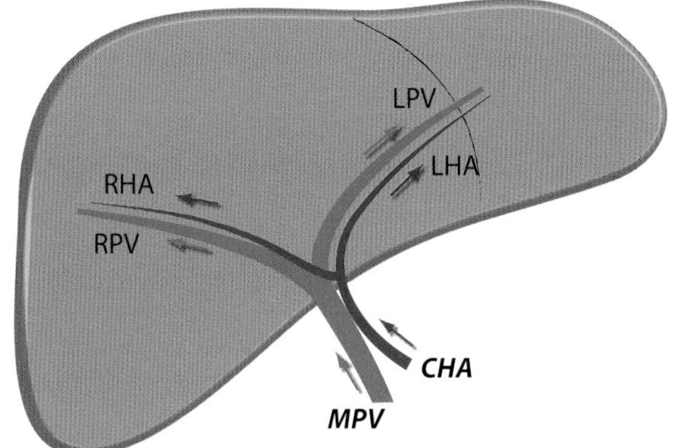

- A pulsatile portal venous waveform is abnormal. The differential diagnosis for a pulsatile portal venous waveform includes tricuspid regurgitation and right-sided CHF. The differential diagnosis for hepatic vein pulsatility is similar, and is discussed in the following section.

- Portal pressure is defined as a direct portal venous pressure of >5 mm Hg, although the portal venous pressure is not measured directly.
- Ultimately, when portal venous pressure is higher than forward pressure, the portal venous flow will reverse, which is diagnostic for portal hypertension. Reversal of portal venous flow is called *hepatofugal* flow (*-fugal* = away, same Latin root as *fugitive*).

reversed = *hepatofugal* flow
hepatic arteries and portal veins flow in opposite directions

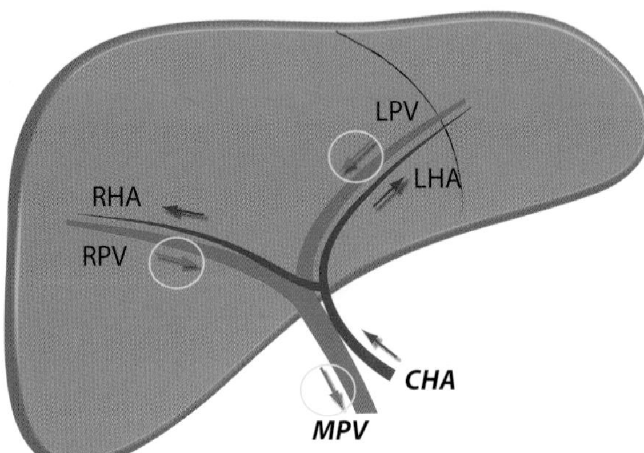

- In addition to flow reversal, there are several secondary findings of portal hypertension:

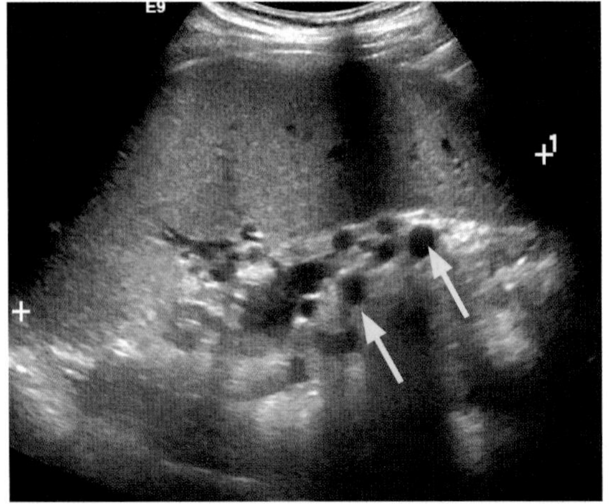

Splenomegaly and splenic varices: Sagittal ultrasound in the left upper quadrant shows an enlarged spleen (calipers) measuring 15 cm in craniocaudal dimension. There are numerous tubular hypoechoic structures (arrows) at the splenic hilum representing varices.

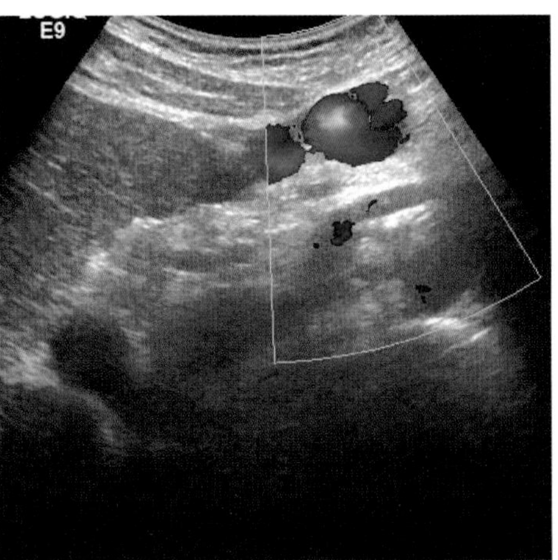

Transverse Doppler ultrasound of the left lobe of the liver shows a recanalized umbilical vein, which is considered diagnostic of portal hypertension.

Case courtesy Julie Ritner, MD, Brigham and Women's Hospital.

Low portal venous velocity (<16 cm/sec).

Dilated portal vein (13 mm is the maximal normal diameter in quiet respiration).

Splenomegaly.

Varices.

Portosystemic shunts are often present, most commonly gastro-esophageal, paraumbilical, or splenorenal. Note that an isolated portosystemic shunt may not be caused by portal hypertension. For instance, isolated obstruction of the splenic vein from pancreatitis or neoplasm may lead to a shunt.

A recanalized umbilical vein is a portosystemic shunt that is diagnostic of portal hypertension.

- Portal hypertension (and reversal of portal flow) can be treated with a transjugular intrahepatic portosystemic shunt (TIPS), which connects a branch of the portal vein to a systemic hepatic vein.
- Ultrasound is used for surveillance of TIPS patency, starting with a post-procedure baseline. Routine follow-up is performed according to the following schedule: In 1 month, every 3 months for the first year, and then every 6 to 12 months.
- Flow in a patent TIPS will be towards the hepatic veins, and flow in the portal veins will be towards the TIPS. Therefore, flow in the main portal vein will be hepatopetal and flow in the right and left portal veins will be hepatofugal (highlighted below with yellow circles).

Patent TIPS:
blood flows through TIPS to hepatic veins
RPV and LPV have reversed flow (toward TIPS)
MPV has hepatopetal flow (toward TIPS)

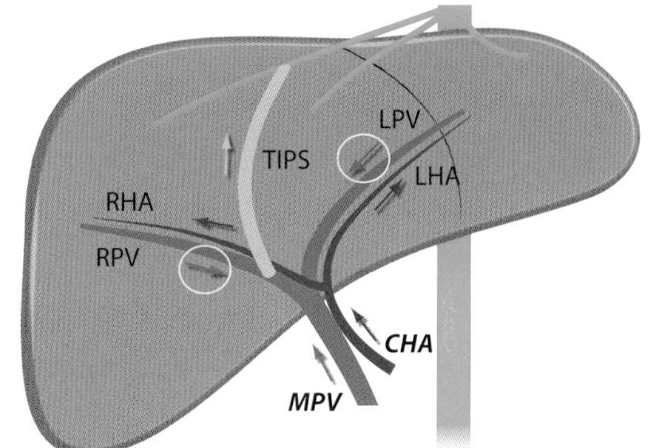

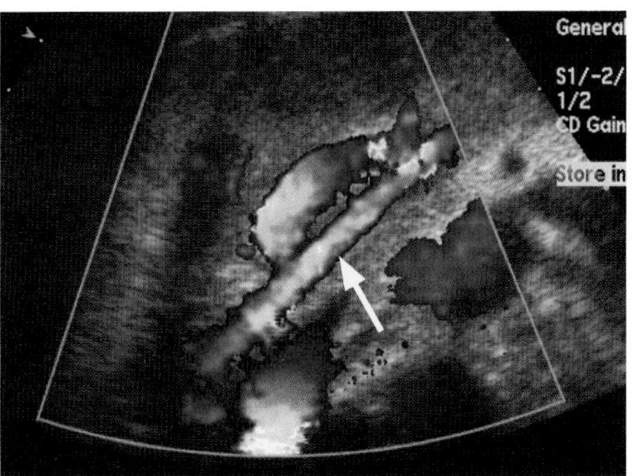

Patent TIPS: Color Doppler of the porta hepatis including the proximal TIPS shows flow within the TIPS (yellow arrow).

Case courtesy Julie Ritner, MD, Brigham and Women's Hospital.

- US can evaluate for stenosis of the TIPS.

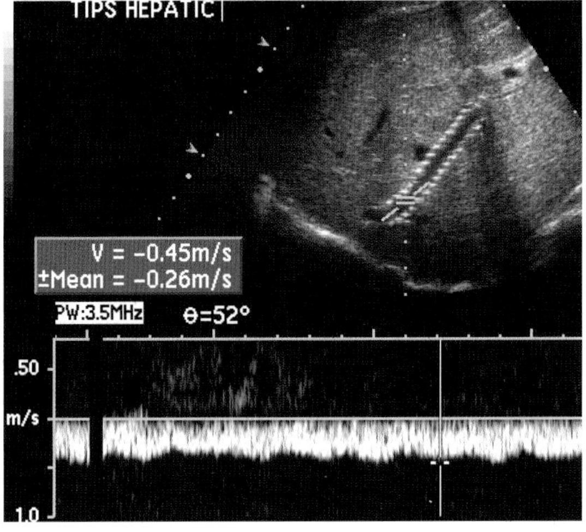

TIPS stenosis: Spectral Doppler of a TIPS shows a velocity of 45 cm/sec, indicative of stenosis due to slow flow.

Case courtesy Julie Ritner, MD, Brigham and Women's Hospital.

High intra-TIPS velocity >190 cm/sec or low intra-TIPS velocity of <90 cm/sec suggests stenosis.

Intra-TIPS velocity change of ±>50 cm/sec since the baseline study is also concerning for stenosis.

Low main portal vein velocity (<30 cm/sec) suggests TIPS stenosis.

- If the TIPS becomes occluded, the right and left portal veins will "re-reverse" and become hepatopetal.

occluded TIPS:
no blood flow through TIPS
RPV and LPV have "re-reversed":
now have hepatopetal flow (away from TIPS)
MPV has hepatopetal flow (towards occluded TIPS)

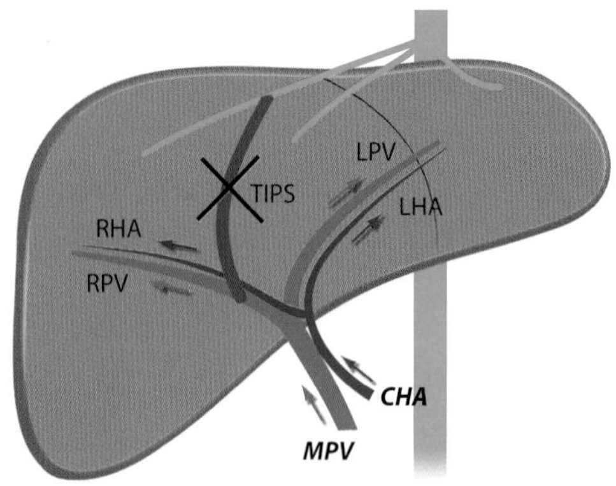

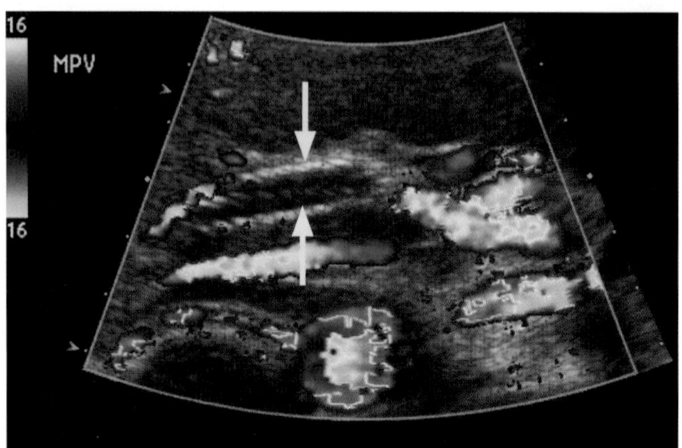

TIPS occlusion: Color Doppler of the porta hepatis including the proximal TIPS shows complete absence of flow within the TIPS (arrows).

Case courtesy Julie Ritner, MD, Brigham and Women's Hospital.

Portal vein thrombosis

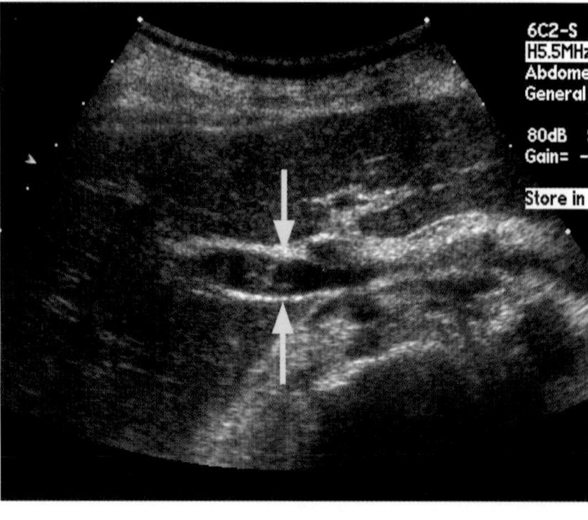

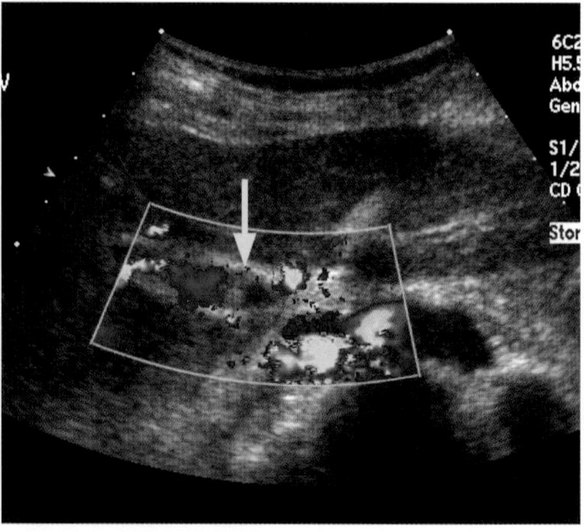

Grayscale transverse image of the porta hepatis shows echogenic debris within the main portal vein (arrows). Color Doppler confirms partial portal vein thrombosis with lack of flow in the proximal portal vein (arrow).

Case courtesy Julie Ritner, MD, Brigham and Women's Hospital.

- Thrombosis of the portal vein can be bland (simple thrombosis) or may be due to tumor invasion.
- Bland portal vein thrombus can be caused by general hypercoagulable state or may be due to local inflammation from pancreatitis or hepatitis.

  In infants, omphalitis or dehydration may also lead to portal vein thrombosis.
- Tumor thrombus is most commonly caused by hepatocellular carcinoma.

- Ultrasound of portal vein thrombosis shows lack of portal venous flow, often with echogenic thrombus within the portal vein.

  Expansion of the portal vein can be seen with either bland or tumor thrombus.

  On color Doppler, flow within the thrombus suggests tumor thrombus.

- One potential pitfall to be aware of is slow (<16 cm/sec) or stagnant portal venous flow in the presence of portal hypertension which may mimic portal vein thrombosis.
- Long-standing portal vein thrombosis leads to *cavernous transformation* of the portal vein, characterized by formation of multiple small periportal collaterals.

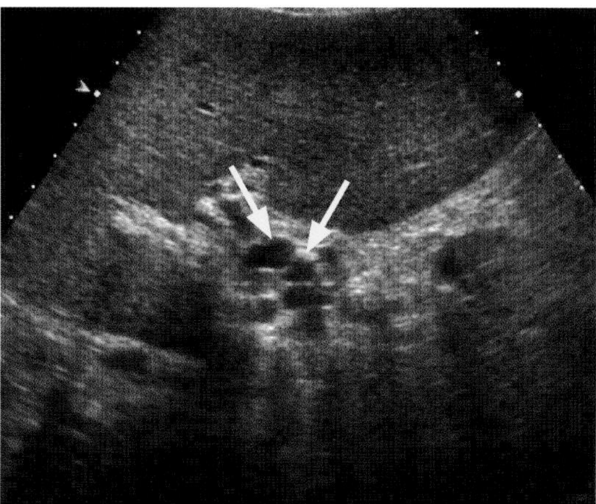

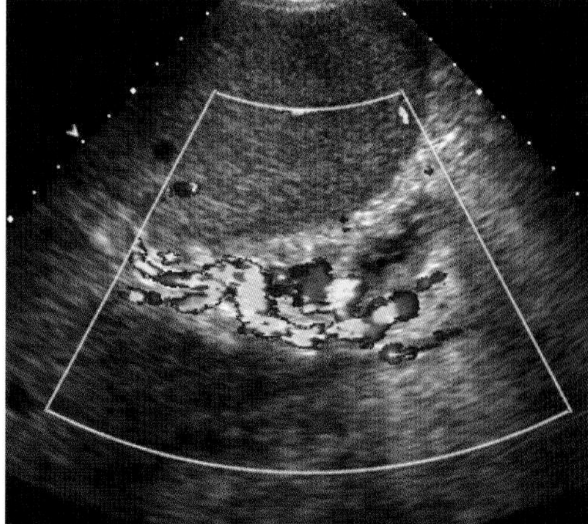

Cavernous transformation of the portal vein: Grayscale transverse image of the porta hepatis shows numerous tubular hypoechoic structures in the expected location of the portal vein (arrows). Color Doppler (right image) demonstrates flow within these collateral vessels, with no identifiable portal vein.

Case courtesy Julie Ritner, MD, Brigham and Women's Hospital.

Portal venous gas

- Portal venous gas is due to abdominal catastrophe (ischemia and infarction) until proven otherwise. If the cause of the portal venous gas is unknown, CT should be performed emergently.
- Grayscale ultrasound shows **peripheral** patchy branching foci of hyperechogenicity that are often transient. Spectral Doppler of the portal vein features numerous characteristic spikes.
- In contrast to portal venous gas, pneumobilia tends to be more central.

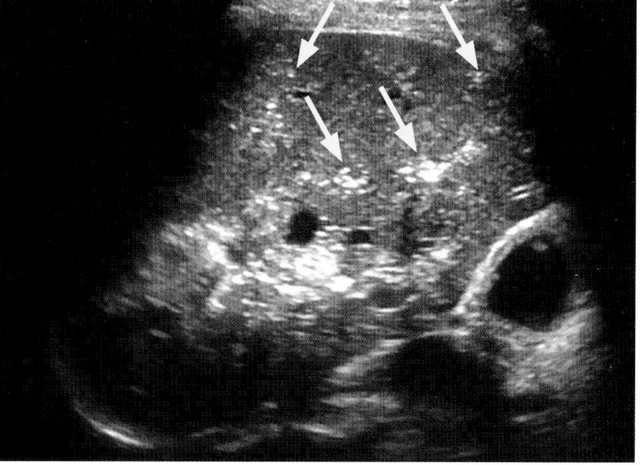

Portal venous gas: Grayscale ultrasound through the liver shows numerous tiny echogenic foci (arrows) in a branching pattern throughout the liver, extending to the periphery.

Case courtesy Julie Ritner, MD, Brigham and Women's Hospital.

Hepatic veins

Normal hepatic vein waveform

- The hepatic veins feed into the IVC and the right side of the heart. The spectral Doppler waveform of the hepatic veins is therefore affected by the cardiac cycle.
- The normal hepatic venous waveform has three distinct components: The A, S, and D waves. Note that *antegrade* flow is defined as forward flow in the normal expected direction.

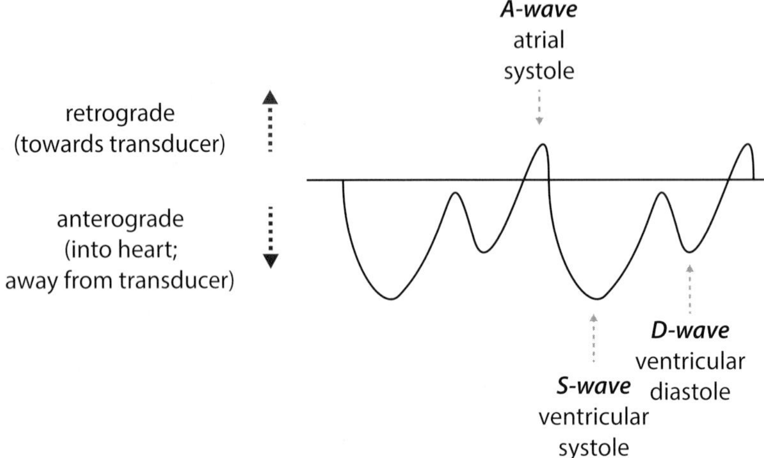

A-wave: Atrial systole, during which blood is forced retrograde (away from the heart) into the liver.

S-wave: Ventricular systole, during which a large volume of blood returns to the right atrium.

D-wave: Ventricular diastole, during which a smaller volume of blood returns to the right atrium.

Increased hepatic vein pulsatility: Accentuated A-wave

- Increased hepatic vein pulsatility is caused by a right-sided cardiac abnormality, either right-sided heart failure or tricuspid regurgitation. Both conditions are characterized by accentuation of the A-wave due to increased retrograde flow during atrial systole.

tricuspid regurgitation

accentuated *A-wave*

short *S-wave*

D-wave

right-sided CHF

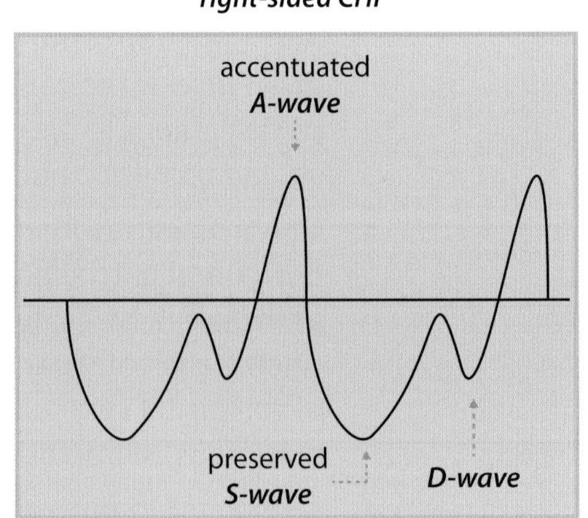

- Normally, the tricuspid valve closes at the beginning of ventricular systole (the beginning of the S-wave).
- In tricuspid regurgitation, there is some degree of blood flow from the right ventricle into the right atrium during ventricular systole, allowing less blood to return to the right atrium from the hepatic veins and IVC during ventricular systole. This results in a decreased or even retrograde S-wave.
- In right-sided heart failure, the tall A-wave is due to increased right atrial pressure; however, in contrast to tricuspid regurgitation, the S-wave is normal since the tricuspid valve remains competent.

Decreased hepatic vein pulsatility

- Decreased hepatic vein pulsatility is seen in cirrhosis, Budd–Chiari (hepatic vein thrombosis), and hepatic veno-occlusive disease.

Pancreas

Pancreatitis

Acute pancreatitis

- Pancreatitis is inflammation of the pancreatic parenchyma, most often caused by alcohol or gallstones.
- Ultrasound is useful in the initial evaluation of pancreatitis to evaluate for gallstones or biliary obstruction.
- Usually, the pancreas appears normal in acute pancreatitis. The pancreas may be diffusely enlarged and relatively hypoechoic due to edema. More severe inflammation may cause the normally hypoechoic pancreas to become isoechoic to liver.
- Ultrasound has limited utility in evaluating complications of pancreatitis such as pancreatic necrosis or peripancreatic fluid collections.

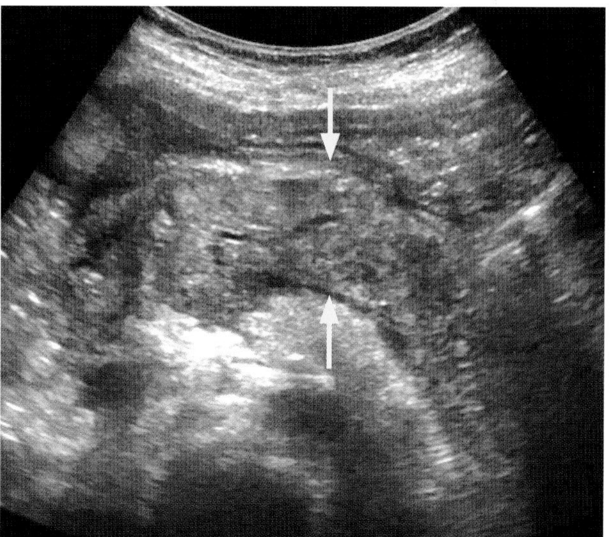

Acute pancreatitis: Transverse ultrasound of the head and body of the pancreas shows a diffusely enlarged, heterogeneous pancreas (arrows) due to pancreatic edema.

Case courtesy Julie Ritner, MD, Brigham and Women's Hospital.

- Complications of acute pancreatitis may be inflammatory, infectious, or vascular.

> A **pancreatic pseudocyst** is usually detectable by ultrasound, although the full extent of large pseudocysts can be difficult to determine by ultrasound alone.
>
> Infectious complications of acute pancreatitis include **peripancreatic abscess**, **infected pseudocyst**, and **infected pancreatic necrosis**.
>
> The two most important vascular complications of pancreatitis are **splenic vein thrombosis** and **splenic artery pseudoaneurysm**, both of which can be characterized by Doppler ultrasound.

Chronic pancreatitis

- Chronic pancreatitis is caused by repeated bouts of acute pancreatitis (most commonly alcoholic).
- The classic ultrasound appearance of chronic pancreatitis is an atrophied gland, with diffuse calcifications and dilated and beaded distal pancreatic duct.
- Calculi within the pancreatic duct may also be seen.

PANCREATIC NEOPLASMS

Pancreatic adenocarcinoma

- Pancreatic adenocarcinoma is the most common pancreatic tumor, and is typically seen in older males.
- Small tumors are hypoechoic, while larger masses may be more heterogeneous. It can be difficult to identify the tumor extent on ultrasound because of infiltrative margins and invasion of the tumor into pancreatic parenchyma and adjacent structures.
- The most common location for a tumor to arise is the pancreatic head, where the mass often presents with ductal obstruction. The *double duct* sign represents dilation of both the pancreatic and common bile ducts caused by malignant obstruction.

Cystic pancreatic neoplasms

- Cystic pancreatic neoplasms are a diverse group of unrelated pancreatic tumors that may appear similar by ultrasound.
- Serous cystadenoma is a benign tumor seen in older females, consisting of multiple tiny cysts. A characteristic calcified scar is not often seen, but is very specific when present.
- Mucinous cystic neoplasm has malignant potential, and is usually seen in middle-aged females. Compared to serous cystadenoma, the cysts are larger in size. The mucin can generate numerous fine echoes.
- Intraductal papillary mucinous neoplasm (IPMN) is a neoplasm of variable and controversial natural history that communicates with either the main pancreatic duct or branch ducts. Demonstration of the ductal communication can be difficult by ultrasound.

Pancreatic endocrine tumors

- Tumors arising from the neuroendocrine cells of the pancreas may be either functioning or nonfunctioning.
- Functioning tumors are usually symptomatic, small at diagnosis, and identified through biochemical testing. In contrast, nonfunctioning tumors may be asymptomatic, and hence, large at the time of diagnosis.
- Intraoperative ultrasound continues to gain ground and is helpful in identifying small tumors at surgery.
- Insulinomas are the most common pancreatic endocrine tumors. Preoperative ultrasound detection is difficult and is successful less than 60% of the time. When seen, insulinomas are hypoechoic, encapsulated pancreatic nodules.
- Gastrinomas are the second most common pancreatic endocrine tumors. Liver metastases are present at the time of diagnosis in 60% of patients.

Pancreatic lymphoma

- B-cell lymphoma is the most common subtype of lymphoma to affect the pancreas, and is almost always associated with adenopathy and multi-organ involvement by the time the pancreas is involved.
- The typical ultrasound appearance of pancreatic lymphoma is a diffusely enlarged, hypoechoic gland.

SPLEEN

PATTERNS OF DISEASE

Splenic calcification

- Granulomatous disease: Calcifications may be scattered or diffuse.
- Splenic infarct.
- Hematoma.
- Calcified splenic artery aneurysm.

Cystic splenic lesion: Color Doppler should always be used to exclude a vascular etiology

- Splenic artery aneurysm or pseudoaneurysm.
- Hematoma.
- Abscess.
- Pancreatic pseudocyst.

Echogenic splenic lesion

- Hemangioma (can also be hypoechoic).
- Hamartoma.
- Lymphangioma.

Hypoechoic splenic lesion

- Laceration (in the setting of trauma).
- Abscess.
- Lymphoma.
- Sarcoidosis.
- Metastasis.
- Infarct (tends to be peripheral).
- Extramedullary hematopoiesis.

Splenomegaly (defined as >14 cm in sagittal plane)

- Mild to moderate splenomegaly:
  - **Portal hypertension** (most common).
  - Infection.
  - AIDS.
- Moderate to marked splenomegaly:
  - Leukemia/lymphoma.
  - Infectious mononucleosis.
- Massive splenomegaly:
  - Myelofibrosis.

KIDNEYS

STONES, OBSTRUCTION, AND HYDRONEPHROSIS

Evaluation of kidney stones

- Ultrasound is an excellent modality for evaluation of nephrolithiasis, which may cause renal obstruction and resultant hydronephrosis.
- An echogenic shadowing focus in the kidney, ureter, or bladder is suspicious for a stone.
- After diagnosing a renal or ureteral calculus, one should always evaluate for the presence of hydronephrosis and perinephric fluid.

Approach to hydronephrosis

- The most common cause of hydronephrosis is an obstructing calculus.

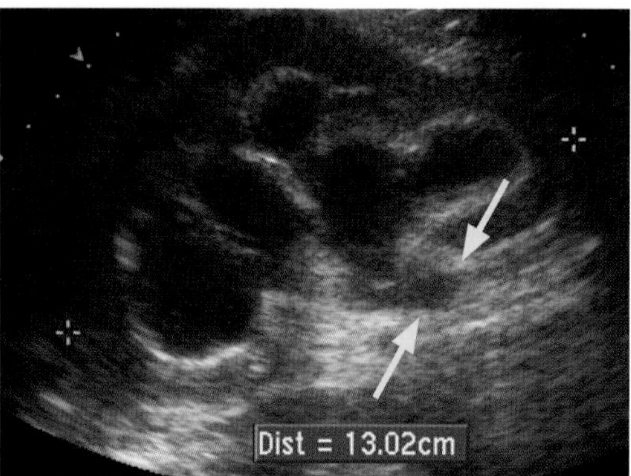

Sagittal view of the left kidney shows marked hydroureteronephrosis (arrows show dilation of the proximal ureter).

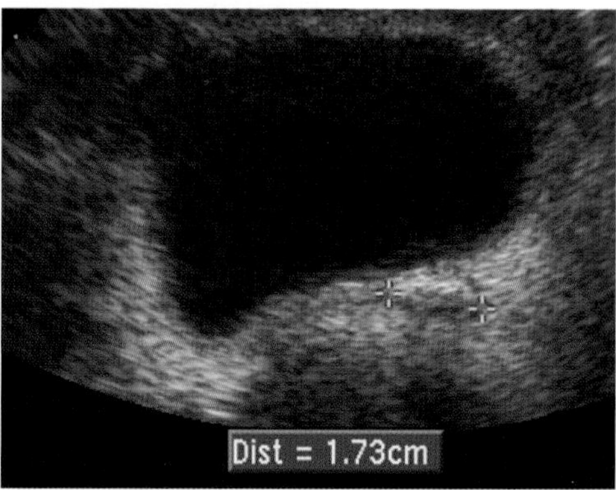

Transverse view of the bladder in the same patient shows a 17 mm shadowing left UVJ calculus (calipers).

- Although hydronephrosis is usually due to ureteral obstruction, it is possible to have hydronephrosis without obstruction. For instance, vesicoureteral reflux or pregnancy may cause a dilated ureter without obstruction. Pregnancy preferentially affects the right side.
- Likewise, obstruction without hydronephrosis may also be seen in:
  - Very acute obstruction.
  - Obstruction with dehydration, where there is insufficient urine production to create a pressure backup.
  - Obstruction with ruptured fornix. Increased pressure from obstruction may cause a fornix to rupture, which would decompress the renal pelvis and spill fluid into the perinephric space.

Pitfalls in diagnosing hydronephrosis

- It can sometimes be difficult to distinguish between hydronephrosis and multiple renal sinus cysts. Renal sinus cysts are subsequently discussed and include peripelvic and parapelvic cysts. On imaging, renal sinus cysts will show a single or multiple discrete cystic lesions that do not communicate with each other.
- In true hydronephrosis, all the dilated fluid-filled spaces are contiguous.

Resistive index (RI) may be helpful in diagnosing obstruction

- The renal resistive index (RI) may be elevated in acute obstruction, thought to be due to cytokine-mediated renal artery vasoconstriction.
  - The resistive index is calculated with pulse-width Doppler of the renal segmental or arcuate arteries.
    - RI = (PSV – EDV)/PSV
    - PSV = peak systolic velocity
    - EDV = end diastolic velocity

Higher resistive indices correlate with higher resistance.

With no diastolic flow, RI = PSV/PSV = 1

Reversal of diastolic flow technically causes RI >1, although in such cases RI is not measured.

- A RI of >0.7 on the affected side, or a difference of >0.1 between kidneys, suggests acute obstruction.

  Bilateral elevated RIs (>0.7) are nonspecific and can be due to any number of medical renal processes.

- The resistive index is not used to diagnose chronic obstruction.

Ureteral jets may be helpful but are controversial

- A ureteral jet is flow of urine into the bladder as seen by color Doppler.
- Flow from the kidney to the bladder would be completely eliminated in complete obstruction, so theoretically the presence of a ureteral jet rules out a complete obstruction. However, ureteral jets are very commonly seen even with stones, and jets are often absent in normal patients.

Solid renal masses

Angiomyolipoma (AML)

- An angiomyolipoma is a benign hamartoma made up of blood vessels (angio), smooth muscle (myo), and fat (lipoma).
- Although benign, there is an increased risk of hemorrhage if >4 cm in size. The hemorrhage may be caused by microaneurysm rupture within the vascular elements of the AML.
- On ultrasound, AML is echogenic due to the fat component. There is considerable overlap between the ultrasound appearance of AML and renal cell carcinoma.

  About one third of AML demonstrate shadowing, which is a specific finding for AML.

  Multiple AML are seen in tuberous sclerosis.

Oncocytoma

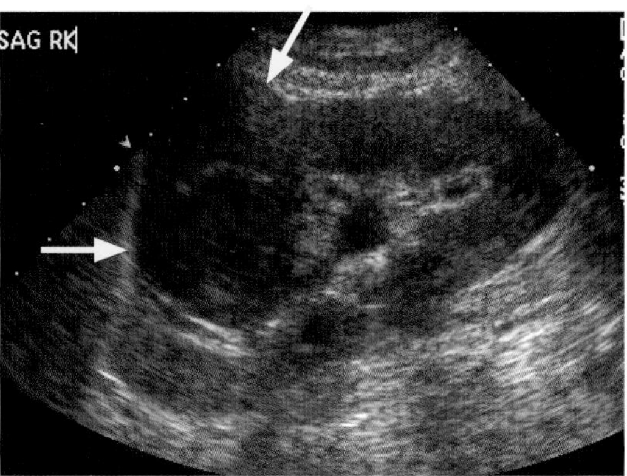

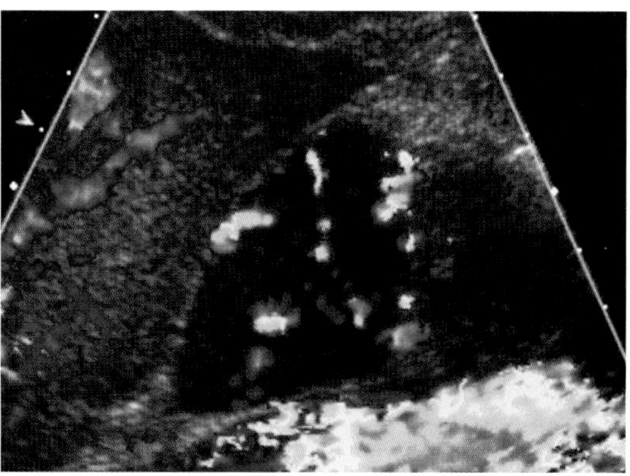

Oncocytoma: Sagittal ultrasound through the right kidney (left image) demonstrates an exophytic solid renal mass (arrows) that is isoechoic to cortex. Color Doppler suggests a *spoke-wheel* pattern of vascularity.

Case courtesy Julie Ritner, MD, Brigham and Women's Hospital.

- Oncocytoma is a benign renal tumor arising from tubular cells.
- On ultrasound, oncocytoma is indistinguishable from renal cell carcinoma (RCC). It may be hypoechoic, isoechoic, or hyperechoic. A spoke-wheel vascular pattern is sometimes seen on color Doppler.
- Due to imaging overlap with RCC, oncocytomas are treated surgically, even if the typical stellate or spoke-wheel vessels are seen.

Renal cell carcinoma (RCC)

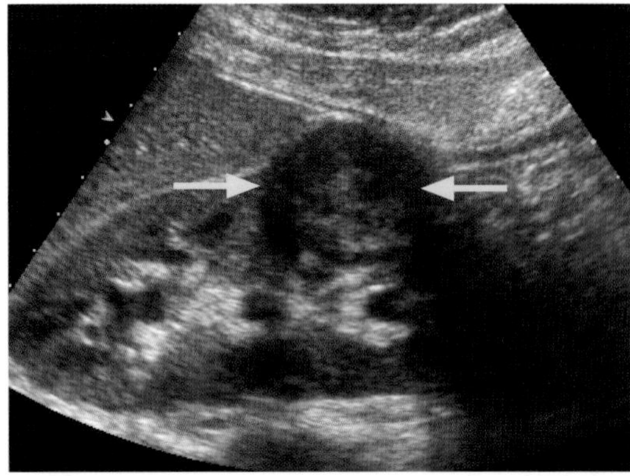

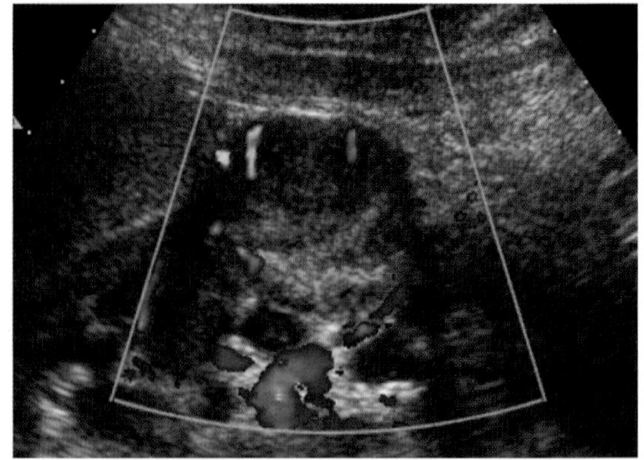

Renal cell carcinoma: Sagittal ultrasound through the kidney shows a hypoechoic solid mass (arrows) with heterogeneous echotexture in the interpolar region. The mass demonstrates vascularity on color Doppler (right image).

Case courtesy Julie Ritner, MD, Brigham and Women's Hospital.

- Renal cell carcinoma (RCC) is the most common solid renal mass.
- The staging of RCC uses the Robson system, which is discussed in the genitourinary section.
- RCC is most often isoechoic to renal cortex, but can occasionally be hypoechoic or even hyperechoic (mimicking AML). A hypoechoic rim and intratumoral cystic changes are typically seen only in RCC, which may help to distinguish it from AML.
- In the presence of a renal mass, the renal veins must be carefully evaluated as RCC has a propensity for venous invasion. Venous invasion is Robson stage IIIA, and the presence of venous invasion has important implications for surgical approach.
- Color and spectral Doppler are helpful in differentiating bland renal vein thrombus (which would not be stage IIIA) from tumor thrombus. Tumor thrombus will have color Doppler flow with an arterial waveform.

Renal lymphoma

- Renal lymphoma (most commonly high-grade B-cell) may disseminate hematogenously or spread directly from the retroperitoneum to the kidney. Primary renal lymphoma is very rare and of uncertain origin as there is no native lymphoid tissue within the kidney.
- The most common imaging presentation of renal lymphoma is multiple hypoechoic renal masses. Retroperitoneal adenopathy is usually present. A solitary mass is an uncommon presentation. Diffuse lymphomatous infiltration producing nephromegaly is rare.

Renal cysts and cystic masses

Potential pitfalls in diagnosing a cystic lesion

- Renal scanning should be performed with multiple angles of insonation to differentiate hydronephrosis from a renal sinus cyst (parapelvic or peripelvic cyst). In hydronephrosis, the dilated spaces will all connect.
- Color Doppler should always be utilized, as a renal artery aneurysm may mimic a cyst in grayscale.

Simple cortical cyst

- A simple renal cyst should have the sonographic hallmarks of a simple cyst, featuring an imperceptibly thin wall, anechoic internal contents, and posterior through transmission.
- Harmonic imaging can be helpful in confirming the diagnosis of simple renal cyst by eliminating artifactual low-level internal echoes.

Renal sinus cyst

- A cyst in the renal sinus may be a peripelvic or parapelvic cyst. Peripelvic cysts are secondary to lymphatic obstruction and are often multiple. In contrast, a parapelvic cyst is a renal parenchymal cyst that herniates into the renal sinus and is usually solitary.
- When multiple renal sinus cysts are present (most commonly peripelvic cysts), the appearance may mimic hydronephrosis. In contrast to hydronephrosis, renal sinus cysts will not be contiguous with each other.

Renal abscess

- Renal infection, discussed below, may appear as a complex cystic renal mass.

Cystic renal cell carcinoma

- Although most cases of RCC present as a solid renal mass, a significant minority may present as a complex cystic lesion. Worrisome ultrasound findings of a complex cystic mass include thick septa, irregular wall thickening, and a mural nodule.
- The Bosniak classification of complex renal masses is based on CT appearance and depends on enhancement. The Bosniak classification is described in the genitourinary imaging section.

Renal infection

Acute diffuse pyelonephritis

- Pyelonephritis is infection of the renal parenchyma, usually by gram-negative urinary tract organisms that ascend from the lower genitourinary tract.
- The most common ultrasound appearance of pyelonephritis is a normal kidney. Occasionally generalized renal edema and engorgement can be seen.

Focal pyelonephritis

- Focal pyelonephritis is a focal or multifocal infection of the renal parenchyma.
- The classic ultrasound appearance is a hypoechoic mass (or masses) with low-amplitude echoes that disrupts the corticomedullary junction. A distinct wall is lacking.

Renal abscess

- A renal abscess is a focal necrotic parenchymal infection with a defined wall. Urinalysis may be negative up to 30% of the time if the infection does not involve the collecting system.
- Small abscesses (<3 cm) often undergo a trial of conservative medical therapy, while larger abscesses are typically drained.
- Ultrasound shows a fluid-filled renal mass with a distinct wall, which may be multiloculated.

Emphysematous pyelonephritis

- Emphysematous pyelonephritis is a complication of acute pyelonephritis characterized by replacement of renal parenchyma by gas. It is caused by gas-forming organisms, most commonly *E. coli*. Emphysematous pyelonephritis is almost exclusively seen in diabetic or immunocompromised individuals.
- Emphysematous pyelonephritis is a surgical emergency requiring broad-spectrum antibiotics and emergent nephrectomy. Mortality can reach 40%.
- Ultrasound shows high-amplitude echoes in the renal parenchyma representing gas locules with posterior dirty acoustic shadowing.

Tuberculous pyelonephritis

- Tuberculous pyelonephritis, caused by hematogenous spread of *M. tuberculosis*, is characterized by focal cavitary renal lesions with calcification.
- *Putty kidney* is an atrophic, calcified kidney seen in end-stage renal tubercolosis.

Xanthogranulomatous pyelonephritis

- Xanthogranulomatous pyelonephritis results from repeated cycles of chronic low-grade infection caused by an obstructing calculus that leads to fibrofatty replacement of renal parenchyma.
- On ultrasound, the kidneys are enlarged with areas of mixed echogenicity. A central stone is nearly universally present, which may be staghorn in morphology.

Pyonephrosis

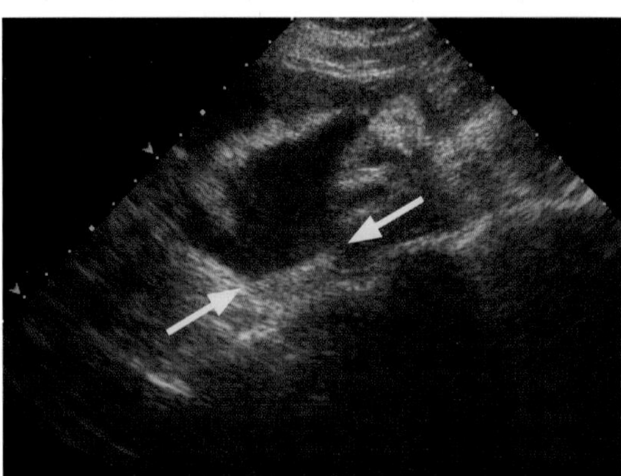
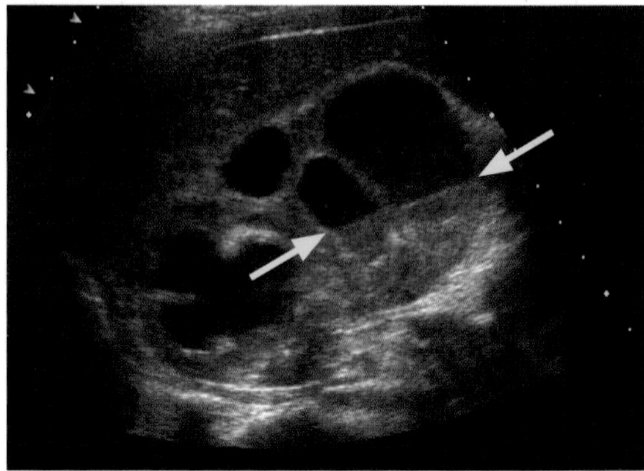

Pyonephrosis due to malpositioned nephroureteral stent: Initial ultrasound (left image) shows moderate hydronephrosis with a subtle echogenic dependent fluid–debris level (arrows). Low-level echoes are present within the collecting system. The nephroureteral stent is not visualized.

Subsequent ultrasound less than 12 hours later (right image) shows marked progression of hydronephrosis, a much larger fluid–debris level (arrows), and low level internal echoes within the dilated collecting system. Scanning of the distal ureter (not shown) revealed a malpositioned nephroureteral stent as the cause of obstruction.

Case courtesy Julie Ritner, MD, Brigham and Women's Hospital.

- Pyonephrosis is infection of an obstructed collecting system and is a surgical emergency. Treatment is emergent relief of obstruction, either with percutaneous nephrostomy or ureteral stent.
- Ultrasound features echoes within a dilated collecting system. A fluid level may be present.

HIV associated nephropathy

- The HIV virus may directly infect the renal parenchyma to produce HIV nephropathy, most commonly resulting in focal segmental glomerulosclerosis (FSGS). HIV nephropathy clinically presents with nephritic renal failure.
- The kidneys are characteristically echogenic. **Enlarged echogenic** kidneys are specific for HIV nephropathy, although the kidneys are enlarged only about 20% of the time.

Multicystic renal disease

Autosomal dominant polycystic kidney disease (ADPKD)

- Autosomal dominant polycystic kidney disease (ADPKD) is the most common cause of multiple renal cysts in adults. ADPKD is associated with cysts in the liver and other visceral organs.
- 15% of patients have saccular cerebral aneurysms.
- The natural history of ADPKD is renal failure by middle age.
- ADPKD does not confer an increased risk of renal cell carcinoma; however, complex cysts with internal hemorrhage are difficult to distinguish from renal cell carcinoma.
- Imaging of ADPKD shows markedly enlarged kidneys with innumerable cysts of varying size and echogenicity.

Autosomal recessive polycystic kidney disease (ARPKD)

- Autosomal recessive polycystic kidney disease (ARPKD) is a diagnosis of infancy. Prognosis is poor. If the child survives infancy, hepatic fibrosis usually develops.
- ARPKD presents in utero as enlarged echogenic kidneys since the cysts are too small to be individually resolved by ultrasound.

Acquired renal cystic disease

- Patients on long-term dialysis often develop many small renal cysts superimposed upon atrophic kidneys. Acquired cystic disease does confer an increased risk of renal cell carcinoma, in contrast to ADPKD.

Imaging of renal transplant

Approach to renal transplant

- The goal of ultrasound evaluation after renal transplant is to determine whether there is a treatable surgical or vascular complication. Ultrasound is not useful for differentiating among the various kinds of parenchymal rejection.
- The transplanted kidney is implanted in the right or left iliac fossa (right more commonly), and is often very well imaged due to its superficial location.
- An elevated RI (>0.7) suggests renal dysfunction, but this finding is nonspecific.

Surgical complications following renal transplant

- **Ureteral obstruction** is apparent on ultrasound as hydronephrosis.
- **Fluid collection** (blood, pus, urine) is highly dependent on timing:

  Immediately postoperative: Hematoma.

  1–2 weeks postoperative: Urinoma.

  3–4 weeks postoperative: Abscess.

  2nd month and beyond: Lymphocele.

Vascular complications following renal transplant

- **Renal vein thrombosis**: The renal *artery* Doppler may show reversal of diastolic flow.
- **Renal artery stenosis**: Elevated flow velocities are seen at the site of stenosis, with a *parvus et tardus* waveform distal to the stenosis. Usually takes several weeks to months to develop.
- **Pseudoaneurysm** is usually due to renal biopsy.

Medical complications

- Medical complications generally cannot be differentiated on ultrasound. Biopsy is necessary for diagnosis, although the time elapsed since the transplant may be a helpful clue.
- Hyperacute rejection: Occurs in first few hours after transplant.

  Hyperacute rejection is very rare, and is due to ABO blood type incompatibility.
- Acute tubular necrosis (ATN): Occurs in the immediate few postoperative days.

  ATN is usually a sequela of pre-implantation ischemia.
- Acute rejection: Occurs within three months of transplant.
- Chronic rejection: Occurs after three months of transplant.
- Drug toxicity may caused by cyclosporine, which is nephrotoxic.

Post-transplant lymphoproliferative disorder (PTLD)

- Post-transplant lymphoproliferative disorder (PTLD) is a type of lymphoma that is thought to be due to immune suppression and Epstein–Barr virus proliferation.
- PTLD can arise anywhere in the body. Any new mass in any organ in a transplant patient should raise concern for potential PTLD.
- Ultrasound of renal PTLD will show an amorphous hypoechoic mass that may simulate a fluid collection on grayscale images. Unlike fluid, PTLD will demonstrate Doppler flow.

Medullary nephrocalcinosis

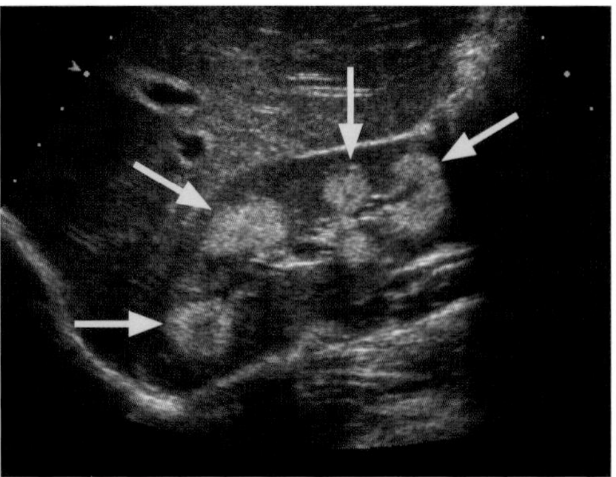

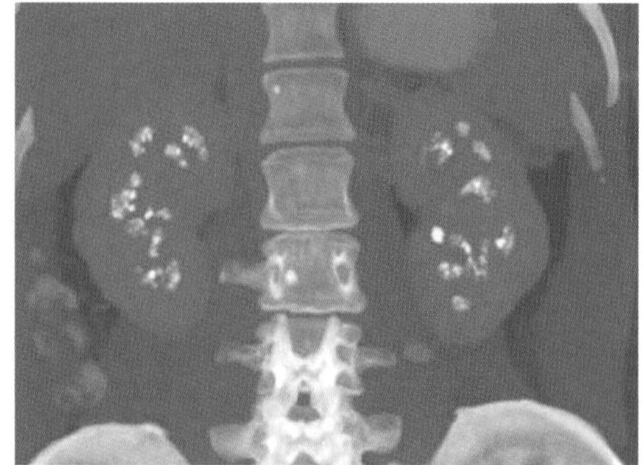

Medullary nephrocalcinosis: Sagittal ultrasound through the right kidney (left image) shows diffusely echogenic renal pyramids (arrows). Coronal CT MIP in bone windows (right image) in a different patient demonstrates symmetric cloud-like renal medullary calcification bilaterally.

Ultrasound case courtesy Julie Ritner, MD, Brigham and Women's Hospital.

- Any cause of hypercalcemia and hypercalciuria can cause medullary calcification.

Differential of medullary nephrocalcinosis

- Hyperparathyroidism is the most common cause of medullary nephrocalcinosis.
- Renal tubular acidosis (distal type).
- Medullary sponge kidney is caused by ectatic tubules in the medullary pyramids leading to stasis and stone formation.
- Papillary necrosis.
- In a child, treatment with furosemide can lead to medullary nephrocalcinosis.

Cortical nephrocalcinosis

- Much more rare than medullary nephrocalcinosis, cortical nephrocalcinosis is due to diffuse cortical injury.

Ddx of cortical nephro-calcinosis

- Acute cortical necrosis.
- Hyperoxaluria (rare).
- Alport syndrome.
- Autosomal recessive polycystic kidney disease.

Echogenic kidneys

- Echogenic kidneys are most commonly due to medical renal disease, such as diabetic nephropathy, glomerulosclerosis, acute tubular necrosis, etc.
- HIV nephropathy causes enlarged and echogenic kidneys.

Echogenic renal mass

Differential of echogenic renal mass

- Angiomyolipoma (AML). A shadowing echogenic renal mass is relatively specific for AML.
- Malignant neoplasm (atypical appearance).
- Renal calculus.
- Intrarenal gas.
- Milk of calcium, caused by crystals precipitating out of supersaturated solution.
- Sloughed papilla, secondary to papillary necrosis, may appear as an echogenic mass in the collecting system.

SCROTAL ANATOMY

Epididymis: Function and anatomy

- The epididymis carries sperm away from the testicle to the vas deferens.
- The epididymis is composed of head, body, and tail. The head may measure up to 10 mm.
- The epididymis is normally hypoechoic and has less blood flow compared to the testicle. Relatively increased epididymal blood flow can be seen in epididymitis.

Mediastinum testis: Function and anatomy

- The mediastinum testis is fibrous tissue in the hilum of the testicle, from which fibrous septa radiate towards the testicular periphery. It provides structural support to the rete testis.

Rete testis: Function and anatomy

- The rete testis is a network of tubules that carries sperm from the seminiferous tubules to the vas deferens. It functions to concentrate sperm.

TESTICULAR MASSES

Approach to a testicular mass

- **Intratesticular** masses are usually **malignant** (90–95%). Conversely, most **extratesticular** masses are benign in an adult, although a pediatric mass in this location may be malignant.
- The retroperitoneum should always be evaluated if an intratesticular mass is seen. Likewise, if retroperitoneal adenopathy is seen in a reproductive-age male, the testicles should always be examined.
- Most scrotal masses are hypoechoic relative to normal testicular parenchyma.
- On Doppler, most masses will have increased vascularity with high diastolic flow, producing a low resistance waveform.

Malignant germ cell tumor (GCT): Seminoma

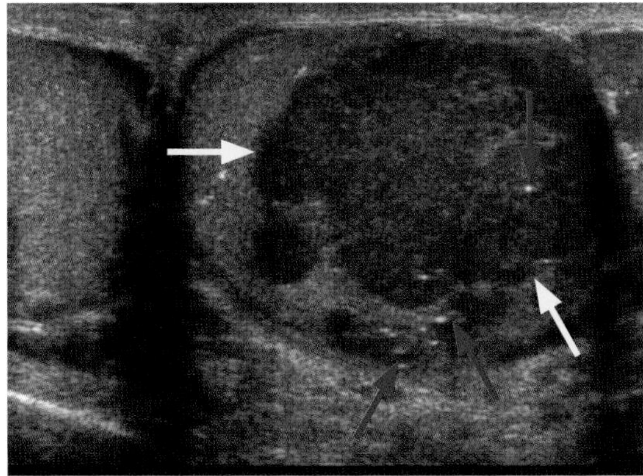

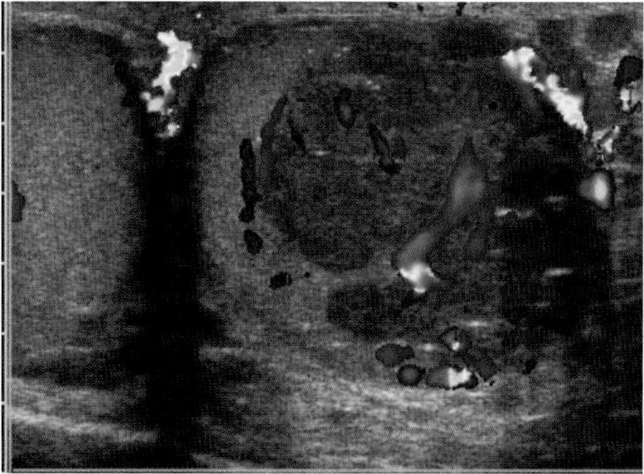

Seminoma: Grayscale (left image) and color Doppler show a heterogeneous hypoechoic vascular mass (yellow arrows) in the left testis. Note the presence of numerous tiny echogenic foci (red arrows) representing microlithiasis.

Case courtesy Julie Ritner, MD, Brigham and Women's Hospital.

- Seminoma is the most common testicular malignancy. It has a favorable prognosis.

  Seminoma typically occurs in middle-aged men. Uncommonly, hCG may be elevated.

  The spermatocytic subtype of seminoma occurs in slightly older men (mid 50s) and has excellent prognosis with orchiectomy only. Tumor markers are not elevated.

Malignant germ cell tumors: Nonseminomatous germ cell tumors (NSGCT)

- Nonseminomatous germ cell tumors (NSGCT) include embryonal carcinoma, teratoma, yolk sac tumor, choriocarcinoma, and mixed subtypes.

  Mixed germ cell tumor is the most common NSGCT, and is the second most common primary testicular malignancy after seminoma. The most common components of mixed NSGCT are embryonal carcinoma and teratoma.

  Embryonal cell carcinoma in its pure form is rare and in adults is typically seen as a component of mixed germ cell tumors. The infantile form, called endodermal sinus tumor or yolk sac tumor, is the most common testicular tumor of infancy. AFP is elevated.

  Teratoma is rare in its pure form in adults, but is seen in 50% of mixed NSGCT. Teratoma is classified as mature, immature, and malignant. In adults, teratomas are usually malignant. In children, teratomas are usually benign, with the mature subtype most commonly seen.

  Choriocarcinoma is the most aggressive and rare NSGCT. Choriocarcinoma metastasizes early, especially to brain and lung. Metastases tend to be hemorrhagic. hCG is always elevated and gynecomastia may result from elevated chorionic gonadotropins.

- NSGCT generally occur in younger patients compared to seminomas, typically in young men in their 20s and 30s. NSGCT tend to be more aggressive than seminomas. Local invasion into the tunica albuginea and visceral metastases are common.
- A heterogeneous testicular mass that contains solid and cystic components and coarse calcification is a typical appearance for a NSGCT. It is not possible to distinguish the various subtypes of NSGCT on sonography.

Burnt-out germ cell tumor

- *Burnt-out* germ cell tumor is a primary testicular neoplasm that is no longer viable in the testicle even though there is often viable metastatic disease, especially retroperitoneal.
- In the testicle, focal calcification with shadowing is characteristic. A mass may or may not be present.
- Treatment is orchiectomy in addition to systemic chemotherapy.

Testicular microlithiasis

- Testicular microlithiasis is multiple punctate testicular calcifications.
- There is a controversial association between microlithiasis and testicular neoplasm. While the overall absolute risk for developing testicular cancer remains very small in the presence of microlithiasis, the relative risk may be increased.
- Current guidelines do not support screening by ultrasound or tumor markers, but patients with microlithiasis may perform self-examinations and be seen in follow-up as needed.
- At least five microcalcifications must be present per image to be called microlithiasis. If there are fewer than five microcalcifications the term *limited microlithiasis* is used.
- Microlithiasis can produce a *starry sky* appearance if calcifications are numerous.

  In the liver, hepatitis can cause a *starry sky* appearance due to increased echogenicity of the portal triads.

Testicular metastases

- The most common metastases to the testicles are leukemia and lymphoma, as the relevant chemotherapeutic agents do not cross the blood–testis barrier.
- Hematologic malignancies typically present in older patients, tend to be bilateral, and may be infiltrative with diffuse testicular enlargement.

Benign testicular tumors

- An **epidermoid** is a keratin-filled cyst with a distinctive *onion-ring* appearance of concentric alternating rings of hypo- and hyperechogenicity. If suspected, local excision is performed instead of the standard orchiectomy typically performed for presumed malignant masses.

- **Sex-cord stromal tumors** are 90% benign but are sonographically indistinguishable from malignant tumors. Orchiectomy is therefore the standard treatment.

  Leydig cell tumor can present with gynecomastia due to estrogen secretion.

  Sertoli cell tumor is associated with Peutz–Jeghers and Klinefelter syndromes.

Sarcoidosis

- Sarcoidosis may involve either the testis, the epididymis, or both. Scrotal involvement is rare, but presents clinically as painless scrotal enlargement.
- The ultrasound appearance of testicular sarcoid is indistinguishable from a solid malignant mass. If sarcoidosis is suggested by clinical history, the testicular mass must be biopsied to exclude malignancy. Without tissue pathology, a mass cannot be assumed to be sarcoid.

Benign testicular tumor mimics

- Congenital adrenal rests are embryologic remnants of adrenal tissue trapped within the testis. These are typically seen in newborns with congenital adrenal hyperplasia.

  Adrenal rests appear as *bilateral* hypoechoic masses and classically enlarge with ACTH exposure.

- Polyorchidism/supernumerary testis: An extra testicle has an identical imaging appearance to normal testicular parenchyma.

  Extranumerary testes carry a slightly increased risk of torsion and testicular cancer.

Extra-testicular masses

- In contrast to intratesticular masses, **extratesticular** masses are usually **benign**. Up to 16% of extratesticular masses may be malignant, however, and ultrasound cannot reliably differentiate benign from malignant masses.

Benign extratesticular masses

- Spermatic cord lipoma is the most common extratesticular neoplasm overall.
- Benign adenomatoid tumor of the tunica albuginea is the most common epididymal neoplasm.

The "-celes" and cystic lesions

Hydrocele

- A hydrocele is excess fluid in the scrotum surrounding the testicle. Most are asymptomatic.
- A hydrocele may be congenital (due to patent processus vaginalis in utero or infancy), idiopathic, or post-inflammatory. Regardless of etiology, there is never fluid at the *bare area* where the testicle is attached to the tunica vaginalis.

Hematocele

- A hematocele is blood in the scrotum due to trauma or torsion.

Varicocele

- A varicocele is a dilated venous pampiniform plexus in the scrotum. A primary varicocele is due to incompetent valves of the internal spermatic vein. A secondary varicocele is due to increased venous pressure caused by an obstructing lesion.
- Varicocele is a common cause of infertility, seen in up to 40% of males presenting to an infertility clinic.
- Varicoceles are much more common on the left as the left testicular vein drains into the left renal vein and the superior mesenteric artery can compress the left renal vein. In contrast, the right testicular vein drains directly into the infrarenal IVC.
- 85% of varicoceles are left-sided and 15% are bilateral. *An isolated right-sided varicocele should prompt a search for a right-sided retroperitoneal mass.*

- On ultrasound, varicoceles appear as multiple tubular and serpentine anechoic structures >2 mm in diameter in the region of the upper pole of the testis and epididymal head. The varicoceles follow the spermatic cord into the inguinal canal and can be compressed by the transducer. Careful optimization of Doppler parameters shows the slow venous flow within the varicocele.

Epididymal cysts and spermatocele

- An epididymal cyst is an anechoic fluid-containing cyst that can occur anywhere in the epididymis.
- A spermatocele is cystic dilation of the epididymis filled with spermatozoa, usually occurring in the epididymal head. Classic ultrasound appearance is an epididymal cyst with internal low-level mobile echoes.
- A simple epididymal cyst and a spermatocele cannot always be reliably distinguished by ultrasound.

Simple testicular cyst

- A simple testicular cyst meets sonographic criteria for a simple cyst (smooth posterior wall, imperceptible wall thickness, completely anechoic, posterior through transmission).

Tubular ectasia of rete testis

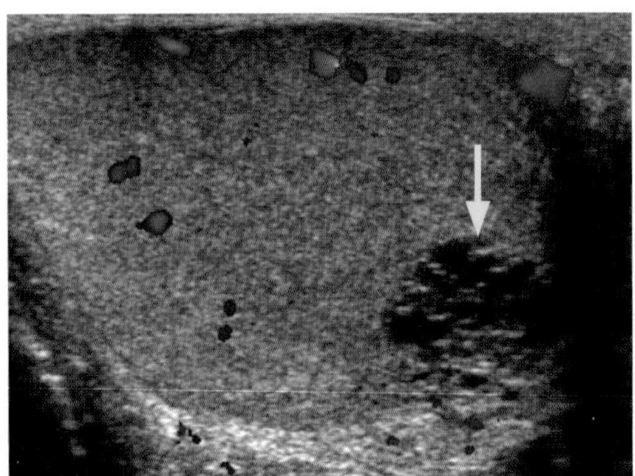
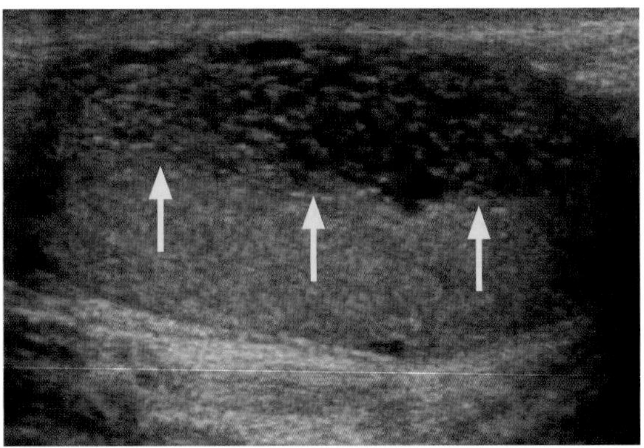

Tubular ectasia of the rete testes:

Transverse color Doppler ultrasound of the right testicle (left image) shows cystic dilation at the mediastinum testes (arrow). There is no flow within the lesion. This appearance is highly suggestive of tubular ectasia, although an avascular mass may rarely have a similar appearance.

Sagittal ultrasound (right image) shows elongation of the cystic dilation (arrows) along the mediastinum testes, which is confirmatory for tubular ectasia.

Case courtesy Julie Ritner, MD, Brigham and Women's Hospital.

- Tubular ectasia of the rete testis is nonpalpable, asymptomatic, cystic dilation of the tubules at the mediastinum testes caused by epididymal obstruction. Tubular ectasia is often accompanied by an epididymal cyst or spermatocele.
- Tubular ectasia of the rete testis is common in older patients and may be bilateral.
- Imaging shows numerous tiny dilated structures in the region of the mediastinum testis, often seen in conjunction with an epididymal cyst/spermatocele.
- Important to be aware of only as a tumor mimic. Tubular ectasia is benign and no treatment is necessary.

Tunical cyst

- The tunica albuginea is the capsule overlying the testis. A cyst of the tunica albuginea presents as a palpable superficial nodule that resembles a BB.
- Sonography shows a typically small, simple, extra-testicular cyst.
- No treatment is necessary.

Vascular disease of the testis

Testicular torsion

- Testicular torsion is twisting of the testicle around the spermatic cord and the vascular pedicle. Torsion presents with acute scrotal pain and is a surgical emergency.
- Torsion may lead to irreversible testicular infarction if not de-torsed within a few hours.

  De-torsion within 6 hours has an excellent prognosis.

  De-torsion after 24 hours has a poor prognosis for testicular salvage.
- *The bell-clapper* deformity predisposes to torsion due to a small testicular bare area. The bare area is the testicular attachment site and normally prevents the testicle from rotation.
- Ultrasound findings of torsion are dependent on the time elapsed since torsion:

> **Hyperacute** (within a few hours): Ultrasound shows a hyperechoic and shadowing *torsion knot* of twisted epididymis and spermatic cord, with no blood flow in the affected testicle.
>
> **Acute** (between a few hours and 24 hours): Affected testicle is enlarged and heterogeneous.
>
> **Missed torsion** (>24 hours): Affected testicle is enlarged and mottled, with scrotal skin thickening and increased flow in the scrotal wall. A complex or septated hydrocele may be present.

Segmental infarction

- Segmental infarction is a focal testicular infarction that can be due to microvascular thrombosis from acute inflammation, vasculitis, or sickle cell disease.
- Patients are typically in their 30s and present with acute pain which may mimic epididymitis or torsion clinically.
- The typical appearance of infarction is a wedge-shaped hypoechoic area with no flow on Doppler.
- The primary differential consideration of infarction is a hypovascular tumor. Infarcted tissue may undergo necrosis, making differentiation from tumor even more difficult. MRI may be helpful to distinguish infarction from tumor in ambiguous cases to potentially spare the patient from orchiectomy.

Scrotal trauma

Hematoma

- The sonographic appearance of an acute scrotal hematoma is an echogenic, extratesticular mass with no Doppler flow. When large, the hematoma can compress the testicle.
- When the hematoma evolves into a complex, multiseptated mass-like lesion, the distinction between the extratesticular hematoma and the testicle may become difficult. Proper distinction is necessary to avoid mistaking the hematoma for a testicular mass.

Testicular contusion

- Testicular contusion produces a peripheral, hypoechoic lesion that may mimic tumor.
- Even with a history of trauma, a suspicious testicular lesion requires further evaluation to exclude malignancy, typically with a short-term follow-up.

Testicular rupture

- Testicular rupture causes capsule disruption, often with protrusion of testicular parenchyma through the defect. Rupture is often associated with a testicular hematoma or contusion.
- Prompt diagnosis is critical, as testicular viability is dependent upon timely repacking of the seminiferous tubules back inside the capsule.
- Testicular rupture results in disruption of the blood–testis barrier and may be associated with future infertility due to the formation of anti-spermatozoa antibodies.

Scrotal infection

Epididymitis

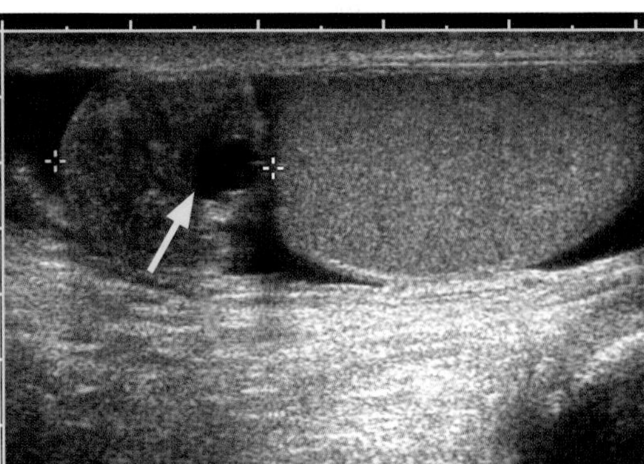

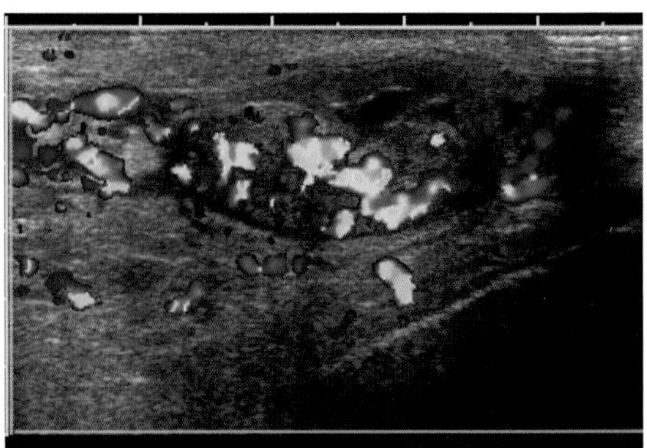

Epididymitis: Sagittal grayscale ultrasound (left image) of the testicle and epididymis shows a markedly enlarged epididymis measuring 1.7 cm (calipers). Incidental note is made of an epididymal cyst (arrow). The testicle has a normal sonographic appearance. Transverse color Doppler of the epididymis (right image) demonstrates markedly increased flow.

Case courtesy Julie Ritner, MD, Brigham and Women's Hospital.

- Epididymitis is infection of the epididymis, almost always ascending from the urinary tract.
- The classic clinical presentation of epididymitis is acute unilateral scrotal pain.
- The main differential based on clinical presentation is testicular torsion. In contrast to torsion, epididymitis features normal testicular blood flow.
- A key ultrasound finding of epididymitis is an enlarged epididymis with increased Doppler flow relative to the testicle (normally, the epididymis has less Doppler flow than the testicle). An associated hydrocele may be present, which often contains low-level echoes.

Epididymo-orchitis

- Epididymo-orchitis is infection that has spread from the epididymis to the testicle.
- Epididymo-orchitis has a similar ultrasound appearance to epididymitis, but blood flow to the testicle will also be increased.
- Infection and secondary inflammation can cause venous hypertension, which is a risk factor for focal testicular ischemia.

Fournier gangrene

- Fournier gangrene is necrotizing fasciitis of the scrotum and perineum, a highly morbid and surgically emergent condition.
- Infection is usually polymicrobial.
- The key imaging finding is subcutaneous gas, which appears on ultrasound as multiple echogenic reflectors in the subcutaneous tissues with dirty shadowing.

VASCULAR ULTRASOUND

GENERAL PRINCIPLES

Angle correction

- The Doppler signal is proportional to cos(θ). There is no Doppler shift at 90°.

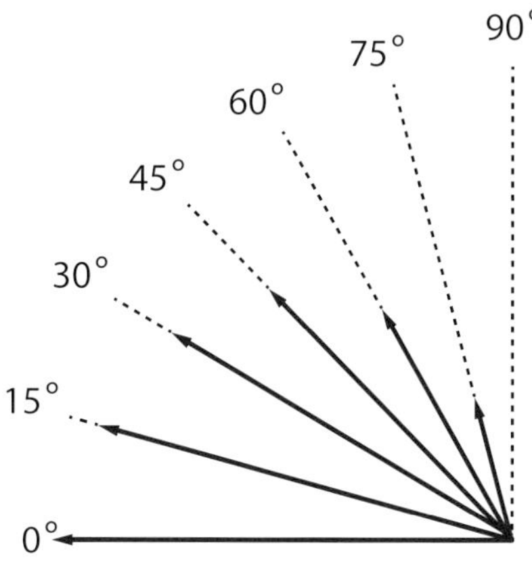

amount of Doppler shift is proportional to cos(θ)

at 90° there is zero Doppler shift

- All measurements of velocity should be made at a consistent angle (typically 60°). Measurements should never be taken at an angle greater than 60°.

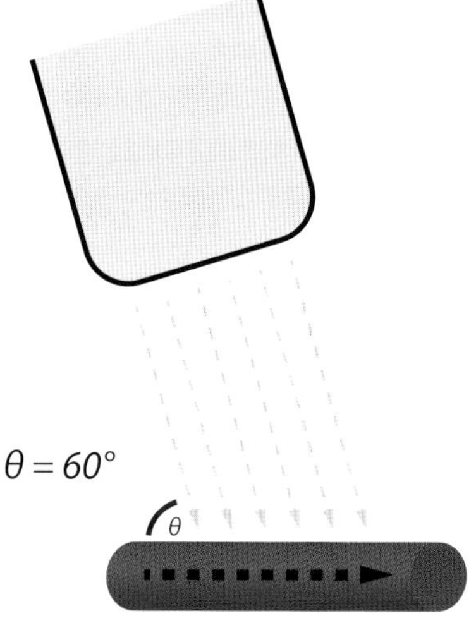

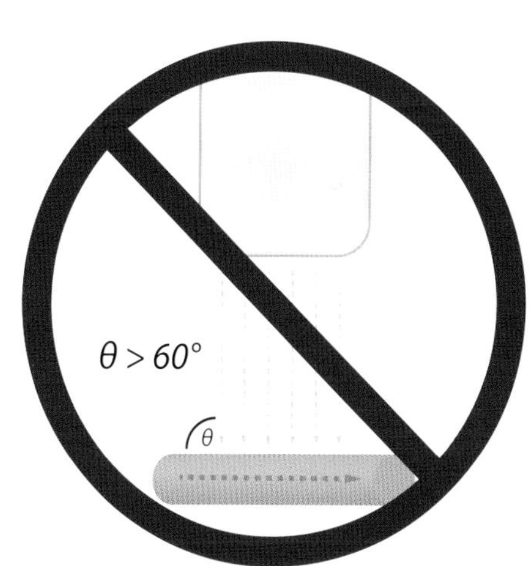

Overview of peak systolic velocity (PSV)

- Peak systolic velocity (PSV) is usually the most accurate method to evaluate the degree of arterial stenosis. PSV is elevated proximal to and at the site of stenosis.
- PSV may be decreased distal to a hemodynamically significant stenosis.
- The differential diagnosis of increased PSV includes:

  Downstream (distal) stenosis.

  Compensatory flow, contralateral to an obstruction or severe stenosis.

  Physiologic hyperdynamic state in a healthy young patient.

- The differential diagnosis of decreased PSV includes:

  Upstream (more proximal) stenosis.

  Poor cardiac pump function.

  Near-total occlusion.

CAROTID ARTERY

Color and spectral Doppler parameters

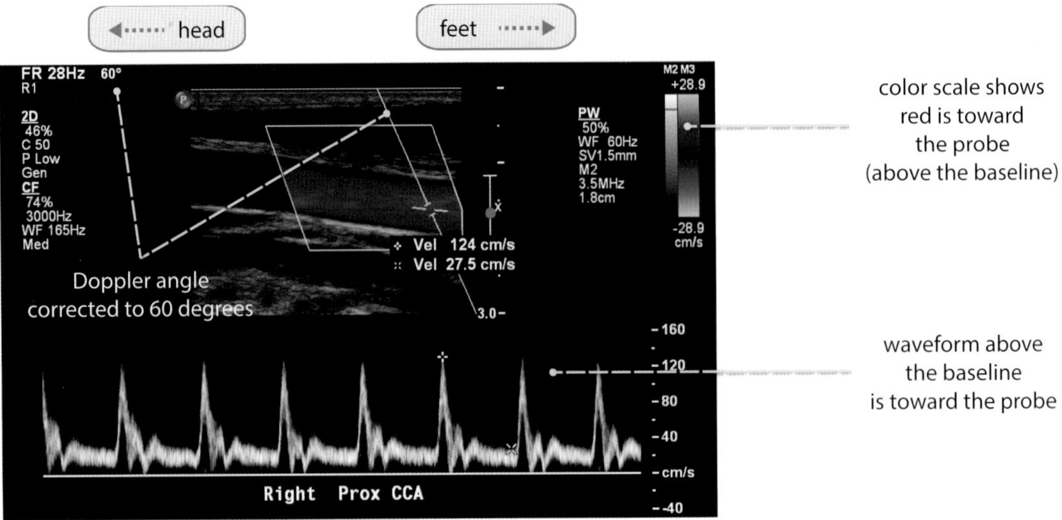

Normal carotid examination: Duplex ultrasound of the right internal carotid artery shows normal spectral waveform. The peak systolic velocity is 124 cm/sec, within the normal range. There is no carotid plaque.

- By convention, for images obtained in the sagittal plane, the patient's head is on the left side of the image and the feet are on the right.
- In general, ultrasound parameters are optimized so that arteries are red and normal arterial flow is above the baseline. Certain parameters need to be adjusted so that arteries above the heart (which are normally heading towards the head) appear similar to arteries below the heart (which normally are heading towards the feet):

  The color scale can be changed: Colors above the baseline go towards the probe.

  Spectral Doppler baseline inversion can be changed: Positive waveforms go towards the probe.

Evaluation of the carotid arteries

- There are three components to the carotid artery exam: Evaluation of plaque morphology, hemodynamic evaluation, and waveform analysis.

Plaque morphology

- Plaque morphology is evaluated on grayscale imaging (without Doppler) and is described in terms of absolute percent stenosis.
- <50% cross-sectional area plaque would not be expected to be hemodynamically significant.
- >50% luminal plaque is expected to show elevation in peak systolic velocity.

Hemodynamic evaluation of stenosis

- Normal peak systolic velocity (PSV) in large arteries is 60–100 cm/sec.
- PSV tends to be elevated at a site of significant stenosis. Per the Society of Radiologists in Ultrasound (SRU) criteria, established in 2003:

  >125 cm/sec suggests >50% stenosis.

  >230 cm/sec suggests >70% stenosis.

  Potential pitfall: An occluded or nearly occluded artery may have no detectable flow.

- An elevated ratio of internal carotid artery to common carotid artery (ICA/CCA) PSV is a useful secondary sign of ICA stenosis.

  <2 is normal.

  >2 suggests >50% ICA stenosis.

  >4 suggests >70% ICA stenosis.

- End diastolic velocity of >100 cm/sec suggests >70% stenosis.
- In high and low flow states, the ICA/CCA ratio is more useful than the absolute PSV.

Waveform analysis

- Stenosis *downstream* (distal) to transducer (outflow lesion): Spectral waveform is high resistance and high velocity in morphology, characterized by decreased diastolic flow. The systolic upstroke is normal and rapid. Spectral broadening and aliasing may be present.

  Spectral broadening describes the widened distribution of RBC velocities due to disruption of laminar flow.

  Aliasing is an artifact where the highest velocities are shown to have a reversed flow.

- Stenosis *upstream* (proximal) to transducer (inflow lesion): Spectral waveform is low resistance and low velocity in morphology, with relatively increased diastolic flow. Systolic upstroke is slowed, producing the *tardus et parvus* waveform.

Carotid stenosis

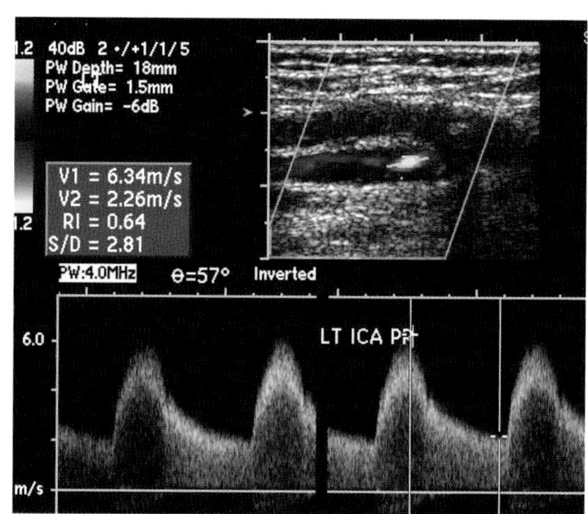

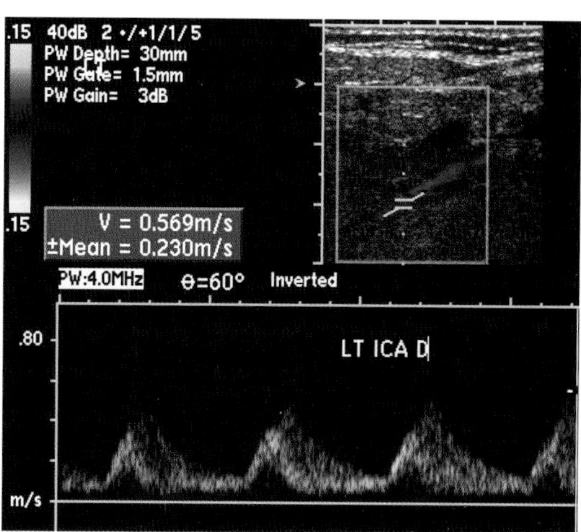

Severe internal carotid artery stenosis: Spectral waveform of the proximal internal carotid artery (left image) shows spectral broadening and markedly elevated peak systolic velocity of 634 cm/sec, consistent with severe stenosis. The grayscale images also show hypoechoic plaque. Evaluation distal to the stenosis (right image) shows a *parvus et tardus* waveform and decreased peak systolic velocity.

Case courtesy Julie Ritner, MD, Brigham and Women's Hospital.

Renal artery stenosis

Renal artery stenosis: Criteria and protocol

- A peak systolic velocity of ≥180 cm/sec is consistent with renal artery stenosis.

  Normal aortic and renal artery velocity is 60–100 cm/sec.

- A renal artery to aortic velocity ratio of >3.5 is also consistent with renal artery stenosis.
- Reduced or absent diastolic flow is suggestive of a stenosis distal to the area of interest.
- As with the carotid artery, a *tardus et parvus* waveform on spectral Doppler is suggestive of a stenosis proximal (upstream) to the transducer, known as an inflow lesion.
- An elevated renal resistive index (>0.7) is nonspecific, but may indicate renal artery stenosis. The resistive index is calculated as follows: RI = (PSV – EDV)/PSV, where PSV is peak systolic velocity and EDV is end-diastolic velocity.

  RI is measured in the segmental arteries of the upper, mid, and lower poles.

  Elevated resistive indices can also be seen in acute urinary obstruction or medical renal disease.

Atherosclerotic renal artery stenosis

- Atherosclerosis is by far the most common cause of renal artery stenosis, typically affecting the ostium of the renal artery.

Fibromuscular dysplasia (FMD)

- Fibromuscular dysplasia (FMD) is a vasculitis that primarily affects the renal and carotid arteries in middle-aged females.
- The most common location of stenosis in FMD is the distal two thirds of the renal artery.
- The classic angiographic appearance of FMD is a *string of pearls* caused by multifocal alternating stenoses and post-stenotic dilations.

Deep venous thrombosis (DVT)

Lower extremity venous system anatomy

- The superficial venous system is composed of the great and small saphenous veins.

  The great saphenous vein drains into the common femoral vein. Although the great saphenous vein is technically part of the superficial system, clots near the saphenofemoral junction are typically treated with anticoagulation because of their propensity to become dislodged.

  The small saphenous vein drains into the popliteal vein (which continues proximally as the femoral vein). Clots in the small saphenous vein are typically not treated.

- Deep venous system anatomy mirrors arterial anatomy:

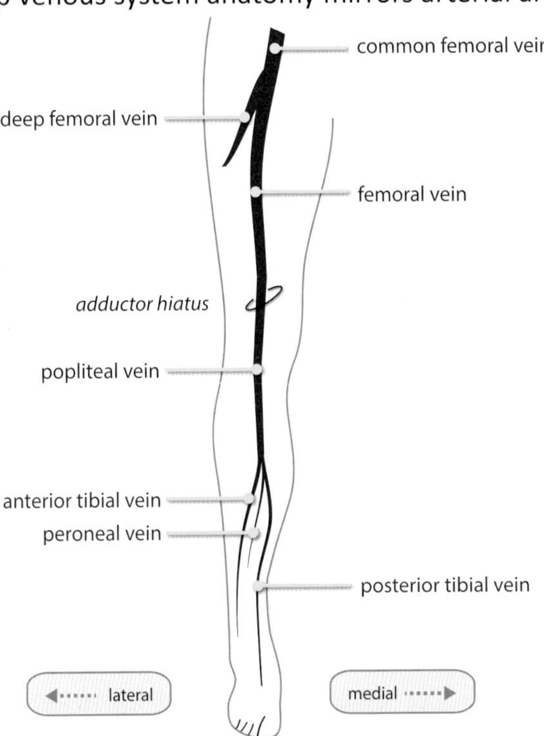

The common femoral vein (CFV) drains into the external iliac vein and begins at the level of the inguinal ligament. The CFV lies medial to the common femoral artery.

CFV tributaries include the deep femoral and femoral veins. The femoral vein was previously called the superficial femoral vein. The term *superficial femoral vein* should be avoided as it wrongly implies that this vein is part of the superficial venous system.

The three calf veins are the anterior tibial vein (lateral), peroneal vein (middle), and posterior tibial vein (medial), which join to form the popliteal vein (PV). The PV continues into the femoral vein.

Overview of the deep venous thrombosis (DVT) examination

- A lower extremity venous ultrasound exam should include venous compression, color and spectral Doppler, and evaluation of venous augmentation and respiratory variation.

  Augmentation is the normal change in waveform when the calf is compressed. Lack of augmentation suggests a distal venous obstruction between the calf and the transducer.

  Respiratory variation is the normal change in waveform when the patient inspires. Lack of respiratory variation suggests a proximal venous obstruction.

- The popliteal, femoral, proximal deep femoral, and common femoral (including the saphenofemoral junction) veins should be imaged every 2–3 cm with and without compression.

Venous compression

- The hallmark sonographic finding of a DVT is a noncompressible vein with or without an intraluminal clot. A partially thrombosed vein may be partially compressible, while a completely thrombosed vein will not be compressible at all.

Color Doppler

- Color Doppler is almost always used to help localize the veins, but it is not necessary for diagnosing DVT.
- Normal color Doppler flow in a noncompressible vein is suspicious for nonobstructing thrombus.

Acute versus chronic deep venous thrombosis

- While the diagnosis of DVT is usually straightforward, distinguishing between acute and chronic thrombus can be difficult. Evaluation of the clot's echogenicity is not a reliable way to determine the acuity of the clot as artifactual echoes within the vein lumen can overlap with the clot.
- Sonographic findings of chronic venous thrombus include clot retraction and poor visualization of the clot, only partial compressibility, irregularly echogenic and thickened vein walls, and prominent collateral veins.

Aortic disease

Abdominal aortic aneurysm (AAA)

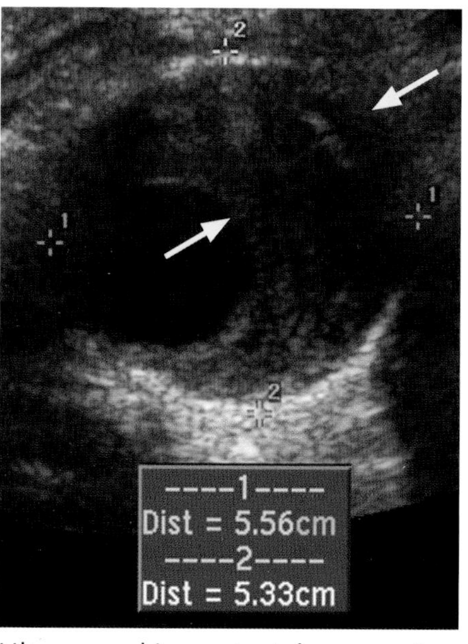

Transverse grayscale ultrasound of the infrarenal abdominal aorta shows an aortic aneurysm measuring 5.6 cm in diameter (calipers), with extensive mural thrombus (arrows).

- Ultrasound is a principle screening modality for abdominal aortic aneurysm, with a proven mortality benefit in 65–79-year-old men who have ever smoked tobacco.
- If an aneurysm is present, the diameter is measured in three orthogonal planes.
- Aneurysms with an axial diameter of >5.5 cm should be considered for elective treatment.
- Aneurysms 3–5.5 cm are typically followed.

Aortic dissection

- In aortic dissection, a tear in the intima allows blood into the media. The characteristic intimal dissection flap is typically echogenic.
- Color Doppler may show flow in both true and false lumens, often with different flow rates.

Thyroid and parathyroid

Diffuse thyroid disease

Hashimoto thyroiditis (chronic lymphocytic thyroiditis)

- Hashimoto thyroiditis is an autoimmune disease that ultimately produces destruction of the thyroid gland parenchyma. It is the most common cause of hypothyroidism.
- Hashimoto thyroiditis can present with a variety of clinical findings, thyroid function test results, and imaging appearances, dependent on the duration and severity of the disease.
- Ultrasound may show either a diffusely nodular gland or a diffusely coarsened gland without a measurable nodule. The isthmus is characteristically thickened.
- Patients with Hashimoto thyroiditis are at increased risk of thyroid lymphoma. Any rapidly growing nodule should raise suspicion for lymphoma.

Graves disease

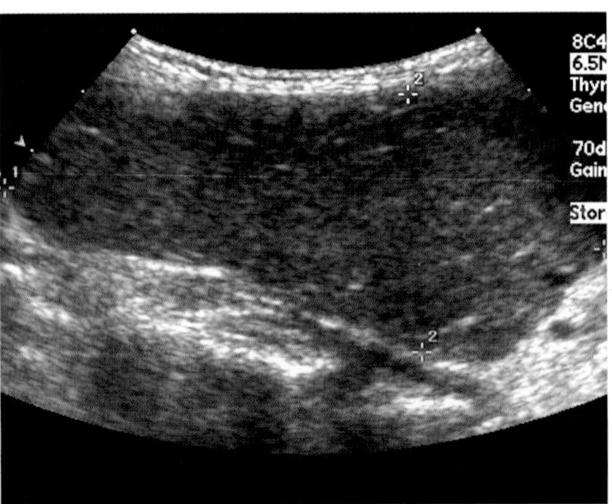

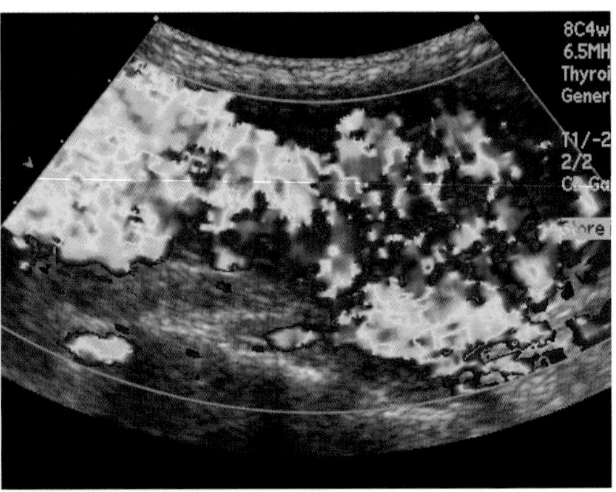

Graves disease: Sagittal grayscale ultrasound of the thyroid (left) demonstrates a diffusely enlarged gland with coarsened, heterogeneous echotexture. Color Doppler (right image) shows markedly increased Doppler flow representing the *thyroid inferno* sign.

Case courtesy Julie Ritner, MD, Brigham and Women's Hospital.

- Graves disease causes autoimmune activation of the TSH receptor, stimulating thyroid hormone synthesis and secretion. Patients clinically present with thyrotoxicosis.
- The typical grayscale sonographic appearance of Graves disease is diffuse enlargement of the gland with a coarsened echotexture. The borders of the gland are often lobulated.
- The key color Doppler finding is the *thyroid inferno* sign, which represents marked hypervascularity caused by arteriovenous shunting and enlarged peripheral vessels.

Subacute thyroiditis (de Quervain thyroiditis)

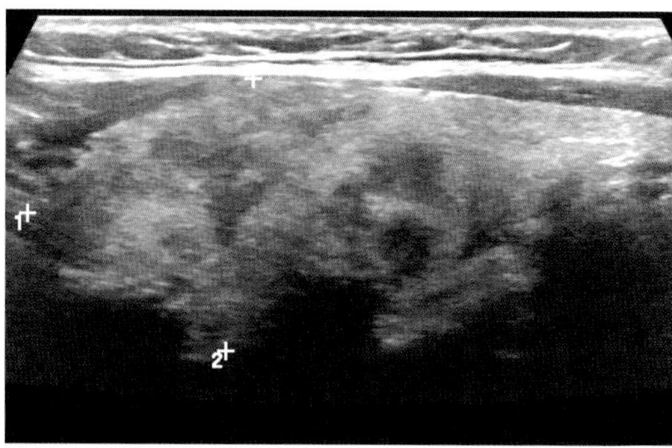
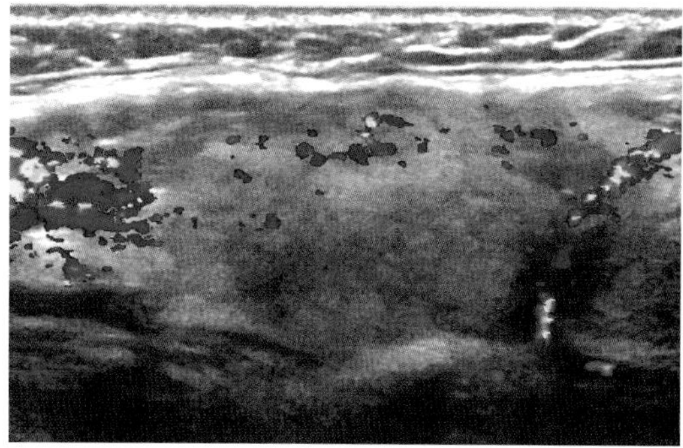

Subacute (de Quervain) thyroiditis: Sagittal grayscale thyroid ultrasound (left image) demonstrates patchy areas of decreased echogenicity with no discrete nodule. Color Doppler (right image) does not demonstrate increased vascularity, in contrast to Graves disease.

Case courtesy Julie Ritner, MD, Brigham and Women's Hospital.

- Subacute (de Quervain) thyroiditis is granulomatous inflammation of the thyroid, thought to be viral in origin. The gland is usually tender and adjacent cervical adenopathy is common.
- Ultrasound findings are non-specific and may feature a heterogeneous gland with patchy areas of decreased echogenicity.
- Subacute thyroiditis is treated with steroids. Follow-up ultrasound appearance can show a dramatic response to treatment.

Multinodular gland

- The term *multinodular gland* is preferred over *multinodular goiter* because *goiter* is a generic term for an enlarged gland, which can have numerous causes.
- On imaging, a multinodular gland will appear enlarged with innumerable mixed cystic and solid nodules.

THYROID NODULE AND THYROID CANCER

Approach to a thyroid nodule

- There are no definitive ultrasound features that distinguish benign from malignant nodules.
- Some institutions biopsy all solid nodules >1 cm by fine needle aspiration.

Thyroid cancer (malignant thyroid nodule)

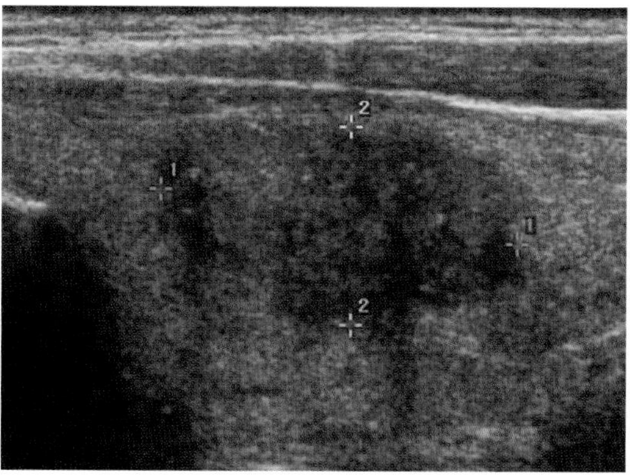
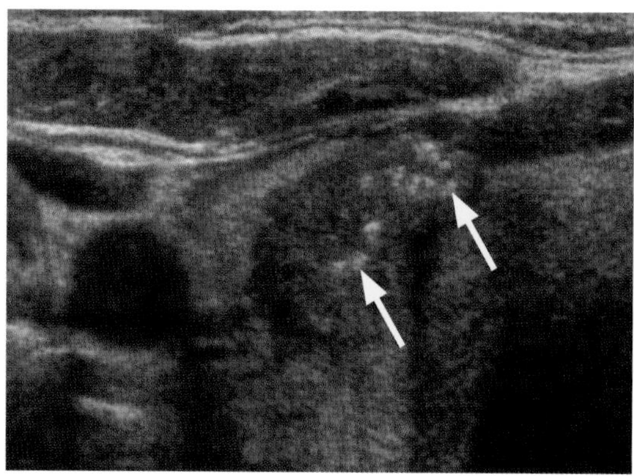

Thyroid carcinoma: Sagittal (left image) and transverse grayscale images through the left lobe of the thyroid demonstrate a solid nodule (calipers) with irregular borders containing punctate calcifications (arrows).

Case courtesy Julie Ritner, MD, Brigham and Women's Hospital.

- A typical ultrasound appearance of a nodule suspicious for malignancy is a solid lesion with punctate calcifications and irregular margins.

  A completely solid nodule is most suspicious. In general, there is decreasing likelihood of cancer with increasing cystic components.

  In general, the likelihood of cancer is dependent on the pattern of calcification. Punctate calcifications are the most suspicious, followed by coarse or rim calcifications. Nodules without any calcification have the least risk of being malignant.

  Taller-than-wide orientation is an ultrasound feature associated with thyroid cancer (analogous to the suspicious breast ultrasound finding of taller-than-wide orientation).

- Papillary cancer is by far the most common histologic subtype of thyroid cancer, and confers the best prognosis.
- Follicular and medullary subtypes are less common and more aggressive. The anaplastic subtype is very rare and has the worst prognosis.
- Thyroid lymphoma can be seen in patients with long-standing Hashimoto thyroiditis.

Malignant adenopathy

- Malignant lymph nodes often appear rounder in morphology than benign lymph nodes, with irregular margins and speckled or central calcifications.
- Metastatic adenopathy from papillary thyroid cancer has a tendency to undergo cystic degeneration. In some cases (especially in young women), a cystic lymph node may be the only presenting feature of thyroid cancer and the thyroid gland may be completely normal by ultrasound.

PARATHYROID IMAGING

Normal parathyroid glands

- The parathyroid glands are normally not visible on ultrasound unless enlarged (due to parathyroid adenoma or hyperplasia).
- The inferior parathyroids are located posterior to the inferior tip of the thyroid.
- The superior parathyroids are located at the posterior aspect of the mid-thyroid.

Parathyroid hyperplasia

- In parathyroid hyperplasia, *all four* parathyroid glands are enlarged and usually visible on ultrasound.

Parathyroid adenoma

- A parathyroid adenoma represents a *single* overactive parathyroid.
- A nuclear medicine Tc-99m sestamibi scan localizes the parathyroid tissue if an adenoma cannot be seen by ultrasound.

UTERUS

PELVIC ANATOMY

Space of Retzius

- The space of Retzius is an extraperitoneal potential space between the pubic symphysis and the bladder.
- A mass in the space of Retzius (such as a hematoma) can displace the bladder posteriorly.
- In contrast, pelvic or abdominal masses will displace the bladder inferiorly or anteriorly.

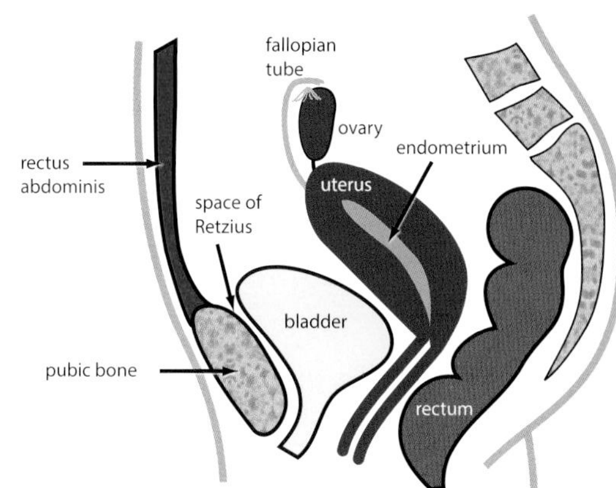

Cervix

- The cervix is seen transvaginally in the sagittal plane as the most proximal portion of the uterus directly posterior to the angle of the bladder.
- The cervix is attached to the posterior edge of the bladder by the parametrium.
- The cervix and uterus normally form a 90-degree angle.
- Nabothian cysts are normal retention cysts due to occlusion of cervical glands.

True and false pelves

- The linea terminalis is a bony landmark separating the true (inferior) pelvis from the false (superior) pelvis. The linea terminalis is a composite of the arcuate line of the ilium, the iliopectineal line, and the pubic crest.
- Normally, the uterus and ovaries are in the true pelvis.
- The dome of a full bladder extends into the false pelvis, pushing small bowel out of the true pelvis. The bladder acts as a sonographic window into the true pelvis.

Normal variant uterine positions

- About 20 degrees of uterine anteflexion is normal. As the bladder fills, the degree of anteflexion decreases.
- Retroversion of the uterus may cause poor visualization of the fundus transabdominally.

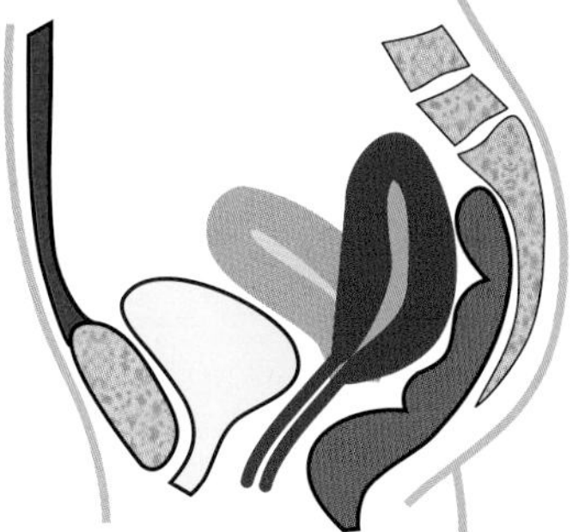

- Retroflexion of the uterus may cause even more severe sound attenuation of the uterine fundus.

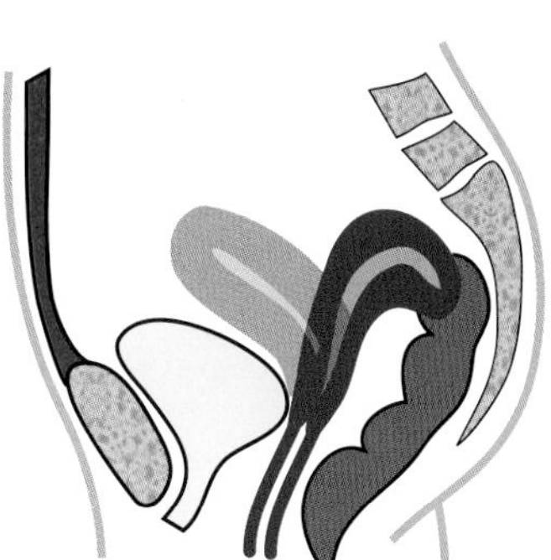

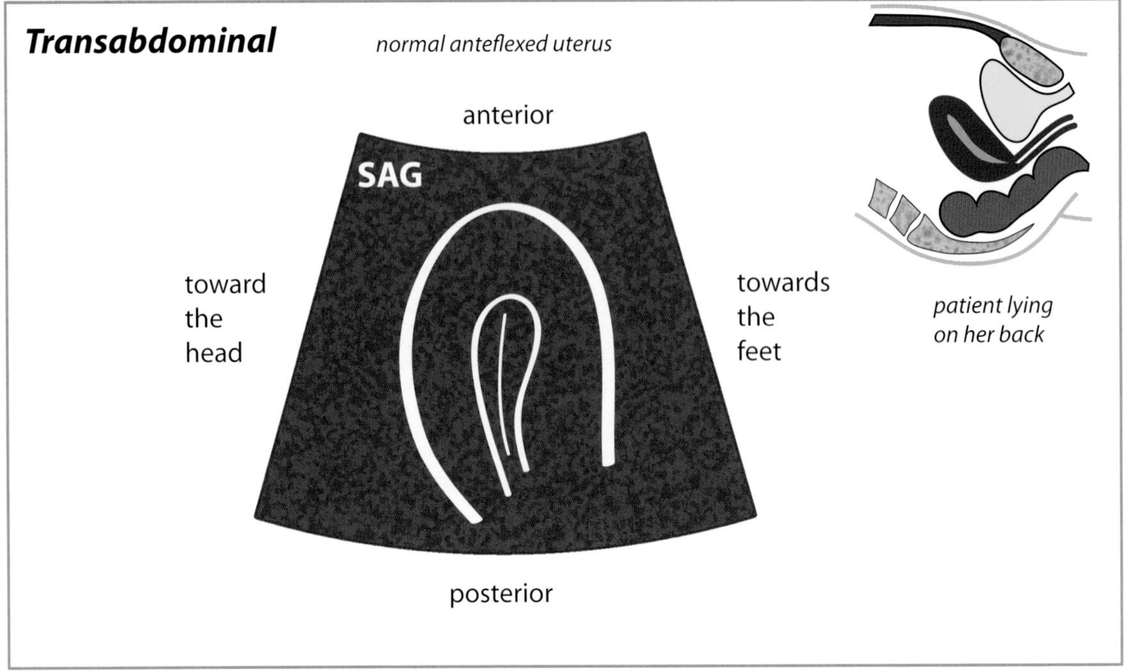

rotate 90 degrees counterclockwise for endovaginal orientation

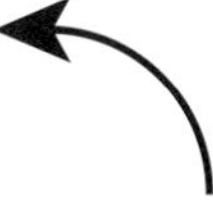

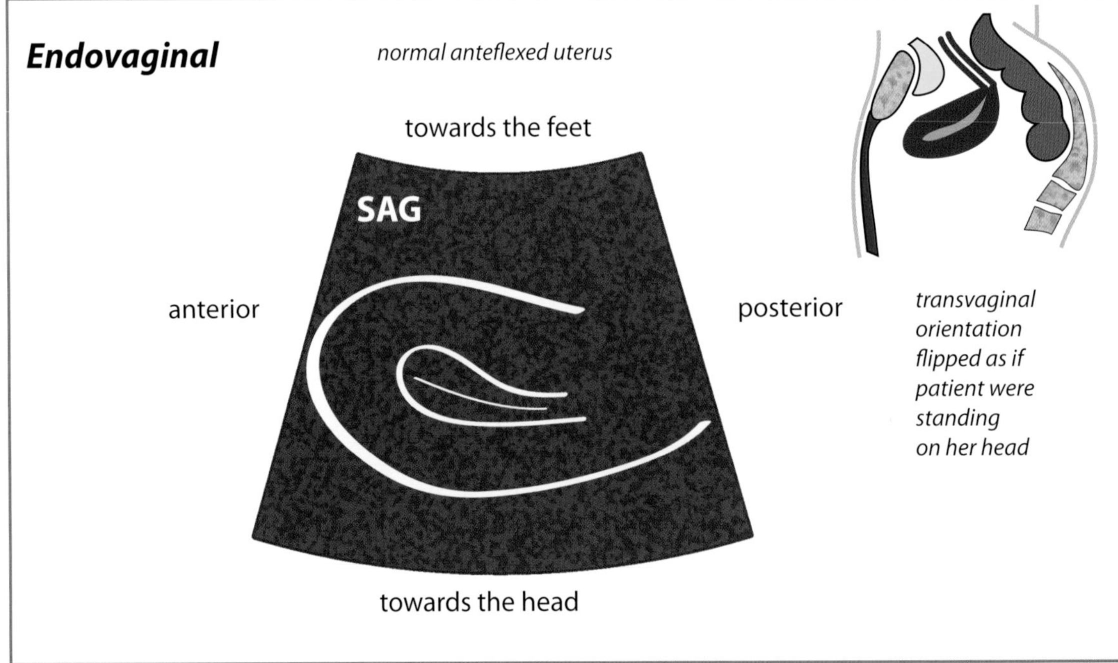

- The sagittal scan plane is rotated 90 degrees between transabdominal and endovaginal orientation. The patient typically empties her bladder prior to endovaginal scanning.

Congenital uterine malformations

Overview of uterine malformations

normal

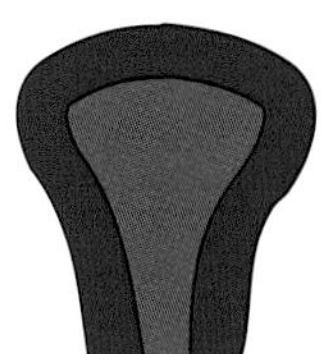

didelphys

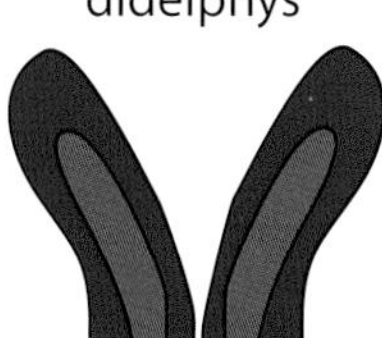

bicornuate

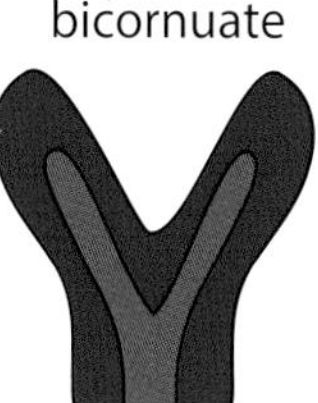

septate

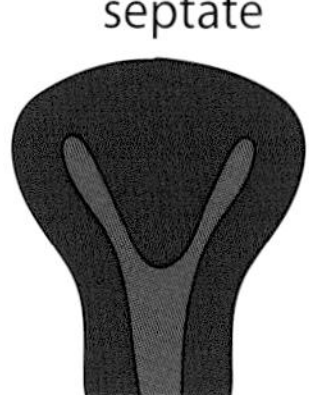

- Uterine malformations are due to abnormal development of the paired Müllerian ducts, which normally fuse during embryogenesis.

> **Complete failure** of fusion → **didelphys** uterus.
>
> **Partial failure** of fusion → **bicornuate** uterus.
>
> **Failure of resorption** of inter-Müllerian septa → **septate** uterus (by far most common uterine anomaly).

- Congenital uterine abnormalities may be associated with urinary tract abnormalities such as renal ectopia or agenesis. The kidneys should be evaluated if a uterine malformation is seen.
- Uterine anomalies increase the risk of reproductive problems since the uterine cavity (or cavities) are abnormally small and/or abnormal in contour.
- The American Fertility Society (now known as the American Society of Reproductive Medicine) classifies Müllerian duct anomalies. Class I is uterine agenesis/hypoplasia, class II is a unicornuate uterus, and classes III through VII represent the anomalies discussed below.

Didelphys uterus (class III)

- A didelphys uterus is two completely separate uteri and cervices, with complete endometrium, myometrium, and serosal surfaces on each side. 75% have a vaginal septum.

Bicornuate uterus (class IV)

- A bicornuate uterus has two uterine fundi, with a shared proximal lower uterine segment.
- A bicornuate uterus may be bicornis bicollis (two cervices) or bicornis unicollis (one cervix).

Septate uterus (class V)

- A septate uterus consists of two uterine cavities, divided by a fibrous or muscular septum.
- Septate uterus is the most likely of all uterine anomalies to be implicated in pregnancy loss since the fibrous septal tissue or myometrium is relatively avascular.

Arcuate uterus (class VI)

- An arcuate uterus is a small inpouching or concave surface of the fundus, which is considered a normal variant rather than an anomaly.

Diethylstilbestrol (DES) uterus (class VII)

- In utero exposure to diethylstilbestrol (DES) causes the fetus to develop a hypoplastic uterus with a T-shaped endometrial contour and is associated with an increased risk of clear cell vaginal cancer. DES hasn't been used since the 1970s.

Endometrium

Measuring the endometrium

- The thickest portion of the endometrium should be measured transvaginally in the sagittal orientation. Ideally, the endometrium should be measured in the *menstrual* phase.
- Endometrial fluid is not included in the measurement: If endometrial fluid is present, the flanking endometrium is measured and the two components are summed.

Cyclical endometrial thickness

- Days 1–4: **Menstrual** phase. Endometrial thickness <4 mm.

  The endometrium is a thin, echogenic stripe in the menstrual phase.

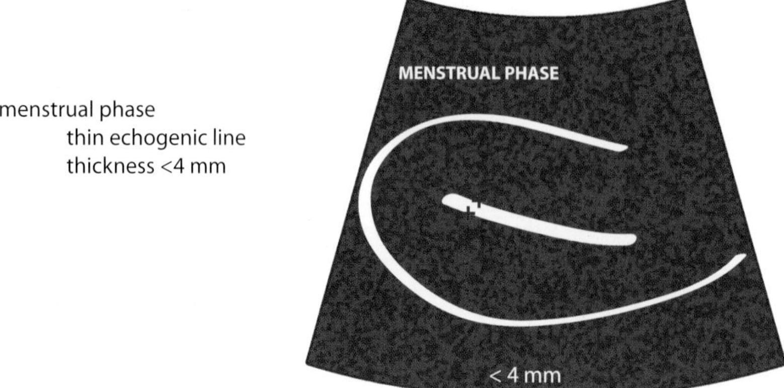

- Days 5–9: **Early proliferative** phase. Endometrial thickness 4–8 mm.
- Days 10–14: **Late proliferative** (periovulatory) phase. Endometrial thickness 6–10 mm.

  Estrogen effects dominate in the proliferative phase, causing increased functional zone thickness.

  The endometrium becomes trilaminar with a hypoechoic zone between the endometrial cavity and the peripheral echogenic endometrium.

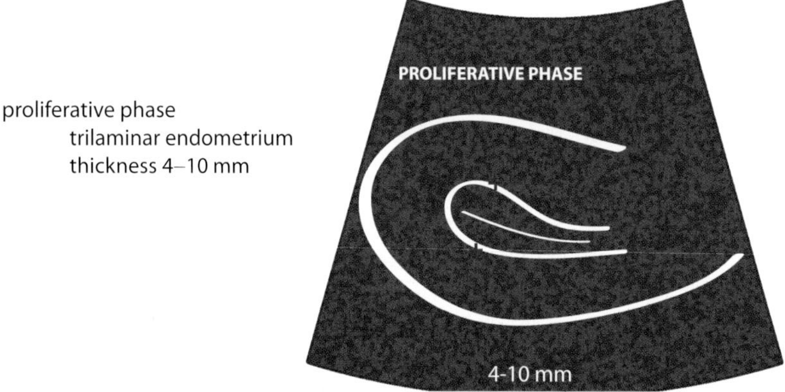

- Days 15–28: **Secretory** phase: Endometrial thickness 7–14 mm.

  Progesterone effects dominate in the secretory phase, causing the functional layer to becomes even thicker, soft, and edematous as the spiral arteries become tortuous. The functional layer increases in echogenicity and becomes isoechoic relative to the basal layer.

  The endometrium reaches its maximum thickness and echogenicity in the late secretory phase.

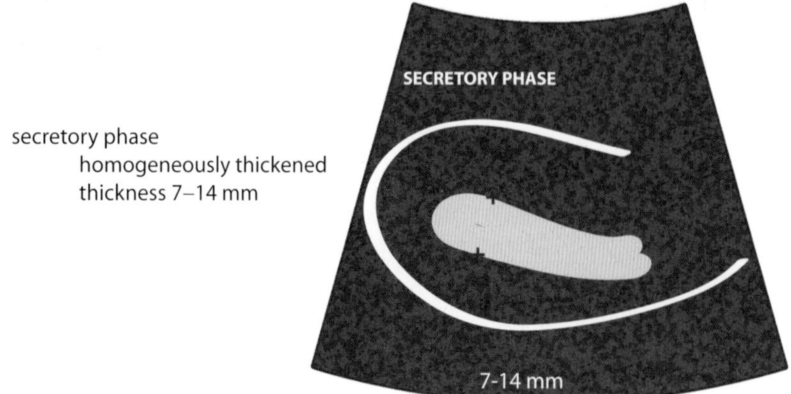

Endometrial polyp

- An endometrial polyp can cause mucous discharge or irregular vaginal bleeding between cycles. Most endometrial polyps are benign, but larger polyps (>1.5 cm) or polyps occurring in postmenopausal patients may have malignant potential.
- Ultrasound shows a focal nodular area of endometrial thickening, often with a feeding vessel by Doppler. A polyp is more definitively diagnosed by sonohysterogram, where saline is instilled into the uterus prior to transvaginal ultrasound.

Tamoxifen effect

- Tamoxifen is an estrogen agonist/antagonist used in the treatment of breast cancer. It acts as an antagonist at the breast and an agonist at the endometrium.
- Tamoxifen can cause endometrial hyperplasia, metaplasia, and carcinoma.
- Ultrasound shows irregular, cystic endometrium, which may simulate endometrial cancer or endometrial cystic atrophy.
- Most women on tamoxifen are screened by ultrasound every 6 months for endometrial carcinoma.

Endometrial cancer and postmenopausal endometrial thickness

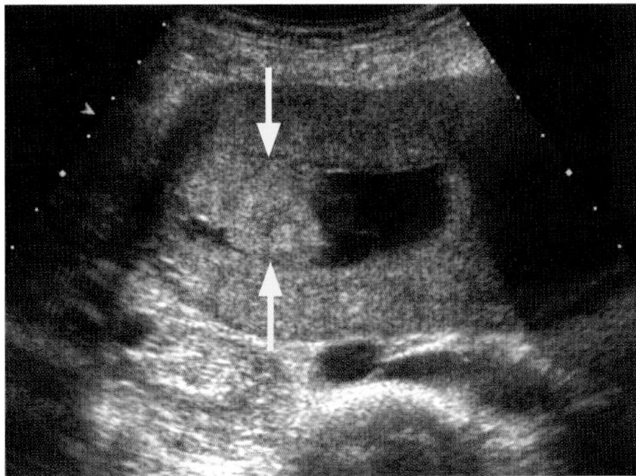

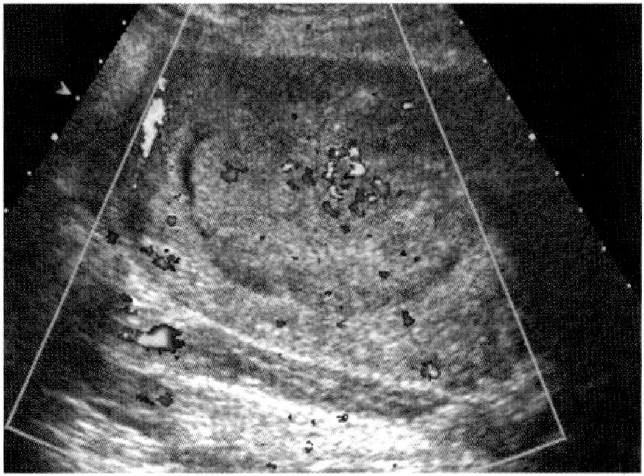

Endometrial cancer: Grayscale ultrasound of the uterus (left image) shows a mildly echogenic, irregular endometrial mass (arrows). Fluid in the endometrial canal has likely accumulated due to cervical stenosis. Color Doppler shows vascularity within the mass.

Case courtesy Julie Ritner, MD, Brigham and Women's Hospital.

- Over 95% of endometrial carcinoma presents with postmenopausal bleeding. The main risk factor for endometrial cancer is prolonged estrogen exposure, which occurs with nulliparity, obesity, late menopause, and tamoxifen.
- If the patient is not bleeding, the postmenopausal endometrium should be <8 mm thick. Although an incidentally thickened endometrium may be a normal hyperplastic response to estrogen exposure, a thickened endometrium should always be regarded with suspicion for malignancy in a postmenopausal woman.

  If the endometrium is thicker than 8 mm in a postmenopausal woman, the patient should be evaluated further, typically via endometrial biopsy with or without hysteroscopy.

  Although uncommonly seen in the absence of bleeding, the finding most suggestive of endometrial carcinoma is the presence of ill-defined margins separating the endometrium and the myometrium.
- If the patient is bleeding and the endometrium is less than 5 mm, the bleeding is caused by endometrial atrophy. There is negligible risk of endometrial cancer if the thickness is less than 5 mm.
- Postmenopausal bleeding with an endometrium thicker than 5 mm may represent endometrial carcinoma and further workup is needed. Note that the average endometrial thickness with endometrial carcinoma is 21 mm.

Ectopic endometrium

Endometriosis

- Endometriosis is ectopic endometrial tissue outside of the endometrial cavity.
- An endometrioma is a hemorrhagic focus of ectopic endometrial tissue.
- The classic ultrasound appearance of an endometrioma is a well-defined complex cyst with **homogeneous low-level internal echoes** and increased through transmission. Small linear echogenic foci are often seen at the cyst periphery. This classic appearance isn't always seen and occasionally an endometrioma may appear similar to a neoplasm.
- While the ovary is the most common site of involvement, endometriosis may affect the adnexa, pelvic viscera, or even organs outside of the pelvis, such as the brain.

Adenomyosis

- Adenomyosis is endometrial tissue within the myometrium. Adenomyosis typically presents with menorrhagia and pain.
- Ultrasound shows heterogeneous myometrium, typically more prominent in the posterior wall, associated with subendometrial cysts. The uterus may be globular and enlarged and there is often poor differentiation of the endometrial–myometrial border. Focal adenomyosis, known as an adenoma, may simulate a fibroid.

Myometrium

Fibroid (leiomyoma)

- Fibroids are extremely common benign tumors of smooth muscle seen in 25% of white women and 50% of black women over age 30.
- The typical ultrasound appearance of a fibroid is a slightly heterogeneous, hypoechoic uterine mass with linear bands of shadowing.
  - Calcification is often seen.
  - May undergo cystic degeneration and appear as an anechoic mass with posterior through transmission.
- Fibroid location:
  - **Intramural**: Location in the myometrium is the most common fibroid location.
  - **Submucosal**: A submucosal fibroid may bulge into the endometrial canal, producing pain and bleeding.
    - A submucosal fibroid can be resected hysteroscopically if >50% of the fibroid is intraluminal.
    - An intracavitary fibroid is a variant of a submucosal fibroid located nearly entirely within the uterine cavity.
  - **Subserosal**: A subserosal fibroid may simulate an adnexal mass if pedunculated, but Doppler will show blood supply coming from uterus.
  - **Cervical**: Rare, may simulate cervical cancer.

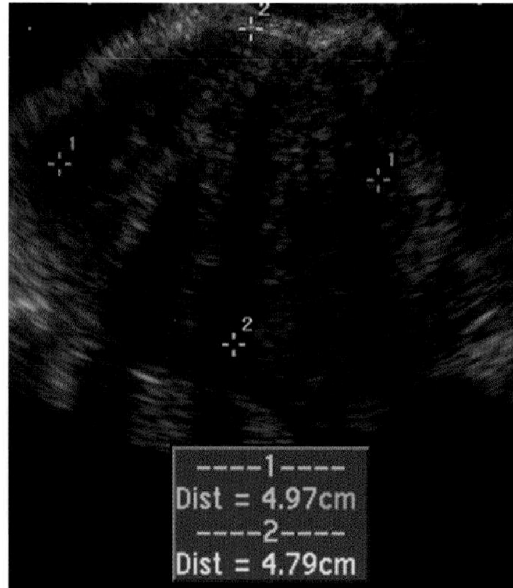

Fibroid: Ultrasound shows a hypoechoic myometrial mass (calipers) with linear bands of shadowing.

- A **lipoleiomyoma** is a variant of fibroid that contains fat and is echogenic.

Leiomyosarcoma

- Malignant transformation of a fibroid to leiomyosarcoma is extremely rare.
- A "funny looking fibroid" is much more likely to be a benign, inhomogeneous fibroid rather than a leiomyosarcoma.
- Tamoxifen increases the risk of leiomyosarcoma in addition to endometrial carcinoma.

Miscellaneous uterine disease

Endometrial fluid

- It is never normal to have more than a tiny amount of fluid in the endometrial canal.
- In a premenopausal woman, endometrial fluid can be due to bleeding from menses or spontaneous abortion.
- In a postmenopausal woman, endometrial fluid can be due to cervical stenosis, and a careful evaluation for cervical malignancy should be performed.

Uterine infections

- **Endometritis** is inflammation or infection of the endometrium, and is commonly seen postpartum, typically with no specific findings on ultrasound. Gas in the uterus may be normal up to 3 weeks postpartum (seen in 7% of normal cases), but gas in the uterus later than 3 weeks after delivery may represent endometritis.
- **Pyometra** (pus within the uterus) is very rare and usually due to outflow obstruction. An evaluation for cervical malignancy should be performed.

Intrauterine device (IUD)

- The ultrasound appearance of an intrauterine device (IUD) is dependent on the type of IUD:
  - Mirena IUD (delivers progesterone): Shadowing structure in endometrial canal.
  - Conventional IUD: Highly echogenic.
- Potential complications of an IUD are rare but serious:
  - Increased risk of infection with prolonged IUD use, especially actinomycosis.
  - When pregnancy occurs in the presence of an IUD, there is increased risk for ectopic pregnancy.
  - Uterine perforation is very rare.

Uterine arteriovenous malformation (AVM)

- Uterine arteriovenous malformation may be congenital (very rare) or acquired iatrogenically (e.g., from a D&C).
- Grayscale and color Doppler appearance shows an enlarged, heterogeneous, and multicystic uterus. The appearance is similar to gestational trophoblastic disease (discussed in the first trimester of pregnancy section), but with negative β-hCG.

Post-Cesarean section complications

- **Bladder-flap hematoma** is a rare complication of a low-transverse Cesarean section, where a postsurgical hematoma forms in the vesicouterine space (posterior to the bladder, between the bladder and the uterus).
  - Ultrasound of a bladder-flap hematoma will show a complex mass posterior to the bladder.
- **Subfascial hematoma** is also a rare complication of Cesarean section due to extraperitoneal hemorrhage within the prevesical space (anterior to the bladder).
  - Ultrasound shows a complex mass anterior to the bladder.
- It is important to distinguish a subfascial hematoma from a bladder-flap hematoma as the surgical approach for repair is different.

ANATOMY AND PHYSIOLOGY

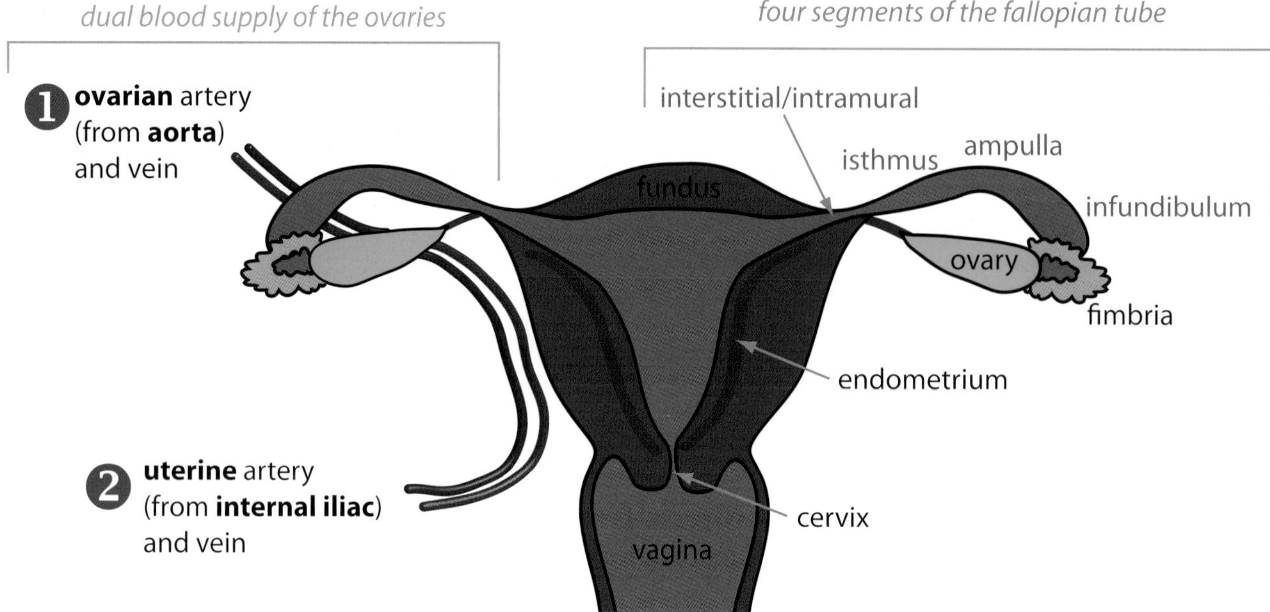

- There is a dual blood supply to the ovary:
  - The ovarian artery comes directly off the aorta to supply the lateral aspect of the ovary.
  - A branch of the uterine artery arises from the internal iliac artery to supply the medial aspect of the ovary.
- The fallopian tube is divided into four segments, from proximal to distal:
  - Interstitial (intramural) is the narrowest segment.
  - Isthmus.
  - Ampulla.
  - Infundibulum.

Cyclical changes in the ovaries

- Day 5–7 of the menstrual cycle: Multiple follicles become apparent in the ovary.
- Day 8–13: One (or more) dominant follicles arise.
  - 4–5 days before ovulation, the dominant follicle grows at the rate of approximately 2–3 mm/day.
  - The maximal diameter of the dominant follicle is approximately 2 cm.
  - The day prior to ovulation, a hypoechoic ring forms around the dominant follicle, which represents the granulosa layer separating from the theca.
- Day 14: **Ovulation.** Physiologic bleeding occurs into the follicle at the time of ovulation, at which point the follicle is called the corpus hemorrhagicum. After ovulation, the corpus hemorrhagicum becomes the corpus luteum.
- Day 15–20: The corpus luteum retains fluid over the next 4–5 days to reach a maximal size of approximately 3 cm.
- Day 20–28. If pregnancy doesn't occur, the corpus luteum involutes to become the corpus albicans, which cannot be seen by ultrasound.
- If pregnancy does occur, the corpus luteum develops into a gland secreting hCG. A prominent corpus luteum may be mistaken for an ectopic pregnancy due to its similar appearance. However, an ectopic pregnancy will only very rarely be *in* the ovary.

OVARIAN CYSTS

Physiologic simple cyst (in a premenopausal patient)

- A simple ovarian cyst is a round or oval anechoic structure with smooth and imperceptibly thin walls, posterior acoustic enhancement, and lack of worrisome features such as solid components, septations, or internal flow on color Doppler.
- A simple ovarian cyst is a follicle that physiologically enlarges from estrogen stimulation as a normal part of the menstrual cycle.
- The Society of Radiologists in Ultrasound (SRU) published a consensus in 2010 regarding management of asymptomatic ovarian and adnexal cysts imaged at ultrasound.

SRU consensus (premenopausal)

- Cysts ≤3 cm do not need to be described in the report, and there is no need for follow-up.
- Cysts >3 and ≤5 cm should be mentioned in the report and described as benign, with no follow-up necessary.
- Cysts >5 and ≤7 cm are almost certainly benign but should be followed annually.
- Cysts >7 cm should be evaluated by MRI or surgery, as a full ultrasound assessment is difficult.

Postmenopausal simple ovarian cyst

SRU consensus (post menopausal)

- Cysts ≤1 cm do not need to be reported or followed.
- Cysts >1 cm and ≤7 cm are almost certainly benign, but should be described and followed annually with ultrasound (similar to premenopausal cysts >5 and ≤7 cm).
- Cysts >7 cm should be evaluated by MRI or surgery, as a full ultrasound assessment is difficult (similar to a premenopausal cyst of the same size).

Functional cyst

- A functional cyst is the result of a follicular cycle that did not execute normally. Functional cysts include follicular cysts, corpus luteal cysts, and theca-lutein cysts.
- A **follicular cyst** is a simple cyst larger than 25 mm, representing a follicle that did not undergo ovulation.
- A **corpus luteal cyst** may grow to greater than 3 cm if it fails to involute normally.

  A corpus luteal cyst can have variable appearances, but will often look like a complex ovarian cyst.

  High diastolic flow is often present, which can also be seen in ovarian cancer.
- **Theca-lutein cysts** are often multiple and arise from elevated hCG. They can be seen in molar pregnancy, multiple gestations, or infertility patients on gonadotropins or clomiphene.
- A **hemorrhagic cyst** is the result of hemorrhage into a functional cyst, most commonly a corpus luteum. Ultrasound findings can be suggestive, although a complex cyst should be followed-up at least once to ensure resolution.

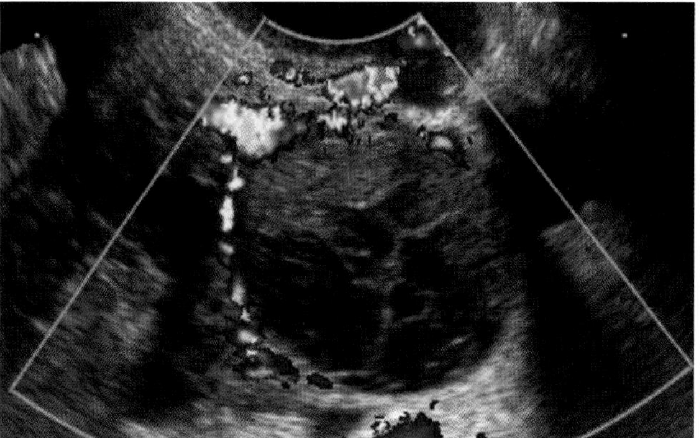

Hemorrhagic cyst: Transvaginal color Doppler of an ovary shows a large complex ovarian cystic mass containing web-like internal echoes, with no flow on color Doppler. Follow-up ultrasound confirmed resolution.

An acutely hemorrhagic cyst may be hyperechoic and potentially mimic a solid mass, but will usually show posterior enhancement. As the clot dissolves, the internal echo pattern becomes more complex to produce characteristic **web-like internal echoes**. Retractile mural clot features concave margins and absent Doppler flow. In contrast, a solid mural nodule features a convex margin and internal flow.

Ovarian hyperstimulation syndrome (OHSS)

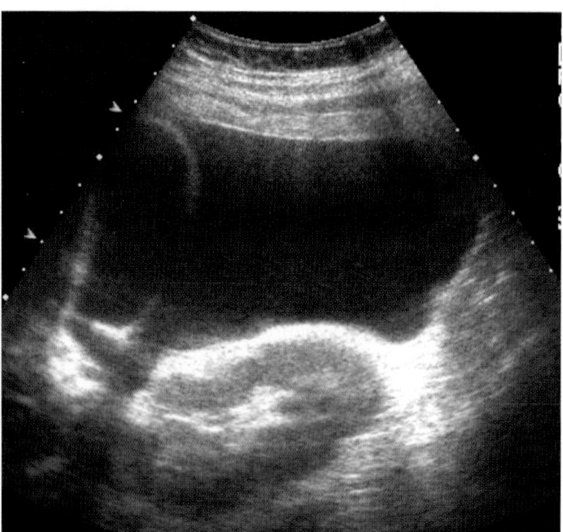

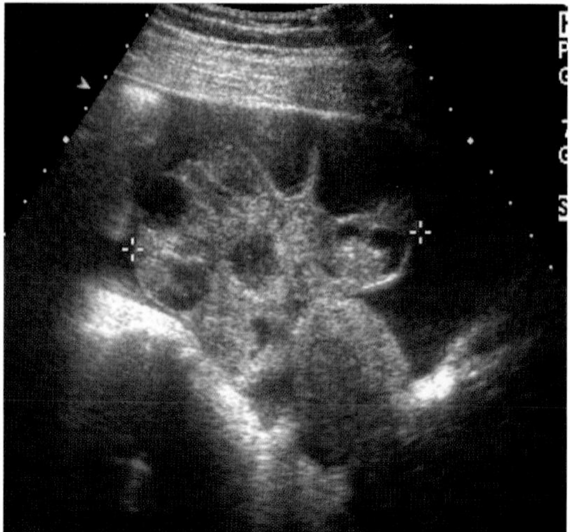

Ovarian hyperstimulation syndrome: Sagittal grayscale ultrasound of the right upper quadrant (left image) shows a large amount of ascites. Right lower quadrant ultrasound (right image) shows a markedly enlarged ovary (calipers measure greater than 8 cm), with numerous enlarged follicles. The patient was receiving infertility treatment.

- Ovarian hyperstimulation syndrome (OHSS) is a complication of fertility treatment, thought to be due to VEGF dysregulation causing capillary leak.
- The criteria for diagnosis of OHSS include abdominal pain, enlargement of the ovary to greater than 5 cm, and presence of either ascites or hydrothorax. At least one additional laboratory or clinical symptom must be met, including elevated hematocrit (≥45%), elevated WBC (>15,000), elevated LFTs, acute renal failure, or dyspnea.
- OHSS increases the risk of ovarian torsion and ectopic pregnancy.

Polycystic ovarian syndrome (PCOS)

- Polycystic ovarian syndrome is a clinical syndrome of obesity, insulin resistance, anovulation, and hirsutism secondary to excess androgens.
- Ultrasound criteria include >12 small follicles (most often arranged around the periphery of the ovary), none greater than 9 mm in diameter, and an ovarian volume >10 mL. Ovarian volume is calculated by multiplying the diameter of three orthogonal planes by 0.52.
- The ovarian stroma is typically very vascular when evaluated by color Doppler.
- A differential consideration is normal ovaries under the influence of oral contraceptives, although contraceptives will not increase the vascularity of the ovary.

Adnexal cystic lesions

Paraovarian cyst

- A paraovarian cyst is a simple cyst separate from the ovary, thought to be developmental in origin.
- Paraovarian cysts are considered normal if <5 cm.
- The main differential is an ovarian cyst. Ovarian cysts should be reported (and followed) if they are greater than 3 cm, while paraovarian cysts do not need to be followed unless they are greater than 5 cm.

Peritoneal inclusion cyst

- A peritoneal inclusion cyst is a septated fluid collection formed by adhesions from prior surgery. The ovary is always closely associated with the peritoneal inclusion cyst, either trapped within or adjacent to it.
- It is important *not* to recommend surgery for treatment of a peritoneal inclusion cyst, as further surgery may create additional adhesions.
- The main differential of a peritoneal inclusion cyst is a cystadenoma, which has thick septations and tends to exert mass effect.

Dilated fallopian tube

- The fallopian tube may become distended due to infection, inflammation, or traction from pelvic adhesions.
- A **hydrosalpinx** is a fluid-filled fallopian tube lacking internal echoes. Ultrasound shows a dilated, anechoic, paraovarian tubular structure with incomplete septations. The incomplete septations represent infoldings of the tubular walls.
- **Hematosalpinx** is a blood-filled fallopian tube that can be seen in the setting of a ruptured ectopic pregnancy or endometriosis. Imaging will show internal echoes within the dilated tube.
- **Pyosalpinx** is a pus-filled fallopian tube resulting from pelvic inflammatory disease. As in hematosalpinx, imaging will show internal echoes within the dilated tube.

VASCULAR ADNEXAL DISEASE

Adnexal torsion

- Adnexal torsion results from twisting of the ovarian vascular pedicle. This results in pain and potential vascular compromise to the ovary.
- Acute pain is usually localized to the affected side. Pain may be episodic, especially if the torsion is intermittent. Torsion occurs mainly in reproductive-age women, and commonly occurs in pregnancy. Torsion occurs more commonly on the right side due to the position of the sigmoid colon, which inhibits free rotation of the left adnexa. Torsion may clinically mimic appendicitis.

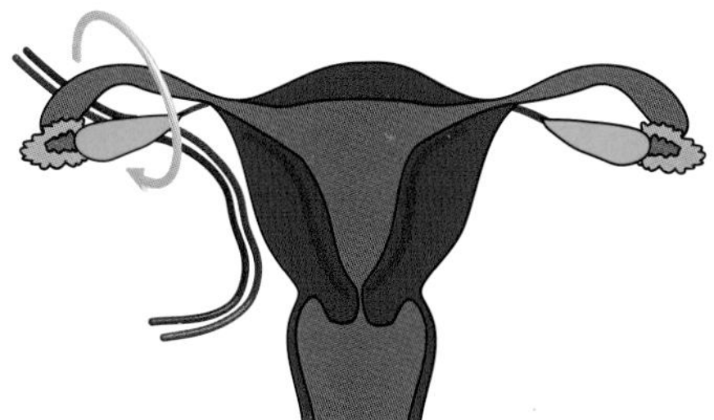

Diagram demonstrates dual blood supply of the ovary, with the yellow curved arrow representing adnexal torsion.

- The ovary may be predisposed to torsion by a lead-point mass, most commonly a dermoid.
- Because of the dual blood supply to the ovary (lateral from the ovarian vessels off the aorta, and medial from the uterine vessels from the internal iliac), flow may still be detectable by color Doppler even with torsion.
- The classic ultrasound presentation of torsion in a patient with acute pelvic pain is an enlarged ovary with free fluid and abnormal ovarian Doppler. The vascular pedicle may be twisted, which is very specific when seen. However, in the real world, the imaging findings tend to be less specific and may include:

  Enlarged ovary >4 cm in diameter.

  Unusual position of the affected ovary, which may even be found on the contralateral side.

  Follicles pushed to the periphery of the ovary.

  Free fluid in the pelvis.

  Variable Doppler findings: Complete lack of flow is concerning, although this is rarely seen. Other Doppler findings include intermittent flow, venous flow on spectral imaging, and even normal flow.

OVARIAN NEOPLASM

Dermoid cyst

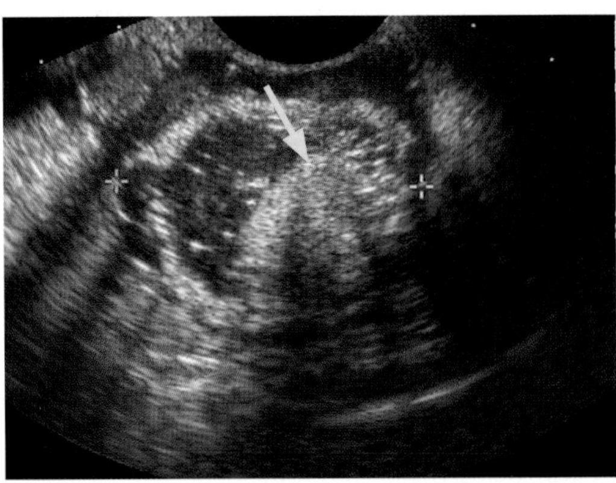

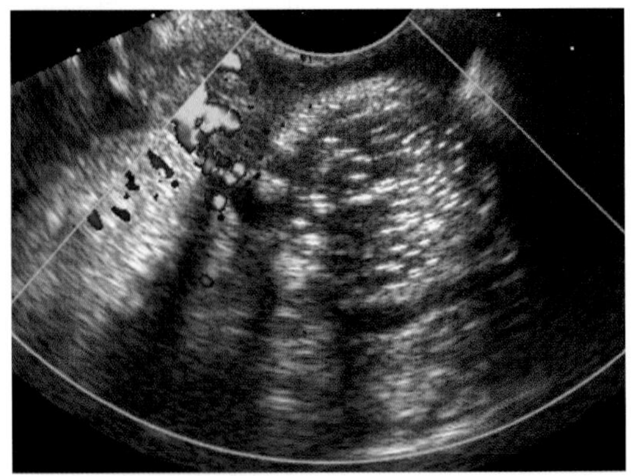

Dermoid cyst: Grayscale ultrasound image of the right ovary (left image) shows a complex ovarian cyst with a densely echogenic, shadowing focus centrally representing the Rokitansky nodule (arrow). Color Doppler shows the *dot-dash* sign, echogenic shadowing, and no significant internal Doppler flow.

- Dermoid cyst, also called a mature cystic teratoma, is the most common ovarian neoplasm. Technically, a *teratoma* contains all three primitive germ cell layers, while a *dermoid cyst* may contain only two. In general use, however, these terms are interchangeable.
- Dermoid cysts are benign. Malignant transformation is very rare and typically occurs in postmenopausal patients.
- A dermoid cyst can act as a lead point for adnexal torsion.
- The classic ultrasound appearance of a dermoid cyst is a complex ovarian cyst with an echogenic *Rokitansky* nodule, a mural nodule containing solid elements. The imaging appearance can be variable, however, and other common imaging features include:

  The *dot-dash* pattern describes interrupted echogenic lines thought to be produced by keratin fibers.

  The *tip of the iceberg* sign describes obscuration of the deeper contents due to high-attenuation material.
- CT or MRI will confirm the presence of fat in ambiguous cases.

Ovarian cancer

- Ovarian cancer is the sixth most common cancer in females, but is the leading cause of death from gynecologic malignancy as it commonly presents at an advanced stage.
- Ultrasound findings suggestive of a malignant mass include:

Mural nodule.	**High flow on color Doppler.**
Thick or irregular walls or septae.	**Presence of ascites.**
Solid components.	**Papillary projections.**

- The four histologic types of ovarian neoplasm are: Epithelial neoplasm (comprises two thirds of all ovarian neoplasms), germ cell tumor, sex cord-stromal tumor, and metastasis.

  The three subtypes of epithelial neoplasm are serous, mucinous, and endometrioid. Endometrioid carcinoma may arise from an endometrioma.

  Teratoma (dermoid cyst), discussed above, is a germ cell tumor. Struma ovarii is a subtype of teratoma that is composed of mature, functioning thyroid tissue.

  Sex cord-stromal tumors include fibroma, thecoma, and fibrothecoma. Meigs syndrome is the triad of benign ovarian fibroma, ascites, and right pleural effusion. Tumors containing thecal cells produce estrogen and may cause endometrial carcinoma.

  Metastasis to the ovary is usually from an extra-pelvic primary. Common extra-pelvic primary cancers that may metastasize to the ovary include gastric and breast cancer. A Krukenberg tumor is an ovarian metastasis of a mucin-producing tumor, typically gastric or colonic. Endometrial cancer may also metastasize to the ovaries.

IMAGING OF THE EARLY PREGNANCY

Gestational sac

- The gestational sac is the earliest imaging finding in early pregnancy.
- The *intradecidual* sign and the *double decidual sac* sign are two findings that may aid in the detection of very early pregnancy.

  The intradecidual sign represents the gestational sac within the thickened decidua, seen at ≤5 weeks.

  The *double decidual sac* sign represents two echogenic rings encircling the gestational sac. It is most useful when seen, where it confirms the presence of an intrauterine pregnancy (IUP). The absence of a double decidual sign is considered indeterminate and may suggest either an IUP or the pseudogestational sac of an ectopic pregnancy.

  A *pseudogestational sac,* in contrast, is an intrauterine fluid collection surrounded by a single decidual layer, seen in the context of ectopic pregnancy.

  Practically, these signs are of limited clinical utility. With a positive pregnancy test and normal adnexae, any fluid collection in the uterus is overwhelmingly likely to represent a very early intrauterine pregnancy (IUP), regardless of the presence of the intradecidual, double decidual sac, or pseuodogestational sac signs.
- A gestational sac should be seen by transvaginal ultrasound if the β-hCG is greater than 1,500. The gestational sac is normally seen by 5 weeks.
- The mean sac diameter (MSD) is the average diameter of the gestational sac measured in three orthogonal planes. The MSD is not routinely measured.

  If the MSD measures 8 mm, a yolk sac should be visible. If a yolk sac is not present, the pregnancy is unlikely to be successful.

  If the MSD measures 16 mm, an embryo should be visible. If an embryo is not seen when the MSD is 16 mm or greater, the pregnancy is unlikely to be successful.
- A subchorionic hematoma is a potential complication of early pregnancy caused by bleeding of the chorionic attachment.

  A small subchorionic hematoma surrounding the gestational sac is of no clinical significance.

  A large subchorionic hematoma will cause an approximately 40% chance of pregnancy failure.

Yolk sac

- Unlike in a chicken's egg, the fetal yolk sac doesn't contain any nutrients. It is a vestigial structure that functions in the early circulation before the development of the heart.
- The yolk sac is normally seen by 5.5 weeks.
- If the yolk sac is abnormally large (>6 mm), the pregnancy has a high chance of failure.

Heartbeat and heart rate

- A heartbeat is almost always detected when the embryo is large enough to be seen. It is unusual to see an embryo with a measurable crown rump length (CRL) without a heartbeat. If no heartbeat is seen in a visible embryo, the pregnancy has a high risk of failure.
- It has long been accepted that a heartbeat should always be seen with a CRL of 5 mm, and lack of a heartbeat was felt to be 100% diagnostic of a failed pregnancy.

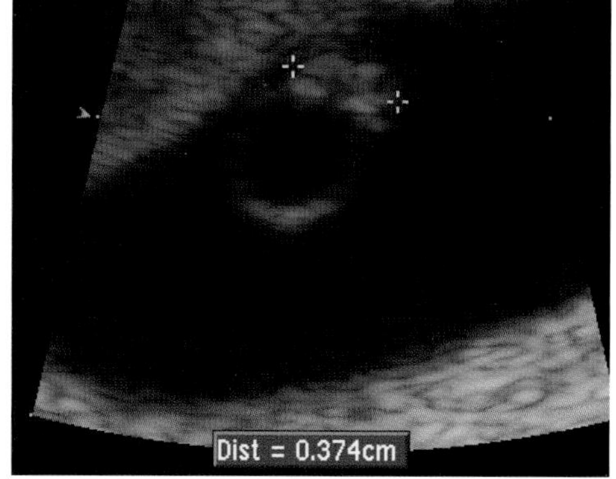

Normal embryo (measuring 3.7 mm) and yolk sac. This embryo had normal heart rate of 112 bpm.

- Recent literature, however, suggests that definitive diagnosis of pregnancy failure based on absent heartbeat be withheld until the embryo has reached a size of 7 mm. Based on this, it may be prudent to recommend follow-up if no heartbeat is seen in an embryo under 7 mm, although the chance of a successful pregnancy in such a case is low.
- Absence of a heartbeat by a gestational age of 6.5 weeks or greater is 100% diagnostic of a failed pregnancy. Note that it is only possible to be certain of pregnancy dating if the patient has had a previous ultrasound to establish early dating, or if the patient underwent IVF with a known transfer date. The date of the last menstrual period is not reliable enough.
- If the early heartbeat is less than 90 bpm, there is very little chance that the pregnancy will be successful. There is no such thing as a "too fast" heart rate. In fact, embryos with a faster heart rate have the highest chance of normal outcome.

  If the CRL is ≤4 mm, ≤90 bpm is considered slow and ≥100 is normal.

  If the CRL is 5–9 mm, ≤110 bpm is considered slow and ≥120 is normal.
- Heart rate is measured using M-mode Doppler.

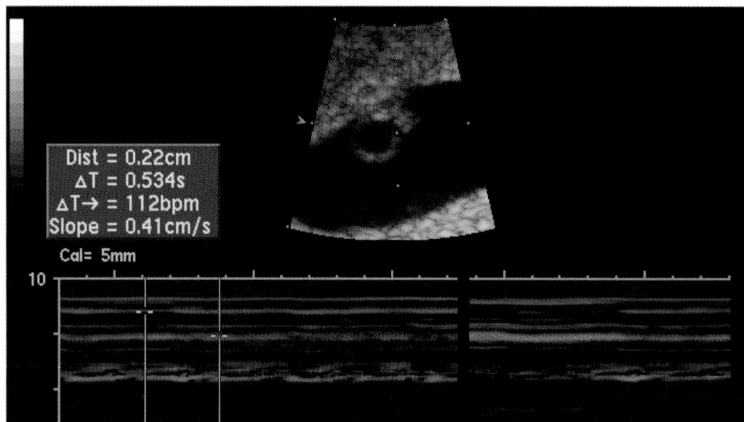

Normal heart rate:

M-mode Doppler shows a calculated heart rate of 112 bpm, which is normal in this 6-week embryo with a 3 mm CRL.

Pregnancy dating

Dating convention

- Early human civilizations may have associated sex with pregnancy, but not until recently has ovulation (occurring approximately 14 days prior to the first day of menses) been associated with conception.
- The modern convention for dating pregnancy is a holdover from ancient times. Gestational age is calculated from the first day of the last menstrual cycle, *not* from conception. Therefore, a "6 week" pregnancy has really only been growing for 4 weeks. For IVF patients with a precisely known implantation date, 2 weeks are added to be consistent with the dating of spontaneous pregnancies.

Assigning gestational age

- Between 5 and 6 weeks gestation, gestational age is determined based on three typical appearances of the early pregnancy.
- Gestational sac only (with or without *double sac* sign): 5.0 weeks.
- Gestational sac with a yolk sac, but without an embryo: 5.5 weeks.
- Gestational sac with an embryo <3 mm and heartbeat: 6 weeks.
- For embryos ≥3 mm in length, the crown rump length is used to assign gestational age using established reference tables. The CRL can estimate gestational age up to 12 weeks. After 12 weeks, dating is estimated using multiple fetal measurements.

guarded pregnancy prognosis: follow-up ultrasound recommended

1

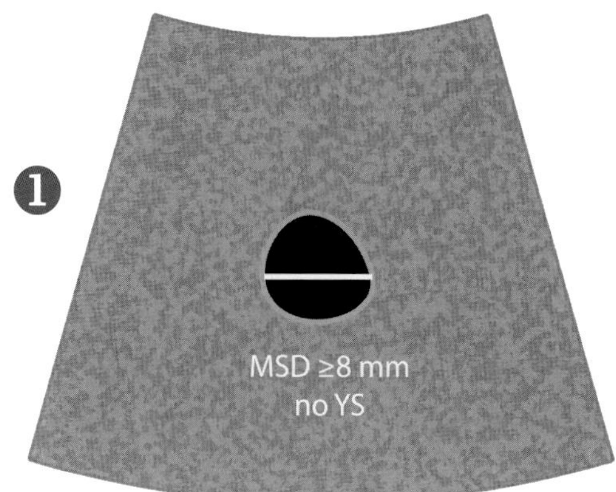

mean sac diameter ≥8 mm
with no yolk sac

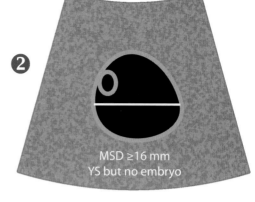

2

MSD ≥16 mm
YS but no embryo

mean sac diameter ≥16 mm
with a yolk sac but no embryo

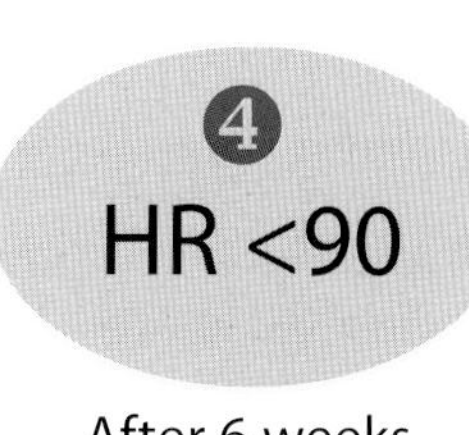

After 6 weeks

3

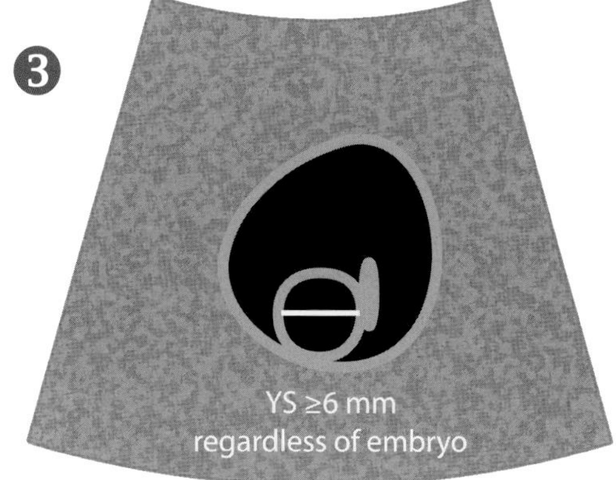

A yolk sac ≥6 mm portends a poor prognosis even if the embryo has a normal heart rate.

5

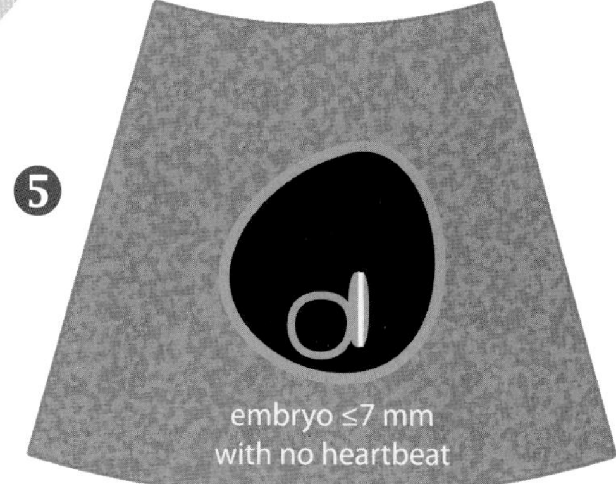

Any visible embryo should have a heartbeat. If the heartbeat is not seen, there is very little chance of successful pregnancy.

definite pregnancy failure:

1 **known gestational age ≥6.5 with no heartbeat.**

The only ways to reliably know a precise gestational age are if a previous ultrasound was performed to establish dating, or the patient underwent in vitro fertilization with a known embryo transfer date.

2

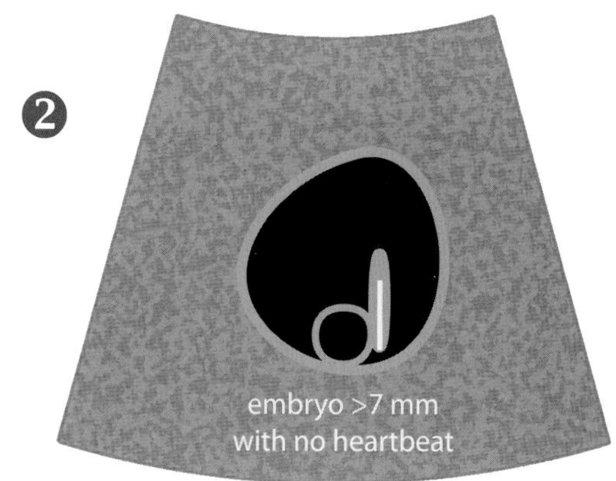

Ectopic pregnancy

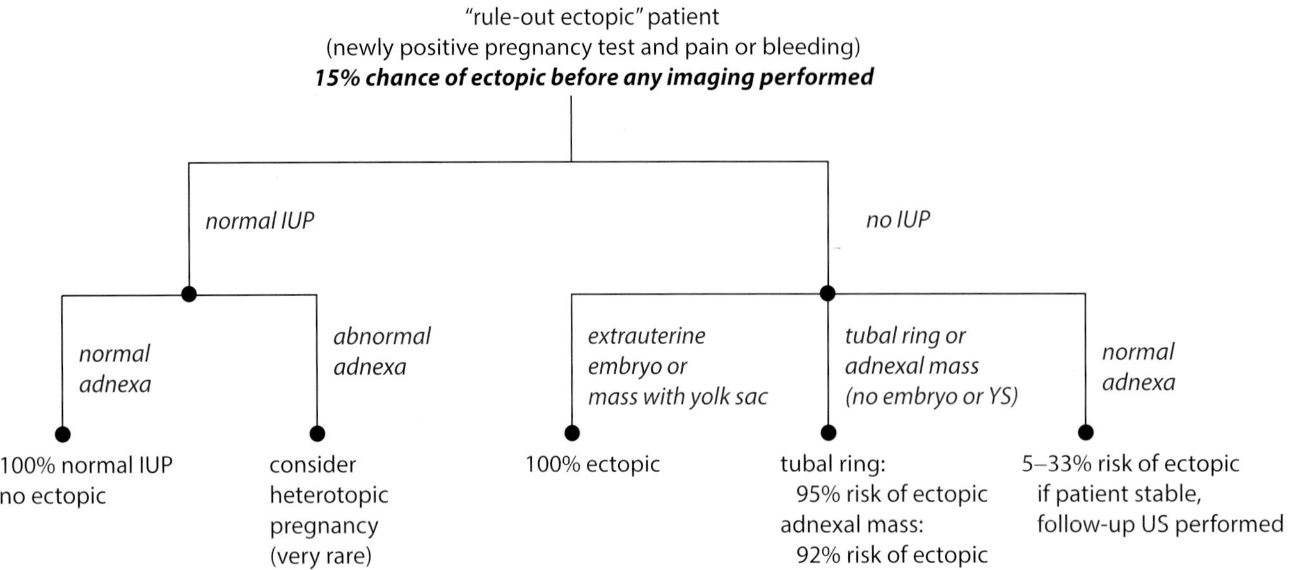

Overview of ectopic pregnancy

- Ectopic pregnancy is defined as a pregnancy outside of the endometrial cavity. Hemorrhage and resultant hypovolemic shock may be life-threatening to the mother.
- The classic clinical presentation of ectopic pregnancy is a positive pregnancy test, vaginal bleeding, pelvic pain, and tender adnexal mass. This presentation is seen in less than 50% of patients.

Risk stratification

- Any woman with a newly positive pregnancy test and either pain or bleeding is classified as a *rule-out ectopic* or *clinically suspected ectopic* patient and has about a 15% chance of having an ectopic pregnancy before any imaging is performed.
- A *rule-out ectopic* patient may have an intrauterine pregnancy (IUP), ectopic pregnancy, or spontaneous abortion. The IUP may be normal, abnormal, or too early to detect.
- The role of imaging is to determine if an IUP is present and to evaluate the common locations (especially the adnexae) where an ectopic may potentially be found.

Definite diagnoses are the exception

- More often than not, it is not possible to definitively diagnose ectopic pregnancy, except in the following situations:

  An extrauterine gestational sac that contains either an embryo or a yolk sac is 100% diagnostic of an ectopic pregnancy.

  A normal IUP, seen in conjunction with normal adnexae, is 100% diagnostic of a normal IUP.
- As previously discussed, the *pseudogestational sac sign* has been reported in the setting of ectopic pregnancy. However, identifying a structure that may be a pseudogestational sac can be a pitfall, as this may represent a very early gestational sac instead. One needs to be very careful before concluding that an ectopic pregnancy is present based solely on the presence of a presumed pseudogestational sac, as incorrect diagnosis may result in administration of cytotoxic therapy that can have disastrous consequences for an intrauterine pregnancy. Careful clinical management and close imaging follow-up should be used if an ectopic is suspected and a pseudogestational sac sign is an isolated imaging abnormality.

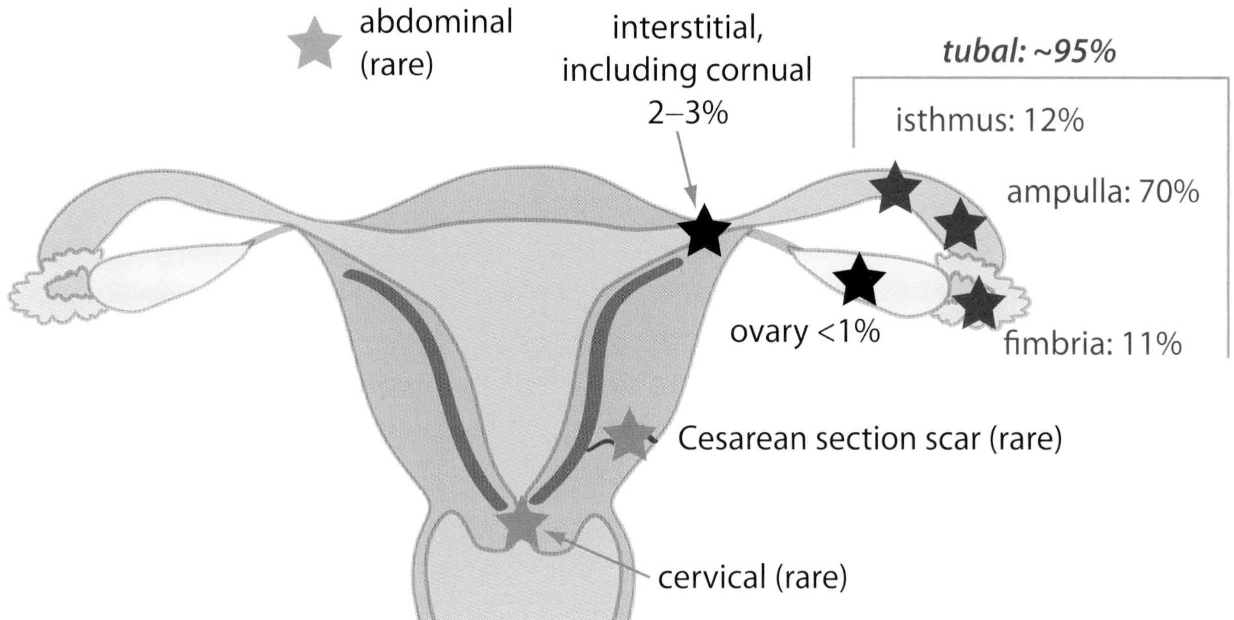

- Most (~95%) ectopic pregnancies occur in the fallopian tube, with the ampullary segment being the most common site.
- It is rare for an ectopic pregnancy to be in the ovary (<1% of all ectopics).
- An especially dangerous location for an ectopic pregnancy is the interstitial portion of the fallopian tube. An interstitial ectopic carries an especially high risk of catastrophic hemorrhage due to its propensity for delayed rupture and proximity to the ovarian vessels.

  Ultrasound of an interstitial ectopic shows absent myometrium along the lateral edge. The *interstitial line* sign represents a thin, echogenic line extending from the endometrial canal to the center of the interstitial ectopic mass. This echogenic line is thought to represent the nondistended, empty endometrial canal.

- A **heterotopic pregnancy** is a simultaneous IUP and ectopic pregnancy. Patients undergoing assistive reproductive techniques are at increased risk for heterotopic pregnancy. Prior to the popularity of these fertilization procedures, heterotopic pregnancies were extremely rare. Given the increased prevalence of assistive reproductive techniques, however, the adnexae must be carefully evaluated even in the presence of an IUP.

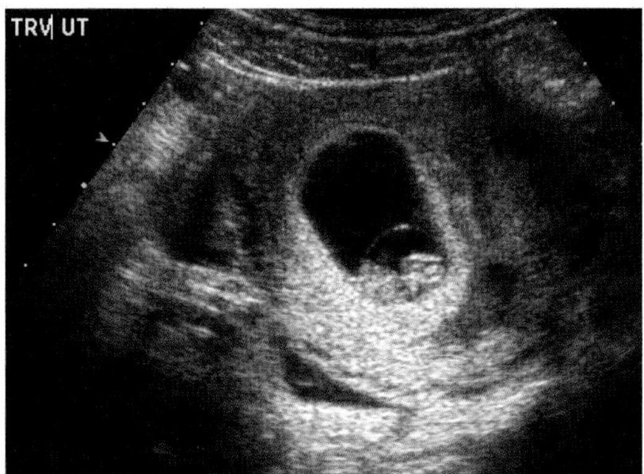

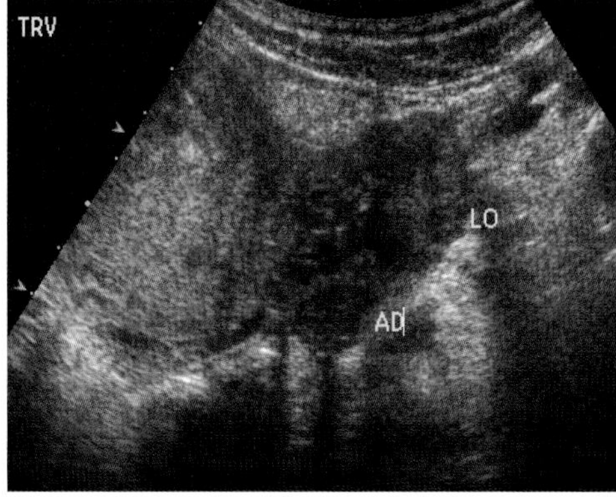

Heterotopic pregnancy: Transverse grayscale ultrasound of the uterus (left image) demonstrates a normal intrauterine pregnancy. Transverse scanning of the left adnexa shows a rounded hypoechoic adnexal mass (AD) distinct from the left ovary (LO).

Case courtesy Julie Ritner, MD, Brigham and Women's Hospital.

- Ectopic pregnancy may also occur (rarely) in a prior Cesarean section scar, in the cervix, or in the abdomen. When in the abdomen, the ectopic pregnancy can become large before causing symptoms.

Imaging findings of ectopic pregnancy

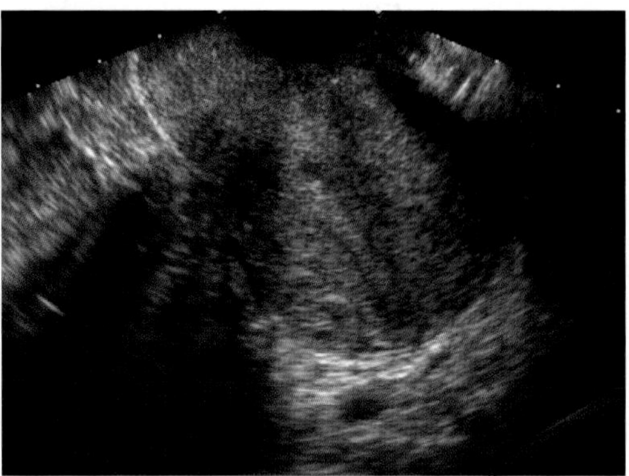

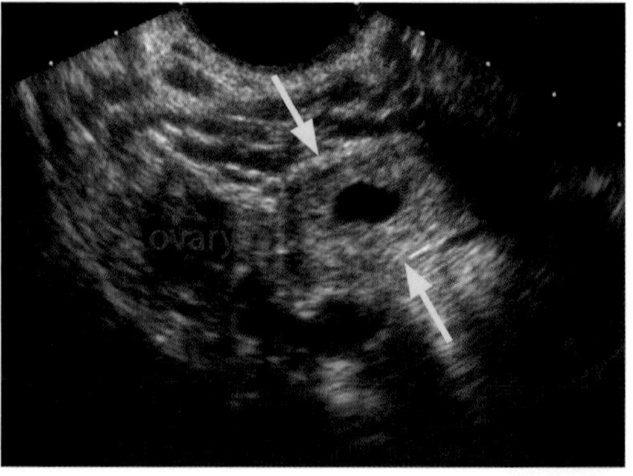

Adnexal ectopic: Sagittal grayscale endovaginal ultrasound of the uterus (left image) shows a normal uterus, with no evidence of intrauterine pregnancy. Ultrasound of the adnexa (right image) shows an adnexal ring (yellow arrows), discrete from the normal ovary. In a patient with a suspected ectopic, the presence of an adnexal ring and no intrauterine pregnancy has a 95% positive predictive value of being an ectopic pregnancy.

Case courtesy Julie Ritner, MD, Brigham and Women's Hospital.

- In the absence of an IUP, an adnexal mass has a 92% positive predictive value of being an ectopic.
- In the absence of an IUP, an adnexal ring has a 95% positive predictive value of being an ectopic.
- An extrauterine embryo (with or without heartbeat) or mass with yolk sac has a 100% predictive value of being an ectopic.
- The nonspecific *ring of fire* sign describes increased peripheral color Doppler flow surrounding an adnexal mass. This sign is rarely helpful as it can be seen in both ectopic pregnancy and corpus luteum.
- In a rule-out ectopic patient, an ovarian mass is overwhelmingly more likely to be a corpus luteum than an ectopic pregnancy unless a definite embryo or yolk sac is identified. In contrast, an extra-ovarian mass would be concerning for ectopic. In ambiguous cases, it may be helpful to gently apply pressure with the ultrasound probe and watch for movement of the mass with respect to the ovary to identify if a mass is ovarian or adnexal in origin.

Following serial hCG

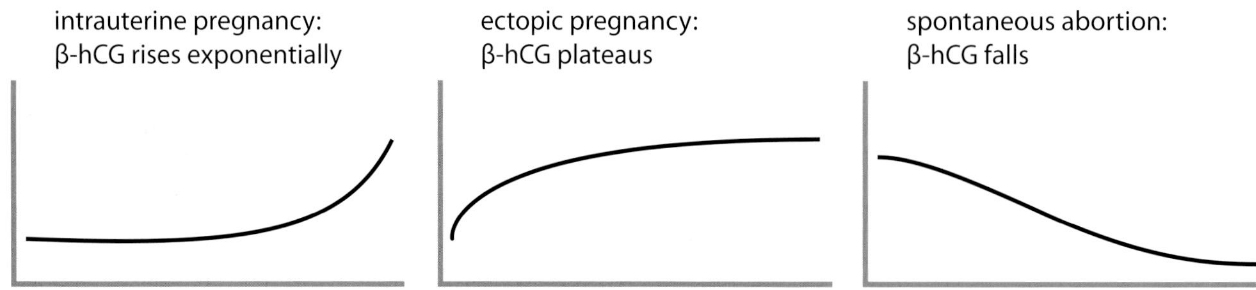

- The pattern of hCG levels over time may be a helpful adjunct to imaging in following-up the *rule-out ectopic* patient.

Gestational trophoblastic disease (hydatidiform molar pregnancy)

- Gestational trophoblastic disease, also called hydatidiform molar pregnancy (or molar pregnancy for short), is invasive neoplastic overgrowth of the trophoblast into the myometrium or beyond. The trophoblast normally develops into the placenta.
- The classic clinical presentation of molar pregnancy is hyperemesis, markedly elevated hCG, and an enlarged uterus. The patient may also present with painless vaginal bleeding.
- Complete hydatidiform mole does not contain any fetal parts. It is caused by loss of the egg's DNA prior to fertilization by the sperm and has a diploid karyotype of 46,XX (most commonly) or 46,XY. A complete mole may progress to metastatic choriocarcinoma.

  Chorioadenoma destruens is a complete mole that invades the myometrium.

  Molar pregnancy is associated with theca lutein cysts, which arise in response to elevated hCG.
- Partial hydatidiform mole is associated with some fetal development. It is usually caused by two sperm fertilizing the same egg and has a triploid karyotype of 69,XXX, 69,XXY, or 69,XYY. Partial mole is less likely to progress to choriocarcinoma.
- On ultrasound, molar disease causes uterine enlargement with a classic heterogeneous and multicystic *snowstorm* appearance. Visualization of fetal parts suggests a partial mole.
- Treatment of a molar pregnancy is endometrial suction curettage and close follow-up of serum hCG levels.

Retained products of conception (RPOC)

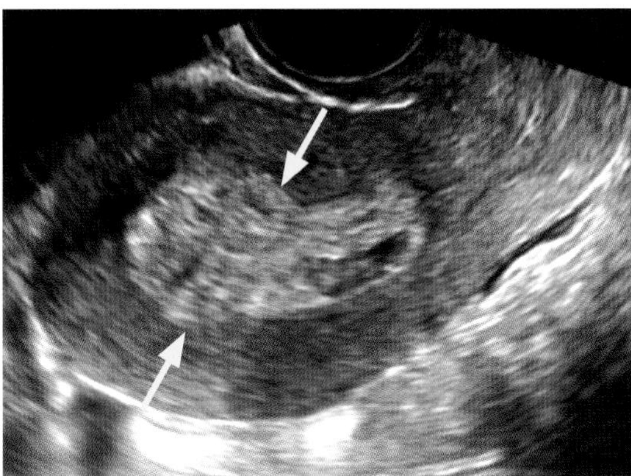

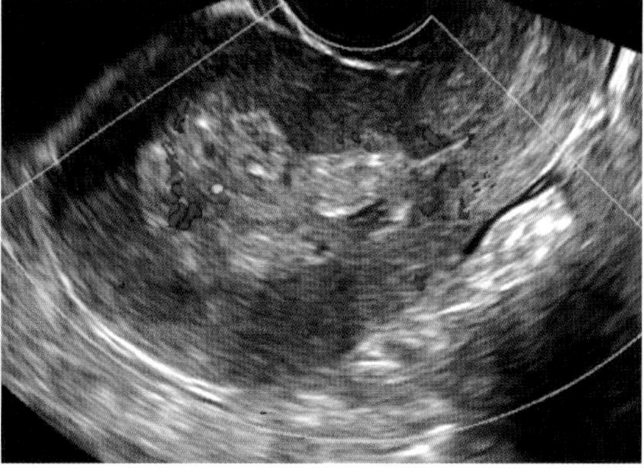

Retained products of conception: Sagittal grayscale ultrasound through the uterus demonstrates a markedly thickened and heterogeneous endometrium (arrows). Color Doppler shows vascularity within the endometrium, especially toward the uterine fundus. These imaging findings are suggestive of, but not diagnostic of, RPOC. Retained products of conception were proven at curettage.

Case courtesy Julie Ritner, MD, Brigham and Women's Hospital.

- Retained products of conception (RPOC) are placental or fetal tissues that remain in the uterus after delivery, miscarriage, or termination.
- Untreated RPOC can lead to continued maternal bleeding and endometritis.
- The sonographic findings of an endometrial blood clot and RPOC overlap and it is often not possible to differentiate between these two entities. An endometrial mass, with or without Doppler flow, in the appropriate clinical context has only about a 50% positive predictive value. The presence of Doppler flow is *not* diagnostic of RPOC, as endometrial color Doppler flow can be detected in the presence or absence of RPOC. Color Doppler flow is seen more commonly with RPOC, however.
- A normal-appearing uterus, with an endometrial thickness less than 10 mm, is highly unlikely to contain RPOC.

- The placentation type (chorionicity and amnionicity) substantially affects the risk for pregnancy complications and influences how closely the pregnancy should be followed. The placentation should always be stated when first describing a multiple gestation.
- The zygosity (number of fertilized eggs) cannot always be determined by ultrasound. Monozygotic twins can have any placentation type, depending on when the developing zygote splits. Dizygotic twins, however, are always diamniotic/dichorionic, and only dizygotic twins can be different sexes.

  Monozygotic ("identical") twins arise from a single egg fertilized with a single sperm.

  Dizygotic ("fraternal") twins arise from two individually fertilized eggs.
- The chorionicity is the number of placentas.

  Monochorionic twins share a single placenta.

  Dichorionic twins each have a separate placenta.
- Amnionicity is the number of amnions.

  Monoamniotic twins share a single amniotic sac.

  Diamniotic twins each have a separate amniotic sac.
- By convention, chorionicity is stated before the amnionicity when stating the placentation. For instance, the abbreviation mono/di refers to monochorionic/ diamniotic twins.

Overview of complications by placentation type

- The more that the twins share, the greater the risk of complications.
- Di/di twins have an increased risk of premature delivery and low birth weight compared to singleton gestations.
- Mono/di twins have an increased risk of complications related to a shared placenta, including twin–twin transfusion, acardiac twin syndrome, and twin embolization.
- In addition to being at risk for the same complications as mono/di twins, mono/mono twins are also at risk for cord entanglement and being conjoined.

Early counting of multiple gestations

- If two separate gestational sacs are identified, the placentation is di/di. The zygosity is indeterminate.

  Although dizygotic twins are always di/di, early splitting of a single fertilized egg can also lead to di/di monozygotic twins.
- If a single gestational sac contains two yolk sacs, the placentation is mono/di, and the twins are monozygotic.

Dizygotic ("fraternal") twins

- Dizygotic twins result when two eggs are each fertilized by a different sperm.
- Dizygotic twins are always dichorionic/diamniotic.

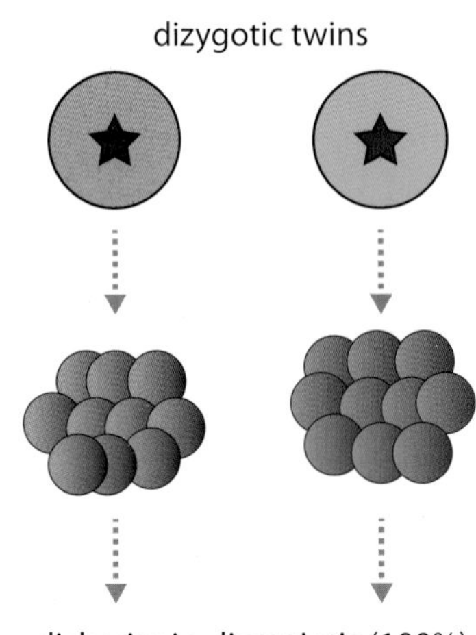

Monozygotic ("identical") twins

monozygotic twins
(single egg fertilized with a single sperm)

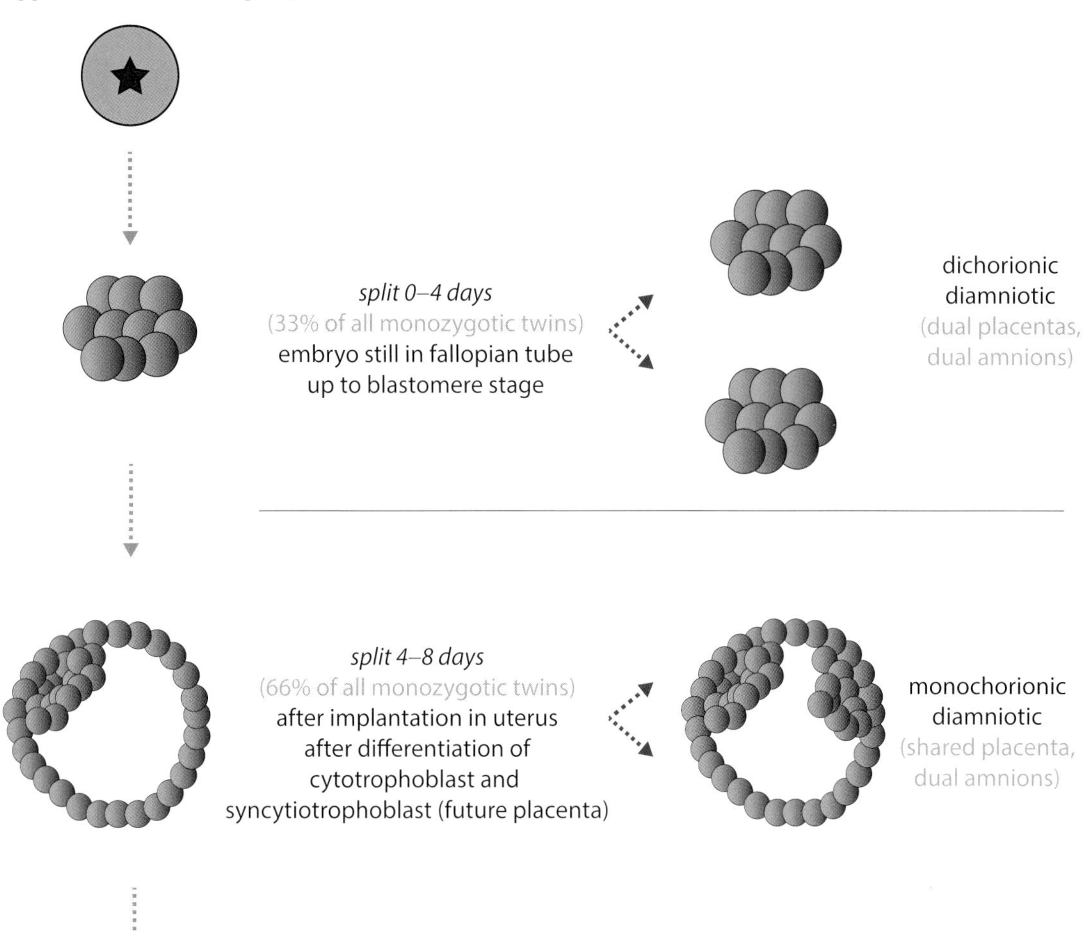

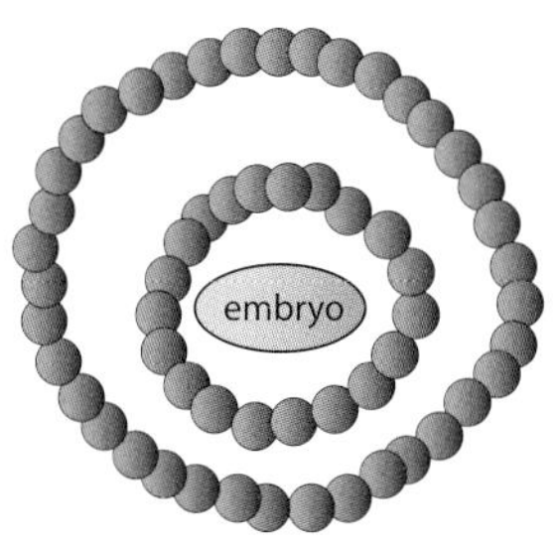

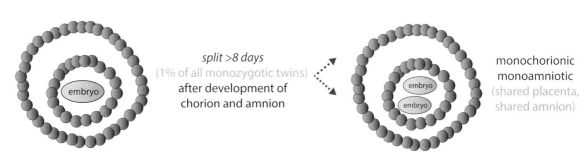

split >8 days
(1% of all monozygotic twins)
after development of
chorion and amnion

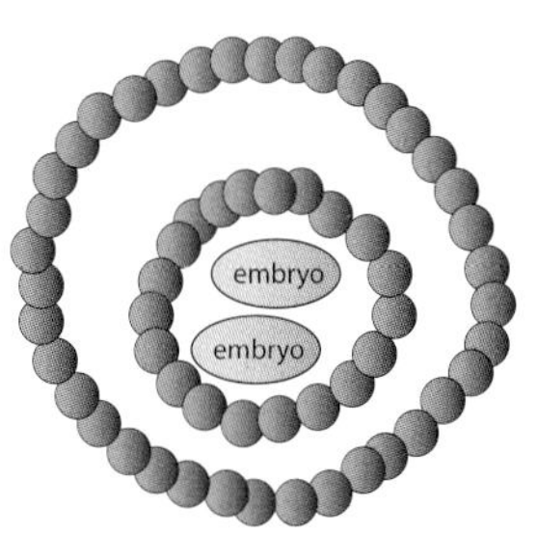

monochorionic
monoamniotic
(shared placenta,
shared amnion)

- Monozygotic twins are the result of splitting of the blastocyst or embryo, formed by fertilization of a single egg by a single sperm. Although "identical" monozygotic twins are always the same sex, they may not be identical phenotypically due to local differences in the uterine and placental environment.
- **33% split early** (0–4 days), before formation of either the placenta or amnion, leading to **dichorionic/diamniotic twins**.
- **66% split intermediate** (4–8 days), after formation of the placenta but before the amnion has developed, leading to **monochorionic/diamniotic twins**.
- **1% split late** (>8 days), after formation of the chorion and amnion, leading to **monochorionic/monoamniotic** twins. Very late splitting may result in conjoined twins, which are always monochorionic/monoamniotic.

Di/di (dichorionic/diamniotic) twins

- Di/di twins each have a separate placenta and amniotic sac.
- On ultrasound, two placentas can usually be separately identified.
- The inter-twin membrane will be relatively thick as there are two layers of chorion and two layers of amnion separating each twin.
- In the second and third trimesters, the thickness of the inter-twin membrane is less reliable to determine chorionicity because the membrane becomes thinner as gestation progresses.
- The *twin peak* sign (also called *lambda* sign) represents a triangle-shaped placental infolding at the interface of the placenta and the thick inter-twin membrane that is seen in di/di twins. The *twin peak* sign is most useful when it is difficult to distinguish two placentas.
- If the twins are different sexes, they must be dizygotic twins, which are always di/di.

Mono/di (monochorionic/diamniotic) twins

- Mono/di twins share a placenta, but have separate amniotic sacs.
- The shared placenta is usually apparent on ultrasound.
- The inter-twin membrane is thin, as it is composed of only two layers of amnion.

Mono/mono (monochorionic/monoamniotic) twins

- Mono/mono twins share both a placenta and a single amniotic sac.
- Mono/mono twins have a shared placenta with no intervening membrane between the twins. Intertwined cords are diagnostic of mono/mono placentation when seen.
- Isolated lack of visualization of an inter-twin membrane is not sufficient to diagnose mono/mono twins. If no inter-twin membrane (or intertwining cord) is seen, then the amnionicity cannot be determined. Because mono/mono twins are so rare, it is more common to have mono/di twins with non-visualization of the inter-twin membrane.

Conjoined twins

- Conjoined twins are caused by late (>13 days) incomplete division of the embryo.

Complications of monochorionic twins

Twin–twin transfusion syndrome (TTTS)

- Twin–twin transfusion syndrome (TTTS) is a complication of monochorionic twins (either mono- or di-amniotic) caused by disproportionate blood flow between the fetuses.
- The *donor* twin transfers excess blood flow to the *recipient* twin. The donor twin is small and has oligohydramnios. The recipient twin is larger and has polyhydramnios.
- There are three criteria to diagnose TTTS by ultrasound:
  1) Disproportionate fetal sizes, with at least 25% discrepancy.
  2) Disproportionate amniotic fluid, with the small twin having oligohydramnios and the large twin having polyhydramnios.
  3) Single shared placenta (monochorionic).
- There is a spectrum of severities of TTTS. In the earliest stages, the donor twin's bladder is still visible and the direction of umbilical artery Doppler flow is normal. Later stages are marked by fetal hydrops or death.
- *A stuck twin* describes severe oligohydramnios in the donor (small) twin. A *stuck* twin has so little amniotic fluid that the amnion is wrapped around the twin like shrink wrap.
- Treatment options of TTTS include laser ablation of placental arteriovenous fistulas, therapeutic amniocentesis from the recipient (large, poly) twin, or selective coagulation of the umbilical cord of the less viable twin.

Acardiac twins

- Acardiac twinning, also called twin reversed arterial perfusion (TRAP) sequence, is a severe variant of twin–twin perfusion syndrome. Similar to TTTS, acardiac twinning is a complication of monochorionic twins (either mono- or di-amniotic).
- In acardiac twins, the donor fetus supplies circulation to itself and an acardiac twin, enabled by placental fistulous connections. The acardiac twin has rudimentary or no development of structures above the thorax.
- Doppler of the umbilical arteries and vein shows reversed flow in the acardiac twin.

  Normally, the umbilical arteries carry deoxygenated blood *out* of the fetus, pumped by the fetal heart. In the acardiac twin, the umbilical arteries carry nutrient-depleted, poorly oxygenated blood *into* the fetus, pumped by the donor twin's heart. Doppler of the acardiac twin's umbilical arteries show an arterial waveform going into the fetus.

  Normally, the umbilical vein carries oxygenated blood *into* the fetus, from the placenta. In the acardiac twin, the umbilical vein carries deoxygenated blood out of the fetus. Doppler of the acardiac twin's umbilical vein shows a venous waveform going out of the fetus.

- Treatment is coagulation of the acardiac twin's umbilical cord.

Twin embolization syndrome

- When one monochorionic twin dies in utero, the surviving twin is at risk for twin embolization syndrome, which can cause CNS, gastrointestinal, or renal infarcts.
- In general, prognosis for a surviving monochorionic twin is very poor when one twin dies in utero. In contrast, prognosis is generally good for a surviving dichorionic twin when one twin dies in utero.

- The first trimester embryo is too small for a complete fetal survey; however, a few key anatomic structures can be identified and evaluated.

Crown–rump length (CRL)

- The crown–rump length (CRL) is used to assign gestational age from 6–12 weeks. Measuring the CRL is straightforward in the first trimester as the fetus cannot flex or extend the neck.

Prosencephalon and rhombencephalon

- By 8 weeks, the forebrain (prosencephalon) can be distinguished from the hindbrain (rhombencephalon). Both prosencephalon and rhombencephalon are hypoechoic, although the rhombencephalon is much more prominent. Absence of these structures may be the earliest finding of anencephaly.

Ventral abdominal wall

- The midgut normally herniates through the ventral abdominal wall in the first trimester. During this herniation, the midgut rotates 270 degrees around the axis of the superior mesenteric artery (SMA).
- Physiologic midgut herniation is usually complete by 12–13 weeks. Therefore, a pathologic ventral wall defect, such as omphalocele or gastroschisis, is generally not diagnosed before 13 weeks.
- It is common to see some fullness at the base of the umbilical cord before 13 weeks, which usually represents physiologic midgut herniation. If the fullness is especially prominent then it may be prudent to bring the patient back for a follow-up at 13 weeks to evaluate for a true ventral wall defect.

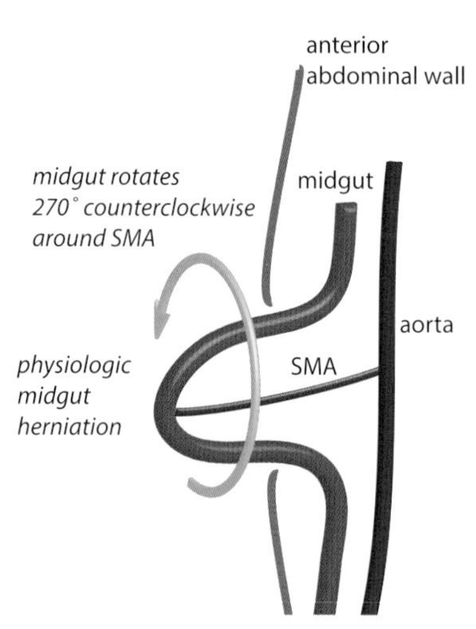

Nuchal translucency

- Increased thickness of the nuchal translucency is associated with increased risk of Down syndrome and other chromosomal abnormalities. With a fixed false-positive rate of 5%, nuchal translucency alone can detect approximately two thirds of cases of trisomy 21.
- The nuchal lucency must be measured properly to obtain an accurate value.

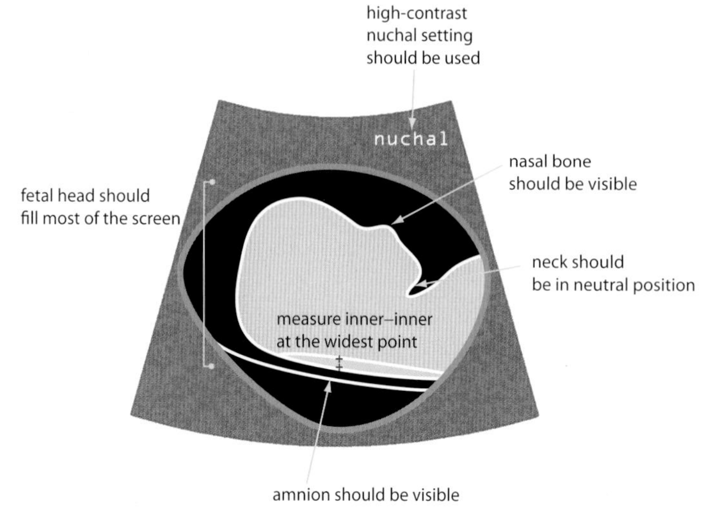

- At 11 weeks, the upper limit of normal is 2.2 mm.
- At 14 weeks (CRL 79 mm), the upper limit of normal is 2.8 mm.
- Nuchal translucency is combined with maternal serum testing to calculate an overall risk of trisomy 21.

SECOND AND THIRD TRIMESTER MEASUREMENTS

Head measurements

- The **biparietal diameter** (BPD) is measured from the outer edge of the skull closest to the transducer to the inner edge of the skull farthest from the transducer.

  The plane of measurement is at the level of the thalami and cavum septum pellucidum. The skull should be completely visualized all the way around.

  The corrected BPD incorporates the occipital frontal diameter (OFD) and a correction factor.

- The **occipital frontal diameter** (OFD) is measured from the middle of the frontal skull to the middle of the occipital skull.

  The measurement plane is the same as that used to measure the BPD, at the level of the thalami and cavum septum pellucidum.

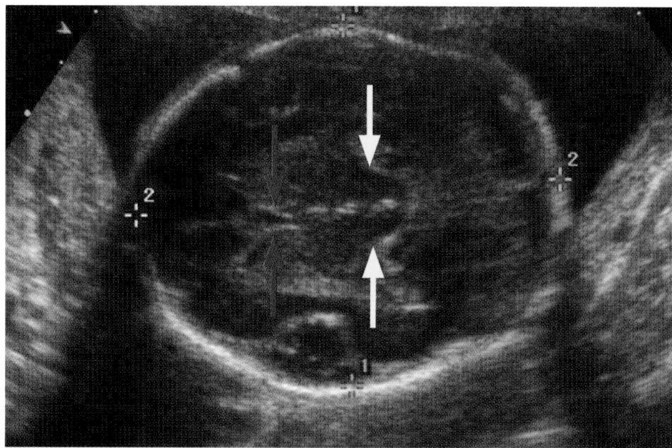

The scanning plane for head measurements is at the level of the thalami (yellow arrows) and cavum septum pellucidum (red arrows).

The BPD (calipers marked 1) is measured from outer edge to inner edge of calvarium.

The OFD (calipers marked 2) is measured from middle to middle edge of calvarium.

Case courtesy Carol Benson, MD, Brigham and Women's Hospital.

Abdomen measurements

- The abdominal diameter is measured from outer skin-to-skin in AP and transverse at the level of the intrahepatic umbilical vein, portal vein, and fetal stomach.
- Ideally, the abdomen should be round, with less than 1 cm difference between the AP and transverse measurements.
- The entire circumference of the skin should be well visualized.
- The best measurements are often obtained if the anterior–posterior axis of the fetal abdomen is angled approximately 45 degrees so that the artifacts from the spine are minimized.

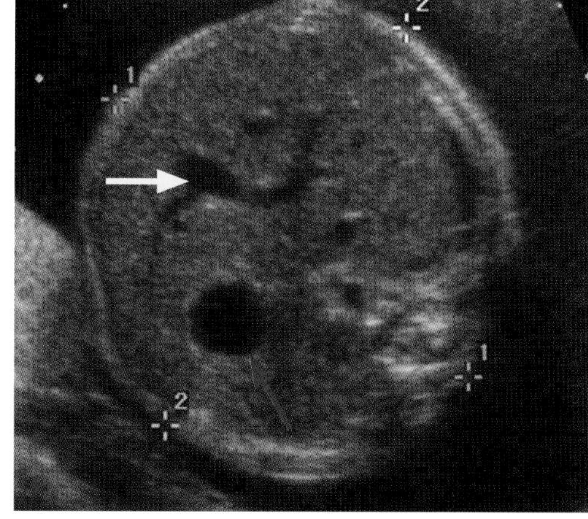

The scanning plane for abdominal diameter is at the junction of the umbilical vein and portal vein (yellow arrow). The stomach (red arrow) should be visualized. Note how the anterior–posterior axis of the abdomen is angled approximately 45 degrees to minimize artifacts from the spine.

Case courtesy Carol Benson, MD, Brigham and Women's Hospital.

Femur length

- The femur length is most accurately measured when the femur is closest to the transducer, perpendicular to the sound beam.

Amniotic fluid index (AFI)

- To quantify the amniotic fluid index (AFI) between 16 and 42 weeks, the largest vertical pocket of fluid is measured (in cm) in each of the four quadrants and summed. AFI varies with gestational age. In borderline cases, the subjective assessment should take precedent. Some references state that an AFI between 7 and 25 is normal, but these cutoffs vary.

  Oligohydramnios: AFI ≤6.3 cm is ≤2.5th percentile. Peaks at 24 weeks: 9.0 cm = 2.5th percentile.

  Polyhydramnios: AFI ≥19.2 cm is ≥97.5th percentile. Peaks at 36 weeks: 27.9 cm = 97.5th percentile.

- The amount of amniotic fluid should always be subjectively assessed.

Nuchal fold (second trimester only)

- A thickened nuchal fold is the most sensitive and specific ultrasound finding to suggest Down syndrome.
- Compared to nuchal lucency, measurement of nuchal fold is performed later in pregnancy. In contrast to the nuchal lucency, the nuchal fold is measured in the axial plane at the level of the posterior fossa.
- The nuchal fold is only measured from 16–20 weeks.

  <5 mm is normal.

  5–5.9 mm is borderline.

  ≥6 mm is a major marker for trisomy 21.

- A very thick nuchal fold may represent a cystic hygroma, which is associated with Turner syndrome (45,X).

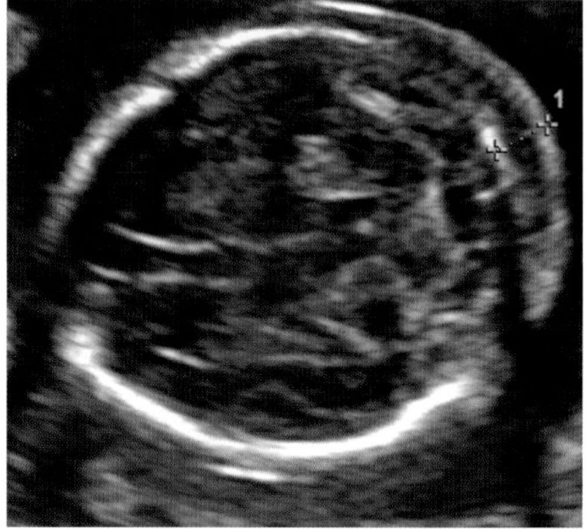

Ultrasound of a 20-week fetus at the level of the brain and posterior fossa demonstrates a thickened nuchal fold >6 mm (calipers).

Case courtesy Beryl Benacerraf, MD, Diagnostic Ultrasound Associates, Boston.

Evaluation of the Cervix in Second and Third Trimesters

Cervical shortening

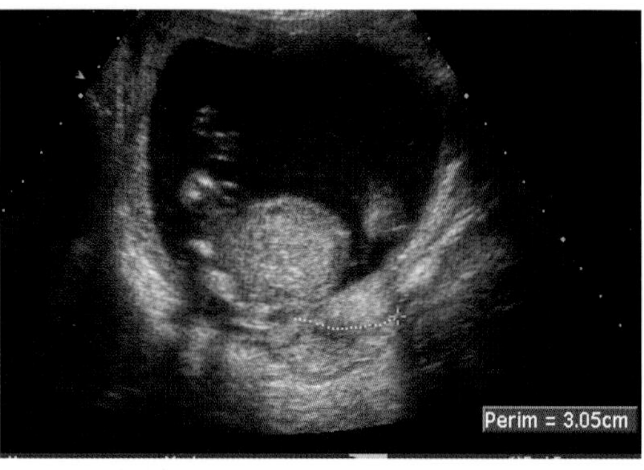

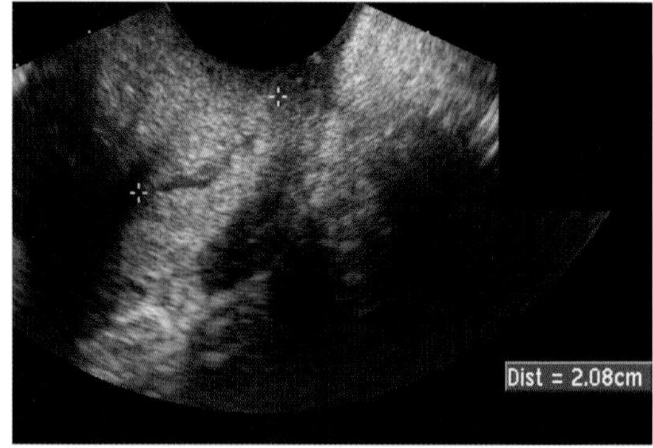

Shortened cervix: Transabdominal grayscale ultrasound (left image) shows a borderline shortened cervix, measuring 3.05 cm. A transvaginal ultrasound more accurately demonstrates the length of the cervix, which is shortened, measuring 2.08 cm in length.

- Shortening of the cervix is a risk factor for pre-term delivery. A cervical length <3 cm is abnormal. The presence of cervical funneling (change in shape) is an ancillary finding.

  The mnemonic ***trust your vaginal ultrasound*** can be used to remember the sequence of cervical funneling. A **T**-shaped cervix is normal. As funneling progresses, the cervix resembles **Y**, **V**, and **U** shapes.

- Prior to viability (24 weeks), treatment is cervical cerclage. After 24 weeks, treatment tends to be conservative (bedrest) due to concern for membrane rupture with any procedure.

Placental embryology and physiology

- The placenta is formed by fetal chorion and maternal endometrium.
- The mature placental circulation allows exchange of oxygen and nutrients between maternal and fetal vessels through a membrane, although the blood does not admix.

Single umbilical artery

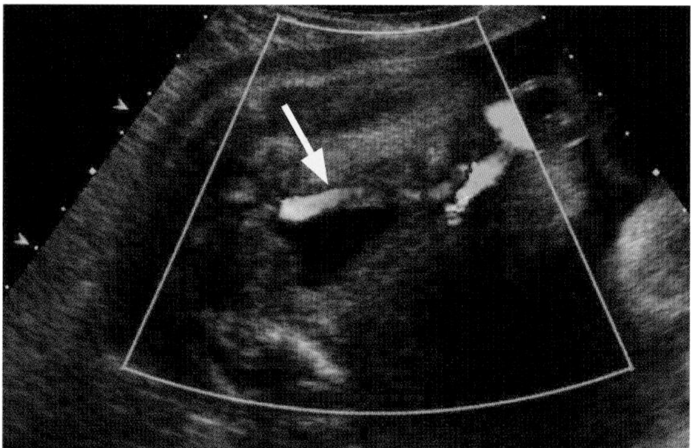

Two vessel cord (single umbilical artery):

Color Doppler through the fetal bladder demonstrates a single umbilical artery (arrow).

Case courtesy Beryl Benacerraf, MD, Diagnostic Ultrasound Associates, Boston.

- The normal umbilical cord has two umbilical arteries and a single umbilical vein. A single umbilical artery is associated with fetal anomalies (most commonly cardiovascular) in up to 50% of fetuses.
- There is an increased incidence of a single umbilical artery in trisomies 13 and 18.

Abnormalities of placental thickness

- Placental thickness is not routinely measured, but in fetal hydrops the placenta may become thickened.
- In polyhydramnios, the placenta usually becomes stretched and thinned. In the presence of polyhydramnios, if the placenta looks normal in thickness, or especially if the placenta looks thickened, concern should be raised for fetal hydrops.

Vasa previa

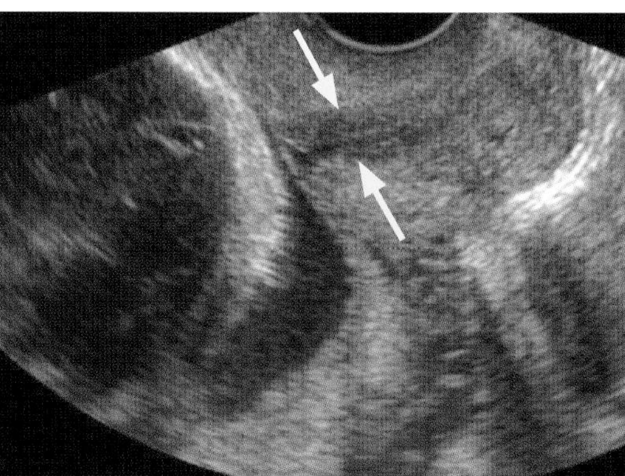

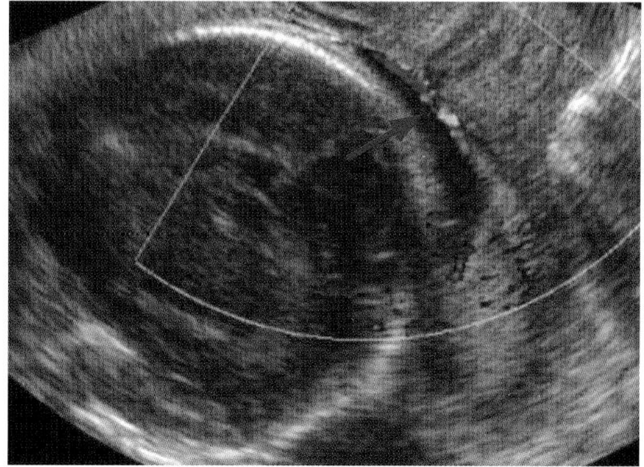

Grayscale ultrasound (left image) in the region of the fetal head and cervix demonstrates the position of the cervix (yellow arrows). Although the grayscale image appeared normal, color Doppler shows a placental vessel (red arrow) traversing the internal cervical os. Spectral Doppler (not shown) confirmed presence of a fetal arterial vessel.

Case courtesy Beryl Benacerraf, MD, Diagnostic Ultrasound Associates, Boston.

- Vasa previa is the traversing of fetal placental vessels across the internal cervical os, which can be caused by velamentous insertion or a placental succenturiate lobe.

  Velamentous insertion is the insertion of the umbilical cord outside the margin of the placenta.

  A **succenturiate lobe** is an island of placental tissue separate from the main placenta, connected to the main placenta by blood vessels.

FETAL HYDROPS

Overview of hydrops

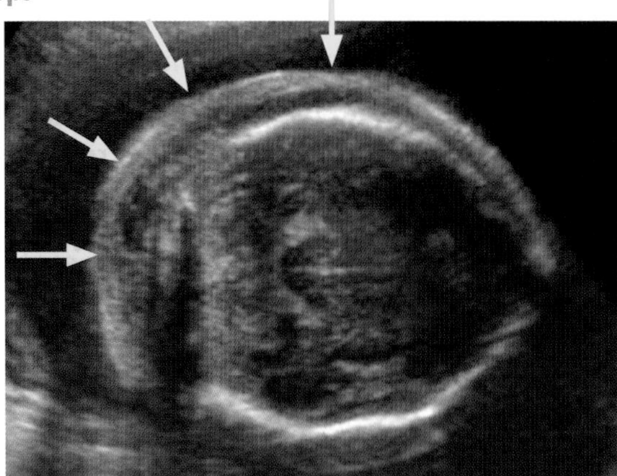

Fetal hydrops:

Transverse ultrasound of a fetal head shows diffuse skin thickening of the scalp (arrows). Polyhydramnios is also present (although incompletely seen on this single image).

Case courtesy Beryl Benacerraf, MD, Diagnostic Ultrasound Associates, Boston.

- Hydrops is a fluid-overload state characterized by at least two of the following: Ascites, pleural or pericardial effusion, skin thickening, polyhydramnios, and placental enlargement.
- Hydrops may be classified as immune or non-immune. Prognosis is variable but tends to be poor for non-immune hydrops.

Immune hydrops

- Immune-mediated hydrops is fetal hemolytic anemia caused by prior maternal exposure to fetal antigens, by far most commonly the Rh antigen.
- Prognosis is good if treated with intrauterine or peripartum fetal blood transfusions.

Non-immune hydrops

- Non-immune hydrops can be due to a diverse array of causes, most of which lead to a common pathway of extracellular fluid overload. Prognosis of non-immune hydrops tends to be poor, as the primary cause is often not effectively treatable.
- Etiologies include (more common causes in bold):

  Primary cardiac abnormalities, including structural abnormalities and arrhythmias.

  Extra-cardiac shunt, including vein of Galen malformation, hepatic hemangioendothelioma, and twin–twin transfusion syndrome, all of which may lead to high-output cardiac failure.

  Infectious, especially parvovirus B19 and TORCH infections.

  Decreased oncotic pressure, due to hepatitis and fetal nephrotic syndrome.

  Increased capillary permeability, which can be due to anoxic injury.

  Venous obstruction, seen in Turner (45,X) syndrome.

Fetal ascites

- When seen with other abnormalities, ascites is one of the criteria for diagnosis of hydrops.
- Isolated fetal ascites may be due to urinary obstruction and resultant calyceal or bladder rupture or meconium peritonitis.

Fetal pleural effusion

- Fetal pleural effusion is a criterion for diagnosis of hydrops.
- When seen in isolation (not a component of hydrops or due to any other abnormality), fetal pleural effusion is mostly commonly caused by congenital chylothorax. Fetal chylothorax is thought to be due to thoracic duct or lymphatic malformation. At birth the pleural fluid is simple, but after the baby begins to drink milk it becomes chylous.
- Fetal pleural effusions can also be seen in Turner or Down syndromes.

AMNIOTIC FLUID

Overview of fetal amniotic fluid

- Amniotic fluid surrounds the fetus and is required for normal development of multiple organ systems, including the lungs.
- The amount of amniotic fluid should routinely be assessed subjectively. It is not necessary to routinely measure the amount of amniotic fluid; however, if a measurement is needed, the amniotic fluid index (AFI) may be used for quantification.
- Amniotic fluid is produced primarily by the fetal genitourinary tract and is excreted by the fetus as urine. A small amount of amniotic fluid is also produced by the fetal lungs and nasopharyngeal cavities.
- Disorders of the fetal genitourinary tract may cause oligohydramnios due to insufficient secretion of fluid.
- Amniotic fluid is absorbed primarily by fetal swallowing.
- Disorders of the gastrointestinal tract or central nervous system may cause polyhydramnios due to impairment of swallowing or absorption of fluid.

Oligohydramnios

- Oligohydramnios is too little amniotic fluid.
- Oligohydramnios may lead to Potter sequence, which describes the typical malformations induced by confinement from oligohydramnios including facial dysmorphism, pulmonary hypoplasia, club feet, and musculoskeletal contractures.
- Most commonly, oligohydramnios is associated with intrauterine growth restriction (IUGR) without a fetal structural anomaly.
- Although malformations are relatively uncommon, the genitourinary system must be carefully evaluated in the setting of oligohydramnios. Several genitourinary anomalies may lead to oligohydramnios, including:

  Renal agenesis – fatal if bilateral.

  Congenital bladder outlet obstruction, including posterior urethral valves.

  Bilateral ureteropelvic junction obstructions.

  Renal dysplasias, including autosomal recessive polycystic kidney disease (ARPKD).

Polyhydramnios

- Polyhydramnios is too much amniotic fluid.
- Greater than half of cases of polyhydramnios are idiopathic, with a normal fetus. The remainder may be associated with chromosomal abnormalities, diabetes, or structural defects (primarily of the gastrointestinal tract), including:

  Primary upper GI obstruction or atresia, such as laryngeal, esophageal or duodenal atresia.

  Secondary obstruction, due to diaphragmatic hernia, gastroschisis, or omphalocele.

  Severe CNS anomalies (which often cause disorders in swallowing).

  Monochorionic twin syndromes, such as twin–twin transfusion syndrome.

  Placental abnormalities, such as chorioangioma. Chorioangioma is a benign placental hemangioma that may cause polyhydramnios when highly vascular.

Ventriculomegaly

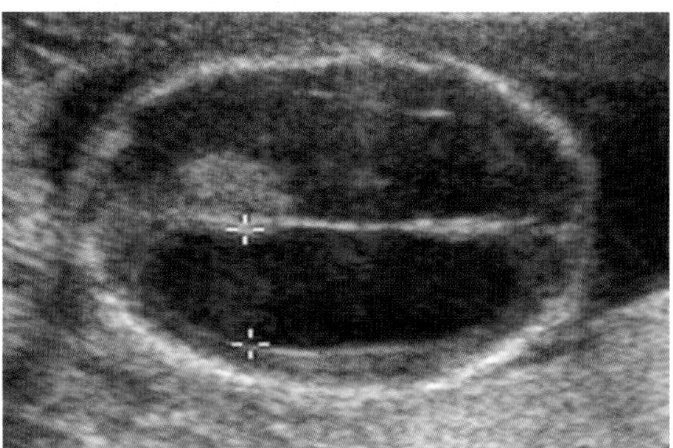

Ventriculomegaly:

Transverse ultrasound of the fetal head shows moderate symmetrical dilation of the lateral ventricles, with the calipers measuring 14 mm. Regardless of the gestational age, the lateral ventricles should always measure <10 mm.

Case courtesy Beryl Benacerraf, MD, Diagnostic Ultrasound Associates, Boston.

- Ventriculomegaly is enlargement of the cerebral ventricles. The term hydrocephalus is usually avoided because that implies ventriculomegaly due to obstruction.
- Throughout gestation, the lateral ventricles should each measure less than 10 mm when measured at the atrium. The atrium is the confluence of the lateral ventricle, temporal horn, and occipital horn. The normal choroid plexus has a rounded border in this location.

  Mild ventriculomegaly: 10–12 mm; moderate: 12–15 mm; marked: >15 mm
- Normally, the choroid plexus fills the lateral ventricle. The *dangling choroid* sign represents the dependent drooping of choroid plexus seen in ventriculomegaly.

  Ventriculomegaly may be present even in a ventricle measuring <10 mm if there is >3 mm of fluid between the medial margin of the ventricle and the choroid.
- Ventriculomegaly is a sign that something else is wrong, with a diverse array of etiologies:

  Primary CNS structural (aqueductal stenosis, Dandy Walker, Chiari II, holoprosencephaly, agenesis of the corpus callosum).

  Genetic (trisomies 13 and 18).

  Destructive (due to infection, hemorrhage, or infarct).

  Idiopathic.

Anencephaly

- Anencephaly is a lethal anomaly with complete lack of development of fetal cerebral cortex and calvarium above the orbits.
- AFP is elevated in anencephaly, as there is direct exposure of neural tissue to the amniotic fluid.
- Anencephaly may cause polyhydramnios due to impairment in swallowing.
- *Angiomatous stroma* is residual neural-type tissue that may be tethered above the head and may be confused with an encephalocele.
- The differential of anencephaly is amniotic band syndrome, which is almost always asymmetric.

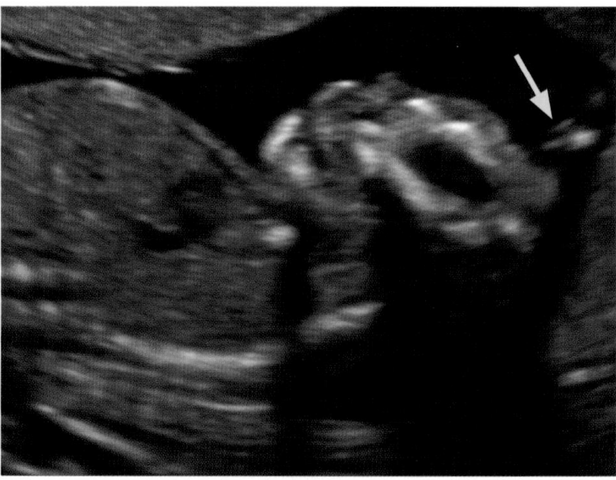

Sagittal paramedian 17-week fetal ultrasound through the head and thorax shows lack of calvarium above the level of the orbits. Echogenic foci superior to the anencephalic head likely represent angiomatous stroma (arrow).

Case courtesy Beryl Benacerraf, MD, Diagnostic Ultrasound Associates, Boston.

Cephalocele

- A cephalocele is a midline neural tube defect characterized by protrusion of intracranial structures outside of the calvarium. The occipital skull is the most common location.
- A meningocele contains only meninges. An encephalocele also contains neural tissue.
- In addition to cephalocele, the primary differential consideration of a mass posterior to the occipital skull is a cystic hygroma, which is a congenital lymphatic malformation and the most common fetal neck mass.

Dandy Walker malformation

- Dandy Walker is a diverse spectrum of diseases characterized by hypogenesis of the cerebellar vermis and resultant fourth ventricular dilation.
- Dandy Walker is associated with agenesis of the corpus callosum.

Chiari II/Myelomeningocele

- Chiari II is the combination of a small posterior fossa and a neural tube defect. By far the most common associated neural tube defect is a lumbar myelomeningocele. A myelomeningocele contains both neural elements and meninges.
- The *banana* sign describes the characteristic flattened cerebellar hemispheres in the small posterior fossa. The banana sign is very specific for Chiari II. In fact, if the banana sign is seen, then a myelomeningocele is presumed to be present even if not identified on ultrasound.
- The *lemon* sign describes flattening of the frontal bones, causing the calvarium to have the morphology of a lemon when seen axially. Unlike the banana sign, the lemon sign is not specific for Chiari II.

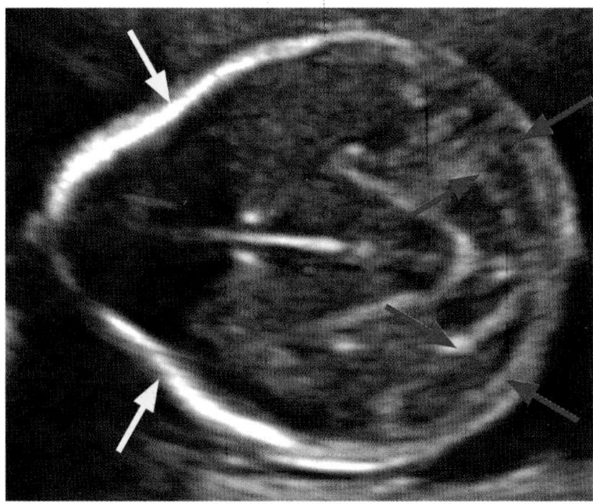

Fetal ultrasound through the brain and posterior fossa demonstrates the *banana* and *lemon* signs. There is flattening of the frontal bones (*lemon* sign, yellow arrows) and flattening of the cerebellar hemispheres (*banana* sign, red arrows). Although the *lemon* sign is nonspecific, the *banana* sign is very specific for Chiari II.

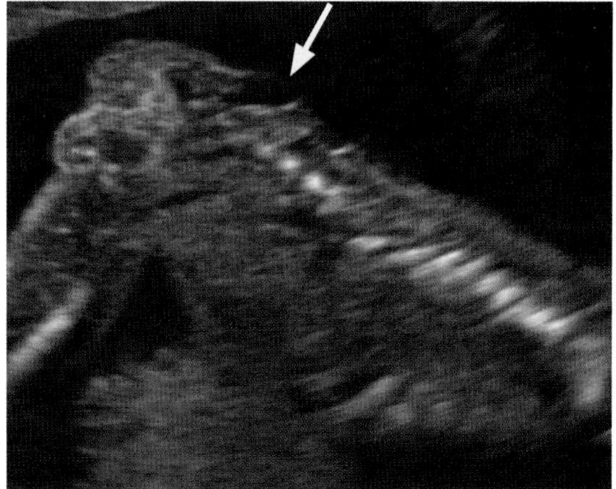

Sagittal ultrasound through the thoracolumbar spine in the same fetus shows a lumbar open neural tube defect (arrow) representing either a meningocele or myelomeningocele.

Case courtesy Beryl Benacerraf, MD, Diagnostic Ultrasound Associates, Boston.

Holoprosencephaly

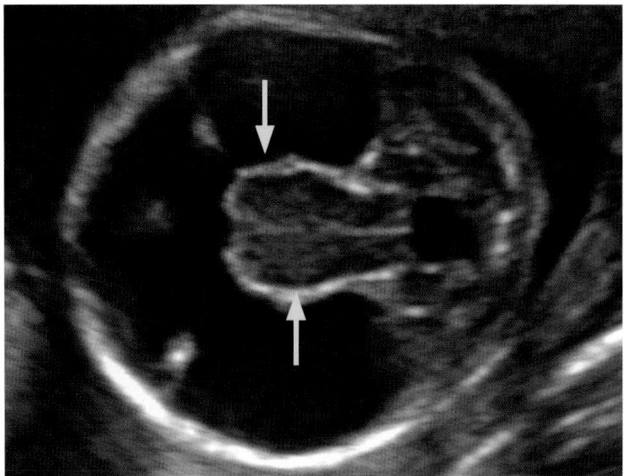

Holoprosencephaly:

Oblique axial/coronal ultrasound through the posterior brain shows fused thalami across the midline (arrows). A large dorsal cyst is present, largely replacing the visualized supratentorial brain. No falx is seen.

Case courtesy Beryl Benacerraf, MD, Diagnostic Ultrasound Associates, Boston.

- Holoprosencephaly is failure of midline cleavage of the primitive prosencephalon in early embryologic development. The most severe form, *alobar* holoprosencephaly, leads to fused thalami and a single monoventricle that may communicate with a large dorsal cyst. Brain tissue surrounds the monoventricle, forming a characteristic *boomerang* shape.
- Holoprosencephaly is associated with trisomy 13, facial hypoplasias, and midline facial anomalies including clefts.

Agenesis of the corpus callosum

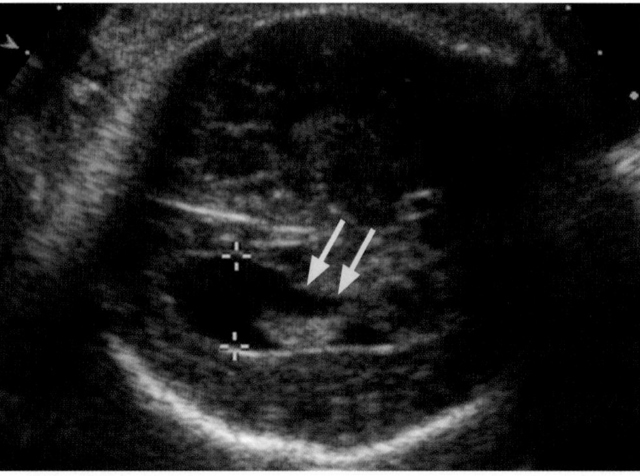

Agenesis of the corpus callosum:

Transverse ultrasound through the fetal head shows ventriculomegaly and a colpocephalic configuration of the lateral ventricle with a dilated teardrop-shaped occipital horn (calipers). There is a concave medial border (arrows) of the lateral ventricle representing protrusion of Probst bundles. The ventricle is oriented parallel to the falx.

Case courtesy Beryl Benacerraf, MD, Diagnostic Ultrasound Associates, Boston.

- Absence of the corpus callosum can be a difficult diagnosis to make. Because the normal corpus callosum is not always visualized on ultrasound, it is often necessary to rely on secondary abnormal morphology of the ventricular system to diagnose absence of the corpus callosum.

> **Absence of the cavum septum pellucidum (CSP)** is associated with agenesis of the corpus callosum.
>
> Abnormal ***teardrop* morphology** of the lateral ventricles with dilated occipital horns, known as *colpocephaly*, is associated with absence of the corpus callosum. Colpocephaly is often seen together with ventriculomegaly.
>
> **Widely separated ventricular frontal horns** and **parallel configuration** of the lateral ventricles both suggest agenesis of the corpus callosum.
>
> The **medial borders of the lateral ventricles may be concave**, due to protrusion of Probst bundles and the cingulate gyrus. Probst bundles are axons that normally constitute the corpus callosum. In agenesis of the corpus callosum, the Probst bundles do not cross the midline. Instead, they pursue an aberrant course parallel to the interhemispheric fissure, indenting the medial margin of the lateral ventricles.
>
> A **midline interhemispheric cyst** may be present, representing superior herniation of the third ventricle.

- A minority of babies with agenesis of the corpus callosum have trisomy 8, 13, or 18.

Absence of the cavum septum pellucidum (CSP)

- The cavum septum pellucidum (CSP) should always be identified in a normal fetus.
- If the CSP is not seen, the primary consideration is agenesis of the corpus callosum, as the cavum septum pellucidum and corpus callosum are formed simultaneously.
- Uncommonly, the CSP may be absent in the presence of a normal corpus callosum. This may represent septo-optic dysplasia and fetal MRI should be recommended.

Hydranencephaly

- Hydranencephaly is complete cortical destruction due to infarct or infection. The brain parenchyma is obliterated and replaced by fluid.
- The most common cause of hydranencephaly is in utero complete occlusion of the MCA.
- In contrast to severe hydrocephalus, a cortical mantle is absent in hydranencephaly.
- In contrast to holoprosencephaly, a falx is typically visualized in hydranencephaly.

Choroid plexus cyst

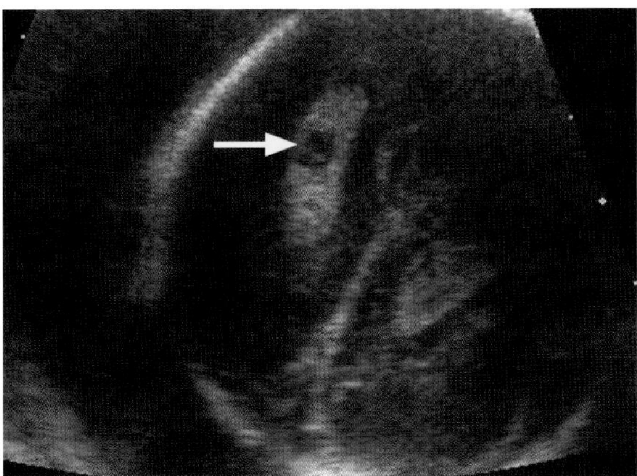

Choroid plexus cyst:

Transverse ultrasound of a fetal head shows a hypoechoic cyst (arrow) located within the echogenic, otherwise normal-appearing choroid.

- Cysts within the choroid plexus are common (seen in 1–5% of fetal surveys). The vast majority of choroid plexus cysts are present in normal fetuses and resolve on follow-up scans. However, up to 50% of trisomy 18 fetuses will have choroid plexus cysts.
- Choroid plexus cysts can be considered an incidental finding in the absence of any other sonographic abnormality and with a normal maternal serum screen.
- A potential mimicker of a choroid plexus cyst is the *spongy choroid*, which describes a heterogeneous echogenic choroid that is a normal variant.

Vein of Galen malformation

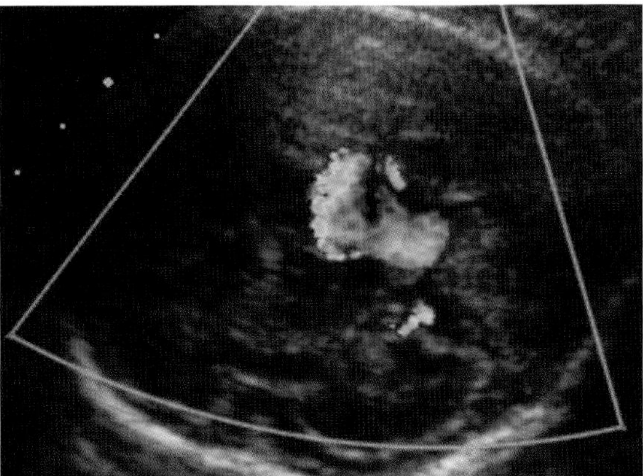

Vein of Galen malformation:

Color Doppler ultrasound of the fetal head shows an enlarged midline vascular structure representing a vein of Galen malformation.

Case courtesy Beryl Benacerraf, MD, Diagnostic Ultrasound Associates, Boston.

- Vein of Galen malformation is dilation of the vein of Galen (in the pineal region) caused by an arteriovenous fistula.
- Vein of Galen aneurysm is a shunt lesion that may cause high-output cardiac failure, leading to hydrops.

Fetal thorax

Evaluation of the fetal thorax

- Abnormal position of the heart in the thorax is an important clue to the possible presence of a thoracic anomaly. Abnormal cardiac position or axis may be secondary to a thoracic mass lesion or pulmonary hypoplasia.

Congenital diaphragmatic hernia (CDH)

- Congenital diaphragmatic hernia (CDH) is herniation of abdominal organs (most commonly bowel) into the thorax through a diaphragmatic defect. CDH is the most common fetal intrathoracic mass lesion.
- Most cases are isolated anomalies; however, a prominent minority of fetuses have other anomalies, most commonly congenital heart disease.
- By far, the most common location for CDH is the left posterior thorax, called a Bochdalek hernia (mnemonic: "back to the left"). A Bochdalek hernia may displace the heart.
- When a CDH occurs on the right it is called a Morgagni hernia. The diaphragmatic defect of a Morgagni hernia tends to be anterior, with the liver the most commonly herniated organ.
- The two classic fetal ultrasound findings of CDH are a cystic intra-thoracic mass representing the stomach and/or bowel, and absence of the stomach bubble below the diaphragm.
- Complications of CHD include pulmonary hypoplasia on the affected side, bowel obstruction with resultant polyhydramnios, and obstruction of venous return due to IVC compression, which may lead to ascites.

Bronchopulmonary foregut malformation

- Bronchopulmonary foregut malformations are a spectrum of congenital abnormalities of the fetal lungs and upper GI tract.
- **Congenital pulmonary airway malformation (CPAM)** is a hamartomatous proliferation of small airways that communicates with the bronchial tree. *Blood supply is from the pulmonary circulation.* CPAM was previously called congenital cystic adenomatoid malformation (CCAM).

  CPAM can be classified into three types based on the size of cysts (Type I – large cysts; Type II – small cysts; Type III – tiny cysts too small to see on ultrasound). Today this classification is not used much because prognosis is dependent on size of the entire lesion rather than the size of the individual cysts.

  CPAM is not associated with other anomalies (unlike CDH).

  CPAM may appear to spontaneously regress on ultrasound, but will remain apparent on CT or MR.
- **Sequestration** is aberrant lung tissue with a *systemic blood supply,* usually from the aorta. The most characteristic location of sequestration is the left lower lobe.

  The classic ultrasound appearance of sequestration is an echogenic mass at the left lung base. The sequestration may occasionally be subdiaphragmatic and simulate an adrenal mass.

  Systemic blood supply should be confirmed with color Doppler. In the absence of the Doppler findings, sequestration may be difficult to differentiate from CPAM. In contrast to the findings of CPAM, cysts are less common, there is less mass effect, and location is almost always in the lower lobes.
- Bronchogenic, gastrointestinal duplication, and neurenteric cysts almost always appear as solitary, simple cysts on ultrasound.

Pulmonary hypoplasia

- Pulmonary hypoplasia is inadequate lung development. Hypoplasia can be due to a thoracic mass lesion (such as CDH), oligohydramnios, or a skeletal dysplasia affecting the ribs.
- It is important to evaluate the size of the fetal thorax in relation to the abdomen on coronal images. A small, *bell-shaped* fetal thorax suggests pulmonary hypoplasia.

Laryngeal or tracheal atresia

- Atresia of the upper airway, otherwise known as congenital high airway obstruction syndrome (CHAOS), is lethal and may cause **bilateral enlarged echogenic lungs**.

Fetal abdomen

- Anomalies of the fetal gastrointestinal tract may cause polyhydramnios due to disruption of swallowing or impaired absorption of swallowed amniotic fluid.

Esophageal atresia

- Esophageal atresia is a blind-ending esophagus, due to incomplete division of the foregut in early embryologic development.
- Esophageal atresia is usually associated with a tracheoesophageal fistula.
- The classic ultrasound findings of esophageal atresia are polyhydramnios and an absent stomach bubble.

Duodenal atresia (DA)

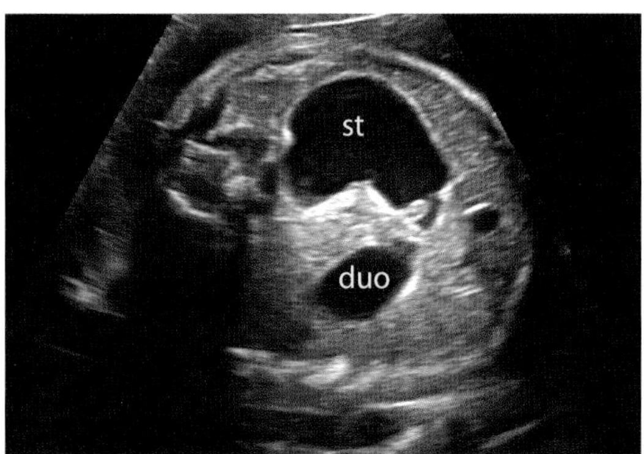

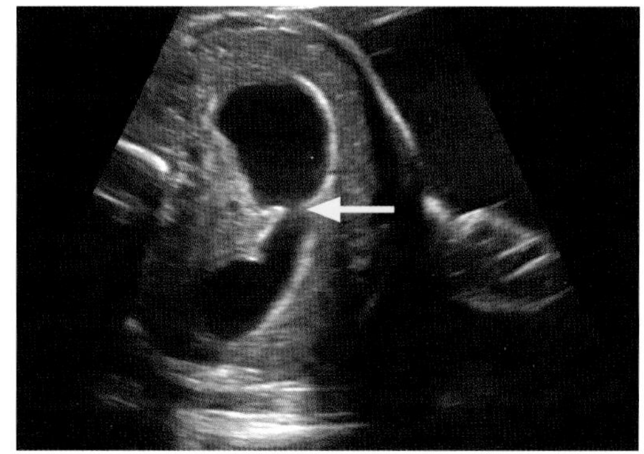

Duodenal atresia: Two transverse images through the fetal abdomen (left image) show the dilated stomach (st) and dilated proximal duodenum (duo) representing the *double bubble* sign. The image on the right confirms that these two dilated structures connect (arrow).

Case courtesy Julie Ritner, MD, Brigham and Women's Hospital.

- Duodenal atresia (DA) causes duodenal obstruction from lack of recanalization of the duodenal lumen. Duodenal atresia is the most common cause of fetal duodenal obstruction.
- Approximately one third of babies with DA will have Down syndrome. If a *double bubble* sign is seen, a careful screen for additional findings of Down syndrome should be performed (e.g., thorough heart exam, nuchal fold if 16–20 weeks, etc.).
- The classic appearance of DA is the *double bubble* sign, representing a dilated stomach and dilated proximal duodenum. The differential diagnosis of the *double bubble* sign includes duodenal web, stenosis, and annular pancreas.

Distal fetal bowel obstruction

- A distal fetal bowel obstruction may be structural or functional.
- Structural causes of distal bowel obstruction include jejunal atresia, ileal atresia, and anorectal malformation.

  Anorectal malformation is commonly associated with additional abnormalities, including the VACTERL association (vertebral, anorectal, cardiac, tracheoesophageal, renal, and limb anomalies).
- Functional bowel obstruction may be due to Hirschsprung disease or meconium ileus.

  Hirschsprung disease results in a functional obstruction due to absent distal enteric ganglion cells.

  Meconium ileus causes obstruction from impaction of meconium in the ileum. Nearly all infants with meconium ileus have cystic fibrosis; however, meconium ileus is rarely identified before the 3rd trimester.

Fetal manifestations of meconium

- **Meconium ileus** is bowel obstruction caused by impacted meconium in a fetus with cystic fibrosis.
- **Meconium peritonitis** is peritoneal inflammation secondary to in utero bowel perforation and resultant spillage of meconium into the peritoneal cavity. This leads to peritoneal adhesions and, ultimately, dystrophic calcifications.
- **Meconium pseudocyst** is a cystic abdominal structure, often with peripheral calcification, representing a walled-off bowel perforation. It is a sequela of meconium peritonitis.

Hyperechoic small bowel

- Hyperechoic or echogenic bowel is a nonspecific finding that is associated with Down syndrome. Other causes of hyperechoic small bowel include TORCH infection, cystic fibrosis, and swallowing of intra-amniotic blood. It may also be associated with intrauterine growth restriction.
- If the bowel is only mildly echogenic (less echogenic than bone) and no mass effect is present, this appearance may represent a normal variant.

Omphalocele

- An omphalocele is a midline anterior abdominal wall defect with resultant herniation of intra-abdominal contents covered by a peritoneal membrane. Omphalocele is the most common anterior abdominal wall defect.
- The key to differentiate omphalocele from gastroschisis (discussed below) is the position of the umbilical cord insertion. In omphalocele, the umbilical cord inserts *centrally* at the base of the herniated sac.
- When small, omphaloceles often contain just bowel. Larger omphaloceles may also contain liver and carry a worse prognosis.
- Omphalocele is associated with other anomalies in 50–75% of cases, including cardiac anomalies, trisomies, and Beckwith–Wiedemann syndrome (a congenital overgrowth syndrome characterized by omphalocele, macroglossia, hemihypertrophy, and visceromegaly).

Gastroschisis

- Gastroschisis is a paraumbilical (usually right-sided) anterior abdominal wall defect, through which bowel herniates without a peritoneal covering. Gastroschisis is the second most common abdominal wall defect.
- Unlike omphalocele, gastroschisis is usually seen as an isolated anomaly.
- Gastroschisis is seen more commonly in very young (teenage) mothers.
- Prognosis is similar to a simple omphalocele (with no other associated abnormalities).

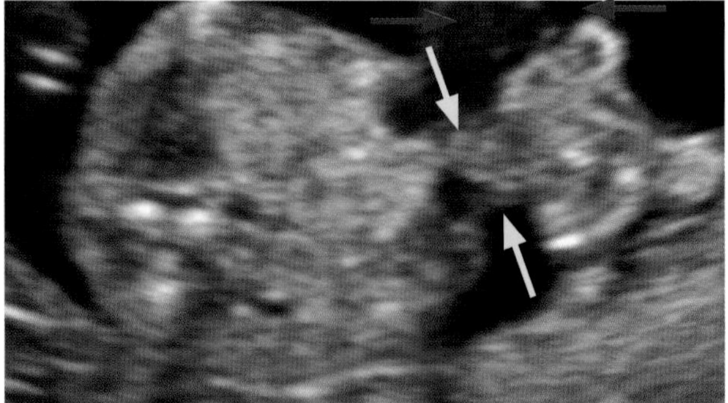

Gastroschisis: Transverse ultrasound through the fetal abdomen shows loops of bowel herniating outside of the anterior abdominal wall (yellow arrows), lateral to the normal midline cord insertion (red arrows). The bowel loops have a lobulated contour because there is no peritoneal covering.

Case courtesy Beryl Benacerraf, MD, Diagnostic Ultrasound Associates, Boston.

Pentalogy of Cantrell

- Pentalogy of Cantrell is a rare disorder consisting of ectopia cordis (extra-thoracic heart), omphalocele, diaphragmatic defect, pericardial defect, and disruption of the sternum.

- Although oligohydramnios may be due to many causes, the complete genitourinary (GU) tract (kidneys, ureters, bladder, and urethra) should be carefully evaluated in every fetus with oligohydramnios.
- Oligohydramnios due to a fetal GU malformation can be divided into three categories:
  - Fetal hydronephrosis (obstructive uropathy).
  - Cystic renal disease.
  - Bilateral renal agenesis.
- If the fetal bladder is not visualized (a bladder not filled with fluid will not be visible on ultrasound) the cause of oligohydramnios is likely a renal anomaly, such as:
  - Bilateral multicystic dysplastic kidneys.
  - Bilateral renal agenesis.
  - Autosomal recessive polycystic kidney disease (ARPKD).
- Normal fetal kidneys grow approximately 1 mm per week of gestation. For instance, a 20 week fetus should have kidneys approximately 2 cm in length.

Fetal hydronephrosis overview

- Screening for fetal hydronephrosis is routinely performed to evaluate for potentially treatable causes, such as obstruction or reflux, which may lead to progressive childhood renal failure if undiagnosed.
- The axial diameter of the renal pelvis is measured to assess for hydronephrosis. The accepted range of normal depends on gestational age. Less than 4 mm is always normal and ≥10 mm is always abnormal.

> **Normal**: <5 mm greater than 20 weeks; <4 mm at 16–20 weeks.
>
> **Equivocal**: 5–9 mm greater than 20 weeks; 4–6 mm at 16–20 weeks.
>
> **Abnormal**: ≥10 mm at 30 weeks; ≥8 mm at 20–30 weeks; ≥6 mm at 16–20 weeks.

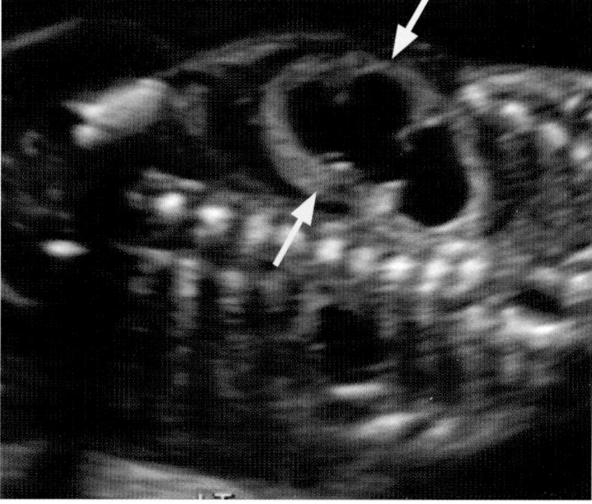

Fetal hydronephrosis: Coronal fetal ultrasound shows bilateral hydronephrosis, severe on the right (arrows). This fetus has trisomy 18, which is associated with hydronephrosis.

Case courtesy Beryl Benacerraf, MD, Diagnostic Ultrasound Associates, Boston.

- Hydronephrosis, hydroureter, and a **normal bladder** may be due to distal ureteral obstruction or reflux.
  - Distal ureteral obstruction from **ectopic insertion of the ureter** into the bladder is often associated with the upper pole moiety of a duplicated collecting system. The most common ectopic insertion of an upper pole moiety is inferior and medial to the normally inserting lower pole ureter.
  - A **ureterocele** is dilation of the intramural portion of the ureter which balloons out into the bladder and causes a functional obstruction at the ureterovesicular junction. Ureterocele is also associated with ectopic insertion of the upper pole moiety of a duplicated system.
  - Although not a physical obstruction, severe **vesicoureteral reflux** may cause hydronephrosis and hydroureter, but the bladder remains normal.
- Bladder outlet obstruction leads to hydronephrosis, hydroureter, and a **dilated bladder**.
  - **Posterior urethral valves** is by far the most common cause of bladder outlet obstruction.
  - **Urethral atresia** is a rare cause of bladder outlet obstruction.
- Hydronephrosis can lead to cystic renal dysplasia, a sign of irreversible renal damage.

Posterior urethral valves

- Posterior urethral valves is congenital obstruction of the posterior urethra due to a membranous flap in the proximal urethra.
- Ultrasound shows severe dilation of the posterior urethra resulting in the *keyhole* sign. The bladder is typically enlarged and thickened. Hydroureteronephrosis and oligohydramnios are usually present.

Autosomal recessive polycystic kidney disease (ARPKD)

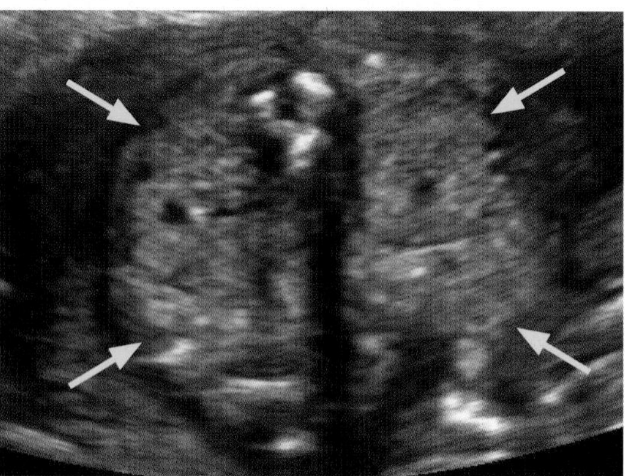

Autosomal recessive polycystic kidney disease:

Transverse ultrasound through the fetal abdomen at the level of the kidneys shows massively enlarged and echogenic kidneys (arrows).

There is complete absence of surrounding amniotic fluid, consistent with severe oligohydramnios.

Case courtesy Beryl Benacerraf, MD, Diagnostic Ultrasound Associates, Boston.

- Autosomal recessive polycystic kidney disease (ARPKD) is a congenital disorder of diffuse collecting tubule dilation, leading to innumerable tiny renal cysts that are too small to be resolved by sonography.
- Ultrasound findings include very large and echogenic kidneys and severe oligohydramnios, caused by markedly reduced renal function.
- Prognosis is poor. ARPKD is associated with hepatic fibrosis if the baby survives infancy.

Multicystic dysplastic kidney (MCDK)

- Multicystic dysplastic kidney (MCDK) is thought to be the end result of fetal obstructive uropathy.
- If MCDK is unilateral and there are no associated abnormalities, the prognosis is excellent. MCDK may be fatal if bilateral, however.
- MCDK may affect only the upper pole of an obstructed duplicated system.
- On imaging, multiple *non-communicating* cysts are interspersed with dysplastic renal parenchyma. In contrast to hydronephrosis, the cysts of MCDK do not connect to the collecting system.
- The natural history of MCDK is gradual involution.

Osteogenesis imperfecta (OI)

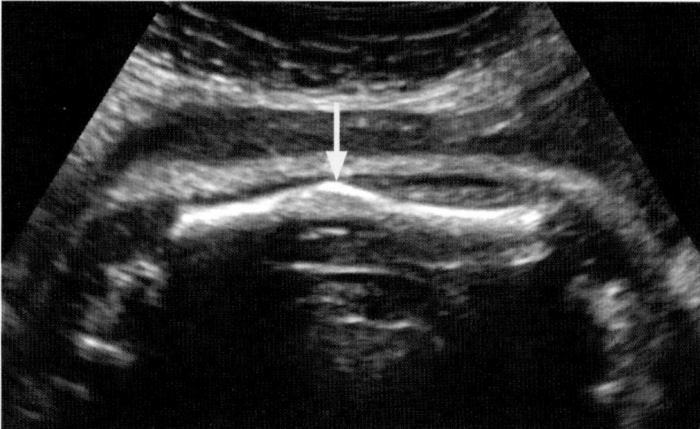

Osteogenesis imperfecta (non-fatal type): Third-trimester fetal survey shows an abnormal kinking (arrow) of the femur from prior in utero fracture.

Case courtesy Julie Ritner, MD, Brigham and Women's Hospital.

- Osteogenesis imperfecta (OI) is a spectrum of congenital bone anomalies characterized by multiple fractures due to abnormal type I collagen. There are several types of OI, with type 2 being lethal. Type 2 can be diagnosed in the second trimester, but types 1, 3, and 4 are not typically diagnosed until the third trimester.
- OI causes severe shortening of the long bones (>3 SD below the mean). The long bones and ribs appear "wrinkled" due to multiple fractures. The thorax is usually small due to broken and structurally soft ribs.
- Unlike thanatophoric dysplasia, bony mineralization is decreased. Decreased calvarial mineralization causes the entire brain (including the nearfield) to be visualized well.

Thanatophoric dysplasia

- Thanatophoric dysplasia is a lethal skeletal dysplasia with characteristic *telephone receiver* femurs, severe limb shortening and bowing, and rib shortening.
- Platyspondyly is characteristic, which is flattening of the ossified portions of the vertebral bodies.
- The classic *cloverleaf skull* is caused by protrusion of the frontal and temporal lobes.
- Bony mineralization is normal.

Sacrococcygeal teratoma

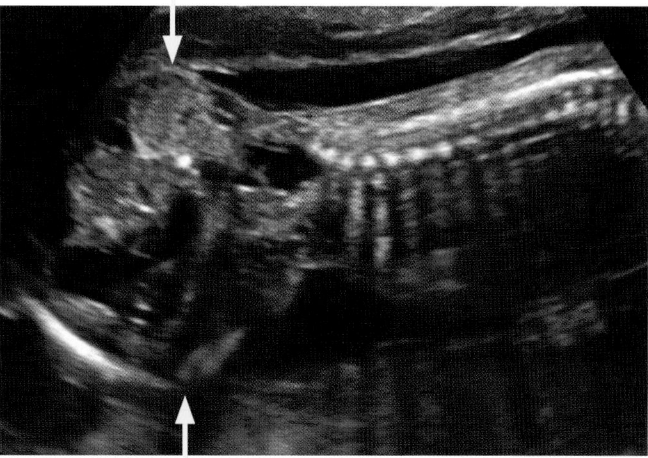

Sacrococcygeal teratoma:

Parasagittal ultrasound of the fetal torso and spine shows a large, heterogeneous, solid and cystic mass (arrows) arising from the sacrum/coccyx.

In contrast to myelomeningocele, the lumbosacral spine demonstrates normal tapering and the overlying skin is intact.

Case courtesy Beryl Benacerraf, MD, Diagnostic Ultrasound Associates, Boston.

- Sacrococcygeal teratoma is a germ cell tumor of the sacrum. It often presents prenatally as a mixed solid and cystic complex mass.
- Sacrococcygeal teratoma may be associated with high output cardiac failure.
- The other primary differential consideration for a distal fetal spinal mass is a myelomeningocele, which is associated with spine abnormalities and a dorsal skin defect.

Trisomies and syndromes

- Fetal anomalies often occur in associations. For instance, omphalocele may be a *sentinel* finding that signifies the presence of trisomy 13, 18, or Beckwith–Wiedemann syndrome. If a sentinel finding is seen, a careful search should be performed for associated anomalies seen in trisomies and syndromes.

Trisomy 13 from head to toe

Trisomy 13

- Holoprosencephaly and midline facial anomalies.
- Encephalocele.
- Congenital heart disease.
- Omphalocele.
- Horseshoe kidney.
- Polycystic kidneys.
- Polydactyly.

Trisomy 18 from head to toe

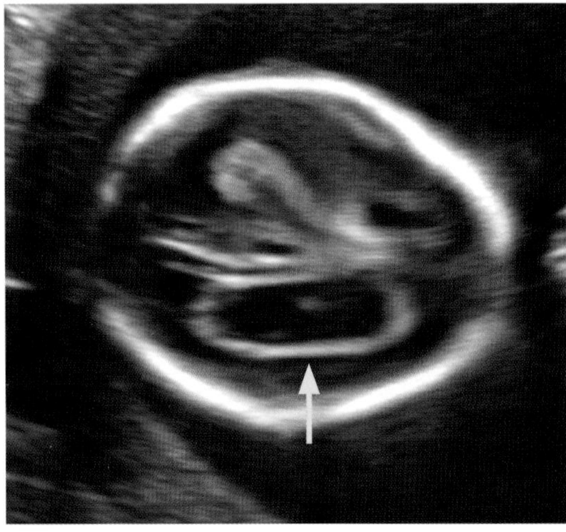

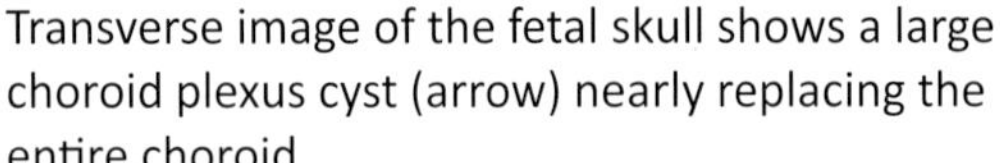

Transverse image of the fetal skull shows a large choroid plexus cyst (arrow) nearly replacing the entire choroid.

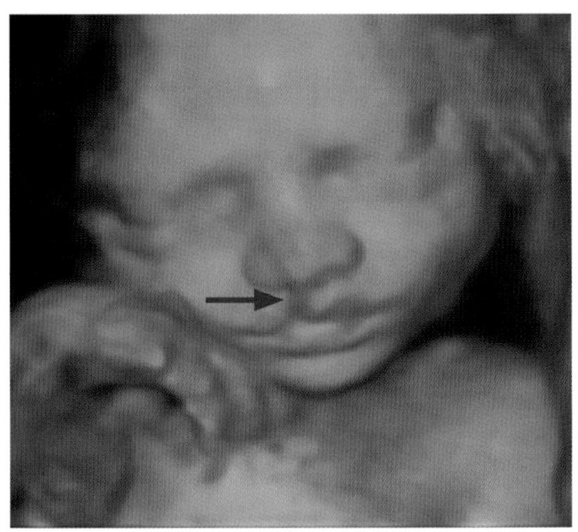

3D ultrasound of the fetal face shows a cleft lip (red arrow).

Trisomy 18: *Case courtesy Beryl Benacerraf, MD, Diagnostic Ultrasound Associates, Boston.*

Trisomy 18

- *Strawberry* sign: Inward bowing of the frontal bones creates a strawberry shape to the calvarium, with the tip of the strawberry projected anteriorly.
- Choroid plexus cysts.
- Facial cleft.
- Micrognathia.
- Cardiac anomalies.
- Omphalocele.
- Congenital diaphragmatic hernia.
- Horseshoe kidney.
- Hydronephrosis.
- Clenched hand that never opens, with overlapping fingers.
- Rocker bottom feet.

Trisomy 21 (Down syndrome) from head to toe

Trisomy 21	• *Increase in* **nuchal fold** *(>6 mm), measured between weeks 15 and 21, is the single most sensitive and specific ultrasound finding for trisomy 21.* • *In contrast,* **nuchal translucency** *is measured earlier in the pregnancy (11–14) weeks, and is less specific for trisomy 21.* • Absent ossification of nasal bone. • Cystic hygroma (although more common in Turner syndrome). • Congenital heart disease: VSD and endocardial cushion defect in particular. • Echogenic bowel. • Duodenal atresia. • Echogenic intracardiac focus. • Shortened femur and humerus. • Hypoplasia of the middle phalanx of the little finger. • Sandal gap toes.

Beckwith–Wiedemann syndrome (BWS)

- Beckwith–Wiedemann syndrome (BWS) is a syndrome of overgrowth that carries an increased risk of childhood cancers. BWS is mostly sporadic, but 10–15% of cases follow an autosomal dominant inheritance.

Beckwith–Wiedemann	• BWS increases the risk of developing Wilms tumor (the most common tumor in BWS), hepatoblastoma, and other childhood tumors. The standard of care is screening with abdominal ultrasound every 3 months until age 8. • Hemihypertrophy, organomegaly. • Macroglossia. • Omphalocele. • Perinatal hypoglycemia.

Meckel–Gruber

- Meckel–Gruber is an autosomal recessive multi-organ syndrome.

Meckel–Grubrer	• Encephalocele. • Renal dysplasia causing multiple tiny renal cysts, which appear as echogenic kidneys, analogous to ARPKD. • Polydactyly.

Neonatal brain imaging

Germinal matrix hemorrhage

- The germinal matrix is the site of neuronal precursor cells located in the caudothalamic groove.
- Grade I: Hemorrhage confined to the germinal matrix.
- Grade II: Hemorrhage extends into the ventricles **without** ventriculomegaly.
- Grade III: Hemorrhage extends into the ventricles **with** ventriculomegaly.
- Grade IV: Hemorrhage extends out of the ventricles into the parenchyma.

References, resources, and further reading

General References:

Middleton, W.D., Kurtz, A.B. & Hertzberg, B.S. Ultrasound: The Requisites (2nd ed.). Mosby. (2003).

Rumack, C.M., Wilson, S.R., Charboneau, J.W. & Levine, D. Diagnostic Ultrasound (4th ed.). Mosby. (2011).

Hepatobiliary and Right Upper Quadrant:

Berk, R., Van der Vegt, J. & Lichtenstein, J. The hyperplastic cholecystoses: cholesterolosis and adenomyomatosis. Radiology, 146(3), 593(1983).

Breda Vriesman, A.C. van. et al. Diffuse gallbladder wall thickening: differential diagnosis. AJR. American Journal of Roentgenology, 188, 495-501(2007).

Chawla, S., Trick, W.E., Gilkey, S. & Attar, B.M. Does Cholecystectomy Status Influence the Common Bile Duct Diameter? A Matched-Pair Analysis. Digestive Diseases and Sciences, 55, 1155-60(2010).

Coss, A. & Enns, R. The investigation of unexplained biliary dilatation. Current Gastroenterology Reports, 11(2), 155-9.

Gallahan, W.C. & Conway, J.D. (2010). Diagnosis and management of gallbladder polyps. Gastroenterology Clinics of North America, 39(2), 359-67, x.

Goyal, N. et al. (2009). Non-invasive evaluation of liver cirrhosis using ultrasound. Clinical Radiology, 64(11), 1056-66(2009).

Hanbidge, A.E. et al. From the RSNA refresher courses: imaging evaluation for acute pain in the right upper quadrant. Radiographics, 24, 1117-35(2004).

McNaughton, D.A. & Abu-Yousef, M.M. Doppler US of the liver made simple. Radiographics, 31, 161-88(2011).

Rosenthal, S.J., Cox, G.G., Wetzel, L.H. & Batnitzky, S. Pitfalls and differential diagnosis in biliary sonography. Radiographics, 10(2), 285-311(1990).

Rybicki, F. The WES Sign. Radiology, 214, 881-2(2000).

Spence, S.C., Teichgraeber, D. & Chandrasekhar, C. Emergent right upper quadrant sonography. Journal of Ultrasound in Medicine, 28, 479-96(2009).

Yarmenitis, S.D. Ultrasound of the gallbladder and the biliary tree. European Radiology, 12(2), 270-82(2002).

Pancreas:

Bruno, C., Minniti, S. & Schenal, G. The Role of Ultrasound in Acute Pancreatitis. In E.J. Balthazar, A.J. Megibow & R.P. Mucelli (Eds.), Imaging of the Pancreas: Acute and Chronic Pancreatitis (pp. 33-47). Springer. (2009).

D'Onofrio, Mirko. The Role of Ultrasound (in Chronic Pancreatitis). In E. Balthazar, A. Megibow & Roberto Pozzi Mucelli (Eds.), Imaging of the Pancreas: Acute and Chronic Pancreatitis (pp. 139-48). Springer. (2009).

Martínez-Noguera, A. & D'Onofrio, M. Ultrasonography of the pancreas. Conventional imaging. Abdominal Imaging, 32(2), 136-49(2007).

Spleen:

Peddu, P., Shah, M. & Sidhu, P.S. Splenic abnormalities: a comparative review of ultrasound, microbubble-enhanced ultrasound and computed tomography. Clinical Radiology, 59(9), 777-92(2004).

Renal:

Mostbeck, G.H., Zontsich, T. & Turetschek, K. Ultrasound of the kidney: obstruction and medical diseases. European Radiology, 11(10), 1878-89(2001).

Paspulati, R.M. & Bhatt, S. Sonography in benign and malignant renal masses. Radiologic Clinics of North America, 44(6), 787-803(2006).

Tublin, M.E., Bude, R.O. & Platt, J.F. The resistive index in renal Doppler sonography: where do we stand? American Journal of Roentgenology, 180(4), 885(2003).

Vourganti, S., Agarwal, P.K., Bodner, D.R. & Dogra, V.S. Ultrasonographic evaluation of renal infections. Radiologic Clinics of North America, 44(6), 763-75(2006).

Scrotum and Testicle:

Cokkinos, D.D., Antypa, E., Tserotas, P., Kratimenou, E., Kyratzi, E., Deligiannis, I. et al. Emergency ultrasound of the scrotum: a review of the commonest pathologic conditions. Current Problems In Diagnostic Radiology, 40(1), 1-14(2011).

Dogra, V., Gottlieb, R., Oka, M. & Rubens, D. Sonography of the scrotum. Radiology, 227, 18-36(2003).

Frates, C., Benson, C.B., Laing, F.C., Disalvo, N. & Doubilet, M. Solic Extratesticular Masses Evaluated with Sonography: pathologic correlation. Radiology, 204, 43-6(1997).

Pearl, M. & Hill, M. Ultrasound of the Scrotum. Seminars in Ultrasound, CT, and MRI, 28(4), 225-48(2007).

Vascular:

Bounameaux, H., Perrier, A. & Righini, M. Diagnosis of venous thromboembolism: an update. Vascular Medicine (London, England), 15(5), 399-406(2010).

Grant, E.G. et al. Carotid artery stenosis: gray-scale and Doppler US diagnosis – Society of Radiologists in Ultrasound Consensus Conference. Radiology, 229(2), 340-6(2003).

Hamper, U.M., DeJong, M.R. & Scoutt, L.M. Ultrasound evaluation of the lower extremity veins. Radiologic Clinics of North America, 45(3), 525-47, ix(2007).

Sidhu, R. & Lockhart, M.E. Imaging of Renovascular Disease. Seminars in Ultrasound, CT, and MRI, 30(4), 271-88(2009).

Spyridopoulos, T.N. et al. Ultrasound as a first line screening tool for the detection of renal artery stenosis: a comprehensive review. Medical Ultrasonography, 12(3), 228(2010).

Thyroid:

Frates, M.C. et al. Management of thyroid nodules detected at US: Society of Radiologists in Ultrasound consensus conference statement. Radiology, 237(3), 794-800(2005).

Female Pelvis:

Goldstein, S.R. Abnormal uterine bleeding: the role of ultrasound. Radiologic Clinics of North America, 44(6), 901-10(2006).

Levine, D. et al. Management of Asymptomatic Ovarian and Other Adnexal Cysts Imaged at US: Society of Radiologists in Ultrasound Consensus Implications for Patient Care. Ultrasound Quarterly, 26, 121-31(2010).

Patel, M.D. Practical approach to the adnexal mass. Radiologic Clinics of North America, 44(6), 879-99(2006).

Potter, A.W. & Chandrasekhar, C. A. US and CT evaluation of acute pelvic pain of gynecologic origin in nonpregnant premenopausal patients. Radiographics, 28(6), 1645-59(2008).

Ectopic and Early Pregnancy:

Bhatt, S., Ghazale, H. & Dogra, V.S. Sonographic evaluation of ectopic pregnancy. Radiologic Clinics of North America, 45(3), 549-60, ix(2007).

Doubilet, P.M. & Benson, C.B. Emergency obstetrical ultrasonography. Seminars in Roentgenology, 33(4), 339-50(1998).

Doubilet, P.M. & Benson, C.B. First, do no harm.. to early pregnancies. Journal of Ultrasound in Medicine, 29(5), 685(2010).

Durfee, S.M., Frates, M.C., Luong, A. & Benson, C.B. The sonographic and color Doppler features of retained products of conception. Journal of Ultrasound in Medicine, 24(9), 1181-6; quiz 1188-9(2005).

Eyvazzadeh, A.D. & Levine, D. Imaging of pelvic pain in the first trimester of pregnancy. Radiologic Clinics of North America, 44(6), 863-77(2006).

Lin, E.P., Bhatt, S. & Dogra, V.S. Diagnostic clues to ectopic pregnancy. Radiographics, 28(6), 1661-71(2008).

Multiple Gestations:

Lewi, L. et al. Monochorionic diamniotic twins: complications and management options. Current Opinion in Obstetrics & Gynecology, 15(2), 177-94(2003).

Shetty, A. & Smith, A.P.M. The sonographic diagnosis of chorionicity. Prenatal Diagnosis, 25(9), 735-9(2005).

Placenta:

Baughman, W.C., Corteville, J.E. & Shah, R.R. Placenta Accreta: Spectrum of US and MR Imaging Findings. Radiographics, 28(7), 1905(2008).

Elsayes, K.M. Imaging of the Placenta: A Multimodality Pictorial Review. Radiographics, 29(5), 1371-91(2009).

Fetal Screening and Anomalies:

Bellini, C. et al. Etiology of nonimmune hydrops fetalis: a systematic review. American Journal of Medical Genetics. Part A, 149A(5), 844-51(2009).

Bethune, M. Time to reconsider our approach to echogenic intracardiac focus and choroid plexus cysts. The Australian & New Zealand Journal of Obstetrics & Gynaecology, 48(2), 137-41(2008).

Biyyam, D., Chapman, T. & Ferguson, M. Congenital Lung Abnormalities: Embryologic Features, Prenatal Diagnosis, and Postnatal Radiologic-Pathologic Correlation1. Radiographics, 98195, 1721-39(2010).

Chen, C.-P. Pathophysiology of increased fetal nuchal translucency thickness. Taiwanese Journal of Obstetrics & Gynecology, 49(2), 133-8(2010).

Chow, J.S., Benson, C.B. & Doubilet, P.M. Frequency and nature of structural anomalies in fetuses with single umbilical arteries. Journal of Ultrasound in Medicine, 17(12), 765-8(1998).

Doubilet, P.M. et al. Choroid plexus cyst and echogenic intracardiac focus in women at low risk for chromosomal anomalies: the obligation to inform the mother. Journal of Ultrasound in Medicine, 23(7), 883-5(2004).

Eik-Nes, S.H. The 18-week fetal examination and detection of anomalies. Prenatal Diagnosis, 30(7), 624-30(2010).

Fong, K.W. et al. Detection of fetal structural abnormalities with US during early pregnancy. Radiographics, 24(1), 157-74(2004).

Goldstein, R.B., & Filly, R.A. Prenatal diagnosis of anencephaly: spectrum of sonographic appearances and distinction from the amniotic band syndrome. AJR. American Journal of Roentgenology, 151(3), 547-50(1988).

Nyberg, D.A., Hyett, J., Johnson, J.-A. & Souter, V. First-trimester screening. Radiologic Clinics of North America, 44(6), 837-61(2006).

Souter, V.L. & Nyberg, D.A. Sonographic screening for fetal aneuploidy: first trimester. Journal of Ultrasound in Medicine, 20(7), 775-90(2001).

7 Nuclear imaging

Contents

PET-CT

Technical considerations

Basic positron emission tomography (PET) physics

- A positron emission tomography (PET) radiotracer emits a positron that travels a small local distance within the tissue. After meeting an electron, both the positron and electron annihilate and create two 511 keV photons travelling nearly 180 degrees apart.
- The two high-energy photons travelling in opposite directions are simultaneously detected by a circular crystal, which can determine that the two photons arrived coincidentally.

Radiotracer: Fluorine-18 FDG

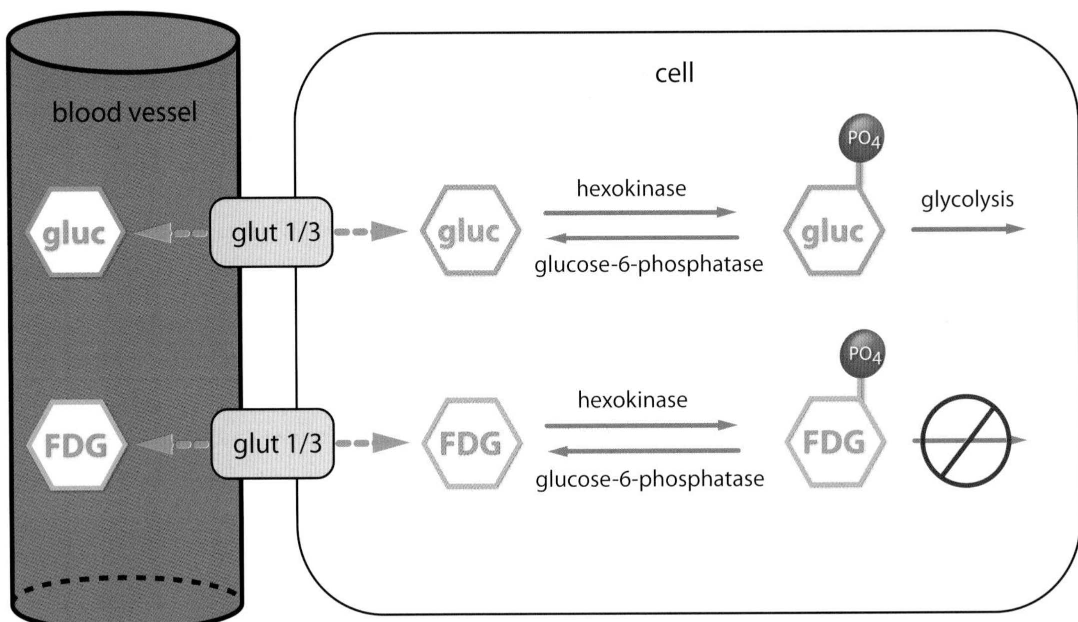

- Fluorine-18 (F-18) is a positron emitter, half-life 110 minutes. F-18-fluorodeoxyglucose (F-18 FDG) is a glucose analog that competes with glucose for transport into cells by the GLUT 1 and 3 transporters. After becoming phosphorylated by hexokinase, FDG-phosphate cannot undergo glycolysis and is effectively trapped in cells.

Radiotracer uptake quantification

- The standardized uptake value (SUV) roughly quantifies FDG uptake.
- SUV is proportional to (ROI activity * body weight) / administered activity.
- SUV of a region of interest can vary significantly depending on numerous factors including specific equipment, time elapsed since FDG administered, amount of tracer extravasation, muscle uptake, glucose and insulin levels at time of injection, etc.
- Malignancy can never be definitively diagnosed or excluded using SUV as the sole criterion.
- A preferred approach to absolute SUV values is to use a ratio of background liver, cerebellum, or basal ganglia to compare with a region of interest.

  For instance, using the basal ganglia uptake as a baseline, relative SUV of a region of interest <20% is "mild"; 20–60% is "moderate"; and >60% is "intense" uptake.

CT correlation

- Most modern PET exams are performed together with a CT as a PET-CT. One important exception is in the pediatric population, where PET may be performed in isolation to reduce the risk of radiation exposure from CT.
- The CT exam is often performed with a lower dose than a diagnostic-quality CT. The CT protocol varies by institution (e.g., whether intravenous contrast is administered).
- The CT is used for anatomic localization and attenuation correction.
- Very dense retained oral contrast (or dense metallic objects such as joint prostheses) may cause artifacts of FDG uptake due to miscalculation of attenuation correction.

Patient preparation

- The uptake of FDG in both normal and pathological tissues is dependent on the serum glucose and insulin levels.
- Elevated insulin levels will cause increased muscle uptake and decreased sensitivity for detecting mildly PET-avid lesions.
- Patients should be NPO for at least four hours to allow insulin to reach a basal level.
- Blood glucose should be below 200 mg/dL, preferably below 150.
- After injection of F-18 FDG, the patient should rest in a quiet room for 60 minutes.

  If the patient talks, the vocal cords may show FDG uptake.

  If the patient walks, the muscles may show FDG uptake.

Normal FDG distribution

- Brain: The brain has intense FDG uptake. Brains love sugar!

  Despite intense uptake, with appropriate windowing, excellent detail of the cortex, basal ganglia, and cerebellum can be seen.
- Kidneys, ureters, and bladder: FDG is concentrated in the urine, with very intense uptake in the renal collecting system, ureters, and bladder.
- Salivary glands, tonsils, thyroid: Mild to moderate symmetric uptake.
- Liver: The liver is moderately FDG avid and typically shows inhomogeneous uptake.
- Bowel: Diffuse mild to moderate uptake is normal. Focal uptake within the bowel, however, should be regarded with suspicion.

  Note that metformin can increase colonic, and to a lesser extent, small bowel FDG uptake.
- Heart: Uptake is totally variable, depending on insulin/glucose levels. The heart prefers fatty acids but will use glucose if available.
- Muscles: FDG uptake is normally low. However, elevated insulin levels or recent exercise can cause increased muscle uptake.
- Brown fat: Brown fat is metabolically active adipose tissue typically found in the supraclavicular region and intercostal spaces that can be mild to moderately FDG avid, especially if the patient is cold.

Lung cancer

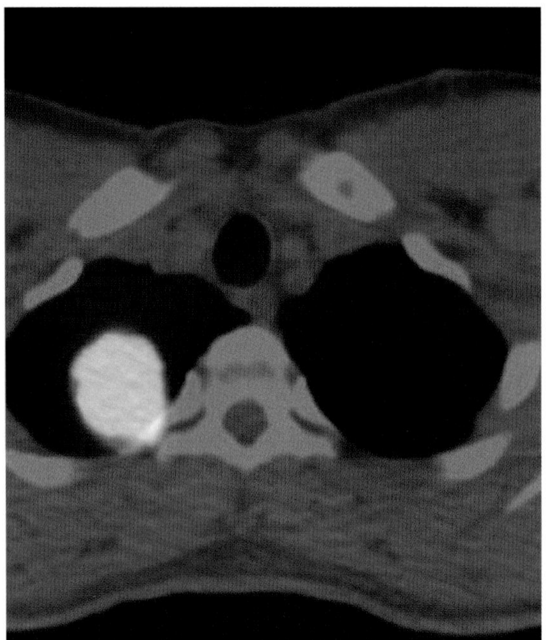

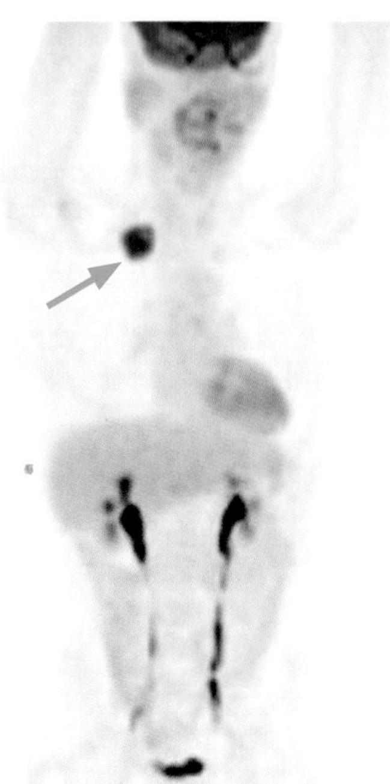

Lung cancer initial staging: Fused axial PET-CT (left image) and coronal PET MIP show an intensely FDG-avid right upper lobe mass (arrow) representing the patient's primary bronchogenic carcinoma. There were no enlarged or FDG avid hilar or mediastinal lymph nodes, and no distant metastases.

- PET-CT plays a role both in the initial staging of patients with lung cancer, and in evaluating response to treatment. Typically, only non small-cell lung cancer is evaluated by PET as small-cell is considered to be metastatic at diagnosis.
- For initial staging, PET-CT is most useful to evaluate local tumor extension and to search for distant metastases. Approximately 10% of patients with a negative metastatic workup by CT will have PET evidence of metastasis.
- PET is very sensitive for detecting malignant lymph nodes; however, it is not specific. A negative PET would allow surgery to proceed without further testing. Mediastinoscopy is the gold standard for lymph node staging. Given the lack of PET specificity, PET-positive mediastinal nodes must be followed by mediastinoscopy before potentially curative surgery is denied based solely on the PET.

Solitary pulmonary nodule (SPN)

- Evaluation of a suspicious solitary pulmonary nodule (SPN) is an indication for PET-CT.
- 8 mm is typically the smallest size nodule that can be reliably evaluated by PET.
- The majority of malignant SPNs are FDG avid. However, low-grade tumors such as bronchioloalveolar cell carcinoma or carcinoid may not be metabolically active and may be falsely negative on PET.
- Conversely, the majority of benign SPNs are not FDG avid. However, active granulomatous disease (including tuberculosis) may take up FDG and represent a false positive on PET.
- It is never possible to definitively diagnose a nodule as benign or malignant based on SUV.
- In general, if a nodule is not FDG avid, short-term follow-up is reasonable. If the nodule is FDG avid then biopsy or resection is preferred.

Colon cancer

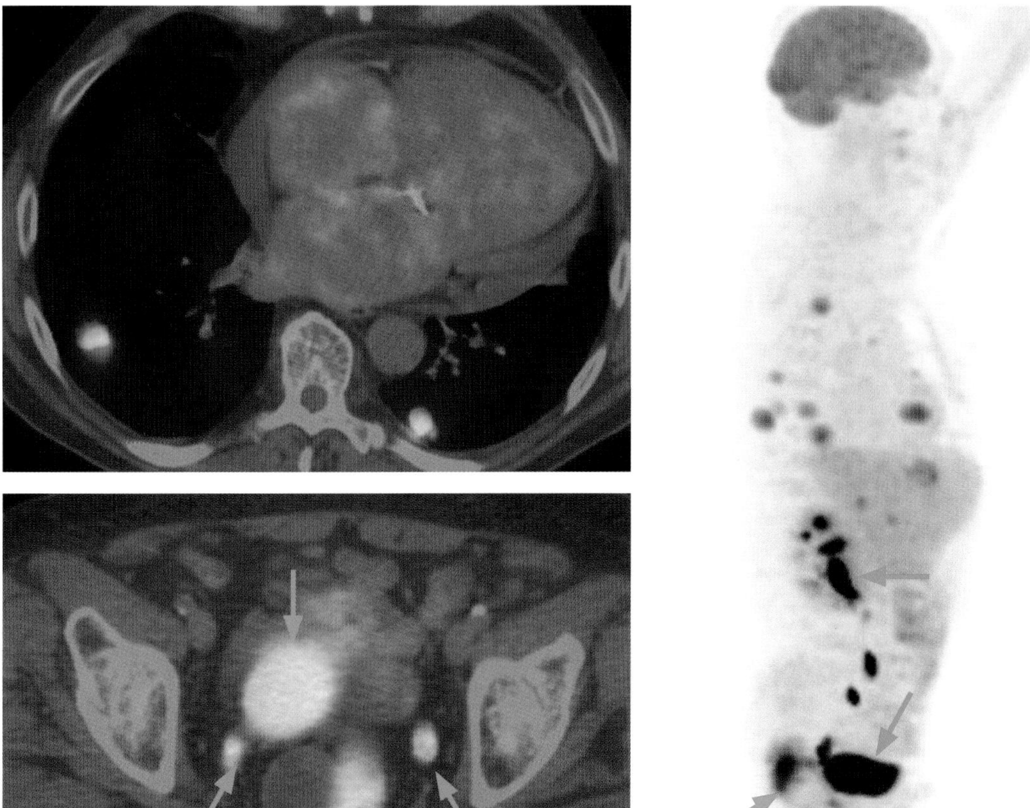

Metastatic rectosigmoid cancer: Fused axial PET-CT through the lungs (top left image), through the pelvis (bottom left image), and a sagittal PET MIP (right image) show the intensely FDG-avid primary rectosigmoid malignancy (blue arrows), with numerous pulmonary metastases. Note the physiologic intense activity in the renal collecting system, bladder and ureters (green arrows).

- PET-CT has a limited role in determining local extent of colon cancer due to poor spatial resolution and physiologic bowel uptake, but PET-CT does play a primary role in evaluating metastatic disease in colorectal malignancies. In particular, since isolated hepatic metastases can be resected or ablated, evaluation for extrahepatic metastases is a common indication for PET-CT.
- After initial treatment, follow-up PET-CT is usually delayed approximately 2 months due to a flare phenomenon of increased FDG uptake in the peritreatment period.

Head and neck cancer

- PET-CT is often used in the initial staging of head and neck squamous cell carcinoma, especially for evaluation of regional nodal metastases.
- Specificity for evaluating recurrent disease after chemoradiation is limited due to altered anatomy and inflammation from treatment. Usually post-treatment scans should be delayed 4 months after treatment to minimize these effects.

Thyroid cancer

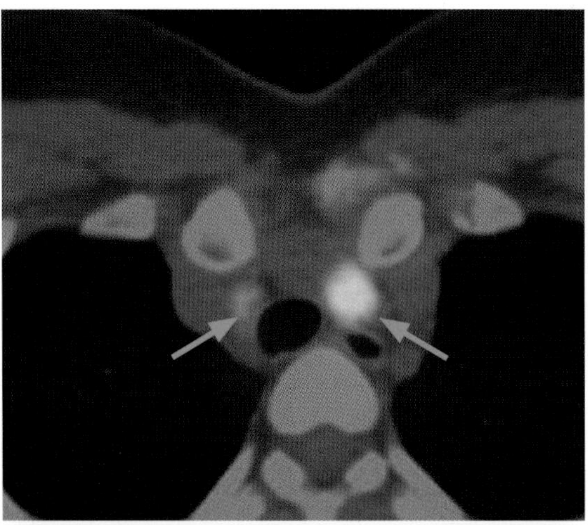

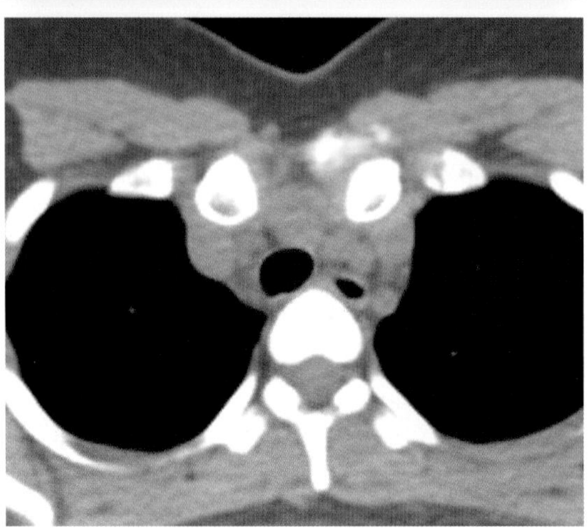

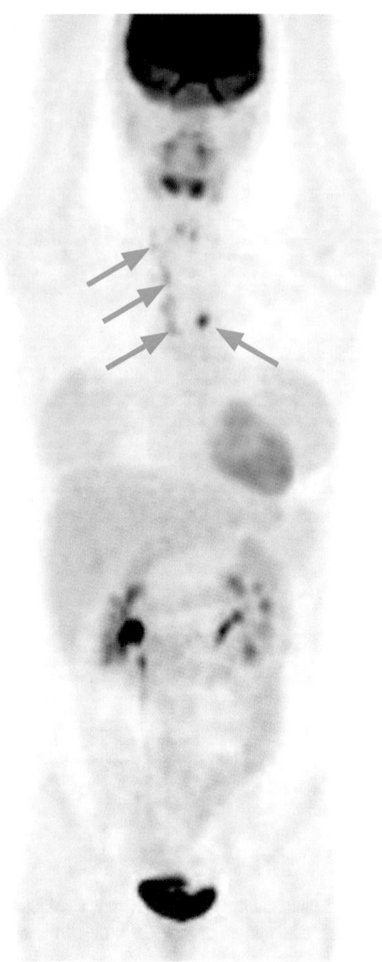

Iodine-resistant thyroid cancer: Fused axial PET-CT (top left image), noncontrast CT (bottom left image), and coronal PET MIP show several moderately FDG-avid right cervical and paratracheal lymph nodes and a single intensely FDG-avid left paratracheal node (arrows). There is symmetric physiologic salivary gland uptake seen on the coronal MIP. The I-131 scan (not shown) was negative.

- Undifferentiated or medullary thyroid cancers may not take up radioiodine but may be FDG avid. PET-CT is used in the clinical setting of a rising thyroglobulin level with negative whole-body radioiodine scans.

Lymphoma

- PET-CT plays a key role in the staging and restaging of patients with lymphoma.
- Most histological types of lymphoma, including Hodgkin and non-Hodgkin lymphoma, are FDG avid. Some low-grade lymphomas, such as small lymphocytic and mantle cell, tend to be less FDG avid, however.
- Increased marrow uptake in lymphoma patients can be difficult to interpret. Diffuse marrow uptake may be due to granulocyte colony-stimulating factor(G-CSF) stimulation, rebound effect from chemotherapy, or malignant marrow infiltration. Focal increased uptake, however, is more likely to represent lymphoma.

Breast cancer

- Although used in the staging and response to therapy of recurrent or stage IV breast cancer, PET-CT is not routinely used for patients with stage I–III breast cancer.

Esophageal cancer

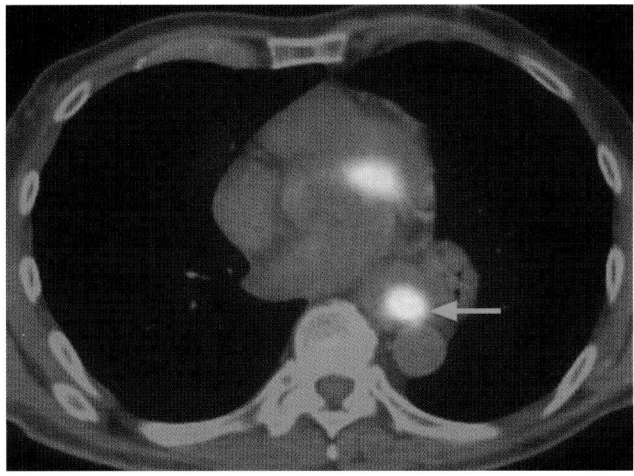

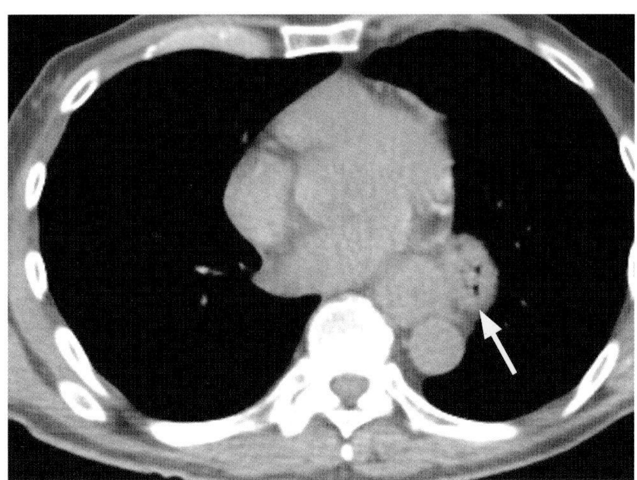

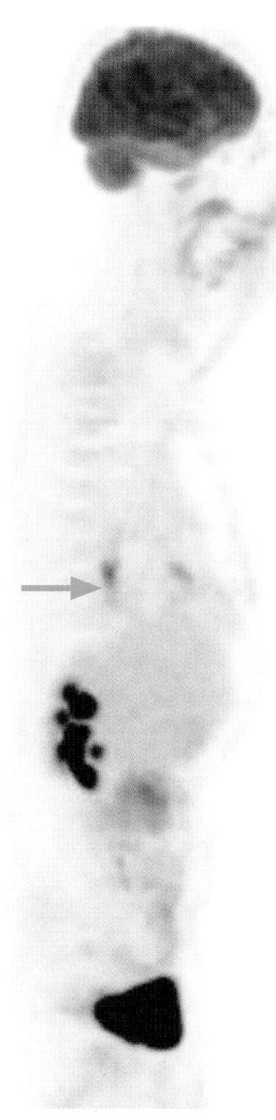

Non-metastatic esophageal cancer: Fused axial PET-CT (top left image) and sagittal PET MIP (right image) show a single focus of intense FDG uptake within the distal esophagus (arrows). Marked esophageal thickening is also apparent on the non-contrast CT (bottom left image). Note the presence of a small paraesophageal hernia (yellow arrow). There is no evidence of metastatic disease. The focus of FDG uptake within the heart on the fused image is physiologic myocardial uptake.

- The primary role of PET-CT in the initial evaluation of patients with esophageal cancer is to identify those with stage IV disease who are not surgical candidates.
- After initial neoadjuvant treatment, a decrease in FDG avidity by at least 30% suggests a more favorable prognosis. In contrast, those patients who do not show a decrease in SUV values can potentially be spared ineffective chemotherapy regimens.

Cancers where PET-CT plays a limited role

Hepatocellular carcinoma (HCC)

- Only 50% of hepatocellular carcinoma (HCC) can be imaged with FDG PET due to high levels of phosphatase, which dephosphorylates FDG and allows it to diffuse out of cells.

Renal cell carcinoma (RCC) and bladder cancer

- Only 50% of renal cell carcinomas are FDG avid, although PET may play a role in detecting metastatic disease.
- Detection of ureteral or bladder lesions is extremely limited due to surrounding high urine FDG uptake.

Prostate cancer

- FDG PET is not used for evaluation of prostate cancer. Recently, carbon-11 choline PET has been FDA approved for imaging prostate cancer, but it is not yet in widespread use.

NUCLEAR CARDIOLOGY

CLINICAL OVERVIEW

Perfusion imaging overview

- Left ventricular perfusion imaging evaluates the blood flow to the myocardium.
- If a perfusion abnormality is present, the following five questions help to characterize the perfusion abnormality:

> **Is the perfusion abnormality reversible** during rest, or is the defect **fixed** at both stress and rest?
>
> **How large is it**: Small, medium, or large?
>
> **How severe is it**: Mild (subendocardial), moderate, or severe (transmural)?
>
> **Where is it**: In which coronary artery territory?
>
> **Are there any associated abnormalities**, such as right ventricular uptake, ischemic dilation, or wall motion abnormalities?

- Each perfusion test has two components: An element of *stress,* and a method of *imaging.*
- The stress component can be physical (treadmill), pharmacologic-adrenergic (dobutamine), or pharmacologic-vasodilatory (dipyridamole or adenosine).
- All perfusion imaging commonly performed uses radionuclides with SPECT imaging. Some protocols include gated SPECT (GSPECT) as well.

  Other types of stress tests performed by cardiologists (EKG stress tests and echocardiographic stress tests) can be performed in lieu of imaging. These non-imaging tests can only detect secondary signs of perfusion abnormalities, such as ischemic EKG changes or wall motion abnormalities.

Clinical applications of myocardial perfusion imaging

- There are several clinical indications for myocardial perfusion imaging.
- **Evaluation of acute chest pain.** Myocardial perfusion imaging is often the gatekeeper to further cardiac workup in patients where there is clinical ambiguity for cardiac ischemia (e.g. chest pain with negative EKG and troponins). A negative myocardial perfusion exam allows safe discharge.

  A normal myocardial perfusion exam is associated with an annual rate of a cardiac event of 0.6%, even among patients with a high pretest likelihood of coronary artery disease.
- **Evaluation of hemodynamic significance of coronary stenosis.** Even with a coronary artery stenosis seen on angiography or CT, patients with a normal nuclear cardiac perfusion exam have a relatively low risk for cardiac events.
- **Risk stratification after MI.** Findings that would classify a patient as high risk include:

> Significant peri-infarct ischemia.
>
> Defect in a different vascular territory (suggesting multi-vessel disease).
>
> Significant lung uptake, suggesting left ventricular dysfunction.
>
> Left ventricular aneurysm.
>
> Low ejection fraction (less than 40% seen) on GSPECT.
>
> Ejection fraction (EF) is calculated as EF = (EDC – ESC)/(EDC – BC)
>
> EDC = end diastolic counts; ESC = end systolic counts; BC = background counts

- **Preoperative risk assessment for noncardiac surgery.**
- **Evaluation of viability prior to revascularization therapy (subsequently discussed).**
- **Evaluation of myocardial revascularization status post CABG.**

Viability imaging overview

- Prior to a revascularization procedure (e.g., CABG or coronary angioplasty/stenting), it is important to know if the hypoperfused myocardium is viable, as the revascularization of scar tissue would not provide a clinical benefit. Hypoperfused myocardium that is viable is known as *hibernating* myocardium.
- Viability imaging can be performed with rest–redistribution thallium-201 perfusion imaging or F-18 FDG PET. F-18 FDG PET is the gold standard for evaluation of myocardial viability, although unlike thallium *FDG-PET does not evaluate perfusion.*
- Static SPECT images from a pure perfusion exam (such as Tc-99m sestamibi, rubidium-82 PET, or N-13 ammonia PET discussed below) cannot distinguish between hibernating myocardium or scar. Both of these entities appear as a fixed (present on both stress and rest images) myocardial perfusion defect.

  Evaluation of gated SPECT (GSPECT) functional data can suggest either hibernating myocardium or scar. Normal or nearly normal wall motion and wall thickening in the area of the perfusion defect suggests viability (hibernating myocardium), while a large defect with abnormal wall motion suggests scar.
- If the region of the perfusion defect takes up FDG (a "mismatch" between FDG PET and perfusion imaging), that region of myocardium is viable and may benefit from an intervention (either CABG or percutaneous intervention).
- In contrast, an FDG PET "match" of a photopenic region corresponding to the perfusion defect is consistent with non-viable scar, and the best treatment is medical therapy only.

Radionuclides used in nuclear cardiology

Thallium-201

- Thallium-201 is a cyclotron-produced radionuclide with a half-life of 73 hours. It decays by electron capture and emits characteristic X-rays of 69–81 keV.

  Relatively low energy characteristic X-rays increase attenuation artifact from chest wall soft tissues.

  It is necessary to administer fairly low doses due to its long half-life, with resultant lower count densities.
- Physiologically, thallium acts like a potassium analog, crossing into the cell via active transport through the ATP-dependent sodium–potassium transmembrane pump.
- Myocardial uptake is directly proportional to myocardial perfusion.
- A 50% stenosis will generally produce a perfusion defect upon maximal exercise.
- Thallium undergoes **redistribution** with simultaneous cellular washout and re-extraction of blood-pool radiotracer. Since ischemic myocardium progressively extracts thallium but washes out more slowly than normal myocardium, post-redistribution images will therefore show normalization of defects in ischemic but viable myocardium. In contrast, a scar will show a persistent defect.

Technetium-99m sestamibi (Cardiolite)

- Unlike thallium, Tc-99m sestamibi **does not undergo redistribution** and remains fixed in the myocardium.
- Sestamibi enters myocardium via passive diffusion and binds to mitochondrial membrane proteins. Similar to thallium, myocardial uptake of sestamibi is proportional to myocardial perfusion.

Rubidium-82

- Rubidium-82 is a positron-emitting PET *perfusion* agent that is generated from strontium-82. A very short half-life of 76 seconds allows high doses to be administered, although such a short half-life precludes the use of exercise stress. Pharmacologic stress is used instead.
- Rubidium-82 acts as a potassium analog, similar to thallium.

Nitrogen-13 ammonia

- Nitrogen-13 ammonia is a positron-emitting PET *perfusion* agent (like rubidium-82) that has a half-life of 10 minutes. Unlike rubidium-82, N-13 is cyclotron-produced and the cyclotron must be on-site due to its short half-life.
- N-13 has excellent imaging characteristics. N-13 positrons have a low kinetic energy and don't travel very far in the tissue before annihilating, which allows relatively high resolution. The short half-life also allows large doses to be given for high counts.
- Like rubidium-82, a relatively short half-life makes use with exercise stress logistically challenging, and N-13 perfusion is almost always coupled with a pharmacologic stress.

F-18 FDG

- F-18 FDG, the same radiotracer used for oncologic imaging, is a positron emitting PET *viability* agent with a half-life of 110 minutes. Unlike rubidium-82 and N-13 ammonia, FDG cannot be used for perfusion.
- F-18 FDG PET images are correlated with a sestamibi perfusion study to evaluate viability. A defect on sestamibi rest perfusion with discordant FDG uptake represents viable *hibernating* myocardium that could potentially be revascularized. In contrast, a sestamibi perfusion defect correlating to lack of F-18 FDG uptake is a scar.

Types of stress – exercise and pharmacologic

- A cardiac perfusion study has two components – *stress* and *imaging.* The stress can be physical or pharmacologic.

General exercise protocol

- Prior to undergoing a myocardial perfusion study, the patient should be NPO for 6 hours to decrease splanchnic blood flow and therefore reduce liver and bowel uptake. Calcium channel blockers and β-blockers should be held to allow patient to reach target heart rate.
- Exercise is performed with a multistage treadmill (Bruce or modified Bruce) protocol. The target heart rate, which is calculated as 85% of maximal heart rate, must be achieved for the study to be diagnostic. The maximal calculated heart rate is 220 bpm – age.

Dipyridamole stress – pharmacologic vasodilator

- Dipyridamole is an adenosine deaminase inhibitor that allows endogenous adenosine to accumulate. Adenosine is a potent vasodilator, increasing coronary blood flow by 3–5 times.
- A critical coronary artery stenosis cannot further dilate in response to adenosine. That coronary artery territory will appear as a relative perfusion defect on stress imaging.
- Unlike a physical stress, a dipyridamole stress does not increase cardiac work or O_2 demand.
- Caffeine and theophylline reverse the effects of dipyridamole and must be held for 24 hours.
- The antidote is aminophylline (100–200 mg), which has a shorter half-life than dipyridamole, so the patient must be continuously monitored.

Adenosine stress – pharmacologic vasodilator

- Adenosine has identical physiologic effects to dipyridamole but a more rapid effect.
- Adenosine half-life is approximately 30 seconds and thus does not require a reversal agent.

Regadenoson – pharmacologic vasodilator

- Regadenoson is an adenosine receptor agonist with a 2–3-minute half-life. It is easier to administer than adenosine with a convenient universal-dose intravenous injection.

Dobutamine stress – pharmacologic stress

- Dobutamine is a β_1 agonist that increases myocardial oxygen demand. Dobutamine is usually reserved for when adenosine is contraindicated (severe asthma, COPD, or recent caffeine).

IMAGING PROTOCOLS

Single-day Tc-99m sestamibi perfusion study

- A single-day Tc-99m sestamibi perfusion study is the most common myocardial perfusion exam performed. Rest images are first obtained after 8–10 mCi Tc-99m sestamibi. Stress images are obtained after an additional 20–30 mCi Tc-99m sestamibi is administered during peak exercise, or after administration of pharmacologic stress.
- Imaging is performed approximately 30 minutes after injection, to allow liver activity to clear. Because there is no redistribution, imaging can be delayed after tracer administration.
- Gated SPECT images show wall motion at time of imaging, while perfusion images show perfusion *at time of injection.*

PET perfusion

- PET rest–stress myocardial perfusion has greater sensitivity, specificity, and accuracy for diagnosis of coronary artery disease compared to SPECT imaging.
- Attenuation-correction CT improves diagnostic accuracy by eliminating attenuation artifact.
- Rubidium-82 and N-13 ammonia are perfusion agents and are imaged on a PET system using coincidence detection. The shorter half-life of these tracers allows higher activities to be administered with lower overall radiation exposure. For quantification of myocardial blood flow, N-13 ammonia is preferred as rubidium has a lower extraction fraction.

Exercise thallium

- Because thallium undergoes redistribution, imaging is performed immediately post-exercise and approximately 3–4 hours later once redistribution has occurred. Thallium is uncommonly used because of the long 73 hour half-life and resultant high patient dose.

IMAGE INTERPRETATION

Key to successful image interpretation is a systematic approach:

- Quality control: Is it a good study?

  For instance, in a single-day rest–stress study, the stress images should have higher signal to noise compared to the rest images since 3x more radiotracer was administered. If not, consider dose infiltration.

- The coronal/rotating MIP can show important ancillary findings:

Is there motion artifact?	Is there breast attenuation artifact?
Is there significant right ventricular uptake? If so, implies right heart disease or pulmonary hypertension.	Is there pulmonary uptake? If so, implies left ventricular dysfunction.

- Gated SPECT (GSPECT) images allow evaluation of wall motion and wall thickening.
- Evaluation of the rest and stress SPECT perfusion images is the core of the exam, with the key question: **Is there a perfusion defect on the stress images?**

  Is the defect reversible on rest images? A fixed defect may represent either myocardial scar or hibernating myocardium, while a reversible defect signifies cardiac ischemia.

  If the defect is reversible, how severe is the defect? Mild, moderate, or severe?

  How large is the defect (number of myocardial segments, described on the next page)?

  Small (1–2 segments); medium (3–4 segments); large (5 or more segments).

  Where is it and in which coronary artery territory?

  Is there dilation of the left ventricle during stress (transient ischemic dilation; **TID**)? If so, may imply three vessel disease, even if there is no focal defect.

  In summary, an example interpretation may be: *There is a medium-sized defect of severe intensity involving the mid and basal inferior wall, corresponding to RCA territory.*

apex ←——————→ base

SA (short axis)

anterior wall

LAD Cx RCA

septum LAD Cx lateral wall RCA

inferior wall

LAD Cx RCA

septum ←——————→ free lateral wall

VLA (vertical long axis)

anterior wall

LAD

LAD apex RCA

inferior wall

Cx

inferior wall ←——————→ anterior wall

HLA (horizontal long axis)

RCA

apex

LAD septum Cx lateral wall

LAD

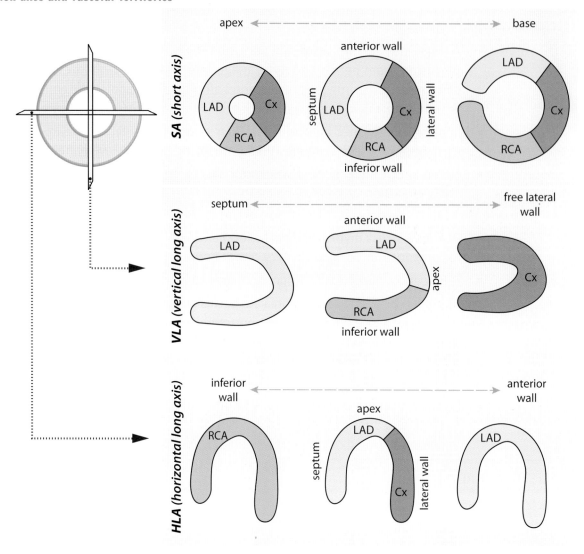

- The heart is reconstructed into short axis (SA, the traditional "donut" view from apex of heart through the base), vertical long axis (VLA, a "U-shaped" view pointing to the left), and the horizontal long axis (HLA, a "U-shaped" view pointing down). The polar plot represents the entire three-dimensional left ventricle unfolded onto a two-dimensional map.

Myocardial segments

17 segment left ventricular segmentation:

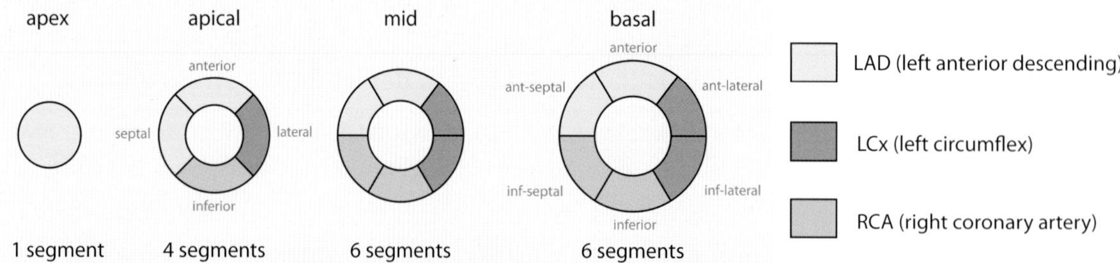

- For evaluation of perfusion defect size, there are 17 standard left ventricular segments, evaluated on the SA ("donut") views. Each segment is usually supplied by the color-coded coronary artery indicated above, although vascular supply is variable between patients.

Normal

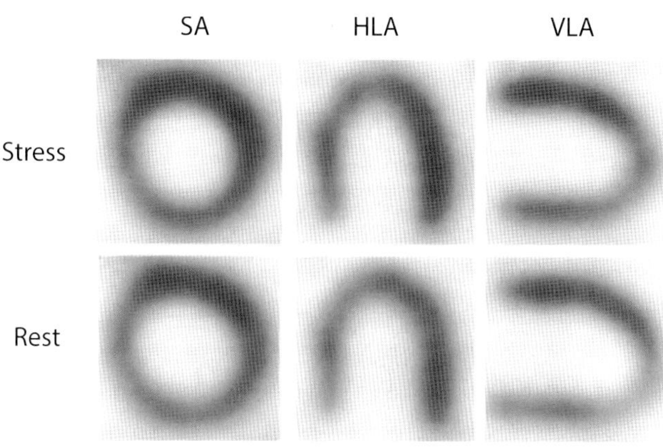

Normal exercise stress sestamibi perfusion study: 5.1 mCi Tc-99m sestamibi was administered and rest SPECT images were obtained. Subsequently 16 mCi Tc-99m sestamibi was administered at peak exercise using a modified Bruce treadmill protocol and the stress SPECT images were obtained.

The rest and stress images are identical and normal.

SA = short axis
HLA = horizontal long axis
VLA = vertical long axis

Fixed defect

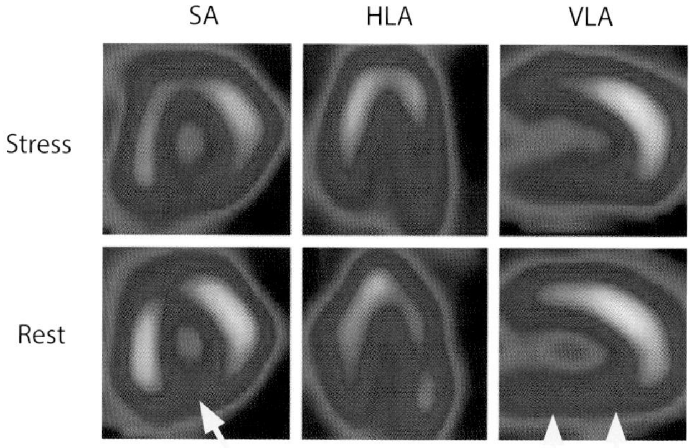

Fixed defect seen on regadenoson sestamibi perfusion study. 7.67 mCi Tc-99m sestamibi was administered and rest SPECT images were obtained. Subsequently 0.4 mg regadenoson was administered intravenously followed by 32 mCi Tc-99m sestamibi and stress SPECT images were obtained. The stress images are displayed above the rest images.

There is a moderate-sized fixed defect involving the mid and basal inferior wall (arrows), in the right coronary artery distribution. This represents either scar or hibernating myocardium.

Reversible defect

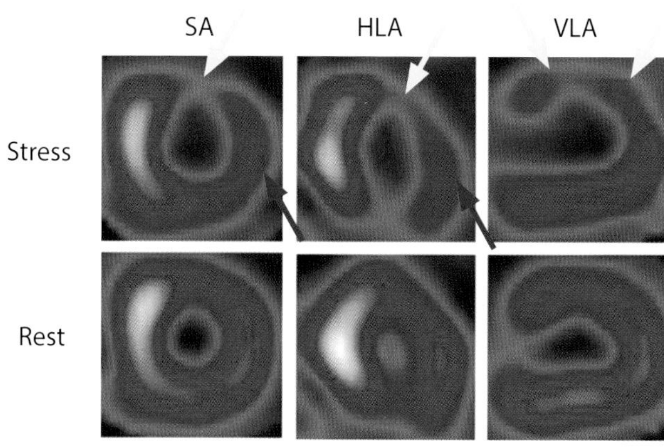

Large reversible defect seen on regadenoson sestamibi perfusion study: 11 mCi Tc-99m sestamibi was administered and rest SPECT images were obtained. Subsequently 0.4 mg regadenoson was administered intravenously followed by 29 mCi Tc-99m sestamibi and stress SPECT images were obtained. The stress images are displayed above the rest images.

There is a large-sized partially reversible defect of severe intensity involving the apical, mid, and basal segments of the anterior (LAD territory, yellow arrows) and lateral (left circumflex territory, red arrows) walls.

Thyroid

Radiotracers

Iodine-131

- I-131 emits both beta particles and 364 keV gamma photons (only the gamma photons are used for imaging). The half-life is 8 days. I-131 is generator produced.
- I-131 is only used for therapy. Indications include treatment of thyroid cancer status post thyroidectomy, and hyperthyroidism from Graves disease or multinodular gland.

Iodine-123

- I-123 decays by electron capture and produces 159 keV gamma photons. It has a half-life of 13 hours. I-123 is expensive as it is produced by cyclotron. It is administered orally.
- I-123 is an excellent radioisotope for thyroid imaging, as it can image in high detail and obtain thyroid uptake values.

Tc-99m pertechnetate

- Technetium-99m emits a 140 keV gamma photon and has a half-life of 6 hours.
- Unlike iodine, pertechnetate is not trapped by the thyroid. After initial uptake it is released into the blood pool. Thyroid uptake is not routinely quantified with Tc-99m (due to its rapid washout), but pertechnetate does provide excellent images of the thyroid gland.
- Because pertechnetate does not specifically localize to the thyroid, high background counts are typical. Only 1–5% of administered activity is taken up by the thyroid.
- In contrast to I-123, the salivary glands are clearly seen with pertechnetate.
- Unlike I-123, Tc-99m is administered intravenously.
- Tc-99m pertechnetate is preferred over I-123 when the patient has received recent intravenous iodinated contrast (iodine in contrast blocks thyroid uptake of additional iodine), when IV medication is necessary, or when a quick study is required.

Pregnancy and breast feeding

- All thyrotropic agents cross the placenta and I-131 is contraindicated in pregnancy. Fetal iodine is taken up beginning at 12 weeks gestation.
- A breast feeding mother who medically requires an I-131 ablative dose must stop breast feeding permanently for the current child.
- For I-123, breast feeding can be resumed 2–3 days after administration.
- For Tc-99m, breast feeding can be resumed 12–24 hours after administration.

Patient preparation

- Patients undergoing I-123 or I-131 imaging/therapy must have non-suppressed TSH, which can be achieved by stopping exogenous thyroid hormone for 4 weeks, or by two intramuscular injections of recombinant TSH (rTSH).

Diagnostic Indications (I-123 or Tc-99m pertechnetate)

Ectopic thyroid

- Either I-123 or Tc-99m can be used to localize suspected ectopic thyroid tissue.
- Lingual thyroid is ectopic thyroid tissue at the base of tongue.
- Functional thyroid tissue may rarely be seen in an ovarian teratoma (struma ovarii).
- Retrosternal thyroid tissue is most often due to a substernal goiter.

Thyroid nodule

- Thyroid nodules are typically only imaged if the cytology is indeterminate.
- Hyperfunctioning nodules are almost always benign adenomas.
- Cold nodules have approximately 20% risk of malignancy, although the most common cold nodule (~70–75%) is a benign colloid cyst.
- A warm nodule usually represents a cold nodule with overlapping thyroid tissue.

  A warm nodule requires further investigation such as biopsy if oblique views are indeterminate.
- A discordant thyroid nodule is "hot" on Tc-99m and "cold" on I-123 as it has maintained the ability to uptake technetium but is unable to trap iodine. Biopsy is usually recommended as a discordant nodule may be malignant.
- Malignancy is relatively uncommon in a multinodular goiter. While a dominant cold nodule should undergo further investigation, smaller cold nodules are unlikely to be malignant.

Graves disease

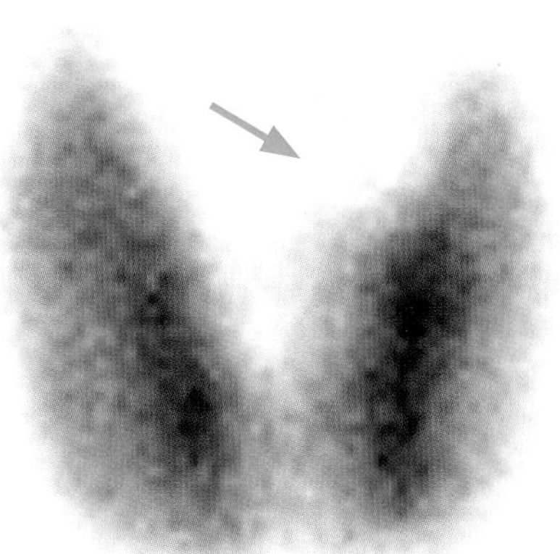

Graves disease: I-123 scan with 0.3 mCi I-123 NaI administered.

There is diffuse uptake throughout the thyroid gland. A faint pyramidal lobe is present (arrow).

24 hour uptake is elevated at 56%.

- Graves disease is an autoimmune disorder characterized by hyperthyroidism, thyromegaly, homogeneously increased thyroid activity, and often a prominent pyramidal lobe.
- Both 6-hour and 24-hour iodine uptake are elevated.

  Normal 6-hour uptake is 6–18% and normal 24-hour uptake is 10–30%.
- Although usually an I-123 and a Tc-99m scan can be differentiated by the presence of salivary uptake with Tc-99m, in Graves disease this distinction is often not possible. In Graves disease, thyroid uptake can be so strong that the salivary glands are often not seen, causing a similar appearance with either radiotracer.
- Definitive treatment of Graves disease is I-131 radiotherapy or (less commonly) surgery. Antithyroid drugs (e.g., methimazole or propylthiouracil) are another option and may achieve a remission after 1–2 years of use.

Hashimoto thyroiditis

- Hashimoto thyroiditis is the most common inflammatory disease of the thyroid.
- Like Graves disease, Hashimoto thyroiditis also clinically presents with thyromegaly. In Hashimoto thyroiditis, however, thyroid hormone levels are variable depending on the disease stage. Most patients with Hashimoto thyroiditis are hypothyroid.
- Appearance on thyroid scan is variable, ranging from diffusely increased activity that resembles Graves disease to patchy uptake similar to a multinodular goiter. The patchiness is thought to be due to cold areas from infiltration by lymphocytes and lymphoid follicles.

Subacute thyroiditis

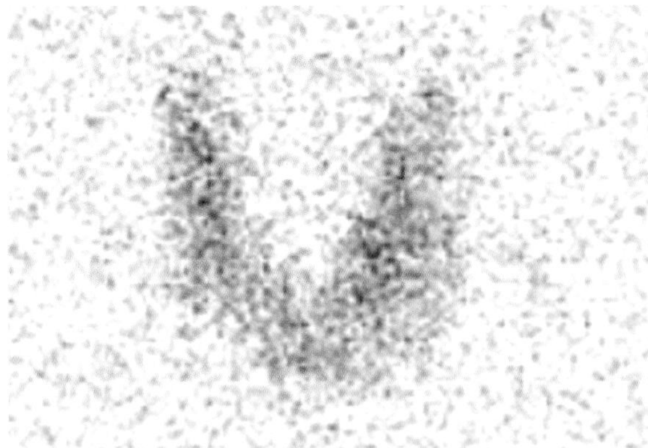

Subacute thyroiditis: I-123 scan with 0.222 mCi administered.

There is diffusely low thyroid uptake with very low background to thyroid uptake ratio. 24-hour uptake was only 4.9%.

- The classical clinical presentation of subacute thyroiditis is a painful swollen gland, although many patients present with silent hyperthyroidism.
- Imaging shows decreased radiotracer uptake and a low 24-hour uptake.
- Subacute thyroiditis is typically a self-limited condition. Treatment is directed towards symptom control with nonsteroidal anti-inflammatory drugs or steroids in severe cases.

THERAPEUTIC INDICATIONS (I-131)

Thyroid carcinoma, post-thyroidectomy

- Approximately 1–2 months after thyroidectomy, I–131 is administered to treat and simultaneously image residual and potential metastatic disease.
- Following thyroidectomy, thyroid replacement therapy is withheld to allow endogenous TSH to increase. This increases uptake of therapeutic I-131 by any residual or metastatic thyroid tissue. The goal TSH is 30–50 μIU/mL.
- The dosing of I-131 is dependent on the oncologic risk:

  Low-risk patient (tumor <1.5 cm, no invasion of thyroid capsule): <30 mCi I-131 administered.

  High-risk patient: 100–200 mCi I-131 administered.

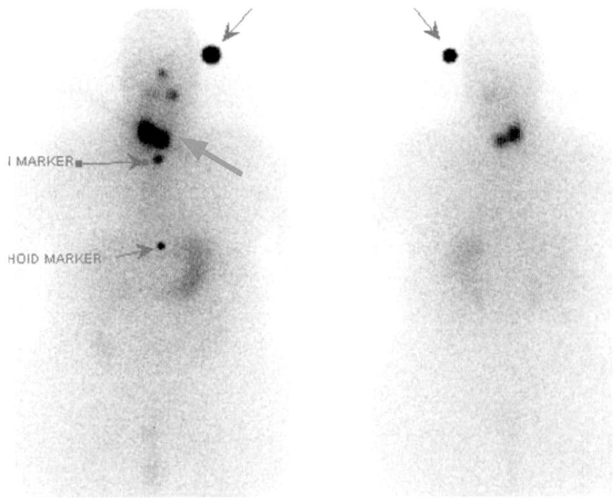

I-131 ablative therapy: 99 mCi I-131 administered orally four days prior to scanning. The gray arrows point to markers.

Anterior and posterior planar imaging shows a large focus of residual uptake in the thyroid bed (blue arrow) and mild symmetric salivary gland uptake. There is physiologic uptake in the stomach, bladder, and bowel.

- A new approach is a standard dose of 30 mCi for treatment of all T1, T2, and N1 cancers.

Thyroid carcinoma, post radioiodine therapy

- After ablation with I-131, patients with thyroid carcinoma are monitored by following thyroglobulin levels. If thyroglobulin levels rise, an I-123 scan is performed to evaluate for disease recurrence or metastasis. If the I-123 scan is positive, repeat I-131 radioiodine is administered for ablation. Note that the presence of anti-thyroglobulin antibodies precludes the ability to monitor the thyroglobulin levels.

Treatment of Graves Disease

- I-131 is administered in a single oral dose to treat Graves disease. Contraindications to I-131 include pregnancy, lactation, and inability to comply with radiation safety guidelines.

- The dosing of I-131 for treatment of Graves varies by institution. Many endocrinologists advocate a calculated dose based on the estimated thyroid weight and 24-hour uptake, while another study has shown one of three fixed doses (up to 15 mCi) to be equally effective.
- Adequate dosing of I-131 can treat greater than 90% of patients with Graves disease.

Treatment of multinodular goiter

- I-131 can be used to reduce goiter size, especially in patients who choose not to undergo surgery. The dose of I-131 to treat toxic multinodular goiter may be higher than that for Graves disease, and multiple treatments may be required.
- 25 mCi is a typical dose administered to treat toxic multinodular goiter.

Parathyroid

Radiotracer

Tc-99m sestamibi

- Tc-99m sestamibi is taken up by parathyroids *and* the thyroid; however, thyroid activity decreases over time. The same agent is used for nuclear cardiology.

Indications

Parathyroid adenoma

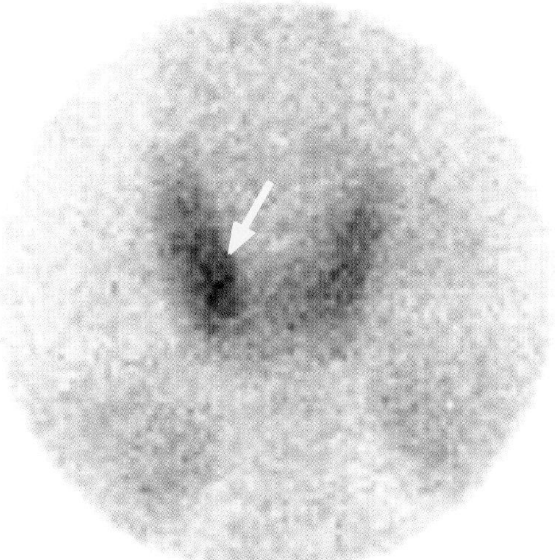

Early anterior pinhole image of the thyroid after the administration of 5 mCi Tc-99m sestamibi shows diffuse uptake throughout the thyroid, with a focal area of increased uptake (arrow) in the lower pole of the right lobe.

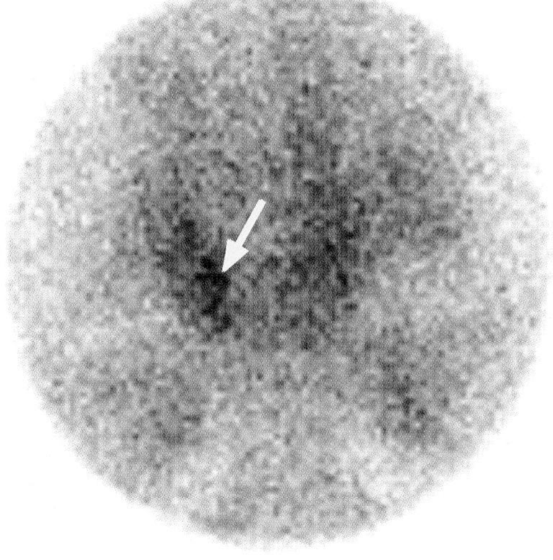

Delayed anterior pinhole image show interval partial washout of Tc-99m sestamibi. There is a persistent focus of radiotracer uptake (arrow) in the right lower pole. A right inferior parathyroid adenoma was confirmed at surgery.

- Dual-phase (early and delayed) imaging with Tc-99m sestamibi can localize a suspected parathyroid adenoma in a patient with elevated parathyroid hormone.
- A parathyroid adenoma shows increased uptake on early images and persistent retained activity on delayed images. In contrast, a thyroid adenoma will also initially show increased uptake but will then wash out on delayed images.
- Parathyroid tissue does *not* take up Tc-99m pertechnetate, which can be administered in indeterminate cases.

GASTROINTESTINAL

LIVER–SPLEEN IMAGING

Radiotracer: Tc-99m sulfur colloid

- Sulfur colloid is taken up by reticuloendothelial cells, which are found in the liver, spleen, and bone marrow. Sulfur colloid is also taken up by Kupffer cells in the liver. Hepatic Kupffer cells make up only approximately 10% of the liver mass.
- 80–90% of sulfur colloid particles are taken up by the liver. Most of the remainder is taken up by the spleen, and a small amount taken up in the bone marrow. The bone marrow is not normally seen at typical windowing levels.
- Although Tc-99m has a physical half-life of 6 hours, sulfur colloid is rapidly cleared with a biologic half-life of 2–3 minutes.

Focal decreased hepatic uptake on sulfur colloid scan

- The most common cause of a photopenic defect (complete absence of radiotracer) is a hepatic cyst. It may be difficult to distinguish focal *decreased* uptake from a *photopenic* defect if the lesion is small.
- Most hepatic masses cause focal decreased radiocolloid uptake, including hepatocellular carcinoma (HCC), adenoma, and abscess. Focal decreased uptake should raise concern for HCC in a patient with any risk factors for HCC such as cirrhosis or chronic hepatitis.

Focal increased hepatic uptake on sulfur colloid scan

- Focal nodular hyperplasia, discussed below, may hyperconcentrate radiocolloid.
- A regenerating nodule in a cirrhotic liver can cause focal increased sulfur colloid uptake.
- Budd–Chiari syndrome (hepatic vein thrombosis) can lead to increased uptake in the caudate lobe in the later stage of disease.

Colloid shift

- Colloid shift is increased sulfur colloid accumulation within the spleen and bone marrow. It suggests liver dysfunction, most commonly due to cirrhosis.

Diffuse pulmonary uptake

- Diffuse pulmonary uptake on a sulfur colloid scan is nonspecific, and can be seen in:

Cirrhosis.

COPD with superimposed infection.

Langerhans cell histiocytosis.

High serum aluminum (either due to antacids or excess aluminum in the colloid preparation).

Focal nodular hyperplasia (FNH)

- Focal nodular hyperplasia (FNH) is a benign liver mass that can have a variable appearance on a sulfur colloid scan. Most commonly, FNH will be indistinguishable from background liver on a sulfur colloid scan due to Kupffer cells within the FNH. FNH may also appear to have increased uptake due to a combination of hypervascularity and Kupffer sulfur colloid uptake. In approximately one third of cases there is insufficient colloid concentration and FNH may appear as a photopenic defect.
- In contrast to FNH, a hepatic adenoma does not contain Kupffer cells and will consistently cause a cold defect.
- An adjunct or alternative to sulfur colloid scan is a HIDA scan. FNH contains biliary ductules so it should be positive on a HIDA scan.

Intrapancreatic spleen

- The presence of an intrapancreatic spleen can be confirmed by sulfur colloid scan in indeterminate cases, where the suspected intrapancreatic spleen will show uptake. A Tc-99m damaged red cell study can also be performed.

Gastrointestinal bleeding

Radiotracer: Tc-99m labeled RBCs

- Technetium-99m labeled red blood cells are prepared in vitro by mixing 1–3 mL of anticoagulated blood with stannous chloride and an oxidizing agent. Tc-99m is added and has a labeling efficiency of 95%. The labeling procedure takes more than 20 minutes.

  An in-vivo technique provides much noisier images due to worse labeling efficiency and resultant free pertechnetate, and is therefore uncommonly performed.

- Alternatively, Tc-99m sulfur colloid can be used. Sulfur colloid does require significant preparation time, but has rapid blood clearance and a vascular half life of 2–3 minutes.

Acute GI bleed

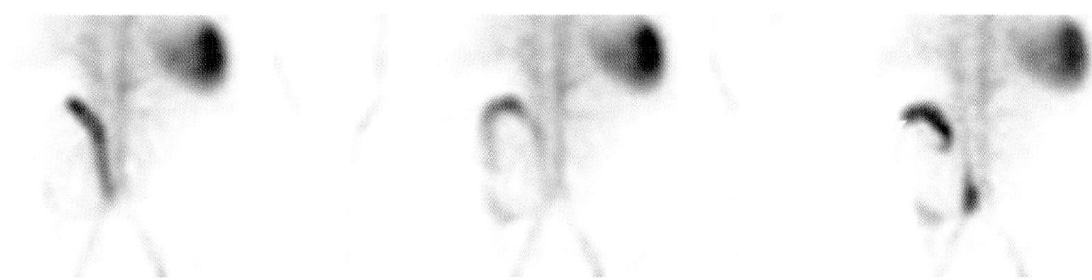

GI bleed: Sequential images of the lower abdomen from a Tc-99m tagged RBC study show a focus of radiotracer uptake in the right lower quadrant, which changes shape and position over time (arrows). This correlates to small bowel in the distribution of the superior mesenteric artery.

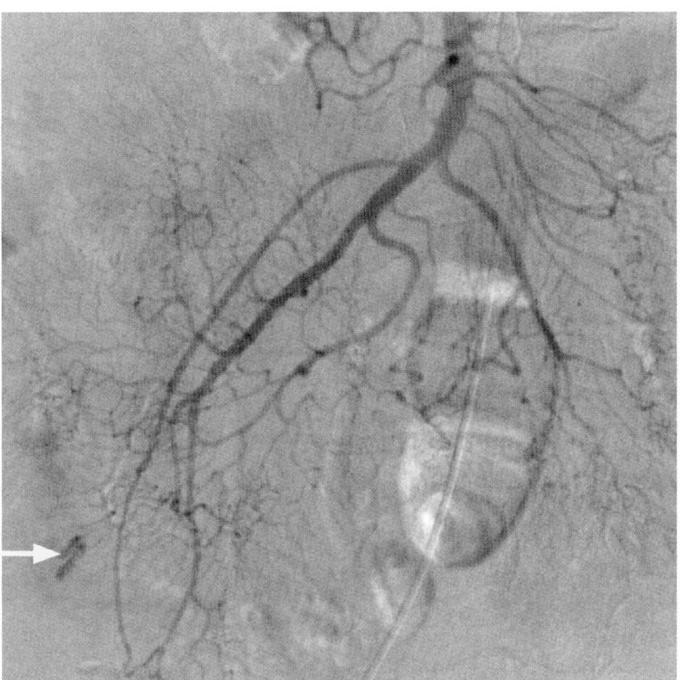

Superior mesenteric artery angiogram in the same patient performed within one hour of the above tagged RBC study shows a focus of contrast extravasation in a distal ileocolic branch (arrow).

This patient was treated with coil embolization of the distal ileocolic branch artery.

- A tagged red cell study can be used to identify patients who may be suitable for angiography versus those who are not. Bleeding rates as low as 0.2 mL/min can be detected with a tagged red-blood cell study compared to 1 mL/min for angiography.
- A positive study shows activity that changes shape and position over time due to peristalsis of intraluminal blood, with a pattern suggestive of either small or large bowel source.

Meckel imaging

Radiotracer: Tc-99m pertechnetate

- Technetium-99m pertechnetate localizes to gastric mucosa.

Meckel diverticulum

- Meckel diverticulum is a remnant of the embryological omphalomesenteric duct, most commonly located in the distal ileum. Approximately 10–60% of Meckel diverticula contain ectopic gastric mucosa, which may result in mucosal damage and GI bleeding.
- A positive Meckel scan demonstrates a focal area of increased activity, typically in the right lower quadrant. A lateral view is often helpful to ensure that activity is anterior and not associated with the ureter.
- Other causes of right lower quadrant pain include appendicitis and intussusception, which can cause more diffuse, regional increased uptake due to hyperemia.

Hepatobiliary imaging (HIDA)

Radiotracers: Tc-99m IDA agents

- Tc-99m-iminodiacetic acid (IDA) analogs are used to image the biliary system. Regardless of the tracer, the test is typically called a "HIDA" scan.
- **Disofenin** allows visualization of biliary system with bilirubin levels as high as 20 mg/dL and has 90% hepatic uptake. **Mebrofenin** allows visualization of biliary system with bilirubin levels as high as 30 mg/dL and has an even higher 98% hepatic uptake. Both are actively transported into hepatocytes but are not conjugated.

HIDA protocol

- Patient must be NPO for 6 hours prior, but must have eaten within 24 hours. If the patient has been NPO for >24 hours, then cholecystokinin (CCK; dose 0.02 μg/kg, given as slow infusion) can be given to empty the gallbladder before radiotracer is administered.

  CCK must be administered slowly or the patient may experience an exacerbation of their symptoms.

  In general, one should wait at least two hours after administering CCK before beginning the exam.

- Dynamic imaging of the right upper quadrant begins immediately after injection of radiotracer. As soon as the gallbladder is visualized, acute cholecystitis is ruled out.
- If the gallbladder is not visualized by one hour, then morphine is given (0.04 mg/kg, up to a maximum dose of 4 mg) and imaging continues for 30 more minutes. Morphine contracts the sphincter of Oddi, redirecting bile into the cystic duct.

  Morphine should only be given if tracer is visualized in the small bowel, otherwise there is the theoretical risk of worsening a potential common bile duct obstruction. However, nonvisualization of tracer in the small bowel is not specific for common bile duct obstruction.

- If the patient has a morphine allergy, an alternative is to image for a total of 4 hours.

Normal HIDA scan

- In a normal HIDA scan, the liver is visible by 5 minutes.
- The gallbladder is typically seen by 15 minutes due to radiotracer flow into the cystic duct.
- Tracer should be seen in the small bowel to ensure a patent common bile duct.

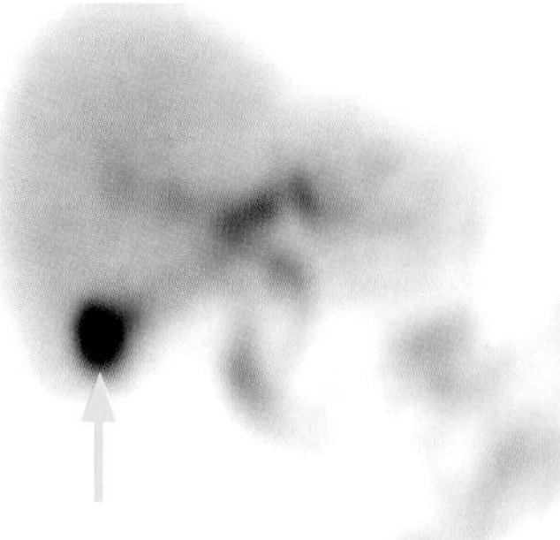

Single image from a HIDA scan 15 minutes after 4.1 mCi Tc-99m disofenin administered shows normal visualization of the liver, gallbladder (arrow), and small bowel.

Acute cholecystitis

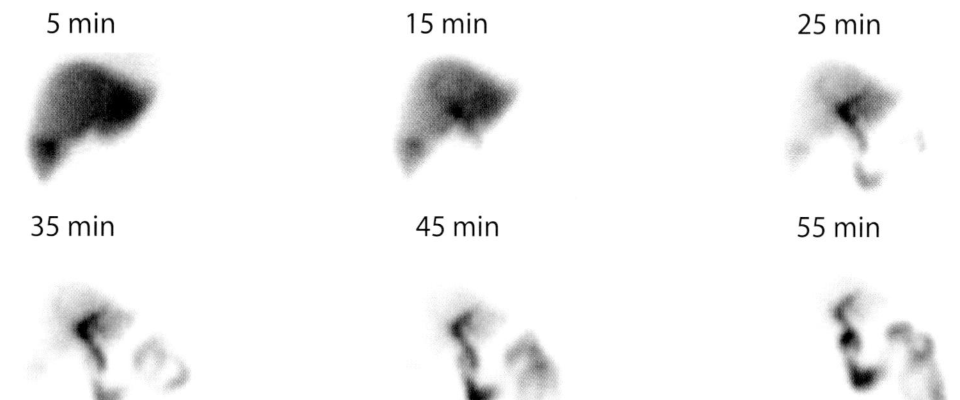

Acute cholecystitis: Sequential images from a HIDA scan with 3.87 mCi Tc-99m disofenin administered shows prompt visualization of the liver. The small bowel is visualized by 25 minutes. There is no visualization of the gallbladder during the course of the exam. The patient had a morphine allergy so 4-hour delayed images were obtained instead (not shown), which also do not demonstrate the gallbladder.

- Almost all patients with acute cholecystitis have cystic duct obstruction.
- Nonvisualization of the gallbladder after 90 minutes of imaging and morphine augmentation is approximately 86–98% sensitive for the diagnosis of acute cholecystitis, with a false-positive rate of approximately 6%, most commonly due to pancreatitis and biliary stasis.
- The *rim* sign describes increased hepatic activity surrounding the gallbladder fossa, thought to be due to hyperemia and possibly gangrenous cholecystitis.
- False positive HIDA (gallbladder non-visualization *without* acute cholecystitis) can be due to:

Recent meal (within 4 hours) or prolonged fasting (greater than 24 hours).	Pancreatitis.
Administration of CCK *immediately* prior to the exam, which can cause persistent sphincter of Oddi relaxation.	Severe illness.
Total parental nutrition.	Chronic cholecystitis.
	Cholangiocarcinoma of the cystic duct (very rare).

- False negative HIDA (gallbladder visualization *with* acute cholecystitis) is very rare and can be due to:

Acalculous cholecystitis with a patent cystic duct.
Duodenal diverticulum simulating the gallbladder; however, a lateral view would differentiate.
Biliary cyst simulating the gallbladder.

Chronic cholecystitis

- Chronic cholecystitis is long-standing gallbladder inflammation causing loss of normal gallbladder function and predisposing to formation of stones.
- Chronic cholecystitis may be a cause of chronic recurrent abdominal pain.
- Diagnosis can be difficult as there is no single pattern that is pathognomonic of chronic cholecystitis based on HIDA. In fact, most cases of chronic cholecystitis have a normal HIDA scan.
- A low gallbladder ejection fraction (GBEF) is thought to be suggestive of chronic cholecystitis. To measure the ejection fraction, pre- and post-CCK injection gallbladder counts are compared. A GBEF <35% suggests chronic cholecystitis, although the reliability of this finding is controversial as ejection fraction is dependent on the rate of CCK injection and standard infusion protocols have not been determined.

Biliary leak

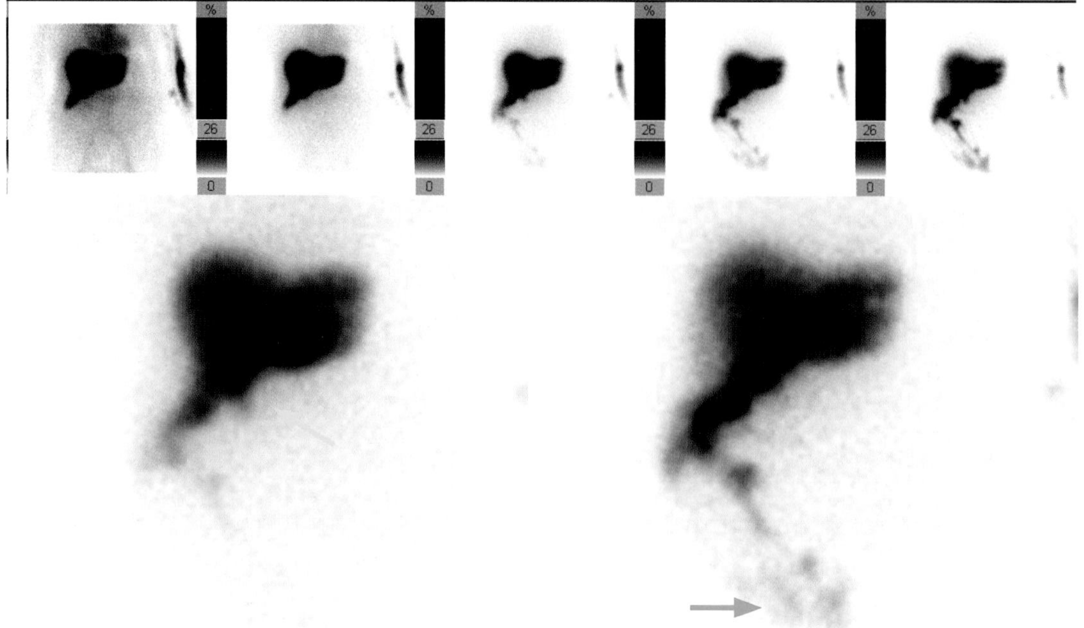

Bile leak: Sequential images (top row) and two enlarged still images (bottom two images) from a HIDA scan with 5.4 mCi Tc-99m disofenin administered to a patient with right upper quadrant pain status post cholecystectomy shows tracer accumulating in the gallbladder fossa (yellow arrow) and pooling in the right paracolic gutter (blue arrow). The gallbladder is surgically absent. The leak was thought to arise from the cystic duct stump.

- A HIDA scan is an accurate method to assess for the presence of a biliary leak.
- Imaging can be performed in the right lateral decubitus position to promote dependent pooling of bile.

Hepatic dysfunction

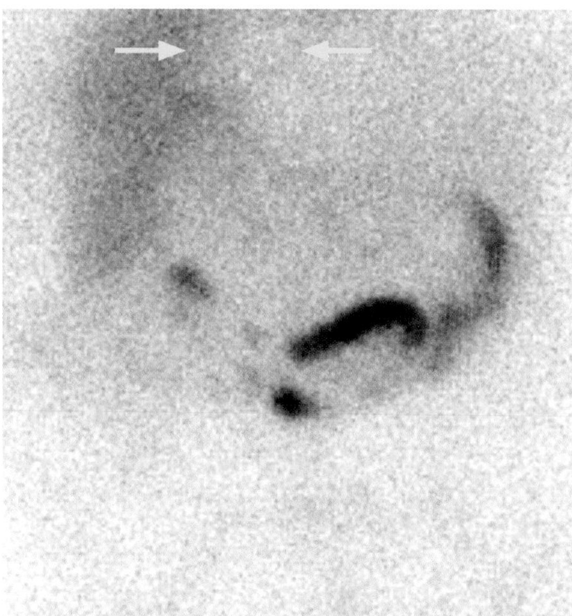

Severe hepatic dysfunction in a patient with cholangiocarcinoma: Single image from a HIDA scan obtained 30 minutes after 6.1 mCi Tc-99m disofenin administered shows a large amount of background and blood pool uptake with minimal tracer in the liver. A large photopenic defect in the left lobe of the liver (arrows) corresponds to the patient's cholangiocarcinoma. There is small bowel tracer excretion.

- Since the IDA tracers are actively transported into hepatocytes and then secreted into the bile, severe hepatic dysfunction will cause very poor hepatic uptake and blood pool clearance will be delayed.
- Since functioning hepatocytes are necessary to extract the tracer, a hepatic mass will appear as a focal photopenic defect.

Radiotracers

Tc-99m-MAA (perfusion)

- Technetium-99m macro-aggregated albumin (MAA) is a particulate radiopharmaceutical that lodges in the pulmonary capillary bed and can therefore be used to evaluate pulmonary perfusion. Most particles are between 10 and 30 μm in size.
- Typically 3 to 5 mCi Tc-99m MAA are administered, comprising between 200,000 and 600,000 particles. Particle fragments begin to break down in approximately 30 minutes. In children, pregnant patients, patients with mild pulmonary hypertension, and patients with a known right-to-left shunt, the dose can be halved to approximately 100,000 particles.
- A relative contraindication to MAA is severe pulmonary hypertension, as obstruction of even a few pulmonary capillaries can cause clinical worsening.
- A right-to-left shunt causes immediate renal and brain uptake after intravenous injection. A Tc-99m MAA study may be able to quantify the shunt fraction in these patients. Note that renal uptake can also be seen if free pertechnetate is present, but evaluation of the head and neck can differentiate free pertechnetate from a right-to-left shunt. Free pertechnetate is taken up by the thyroid, but not the brain. A right-to-left shunt, in contrast, demonstrates immediate brain uptake and no significant uptake in the neck.
- Clumping of MAA can be seen when MAA is inadvertently drawn back into the injection syringe, causing coagulation with the patient's blood.

Xenon-133 (ventilation)

- Xenon-133 is an inhaled gas with a physical half-life of 5.3 days, which emits 81 keV gamma photons and is also a beta-emitter. The critical organ is the trachea. The biologic half life is very short because the vast majority of the gas is exhaled. Although 10–20 mCi is administered, there is very little radiation exposure.
- Xenon-133 is imaged posteriorly to avoid breast artifacts, as the relatively low keV is easily attenuated by soft tissue. Washin–washout imaging can be performed to evaluate for air trapping, which is seen in COPD.
- Xenon-133 requires good patient cooperation as the patient must breathe on a closed spirometer for several minutes. Exhaled Xenon-133 must be carefully disposed of, either exhausted to the atmosphere or trapped in a charcoal trap until it decays. Xenon-133 must be administered in a negative pressure room to prevent accidental leakage.

Tc-99m DTPA (ventilation)

- Tc-99m DTPA is a technetium-labeled aerosol. Unlike Xenon-133, DTPA does not allow for dynamic washin–washout imaging. Once inhaled, the particles remain in place for approximately 20–60 minutes. 30 mCi is typically administered.
- Compared to Xenon, DTPA has greater ease of use. Specific advantages include the ability to image in multiple projections, no need for exhaust systems, and ability to use portably.

Clinical VQ Scanning in the era of CT pulmonary angiography

Diagnosis of pulmonary embolism in pregnancy

- Pulmonary embolism is the leading cause of death in pregnancy in the developed world, and diagnosis must be weighed against radiation exposure to the mother and the fetus.

Pulmonary embolism CT angiogram: Maternal breast dose approximately 10–70 mGy (much greater than ACR mammography guidelines of 3 mGy/breast). Fetal dose 0.1–0.66 mGy.

Perfusion scanning: Maternal breast dose <0.31 mGy. Fetal dose 0.1–0.37 mGy.

- Technique: In most cases, only perfusion (Q) scanning is necessary and ventilation scanning is not commonly performed. The administered dose of Tc-99m MAA is typically one half of the standard dose, or approximately 100,000 particles.
- Diagnostic accuracy for PE has been shown to be equivalent between PE-CT and Q scanning.
- The primary advantage of PE-CT is the demonstration of an alternative diagnosis not seen on plain radiographs approximately 5% of the time, at the expense of 100x increase in breast radiation exposure and slightly higher fetal dose.
- Nuclear medicine perfusion scanning is recommended in suspected pulmonary embolism in a pregnant patient with a normal chest radiograph. In clinical practice, PE-CT is often more readily available, which may influence the choice of exam performed.

Diagnosis of pulmonary embolism with PIOPED II

High probability: Specificity for pulmonary embolism 97%, positive predictive value 88%

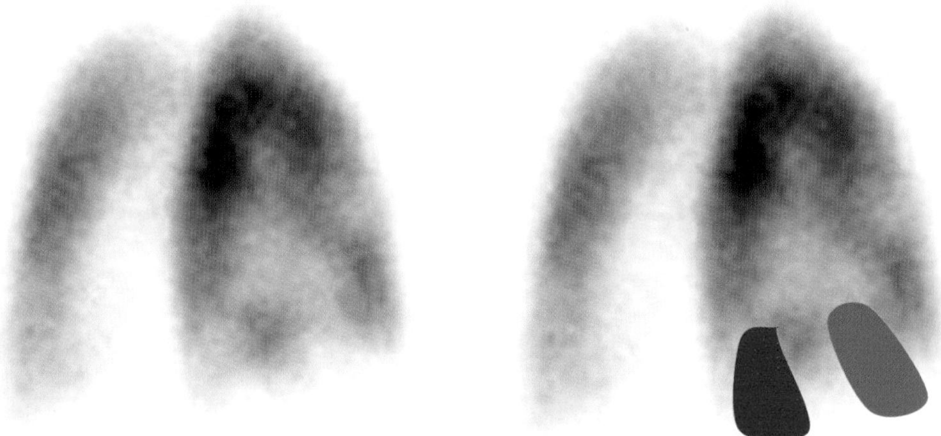

High probability for pulmonary embolism: RPO perfusion images (same image, without and with annotations) after 4.7 mCi Tc-99m MAA administered show two large segmental defects in the posterior basal (red) and anterior basal (brown) segments of the right lower lobe. The ventilation scan (not shown) was normal.

- Two or more large (>75% of a segment) mismatched segmental defects without associated radiographic abnormality is high probability for pulmonary embolism.

Intermediate probability: Not clinically helpful, further imaging is required

- One large segmental mismatched perfusion defect is intermediate probability.
- A triple match in the *lower lung* is intermediate probability. A triple match describes a defect on perfusion, a matched defect on ventilation, and a corresponding abnormality on the chest radiograph.

Low probability: Negative predictive value 84%

- A single large or moderate matched VQ defect is low probability of pulmonary embolism.
- Other low probability findings include absent perfusion of an entire lung, or more than three small segmental lesions.

Very low probability

- Nonsegmental lesions are very low probability.
- *The stripe* sign peripheral to a perfusion defect is very low probability for pulmonary embolism. The *stripe* sign represents a thin line of MAA uptake between a perfusion defect and the adjacent pleural surface, representing intervening perfused lung.

- A solitary triple-matched defect in the *mid–upper* lung is very low probability. In contrast, the previously mentioned lower lung triple-match is more likely to represent PE and is intermediate probability.

Normal

- If the perfusion scan is normal, the exam is normal and the ventilation study is not required.

MUSCULOSKELETAL

RADIOTRACERS

Tc-99m MDP

- Tc-99m MDP is a technetium-labeled diphosphonate. 20 mCi is typically administered, with imaging performed 2–4 hours later.
- Rapid renal excretion is normal. Diffuse soft tissue uptake can be seen in renal failure.
- Patients should void before imaging to prevent the bladder from obscuring a pelvic lesion.
- A three-phase study incudes:

> 1) Radionuclide **angiogram (flow)** evaluates blood flow, with images taken every few seconds. Increased flow suggests hyperemia.
>
> 2) **Blood pool** evaluates the extracellular distribution immediately following the blood flow phase.
>
> 3) Standard **delayed** (skeletal) images are performed approximately 3 hours after injection.

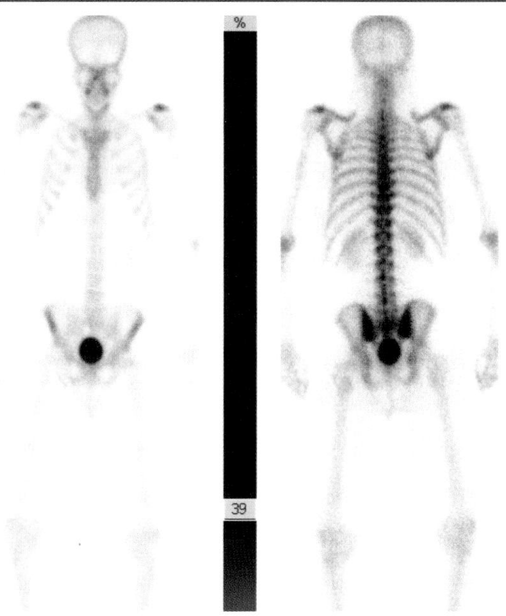

Normal Tc-99m MDP bone scan, with 20 mCi administered in anterior and posterior projections. Note the normal renal and bladder uptake.

COMMON PATTERNS AND CLINICAL APPLICATIONS

Patterns with low probability of metastatic disease (in a patient with a known malignancy)

- A single focus of uptake in a rib is thought to represent malignancy only ~10% of the time.
- Uptake in similar locations in two adjacent ribs is almost always due to trauma.
- Multiple adjacent photopenic bony lesions are unlikely to be metastases, but may represent infarction, avascular necrosis, or sequela of radiation therapy.

Patterns with high probability of metastatic disease

- A single sternal lesion in a patient with breast cancer is due to metastasis ~80% of the time.
- Multifocal areas of increased activity in nonadjacent ribs are suspicious for metastases.
- A single photopenic lesion in patients with a known malignancy (especially neuroblastoma, renal cell carcinoma, and thyroid cancer) is due to metastasis 80% of the time.

Increased soft tissue uptake

- Increased uptake in the brain or heart may be due to recent infarction.
- Malignant pleural effusion or ascites can cause increased uptake.
- Soft-tissue metastases containing calcium, including osteosarcoma, neuroblastoma, or mucin-producing tumors (gastrointestinal and ovarian) can cause soft tissue uptake.

- In the breasts, faint uptake can be normal, but focal intense uptake suggests breast carcinoma. Tracer uptake can be seen at site of recent breast procedure (e.g., biopsy).
- Inflammatory disease, such as myositis ossificans, dermatomyositis, and rhabdomyolysis, can cause radiotracer uptake in the soft tissues and muscles.

Superscan

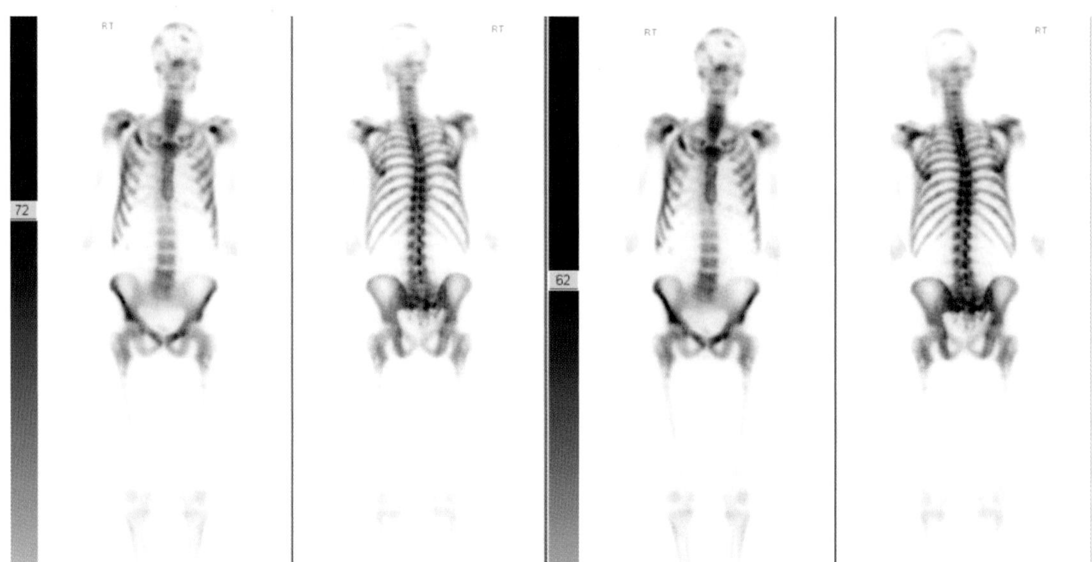

Superscan: Anterior and posterior whole body bone scan at two different windowing levels after 21 mCi Tc-99m MDP administration shows diffusely increased skeletal uptake in the axial skeleton and proximal femurs. There are scattered foci of uptake in the calvarium. No renal uptake is seen.

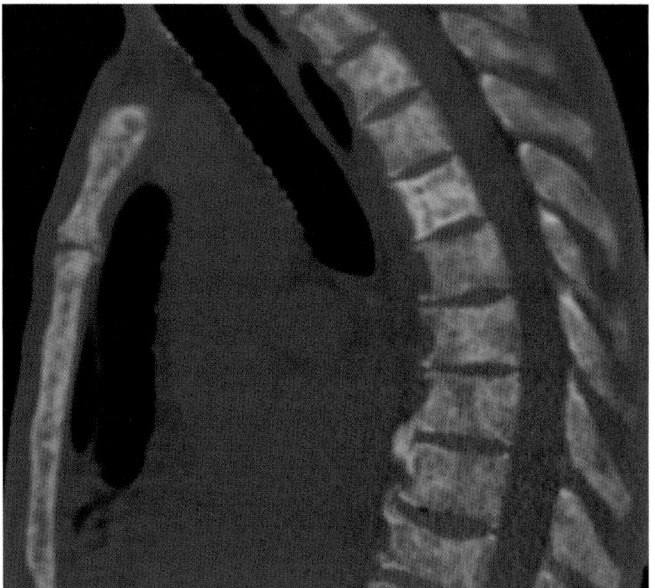

Sagittal CT in the same patient shows diffuse sclerotic appearance of the entire skeleton. This patient had metastatic prostate carcinoma.

- A *superscan* represents diffusely increased osseous uptake. Sometimes the uptake can be so diffuse that it may look normal on first glance. The clue to the presence of a superscan will be nonvisualization (or very faint visualization) of the kidneys. Renal failure may also cause lack of visualization of the kidneys, although the typical diffuse soft tissue uptake seen in renal failure helps distinguish renal failure from a superscan.
- A superscan is most commonly due to metastatic prostate cancer. Other malignancies producing a superscan include breast cancer and lymphoma.
- A superscan can also be caused by metabolic bone disease in primary and secondary hyperparathyroidism. If the cause for the superscan is metabolic, then the long bones tend to be seen very well. In contrast, with metastatic disease the axial skeleton and proximal humeri and femora are primarily affected.

Primary bone tumors

- **Osteosarcoma** typically causes markedly increased uptake, often with increased uptake in the entire affected limb.
- **Ewing sarcoma** features intense and homogeneous activity. It may be positive on all three phases of a three-phase bone scan, mimicking osteomyelitis.
- **Osteoid osteoma** features a vascular central nidus, which demonstrates intense activity. The *double density* sign describes an intense focus of uptake corresponding to the nidus, surrounded by relatively increased uptake representing hyperemia. The differential of the *double density* sign includes osteoid osteoma, Brodie abscess, less likely stress fracture.

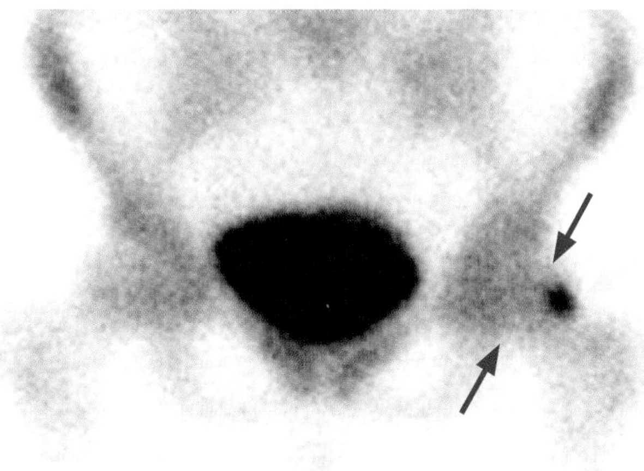

Double density sign of osteoid osteoma: Tc-99m MDP bone scan (25.9 mCi administered) shows asymmetric regional uptake in the left femoral head (red arrows), with a focus of intense uptake at the left lateral head/neck junction (yellow arrow).

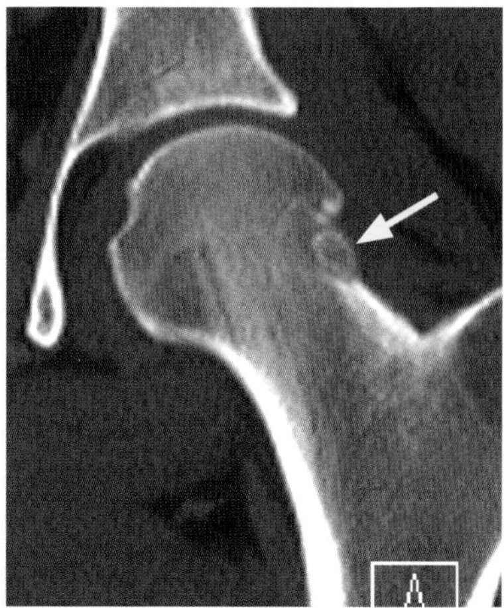

Coronal CT of the left hip shows a well circumscribed lucent lesion (arrow) with a sclerotic rim and lucent nidus, with mild surrounding osteopenia, consistent with osteoid osteoma.

Case courtesy Roger Han, MD, Brigham and Women's Hospital.

Fracture

- An acute fracture (from the initial injury up to 3–4 weeks) will show increased radiotracer uptake surrounding the fracture site. 95% of fractures are positive after one day in patients under 65 years old. Note that skull fractures rarely show activity.
- In the subacute phase (until 2–3 months) radiotracer activity becomes more focal at the fracture.
- In the healing phase (variable time course, with ~40% remaining abnormal after one year) there is a gradual decrease in radiotracer activity.
- Toddler's fracture represents a spiral fracture of the tibia and occurs in recently ambulatory children. Skeletal scintigraphy is sensitive and specific, and routinely used in workup of a limping child if the radiographs are negative.

Stress fracture

- A stress fracture represents a fracture due to abnormal stress in a normal bone.
- Common sites of stress fractures include the tibial diaphysis, the femoral neck, and the metatarsals. Metatarsal stress fractures are the most common stress injury in the foot/ankle, with 90% occurring in the 2nd or 3rd metatarsals.
- The bone scan is typically positive by the time the patient has pain. A stress fracture is positive on all three phases of the bone scan.

Shin splints

- Shin splints cause pain from periostitis at the tibial insertions of the anterior tibialis and soleus muscles.

- A three-phase bone scan shows *normal* blood flow and blood pool images, with linearly increased uptake in the posteromedial tibia on delayed (skeletal) phase.

Insufficiency fracture

- An insufficiency fracture represents a fracture in response to normal stress in an abnormal bone due to underlying osteoporosis.
- A sacral insufficiency fracture typically shows "H" shaped uptake in the sacrum, often referred to as the *Honda* sign.

Prosthesis evaluation

- Evaluation of a painful hip or knee prosthesis for loosening or infection is a common indication for a bone scan.
- In a cemented prosthesis, it is normal to see activity surrounding the prosthesis up to 12 months. In a non-cemented prosthesis, activity may remain increased up to 2 years as bony ingrowth continues.
- In evaluation of a hip prosthesis, *focal* activity at the lesser trochanter (which acts as a fulcrum site) and distal femoral prosthetic tip seen >1 year for cemented or >2 years for non-cemented prosthesis suggests loosening. In contrast, *generalized* increase in radiotracer activity surrounding the prosthesis may suggest osteomyelitis.
- Mild to moderate activity that is limited to the greater trochanter/intertrochanteric region is often due to heterotopic ossification.

Osteomyelitis and musculoskeletal infection

- Osteomyelitis is positive on all three phases of a bone scan. A positive three-phase bone scan is very specific for osteomyelitis in the presence of a normal radiograph (confirming that no fracture is present).
- To evaluate for osteomyelitis in the presence of an underlying abnormality, such as a fracture or prosthesis, WBC imaging (indium-111 or Tc-99m labeled WBCs) combined with a Tc-99m sulfur colloid marrow scan can increase specificity for osteomyelitis. Focal WBC activity in a region devoid of colloid marrow activity is suggestive of osteomyelitis.
- Although rarely performed, gallium-67 scan can also increase specificity for osteomyelitis if the gallium uptake exceeds the bone scan uptake in the area of concern.
- Cellulitis shows increased MDP activity during the blood flow and soft tissue phases, but the skeletal phase is negative.
- Septic arthritis is positive on all three phases of the bone scan on *both* sides of the joint.
- Discitis shows increased skeletal activity in two adjacent vertebral bodies.

Hypertrophic pulmonary osteoarthropathy

- Hypertrophic pulmonary osteoarthropathy is long bone diaphyseal periosteal reaction due to pulmonary disease, most commonly caused by lung cancer.
- Bone scan shows increased parallel lines of activity along the cortex of long bones.

Avascular necrosis (AVN)

- Avascular necrosis (AVN) initially shows decreased radiotracer activity in the affected region, followed by a hyperemic phase with increased uptake.
- SPECT imaging of AVN (especially of the hips) will often show a rim of increased uptake with central photopenia, thought to represent revascularization progressing from outside in.
- Spontaneous osteonecrosis of the knee (SONK) is a cause of atraumatic knee pain in the elderly. It typically appears as intensely increased radiotracer activity in the medial femoral condyle.

Paget disease

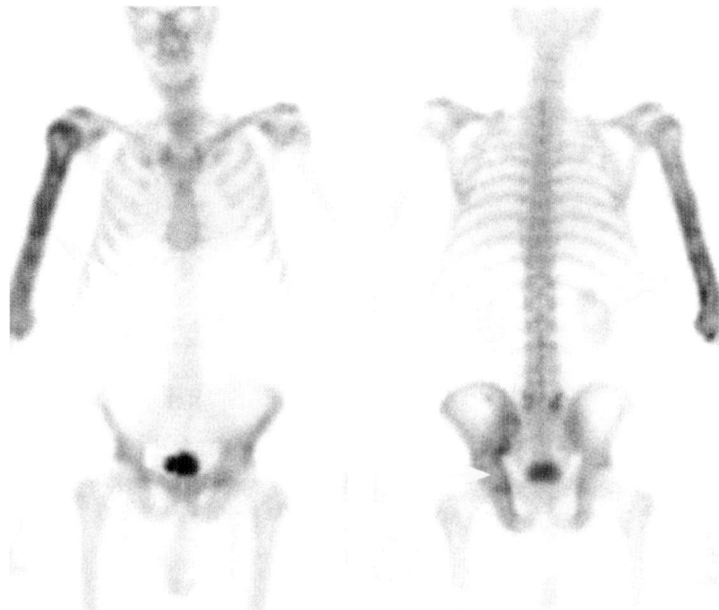

Paget disease: Anterior (left image) and posterior projections from a Tc-99m MDP bone scan (20 mCi administered) show heterogeneously increased radiotracer uptake involving the right humerus, and to a lesser extent the left hemipelvis, best seen on the posterior projection (arrows).

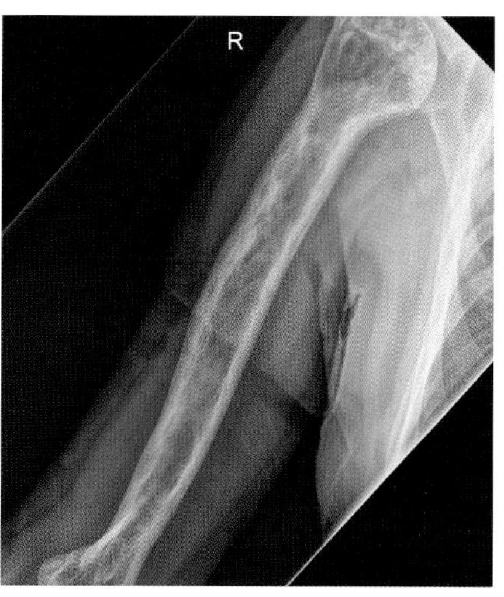

Radiograph of the right humerus shows cortical and trabecular thickening.

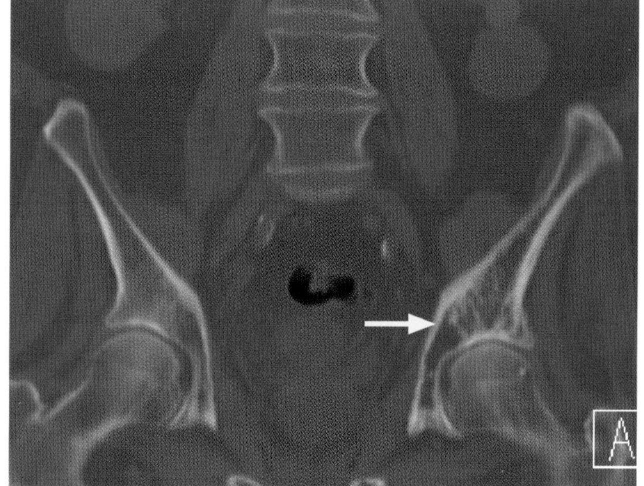

Coronal CT of the pelvis shows asymmetric coarsened trabecular thickening of the left ilium (arrow).

- Paget disease is an idiopathic disturbance of osteoclastic and osteoblastic regulation. Paget has three discrete phases: lytic, mixed, and sclerotic. The lytic (early) phase is typically positive on bone scan and often negative on radiography. The mixed phase is abnormal on bone scan and radiography. The sclerotic phase shows persistent radiographic changes, but the bone scan activity may subside.
- One complication of Paget disease is malignant degeneration to osteosarcoma. A focal cold lesion should raise concern for necrosis in a region of malignant degeneration, although this may be best appreciated by evaluating serial studies.

Complex regional pain syndrome (reflex sympathetic dystrophy)

- Complex regional pain syndrome, previously called reflex sympathetic dystrophy, causes persistent pain, tenderness, and swelling often due to minor trauma.
- Bone scan shows diffusely increased juxta-articular activity in multiple small joints of the hand or foot on delayed (skeletal) images. Blood pool and soft tissue phase uptake is variable, but most commonly both phases are increased.

RADIOTRACERS

Tc-99m DTPA

- DTPA can measure glomerular filtration rate (GFR) and evaluate renal perfusion.
- DTPA is excreted by glomerular filtration. Approximately 20% is extracted by the glomerulus into the tubules with each pass. This is the identical extraction fraction as inulin, which is used to measure GFR exactly.

Tc-99m MAG3

- MAG3 can estimate renal plasma flow and evaluate renal perfusion; however, MAG3 cannot measure GFR.
- MAG3 is filtered and excreted by the tubules. Greater than 50% is extracted by the glomerulus into the tubules with each pass. MAG3 is cleared predominantly by the proximal tubules with minimal filtration. It has a higher extraction fraction than DTPA, which provides better images in patients with renal insufficiency or obstruction.

Tc-99m DMSA

- DMSA scanning is performed in children to evaluate for the presence of renal scarring associated with pyelonephritis. The collecting system is not imaged.
- DMSA is a specialized cortical agent. It is bound in the renal tubules, which allows anatomic imaging of the cortex. It is the only renal tracer where SPECT imaging is performed.

CLINICAL APPLICATIONS OF RENAL IMAGING

Renogram

- A nuclear renogram is a time–activity curve that provides a graphical representation of renal uptake and excretion. Approximately 10 mCi Tc-99m MAG3 (most commonly) or DTPA is administered. A normal renogram has three phases: The flow phase (sharp upslope), cortical function phase (defined peak), and clearance phase (rapid excretion).

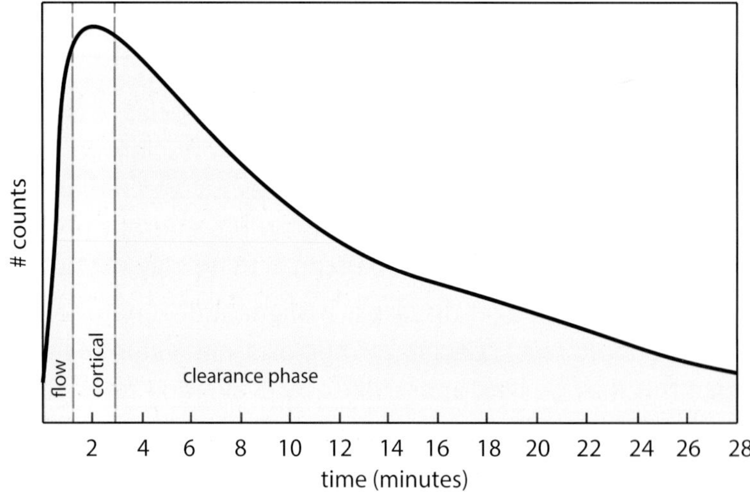

A slow upslope of the flow phase suggests decreased perfusion.

The cortical function phase is the peak of the renogram, and usually occurs in the first 1–3 minutes. Decreased renal function produces delayed cortical uptake.

The clearance phase is characterized by urine excretion into the pelvicalyceal and collecting system, which usually begins after 3 minutes. Lack of pelvicalyceal clearance suggests hydronephrosis.

- A positive ACE renogram is relatively specific for renal artery stenosis, which may be a cause of hypertension. The radiotracer is Tc-99m MAG3, much less commonly Tc-99m DTPA.
- In compensated renal artery stenosis, decreased blood to the glomerulus stimulates renin → angiotensin I → angiotensin II. Angiotensin II constricts the efferent (outgoing) arterioles to restore GFR. Angiotensin I is converted to angiotensin II by angiotensin converting enzyme.

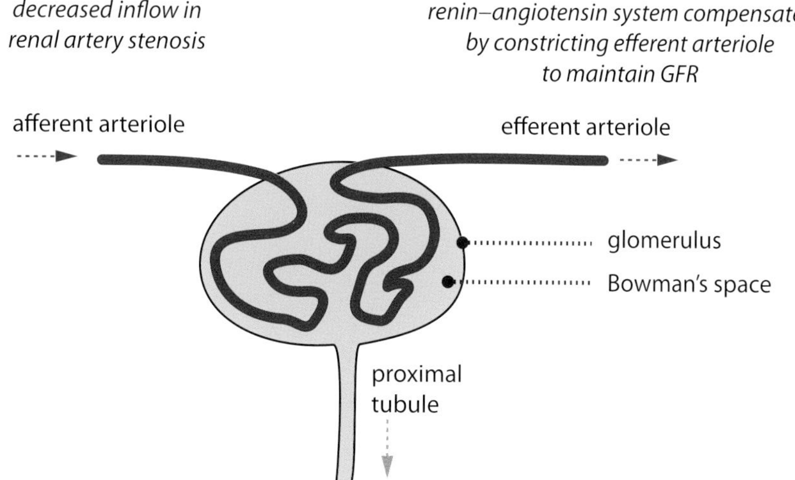

- After administration of an ACE inhibitor (typically captopril, 25–50 mg), the efferent arterioles will relax and GFR will decrease.

  If a patient is already on an ACE inhibitor, it should be stopped for 48 hours to 1 week prior to the exam.

  Intravenous access should be maintained in case fluid resuscitation is needed to treat hypotension.

- A positive study depends on radiotracer (MAG3 or DTPA), but the hallmark is a post-ACE inhibitor renogram that becomes abnormal or more abnormal.

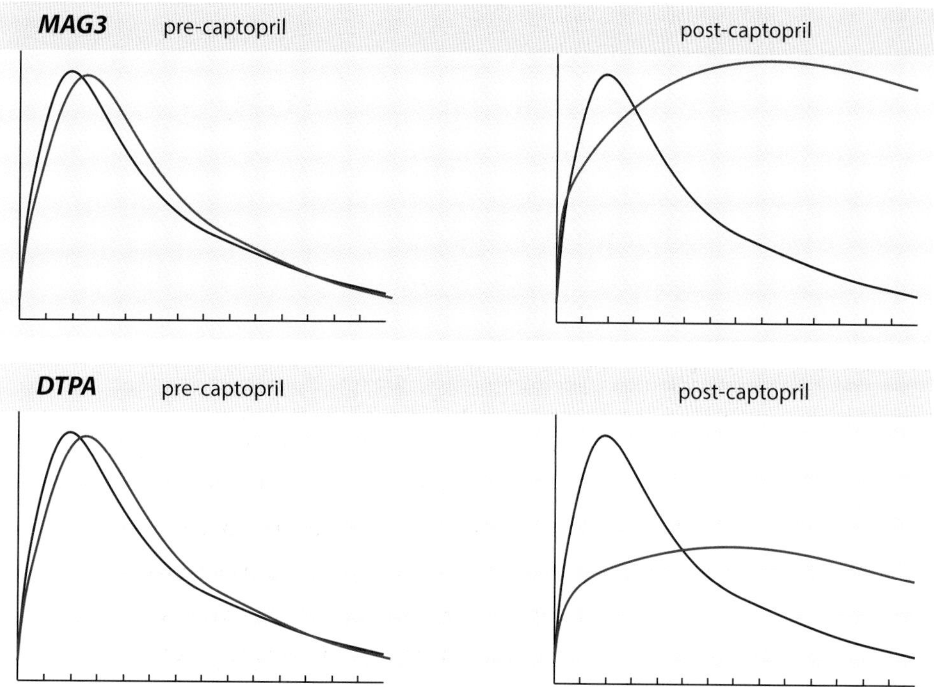

MAG3 (tubular agent): Uptake and secretion are generally preserved even with a reduced GFR, but further ↓ GFR results in ↓ urine production and ↓ washout of secreted agent from collecting system.

Positive criteria for MAG3 study include: <40% uptake by one kidney at 2–3 minutes; difference in cortical activity by 20%; or delay in time to peak activity of more than 2 minutes (compared to pre ACE inhibitor).

DTPA (glomerular agent): Unlike MAG3, ↓ GFR causes diminished uptake and excretion of DTPA.

Diuretic renogram

- If hydronephrosis is present, a diuretic renogram can distinguish between obstruction and a nonobstructive cause of collecting system dilation. Both renal function and urodynamics are evaluated. The radiotracer is Tc-99m MAG3, much less commonly Tc-99m DTPA.
- After approximately 20 minutes of imaging, 40 mg IV lasix is administered. A higher dose of lasix may be needed in patients with renal insufficiency. After administration of lasix, a fixed mechanical obstruction will show no change in the renogram curve. However, in causes of non-obstructive hydronephrosis, the additional pressure of the diuresed kidney will open up the collecting system and allow drainage of radiotracer from the kidney.

  After administration of lasix, a clearance half-time <10 minutes is normal, 10–20 minutes is borderline, and >20 minutes suggests obstruction.
- False positives (diuretic renogram is positive for obstruction in the absence of a true obstruction) can be seen in dehydration, distended bladder, or renal failure (decreased response to diuretics).

Renal cortical imaging

- Renal cortical imaging is limited to renal imaging in children to evaluate for pyelonephritis or scarring. The radiotracer is Tc-99m DMSA.
- A normal DMSA study excludes the diagnosis of acute pyelonephritis.
- A positive study for pyelonephritis can have three patterns:

  Focal cortical defect, multifocal cortical defects, or diffusely decreased radiotracer.

Radionuclide cystography (RNC)

- Radionuclide cystography (RNC) is the most sensitive test for evaluation of pediatric reflux, with less radiation exposure compared to voiding cystourethrogram.
- The radiotracer chosen is variable. Tc-99m pertechnetate, Tc-99m DTPA, and Tc-99m sulfur colloid work well. Regardless of radiotracer chosen, the radionuclide is injected retrograde into the catheterized bladder.
- Grading of reflux:

  Minimal (RNC grade I): Reflux is confined to the ureter.

  Moderate (RNC grade II): Reflux extends superiorly to the pelvicalyceal system.

  Severe (RNC grade III): Severe reflux causing a tortuous ureter and/or dilated intrarenal system.

Whole-body imaging of neoplasm, infection, and inflammation

Radiotracers

I-123 MIBG

- I-123 MIBG is used to image pheochromocytoma in adults and neuroblastoma in children. To a lesser extent, MIBG is taken up by carcinoid, medullary thyroid carcinoma, and paraganglioma. I-131 MIBG can be used for therapy of neuroblastoma in children.
- Normal distribution is areas of sympathetic innervation, including salivary glands, heart, thyroid (although this is typically intentionally blocked with Lugol's solution to reduce thyroid dosimetry), liver, kidney, and bladder.

Indium-111 pentetreotide (Octreoscan)

- An Octreoscan study is primarily used to image carcinoid. Indium-111 is cyclotron-produced and decays by electron capture, emitting two photons at 173 and 247 keV. Its half-life is 67 hours. Pentetreotide is an analog of octreotide used to detect tumors with somatostatin receptors, including amine precursor uptake and decarboxylation (APUD) tumors.

- In clinical use, the most common applications of Indium-111 pentetreotide are evaluation of carcinoid or islet cell tumors. Pentetreotide is quite good for imaging gastrinoma, with relatively reduced sensitivity for insulinoma.
- Although uncommonly performed, glomus tumors of the head and neck (extra-adrenal pheochromocytomas) are seen better with Indium-111 pentetreotide compared to MIBG.
- Normal distribution is intense renal and splenic uptake, with slightly less hepatic uptake.

MIBG versus pentetreotide (octreotide)

- MIBG is generally considered the first line agent for adrenal pheochromocytoma, as the normal renal uptake of pentetreotide may obscure an adrenal lesion. Pentetreotide can be considered as a second line agent for pheochromocytoma if the MIBG scan is negative.
- For evaluation of extra-adrenal pheochromocytoma (i.e., paraganglioma or glomus tumor), MIBG and pentetreotide are roughly equivalent.

Gallium-67

- Gallium-67 is cyclotron-produced and decays by electron capture, with a half-life of 78 hours. It emits multiple gamma rays at 93, 184, 296, and 388 keV (easier to remember as 90, 190, 290, and 390 keV). Gallium binds to transferrin, which is found in infection, inflammation, and neoplasm.
- Normal gallium distribution is high activity in bowel and colon, and less in liver, skull, bone marrow, and salivary glands. Use is limited in the abdomen due to high bowel and liver activity.
- Persistent gallium in the kidneys is never normal after 24 hours and signifies renal disease.
- Diffuse pulmonary uptake is also not normal, with a wide differential of infectious and inflammatory conditions:

  Pneumocystis pneumonia, idiopathic pulmonary fibrosis, sarcoidosis, lymphangitic carcinomatosis, miliary tuberculosis, and fungal infection.
- The *panda* sign represents increased uptake of gallium in the nasopharynx, parotid glands, and lacrimal glands due to inflammation, resembling the dark markings on a panda's face. Classically the *panda* sign is due to sarcoidosis.

  The panda sign is not specific for sarcoidosis, although it strongly suggests sarcoid when the λ sign is also seen (due to bilateral hilar and right paratracheal adenopathy). Sarcoid is also the most common disorder to affect the salivary and lacrimal glands symmetrically.

  The differential diagnosis of the panda sign includes Sjögren syndrome, lymphoma after irradiation, and AIDS.

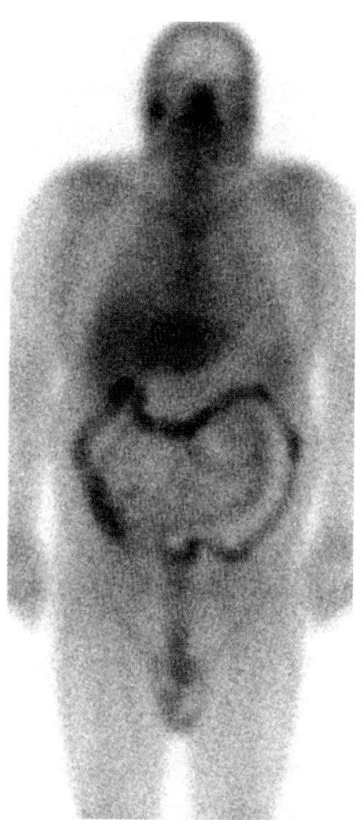

Normal Gallium-67 scan (5.25 mCi administered) shows high uptake in the bowel and salivary glands, moderate uptake in the liver and bone marrow, and faint uptake in the lungs.

- Gallium scans have been largely replaced by PET-CT. A residual first-line application of gallium scan is the evaluation of spinal osteomyelitis.

Thallium-201

- Thallium-201 is cyclotron-produced, decays by electron capture, and produces relatively low-energy characteristic X-rays of 69–81 keV. Its half-life is 73 hours. The normal distribution of thallium demonstrates prominent uptake in the kidneys, heart, liver, thyroid, and bowel.

- Thallium imaging is infrequently used due to its long-half life and resultant high radiation exposure. Historically, thallium has been used in combination with a gallium scan to distinguish between Kaposi sarcoma, lymphoma, and tuberculosis in immunocompromised patients. Thallium was also historically used as a myocardial agent, as previously discussed.

Indium-111 oxine leukocytes (WBCs)

- The normal distribution of indium-111 labeled WBCs is spleen > liver >> bone marrow.
- Infection imaging with an indium-111 WBC scan is performed at 24 hours.
- The key advantage of indium-111 oxine WBCs compared to gallium is the lack of physiologic bowel accumulation, which allows evaluation of abdominal or bowel infection/inflammation.
- Disadvantages compared to gallium include a tedious labeling procedure, higher radiation dose, and less accuracy in diagnosing spinal osteomyelitis.
- Advantages of indium-111 white blood cell scan compared to Tc-99m HMPAO include absence of interfering bowel and renal activity, ability to perform delayed imaging, and ability to perform simultaneous Tc-99m sulfur colloid or Tc-99m MDP bone scan. These combined approaches are very helpful for evaluation of osteomyelitis in the setting of a baseline abnormal bone scan (e.g., prosthesis evaluation), discussed below.

Tc-99m HMPAO leukocytes (WBCs)

- The advantages of a white blood cell scan labeled with Tc-99m HMPAO compared to indium-111 are related to the shorter half-life of Tc-99m, which allows a higher administered activity, better counts, a lower absorbed dose, and ability to perform earlier imaging. For these reason, Tc-99m is often preferred in children in appropriate cases.
- However, a major disadvantage is physiologic uptake within the gastrointestinal and genitourinary tracts due to unbound Tc-99m HMPAO complexes, which limits bowel evaluation. Renal activity occurs early, while bowel activity is seen after 1–2 hours. Additionally, delayed imaging is less practical with Tc-99m due to its shorter half-life.

Clinical Applications

Hepatocellular carcinoma (HCC)

- Historically, increased focal gallium uptake in the liver suggests hepatocellular carcinoma (HCC). Conversely, HCC is extremely unlikely if gallium uptake is diminished.

Combined gallium and thallium imaging

- Kaposi sarcoma is thallium avid, but does not take up gallium. *Mnemonic: KaT (Kaposi is Thallium avid).*
- Tuberculosis and atypical mycobacteria take up gallium but not thallium. This is the opposite of Kaposi sarcoma. *Mnemonic: TuG (Tuberculosis is Gallium avid).*
- Lymphoma takes up both gallium and thallium. *Mnemonic: Lymphoma likes both.*

Osteomyelitis

- A positive triple-phase Tc-99m MDP bone is only specific for osteomyelitis if the radiograph is normal. If there is an underlying abnormality, gallium or WBC scan can increase specificity.
- Gallium imaging can increase specificity of a positive bone scan, especially for vertebral osteomyelitis and discitis.
- A WBC scan (typically with indium-111) can increase specificity in evaluation of an infected orthopedic prosthesis, where scanning is typically performed in conjunction with Tc-99m sulfur colloid. When comparing the two scans (WBC and sulfur colloid),

a discordant region with increased WBC tracer uptake and decreased sulfur colloid uptake is suggestive of marrow replacement by WBCs, consistent with osteomyelitis. Conversely, a region of normal marrow would be expected to demonstrate uptake both by WBCs and sulfur colloid.

Extra-adrenal pheochromocytoma

- The sensitivity of I-123 MIBG for detection of extra-adrenal pheochromocytoma ranges from 63–100%, with potential loss of MIBG uptake seen in tumor cell dedifferentiation, altered membrane transport proteins, or interference by medications. Indium-111 pentetreotide is also an option.
- The role of F-18 FDG PET in the evaluation of metastatic extra-adrenal pheochromocytoma is evolving. Most tumors are FDG avid.

Metastatic carcinoid/neuroendocrine tumor

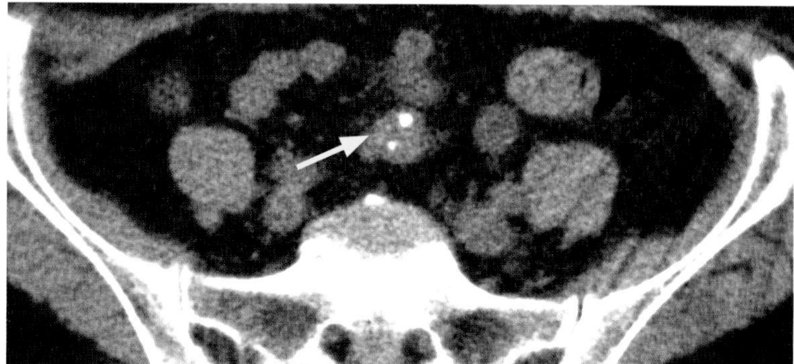

Metastatic carcinoid: Axial non-contrast CT shows a mesenteric mass containing coarse calcification (arrow) in the central lower-abdomen, which has a typical appearance for carcinoid.

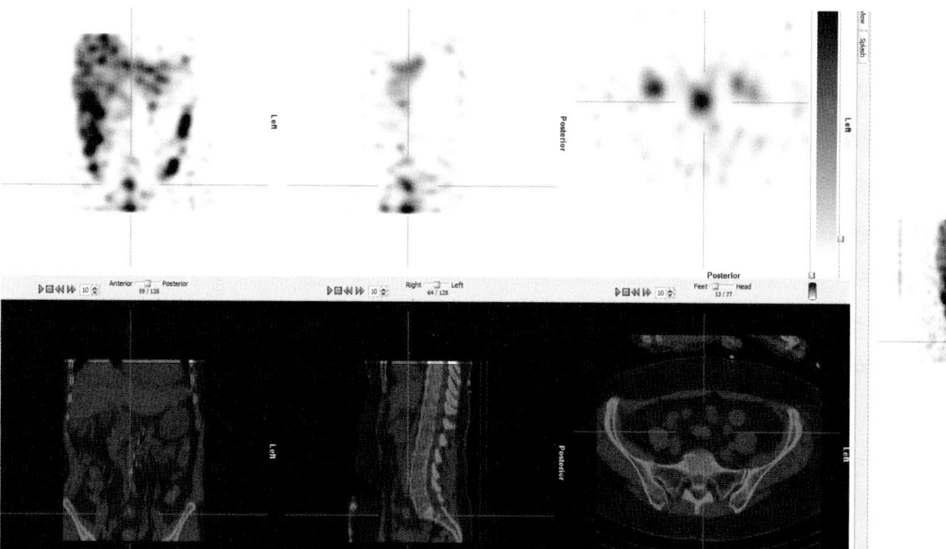

Fused multiplanar SPECT (top row) from an indium-111 pentetreotide scan and CT (bottom row) correlate a focus of increased uptake in the lower abdomen with the calcified mesenteric mass on CT, confirming the diagnosis of neuroendocrine tumor/carcinoid. All other foci of tracer uptake seen on SPECT are localized to bowel, representing physiologic bowel uptake.

- Indium-111 pentetreotide (Octreoscan) is the tracer of choice for evaluation of carcinoid tumor. SPECT is almost always performed.
- The sensitivity for detecting neuroendocrine tumors is 82–95%; however, specificity is only around 50%, especially when a "hot spot" is found near a region of physiologic uptake in the pituitary, thyroid, liver, spleen, urinary tract, or bowel. False positives can also occur in benign processes such as inflammation, Graves disease, and sarcoidosis. These inflammatory false positives are thought to be due to octreotide receptors expressed in activated lymphocytes.

Cerebrovascular

Radiotracers

Tc-99m DTPA

- Tc-99m DTPA is a transient perfusion agent. There is no uptake within the brain parenchyma as it does not cross the blood brain barrier. DTPA is used for planar imaging only and is uncommonly used.

Tc-99m HMPAO/Tc-99m ECD

- Both HMPAO and ECD are perfusion agents that cross the blood brain barrier. To be retained in the cell, ECD is enzymatically modified. In contrast, HMPAO simply needs to be protonated to be trapped. Thus, ECD is only taken up by living cells while HMPAO uptake is a marker of perfusion. In the evaluation of subacute infarct, the phenomenon of luxury perfusion can cause HMPAO uptake to increase (due to increased perfusion), while ECD will show the true defect representing the infarct core.
- Of these two agents, ECD is generally preferred for brain imaging. Compared to HMPAO, ECD has more rapid blood pool clearance, better shelf life, more accurate characterization of perfusion, and is only taken up by living cells.
- Both tracers are used for SPECT imaging.

Clinical applications of cerebrovascular imaging

Brain death

- In brain death, intravenously injected radiotracer is unable to enter the cranial cavity due to increased intracranial pressure.
- Planar imaging is typically performed with either Tc-99m pertechnetate or Tc-99m DTPA. SPECT imaging may also be performed, either with HMPAO or ECD-labelled Tc-99m.
- Imaging shows no tracer perfusing the brain.
- The *hot-nose* sign represents increased collateral flow seen in brain death, but is not specific and may be seen in other abnormalities of cerebral perfusion.

Evaluation of cerebral perfusion

- Evaluation of cerebral perfusion reserve can be performed with an acetazolamide challenge. Normally, cerebral blood flow increases after administration of 1,000 mg acetazolamide, a carbonic anhydrase inhibitor.
- Areas of the brain that already have maximized their autoregulatory mechanisms will not show an increase in perfusion after acetazolamide administration. These areas will have relatively reduced activity compared to the rest of the brain.

Seizure imaging

- In general, seizure foci are hypermetabolic during a seizure (ictal imaging), and hypometabolic between seizures (inter-ictal imaging).
- Neither Tc-99m HMPAO nor ECD undergo redistribution. Either radiotracer can be injected during the seizure or up to 30 seconds after the end of the seizure.

Dementia imaging

- Alzheimer disease typically shows symmetrically ↓ SPECT tracer in the posterior temporal and parietal lobes.
- Lewy body dementia appears similar to Alzheimer but also involves the occipital calcarine cortex.

- Multi-infarct dementia shows multiple asymmetric foci of decreased metabolism.
- Pick disease is characterized by decreased uptake in the frontal lobes and anterior portion of the temporal lobes.

Brain tumor recurrence versus radiation necrosis

- Nuclear medicine can aid in the differentiation of tumor recurrence versus radiation necrosis. Several protocols have been described. Regardless of the nuclear medicine tracer involved, image fusion with MRI is usually performed.
- Thallium-201 generally accumulates in malignant gliomas and not in post-treatment granulation tissue (i.e., thallium is not taken up by radiation necrosis). Thallium-201 uptake requires a living cell and blood brain barrier disruption. The degree of thallium-201 uptake can be graded in comparison to the scalp activity:

  Uptake <scalp is low; uptake between scalp and 2x scalp is moderate; and uptake >2x scalp is high.

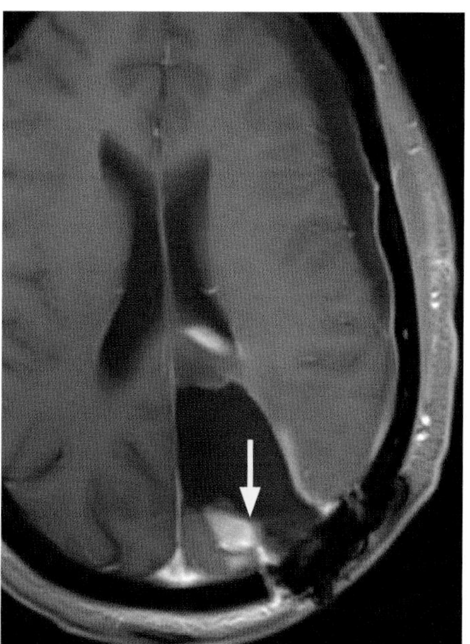

Axial T1-weighted post-contrast MRI shows a left parietal resection cavity with an enhancing nodule (arrow) along the posteromedial aspect of the resection cavity.

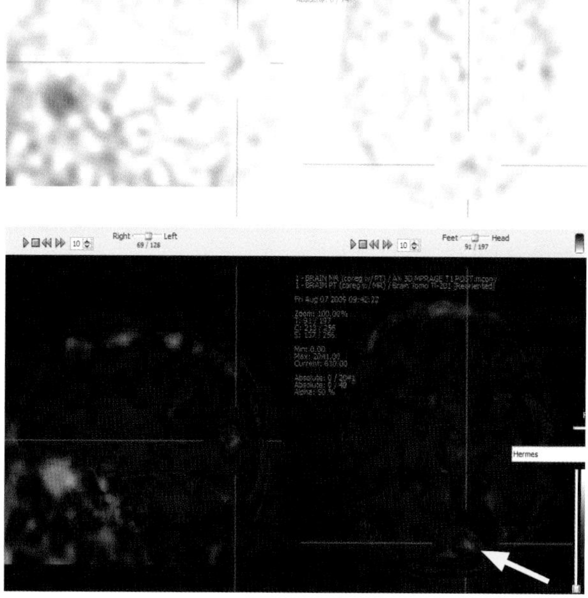

SPECT thallium-201 (top image) and fused SPECT-MRI (bottom image) show thallium uptake in the posteromedial aspect of the resection cavity correlating with the enhancing nodule seen on MRI (arrow). This pattern is suggestive of tumor recurrence.

Single-isotope thallium scan suggestive of tumor recurrence, with 4.4 mCi thallium-201 administered.

- Dual-phase F-18 FDG PET employs early and delayed imaging to evaluate a region of suspected tumor recurrence versus radiation necrosis. PET scanning is performed at 1 hour and 4 hours. Dual-phase PET has been shown to have increased accuracy for the assessment of recurrence versus post-treatment changes in metastatic disease compared to single-phase PET.

Crossed cerebellar diaschisis

- Crossed cerebellar diaschisis is a commonly encountered phenomenon in the presence of a supratentorial lesion (seen in tumors, stroke, and trauma), where the cerebellar hemisphere contralateral to the lesion shows decreased radiotracer uptake. This phenomenon is thought to be due to interruption of corticopontine–cerebellar pathways.

References, resources, and further reading

General Reference:

Mettler, F. and Guiberteau, M. Essentials of Nuclear Medicine Imaging, (5th ed.) Saunders/Elsevier. (2006).

PET-CT:

Adams, M.C. et al. A systematic review of the factors affecting accuracy of SUV measurements. AJR. American Journal of Roentgenology 195, 310-20(2010).

Bomanji, J.B., Costa, D.C. & Ell, P.J. Clinical role of positron emission tomography in oncology. The Lancet Oncology 2, 157-64(2001).

Kumar, R., Halanaik, D. & Malhotra A. Clinical applications of positron emission tomography-computed tomography in oncology. Indian Journal of Cancer 47, 100-19(2010).

Langer, A. A systematic review of PET and PET/CT in oncology: a way to personalize cancer treatment in a cost-effective manner? BMC Health Services Research 10, 283(2010).

Maisey, M.N. Overview of clinical PET. The British Journal of Radiology 75 Spec No, S1-5(2002).

Poeppel, T.D. et al. PET/CT for the staging and follow-up of patients with malignancies. European Journal of Radiology 70, 382-92(2009).

Saif, M.W. et al. Role and cost effectiveness of PET/CT in management of patients with cancer. The Yale Journal of Biology and Medicine 83, 53-65(2010).

Nuclear Cardiology:

Al-Mallah, M.H. et al. Assessment of myocardial perfusion and function with PET and PET/CT. Journal of Nuclear Cardiology 17, 498-513(2010).

Berman, D.S. et al. Comparative use of radionuclide stress testing, coronary artery calcium scanning, and noninvasive coronary angiography for diagnostic and prognostic cardiac assessment. Seminars in Nuclear Medicine 37, 2-16(2007).

Javadi, M.S. et al. Definition of vascular territories on myocardial perfusion images by integration with true coronary anatomy: a hybrid PET/CT analysis. Journal of Nuclear Medicine 51, 198-203(2010).

Thyroid Nuclear Imaging:

Griggs, W.-S. & Divgi, C. Radioiodine imaging and treatment in thyroid disorders. Neuroimaging Clinics of North America 18, 505-15, viii(2008).

GI Nuclear Imaging:

Chamarthy, M. & Freeman, L.M. Hepatobiliary scan findings in chronic cholecystitis. Clinical Nuclear Medicine 35, 244-51(2010).

Howarth, D.M. The role of nuclear medicine in the detection of acute gastrointestinal bleeding. Seminars in Nuclear Medicine 36, 133-46(2006).

Johnson, H. & Cooper, B. The value of HIDA scans in the initial evaluation of patients for cholecystitis. Journal of the National Medical Association 87, 27-32(1995).

Kalimi, R. et al. Diagnosis of acute cholecystitis: sensitivity of sonography, cholescintigraphy, and combined sonography-cholescintigraphy. Journal of the American College of Surgeons 193, 609-13(2001).

Pulmonary Nuclear Imaging:

Durán-Mendicuti, A. & Sodickson, A. Imaging evaluation of the pregnant patient with suspected pulmonary embolism. International Journal of Obstetric Anesthesia 20, 51-9(2011).

Kluetz, P.G. & White, C.S. Acute pulmonary embolism: imaging in the emergency department. Radiologic Clinics of North America 44, 259-71, ix(2006).

Shahir, K. et al. Pulmonary embolism in pregnancy: CT pulmonary angiography versus perfusion scanning. AJR. American Journal of Roentgenology 195, W214-20(2010).

Musculoskeletal Nuclear Imaging:

Helms, C., Hattner, R. & Vogler, J. Osteoid Osteoma: Radionuclide Diagnosis. Radiology 151, 779-84(1984).

Palestro, C.J., Love, C. & Schneider, R. The evolution of nuclear medicine and the musculoskeletal system. Radiologic Clinics of North America 47, 505-32(2009).

Van der Wall, H. et al. Radionuclide bone scintigraphy in sports injuries. Seminars in Nuclear Medicine 40, 16-30(2010).

Zuckier, L.S. & Freeman, L.M. Nonosseous, nonurologic uptake on bone scintigraphy: atlas and analysis. Seminars in Nuclear Medicine 40, 242-56(2010).

Brain Nuclear Imaging:

Fougère, C. et al. PET and SPECT in epilepsy: a critical review. Epilepsy & Behavior 15, 50-5(2009).

Silverman, D.H.S. et al. Positron emission tomography scans obtained for the evaluation of cognitive dysfunction. Seminars in Nuclear Medicine 38, 251-61(2008).

8 Breast imaging

Contents

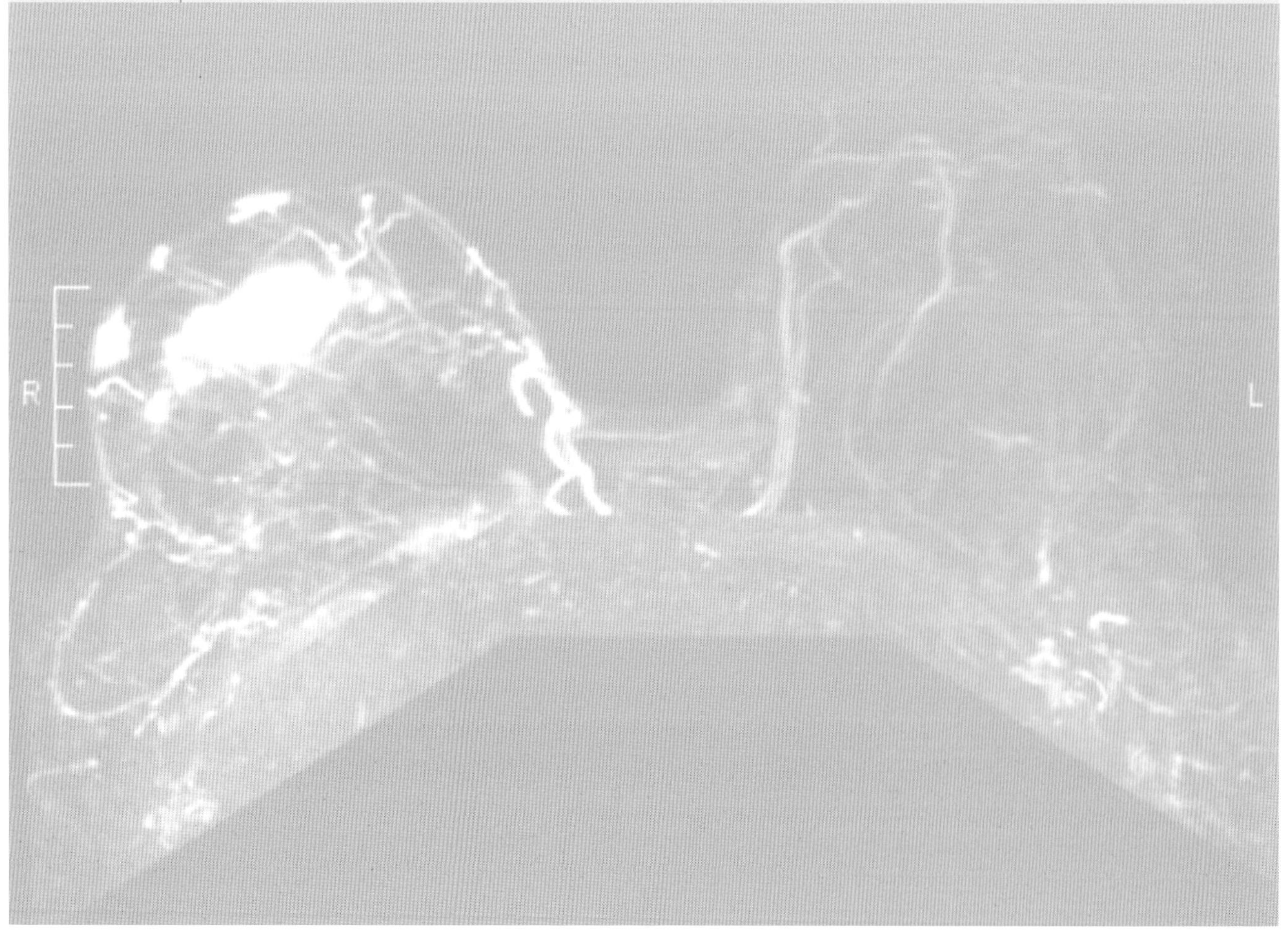

Imaging breast cancer: Key facts

- Breast cancer is the most common female cancer in the United States. The average woman has a one in eight chance of being diagnosed with breast cancer during her lifetime.
- Mammography is the first-line tool for detection of breast cancer; however, the sensitivity of screening mammography for detecting cancer has been estimated at between 68% and 90%, with the lower range of this scale true for mammographically dense tissues.

  Of note, diagnostic mammography (used to evaluate a patient with signs or symptoms suggestive of breast cancer) has a higher sensitivity, up to 93%.
- Ultrasound is a critical adjunct imaging modality to mammography, but ultrasound is not used for screening. The indications for performing breast ultrasound are characterization of palpable abnormalities, further characterization of mammographic findings, first-line evaluation of a breast abnormality in a young (under age 30), pregnant, or lactating woman, guidance for interventional procedures, and evaluation of breast implants.
- MRI is an established breast imaging modality. The indications for breast MRI include screening in high-risk patients (greater than 20% lifetime risk of developing breast cancer), evaluation of extent of disease in a patient newly diagnosed with breast cancer, evaluation of neoadjuvant chemotherapy response, assessment for residual disease after positive surgical margins, evaluation for tumor recurrence, and evaluation for occult breast cancer in a patient with axillary metastases.

The pathway of invasive ductal breast cancer progression

- The current understanding of progression of ductal breast cancer is a multi-step transformation from normal cells to flat epithelial atypia (FEA), to atypical ductal hyperplasia (ADH), to ductal carcinoma in situ (DCIS), to invasive ductal carcinoma (IDC).

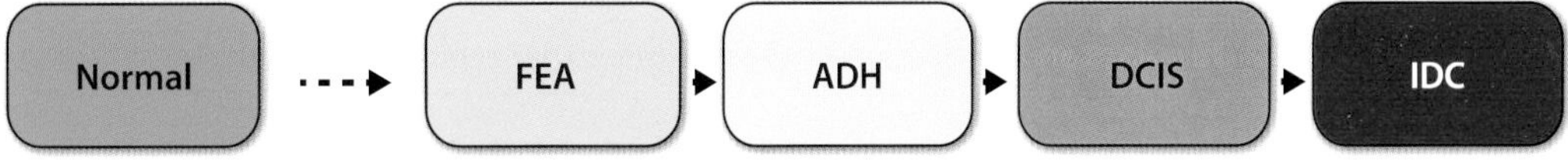

Although controversial, it has been suggested that some steps in this pathway may be reversible.

- ADH is intraductal proliferation with cytological atypia but without the definitive architectural or cytological abnormalities of DCIS. FEA is related to ADH and is characterized by abnormal ductal cells. FEA and ADH are considered non-obligatory precursor lesions; that is, the presence of ADH or FEA is an indicator of a higher risk of developing breast cancer, rather than an obligatory precursor towards invasive cancer.
- If a core biopsy shows FEA, excisional biopsy is advocated by several authors. 14% of patients with a core needle biopsy of FEA will be upstaged to DCIS or invasive carcinoma upon surgical excision.
- A core biopsy with pathology of atypical ductal hyperplasia (ADH) is followed by surgical excision. Approximately 18% of ADH diagnosed by core needle biopsy will be upstaged to either invasive carcinoma or DCIS upon surgical excision.
- Ductal carcinoma in situ (DCIS) is most often occult cancer detected mammographically and is treated surgically. Breast imaging plays an essential role in the diagnosis of DCIS as DCIS is typically asymptomatic and nonpalpable. Histologically, DCIS represents carcinoma contained within the duct, with an intact basement membrane surrounding the duct. Between 30% to 50% of patients with DCIS will develop invasive carcinoma within 10 years. Approximately 43% of DCIS diagnosed by ultrasound-guided core needle biopsy is upstaged to invasive carcinoma upon surgical excision.

Risk factors for developing breast cancer

- The two most important risk factors for breast cancer are female sex and advancing age. Other important risk factors for breast cancer include:

Risk factors for developing breast cancer

- Inherited BRCA1 or BRCA2 mutation. Women with an inherited mutation have greater than 50% chance (some believe as high as 80% chance) of developing breast cancer by age 80.
- First degree relative with breast cancer. In contrast, a non-first degree relative with postmenopausal breast cancer is not considered an increased risk.
- Prior chest radiation for Hodgkin or non-Hodgkin lymphoma.
- Long-term estrogen exposure, such as early menarche, late menopause, late first pregnancy, nulliparity, or obesity (through increased estrogen production by adipocytes).
- Prior biopsy result of a high risk lesion in the lobular neoplasia spectrum, including atypical lobular hyperplasia (ALH) and lobular carcinoma in situ (LCIS).

  Unlike ADH and FEA, which are high risk lesions in the ductal neoplasia spectrum, the high risk lesions in the lobular neoplasia spectrum are not treated with surgical excision.

  ALH and LCIS arise from the terminal duct lobule, can be distributed diffusely throughout the breast, and are considered a marker of increased risk rather than a precursor to invasive carcinoma. Women with LCIS have a 30% risk of developing invasive cancer (usually invasive ductal), which may occur in either breast.

Special histologic subtypes of invasive ductal carcinoma

- Breast cancer is a diverse spectrum of disease with varying histopathology and prognosis.
- The most common subtype of breast cancer is invasive ductal carcinoma (IDC), representing 70–80% of cases. It often presents as a palpable mass, usually with a classic mammographic appearance of a spiculated mass, architectural distortion, and pleomorphic calcifications.
- Combined, a number of less common subtypes make up less than 10% of all breast cancers. In general, these special subtypes have better prognosis than invasive ductal carcinoma not otherwise specified (IDC NOS).

Special subtypes of ductal breast cancer

- **Tubular carcinoma** is a low grade cancer that typically presents as a small spiculated mass. Prognosis is better than IDC NOS.

  It may be difficult for the pathologist to distinguish between radial scars/complex sclerosing lesions and tubular carcinoma, and it is thought that radial scar may be a precursor to tubular carcinoma.
- **Mucinous carcinoma** (synonyms: colloid carcinoma, mucoid carcinoma, and gelatinous carcinoma) typically is a low-density circumscribed mass that can mimic a fibroadenoma on ultrasound. On MRI, mucinous carcinoma usually appears hyperintense on T2-weighted images.
- **Medullary carcinoma** is a rare variant of breast cancer, typically seen in younger women, often with BRCA1 mutation. Medullary carcinoma is locally aggressive, but has a better prognosis than IDC NOS.
- **Papillary carcinoma** is the malignant form of an intraductal papilloma.
- **Adenoid cystic carcinoma** is a very rare breast cancer that presents as a palpable firm mass. Prognosis is excellent with complete resection.

Invasive lobular carcinoma

- Invasive lobular carcinoma comprises approximately 5–10% of breast cancer cases. Compared to invasive ductal carcinoma, invasive lobular is typically much more difficult to diagnose mammographically and clinically due to its tendency to spread through the breast tissue without forming a discrete mass.
- Invasive lobular carcinoma presents an imaging challenge due to its elusive appearance, which ranges from a one-view asymmetry to architectural distortion to a spiculated mass.

Inflammatory carcinoma

- Inflammatory carcinoma represents tumor invasion of dermal lymphatics.
- Clinically, inflammatory carcinoma presents with breast erythema, edema, and firmness.
- On mammography, the affected breast is larger and denser, with trabecular thickening and skin thickening. Occasionally, no discrete mass will be apparent. The primary differential consideration is a breast abscess; however, the clinical setting and exam will usually be able to differentiate.

Paget disease of the nipple

- Paget disease of the nipple is a form of DCIS that infiltrates the epidermis of the nipple.
- Clinically, Paget disease of the nipple presents with erythema, ulceration, and eczematoid changes of the nipple.

Breast cancer prognosis

- In non-metastatic breast cancer, axillary lymph node status is the most important prognostic factor, with the absence of nodal involvement offering the highest likelihood of cure. Similarly, survival is progressively worse with increased number of involved axillary nodes.

  The primary method to detect axillary involvement is a surgical sentinel lymph node biopsy, with a sensitivity of 93%. Sentinel lymph node biopsy is not routinely performed for DCIS unless necrosis or microinvasive disease is present.

  Surgical axillary lymph node dissection has a 99% sensitivity for detecting lymph node involvement. Lymph node dissection is performed if the sentinel lymph node is positive or not identified.

  Women with positive lymph nodes or with large tumors may benefit from neoadjuvant chemotherapy.

- The presence of tumor receptors affects prognosis. Patients with estrogen receptor (ER) and progesterone receptor (PR) positive tumors have longer disease free survival.

  Cancers with HER2/neu overexpression may respond to the monoclonal antibody trastuzamab (brand name Herceptin) or tyrosine kinase inhibitors such as lapatinib.

- Triple-negative cancers are ER, PR, and HER2/neu negative, are biologically aggressive, and portend a poor prognosis. Triple-negative cancers are seen most often in patients with BRCA1 mutation. It has been suggested that triple-negative cancers are a distinct phenotype of breast cancer. On imaging, triple-negative cancers may show benign features on mammography and ultrasound despite their aggressive nature. They are often round with smooth margins, without spiculations and calcifications, and are located posteriorly in the breast.

- There are several histologic subtypes of DCIS, with varying prognosis. A key factor to determine the prognosis of DCIS is the presence of necrosis.

  DCIS without necrosis (cribriform and micropapillary subtypes) is lower grade. Sentinel node evaluation is usually not indicated.

  DCIS with necrosis (poorly differentiated, comedo, and large cell subtypes) is higher grade. On mammography, the typical manifestation of high-grade DCIS is pleomorphic or fine linear branching calcifications, which are caused by calcification of necrotic debris in the duct lumen. Sentinel lymph node biopsy is often performed for high-grade DCIS.

Benign breast disease

Cyclical and proliferative breast disease

Fibrocystic change

- Fibrocystic change is an essentially normal pattern of breast physiology.
- Clinically, fibrocystic change presents as cyclical breast pain, sometimes with a palpable lump. Fibrocystic change is almost always seen in pre-menopausal women.
- Imaging findings are not specific and fibrocystic change is not ever a diagnosis made on imaging. Its only significance is that it may cause certain imaging abnormalities that instigate further workup, such as cysts and calcifications.

Sclerosing adenosis

- Sclerosing adenosis is a benign proliferative lesion caused by lobular hyperplasia and formation of fibrous tissue that distorts the glandular elements.
- Similar to fibrocystic change, the imaging importance of sclerosing adenosis is that it can mimic DCIS with microcalcifications.

Infectious and inflammatory breast disease

Mastitis

- Mastitis is infection of the breast, most commonly by *Staphylococcus aureus.* It is typically seen in nursing mothers (called *lactational* or *puerperal* mastitis) or in diabetic patients.
- Clinically, mastitis presents with breast pain, induration, and erythema.
- Imaging is usually not performed, but mammography or ultrasound can show focal or diffuse skin thickening, breast edema, and adenopathy.
- Treatment is antibiotics. If inadequately treated, mastitis can develop into a breast abscess.

Breast abscess

- A breast abscess is a walled-off purulent collection, typically from *S. aureus.*
- Clinically, breast abscess presents with focal breast pain, erythema, fluctuance, and fever, most commonly subareolar in location.
- On mammography, breast abscess appears as an irregular mass, which can mimic carcinoma based on imaging appearance alone.
- Ultrasound shows an ill-defined mass with heterogeneous echoes and irregular margins. An internal fluid level may be present. The primary differential consideration is inflammatory carcinoma; however, the clinical setting and exam will usually be able to differentiate.
- Treatment is ultrasound-guided aspiration in addition to antibiotics.

Granulomatous mastitis

- Granulomatous mastitis is a rare idiopathic noninfectious cause of breast inflammation that occurs in young women after childbirth.
- Granulomatous mastitis may be associated with breast feeding or oral contraceptives.
- The mammographic and sonographic features of granulomatous mastitis may mimic breast cancer and biopsy is usually warranted.

Periductal mastitis

- Periductal mastitis, also known as plasma cell mastitis, is caused by the irritating contents of intraductal lipids. It is seen in post-menopausal women and produces the classic mammographic appearance of large, rod-like secretory calcifications.

Diabetic mastopathy

- Diabetic mastopathy is a sequela of long-term insulin-dependent diabetes. An autoimmune reaction to matrix proteins from chronic hyperglycemia causes a firm and sometimes painful mass.
- On mammography, diabetic mastopathy can appear as an ill-defined, asymmetric density without microcalcifications.
- Ultrasound typically shows a hypoechoic mass or regional acoustic shadowing, mimicking the appearance of a scirrhous breast cancer.
- Because the mammographic and sonographic appearance can mimic breast cancer, core biopsy is required.

Mondor disease

- Mondor disease is thrombophlebitis of a superficial vein of the breast, most commonly the thoracoepigastric vein.
- Clinically, Mondor disease presents with pain and tenderness in the region of the thrombosed vein. A cordlike, elongated superficial mass may be present.
- Ultrasound shows a dilated, "bead-like" tubular structure with no flow on color Doppler.

Mammography

Screening mammography

- The goal of screening mammography is to detect pre-clinical breast cancer in asymptomatic women. Screening mammography detects 2 to 8 cancers per 1,000 women screened.
- Since 1990, the mortality from breast cancer has been steadily declining at a rate of approximately 2.2% per year, thought to be due to improvements in adjuvant therapy and screening mammography. The current American Cancer Society guidelines (2010) for screening mammography recommend annual screening for women over age 40 (or 10 years younger than a first degree relative with breast cancer).
- In 2009, the US Preventative Services Task Force (USPSTF) reclassified the evidence for screening of women age 40–49 from a class B (moderately strong evidence) to a class C (based on individual factors) recommendation, and also recommended reducing the screening interval between ages 50–74 to biannually. This has caused considerable controversy.
- Statistical models show that screening starting at age 40 (instead of age 50) would avert one additional death from breast cancer for every 1,000 women screened, with a resultant average of 33 life-years gained per 1,000 women screened.
- The potential concerns for mammographic screening include a very small risk of inducing breast cancer from radiation exposure, and risks of over-diagnosis including anxiety from false positives and unnecessary biopsies.
- No single randomized trial has shown a mortality reduction due to mammographic screening in women age 40–49; however, several meta-analyses *have* shown a reduction in breast-cancer specific mortality of 15–20%.
- It is generally accepted that women at 50–69 benefit from annual screening mammography, with a 14–30% reduction in breast-cancer mortality in those women participating in screening mammography.
- There are no strong data to support screening mammography in women over age 70.

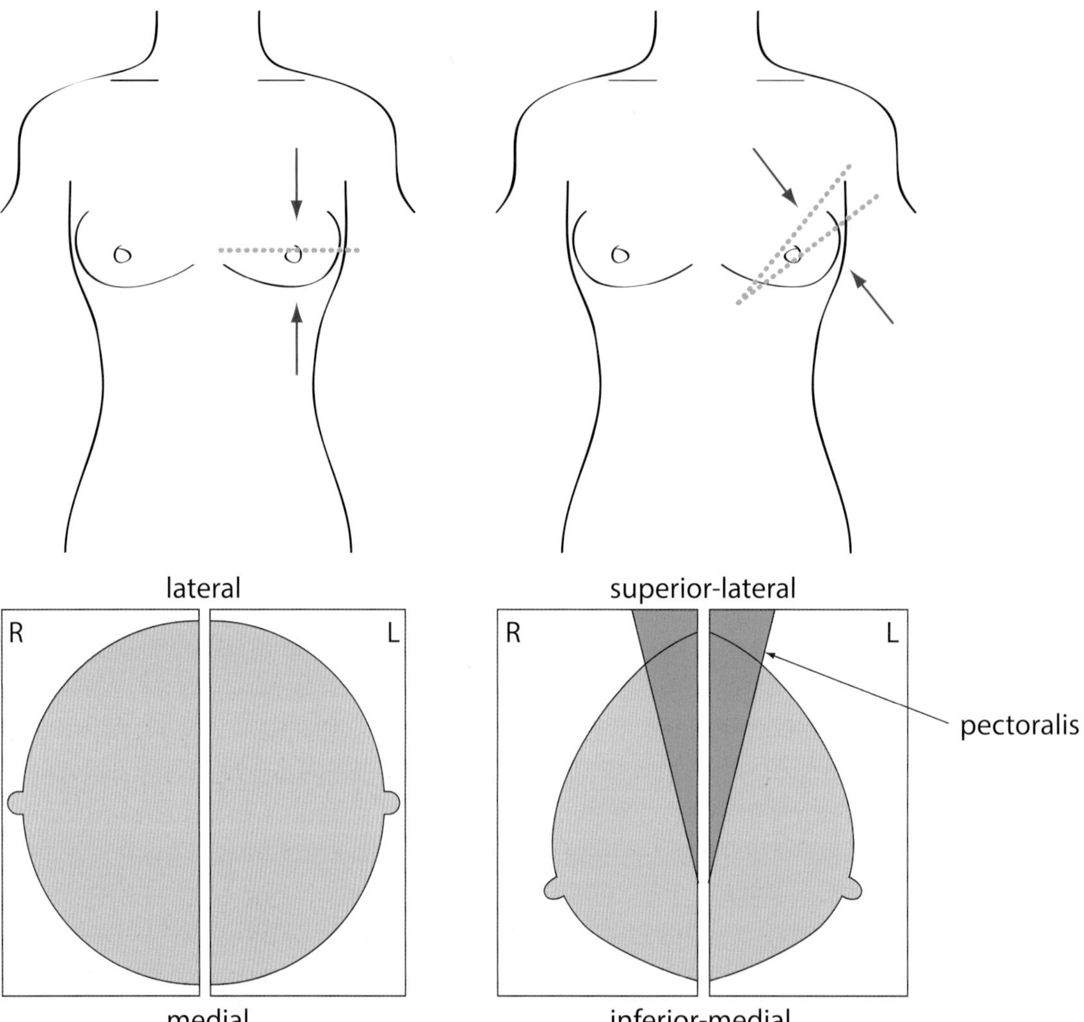

- The two standard mammographic views are cranio-caudal (CC) and medial-lateral-oblique (MLO).
- The cranio-caudal (CC) image plane is transaxial.
- The medial-lateral-oblique (MLO) image plane is approximately 45 to 60 degrees from the axial plane, paralleling the course of the pectoralis muscle heading into the axilla.

  The MLO view is ideal for screening, as it captures most of the breast tissue in a single view.

  Note that the superior-medial breast tissue may be excluded on the MLO view.
- At the technologist's discretion, additional views may be performed to image all of the fibroglandular tissue:

  Cleavage view (CV) images the medial breast tissue of both breasts.

  The **exaggerated CC (XCC)** view pulls either lateral or medial tissue into the imaging detector.

Online and offline screening

- Typically, most screening mammography is interpreted *offline,* where a batch of exams are reviewed in bulk some time after the films were taken.
- *Online* screening, where women have mammography performed and then wait to get a final report from the radiologist, leads to more imaging being performed and more false positives, with the same cancer detection rate.
- In contrast to screening mammography, all diagnostic mammography is performed "online" as a monitored exam with the patient staying for all possible imaging and the final results/recommendations before leaving.

Diagnostic mammography

Indications for diagnostic mammography

- Diagnostic mammography is usually performed for a breast problem (pain, lump, skin thickening, nipple discharge).
- Other indications of diagnostic mammography include annual mammography in an asymptomatic woman with a past history of breast cancer, short interval follow-up (following of BI-RADS 3 lesions), and evaluation of an abnormality found on screening mammogram.

Diagnostic mammography procedure

- Any mammographic abnormality is first localized in three-dimensional space, then worked-up with special problem-solving techniques, which are discussed later in this section.
- Often, ultrasound is added at the radiologist's discretion.
- Each patient waits until all imaging is completed before receiving a summary of the final interpretation and recommendations from the radiologist.

Approach to interpreting a mammogram

Evaluate image quality and adequacy

- The first step in evaluating a mammogram is to determine if the study is technically adequate.
- There should be adequate tissue imaged on both the CC and MLO views. The posterior nipple line is a line drawn from the posterior nipple to the pectoralis muscle – or edge of the film on the CC view if the pectoralis is not visualized. The posterior nipple lines drawn on the CC and MLO views should be within 1 cm of each other.

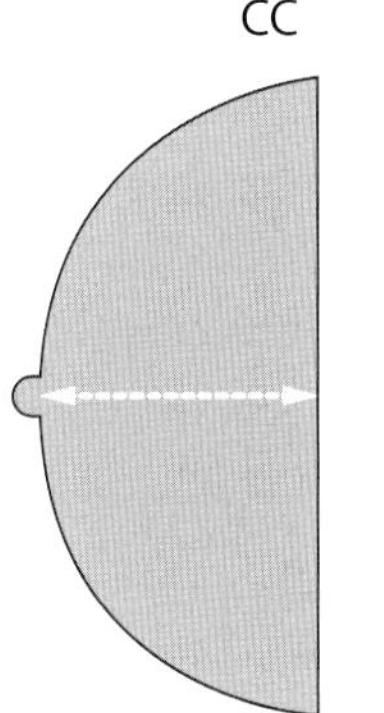

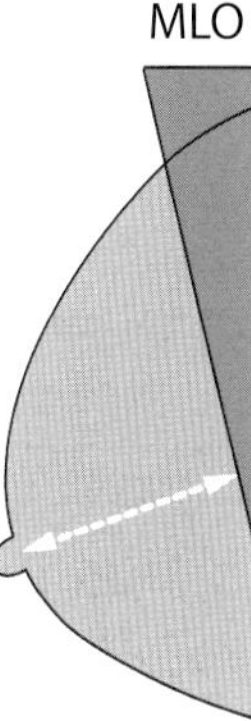

On the MLO view, the pectoral muscle should be visible at least to the level of the nipple.

- The image must be free from blur and artifacts. The trabeculae should be sharp; if blur is present, then benign calcifications can be mistaken for suspicious amorphous calcifications, and subtle calcifications can be missed entirely.
- The nipple of each breast should be in profile in at least one view.

Compare each side

- Each projection should be globally compared side-to-side to evaluate for symmetry.

Evaluate and magnify each image

- Each image should be carefully evaluated for signs of malignancy. The mammographic signs of malignancy are mass, calcification, architectural distortion, and asymmetry. Calcifications are best viewed at 1:1 or higher magnification, while architectural distortion is best seen when the whole breast is visualized.
- When viewing a digital mammogram, every portion of the image should be carefully evaluated at 1:1 zoom.

Compare to prior studies

- Even if a study appears unremarkable at first glance, comparison to prior exams can often reveal a subtle progressive change. For instance, an apparently normal island of parenchymal tissue may be slowly growing and represent malignancy.
- In general, it is best to carefully compare the previous exam from at least two years prior, to appreciated slowly growing changes.

THE MAMMOGRAPHIC REPORT

BI-RADS overview

- The breast imaging and reporting data system (BI-RADS) is a system for standardizing mammography reports that incorporates a strict lexicon, structured reporting, and clearly defined assessment categories.
- All mammographic, ultrasound, and breast MRI findings and reports should closely adhere to the BI-RADS lexicon and assessment categories.

Structure of the mammographic report:

- 1) History and indication for examination with patient risk factors stated.
- 2) List of comparison studies.
- 3) Description of the overall breast composition, using the following categories:

  The breast is almost entirely fat (<25% glandular).

  There are scattered fibroglandular densities (approximately 25%–50% glandular).

  The breast tissue is heterogeneously dense, which could obscure detection of small masses (approximately 51%–75% glandular).

  The breast tissue is extremely dense. This may lower the sensitivity of mammography (>75% glandular).

- 4) A clear description of any significant findings, including location.
- 5) Overall impression, with BI-RADS assessment category and course of action when appropriate.

BI-RADS ASSESSMENT CATEGORIES

Category 0: Need additional imaging

- Additional imaging evaluation (such as spot compression, magnification, special mammographic views, or ultrasound) and/or prior mammograms are necessary before a final assessment can be assigned.
- Category 0 is only appropriate for screening. All diagnostic mammography must conclude with a final assessment from 1–6.

Category 1: Negative

- Breasts are normal.
- Strictly speaking, if a finding is mentioned in the body of the report, then the final assessment should not be BI-RADS 1, no matter how benign the finding. Practically speaking, there is no management difference between BI-RADS 1 and 2, and often an insignificant finding (such as a past biopsy clip, breast implants, or some clearly benign calcifications) would not disqualify a report from being BI-RADS 1.

Category 2: Benign finding(s)

- A finding that is mentioned in the impression but that is definitely benign should technically be BI-RADS 2. No additional workup or follow-up is needed.

Category 3: Probably benign finding – short-interval follow-up recommended

- A finding placed in BI-RADS 3 should have <2% risk of malignancy.
- It is necessary to conduct a complete diagnostic imaging evaluation using diagnostic views (e.g., spot compression magnification, etc.) and/or ultrasound before assigning a probably benign (Category 3) assessment. Category 3 is never appropriate for screening mammography.
- According to the 4th Edition of BI-RADS (2003), Category 3 is not for palpable lesions. However, more recent data suggest that it is acceptable to assign appropriate palpable lesions as BI-RADS 3 after a full imaging workup.
- Action required: Short interval follow-up, typically 6 months. In general, if a benign-appearing lesion demonstrates 2 years of stability it can be considered benign (BI-RADS 2). Any interval change is suspicious and may warrant biopsy.

Category 4: Suspicious abnormality – biopsy recommended

- Findings are suspicious of malignancy, with a probability of being malignant >2% and <95%.
- Category 4 can be subdivided into Category 4A, 4B, and 4C, with 4A being least suspicious, and 4C being most suspicious.
- All recommendations for breast interventional procedures must be at least BI-RADS 4, including cyst or abscess aspiration.
- Action required: Biopsy or aspiration.

Category 5: Highly suggestive of malignancy – biopsy or direct surgical treatment recommended

- These lesions have a high probability (>95%) of being cancer. A lesion that a radiologist describes as "I'll eat my hat if that's not cancer!" should be classified as BI-RADS 5. The prototypical BI-RADS 5 cancer would look like a spiculated mass with fine pleomorphic/linear-branching calcifications.
- Action required: Biopsy or surgery.

Category 6: Known biopsy – proven malignancy – appropriate action should be taken

- This category is reserved for lesions identified on the imaging study with prior biopsy proof of malignancy. Typically, a plan of action is already in place.

Fibroglandular density

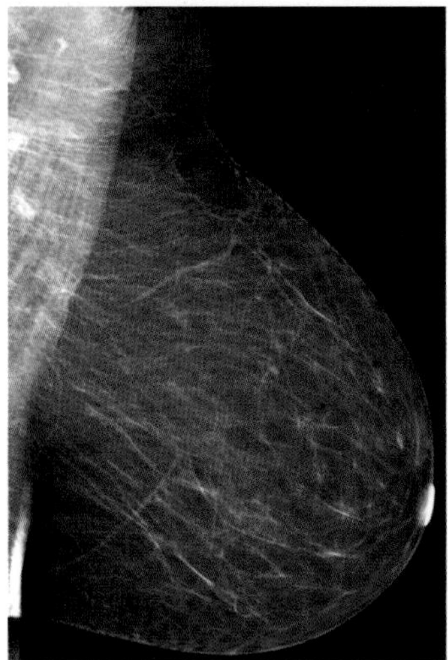

Almost entirely fat
(≤25% fibroglandular)

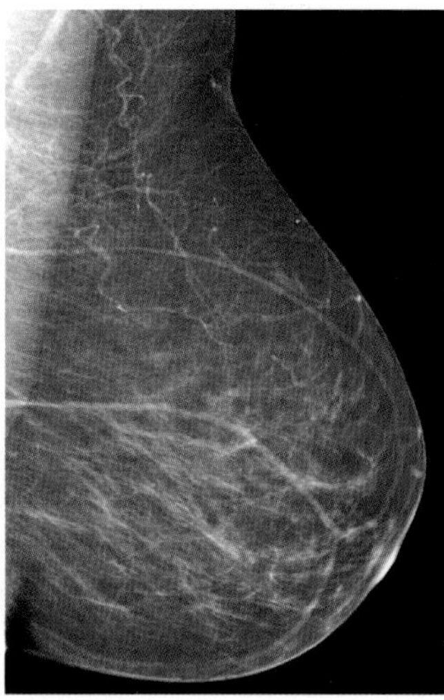

Scattered fibroglandular densities
(25%–50% fibroglandular)

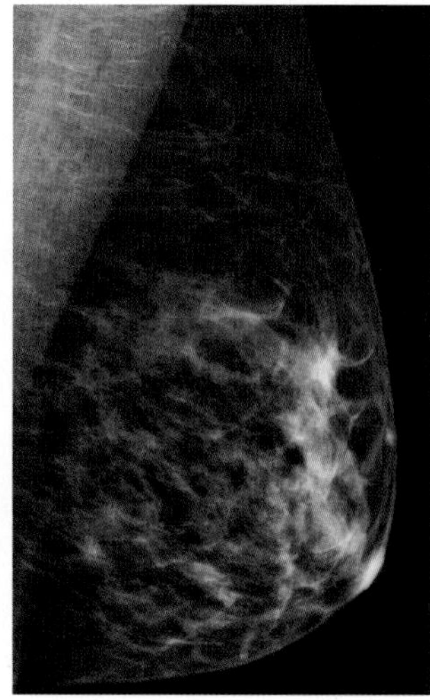

Heterogeneous fibroglandular densities
(51%–75% fibroglandular)

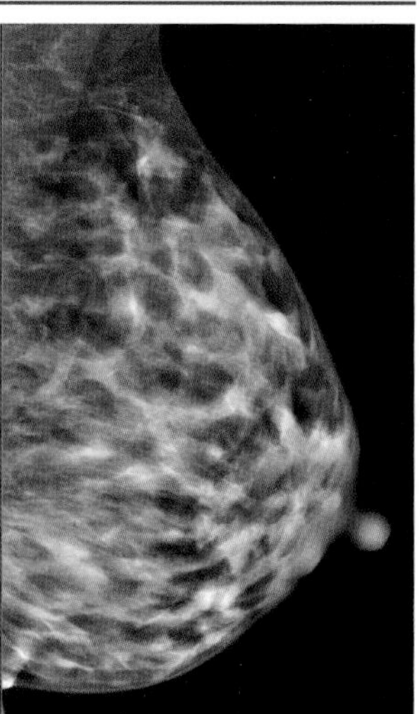

Extremely dense
(>75% fibroglandular)

- In every mammographic report, the mammographic pattern of fibroglandular density should be characterized into one of the above quartiles.
- Women with dense fibroglandular tissue have an increased risk of developing breast cancer, and detection of early cancer can be obscured by the fibroglandular tissue. A woman with extremely dense breasts has a 5x relative risk of breast cancer compared to a woman with almost entirely fatty breasts.
- Bilateral interval increase in fibroglandular density is usually benign and may be caused either by hormonal effects or breast edema. A unilateral increase in fibroglandular density is worrisome for lymphatic obstruction, which may be malignant.
- Edema due to systemic causes, such as congestive heart failure, typically causes bilateral trabecular blurring and skin thickening.
- Hormone therapy may cause an increase in fibroglandular density, without skin thickening. Proliferation of cysts and fibrocystic change can be seen, even in postmenopausal women.
- Pregnancy, lactation, and weight loss may all cause an interval increase in fibroglandular density.

Skin thickening

- Unilateral skin thickening can be due to either benign or malignant causes. Similar to changes in fibroglandular density, bilateral skin thickening is usually benign and the result of a systemic process.

Skin thickening: Benign causes

- Radiation therapy (usually unilateral).
- Acute mastitis (usually unilateral).
- CHF (fluid overload), renal failure (fluid overload due to protein wasting), and liver failure (fluid overload due to hypoalbuminemia) may all produce unilateral or bilateral skin thickening.

Skin thickening: Malignant causes

- Inflammatory carcinoma, which represents invasion of dermal lymphatics by cancer. A mammographic mass may be present.
- Locally advanced carcinoma.
- Lymphatic obstruction from axillary adenopathy.

MAMMOGRAPHIC MASSES USING THE BI-RADS LEXICON

Is the mass seen in more than one view?

- A mammographic mass is a space-occupying lesion with convex borders seen in two different projections. In contrast, an asymmetry is seen in one view only.

Evaluate past films: is it new?

- There are many different descriptors to characterize a mammographic mass using the BI-RADS lexicon, but regardless of morphology, the presence of a new mass is suspicious and must be evaluated fully.
- Conversely, a malignant-looking mass should still be regarded with suspicion even if it hasn't changed. Slow growing carcinomas, such as tubular carcinoma, can stay stable for years.
- A stable mass with all benign features is almost always regarded as benign.

Evaluate the margins, using the BI-RADS lexicon

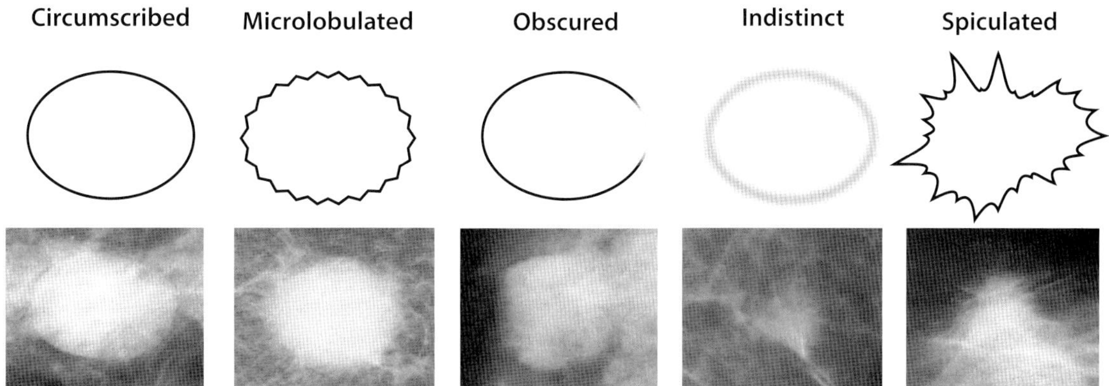

All images courtesy Christine Denison MD, Brigham and Women's Hospital.

- Careful evaluation of the margins of a mammographic mass at the interface with surrounding tissue is key to stratifying the suspicion for malignancy. The five BI-RADS terms used to describe the margins are circumscribed, microlobulated, obscured, indistinct, and spiculated.
- **Circumscribed**: At least 75% of the margin must be well-defined, while the remainder may be obscured with overlying tissue.

  In general, unless a mass is new, a circumscribed mass is benign and a non-circumscribed mass is suspicious. Of course, there are exceptions to this (abscesses can appear malignant and some indolent cancers in elderly women can appear benign).

- **Microlobulated**: A microlobulated mass has a finely irregular or serrated edge.
- **Obscured**: A margin is obscured if it is greater than 25% hidden by superimposed or adjacent normal tissue. The term obscured implies that the radiologist believes that the mass may be circumscribed, but the margin is hidden by overlying tissue.
- **Indistinct**: A poorly defined margin (or portion of the margin) raises concern that the lesion may be infiltrating.
- **Spiculated**: Linear densities radiate from a mass. A spiculated mass is malignant until proven otherwise.

Describe the density

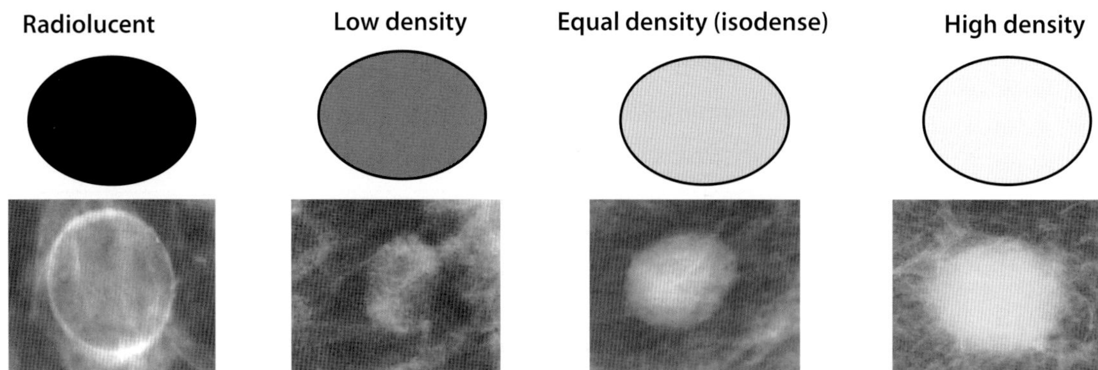

All images courtesy Christine Denison MD, Brigham and Women's Hospital.

- Most breast cancers that form a visible mass are of equal or higher density than the surrounding fibroglandular tissue. Cancers never contain fat, although theoretically it's possible for a breast cancer to engulf a benign fat-containing lesion.
- The BI-RADS lexicon for density includes **radiolucent** (fat density), **low density**, **equal density**, and **high density**. A circumscribed radiolucent mass is benign.

Describe the shape

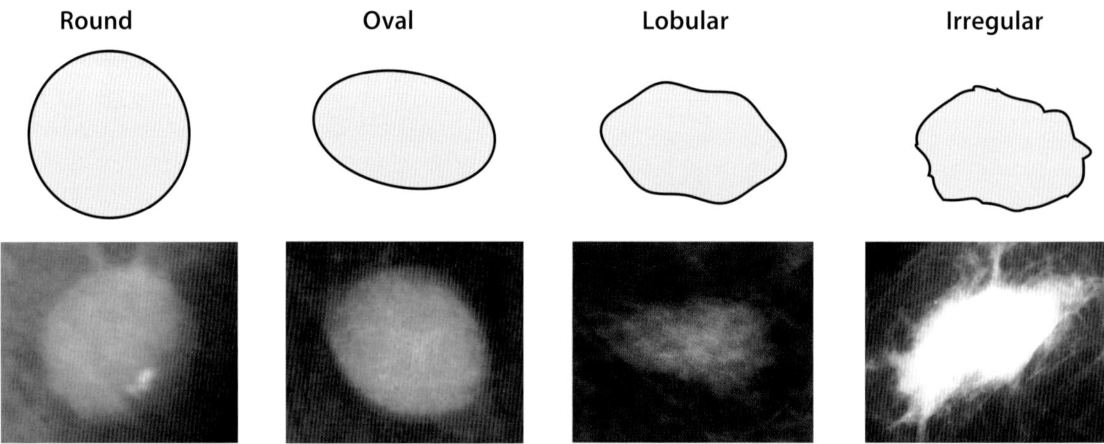

All images courtesy Christine Denison MD, Brigham and Women's Hospital.

- The BI-RADS lexicon for shape includes **round**, **oval**, **lobular** (undulating contour), and **irregular**. Although malignancy may be any form, an irregular mass is most suspicious for malignancy.

Describe the location, by naming the quadrant and (optionally) the depth

- The four quadrants of each breast are: Upper outer quadrant, upper inner quadrant, lower outer quadrant, and lower inner quadrant.
- When referring to the opposite breast, the *mirror opposite* quadrant is the contralateral quadrant with the same name. For instance, the upper outer quadrant of the left breast is the mirror opposite quadrant of the upper outer quadrant of the right breast.
- If *subareolar* or *axillary tail* are used to localize a lesion, then it is not necessary to specify a quadrant.
- Although clockface is used for ultrasound location, quadrant is preferred for mammography.

Measure the size

- Size alone is a poor predictor of malignancy, but determines whether a lesion is growing.

Look for associated features

- **Architectural distortion** represents radiating linear densities emanating from a central point, without a definite mass visible. Architectural distortion is caused by tethering of the normal fibroglandular tissue and is highly concerning for a cancer, although there are some benign causes. If there is no history of surgery or trauma, biopsy is appropriate.
- **Microcalcifications** may be associated with malignant ductal calcification.
- **Skin retraction** is most commonly postsurgical but may represent desmoplastic tumor reaction.
- **Nipple retraction** is tethering or angulation of the nipple. Retraction should not be confused with inversion (where the whole nipple points inwards). Nipple inversion may be developmental, bilateral, and is not necessarily a sign of malignancy if stable.
- **Skin thickening** may represent edema or may be secondary to prior radiation therapy.
- **Trabecular thickening** represents thickening of the fibrous septa of the breast, which can be seen in edema or in patients who have received radiation therapy.
- **Axillary adenopathy** may be normal or suspicious, depending on the morphology of the lymph nodes. Although it is normal for a few nodes to be present in the axilla, nodes with replacement of the normal fatty hilum may warrant evaluation, especially if new.

Example

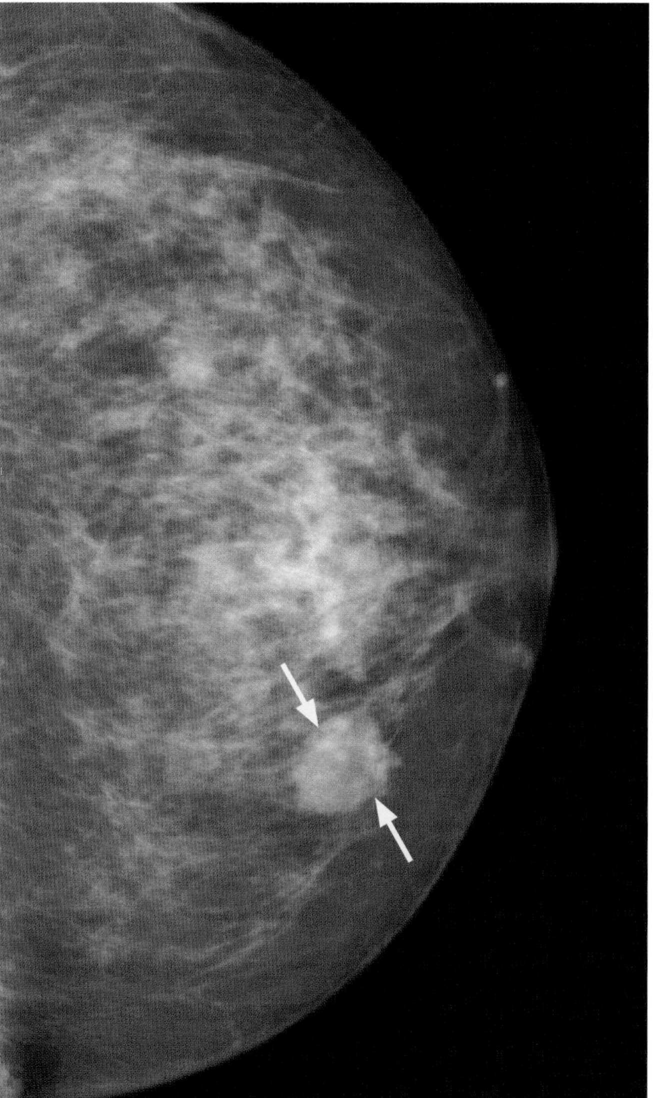

A new, equal density, round 2 cm mass (arrows) with microlobulated margins is seen in the medial breast on the CC view. There are no associated microcalcifications or architectural distortion.

The apparent microlobulated margin was shown to represent overlapping fibroglandular tissue on spot compression and ultrasound, and the true margins of the mass were felt to be circumscribed.

This mass was biopsied and was a benign fibroadenoma.

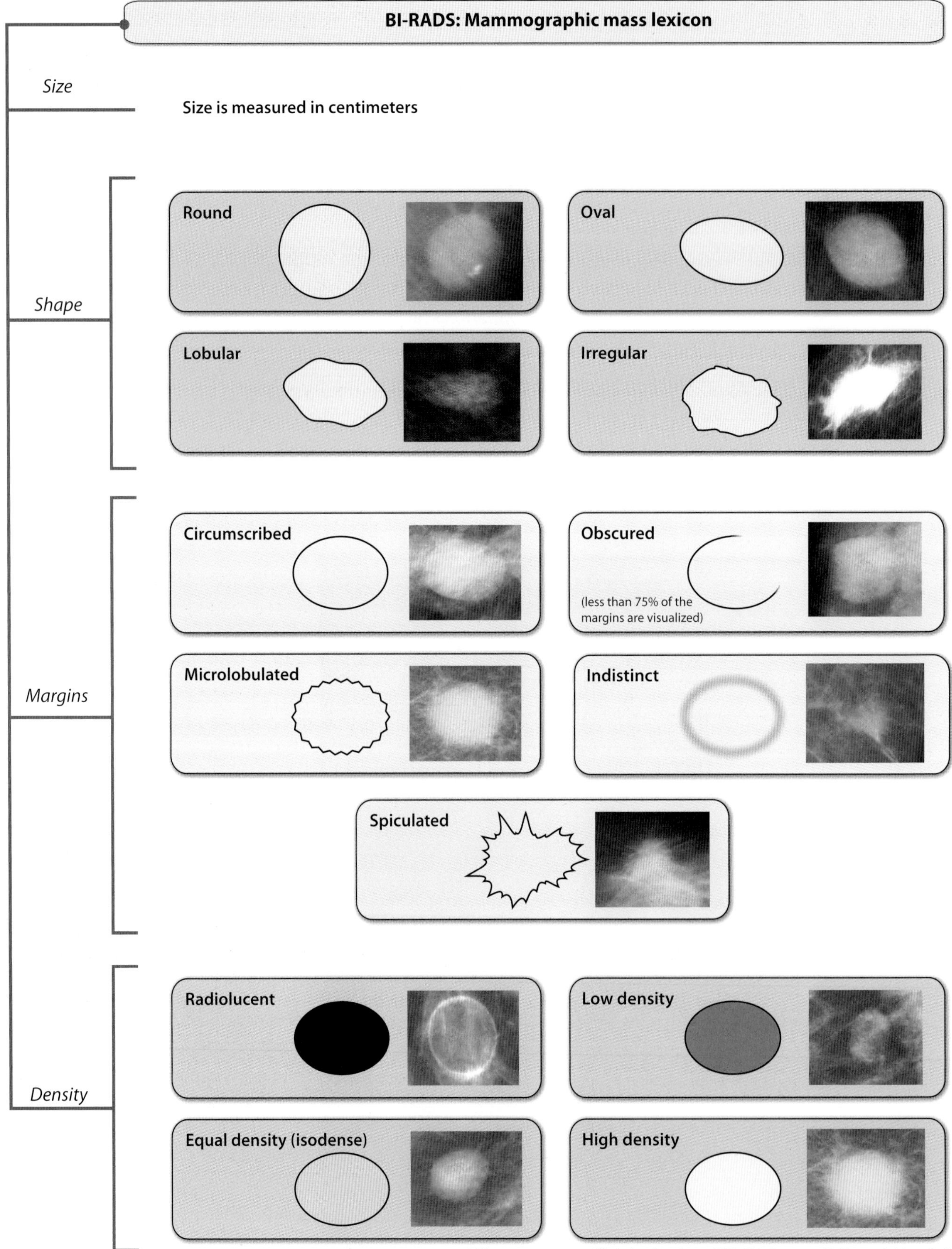

All images courtesy Christine Denison, MD, Brigham and Women's Hospital.

Overview of mammographic calcifications

Significance of mammographic calcifications

- Most mammograms will show calcifications, which are overwhelmingly likely to be benign. However, careful analysis of breast calcifications is essential. Abnormal calcification may be the earliest, and possibly the only, mammographic manifestation of cancer.
- Certain types of calcifications can be definitively characterized as benign, while some are highly suspicious for malignancy. Other morphologies are indeterminate.

Mammographic technique

- It is almost always necessary to perform spot compression *magnification* to characterize calcifications as either indeterminate or suspicious for malignancy. In contrast, most types of benign calcification can be described on routine full-field views (an exception would be milk of calcium calcifications, which generally require a true lateral view with magnification).
- Magnification employs air-gap technique and a small (0.1 mm) focal spot.

Benign calcifications (BI-RADS 2)

Skin calcifications

- Skin calcifications are associated with sweat glands, are usually punctate or lucent-centered, and are most common medially, where the concentration of sweat glands is higher.
- Skin calcifications in a small cluster may project over the breast and resemble suspicious calcifications. If skin calcifications are suspected, a tangential view should be performed. To perform a tangential view, the calcifications should be imaged using the alphanumeric needle localization grid. A BB is then placed over the calcifications as guided by the grid, and then the BB is imaged in tangent. On the tangential view, skin calcifications should be seen in the dermis immediately deep to the BB marker.

Vascular calcifications

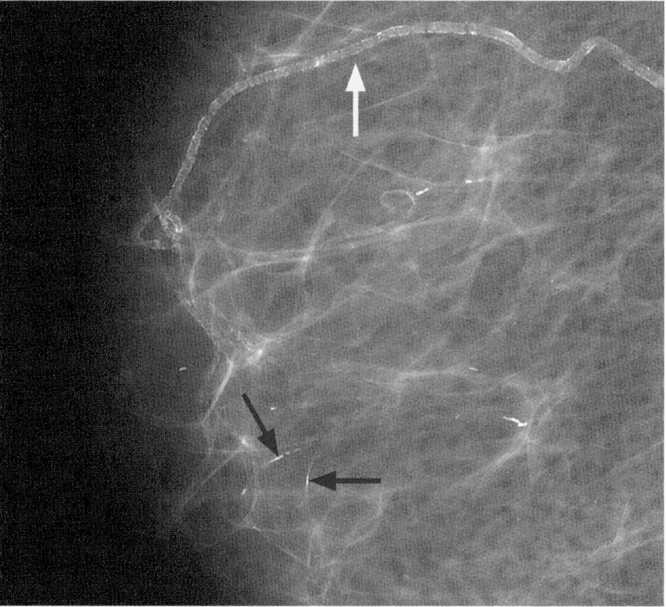

Vascular and secretory calcifications:

Arterial vascular calcifications are present in the upper portion of the image (yellow arrow), while large rod-like calcifications are present in the inferior portion of the image (red arrows).

Case courtesy Sughra Raza, MD, Brigham and Women's Hospital.

- Arterial vascular calcifications within the breast have a distinctive morphology and are typically not mentioned in the body of the report unless they are very extensive or the patient is very young.
- Early or incomplete vascular calcifications may pose a potential problem as they may appear similar to fine linear calcifications, which are suspicious.

Coarse or "popcorn" calcifications

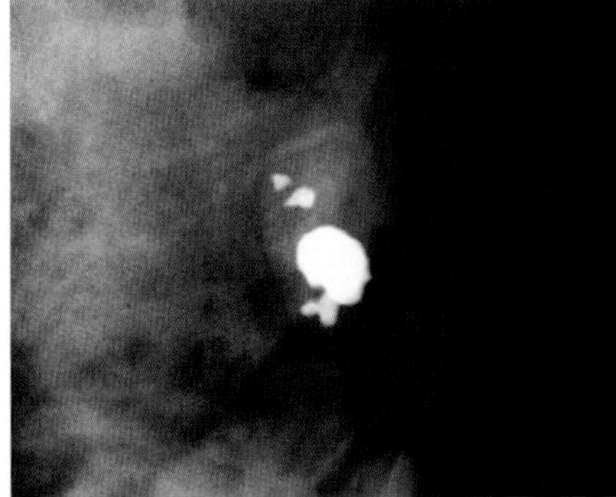

Popcorn calcifications in a hyalinizing fibroadenoma:

Mammogram shows a circumscribed, lobulated mass with associated "popcorn" calcifications, diagnostic of a hyalinizing fibroadenoma.

- "Popcorn" calcifications are caused by an involuting or hyalinizing fibroadenoma.
- Not all fibroadenomas calcify. However, when calcification does occur, it starts as *peripheral* calcification and progresses to the classic chunky popcorn-like appearance.
- At an early stage, the small calcifications of a fibroadenoma may resemble those of cancer and prompt biopsy; however, a benign fibroadenoma can be diagnosed with confidence when the calcifications have the typical popcorn morphology.

Large rod-like calcifications

- Large rod-like calcifications are caused by secretory disease (also called plasma cell mastitis or duct ectasia), which is a benign, inflammatory, asymptomatic process seen in postmenopausal women.
- These calcifications follow a ductal distribution, similar to DCIS; however, the calcifications of secretory disease are large and rod-like as opposed to the fine crushed stone-type calcifications of DCIS.

Milk of calcium calcifications

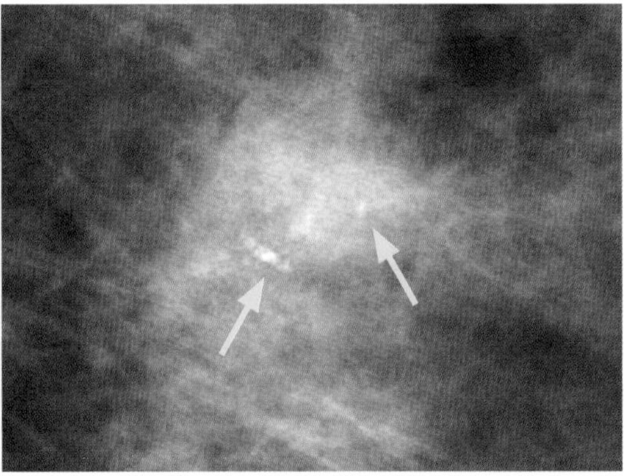

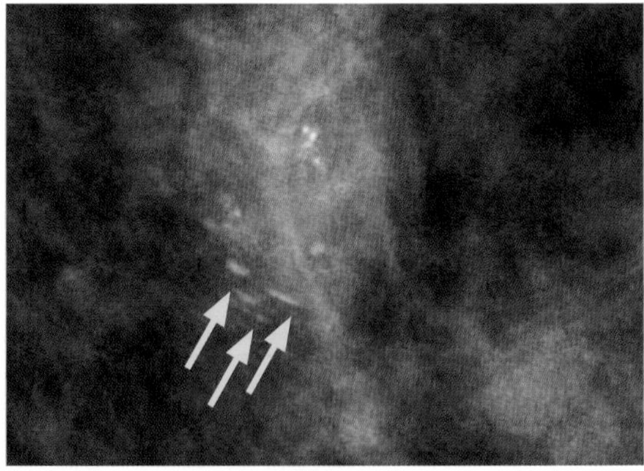

Milk of calcium: CC spot-magnification view (left image) shows amorphous calcifications (arrows). A true lateral spot-magnification view (right image) shows layering of the calcific sediment (arrows), diagnostic of milk of calcium.

- Milk of calcium represents free-floating calcium in tiny benign cysts.
- The most important feature of these calcifications is the apparent change in shape of the calcium particles between the CC and lateral projections.
- On the CC view the calcifications are often indistinct and appear as fuzzy, round, amorphous deposits. On the 90 degree lateral, they are more clearly defined, semilunar or crescent-shaped in morphology due to dependent layering.

Sutural calcifications

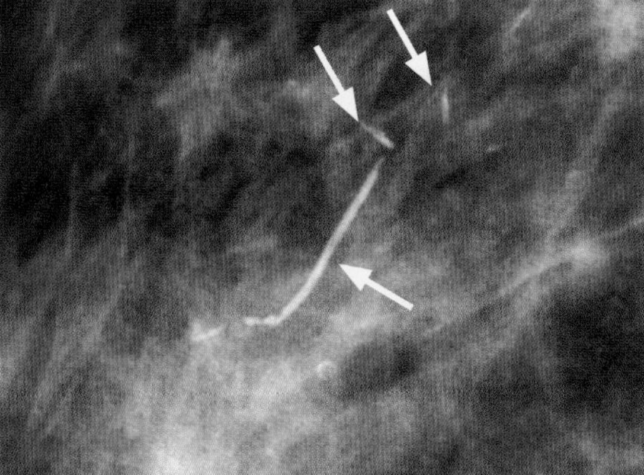

Sutural calcifications:

Curvilinear calcifications of variable lengths (arrows) are present, representing calcification of surgical suture material.

- Sutural calcifications represent calcium deposited on suture material, usually after radiation therapy.
- Sutural calcifications are uncommonly seen due to changes in modern surgical technique.

Dystrophic calcifications

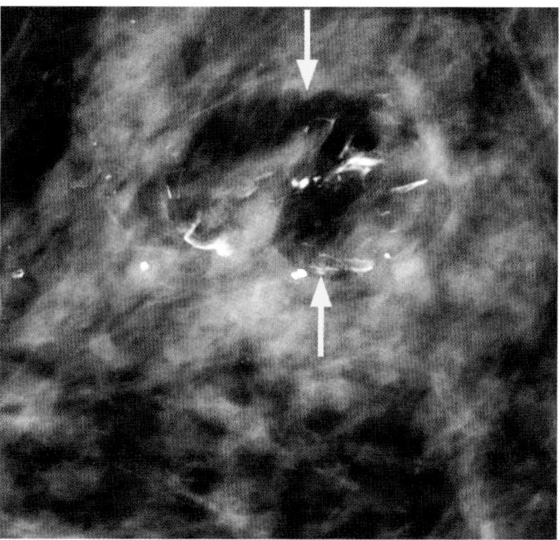

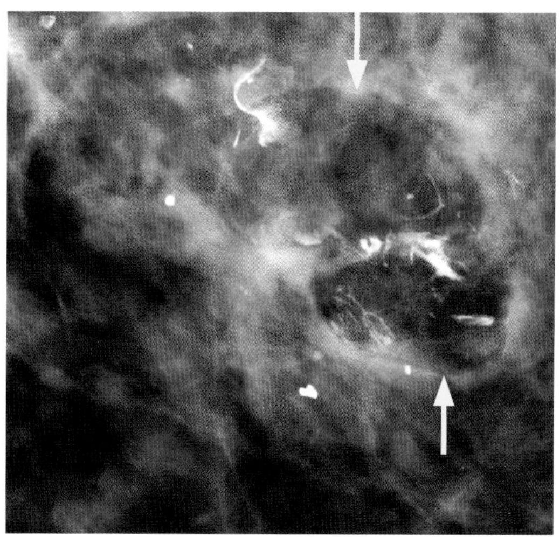

CC and MLO views show a lucent lesion with a bizarre whorled appearance and geometric calcifications (arrows), typical of fat necrosis.

- Dystrophic calcifications may occur as a sequela of surgery, biopsy, trauma, or irradiation.
- Usually the appearance of dystrophic calcification is distinctive, but may pose a diagnostic challenge when new or evolving.

Round calcifications

- Round calcifications are due to various etiologies and are benign.

Punctate calcifications

- Punctate calcifications are round and smaller than 0.5 mm.
- Even though these are considered benign, an isolated cluster of punctate calcifications may warrant close surveillance or even biopsy if new or ipsilateral to a cancer.

Lucent-centered calcifications

- Benign, smooth calcifications with a lucent center can range in size from less than 1 mm to greater than 1 cm in diameter.

"Eggshell" or "rim" calcifications

- Fine peripheral calcification represents calcium deposited on the surface of a sphere, usually occurring in an area of fat necrosis or a cyst with calcified walls.

Intermediate concern calcifications (BI-RADS 4)

Amorphous or indistinct calcifications

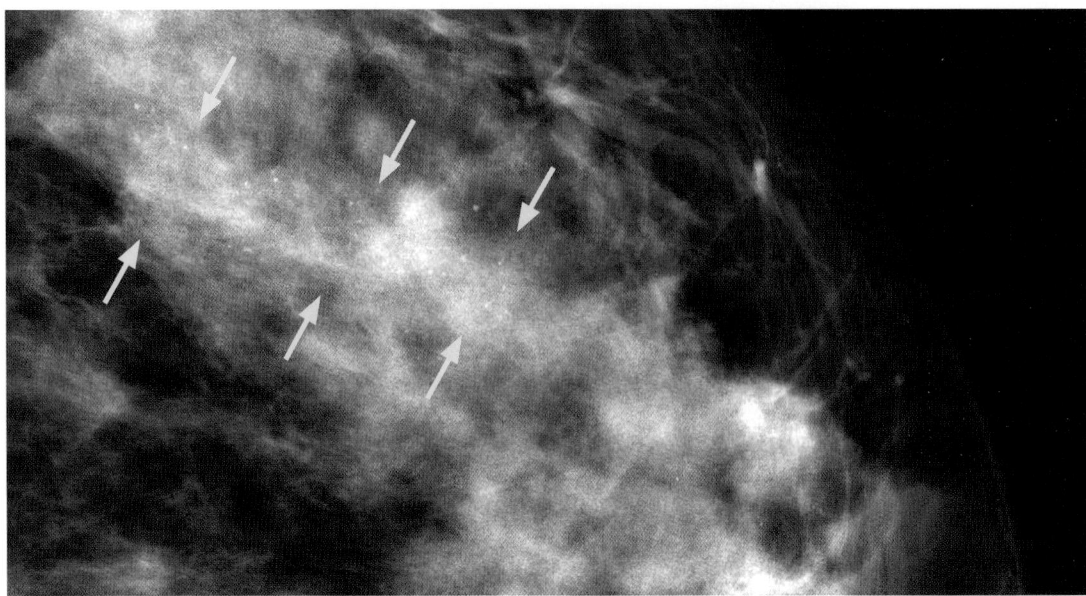

Amorphous calcifications: Numerous amorphous calcifications are present in a dense breast in a segmental distribution (arrows). This pattern is suspicious for malignancy and biopsy is warranted.

- Amorphous calcifications are too small or hazy to ascertain the detailed morphologic appearance.
- Diffuse scattered amorphous calcifications are usually benign, although magnification views are important to rule out any suspicious clusters.
- Amorphous calcifications in a clustered, regional, linear, or segmental distribution are more suspicious and warrant biopsy.

Coarse heterogeneous calcifications

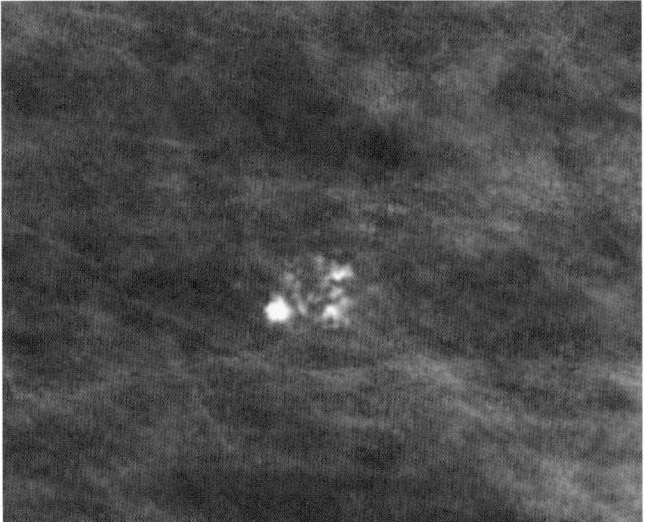

Coarse heterogeneous calcifications:

Coned-down image from a spot magnification mammogram shows a cluster of coarse heterogeneous calcifications. These are intermediate in suspicion and biopsy is warranted.

- Coarse heterogeneous calcifications are irregular calcifications that are generally larger than 0.5 mm, but smaller than dystrophic calcifications.
- Evolving dystrophic calcifications or early calcifications associated with hyalinizing fibroadenomas or fat necrosis may appear as coarse heterogeneous and pose a diagnostic challenge.
- Coarse heterogeneous calcifications may be associated with malignancy and biopsy is often warranted, especially when new.

Higher probability of malignancy calcifications (BI-RADS 4 or 5)

Fine pleomorphic calcifications

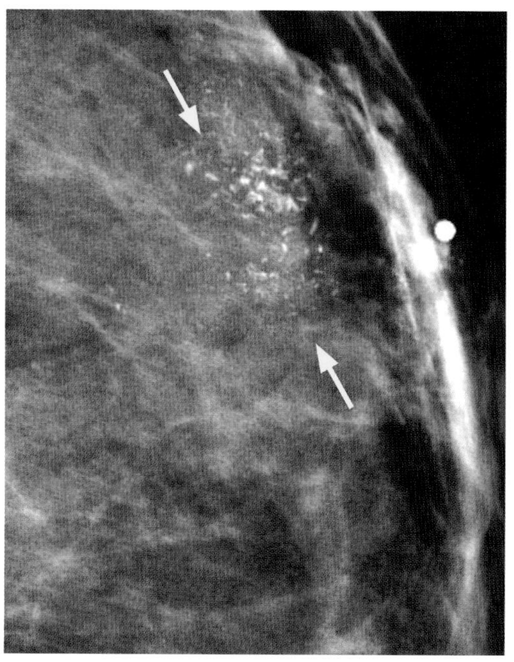

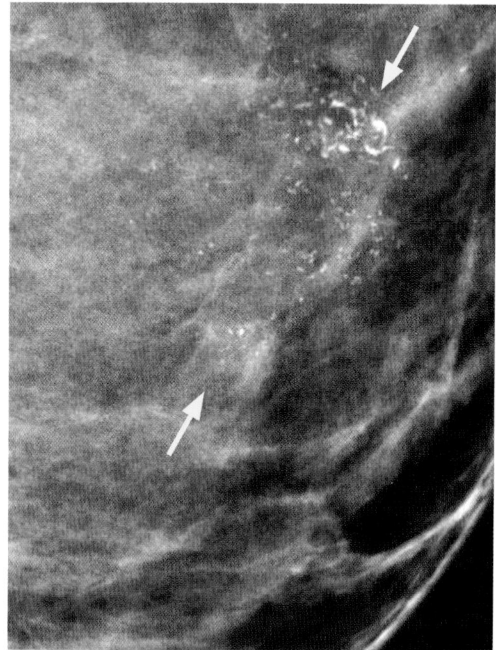

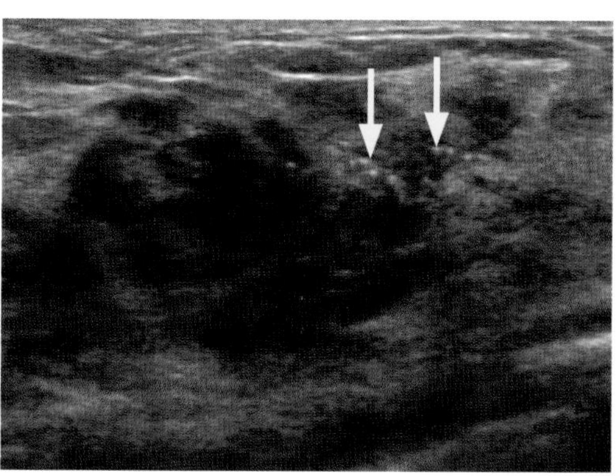

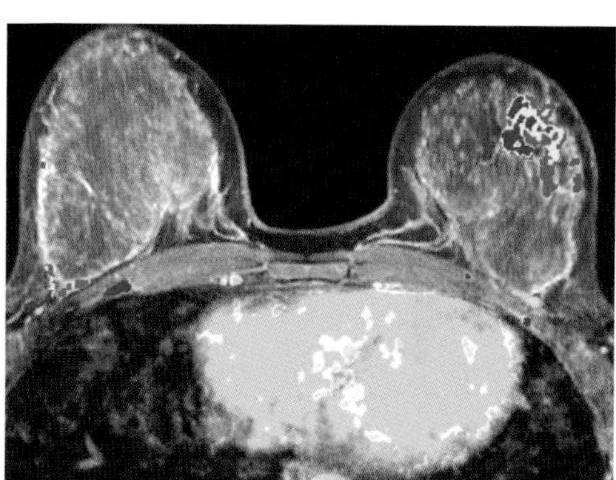

Fine pleomorphic calcifications: CC and MLO mammograms (top images) demonstrate a large cluster of fine pleomorphic calcifications (arrows). Ultrasound (bottom left image) shows an ill-defined hypoechoic mass, with the calcifications evident as punctate echogenic foci (arrows). Color CAD angiomap from the patient's breast MRI shows the segmental, non-masslike enhancement in a clumped distribution in the left breast, with the red color map corresponding to malignant-type washout kinetics. This lesion is highly suspicious for malignancy (BI-RADS 5).

- By definition, fine pleomorphic calcifications vary in shape and size, producing a characteristic *dot–dash* appearance.
- Fine pleomorphic calcifications are highly suspicious for malignancy, most commonly seen in DCIS or invasive ductal carcinoma.
- When evaluating any group or cluster of calcifications, one should always ask, "can these be pleomorphic?" If so, biopsy should be obtained.

Fine linear or fine-linear branching calcifications

- Fine linear and fine-linear branching calcifications are similarly highly suspicious for malignancy. The branching distribution suggests filling of the lumen of a duct system involved by DCIS.

Distribution of calcium

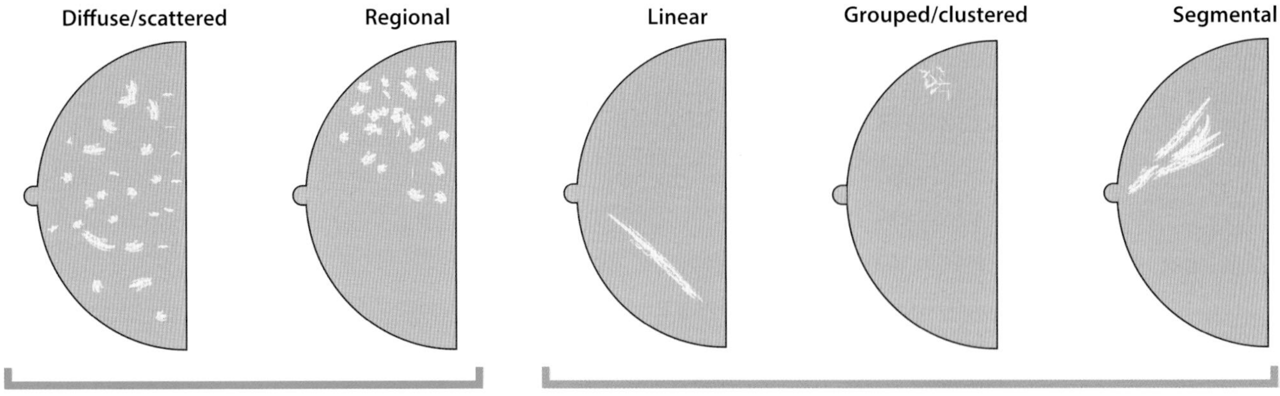

- The distribution of calcification can greatly affect the suspicion of malignancy.
- Although diffuse/scattered and regional calcifications are usually considered benign, the morphology of the calcifications in question is also important. A diffuse/scattered or regional distribution of suspicious fine pleomorphic or fine-linear branching calcifications may represent multicentric cancer.
- Similarly, a more suspicious distribution (linear, grouped/clustered, or segmental) of calcifications with a typically benign morphology may warrant further workup.

Diffuse/scattered calcifications

- Diffuse or scattered calcifications are distributed randomly throughout the breast.
- Punctate and amorphous calcifications in a diffuse or scattered distribution are usually benign and often bilateral, typically associated with fibrocystic change or sclerosing adenosis.

Regional calcifications

- Regional calcifications are distributed in a large volume (>2 cc) of breast tissue not conforming to a ductal distribution. Since this distribution may involve most of a quadrant or more than a single quadrant, malignancy is less likely.

Linear

- Linear calcifications are arrayed in a line.
- Linear distribution of calcifications elevates suspicion for malignancy as this suggests calcium deposits within a duct.

Segmental

- Segmental calcifications suggest calcium deposited in a ductal system, which is worrisome.
- When the morphology is clearly secretory (rod-like), a segmental distribution can be benign.
- When intermediate-suspicion (such as amorphous) or typically benign (such as round or punctate) calcifications are seen in a segmental distribution, concern should be raised for malignancy.

Grouped or clustered

- A cluster is defined as at least five small calcifications in <1 cc of tissue.
- Grouped or clustered calcifications raise suspicion for malignancy.
- The use of the word *clustered* should be reserved for more suspicious calcifications that will be biopsied. The slightly less worrisome *grouped* descriptor is generally used for calcifications that may be able to be followed as BI-RADS 3 rather than immediately biopsied.

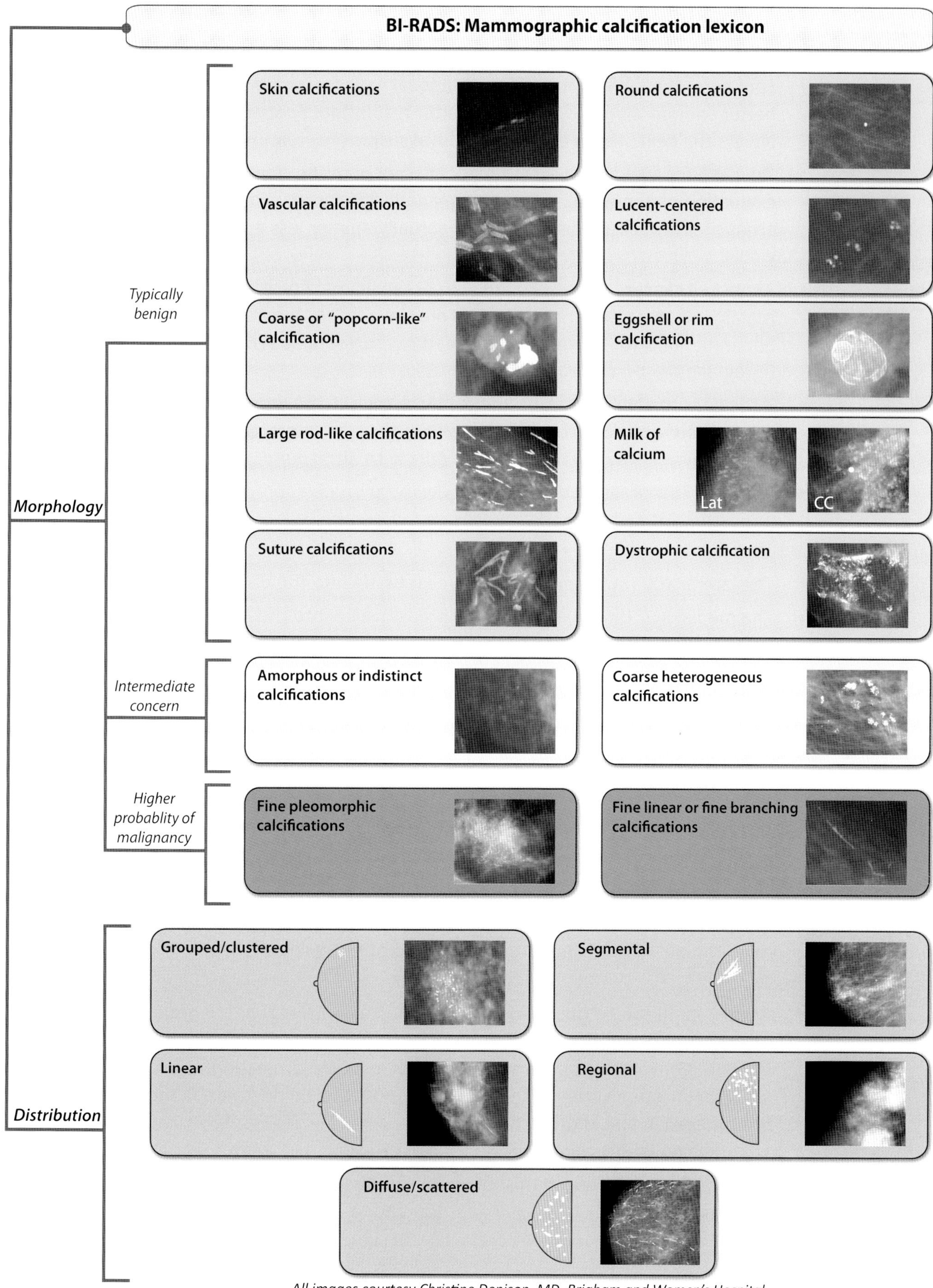
BI-RADS: Mammographic calcification lexicon
Morphology
Typically benign
Skin calcifications
Round calcifications
Vascular calcifications
Lucent-centered calcifications
Coarse or "popcorn-like" calcification
Eggshell or rim calcification
Large rod-like calcifications
Milk of calcium
Lat
CC
Suture calcifications
Dystrophic calcification
Intermediate concern
Amorphous or indistinct calcifications
Coarse heterogeneous calcifications
Higher probablity of malignancy
Fine pleomorphic calcifications
Fine linear or fine branching calcifications
Distribution
Grouped/clustered
Segmental
Linear
Regional
Diffuse/scattered

All images courtesy Christine Denison, MD, Brigham and Women's Hospital.

Spot compression (with or without magnification)

- Spot compression is compression of a focal region of the breast, which allows for better compression and therefore better resolution. Spot compression is almost always the next step in evaluating a focal suspicious mammographic abnormality.
- Typically, for evaluation of calcifications, spot compression *magnification* is used. For evaluation of a mass or asymmetry, magnification is usually not needed. Note that areas of architectural distortion may actually appear less apparent on magnification views.
- Almost all cancers are associated with parenchymal fibrosis due to a desmoplastic reaction. If an apparent asymmetry "presses out" with focal compression, then the apparent abnormality can be presumed to represent superimposed normal pliable fibroglandular tissue.
- If the abnormality does not significantly change shape when compressed, then it is suspicious and spot compression allows the best characterization of its margins. Further evaluation is warranted, typically with ultrasound.
- A smaller compression device will allow more precise compression, with the downside of possibly losing landmarks.

XCC (exaggerated cranio-caudal)

- The lateral XCC (XCCL) pulls lateral breast tissue into the detector.
- The medial XCC (XCCM) pulls medial breast tissue into the detector.

Rolled views (CC variant)

- Rolled views are obtained by moving the top and bottom of the breast in opposite directions. Rolled views are helpful to localize a lesion that is seen on the CC view only.
- Two rolled views are typically obtained. A view is obtained with the top of the breast rolled medially (RCCM) and a second view with the top rolled laterally (RCCL).

  If a lesion moves medially with an RCCM view, then it's in the superior breast.

  If a lesion moves laterally with an RCCM view, then it's in the inferior breast.
- The lateral view can also be rolled, although this is less commonly performed.

Reduced compression

- Images with reduced compression can be obtained to image far posterior lesions that may "slip out" of the detector when full compression is applied.

True lateral view (ML or LM)

- A true lateral can be obtained in an ML (most commonly) or LM projection. In an ML view, the X-rays first travel through the medial breast, with the detector placed laterally. Conversely, the detector is medial in an LM projection. It is ideal to place the lesion in question closer to the detector if possible. For instance, a medial lesion is best imaged in an LM projection.
- The true lateral is used to diagnose milk of calcium. In addition, to spot compression magnification, magnification spot views should also be obtained in the true lateral projection when milk of calcium is suspected.

  In the true lateral view, the precipitated calcium sinks to the bottom of the small cysts, where it is seen mammographically as tiny crescents (versus the fuzzy round appearance of the CC view).
- The true lateral view is helpful to triangulate a lesion seen in the MLO view but not CC.
- The true lateral can be helpful for planning a stereotactic procedure.

Triangulation

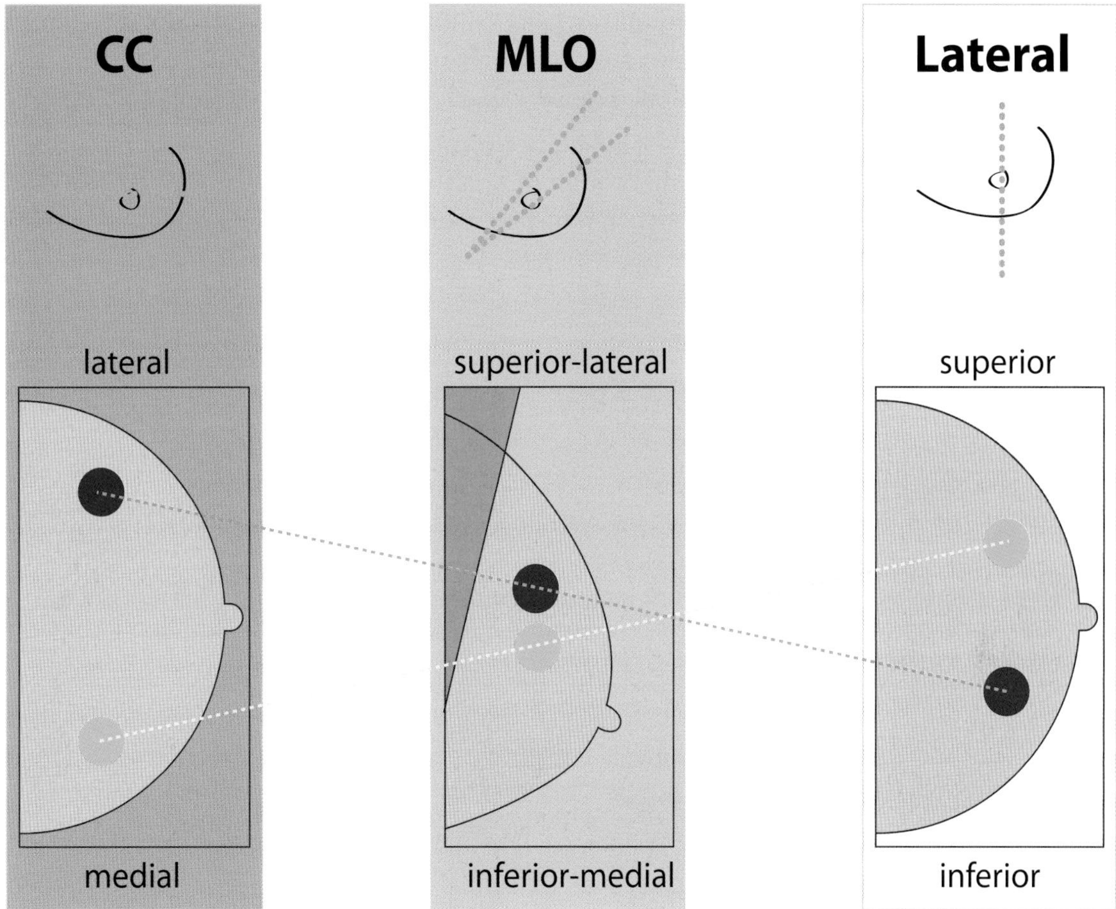

- A true lateral view is helpful to triangulate a lesion seen only on the MLO view.
- If the lesion rises on the lateral compared to the MLO, the lesion is located in the medial breast (**m**edial:**m**uffins rise); If the lesion sinks, it is lateral (**l**ateral:**l**ead sinks).

Mass or focal asymmetry seen on screening mammography

- A screening mammogram can only receive the BI-RADS 1, 2, or 0 assessments. If screening mammogram findings are concerning, the patient is assessed as BI-RADS 0 and is recalled for additional evaluation.
- When the patient returns for the diagnostic workup, spot compression views of the area in question should be obtained. If spot compression shows only normal pliable fibroglandular tissue, then no further workup is needed (BI-RADS 1).
- If an asymmetry persists on spot compression then it needs to be localized on two orthogonal views. When correlating a lesion on two views, it is important to remember that the lesion should be located at approximately the same distance (within 1 cm) from the nipple on each view. This rule may prevent mistaken localization of different lesions on each projection.
- If the lesion is seen only on the MLO, a lateral view should be subsequently obtained to triangulate the lesion as described above. A lesion seen on the MLO view but not the CC view may be located far laterally. An exaggerated CC lateral (XCCL) view can better image the far lateral tissue. Rolled CC views may also help to visualize the lesion.
- A lesion seen only on the CC may be in the upper-inner quadrant and not included in the MLO view. Rolled views are typically performed to localize lesions seen only in the CC view.
- Once a lesion is localized to a quadrant, targeted ultrasound should be performed.

- If a suspicious single-view finding still cannot be localized despite a thorough mammographic and ultrasound evaluation, MRI can be helpful as a problem-solving tool. Mammographic stereotactic biopsy is also an option to biopsy a one-view finding (although stereotactic biopsy is used much most commonly to biopsy calcifications).
- In general, biopsy should be performed for a mass with *any* suspicious feature either on ultrasound or mammography. For instance, a well-circumscribed mammographic mass that has an irregular border on ultrasound is suspicious despite its mammographic appearance.
- Most new findings are suspicious, with a notable exception being a well-circumscribed mammographic mass shown definitively to be a simple cyst on ultrasound.
- Two years of stability is generally considered adequate to call a benign-appearing mass benign.

Palpable mass

- The mammographic workup for a palpable abnormality is similar to that of an asymptomatic lesion found on mammography, with one key difference: In general, all palpable findings are evaluated by ultrasound, even if the mammogram is negative.

Mammographic use of BI-RADS 3

- There are data to support the assignment of BI-RADS 3 in the following three situations, which are not definitively benign but have been shown to have less than 2% risk of cancer.

Circumscribed, benign-appearing solid mass

- A probably benign solid mass must have a benign mammographic appearance. Its shape must be round, oval, or lobulated, and its margins must be circumscribed. The mass must also lack any suspicious microcalcifications. Any new mass should also undergo ultrasound evaluation. If the ultrasound findings are also benign, that mass may be assigned BI-RADS 3 (or BI-RADS 2 if the ultrasound showed a simple cyst).
- A probably benign solid mass that has demonstrated at least two years of stability can usually be considered benign (BI-RADS 2).

Cluster of tiny round calcifications

- The two BI-RADS descriptive terms for round calcifications (which are usually benign) are *punctate* (<0.5 mm in size) and *round* (>0.5 mm in size). It is usually necessary to use spot-compression magnification views to accurately characterize calcifications.
- Punctate or round calcifications in a cluster (≥5 calcifications/cc) can be diagnosed as probably benign (BI-RADS 3). Note that the morphology must be clearly punctate or round, and the distribution must be in a cluster. For instance, a cluster of amorphous calcifications is indeterminate and usually warrants biopsy. Similarly, although rare, punctate or round calcifications in a linear or segmental distribution would be suspicious.

  Some authors advocate using grouped as the BI-RADS distribution descriptor for calcifications that are followed as a BI-RADS 3 and clustered for calcifications that should be biopsied.

Focal asymmetry

- A focal asymmetry is a non-palpable lesion seen on two projections. Unlike a mass, a focal asymmetry does not have outwardly convex margins, and usually is interspersed with fat.
- Assuming no ultrasound correlate is seen, a focal asymmetry can be assessed as probably benign (BI-RADS 3) after a thorough imaging workup.
- In contrast, a *developing asymmetry* is a focal asymmetry that has increased in size. It is suspicious and requires further workup.

Zonal anatomy and pathology

Normal zonal anatomy

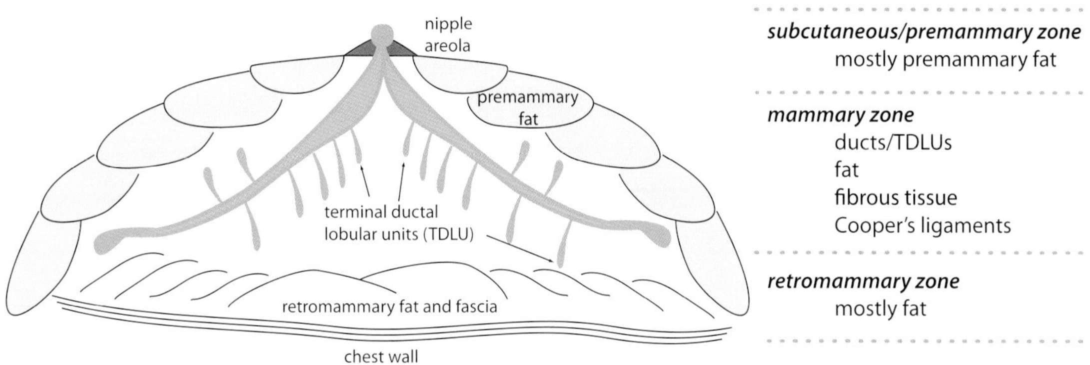

subcutaneous/premammary zone
mostly premammary fat

mammary zone
ducts/TDLUs
fat
fibrous tissue
Cooper's ligaments

retromammary zone
mostly fat

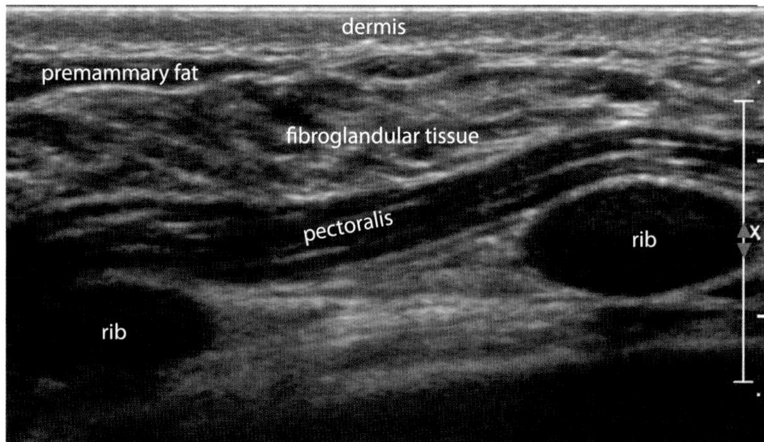

Subcutaneous zone and skin lesions

- The subcutaneous (premammary) zone of the breast contains skin and dermis, subcutaneous fat, and some suspensory Cooper's ligaments. The subcutaneous zone is the site of skin lesions, including benign skin cysts. Dermal lesions are almost always benign and include epidermal inclusion cysts and sebaceous cysts.
- Epidermal inclusion cysts arise from a hair follicle and are filled with keratinous debris. On ultrasound imaging, an epidermal inclusion cyst appears as a circumscribed lesion with variable internal echotexture ranging from anechoic to heterogeneous, depending on the amount of internal keratinous debris.
- Sebaceous cysts are indistinguishable from epidermal inclusion cysts on clinical and imaging findings. Sebaceous cysts arise from the outer sheath of the hair follicle.
- A lesion can be confidently diagnosed as a benign epidermal inclusion cyst or sebaceous cyst when it is located completely within the echogenic dermis.
- In contrast, lesions arising from the hypodermis (subcutaneous fat) can include a broader range of pathologies, including papilloma, fibroadenoma, and breast cancer. It is therefore critical to identify the anatomic site of origin as best as possible.
- Superficial breast lesions that are not entirely within the dermis can pose a diagnostic challenge, as the differential would include a possibly malignant hypodermal lesion. Two clues can be helpful to establish dermal origin:
  1) Visualization of a claw of dermal tissue wrapping around the lesion.
  2) Visualization of a tract connecting the lesion to the epidermal skin surface.

Mammary zone

- The mammary zone is the site of most breast pathology, and includes ducts and terminal ductal lobular units (TDLUs), fat, fibrous tissue, and Cooper's ligaments.

Retromammary zone

- The retromammary zone is just superficial to pectoralis and contains fat and a few Cooper's ligaments.

Imaging fat in the breast

- Parenchymal breast fat is hypoechoic, unlike ultrasound imaging of fat elsewhere in the body.
- In contrast, fat in a lymph node hilum, fat in a lipoma, and fat necrosis may all appear hyperechoic.

Ultrasound technique

Scanning planes

- Ultrasound scanning can be performed in radial/antiradial or transverse/longitudinal planes.
- Radial/antiradial scanning has been advocated as superior because ductal anatomy is oriented radially.

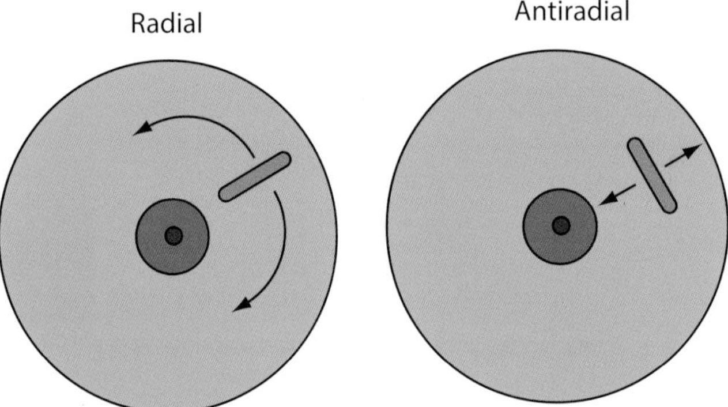

- Transverse/longitudinal orientation is less suited to the centripetal breast anatomy but is familiar from body ultrasound imaging.

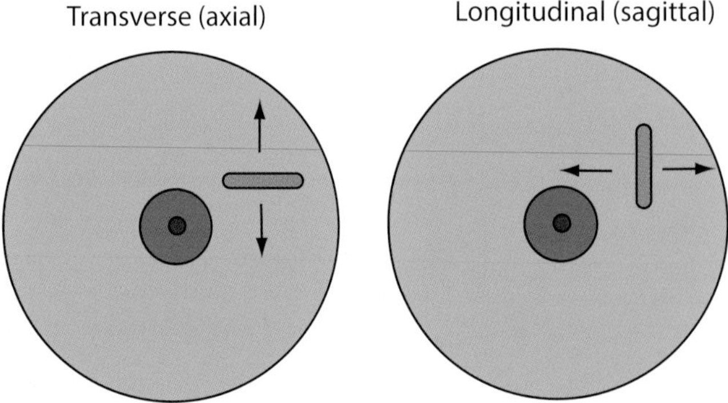

Annotation

- Full annotation is mandatory, including the side, the clock face position, the distance from the nipple, and the orientation (radial/antiradial or transverse/longitudinal).
- Alternatively, some ultrasound systems allow graphical annotations. Documenting the distance from the nipple in addition to the graphic is recommended.

BI-RADS LEXICON TO DESCRIBE ULTRASOUND MASSES

- Similar to the evaluation of mammographic masses, the BI-RADS lexicon provides a framework to describe ultrasound masses. Use of the lexicon allows one to stratify masses on a spectrum from benign to malignant based solely on the report wording.

Size and position

- A mass should be measured in all three orthogonal planes, with position labelled in terms of clockface and distance from the nipple.

Shape

- The BI-RADS lexicon for the shape of an ultrasound mass includes **oval**, **round**, and **irregular**. Unlike the mammographic lexicon, *lobular* is not in the ultrasound lexicon for shape.

Orientation

- The orientation of the long axis of a mass (relative to the skin) is unique to ultrasound.
- A mass that is **parallel** in orientation is more likely to be benign.
- In contrast, a **non-parallel** mass (known informally as "taller-than-wide") is oriented with the long axis vertical and is suspicious for malignancy. This finding is based on the propensity of a malignant process to violate tissue planes.

Margin

- Similar to mammography, benign masses are typically **circumscribed.**
- If the margins of a mass are not circumscribed, they can be characterized as **indistinct**, **angular**, **microlobulated**, or **spiculated**.

> **Indistinct**: No clear boundary between the mass and its surrounding tissue.
>
> **Angular**: Featuring sharp corners.
>
> **Microlobulated**: Serrated appearance of the margins.
>
> **Spiculated**: Linear projections emanating from the mass.

Internal echo pattern

- The internal echo pattern describes the internal texture of an ultrasound lesion. The two types of discrete ultrasound lesions are solid masses and cysts. A cyst can be a simple cyst, a complicated cyst, or a complex mass, which are discussed in detail later. The internal echo pattern helps to differentiate between cystic and solid lesions.
- An **anechoic** structure has no internal echoes and most commonly (but not always) represents a simple cyst.
- A **hypoechoic** structure is characterized by low-level internal echoes, such as seen in a complicated cyst or fibroadenoma.
- An **isoechoic** structure has the same echogenicity as surrounding fat per the BI-RADS definition, although some authors propose that an isoechoic structure is defined relative to surrounding breast tissue. An isoechoic lesion can be challenging to visualize.
- A **hyperechoic** structure is more echogenic than fat. It may be either equal or greater in echogenicity compared to fibroglandular tissue.
- A **complex** echo pattern represents a combination of internal echogenicities, such as seen in a complex mass or necrotic tumor.

Lesion boundary

- The lesion boundary describes the transition between the mass and the surrounding tissue.
- An **abrupt interface** is a clean demarcation between the lesion and surrounding tissue.
- An **echogenic halo** is an echogenic transition zone, which can be seen in cancer or abscess.

Posterior acoustic features

- The posterior acoustic features of a lesion describe the attenuation characteristics of the sound beam deep to the lesion.
- Acoustic **enhancement** (also called posterior through transmission) refers to a column of increased echogenicity posterior (deep) to the mass. Posterior enhancement is one of the characteristics of a simple cyst, although on its own posterior enhancement is not specific.
- **Shadowing** is attenuation of the sound beam as it passes through the lesion. Shadowing is associated with fibrosis, such as from a neoplastic desmoplastic reaction or surgical scar.
- If a lesion has **no posterior acoustic features**, then the echogenicity of the area immediately deep to the mass is the same as adjacent tissue.
- A lesion can also have a **combined pattern** of posterior acoustic features, such as a fibroadenoma containing a large, coarse, shadowing calcification.

Ultrasound differentiation of benign and malignant solid masses

- Certain ultrasound features are associated with benign or malignant lesions. In some circumstances, a solid mass that demonstrates only benign ultrasound findings may be able to be classified as BI-RADS 3 and followed. There is a trend in several institutions, however, to biopsy most or all solid masses, especially if new.

Ultrasound features of a benign mass

- *Lack of any malignant findings: If even a single malignant feature is present then a lesion is indeterminate or suspicious and should be biopsied.*
- Marked hyperechogenicity (relative to fat).
- Circumscribed margins.
- Parallel orientation to the skin (wider-than-tall; width:height >1.4).
- Ellipsoid shape.
- Few gentle macrolobulations.
- Thin echogenic pseudocapsule.

Ultrasound features of a malignant mass

- Spiculated margins, which is the most specific sign of malignancy.
- Non-parallel (taller-than-wide) orientation, the second most specific sign.
- Angular or microlobulated margins.
- Posterior shadowing.
- Markedly hypoechoic echotexture.
- Associated calcifications (visible on sonography as echogenic foci).
- Lesion boundary with wide zone of transition.

Indeterminate ultrasound features

- The following features are not helpful in differentiating between benign and malignant masses: Lesion size, iso- or mild hypoechogenicity, posterior acoustic enhancement, and heterogeneous or homogeneous texture.

Ultrasound use of BI-RADS 3

- There are data to support classification of the following lesions into the BI-RADS 3 (probably benign) category, with less than 2% risk of cancer:
- **Complicated cyst** or **clustered microcysts**.
- **Oval, hypoechoic, circumscribed, parallel mass** (consistent with fibroadenoma).

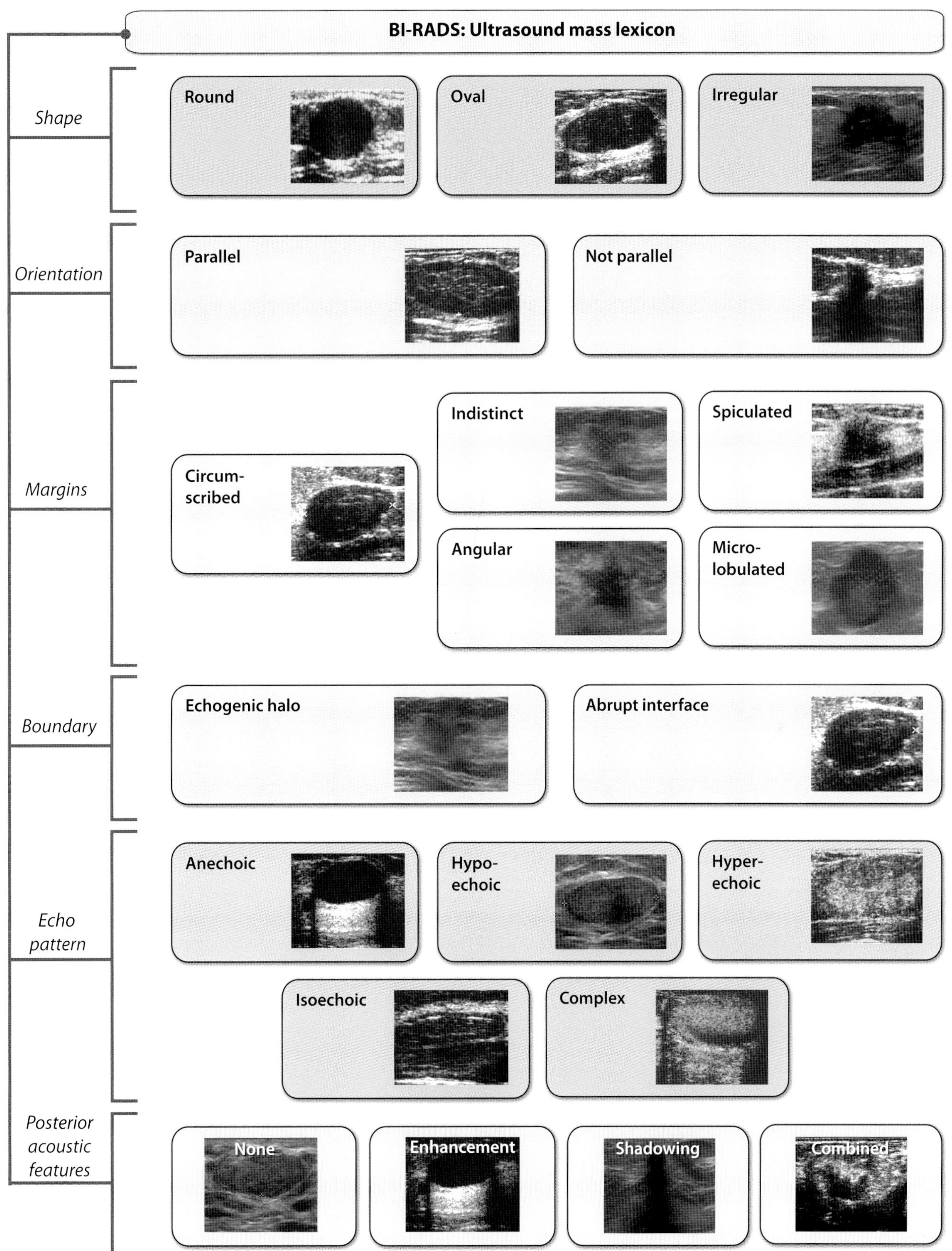

All images courtesy Christine Denison, MD, Brigham and Women's Hospital.

FATTY MASSES

- All fat-density circumscribed masses are benign (BI-RADS 2).

Lipoma

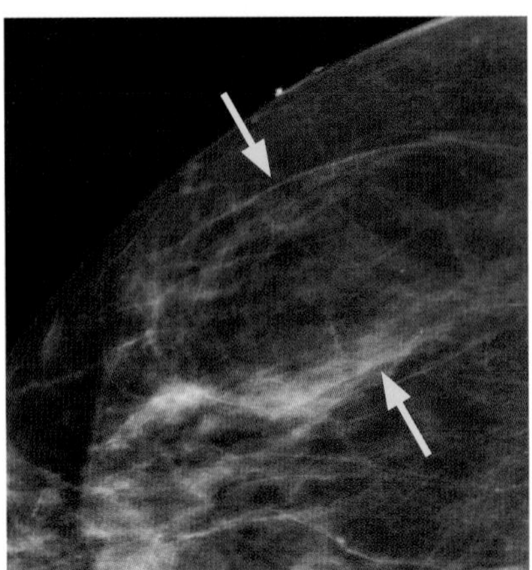

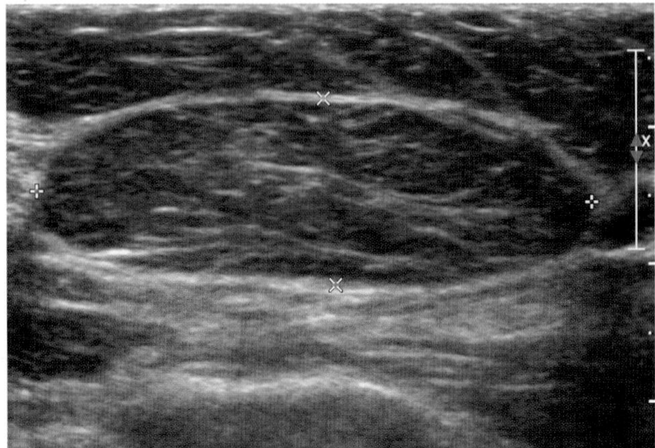

Lipoma: Mammogram shows a circumscribed oval mass that is almost entirely lucent (arrows). Ultrasound shows a circumscribed oval mass (calipers) with internal echotexture identical to the surrounding fat.

Case courtesy Christine Denison, MD, Brigham and Women's Hospital.

- A lipoma is a benign lesion composed of mature adipocytes.
- A lipoma may present clinically as a palpable mass when the normal breast is displaced.
- A lipoma is a benign diagnosis that can be made entirely by mammography, where a lipoma will be seen as a radiolucent mass that may have a thin discrete rim. In contrast to an oil cyst, a lipoma will not have peripheral calcification.
- Ultrasound is not typically used in the evaluation of a suspected lipoma; however, ultrasound of a lipoma would show a circumscribed oval mass isoechoic to fat.

Oil cyst (fat necrosis)

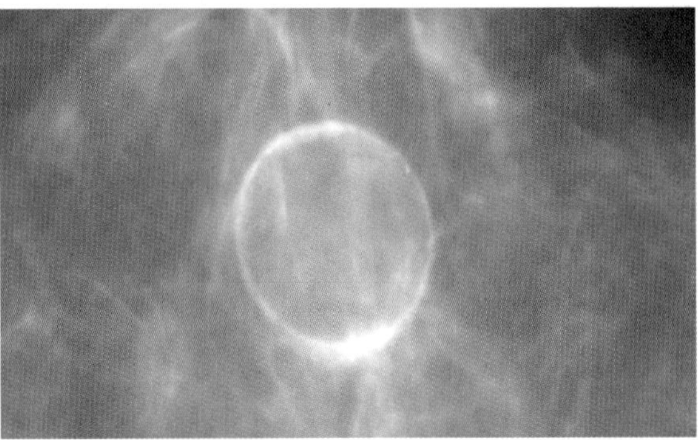

Oil cyst: Mammogram shows a radiolucent mass with a fine peripherally calcified rim.

Case courtesy Christine Denison, MD, Brigham and Women's Hospital.

- An oil cyst is one possible sequela of fat necrosis and can occur post trauma or surgery. Fat necrosis can have many imaging appearances, most commonly dystrophic calcification. The formation of an oil cyst following fat necrosis is less common but has a very distinctive appearance.
- When an oil cyst forms after fat necrosis, fat saponification leads to a circumscribed, lucent lesion that can peripherally calcify.
- Ultrasound is not ideal for further evaluation, because fat necrosis can have a variable appearance on ultrasound.

- Like purely fatty masses, all fat-*containing* circumscribed masses are benign (BI-RADS 2).

Hamartoma (fibroadenolipoma)

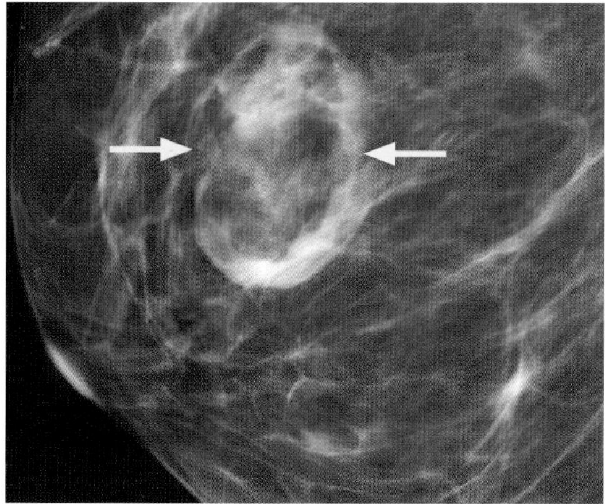

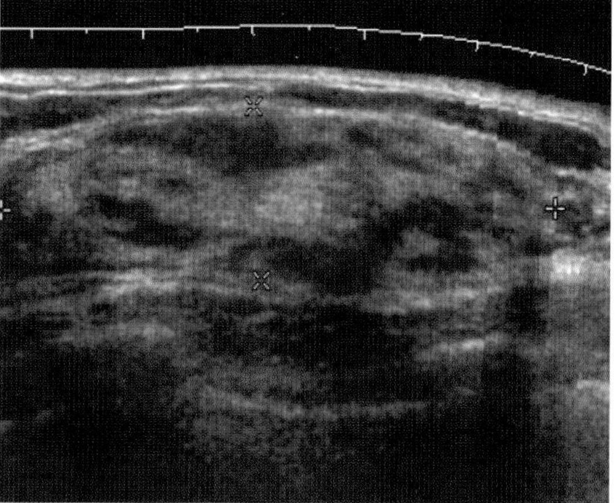

Hamartoma: Mammogram (left image) demonstrates an oval mass containing fat and glandular elements, surrounded by a thin pseudocapsule (arrows). Ultrasound of the same area demonstrates an oval, circumscribed region of normal-appearing fibroglandular tissue and hypoechoic fat (calipers).

Case courtesy Christine Denison, MD, Brigham and Women's Hospital.

- A hamartoma, also known as a fibroadenolipoma, is a benign mass containing fat and glandular tissue elements.
- The classic mammographic appearance of a hamartoma is a "breast within a breast," which displaces normal breast tissue. A pseudocapsule is typically seen surrounding the hamartoma. Mammography is almost always diagnostic. Ultrasound is typically not indicated but would show normal fibroglandular tissue and fat.
- Because fibroglandular elements are present within a hamartoma, it is possible (but rare) for breast cancer to occur within a hamartoma. Any suspicious mass or calcifications within the hamartoma should be worked up.

Galactocele

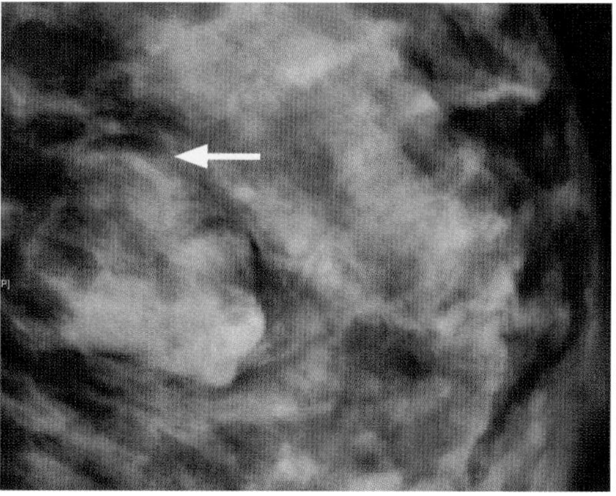

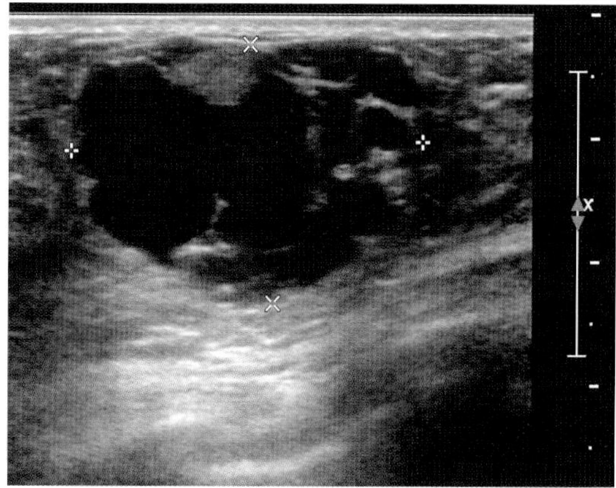

Galactocele: Lateral mammogram (left image) shows a circumscribed, lobulated mass containing both high density and fat. A fluid level is present (arrow), which is very specific for a galactocele. Ultrasound (right image) shows a complex mass (calipers).

Case courtesy Christine Denison, MD, Brigham and Women's Hospital.

- A galactocele is a cystic collection of milk that can present as a palpable mass in a lactating woman.

- On mammography, a galactocele appears as a well-circumscribed, macrolobulated mass containing mixed high density and fat. The classic mammographic finding (although uncommonly seen) is a fat/fluid level seen on the true lateral view.
- On ultrasound, a galactocele typically appears as a cyst-like mass. If aspiration is performed, the cyst fluid would be milky.

Intramammary lymph node

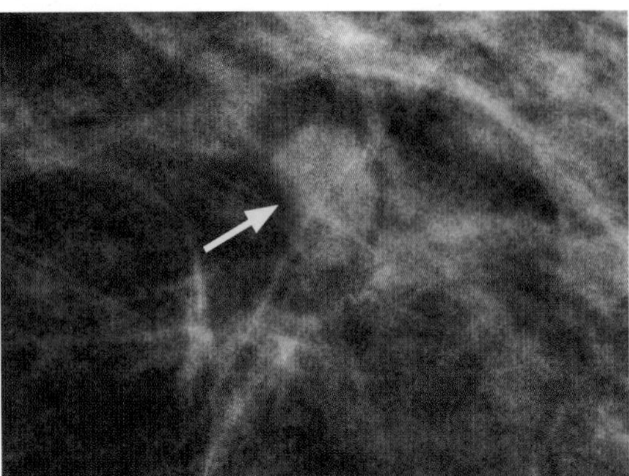
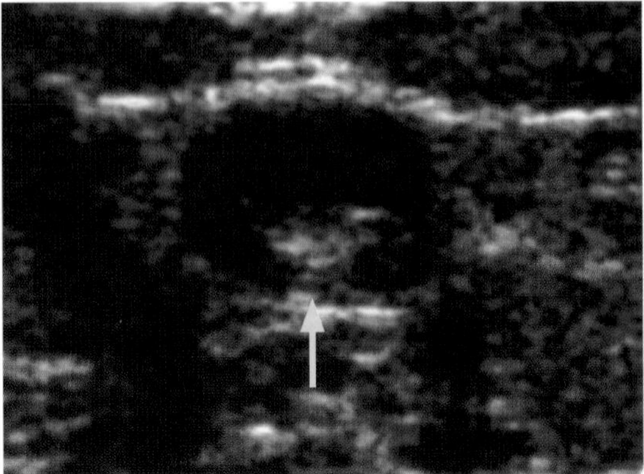

Intramammary lymph node: Mammogram (left image) shows a circumscribed, reniform mass (arrow), highly suggestive of an intramammary lymph node. Ultrasound (in a different patient) of an intramammary lymph node shows an oval, circumscribed mass with a central echogenic fatty hilum (arrow).

Ultrasound case courtesy Christine Denison, MD, Brigham and Women's Hospital.

- An intramammary lymph node is benign. The vast majority of intramammary lymph nodes occur laterally, typically in the upper outer quadrant adjacent to a vessel. A lesion that appears like an intramammary lymph node but is in the medial breast should be carefully evaluated and should be considered suspicious until proven otherwise.
- On mammography, an intramammary lymph node should have a characteristic reniform shape with a fatty hilum (a lucent notch in the middle). If the hilum is not visible, a full workup should be performed including spot compression and/or ultrasound.
- Typically, a normal intramammary lymph node with a fatty hilum can be diagnosed with confidence on mammography, but ultrasound can be useful as a problem solving tool.
- Ultrasound will show a hypoechoic mass with central echogenicity that represents the fatty hilum. Color Doppler imaging would show vessels coming into the hilum.
- Note that while normal intramammary lymph nodes are only sometimes seen within the breast, there are *almost always* lymph nodes present in the axilla. If there is unilateral axillary lymph node enlargement and/or abnormal morphology, concern should be raised for ipsilateral breast cancer. Bilateral enlarged axillary lymph nodes are unlikely to be caused by breast cancer and may be due to systemic inflammatory or neoplastic disease, such as chronic lymphocytic leukemia or lymphoma.

Fibroadenoma

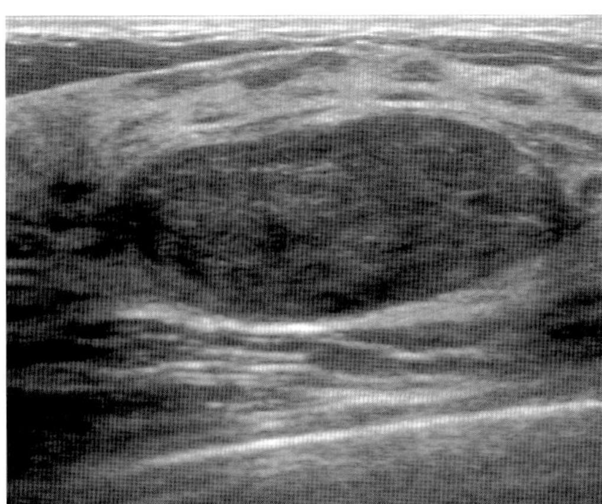

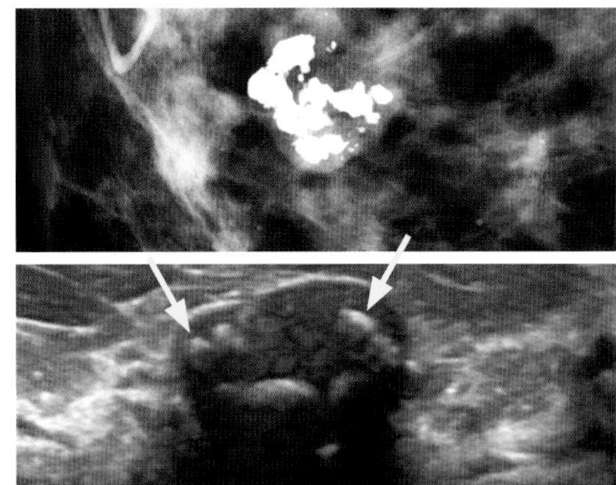

Two different patients with fibroadenomas: On the left is an ultrasound image demonstrating the typical appearance of a fibroadenoma in a young woman, as a circumscribed, oval, parallel, hypoechoic mass with mild posterior enhancement.

On the right is the characteristic mammographic appearance of a hyalinized fibroadenoma in an older woman (top right), as a circumscribed mass with coarse "popcorn" calcifications. This appearance is completely diagnostic and no further workup is necessary. Ultrasound (below right) was performed as this lesion was palpable, as evident by the triangular skin marker on the mammogram. Note the calcifications within the mass (arrows).

Hyalinized fibroadenoma case courtesy Christine Denison, MD, Brigham and Women's Hospital.

- Fibroadenoma is a benign neoplasm seen in young women and is the most common palpable mass in this age group.
- Clinically, a fibroadenoma will present as a firm, mobile mass.
- The classic mammographic appearance of a fibroadenoma is an oval or lobular equal density circumscribed mass, although this imaging appearance is nonspecific. A hyalinizing fibroadenoma, typically seen in older women, has a definitively benign mammographic appearance containing coarse "popcorn" calcification, as in the case above right.
- The typical ultrasound appearance of a fibroadenoma is an oval, circumscribed mass with homogeneous hypoechoic echotexture. Occasionally, a histologically benign fibroadenoma may have suspicious features on ultrasound including irregular borders, heterogeneous internal echotexture, or shadowing, prompting biopsy in these cases.
- A fibroadenoma is benign, but these are often either followed (BI-RADS 3) or biopsied (BI-RADS 4), depending on the imaging characteristics or clinical context.
- If the following ultrasound features are met, the presumed fibroadenoma can be classified as BI-RADS 3, with a false negative rate of 0.5%:

  Ovoid shape, parallel orientation with an width to height ratio of >1.4 (wider-than-tall).

  All margins circumscribed.

  Not highly hypoechoic.
- Variants of fibroadenoma include complex fibroadenoma, juvenile fibroadenoma, and giant fibroadenoma.

  A complex fibroadenoma contains proliferative elements and internal cysts, and confers a slightly increased risk of breast cancer.

  A juvenile fibroadenoma is seen in adolescents and is characterized by very rapid growth.

  A giant fibroadenoma is a fibroadenoma greater than 8 cm in size.
- Fibroadenoma may appear identical to a phyllodes tumor, especially when larger.

Intraductal papilloma/papillary carcinoma

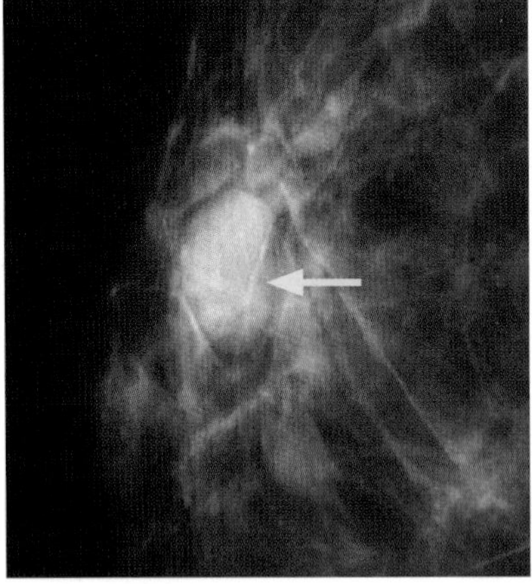

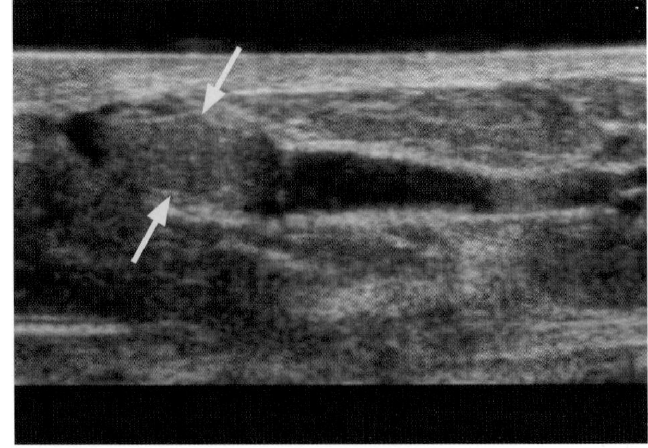

Intraductal papilloma: Spot-compression CC mammogram (left image) shows a lobulated, circumscribed, equal density mass (arrow) in the periareolar region. Ultrasound of the mass shows an oval, isoechoic, circumscribed mass (arrow) within a dilated duct.

Case courtesy Christine Denison, MD, Brigham and Women's Hospital.

- A papilloma is a benign tumor of lactiferous ducts, usually seen in women between age 30 and 50.
- Papilloma is the most common cause of pathologic (bloody, serous, or serosanguinous) nipple discharge. Papilloma grows on a fibrovascular stalk and torsion of the stalk can cause pain and bleeding. Note that DCIS may also present with bloody nipple discharge.
- The typical mammographic appearance of a papilloma is a round or oval, circumscribed or irregular mass, usually located in the subareolar region.
- Although uncommonly performed today, galactography shows an intraductal filling defect.
- On ultrasound, a papilloma appears as a solid round or oval mass. When causing nipple discharge, the papilloma may be evident as a mass in a fluid-filled duct.
- Once biopsied, papillomas are typically treated with surgical excision as papillary carcinoma may appear identical on imaging, especially when atypia is seen histologically.

Pseudoangiomatous stromal hyperplasia (PASH)

- Pseudoangiomatous stromal hyperplasia (PASH) is a rare entity of unknown etiology composed of stromal and epithelial proliferation, thought to be under hormonal control.
- On mammography, PASH appears as an ill-defined, round or oval mass. Occasionally it may be circumscribed.
- Ultrasound shows a hypoechoic or mixed echogenicity, oval or irregular mass.
- Pathologically, PASH may mimic a low-grade angiosarcoma, so excisional biopsy is usually performed if a mass diagnosed as PASH shows interval growth.

Breast cancer

- It is uncommon for breast carcinoma to be circumscribed, but a new circumscribed mass must prompt suspicion, especially in a postmenopausal woman.
- In particular, medullary and mucinous carcinoma are histologic subtypes of breast cancer that can present as a circumscribed round mass on mammography and as a hypoechoic mass on ultrasound. These cancers can be so hypoechoic that they may mimic a benign cyst at first glance. In contrast to a cyst, however, internal vascularity is often present.

LARGE SOLID MASSES, GREATER THAN 3 CM

- Size is a poor predictor of malignancy for solid circumscribed masses.

Giant fibroadenoma

- A giant fibroadenoma is simply a large fibroadenoma >8 cm in size. A giant fibroadenoma has a similar appearance to fibroadenoma excepting its larger size.
- A juvenile fibroadenoma is a rapidly growing fibroadenoma variant seen in adolescents, which may become giant.

Phyllodes tumor

- A phyllodes tumor (previously called cystosarcoma phyllodes) is a rare, rapidly growing tumor that is typically large when first detected.
- Phyllodes tumors occur in an older population compared to fibroadenomas, typically in women age 40–50.
- The majority of phyllodes tumors are benign, although approximately 25% are malignant, and 20% of those may metastasize. Since imaging cannot distinguish between benign and malignant phyllodes, treatment is wide surgical excision. Incomplete excision leads to recurrence.
- The typical mammographic appearance of phyllodes tumor is a large, oval or lobular, circumscribed mass.
- On ultrasound, phyllodes tumor appears as a smoothly marginated mass with heterogeneous internal echotexture. The imaging differential of such a mass includes a large fibroadenoma or cancer.

Lactational adenoma

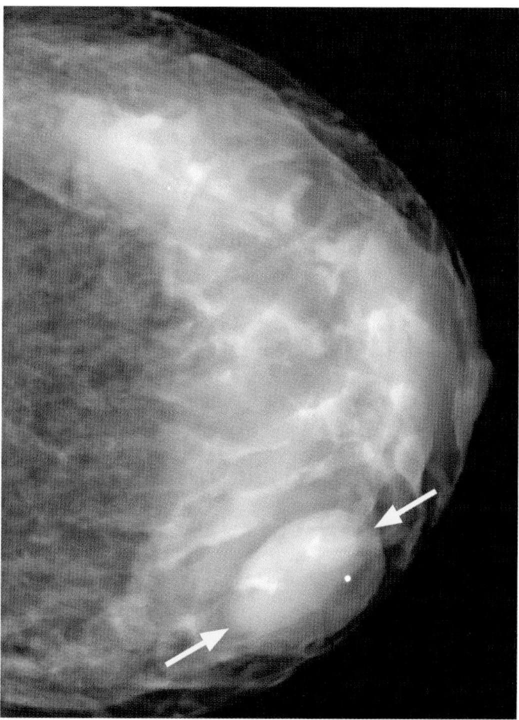

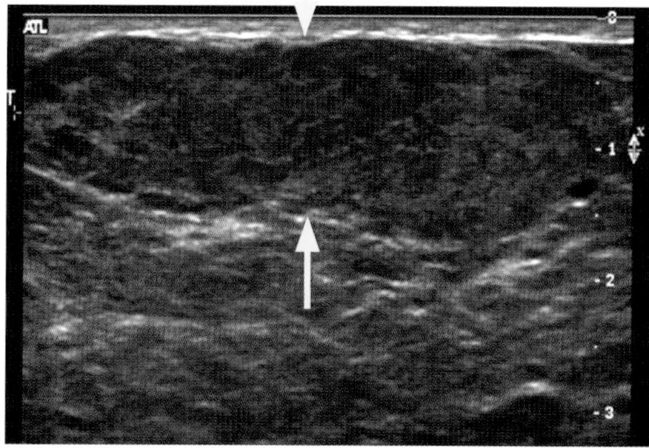

Lactational adenoma:

CC mammogram in a patient with diffusely dense breasts due to lactational change demonstrates a circumscribed, oval, isodense mass in the medial breast (arrow), marked with a BB.

Ultrasound demonstrates a large, circumscribed, macrolobulated, parallel, hypoechoic mass extending the entire width of the field of view (arrows).

Case courtesy Christine Denison, MD, Brigham and Women's Hospital.

- Lactational adenomas are seen in the second or third trimester of pregnancy or the postpartum period.
- Patients present with a freely mobile mass, which may be tender if it has rapidly enlarged.
- A lactational adenoma is benign and does not need excision after biopsy. It regresses when the patient is no longer lactating.

Multiple solid masses

Multiple intraductal papillomas

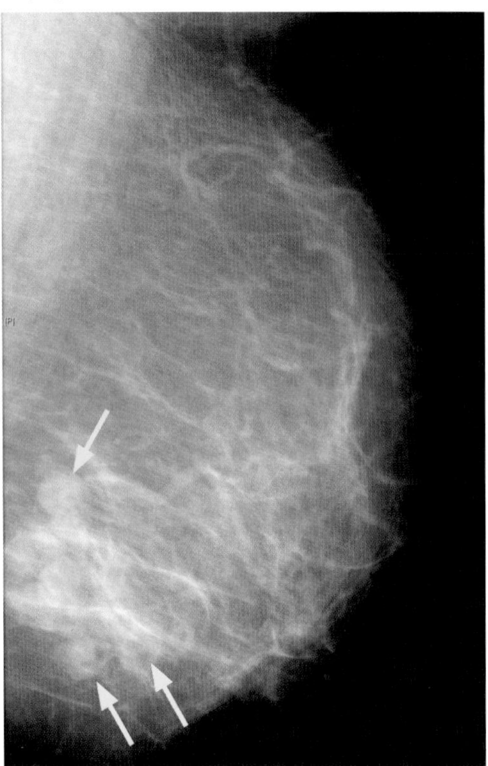

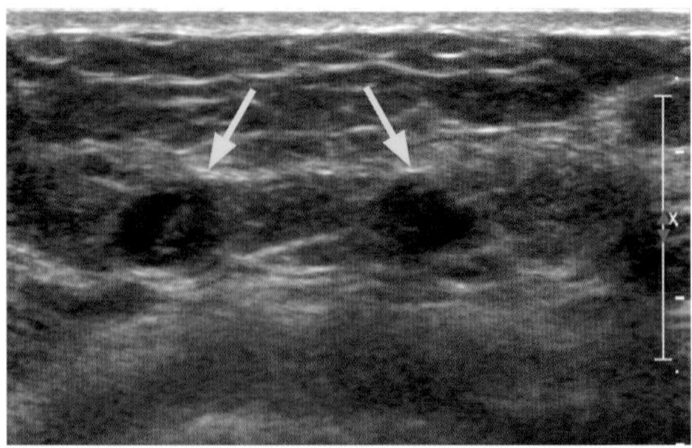

Multiple intraductal papillomas: Mammogram shows numerous round, circumscribed masses (arrows) in the inferior breast on this MLO view.

Ultrasound shows two of these round, hypoechoic, circumscribed, macrolobulated masses on a single frame (arrows); multiple adjacent similar lesions were also present (not shown).

Case courtesy Christine Denison, MD, Brigham and Women's Hospital.

- Multiple intraductal papillomas tend to occur in younger patients compared to solitary papillomas. When multiple, papillomas tend to be more peripheral in location and bilateral. In contrast to solitary papillomas, multiple papillomas are infrequently associated with pathologic nipple discharge.
- Multiple intraductal papillomas confer an increased risk of breast cancer.
- The mammographic appearance of multiple papillomas is of multiple well-circumscribed masses located in the peripheral breast.
- Two similarly named entities have potentially confusing terminology.

  Papillomatosis is a term that is frequently mistaken with multiple intraductal papillomas. Papillomatosis represents microscopic foci of intraductal hyperplasia with a papillary architecture. It is a pathologic diagnosis rather than an imaging finding.

  Juvenile papillomatosis is a rare cause of a mass that resembles a fibroadenoma in adolescents or younger women up to age 40.

Multiple skin masses

Neurofibromatosis

- Neurofibromatosis type 1 (NF1) is an autosomal dominant neurocutaneous disease that features pigmentary changes (e.g., café au lait spots and Lisch nodules) and neurofibromas.
- Cutaneous neurofibromas are the hallmarks of NF1, thought to arise from small nerve tributaries of the skin.
- On mammography, multiple cutaneous neurofibromas may appear as multiple skin masses outlined by air.

Steatocystoma multiplex

- Steatocystoma multiplex is a rare, autosomal dominant disease of multiple intradermal oil cysts. When the skin over the breasts is involved, mammography shows innumerable fat-density masses.

- Note that it is not possible to reliably differentiate cystic versus solid on mammography. However, a cyst may become less dense on spot compression owing to its compressibility.

Simple cyst

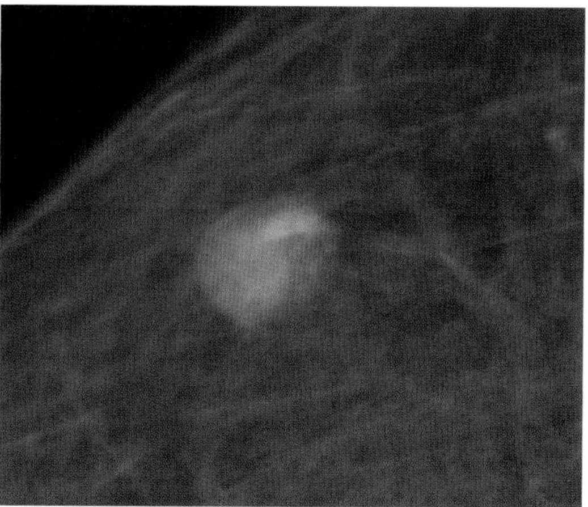

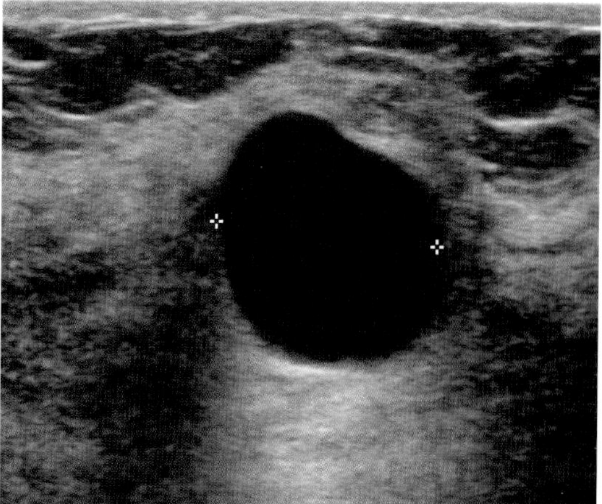

Simple cyst: Mammogram (left image) shows a circumscribed, round, isodense mass. Ultrasound shows an anechoic, gently lobulated, circumscribed structure with an imperceptibly thin wall and increased through transmission.

Case courtesy Christine Denison, MD, Brigham and Women's Hospital.

- A simple cyst is a benign, fluid filled structure that is round, oval, or gently lobulated in shape, with circumscribed margins and anechoic internal echo pattern. A cyst features an imperceptibly thin wall and posterior through transmission (posterior enhancement).
- A cyst that meets all the above criteria is benign and can be classified as BI-RADS 2.
- A simple cyst causing pain or discomfort may be aspirated.

Complicated cyst

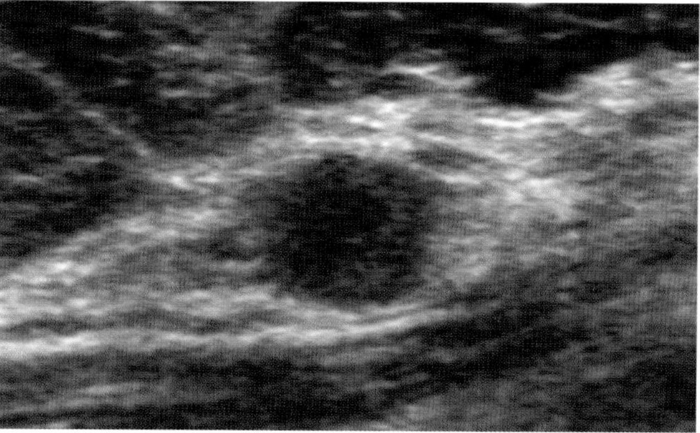

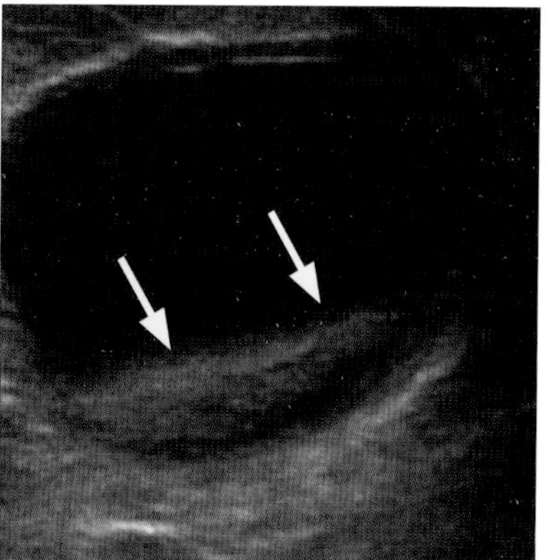

Complicated cysts in two different patients: The complicated cyst on the left features low-level internal echoes, while the complicated cyst on the right demonstrates layering debris with a fluid level (arrows).

Right case courtesy Christine Denison, MD, Brigham and Women's Hospital.

- A complicated cyst is a cyst that contains low-level internal echoes or layering debris.
- A complicated cyst is considered benign, although the risk of malignancy is not negligible. When new, complicated cysts are typically either classified as probably benign (BI-RADS 3) or aspirated. If the aspirated fluid is white, clear, or yellow, the fluid is presumed to be benign and discarded. Bloody fluid is sent for cytology.
- Occasionally, a complicated cyst can appear identical to a solid mass with homogeneous internal echoes. In such a case, core biopsy is typically performed.

Complex mass

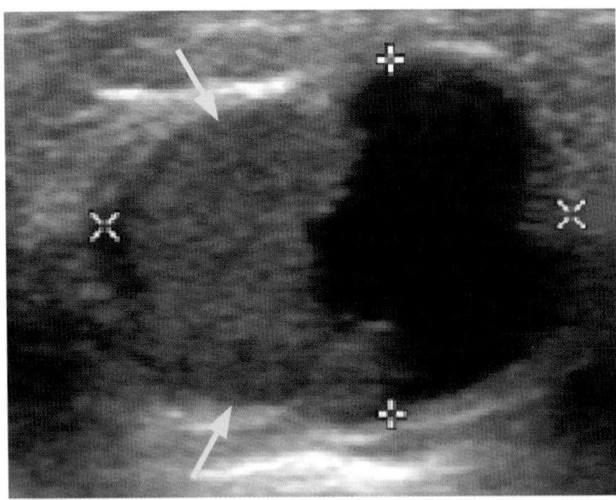

Complex mass:

Ultrasound shows a mixed cystic and solid lesion (calipers) with an irregular solid component (arrows). Although the mass is macrolobulated in shape and has circumscribed margins, the solid component makes this lesion suspicious for malignancy.

Case courtesy Christine Denison, MD, Brigham and Women's Hospital.

- The BI-RADS term *complex mass* describes a cyst with any complex feature, including thick walls or septations, or any solid or nodular element.
- A complex mass is a suspicious BI-RADS 4 lesion that should be biopsied. The solid component should be targeted with a core needle and a post-biopsy tissue marker should be placed.
- 36% of complex masses will be cancer upon biopsy.
- Malignancies that may appear as a complex mass includes intracystic carcinoma, intracystic papilloma, cystic phyllodes tumor, and a solid cancer with central necrosis.

  Intracystic carcinoma is an uncommon presentation of breast cancer, defined as cancer arising from the walls of a cyst. The typical ultrasound appearance of an intracystic carcinoma is a solid mural nodule projecting into the cyst fluid.
- Benign causes of a complex mass include hematoma, abscess, fat necrosis, galactocele, and benign cyst with adherent debris.

Clustered microcysts

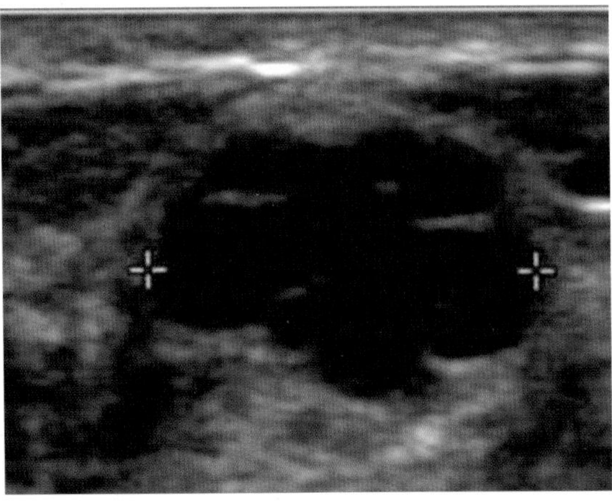

Clustered microcysts:

Ultrasound shows a cystic lesion (calipers) composed of several small 2–3 mm cysts with thin septations and no solid component.

Case courtesy Christine Denison, MD, Brigham and Women's Hospital.

- Thought to be due to apocrine metaplasia or fibrocystic change, clustered microcysts are composed of several adjacent tiny 2–5 mm cystic spaces separated by thin (<0.5 mm) septae.
- Clustered microcysts are a special class of benign cystic lesion. They can be classified as BI-RADS 2 if clearly seen and nonpalpable.
- Clustered microcysts may eventually evolve into a simple benign cyst.

Invasive ductal carcinoma (IDC)

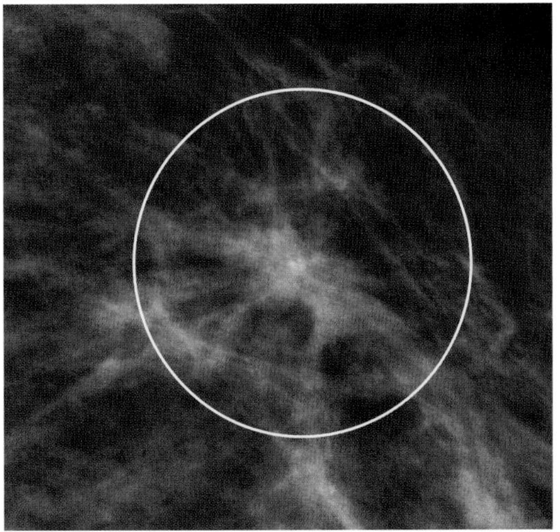

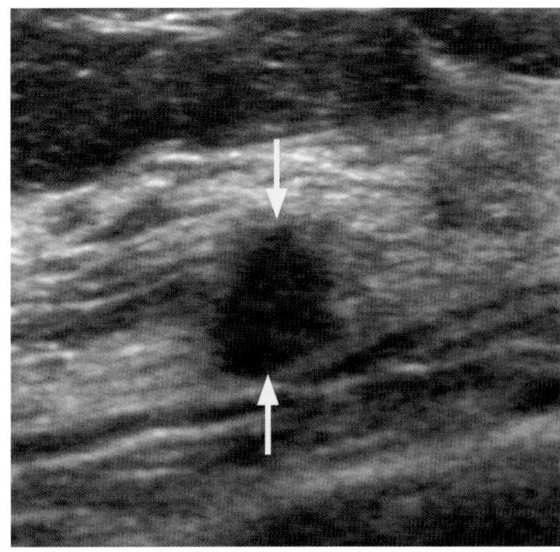

Invasive ductal cancer: Spot compression mammography (left image) demonstrates a high density, irregular mass with spiculated margins and associated architectural distortion (circle). Targeted ultrasound shows an irregular, hypoechoic mass (arrows) with indistinct margins and taller-than-wide orientation.

Case courtesy Christine Denison, MD, Brigham and Women's Hospital.

- Invasive ductal carcinoma (IDC) is the most common form of breast cancer. A typical mammographic appearance of IDC is a high density, spiculated mass. Malignant-type (pleomorphic or fine linear branching) calcifications are often present within the mass.
- It is important to remember that IDC can have a variable imaging appearance and may also present as a round mass, as isolated calcification, as architectural distortion, or any combination of these findings.

Invasive lobular carcinoma

- Invasive lobular carcinoma represents approximately 10% of all breast cancers and can be challenging to diagnose, with a false-negative mammography rate as high as 21%. Invasive lobular carcinoma tends to spread in an infiltrating pattern surrounding the glandular tissue, thus making its detection by mammogram or physical exam often quite difficult.
- The imaging appearance of invasive lobular carcinoma is variable. Similar to invasive ductal carcinoma, invasive lobular carcinoma may present as a mass (with or without spiculation) or subtle architectural distortion (which may be seen in one view only). In contrast to IDC, invasive lobular carcinoma rarely contains microcalcifications.
- Invasive lobular carcinoma is more often multifocal or bilateral compared to IDC.

Tubular carcinoma

- Tubular carcinoma is a slow-growing cancer that typically presents as a small, spiculated mass. The imaging appearance may remain stable across several prior mammograms, which emphasizes the fact that a malignant-appearing finding must be fully evaluated even if stability is demonstrated.
- Prognosis of tubular carcinoma is more favorable compared to IDC NOS.
- It is thought that radial scar may be a precursor to tubular carcinoma.

Radial scar (complex sclerosing lesion)

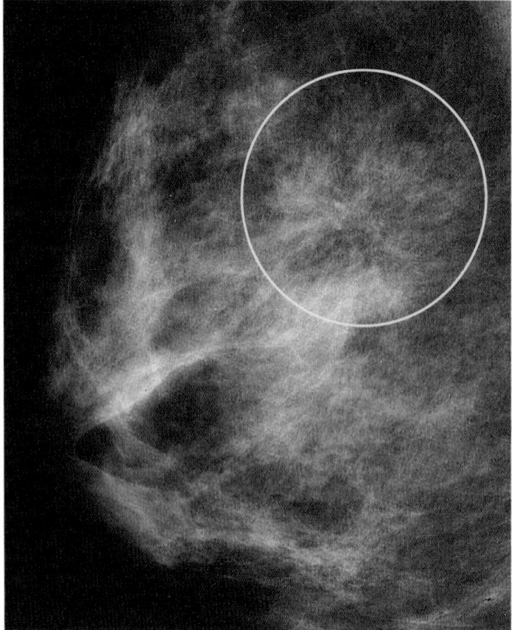
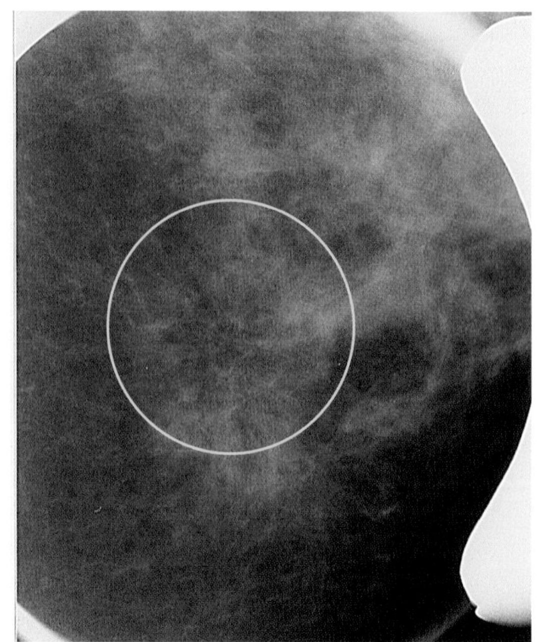

Radial scar: MLO mammogram (left image) shows subtle architectural distortion in the upper breast at middle to posterior depth (circle). Spot compression (right image) better shows architectural distortion (circle).

Case courtesy Christine Denison, MD, Brigham and Women's Hospital.

- A radial scar is a benign lesion of uncertain etiology that appears as a spiculated mass or architectural distortion. Despite the name, a radial scar has nothing to do with a post-traumatic or post-surgical scar. A complex sclerosing lesion is histologically identical but larger (>1 cm); however, recent literature suggests that these two names describe the same entity.
- Histologically, a radial scar is characterized by adenosis, hyperplasia, and central atrophy resulting in pulling-in of adjacent tissue and formation of a spiculated mass and architectural distortion.
- The mammographic and ultrasound appearance of a radial scar may be identical to cancer, appearing as a spiculated mass or architectural distortion on mammography and a hypoechoic shadowing mass on ultrasound.
- Radial scar may be associated with tubular carcinoma and high-risk lesions such as atypical ductal hyperplasia and lobular carcinoma in situ. Treatment is surgical excision.

Post-lumpectomy or post-excisional biopsy scar

- A postsurgical scar, either due to prior lumpectomy or excisional biopsy, may be indistinguishable on mammography from cancer in the absence of clinical history.
- Additional postsurgical changes are often present to aid in the diagnosis, including volume loss in the treated breast and skin retraction. Additionally, unlike recurrent tumor, a postsurgical scar should not get larger over time.
- If the patient was treated with radiation therapy, dystrophic calcification and skin thickening/retraction may also be present.

Abscess

- Although usually apparent clinically, an abscess can appear as an irregular or spiculated mass.

Benign breast fibrosis (sclerosing adenosis and fibrous mastopathy)

- Sclerosing adenosis and diabetic mastopathy are benign conditions that may mimic cancer on imaging.
- Sclerosing adenosis is a benign proliferative breast lesion caused by lobular hyperplasia. Fibrous tissue envelops and distorts the glandular elements, with resultant sclerosis of the affected tissue. Microcalcifications may be present, which mammographically may be indistinguishable from malignancy.
- Diabetic mastopathy is a benign disorder seen in long-term insulin-dependent diabetics that clinically presents as a large, painless, firm breast mass that may be indistinguishable from cancer. It is pathologically associated with inflammatory lymphocytes and fibrosis. Mammography shows an ill-defined mass or asymmetric density, which appears as a hypoechoic shadowing mass on ultrasound.

AXILLARY MASS

Breast cancer nodal metastasis

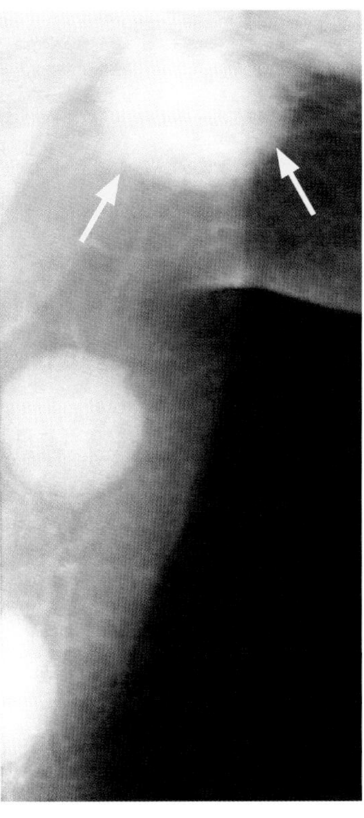

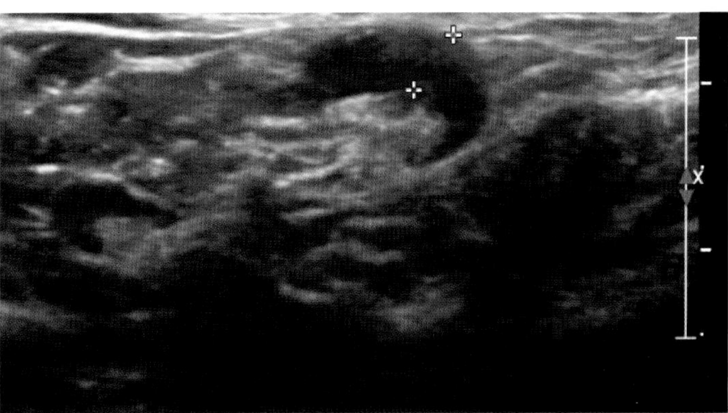

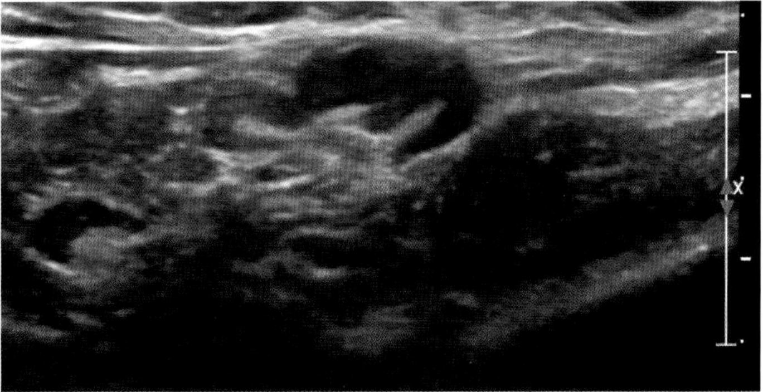

Malignant adenopathy: MLO mammogram (left image) shows numerous rounded, dense masses in the axilla, with the suggestion of indistinct margins of the superiormost mass (arrows). Ultrasound demonstrates several enlarged lymph nodes with asymmetrically thickened cortex measuring up to 1 cm (calipers).

- Unilaterally enlarged axillary lymph nodes are suspicious for breast cancer metastasis, although size alone is nonspecific for determining metastatic involvement.
- Sonographic features suspicious of lymph node metastasis include:

Round shape.	**Focal outwards cortical bulge.**
Thickened (>3 mm) cortex.	**Hilar indentation** or **obliteration of the hilum** by thickened cortex.
Eccentrically thickened cortex.	

- Bilateral adenopathy is more likely to be due to a systemic process, including collagen vascular disease, lymphoma, and leukemia.

Lymphoma

- Lymphoma involving the breast can have a variable appearance. Usually, primary breast lymphoma is caused by diffuse large B-cell lymphoma. Most B-cell lymphomas affecting the breast present as a palpable mass. Axillary adenopathy may be present.
- On mammography, lymphoma may present as a mass with indistinct margins. On ultrasound, lymphoma typically appears as a hypoechoic mass. In contrast to epithelial cancers such as invasive ductal carcinoma, calcifications are rarely seen in breast lymphoma.
- In a patient with a known diagnosis of lymphoma and a new breast mass, the primary consideration remains breast cancer. Histologic sampling is essential as lymphoma is treated with chemoradiation, not surgery.

Angiosarcoma

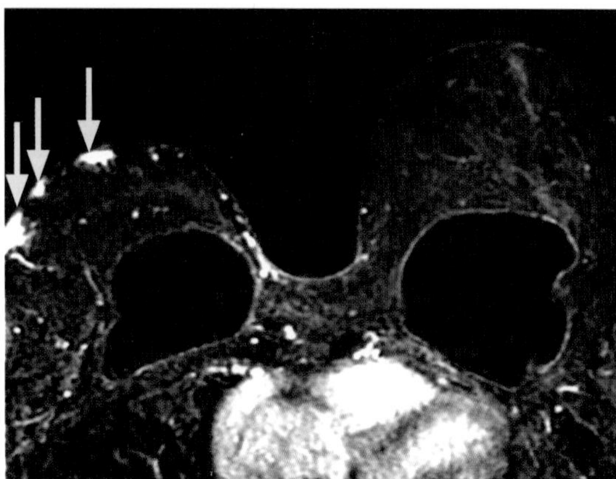

Axial post-contrast subtraction.

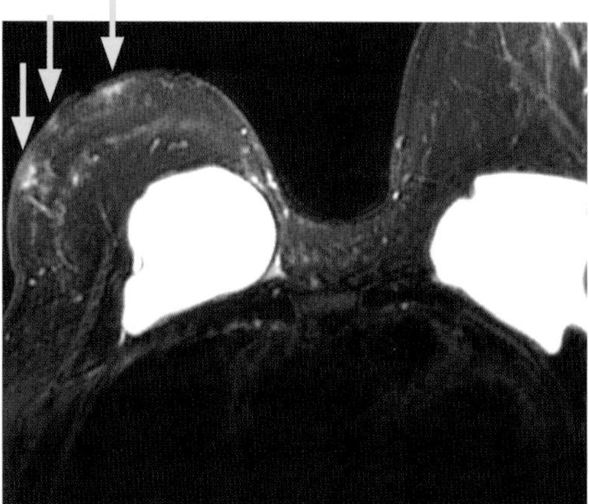

Axial T2-weighted image with fat suppression.

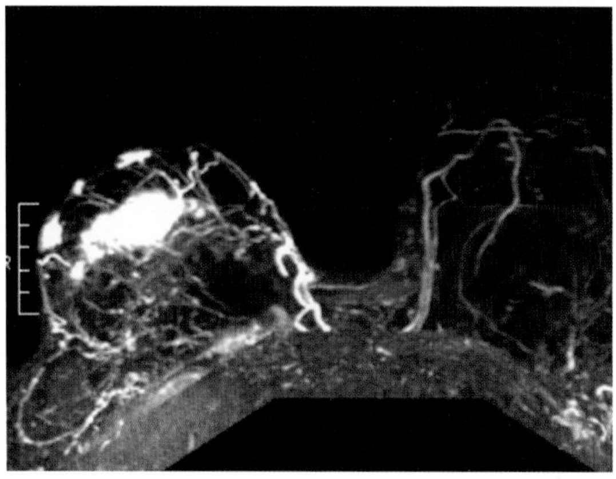

Maximum intensity projection (MIP).

Angiosarcoma:

Axial post-contrast subtraction demonstrates superficial nodular areas of enhancement in the right breast that are contiguous with the skin (arrows).

Axial T2-weighted image shows these superficial enhancing regions are hyperintense (arrows).

Axial MIP shows the extent of the abnormality involving both the skin and the deeper tissues of the right breast.

The patient was previously treated for breast cancer on the right and has bilateral implants.

Case courtesy Lorraine B. Smith, MD, Brigham and Women's Hospital.

- Angiosarcoma of the breast is a rare malignancy that may be primary or secondary to prior breast conservation therapy with radiation therapy.
- On MRI, angiosarcoma is hyperintense on T2-weighted images and demonstrates intense enhancement.

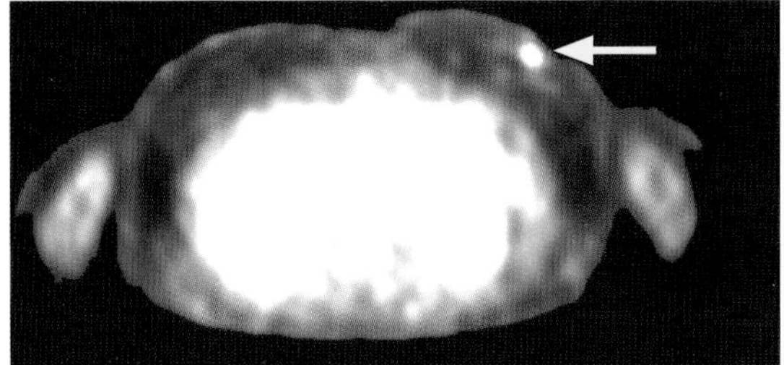

Initial staging FDG-18-PET in a patient with newly diagnosed cutaneous melanoma showed a focus of FDG uptake (arrow) in the left breast, without CT correlate (CT not shown).

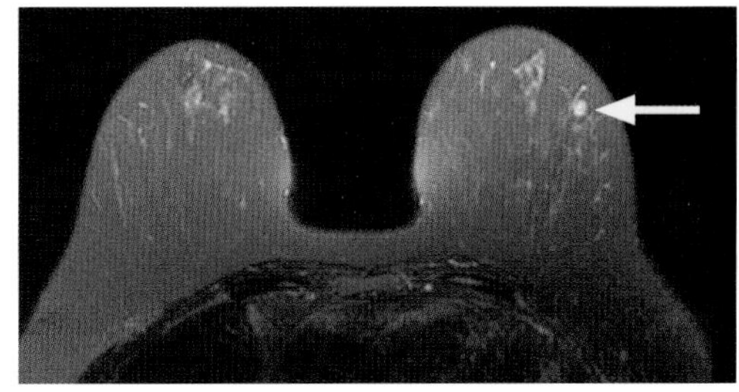

Initial mammogram and ultrasound were negative (not pictured) so an MRI was performed. This T2-weighted sequence shows a round, hyperintense mass in the outer left breast (arrow).

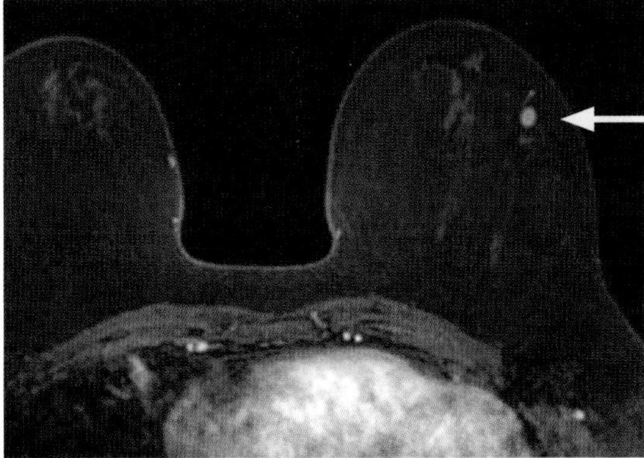

Post-contrast T1-weighted fat suppressed MRI shows enhancement of the circumscribed mass (arrow).

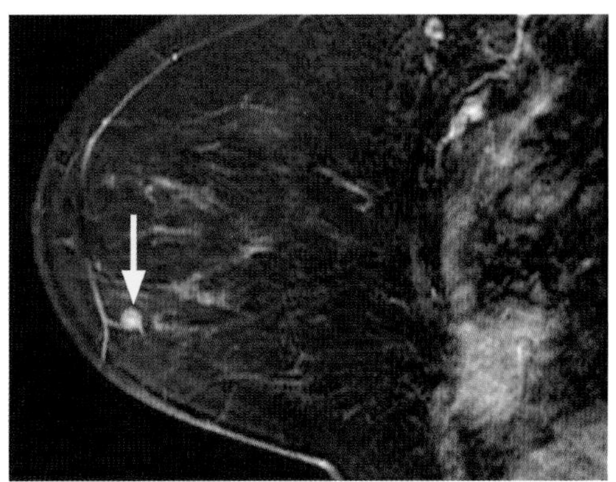

The location of the mass in the lower outer quadrant is confirmed on this post-contrast sagittal image.

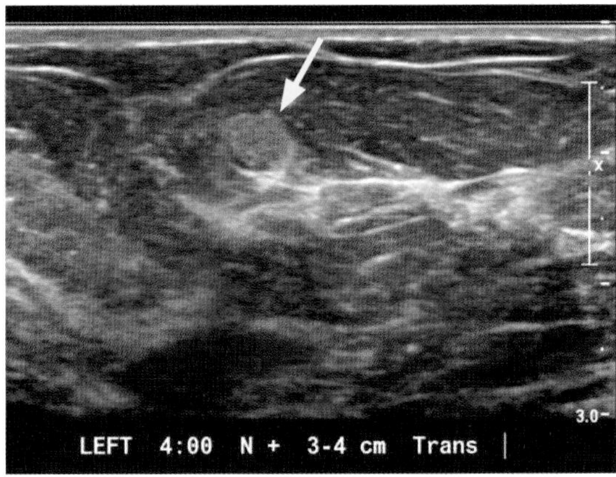

Second-look targeted ultrasound shows a lower-outer quadrant, circumscribed, round, hyperechoic mass (arrow) correlating to the mass seen on MRI.

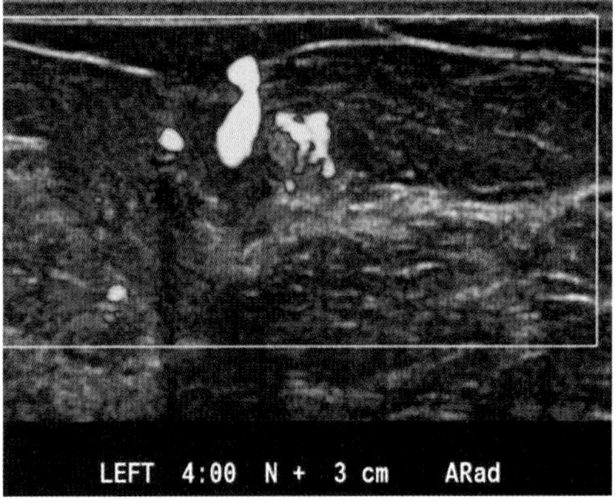

Power Doppler of the mass demonstrates marked vascularity. The MRI allowed localization of this mass, which was subsequently biopsied using US guidance.

Melanoma metastatic to the breast: In comparison to breast cancer, the unusual imaging features of this case are the hyperintense appearance of the metastasis on T2-weighted MRI and homogeneous hyperechogenicity on ultrasound, both of which are considered less suspicious findings for breast cancer (although the relatively rare mucinous carcinoma also typically appears hyperintense on T2-weighted images, it characteristically is isoechoic or hypoechoic on US).

Case courtesy Lorraine B. Smith, MD, Brigham and Women's Hospital.

- Hematogenous metastases to the breast have a variable appearance but are usually circumscribed round masses. Multiple new masses in a non-ductal distribution are especially worrisome for hematogenous metastases.
- Melanoma and renal cell carcinoma have a propensity to metastasize to the breast.

Asymmetry

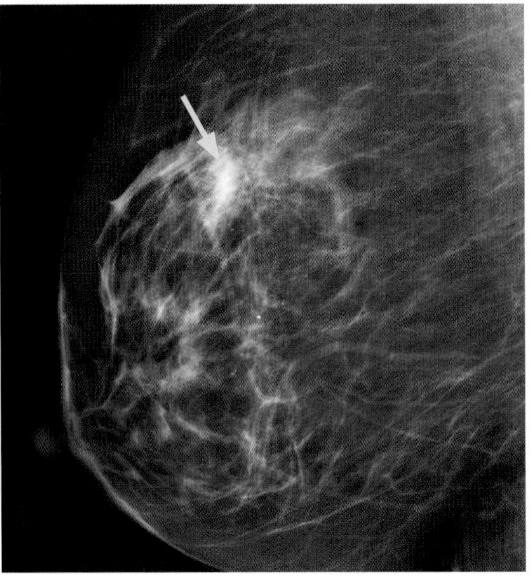

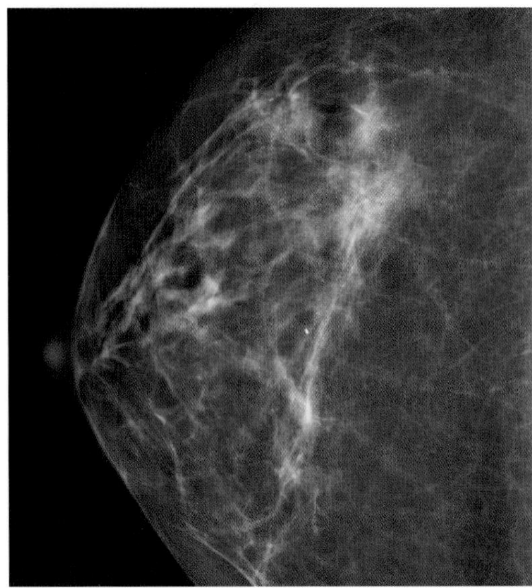

Asymmetry: MLO (left image) and CC views show an asymmetry on the MLO only (arrow), which is shown to represent superposition of fibroglandular tissue at middle to posterior depth on the CC view.

- An *asymmetry* is a region of breast tissue that is prominent on one view only and most commonly represents superposition of glandular tissue.

Global asymmetry

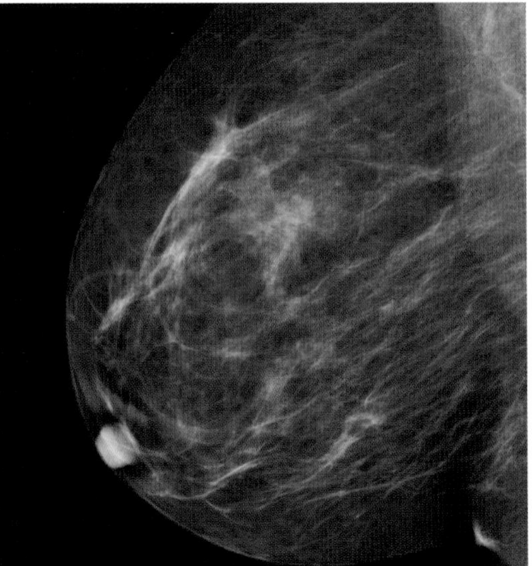

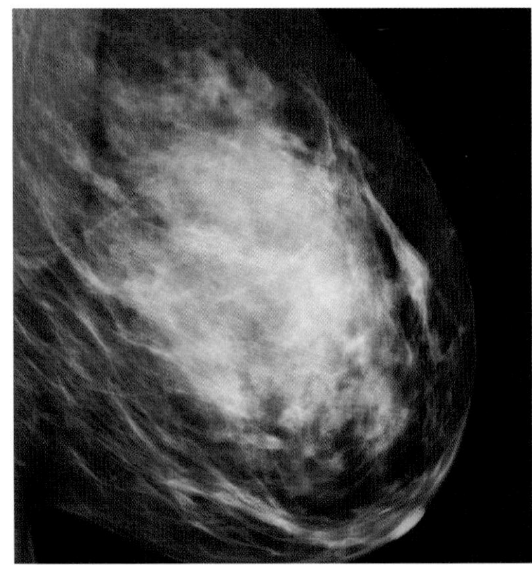

Global asymmetry: Bilateral MLO mammograms show scattered fibroglandular densities in the right breast (image on the left) and a extremely dense pattern in the left breast, with the increased density on the left occupying more than one quadrant. There is no associated mass, calcification, architectural distortion, or skin thickening.

- *Global asymmetry* is an asymmetric amount or density of breast tissue involving the majority of one breast only, most commonly due to greater volume of parenchyma in one breast compared to the other. More than one quadrant must be involved.
- Although global asymmetry is usually a normal variant, when associated with a concerning finding such as a mass, architectural distortion, skin thickening, or any palpable abnormality, then further workup is warranted.

Focal asymmetry

- A *focal asymmetry* is an abnormality involving less than one quadrant seen on two views (in contrast to an asymmetry) but that does not meet the criteria for a mass. A mass will have distinct borders and convex contours, while a focal asymmetry will have concave contours.
- A focal asymmetry usually represents a prominent area of normal breast tissue, particularly when there is interspersed fat, but further evaluation may be warranted.
- After a complete workup (including additional mammographic views with spot compression and targeted ultrasound), a nonpalpable focal asymmetry has <1% chance of being malignant and can be placed in BI-RADS 3. The lesion can be called benign after two years of stability.

Architectural distortion

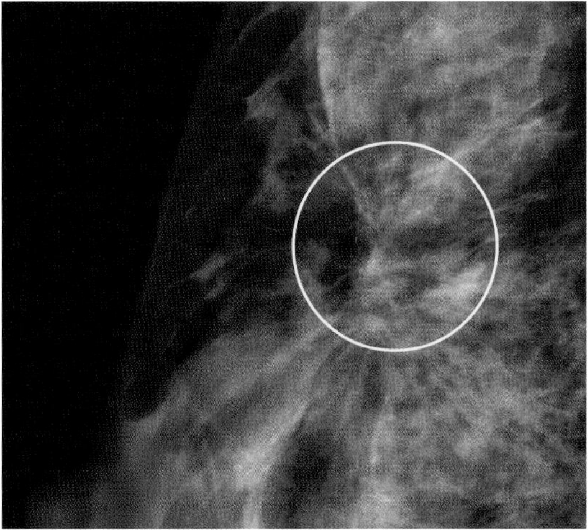

Patient A: Architectural distortion is caused by a scar from prior excisional biopsy (circle).

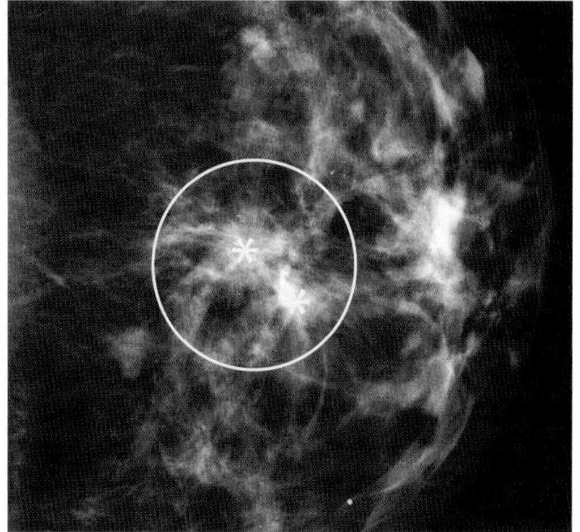

Patient B: Multifocal breast cancer causes architectural distortion (circle), associated with two adjacent spiculated masses (asterisks).

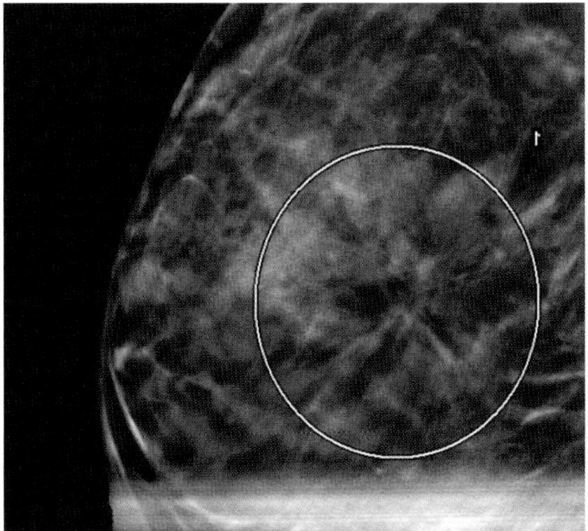

Patient C: Single slice from a mammographic tomogram shows architectural distortion (circle), which was invasive ductal carcinoma on biopsy.

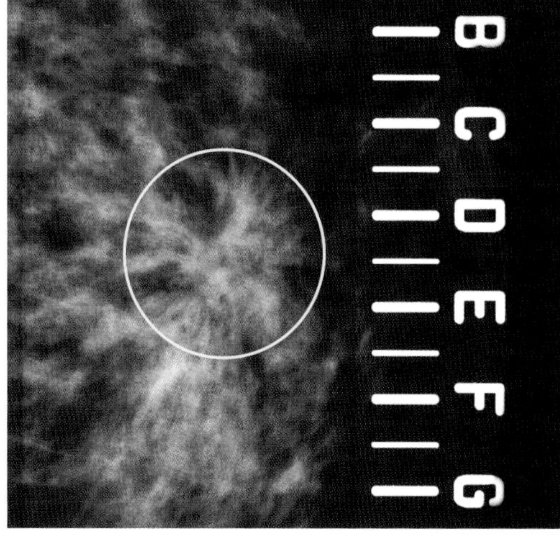

Patient D: Radial scar causing architectural distortion (circle), with an alphanumeric grid in place for wire localization prior to excisional biopsy.

Four different patients with architectural distortion.

- Architectural distortion describes lines radiation from a central point with no central mass visible, producing tethering and indentation of the breast tissue.
- Architectural distortion is suspicious for malignancy. The differential for architectural distortion is similar to the differential for a spiculated mass discussed previously.

Sternalis muscle

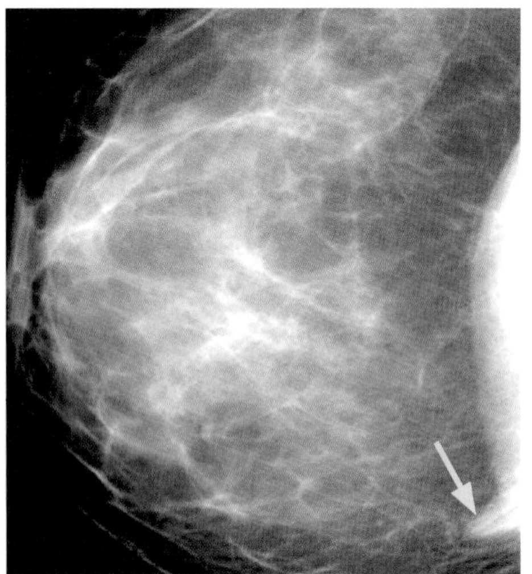

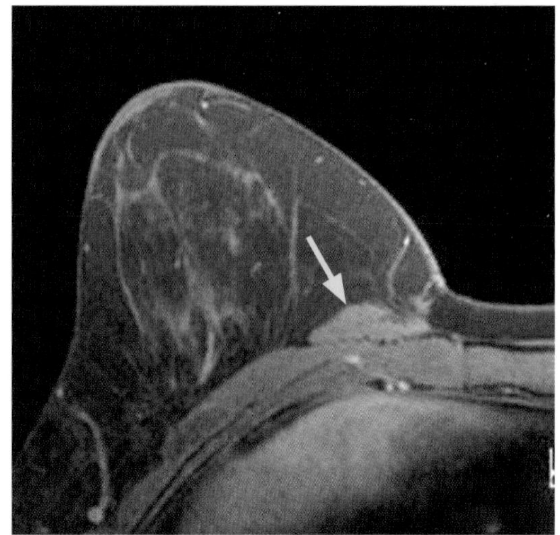

Sternalis muscle: CC mammogram (left image) shows a triangular-shaped density medially (arrow) at far posterior depth, overlying the pectoralis. No abnormality was seen on the MLO view (not shown). The mammographic findings are diagnostic. Axial post-contrast T1-weighted MRI in the same patient (performed for an unrelated reason) confirms an accessory muscle lying anterior to the pectoralis (arrow).

Case courtesy Christine Denison, MD, Brigham and Women's Hospital.

- The sternalis muscle is an accessory parasternal chest wall muscle present in less than 10% of patients. It is either triangular or rounded in shape and seen only on the CC view medially at far-posterior depth. It is more commonly unilateral.
- The main differential consideration is a medial mass; however, the characteristic shape and lack of corresponding finding on the lateral or MLO views is usually sufficient to diagnose a sternalis muscle. MRI can be performed in ambiguous cases.

Accessory nipple (polythelia)

- An accessory nipple (polythelia) is seen in approximately 2% of neonates and may present on mammography as a rounded mass along the mammary crest.
- Physical exam is diagnostic.

Poland syndrome

- Poland syndrome is a congenital disorder characterized by unilateral absence of the pectoralis major muscle, often associated with ipsilateral absence of breast tissue and syndactyly.

Accessory breast tissue

- Accessory or ectopic breast tissue occurs most commonly in the axillary tail.

BREAST MRI

INTRODUCTION

Overview of clinical role of breast MRI

- Breast MRI plays a complementary role to mammography in the evaluation of breast cancer. Contrast-enhanced breast MRI features excellent soft tissue contrast and high sensitivity for the detection of cancer. Although the distinction between normal or benign structures and malignancy is often not apparent using standard T1 and T2-weighted sequences, the addition of dynamic contrast enhancement greatly increases the accuracy for detection of malignancy. However, one of the greatest challenges facing the evolving field of breast MRI is the overlap in imaging findings between benign and malignant lesions. Both tumors and benign lesions may enhance and may exhibit similar morphologic characteristics. Strategies such as the characterization of enhancement kinetic curves and development of a stringent BI-RADS lexicon help to tackle this problem.

  One relative weakness of MRI compared to mammography is the lack of sensitivity to microcalcifications. While some larger calcifications can be detected as susceptibility artifact, mammography is superior to MRI for detection of small calcifications.

- In clinical use to evaluate for breast cancer, standard 1.5 Tesla breast MRI has been shown to have a negative predictive value of 98.9% and a relatively low false positive rate (49.7% positive predictive value for malignancy).

Breast MRI technique

- The risk stratification of an enhancing lesion involves separate evaluation of the lesion morphology (including morphologic description of the enhancement pattern) and the kinetic pattern of enhancement. Thus, both high spatial and temporal resolution is required, which is achieved using modern MRI equipment and protocols.
- Breast MRI is performed with the patient prone using a dedicated breast coil. Imaging of both breasts should be performed unless the patient has had a previous mastectomy. Bilateral imaging is very helpful to distinguish background parenchymal enhancement from pathological enhancement. Both breasts are imaged simultaneously.
- Standard sequences include T1- and T2-weighted images, with and without fat saturation. The crux of the breast MRI exam is the pre- and post-contrast sequences, which are obtained using fat saturation. Dynamic enhanced images are obtained sequentially to evaluate for enhancement over time. Although protocols vary by institution, three-dimensional fat-suppressed high-resolution spoiled gradient-echo T1-weighted images are commonly used for both pre- and post-contrast imaging (GE: VIBRANT; Siemens: VIEWS; Philips: BLISS).
- Intraductal fluid may be hyperintense on T1-weighted images, complicating the evaluation of enhancement. Post-processing is required to evaluate for true enhancement.
- The simplest form of post-processing is subtraction, where the dynamic post-contrast images are subtracted from the initial T1-weighted fat-saturated images.
- The maximum-intensity projection (MIP) image is a useful post-processing tool based on the subtraction images. A MIP highlights the brightest pixel along each parallel ray to create a volumetric data set where the enhancement can easily be seen in three dimensional space.
- Computer-aided detection (CAD) is a helpful adjunct for analysis of contrast-enhanced MRI sequences. CAD allows creation of a color angiomap, where the colors correspond to different temporal patterns of enhancement. These temporal enhancement curves allow further characterization of a lesion to determine the level of suspicion for malignancy.

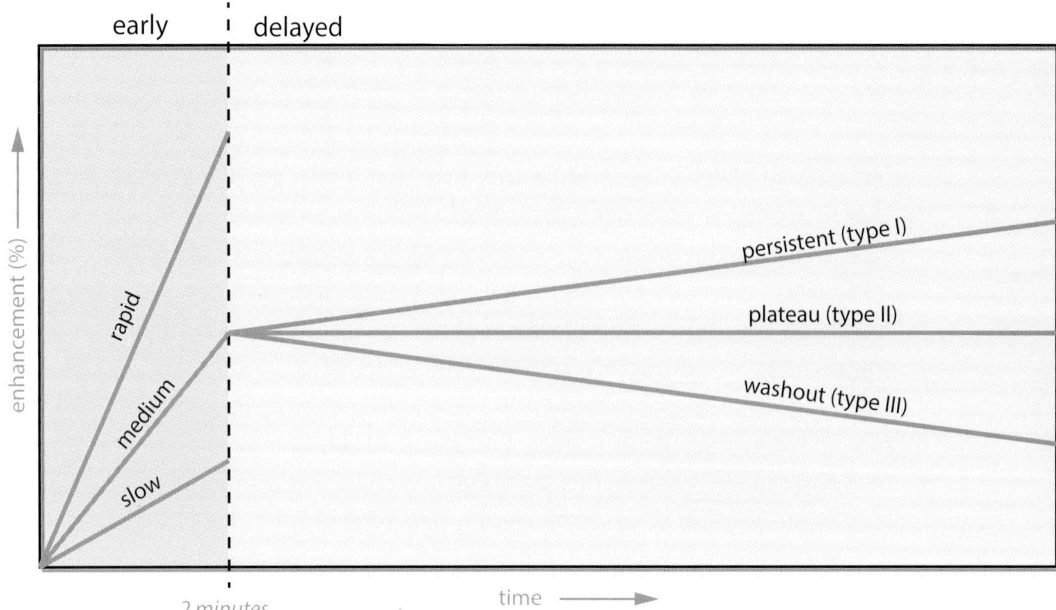

- Tumor angiogenesis and resultant capillary permeability allows early detection of cancer by contrast-enhanced MRI. Because tumor-associated vessels are thought to be relatively large and leaky, quantification of enhancement kinetics would be expected to show rapid enhancement and washout. This principle is the foundation for kinetic analysis in dynamic contrast-enhanced breast MRI.
- Dynamic contrast-enhanced breast MRI repeatedly images the breast at multiple time points. Enhancement curves can be generated by plotting percent relative enhancement (compared to the unenhanced image) against time. The enhancement curve can be divided into *early* (within the first two minutes) and *delayed* phases.
- Per the BI-RADS lexicon, the kinetics of early enhancement can be characterized as slow, medium, and rapid. A malignant lesion would be expected to have rapid early enhancement.
- Analysis of the delayed phase of enhancement allows one to further stratify the risk of malignancy. The BI-RADS lexicon describes three kinetic patterns of delayed enhancement: Persistent (type I), plateau (type II), and washout (type III).
- A **type I (persistent)** curve shows continuously increasing (>10%) enhancement in the delayed phase. Although a type I curve is associated with a benign finding in 83% of cases, up to 9% of malignant lesions may feature a type I curve.
- A **type II (plateau)** curve has an early rise in enhancement, but levels off (within 10%) in the delayed phase. A type II curve is suspicious, although less strongly so than a type III curve. Type II curves have been reported to have a positive predictive value between 64 and 77%.
- A **type III (washout)** curve has a >10% decrease in signal intensity in the delayed phase and is suspicious for malignancy. A type III curve has a positive predictive value of 87–92%, but is seen in only 21% of malignant lesions. False positive benign lesions that may show washout kinetics include lymph nodes, adenosis, and papillomas.
- In the evaluation of a lesion, morphology is much more important than the pattern of enhancement. If a mass with malignant morphology (e.g., spiculated margins or rim enhancement) demonstrates type I enhancement, it remains just as suspicious for cancer. Similarly, a small, circumscribed, reniform mass adjacent to a vessel with type III kinetics is a typical appearance for a benign intramammary lymph node and should not be biopsied.

MRI MASSES

Overview of BI-RADS lexicon for MRI masses

- The mammographic and MRI lexicons have several terms in common to describe mass shape and margin. However, since MRI incorporates dynamic contrast enhancement, new terminology was developed to describe a mass's internal pattern of enhancement.
- A *mass* is defined as a space-occupying lesion that displaces normal breast parenchyma.

Mass shape

- The MRI lexicon for mass shape is identical to that of mammography.
- **Round**: Spherical in shape.
- **Oval**: Elliptical or oblong in shape.
- **Lobular**: Undulating or scalloped contour.
- **Irregular**: Uneven shape. An irregular shape is suspicious for malignancy.

Mass margin

- Evaluation of the margin of an enhancing mass is the most predictive MRI imaging feature. Similar to mammography, the BI-RADS lexicon for mass margin includes **smooth**, **irregular**, and **spiculated.** Smooth margins are more suggestive of benignity, while irregular or spiculated margins are more suspicious for malignancy. A mass with spiculated margins is thought to represent cancer 84–91% of the time.
- The shape and margin of a mass are best evaluated in the early post-contrast sequences. Progressive enhancement of the normal surrounding breast parenchyma on the subsequent post-contrast sequences may obscure the true margins of a mass.

Internal enhancement

- Several descriptive terms unique to breast MRI are used to describe the internal enhancement pattern within a mass.
- **Homogeneous** internal enhancement is uniform and suggestive of a benign lesion.
- **Heterogeneous** internal enhancement describes non-uniform enhancement within the lesion and is suspicious, especially in the presence of rim enhancement.
- **Rim enhancement** is a highly suspicious finding for cancer, representing malignancy in up to 84% of cases, although this finding is only seen in 16% of cancers. Potential pitfalls are a peripherally enhancing inflammatory cyst or fat necrosis, both of which can demonstrate rim enhancement. Note that a cyst will be water-signal on T1- and T2-weighted images with a diagnostic ultrasound appearance, while fat necrosis will have central high signal on the non fat-suppressed T1-weighted images and a characteristic mammographic appearance.
- **Enhancing internal septations** and **central enhancement** are also suspicious for malignancy, although these patterns are less commonly seen compared to rim enhancement. Enhancing internal septations have a positive predictive value for malignancy of >95%.
- **Dark internal septations** are highly specific for a benign fibroadenoma (>95% positive predictive value). A hyalinizing fibroadenoma, typically seen in older women, rarely enhances.

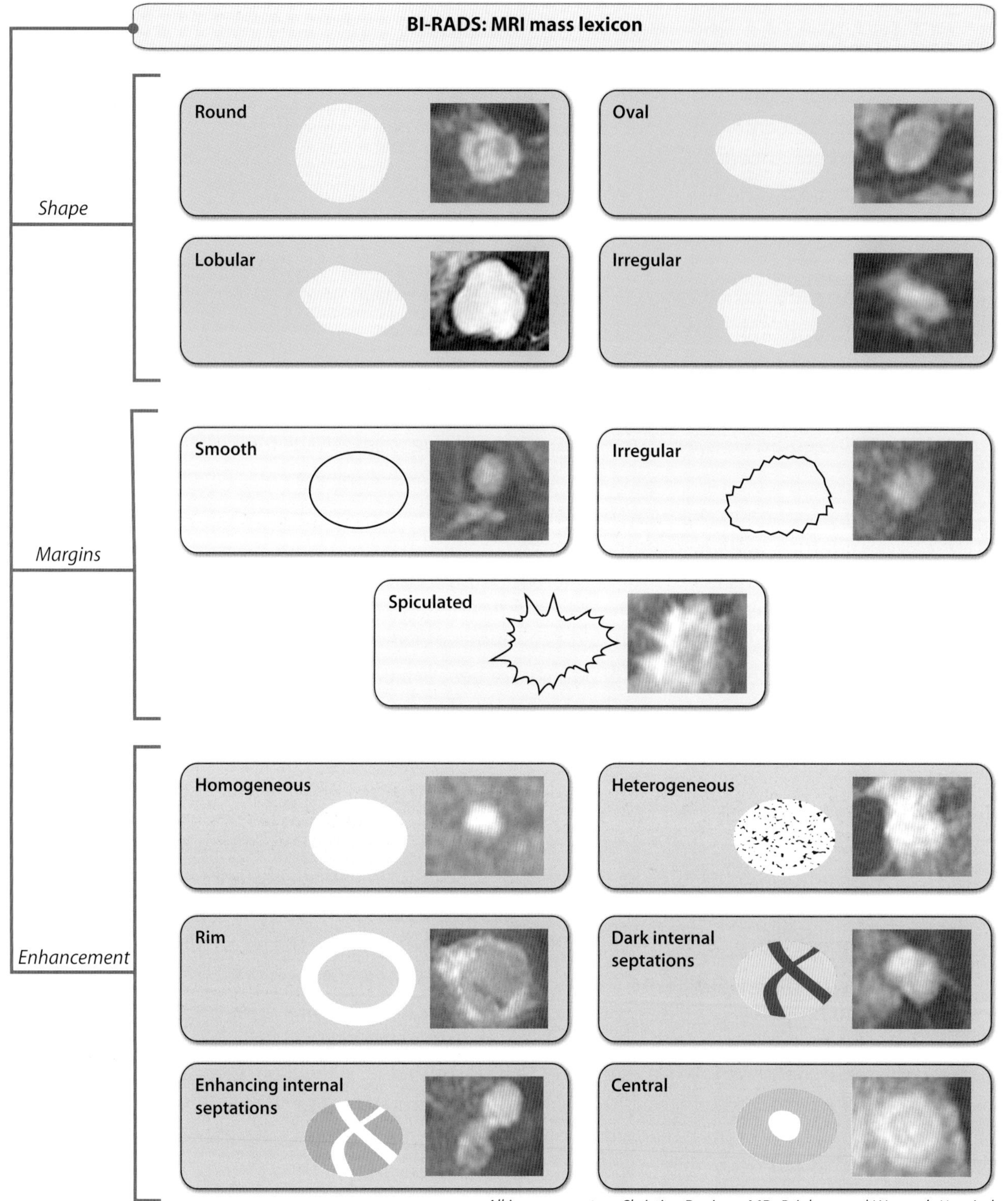

All images courtesy Christine Denison, MD, Brigham and Women's Hospital.

MRI FOCUS

- A *focus* is a small dot of enhancement <5 mm in size that does not have any mass effect or correlate to any abnormality on the precontrast images. A focus is too small for accurate assessment of margins or internal enhancement characteristics. Between 3 and 15% of foci are thought to represent cancer.

  The degree of suspicion for malignancy of a focus or foci depends on multiplicity and menstrual status. For instance, multiple bilateral foci in a premenopausal patient would be much less concerning than a solitary focus in a postmenopausal patient, especially if new.

Non-masslike enhancement (NMLE)

Overview of non-masslike enhancement (NMLE)

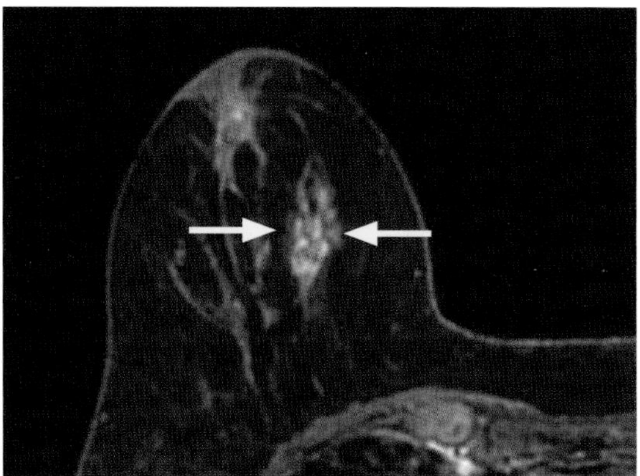

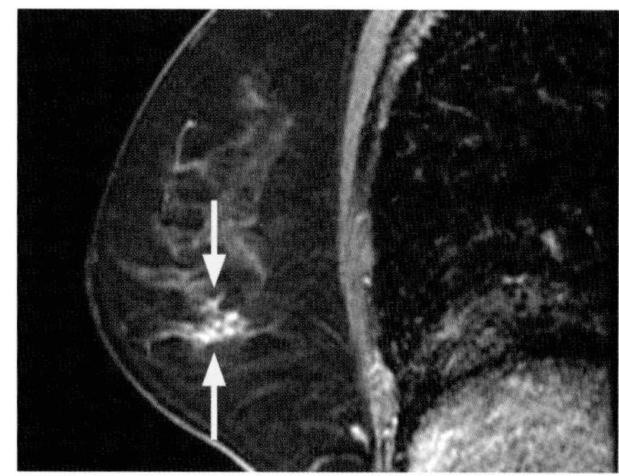

Non-masslike enhancement (NMLE) suggestive of DCIS: Axial (left image) and sagittal fat-saturated T1-weighted postcontrast images show an area of non-masslike enhancement in the lower inner quadrant of the right breast (arrows) with clumped morphology and segmental distribution.

Case courtesy Christine Denison, MD, Brigham and Women's Hospital.

- Non-masslike enhancement (NMLE) is an enhancing region that is not a mass or a focus.
- Similar to mammographic calcifications, non-masslike enhancement is described both in terms of distribution and morphology. The purpose of the lexicon for NMLE is to distinguish between malignancy and benign parenchymal enhancement or fibrocystic changes.

NMLE distribution

- **Linear/ductal**: The distribution is arranged in a line or branching pattern pointing to the nipple, conforming to a duct. Linear/ductal distribution is up to 26% malignant, typically seen with a clumped enhancement morphology.
- **Segmental**: Triangular-shaped distribution of enhancement points towards the nipple. Similar to linear/ductal, segmental distribution suggests a ductal etiology. Segmental distribution is the most common distribution of DCIS (42% of DCIS cases).
- **Focal area:** Distribution is <25% of a quadrant and contains interspersed fat/glandular tissue.
- **Regional**: Geographic distribution is ≥25% of a quadrant.
- **Multiple regions**: At least two regions of NMLE are present.
- **Diffuse**: Uniform NMLE is present throughout the breast. A diffuse distribution of NMLE may be difficult to distinguish from background parenchymal enhancement.

NMLE internal enhancement

- **Heterogeneous**: Enhancement is confluent and non-uniform in morphology. Heterogeneous NMLE is seen in 21% of cases of DCIS.
- **Homogeneous**: Enhancement intensity is uniform throughout the NMLE. This pattern is more suggestive of a benign lesion compared to heterogeneous, but small cancers may enhance homogeneously.
- **Clumped**: The enhancement resembles a cobblestone pattern, also described as a "bunch of grapes." Clumped enhancement is most suggestive of DCIS, especially in a linear/ductal or segmental distribution. Clumped NMLE is seen in 51% of cases of DCIS.
- **Stippled/punctate**: Enhancement features tiny round dots and is associated with benignity.
- **Reticular/dendritic**: Enhancement is strand-like. Reticular/dendritic morphology may be associated with inflammatory carcinoma. The clinical use of this internal enhancement descriptor is not in widespread use and it may be removed from future versions of BI-RADS.

Summary of NMLE

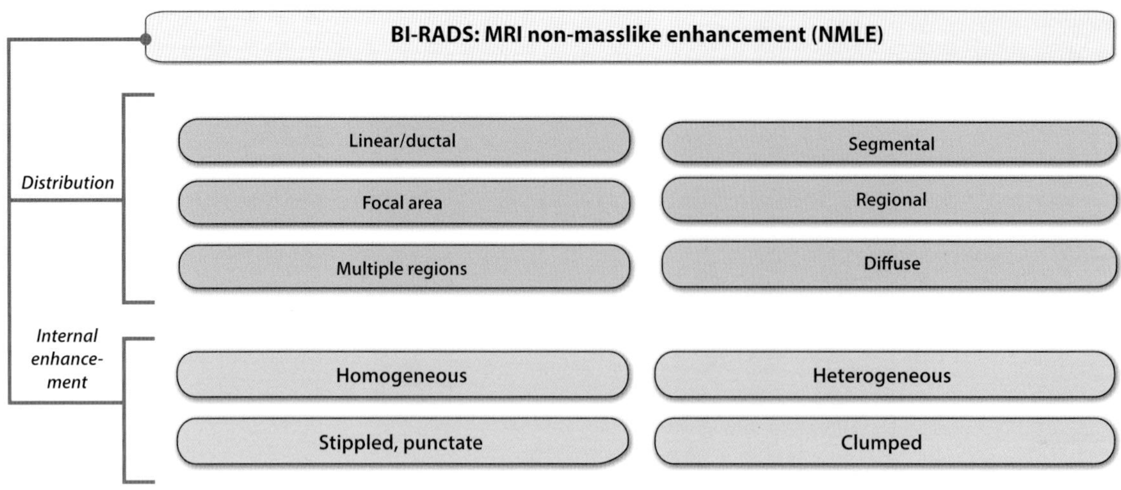

Interpreting breast MRI

- Initial evaluation of the post-processed CAD angiomap or MIP images can give a global overview of any abnormal enhancement.
- The T2-weighted images are evaluated for the presence of hyperintense lesions. Although no specific BI-RADS nomenclature exists to describe the T2 characteristics of a mass, T2 hyperintensity within the enhancing portion of a mass is highly suggestive of a benign lesion. For instance, in younger women, myxoid fibroadenomas are typically hyperintense on T2-weighted images.
- Isolated evaluation of the signal characteristics on T2-weighted images is not a reliable method to classify a lesion as benign. For instance, mucinous carcinoma is typically hyperintense on T2-weighted images. The assessment of the T2-weighted images should be used as a secondary criterion to confirm benignity in a lesion that appears morphologically benign.
- T1-weighted images best show susceptibility artifact from biopsy clips or calcifications, and demonstrate hyperintense hemorrhagic cysts and proteinaceous ductal fluid.
- The principal aspect of the exam is the dynamic post-contrast images with post-processing to evaluate for the presence, morphology, and kinetics of any enhancing masses, foci, or NMLE.

Management guidelines

- Mass or NMLE with a type I kinetic curve and benign morphology:

  BI-RADS 2: Bilateral stippled foci of enhancement, without a dominant mass or suspicious focal NMLE.

  BI-RADS 3: Mass or NMLE with benign morphology and enhancement kinetics, and negative targeted ultrasound. In order for follow-up to be appropriate (rather than biopsy), the lesion must demonstrate only benign features on MRI. It is specifically these benign features, rather than the negative targeted ultrasound, that allow a lesion to be classified as BI-RADS 3.

  BI-RADS 4: Solitary, dominant, or asymmetric NMLE in a high risk patient.
- Mass or NMLE with type II or III kinetic curve and benign morphology:

  BI-RADS 4: A notable exception is a benign intramammary lymph node, which is typically located in the lateral breast adjacent to a vessel, and is reniform in shape.
- Mass or NMLE with type I kinetic and malignant morphology is generally classified as BI-RADS 4.
- A mass or NMLE with a type II–III kinetic curve and malignant morphology may be classified as BI-RADS 4 or 5.

Screening

- Screening for cancer in high-risk patients is an accepted indication for breast MRI. High risk is defined as a 20% or greater lifetime risk of developing breast cancer. There are several models for risk prediction taking into account family history, gene mutations, and exposures such as thoracic radiation (typically administered for treatment of lymphoma). BRCA1 or BRCA2 gene mutation carriers (or untested first-degree relatives of a confirmed carrier) are high risk, with 50–85% lifetime risk of developing breast cancer.
- MRI has been shown to detect occult breast cancer in 2–5% of high-risk women.
- There are no data to support screening breast MRI in women at average risk for breast cancer, even with dense breasts.

Evaluating extent of disease in the ipsilateral and contralateral breast

- In patients with an established diagnosis of breast cancer, MRI can be helpful to evaluate the extent of disease and can change clinical management.
- The presence of two or more sites of cancer in one quadrant (*multifocal* disease) may preclude breast conservation, depending on the size of the breast. MRI has been reported to find additional cancer in the same quadrant in 1–20% of women.
- The presence of cancer in more than one quadrant (*multicentric* disease) usually requires mastectomy. Unsuspected multicentric disease was found by MRI in 2–24% of women.
- MRI is highly accurate to measure tumor size. Compared to ultrasound and mammography, the tumor measurements determined by MRI have the highest correlation with pathology specimens. Ultrasound and mammography tend to underestimate the true size.
- MRI can assess for the presence of enlarged or abnormal axillary lymph nodes to suggest nodal metastasis.
- MRI can evaluate for pectoralis invasion.

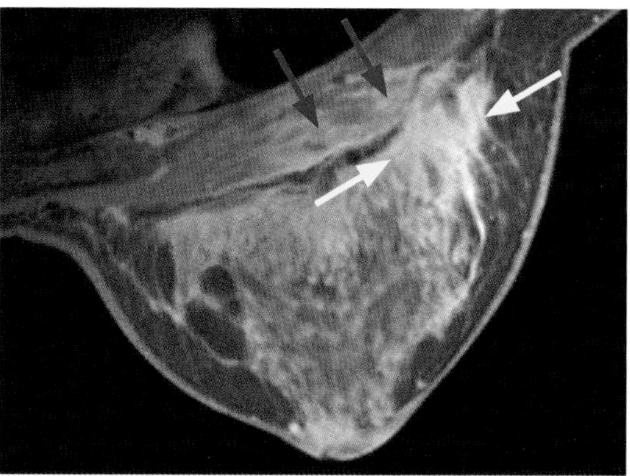
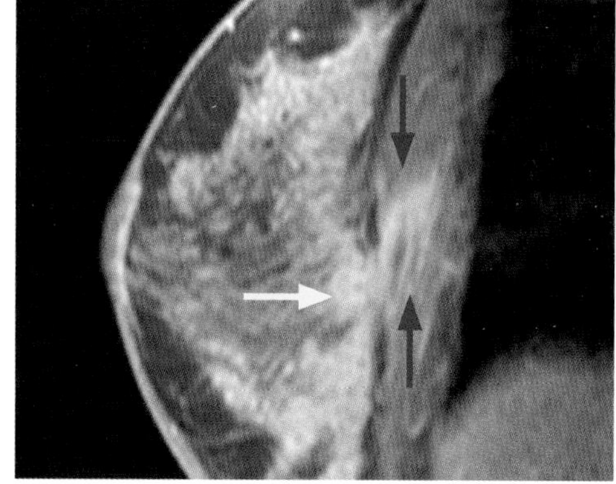

Pectoralis muscle invasion: Axial (left image) and sagittal contrast-enhanced fat-suppressed MRI shows an ill-defined enhancing mass (yellow arrows) in the far posterior breast with loss of normal fat plane separating the posterior fibroglandular tissue from the pectoralis muscle. There is associated abnormal enhancement of the pectoralis muscle itself (red arrows).

Case courtesy Christine Denison, MD, Brigham and Women's Hospital.

- The presence of an enhancing lesion in the contralateral breast has been shown to have a relatively low positive predictive value for malignancy, of approximately 20%. For this reason, there has recently been a trend away from routine MRI screening of the contralateral breast due to the high number of false positives.

Assessment of residual disease

- Breast conservation therapy combines lumpectomy with radiation therapy and is the treatment of choice for most early stage breast cancers. Negative surgical margins are required, and if the margins are positive then re-excision or mastectomy is indicated.
- MRI can evaluate for the extent of residual disease, which may manifest as small nodular areas of enhancement around the lumpectomy site.

Screening for recurrence or new malignancy

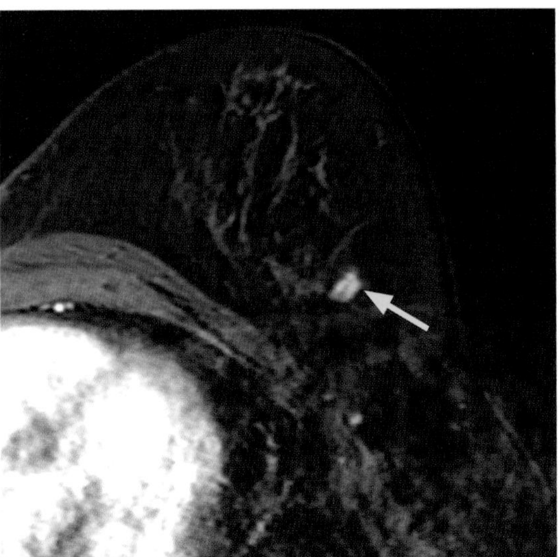
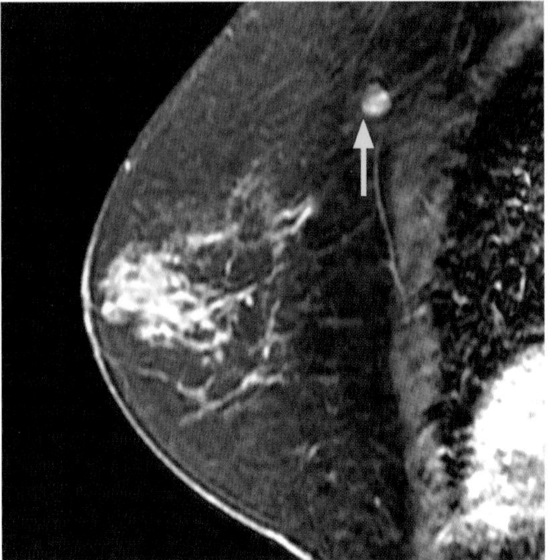

Contralateral second primary after mastectomy: Unilateral contrast-enhanced fat-saturated T1-weighted MRI of the left breast in a patient with previous mastectomy shows a new, irregular, enhancing mass with irregular margins (arrows).

- Breast MRI is commonly performed in patients with treated breast cancer to evaluate for local recurrence or a metachronous primary in the ipsilateral or contralateral breast.
- Local recurrence rates at 15 years are 12% for women who received radiation and 36% for women who did not receive radiation.
- Following lumpectomy, normal enhancement at the lumpectomy site can be seen for up to 6–18 months due to granulation tissue. Enhancement at the lumpectomy scar beyond 18 months may no longer be normal. Of particular concern for recurrence is the reappearance of enhancement after the initial postoperative enhancement has subsided.

Following response to treatment in a patient on neoadjuvant chemotherapy.

- Neoadjuvant therapy is employed to reduce the size of large tumors prior to resection. Follow-up MRI performed even after one or two cycles of chemotherapy can evaluate whether the patient has responded to chemotherapy.
- Cytotoxic therapy may reduce tumor vascularity, which will often alter the enhancement kinetics of a lesion.
- After completion of neoadjuvant therapy, MRI can detect the location and extent of residual disease to guide surgical planning.

Diagnostic problem solving

- In certain situations, MRI can be useful for problem solving after a thorough mammographic and ultrasound workup remains indeterminate. For instance, an asymmetry that persists after spot compression but is not localizable on an orthogonal view or by ultrasound may be assessed by MRI.

Evaluation of silicone implants

- MRI has the highest sensitivity and specificity for evaluation of silicone implant rupture. Unlike the standard breast mass protocol, no gadolinium is administered for an implant evaluation and this exam does not evaluate for cancer.
- Saline implants are typically evaluated by physical exam, mammography, and ultrasound. MRI is not indicated.

POST-SURGICAL IMAGING

IMAGING IMPLANTS

Overview of implants

- Implants can be used either for cosmetic reasons or for breast reconstruction after mastectomy. The two types of implants in common use are filled with either silicone or saline. Silicone implants are comprised of a silicone gel and come in pre-manufactured sizes. Saline implants contain a valve that allows filling of the implant during surgery.
- Regardless of the type of implant, a fibrous capsule is gradually formed as a reaction to the foreign body. The capsule may become calcified. Over time, the implant may partially herniate through the capsule without rupturing, causing a palpable contour deformity.
- Implants can be placed either behind the pectoralis (retropectoral) or directly in front of the pectoralis/behind the fibroglandular tissue (prepectoral/retroglandular).

Mammographic imaging of implants

- When implants are imaged with mammography, standard views are difficult to interpret because the high-attenuation implant can obscure breast tissue. Implant-displaced views (also called Eklund views) displace the implant posteriorly and pull the native breast tissue anteriorly to allow for improved compression and visualization of the breast tissue.
- A saline implant can be identified on mammography due to the presence of its valve. Additionally, the wall of the implant will be denser than the center because the wall is made of silicone elastomer that is denser than saline.
- In contrast, a silicone implant will be uniformly dense and no valve will be present.

Overview of implant rupture

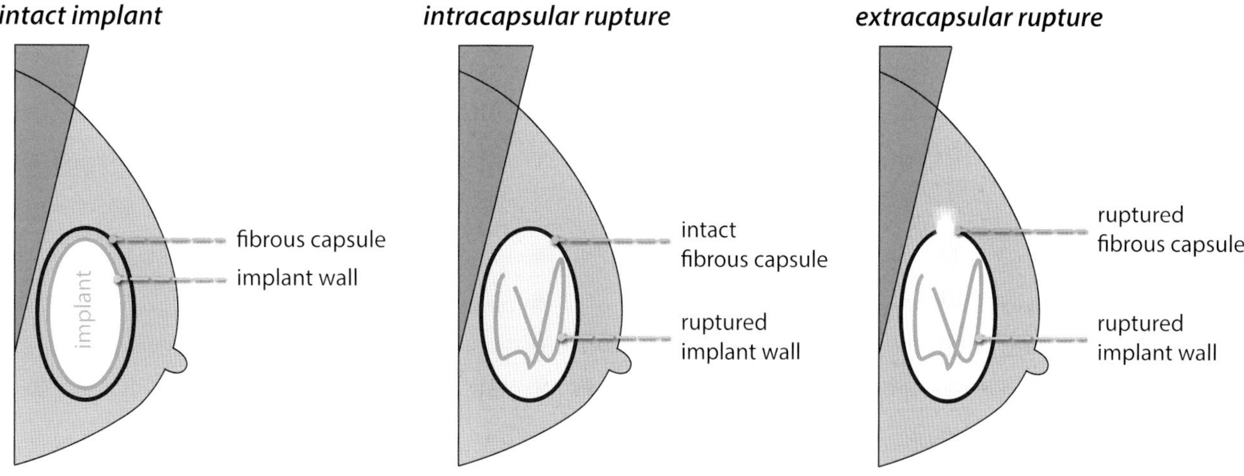

- Rupture of an implant can be contained within the fibrous capsule (intracapsular rupture) or may extend out of the fibrous capsule (extracapsular rupture).
- In general, the distinction between intra- and extracapsular rupture is most important for silicone implants.

Saline implant rupture

- Rupture of a saline implant is usually evident clinically. Rupture causes sudden collapse and resultant instantaneous decrease in breast size. The residual implant wall collapses on itself and the saline is absorbed.

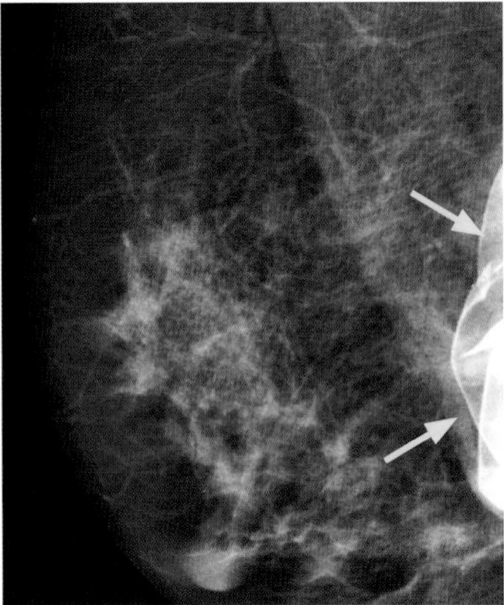

Saline implant rupture:

MLO mammogram partially shows a collapsed retropectoral implant (arrows) at the posterior aspect of the image.

Intracapsular silicone implant rupture

- Intracapsular rupture of a silicone implant may manifest clinically as a subtle change in the implant contour but without significant change in the size or even shape of the breast. Rupture of a silicone implant can be challenging to diagnose clinically.
- Mammography is often normal, and ultrasound or MRI is usually necessary to diagnose silicone implant rupture.
- MRI of intracapsular silicone implant rupture shows the classic *linguine* sign, which describes the fragmented elastomer shell that is freely floating within the silicone contained within the fibrous capsule.

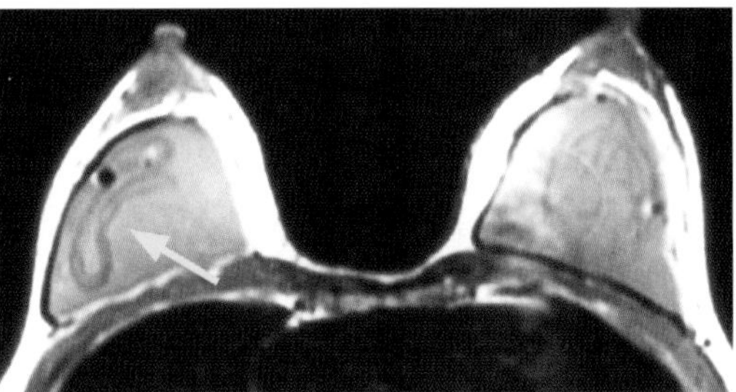

Intracapsular rupture of a silicone implant:

Axial T1-weighted MRI without fat saturation shows the curvilinear undulating contour of the disrupted and collapsed implant wall in the right breast (arrow), representing the *linguine* sign. The fibrous capsule is intact.

Case courtesy Christine Denison, MD, Brigham and Women's Hospital.

- Ultrasound of intracapsular silicone implant rupture shows segments of broken and collapsed implant wall floating within intracapsular silicone.

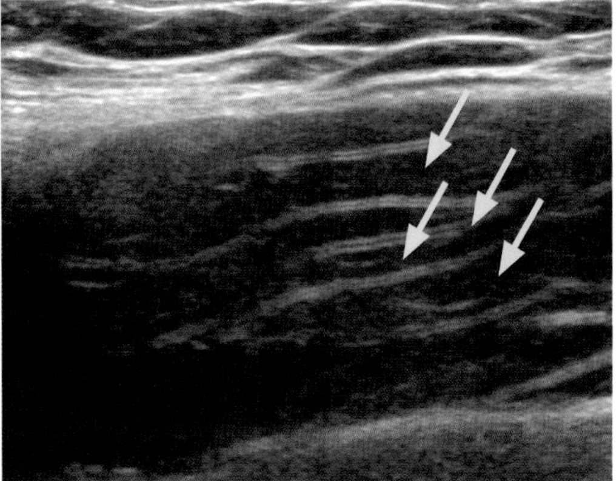

Intracapsular rupture of a silicone implant:

Ultrasound shows a stair step pattern of the echogenic silicone implant wall (arrows). The implant wall is floating within a lake of fluid containing low-level internal echoes, representing silicone.

Case courtesy Christine Denison, MD, Brigham and Women's Hospital.

Extracapsular silicone implant rupture

- Extracapsular rupture of a silicone implant may be evident on mammography as high density silicone extending beyond the edge of the capsule into the breast parenchyma.

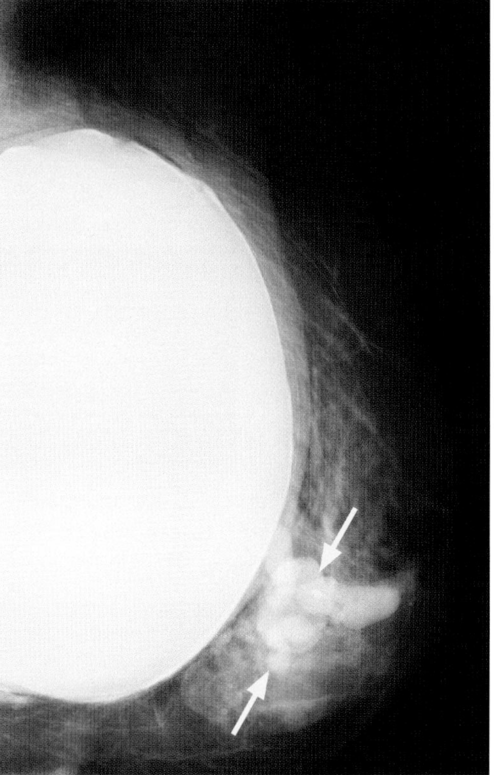

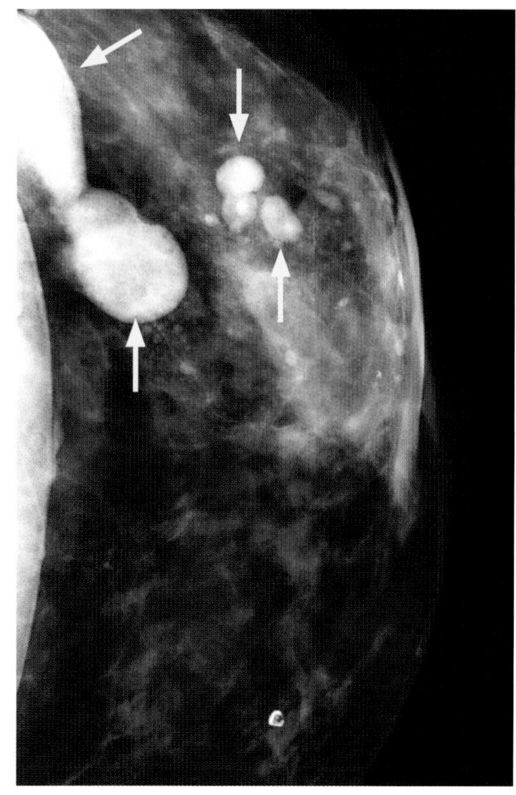

Extracapsular rupture: Standard MLO mammogram (left image) shows a retropectoral implant and frank extravasation of high density silicone into the breast parenchyma (arrows). The implant-displaced CC mammogram better shows the extent of the high density intraparenchymal silicone granulomas.

- On ultrasound, extracapsular silicone rupture causes free silicone to appear in the breast parenchyma, which has a classic *snowstorm* appearance on ultrasound.

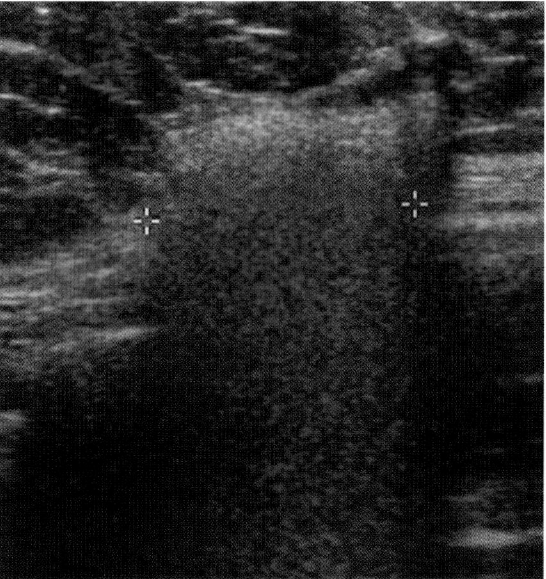

Extracapsular rupture of silicone implant:

Ultrasound shows an echogenic, shadowing mass with a classic *snowstorm* appearance (calipers), suggestive of silicone granuloma from extracapsular rupture.

Case courtesy Christine Denison, MD, Brigham and Women's Hospital.

Reduction mammoplasty

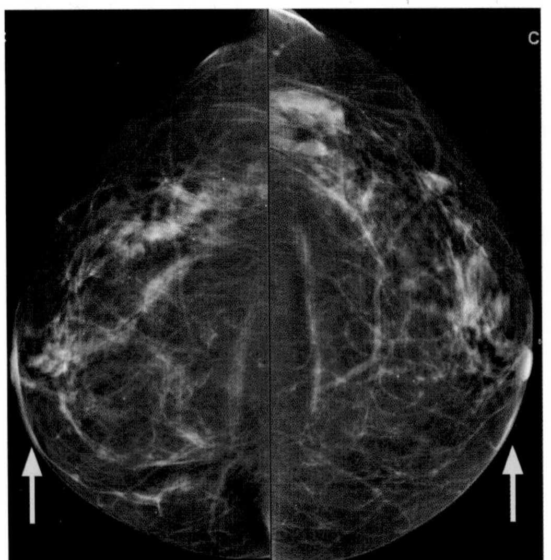

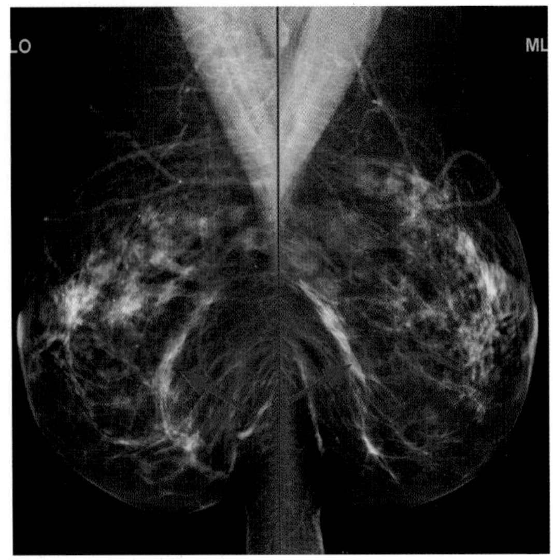

Reduction mammoplasty: Bilateral CC (left images) and MLO mammograms show subtle skin thickening of the lower medial breasts (yellow arrows). Symmetric distortion of the fibroglandular tissue (red arrows) in the lower breast is best seen on the MLO views. The nipples are superiorly displaced.

- Reduction mammoplasty is performed for aesthetic reasons or to reduce back pain caused by large breasts.
- The surgeon removes breast parenchyma and skin from the inferior breast and relocates the nipple to a more superior location.
- The mammographic findings of reduction mammoplasty include skin thickening over the lower breast corresponding to the surgical scars. The lower breast features curvilinear architectural distortion. Fat necrosis may be present.

Gynecomastia

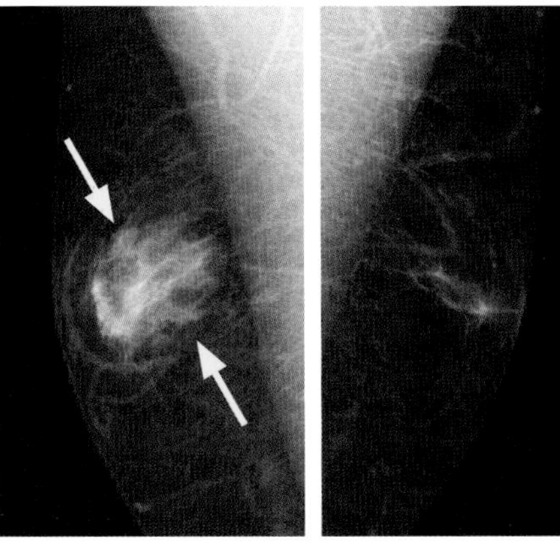

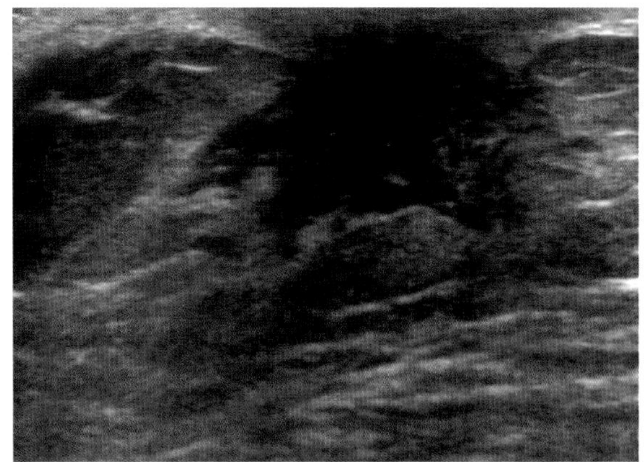

Gynecomastia: Bilateral MLO mammogram (left image) shows a flame-shaped density in the right breast (arrows) in the subareolar region. The left breast is normal. Ultrasound shows a fan-shaped geographic region of subareolar shadowing surrounded by normal breast tissue.

- Gynecomastia is the benign development of glandular tissue in a male. It is the most common diagnosis of males evaluated for a focal breast complaint and clinically presents with a subareolar palpable abnormality.
- Gynecomastia may be due to cirrhosis, drugs (including antihypertensives and antidepressants), marijuana, pituitary hormone dysfunction, or a hormone-producing tumor.
- The typical mammographic appearance is a flame-shaped or triangular subareolar density. Mammography is sufficiently diagnostic. The ultrasound appearance is variable and may be misleading. Ultrasound is generally avoided if the mammographic views are diagnostic.

Male breast cancer

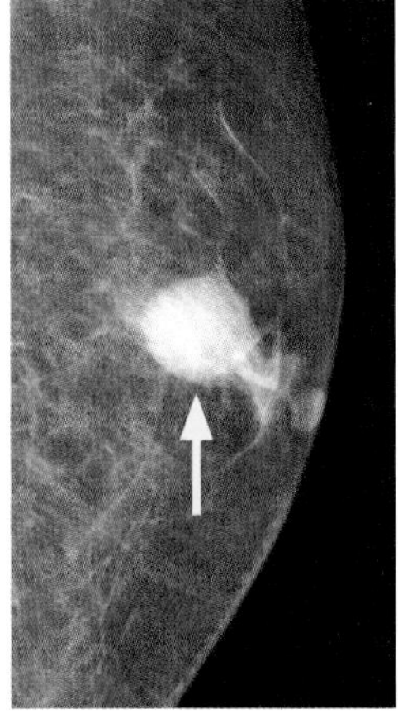

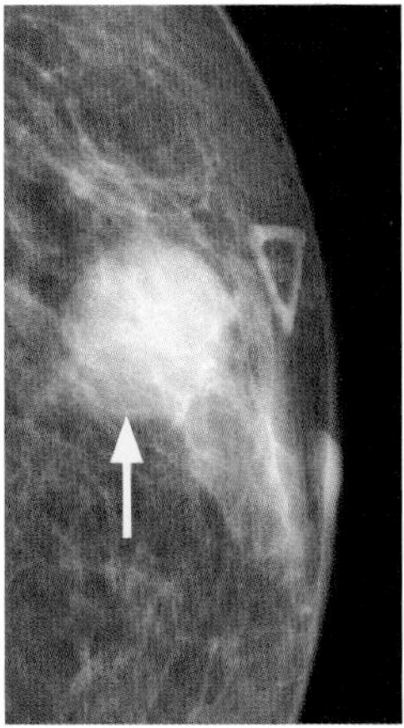

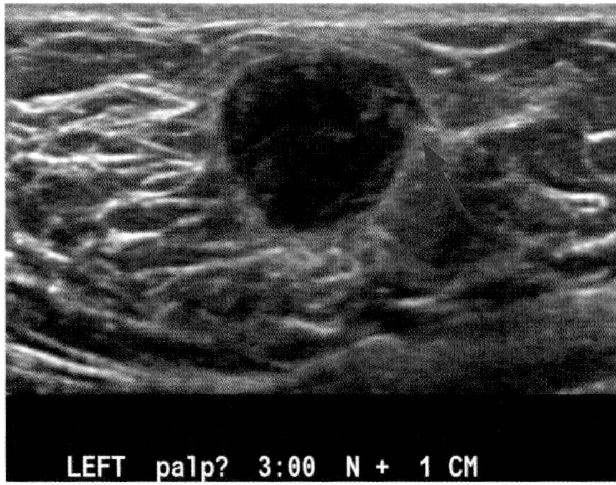

Male breast cancer: Left MLO and CC views to evaluate a palpable finding (marked cutaneously by the triangle) show a round mass (arrows) with obscured margins in the slightly upper outer breast. Ultrasound shows a round mass with an angular margin (red arrow) and heterogeneous internal echoes.

Case courtesy Christine Denison, MD, Brigham and Women's Hospital.

- Male breast cancer accounts for less than 1% of all breast cancers. It tends to affect men greater than 60 years of age and clinically presents as a palpable mass.
- While the typical appearance of male breast cancer is a spiculated mass, it is important to remember that a benign male breast mass is very rare and any breast mass in a male should be regarded with suspicion. Breast cancer may occasionally present as a round, circumscribed mass, which is just as suspicious as a spiculated mass.

Overview of breast interventions

- Regardless of the method of biopsy, the radiologist must perform a radiology–pathology correlation of every case to ensure that the pathologic diagnosis is concordant with the imaging findings. Discordant findings should receive further workup, typically requiring repeat biopsy, either core or excisional. An example of a discordant finding is benign pathology (e.g., fragments of a fibroadenoma) for a highly suspicious, spiculated mass.

Ultrasound-guided core needle biopsy

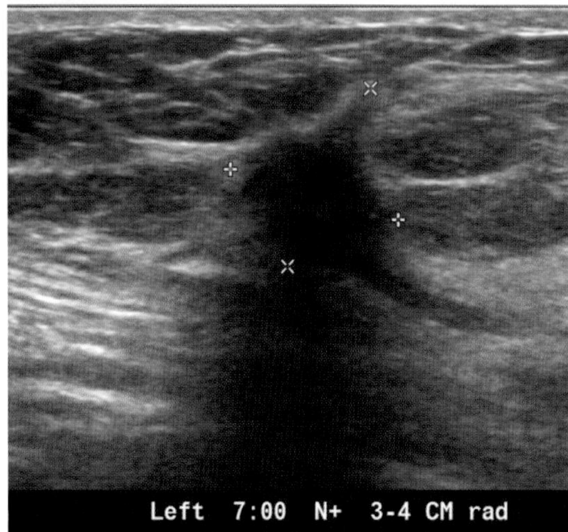

Pre-procedure ultrasound demonstrates a shadowing, spiculated mass (calipers) with taller-than-wide orientation that is highly suspicious.

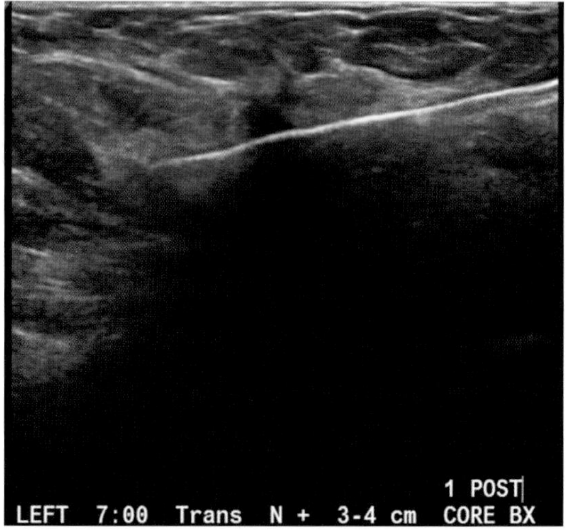

Post-fire image from an ultrasound-guided core needle biopsy shows the core needle traversing the lesion with an appropriate shallow angle of approach.

- Ultrasound-guided core needle biopsy is the preferred approach for a lesion which is well seen on ultrasound. Ultrasound-guided biopsy using standard freehand technique and a 14-gauge spring-loaded needle is a highly accurate method to biopsy breast masses.
- Ultrasound-guided interventions are the most user dependent and take time to master. Appropriate initial positioning of the patient and planning of the approach allows a smooth procedure. Some practitioners always hold the ultrasound probe in the non-dominant hand to allow the dominant hand control over the needle. Others take an ambidextrous approach.
- It is critical when performing an ultrasound-guided procedure to always keep the biopsy device parallel to the chest wall, or at a very shallow angle of obliquity. A standard breast biopsy needle advances approximately 2 cm when sampling. Far posterior lesions can be entered with the tip of the biopsy device and lifted anteriorly off the chest wall before sampling.
- A lateral approach to the lesion is generally preferred.
- The skin entry site should be an appropriate distance from the lesion, with posterior lesions requiring a larger distance between the lesion and the entry site to maintain a nearly parallel biopsy needle course. Once an entry site is chosen, cutaneous and subcutaneous anesthesia is administered under ultrasound guidance and a small dermatotomy is made. Multiple samples are obtained; each needle pass should be documented and needle positioning within the target demonstrated in an orthogonal plane for 1–2 passes.
- After adequate sampling, a titanium tissue marker clip is typically placed and post-procedure mammography is performed to confirm marker position.

Ultrasound-guided cyst aspiration

- The procedure for ultrasound-guided cyst aspiration is similar to that of a core needle biopsy. Instead of employing a spring-loaded biopsy gun, a standard syringe is attached to a 20- or 18-gauge needle and the targeted cyst is aspirated.
- The cyst aspirate should be sent for cytology if bloody or clear. Benign-appearing aspirate, which may be green, grey, yellow, or cloudy, may be discarded. Note that only benign-appearing cysts should be aspirated. A complex mass should be biopsied with a core device.

Stereotactic-guided core biopsy

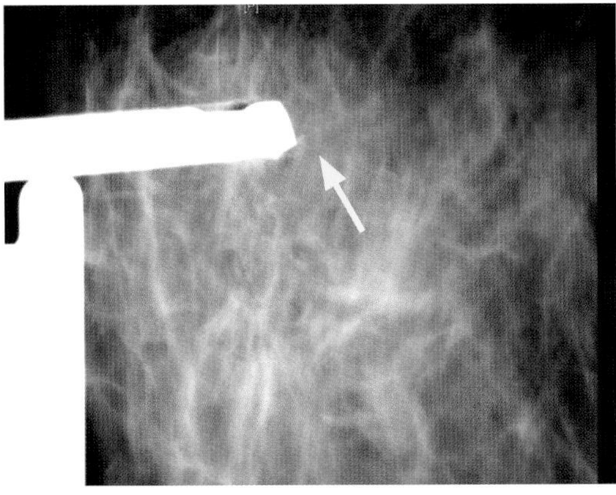

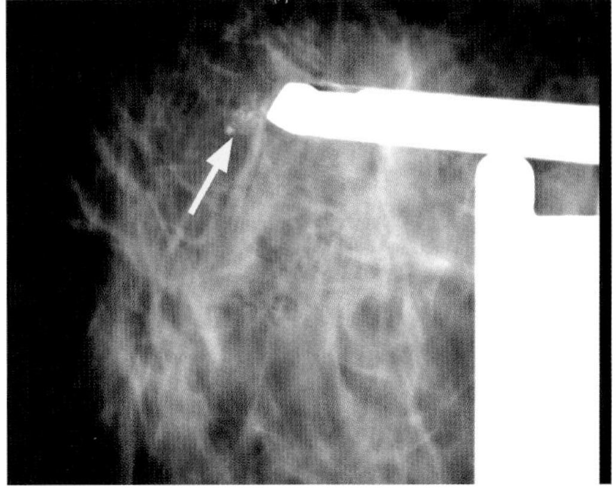

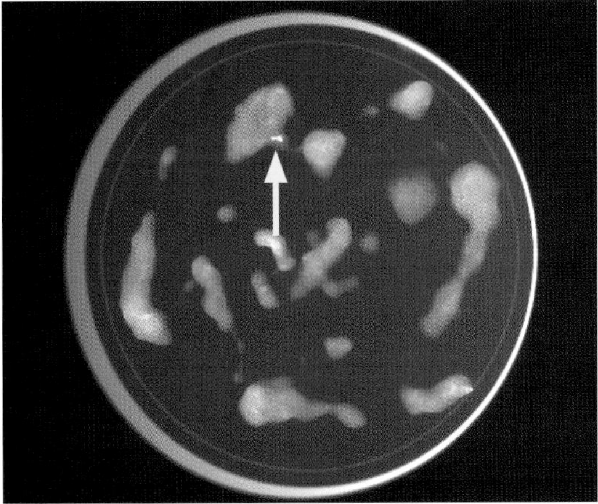

Stereotactic biopsy of calcifications:

Paired 15-degree oblique pre-fire images (top images)show the targeted calcifications (arrows) with appropriate position of the biopsy device.

Specimen radiograph confirms that the targeted calcifications are present within the specimen (arrow).

- Stereotactic guidance is employed most commonly to biopsy calcifications. Less commonly, a stereotactic approach can be used to sample a mammographic finding seen only in one view or a mammographic mass not seen on ultrasound.
- Stereotactic biopsy tables can be prone or seated upright. The advantage of a prone table is elimination of risk from vasovagal syncope. The seated stereotactic apparatus is less expensive and may offer greater patient comfort.
- Contraindications to stereotactic biopsy include a very thin breast measuring <3 cm compressed (although petite needles are available to sample lesions in breasts as thin as 22 mm), far posterior or subareolar location, inability to be positioned on the stereotactic table, and uncontrolled coagulation abnormality. Routine aspirin or clopidogrel use is not a contraindication.
- The breast is immobilized in compression during the entire procedure.
- Paired stereo spot views of the target are obtained 15° to each side (30° apart) relative to the needle path. Once targeting is confirmed by the radiologist, the actual needle path in three-dimensional space is calculated by computer.

- Generous local anesthesia is administered without and with epinephrine (both without imaging guidance) and a small dermatotomy is made at the biopsy needle entrance site.
- A vacuum-assisted 11-gauge biopsy needle is employed and multiple samples are obtained. After the samples are obtained, the specimen must be radiographed to confirm that the targeted calcifications are present.
- Once the presence of calcification is confirmed in the sample, a marker clip is placed, and post-procedure 2-view mammograms are obtained to confirm clip position. Often, small calcifications will be completely removed by the vacuum-assisted biopsy and correct position of the clip is essential if the lesion requires subsequent surgical treatment.

MR-guided biopsy

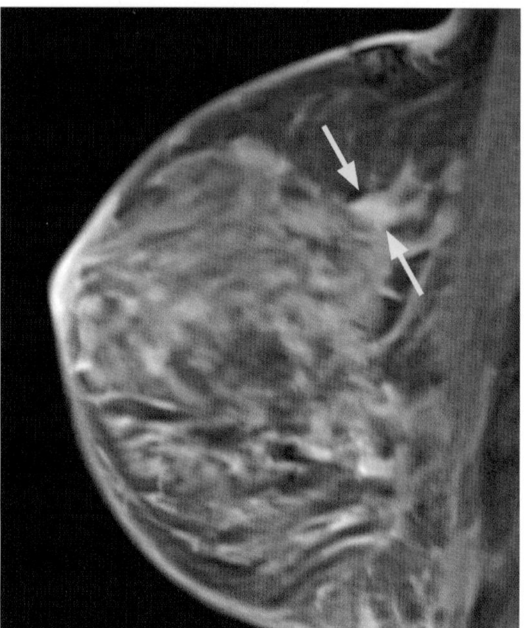

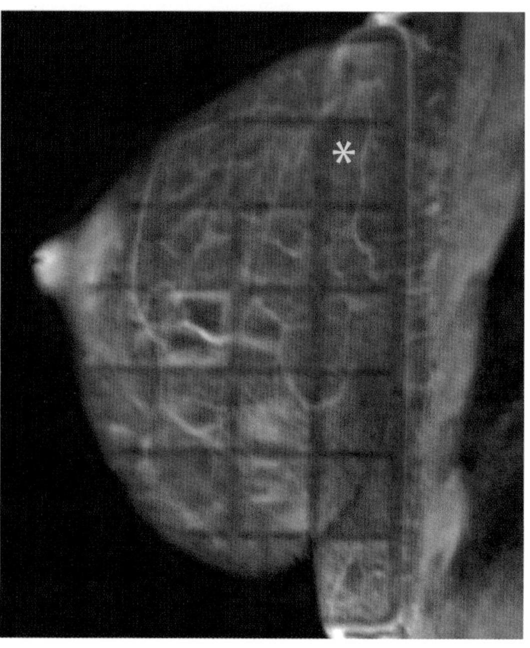

MR images obtained during an MRI-guided biopsy. Post-contrast image through the mid breast (left image) shows the targeted abnormal enhancement (arrows). The lesion is not very conspicuous because the patient had to be repositioned and delayed parenchymal enhancement partially obscures the lesion. The image on the right shows the grid applied to the lateral breast, and the star marks the position of the targeted lesion on the grid. Note that despite the sagittal orientation of these images, the patient is positioned prone.

- MR-guided biopsy can be performed for lesions seen only on MRI. It is common to perform a second-look ultrasound targeted towards the MRI abnormality, which is seen on ultrasound 57% of the time. Second-look ultrasound is performed both for further lesion characterization and to potentially provide a less-expensive biopsy guidance modality, assuming the lesion is visualized and accurately correlates to the MRI finding.
- MR-guided biopsy almost always requires intravenous gadolinium. Time is of the essence during the procedure because the lesion must be targeted before contrast washes out or the lesion becomes obscured by delayed parenchymal enhancement.
- The grid-coordinate method allows accurate biopsy of an abnormality seen only on MRI. This method is most analogous to a grid-based CT-guided biopsy elsewhere in the body.
- With the patient lying prone, a grid is applied to either the medial or lateral breast. A lateral approach is preferred whenever possible. After initial images are obtained, the targeted lesion is localized on the grid. Local anesthesia is administered without imaging guidance. During the biopsy, the core needle device is inserted exactly perpendicular to the breast to a pre-measured depth, similar to stereotactic biopsy. Multiple 9–11-gauge vacuum-assisted samples are obtained. Finally, a post-biopsy marker is deployed.

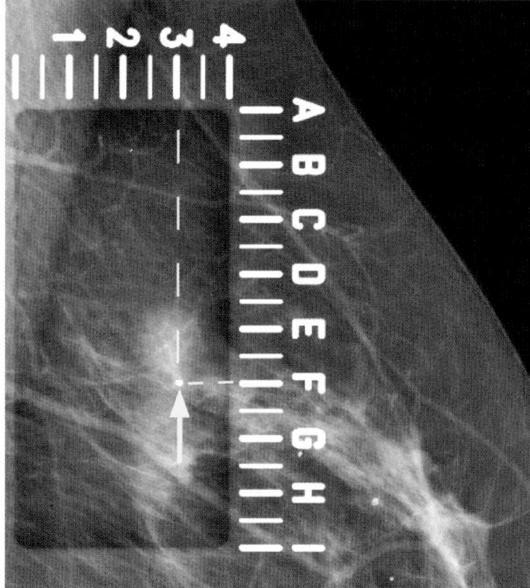

Step 1: Imaging is performed with the alphanumeric localization grid in place. The clip (arrow) is the target of the localization wire (F3 on the grid; dashed lines). The clip is associated with an ill-defined mass, which was previously biopsied as malignant.

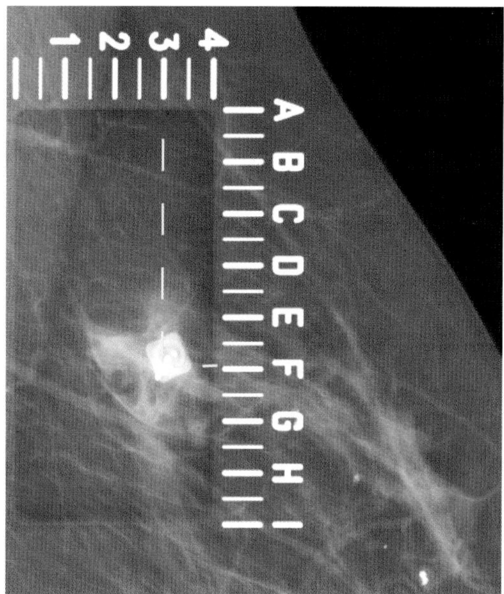

Step 2: After local anesthesia, the needle is inserted into the skin entry site based on the grid and advanced towards the target. Ideally the needle shaft should be exactly in line with the x-ray beam.

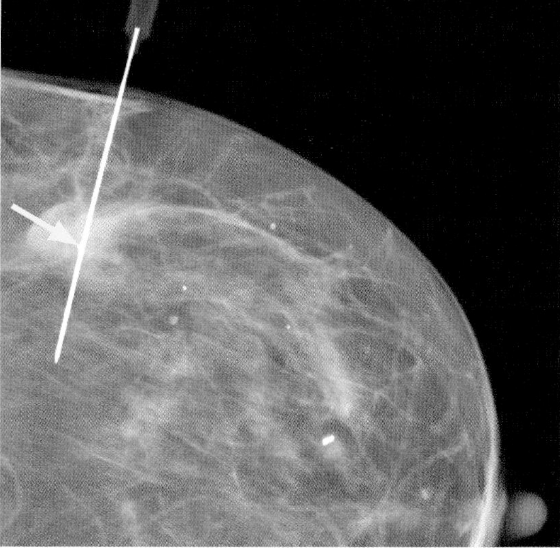

Step 3: Orthogonal imaging is obtained. If necessary, the needle can be advanced or pulled back. The mass is more evident on this orthogonal view. Note the clip location in the epicenter of the mass (arrow).

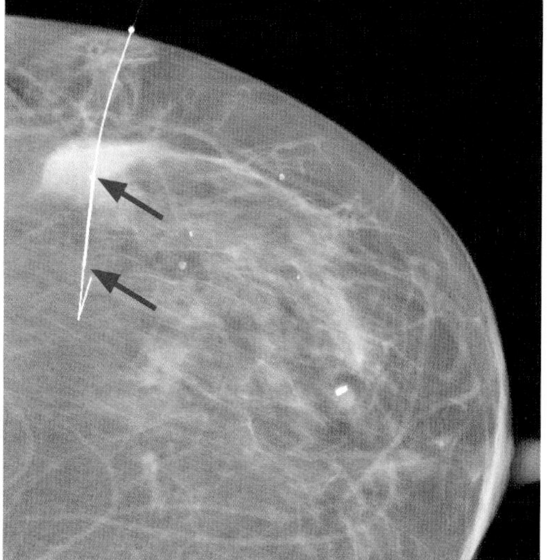

Step 4: Once satisfactory position is confirmed, the wire hook is unsheathed. Note the thickened distal segment (red arrows), which begins 1 cm from the hook and is 2 cm in length. The thickened segment gives the surgeon tactile feedback.

- Mammographic-guided wire localization allows pre-operative localization of a mammographic lesion prior to excisional biopsy or lumpectomy.
- The shortest approach to the lesion should be used and an appropriate wire length should be chosen (typically 5, 7, or 9 cm).
- After the lumpectomy or excisional biopsy, specimen radiographs are obtained to confirm that the targeted lesion and the intact hook wire are contained within the specimen.

References, resources, and further reading

General References:

de Paredes, E.S. Atlas of Mammography (3rd ed.). Lippincott Williams & Wilkins. (2007).

D'Orsi, C.J. et al. ACR BI-RADS Breast Imaging and Reporting Data System (4th ed.). Reston, VA: American College of Radiology. (2003).

Ikeda, D.M. Breast Imaging: The Requisites (2nd ed.). Mosby. (2011).

Breast Cancer Pathology:

Allred, D.C. Ductal carcinoma in situ: terminology, classification, and natural history. Journal of the National Cancer Institute. Monographs, 2010(41), 134-8(2010).

Bombonati, A. & Sgroi, D.C. The molecular pathology of breast cancer progression. The Journal of Pathology, 223(2), 308-18(2011).

Kerlikowske, K. Epidemiology of ductal carcinoma in situ. Journal of the National Cancer Institute. Monographs, 2010(41), 139-41(2010).

Sewell, C.W. Pathology of high-risk breast lesions and ductal carcinoma in situ. Radiologic Clinics of North America, 42(5), 821-30, v(2004).

Virnig, B.A. et al. Ductal carcinoma in situ: risk factors and impact of screening. Journal of the National Cancer Institute. Monographs, 2010(41), 113-6(2010).

Breast Cancer Screening:

Berg, W.A. Beyond standard mammographic screening: mammography at age extremes, ultrasound, and MRI imaging. Radiologic Clinics of North America, 45(5), 895-906, vii(2007).

Feig, S. Cost-effectiveness of mammography, MRI, and ultrasonography for breast cancer screening. Radiologic Clinics of North America, 48(5), 879-91(2010).

Hendrick, R.E. & Helvie, M.A. United States preventive services task force screening mammography recommendations: science ignored. AJR. American Journal of Roentgenology, 196(2), W112-6(2011).

Quanstrum, K.H. & Hayward, R.A. Lessons from the Mammography Wars. New England Journal of Medicine, 363, 1076-9(2010).

Tabár, L. et al. Swedish Two-County Trial: Impact of Mammographic Screening on Breast Cancer Mortality during 3 Decades. Radiology, 260(3), 658-63(2011).

Warner, E. Breast-Cancer Screening. New England Journal of Medicine, 365(11), 1025-32(2011).

Benign Breast Disease:

Cao, M. Mammographic signs of systemic disease. Radiographics, 31(4), 1085-100(2011).

Evans, W. et al. Invasive Lobular Carcinoma of the Breast: Mammographic Characteristics and Computer-aided Detection 1. Radiology, 225(1), 182(2002).

Gouveri, E., Papanas, N. & Maltezos, E. The female breast and diabetes. Breast, 20(3), 205-11(2011).

Santen, R.J. & Mansel, R. Benign breast disorders. New England Journal of Medicine, 275-85(2005).

Mammography:

Bartella, L., Smith, C.S., Dershaw, D.D. & Liberman, L. Imaging breast cancer. Radiologic Clinics of North America, 45(1), 45-67(2007).

Doshi, D., March, D., Crisi, G. & Coughlin, B. Complex Cystic Breast Masses: Diagnostic Approach and Imaging–Pathologic Correlation. Radiographics, 27, S53-65(2007).

Giess, C., Raza, S. & Birdwell, R. Distinguishing Breast Skin Lesions from Superficial Breast Parenchymal Lesions: Diagnostic Criteria, Imaging Characteristics, and Pitfalls, Radiographics, 31(7), 1959-73(2011).

Harvey, J.A., Nicholson, B.T. & Cohen, M.A. Finding Early Invasive Breast Cancers: A Practical Approach. Radiology, 248(1), 61(2008).

Leung, J.W.T. & Sickles, E.A. The probably benign assessment. Radiologic Clinics of North America, 45(5), 773-89, vi(2007).

Sickles, E.A. The spectrum of breast asymmetries: imaging features, work-up, management. Radiologic Clinics of North America, 45(5), 765-71, v(2007).

Breast Ultrasound:

Mendelson, E.B. Problem-solving ultrasound. Radiologic Clinics of North America, 42(5), 909-18, vii(2004).

Raza, S. et al. BI-RADS 3, 4, and 5 Lesions: Value of US in Management—Follow-up and Outcome 1. Radiology, 248(3), 773(2008).

Stavros, A. et al. Solid breast nodules: use of sonography to distinguish between benign and malignant lesions. Radiology, 196, 123-34(1995).

Yang, W. & Dempsey, P.J. Diagnostic breast ultrasound: current status and future directions. Radiologic Clinics of North America, 45(5), 845-61, vii(2007).

Breast MRI:

Argus, A. & Mahoney, M.C. Indications for breast MRI: case-based review. AJR. American Journal of Roentgenology, 196(3 Suppl), WS1-14(2011).

Kuhl, C.K. et al. Dynamic breast MRI imaging: are signal intensity time course data useful for differential diagnosis of enhancing lesions? Radiology, 211(1), 101-10(1999).

Lee, C.H. Problem solving MRI imaging of the breast. Radiologic Clinics of North America, 42(5), 919-34, vii(2004).

Lehman, C.D. Magnetic resonance imaging in the evaluation of ductal carcinoma in situ. Journal of the National Cancer Institute. Monographs, 2010(41), 150-1(2010).

Macura, K.J., Ouwerkerk, R., Jacobs, M.A. & Bluemke, D.A. Patterns of enhancement on breast MRI images: interpretation and imaging pitfalls. Radiographics, 26(6), 1719-34 (2006); quiz 1719.

Molleran, V. & Mahoney, M.C. The BI-RADS breast magnetic resonance imaging lexicon. Magnetic Resonance Imaging Clinics of North America, 18(2), 171-85, vii(2010).

Morris, E.A. Diagnostic breast MRI imaging: current status and future directions. Radiologic clinics of North America, 45(5), 863-80, vii(2007).

Raza, S. et al. Breast MRI - A Comprehensive Imaging Guide. Amirsys. (2009).

Raza, S., Vallejo, M., Chikarmane, S.A. & Birdwell, R.L. Pure ductal carcinoma in situ: a range of MRI features. AJR. American Journal of Roentgenology, 191(3), 689-99(2008).

Thomassin-Naggara, I. Non-masslike enhancement in breast MRI: the pearls of interpretation? Journal of Radiology, 90, 269-75(2009).

Weinstein, S. & Rosen, M. Breast MRI imaging: current indications and advanced imaging techniques. Radiologic Clinics of North America, 48(5), 1013-42(2010).

Yoo, J., Woo, O., Kim, Y. & Cho, K. Can MRI Imaging Contribute in Characterizing Well-circumscribed Breast Carcinomas? Radiographics, 30, 1689-703(2010).

Breast Interventions:

Bassett, L.W., Mahoney, M.C. & Apple, S.K. Interventional breast imaging: current procedures and assessing for concordance with pathology. Radiologic Clinics of North America, 45(5), 881-94, vii(2007).

Berg, W.A. Image-guided breast biopsy and management of high-risk lesions. Radiologic Clinics of North America, 42(5), 935-46, vii(2004).

Helbich, T.H., Matzek, W. & Fuchsjäger, M.H. Stereotactic and ultrasound-guided breast biopsy. European Radiology, 14(3), 383-93(2004).

Kaiser, W.A., Pfleiderer, S.O.R. & Baltzer, P.A.T. MRI-guided interventions of the breast. Journal of Magnetic Resonance Imaging, 27(2), 347-55(2008).

Liberman, L. Percutaneous image-guided core breast biopsy. Radiologic Clinics of North America, 40(3), 483-500, vi(2002).

O'Flynn, E.A.M., Wilson, A.R.M. & Michell, M.J. Image-guided breast biopsy: state-of-the-art. Clinical Radiology, 65(4), 259-70(2010).

9 Cardiovascular imaging

Contents

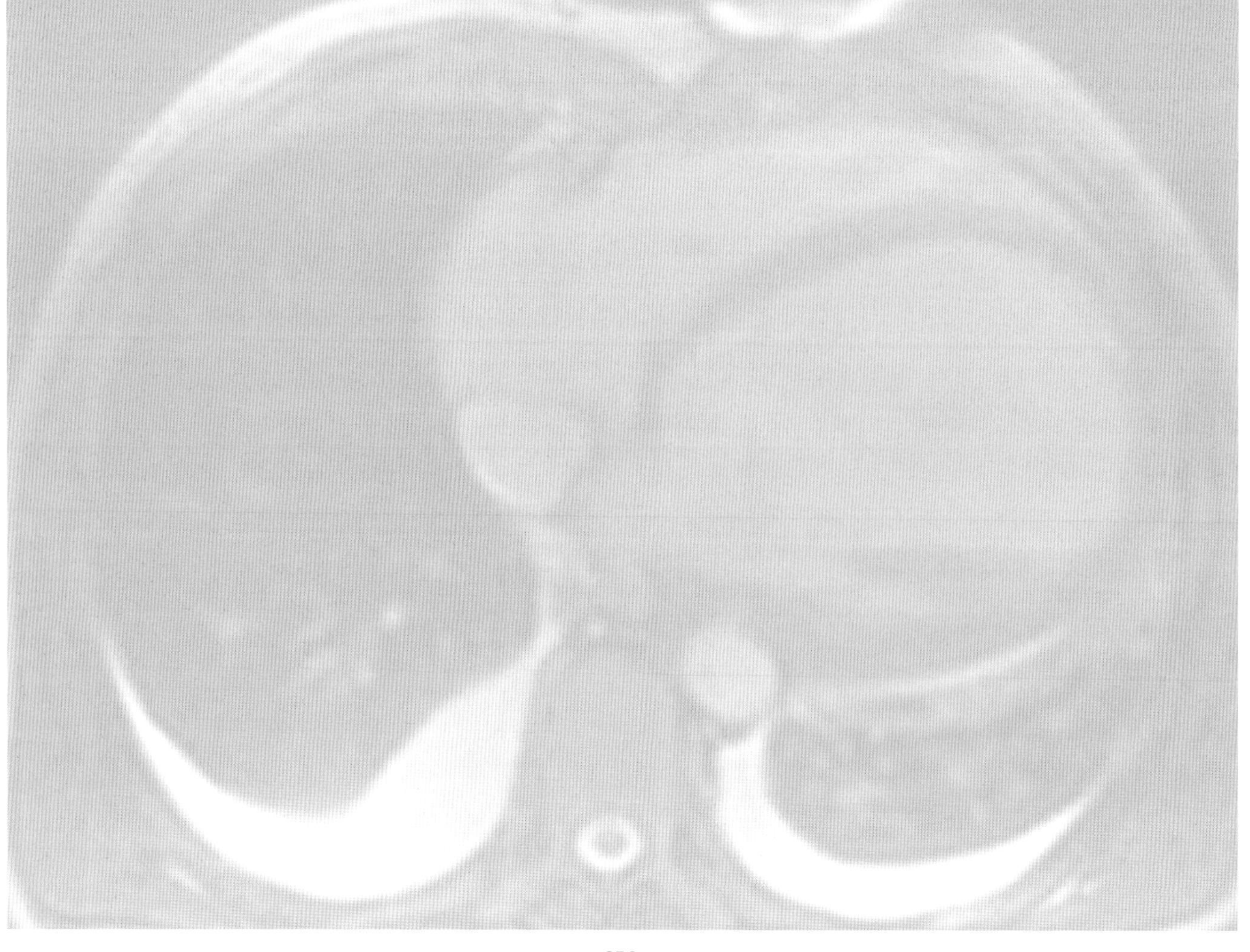

AORTIC ARCH AND VARIANTS

Normal aortic arch branching

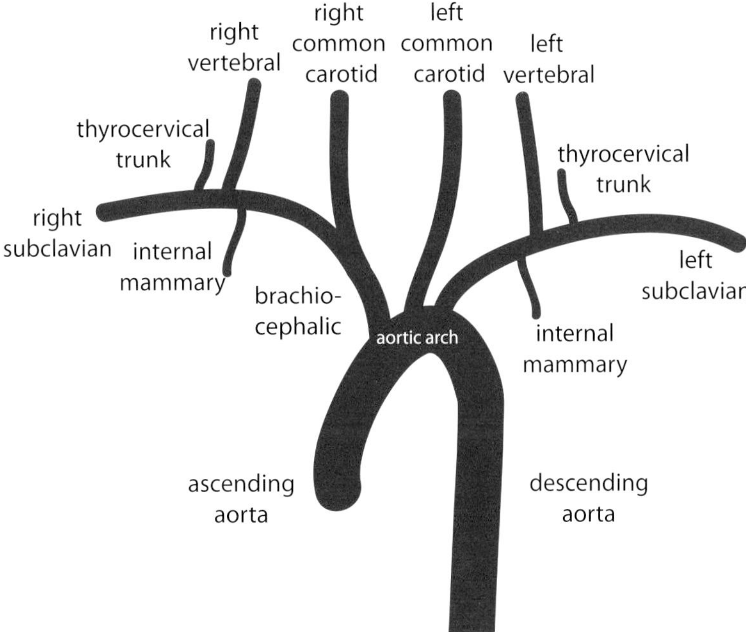

- The normal aortic branching pattern is seen 66% of the time and features three arteries arising from the aortic arch: Brachiocephalic trunk (inominate artery), left common carotid, and left subclavian artery.

Common origin of the brachiocephalic artery and left common carotid artery

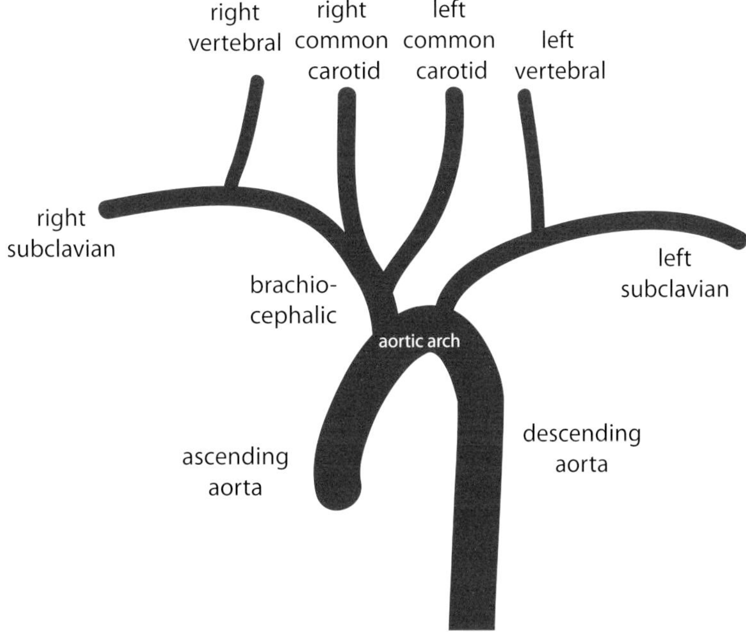

- A common origin of the brachiocephalic artery and left common carotid artery is seen in 13% of patients (more commonly in blacks) and is often incorrectly referred to as a "bovine aortic arch." The term "bovine aortic arch" is a misnomer and is not the preferred description of this anomaly, as a true bovine arch in cattle features a single great vessel arising from the aortic arch.

Aberrant right subclavian

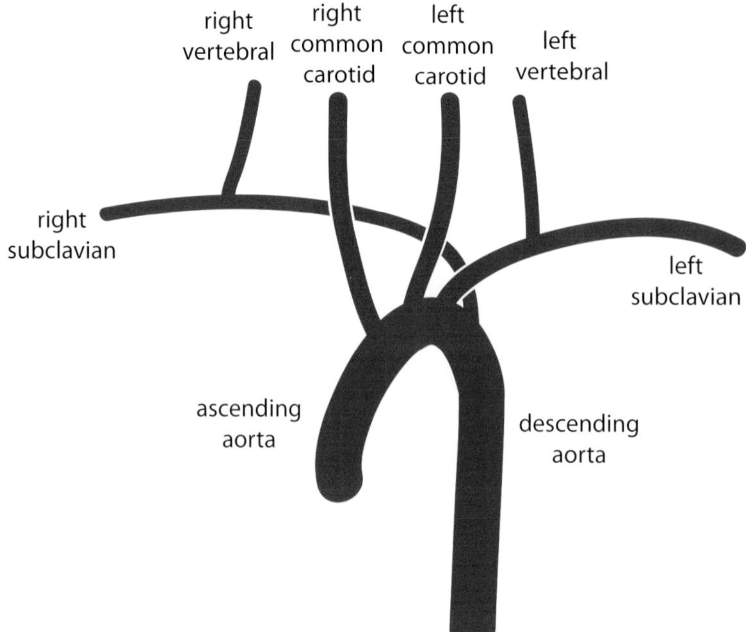

- An aberrant right subclavian is seen in 1% of patients. The right subclavian artery arises directly from the aortic arch distal to the left subclavian and loops behind the esophagus on its way into the right arm.
- It is very uncommon for an aberrant right subclavian artery to cause symptoms, but this anomaly may rarely be a cause of dysphagia via esophageal compression, called dysphagia lusoria. Barium esophogram features a posterior indentation on the esophagus.

  Although usually incidental, it is important to mention the presence of an aberrant right subclavian artery when reading a neck CT. If thyroid surgery is planned, then the recurrent laryngeal nerve will not be in its usual location.
- A diverticulum of Kommerel represents a small bulge at the origin of the aberrant subclavian artery.

Left vertebral origin off aorta

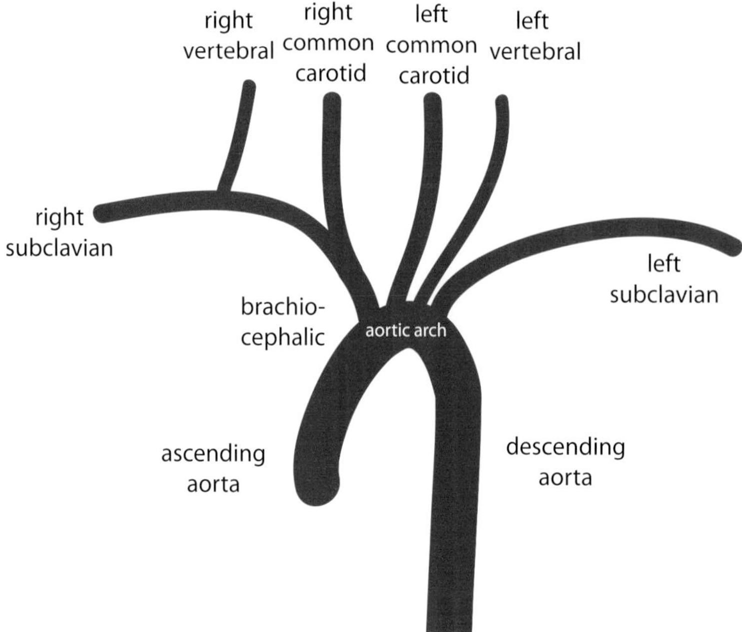

- A four vessel arch with direct origin of the vertebral artery off of the aorta is seen in 6% of the population. The left vertebral is the third aortic branch, proximal to the left subclavian.

Acute aortic syndrome

Overview of acute aortic syndrome

- Acute aortic syndrome represents a clinical spectrum of three related diseases that are characterized by damage to at least one component of the aortic wall, and presents as severe chest pain.
- A defect primarily in the intima is seen in penetrating atherosclerotic ulcer (PAU).
- A defect in the media only describes intramural hematoma (IMH).
- A defect in the intima extending to media is the hallmark of aortic dissection.
- A defect in all three layers (aortic transection) is almost always due to trauma and is considered a separate entity.
- The treatment of acute aortic syndrome depends primarily on the location (ascending versus descending aorta) and is often the same regardless of the underlying etiology.

> **Ascending aorta**: Treatment is most commonly surgical.
> **Descending aorta**: Treatment is most commonly medical (blood pressure control).

- Imaging of the full aorta is generally required in any acute aortic pathology.

Aortic dissection

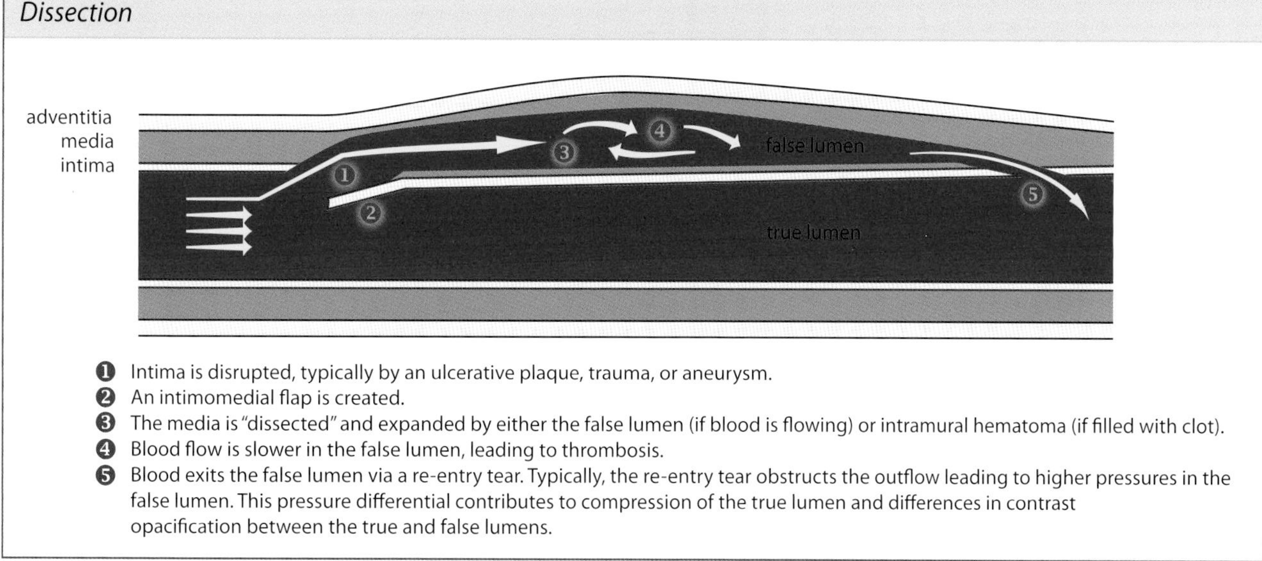

❶ Intima is disrupted, typically by an ulcerative plaque, trauma, or aneurysm.
❷ An intimomedial flap is created.
❸ The media is "dissected" and expanded by either the false lumen (if blood is flowing) or intramural hematoma (if filled with clot).
❹ Blood flow is slower in the false lumen, leading to thrombosis.
❺ Blood exits the false lumen via a re-entry tear. Typically, the re-entry tear obstructs the outflow leading to higher pressures in the false lumen. This pressure differential contributes to compression of the true lumen and differences in contrast opacification between the true and false lumens.

- The key feature of dissection is a disruption in the intima, which allows high-pressure blood to infiltrate and expand the media.
- The most common risk factor for aortic dissection is hypertension, but other risk factors include connective tissue disorders (especially Marfan syndrome), cocaine use, aortopathy associated with a bicuspid aortic valve, weight lifting, and sudden deceleration injury.
- The classification of aortic dissection is the Stanford classification, which divides dissection into types A (ascending aorta) and B (non-ascending aorta). Type A is typically treated surgically, and type B is typically treated medically.

  Aortic dissection secondary to atherosclerosis is more commonly type B (descending aorta).

Stanford A aortic dissection:
Ascending aorta, ±descending aorta
Typically treated surgically

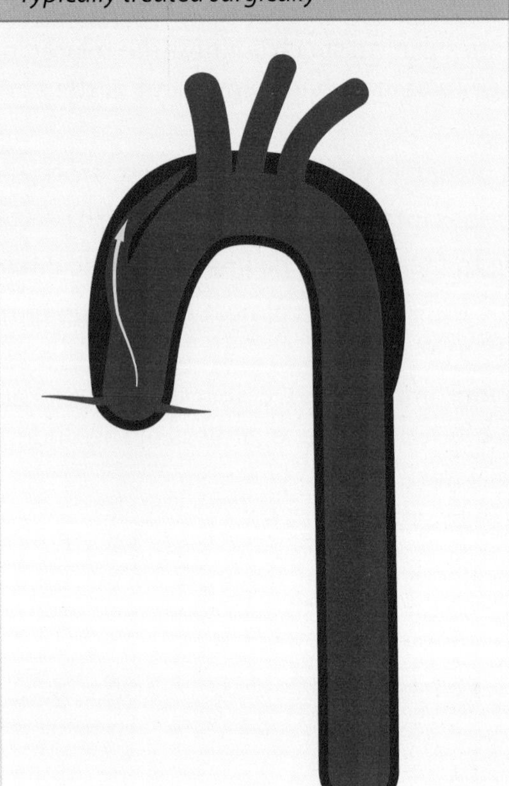

Stanford B aortic dissection:
Descending aorta only
Typically treated medically

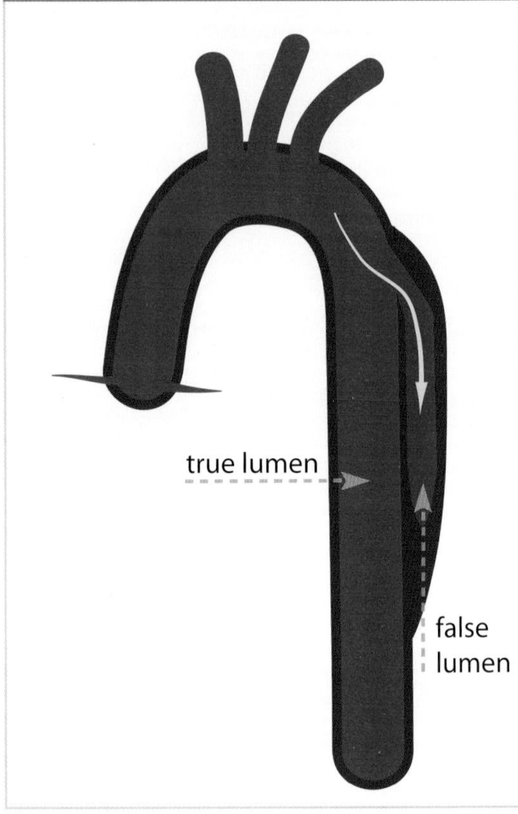

- Stanford A

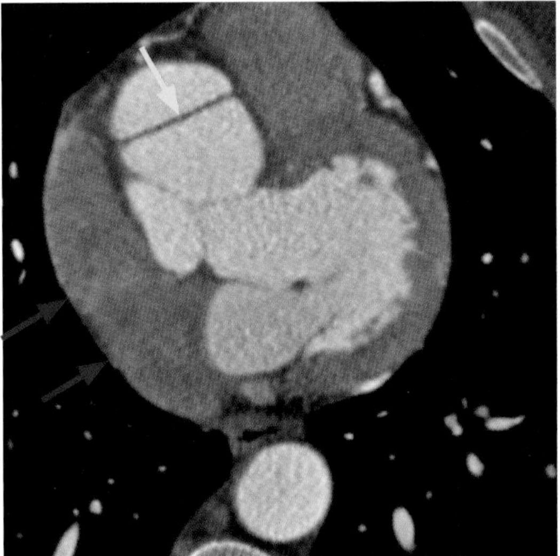

Axial contrast-enhanced gated CT shows a dissection flap in the ascending aorta only (yellow arrow). The descending aorta appears normal. There is a moderate hemopericardium consistent with rupture (red arrows).

- Stanford B

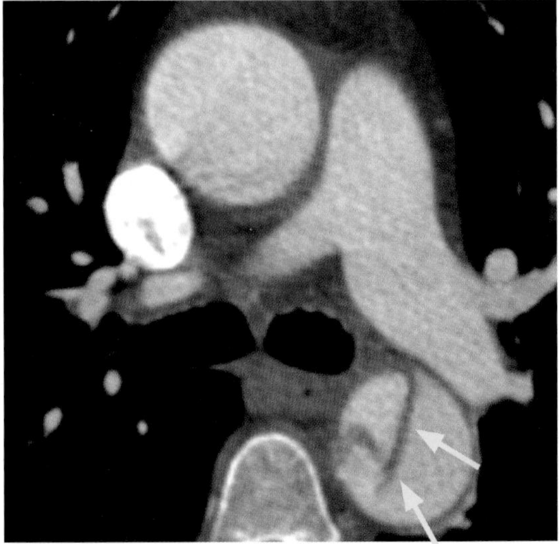

Axial contrast-enhanced gated CT in a different patient shows a dissection flap in the descending aorta only (arrows).

INTRAMURAL HEMATOMA (IMH)

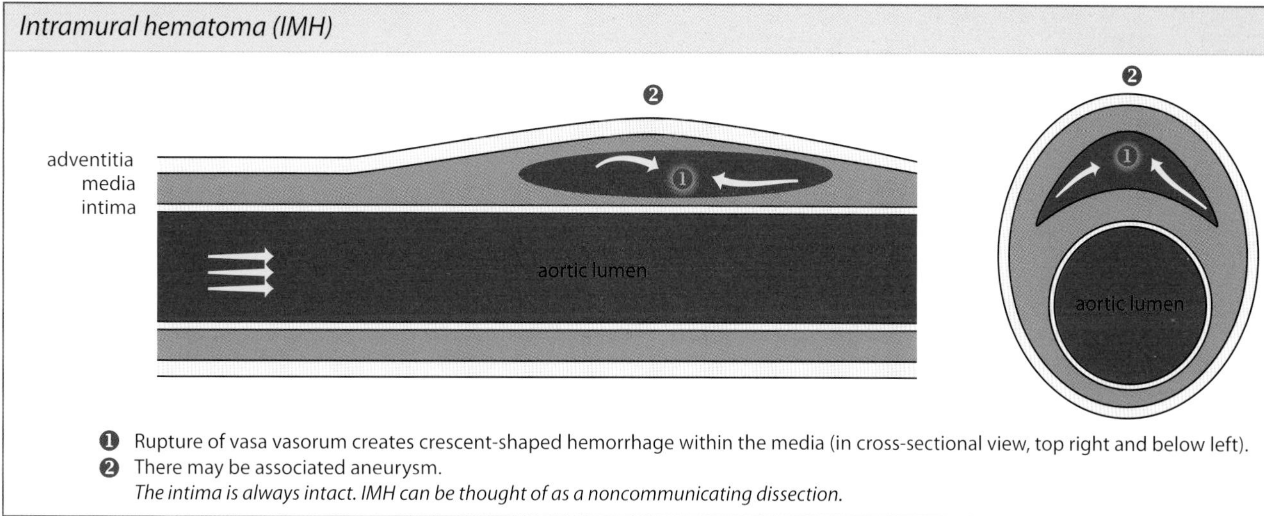

❶ Rupture of vasa vasorum creates crescent-shaped hemorrhage within the media (in cross-sectional view, top right and below left).
❷ There may be associated aneurysm.
The intima is always intact. IMH can be thought of as a noncommunicating dissection.

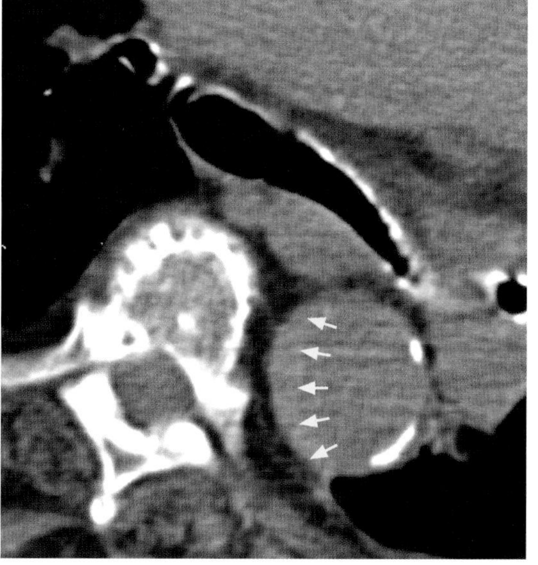

Intramural hematoma on non-contrast CT: Unenhanced CT shows very faint crescent of hyperdense (50 HU) hemorrhage in the descending aorta (arrows).

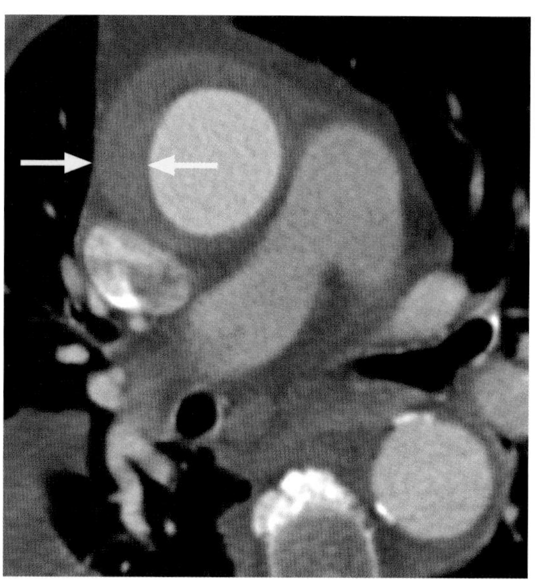

Intramural hematoma on contrast-enhanced CT: Contrast-enhanced CT in a different patient shows a crescentic hyperattenuating (50 HU) rim reflecting intramural hematoma (arrows). There is no disruption of the aortic lumen.

- Intramural hematoma (IMH) is a variant of dissection where blood collects within the media, without an intimal flap to connect the intramural hematoma with the aortic lumen. IMH is thought to be due to rupture of the vasa vasorum, which are small blood vessels that supply the aortic wall.
- Similar to dissection, IMH may be secondary to hypertension or trauma.
- Clinically, IMH can present identically to aortic dissection with acute tearing back pain. The treatment recommendations for IMH are the same as dissection regarding involvement of the ascending versus descending aorta.
- The key imaging finding of IMH is a faint peripheral hyperattenuating (45–50 HU) crescent within the aorta, best seen on noncontrast CT. In high-risk patients, the aortic dissection CT protocol typically includes an unenhanced CT prior to CTA to evaluate specifically for IMH. An alternative strategy in low-risk patients is to perform unenhanced CT only if there is suspicion of IMH on the CTA in order to decrease radiation exposure.

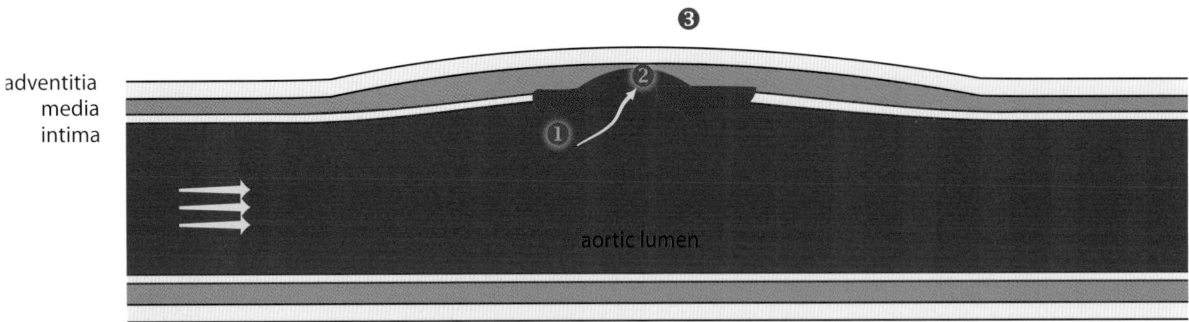

1. Atherosclerotic plaque penetrates the intima.
2. Atherosclerotic plaque ulcerates, allowing blood to extend into the media.
3. PAU may cause the media to enlarge, leading to an aneurysm formation.

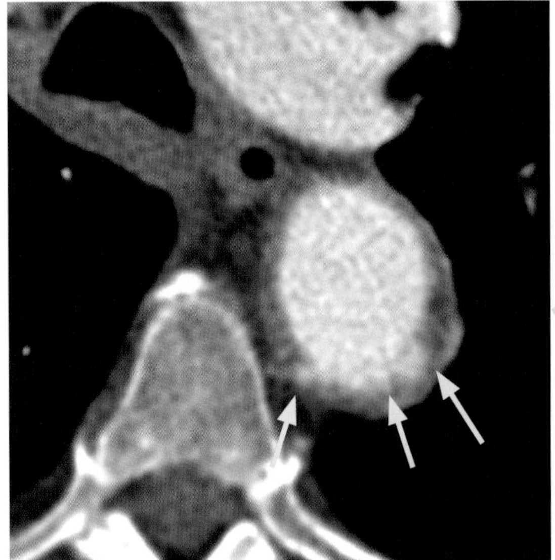

Axial contrast-enhanced CT shows multiple penetrating ulcers (arrows) in the descending aorta, extending beyond the expected contour of the aortic lumen.

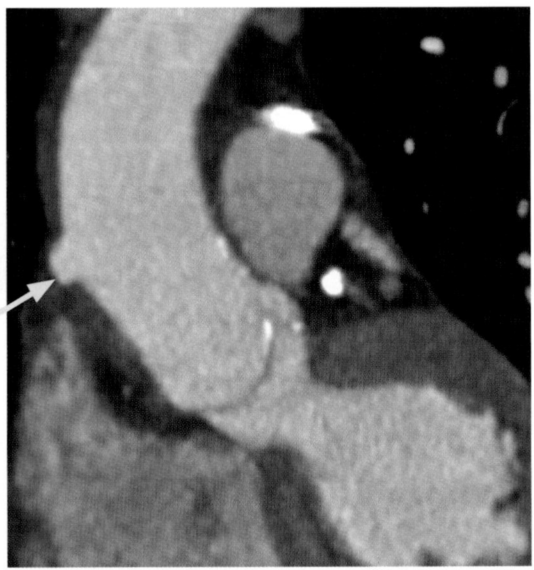

Sagittal oblique gated contrast-enhanced CT in a different patient shows a penetrating atherosclerotic ulcer (arrow) of the ascending aorta, extending beyond the expected contour of the lumen.

- Penetrating atherosclerotic ulcer (PAU) is a focal defect in the intima that occurs at the site of an atherosclerotic plaque. PAU may lead to saccular aneurysm formation.
- In contrast to dissection and IMH, PAU tends to be caused by atherosclerosis rather than hypertension. One of the theories of dissection secondary to atherosclerosis is that it begins as a penetrating ulcer.
- On imaging, PAU appears as contrast ulcerating beyond the expected contour of the aortic wall. The primary differential would be a simple ulcerated atherosclerotic plaque, which would not extend beyond the expected contour of the aortic wall. Atherosclerotic plaque represents chronic atherosclerotic disease and is not an acute aortic syndrome.
- Multiple ulcers may be present throughout the thoracoabdominal aorta, and as with all acute aortic pathologies, imaging of the full aorta is recommended if a PAU is seen.

Aortic trauma

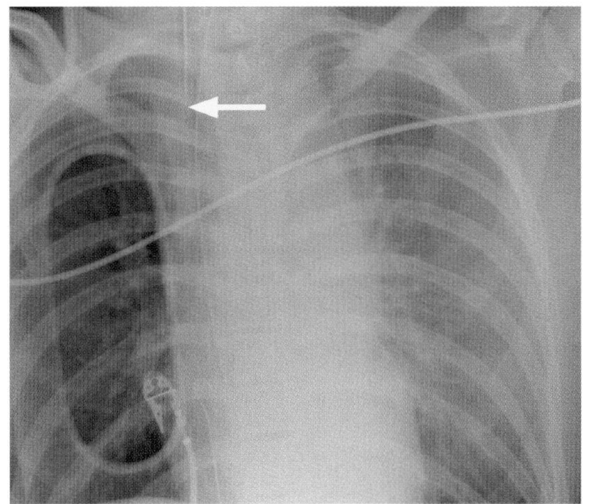

Chest radiograph in a trauma patient shows indistinct widening of the mediastinum. The endotracheal tube is displaced to the right (arrow).

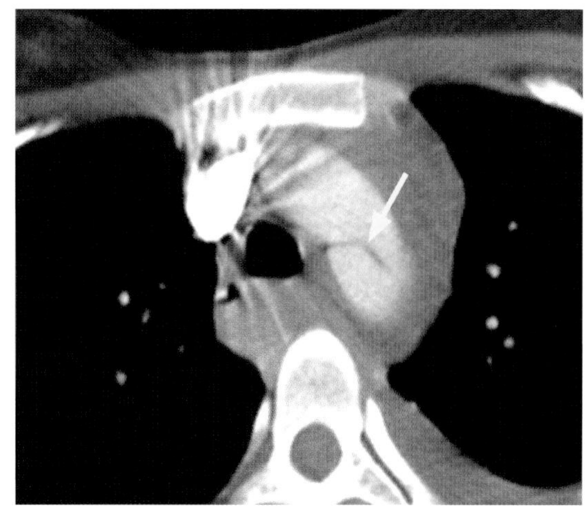

Contrast-enhanced CT shows a mediastinal hematoma and traumatic aortic dissection (arrow). Indistinctness of the lateral arch of the aorta is concerning for tear.

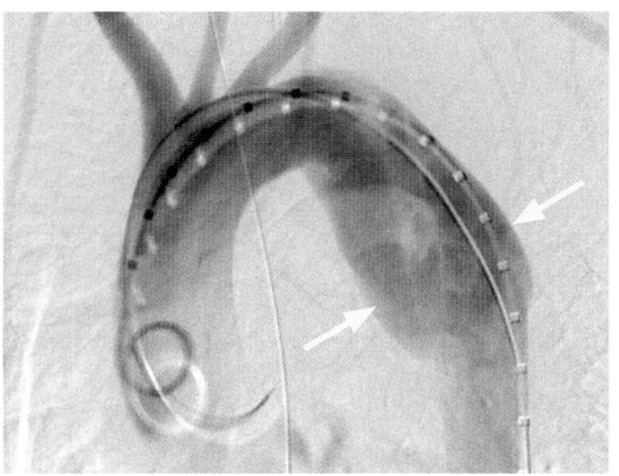

Catheter aortogram shows a large, fusiform pseudoaneurysm (arrows) of the aortic isthmus, distal to the brachiocephalic artery.

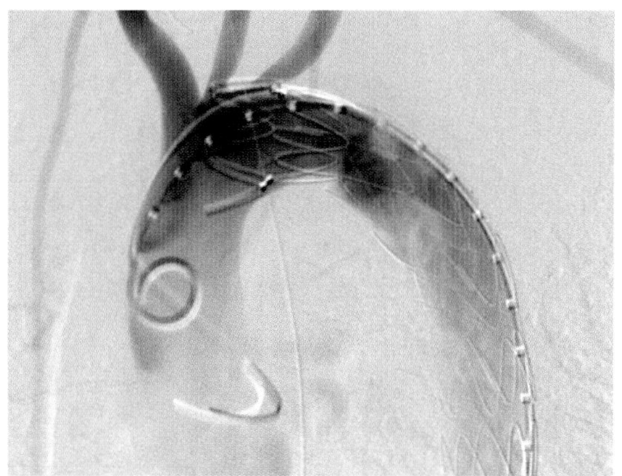

Post repair aortogram shows stent graft in place with good opacification of the arch vessels.

Aortic trauma: *Case courtesy Michael Hanley, MD, University of Virginia Health System.*

- There are three relatively fixed levels of the aorta where traumatic aortic injuries occur secondary to deceleration injury, which are the aortic root, isthmus, and hiatus. The resulting pseudoaneurysm is held in place by the surrounding connective tissues. In the small percentage of patients who survive blunt aortic trauma, injury occurs at the isthmus in 95% of cases.

  Associated injury to the origins of the brachiocephalic, left carotid, or left subclavian arteries is frequently present.

- CTA is the gold standard for evaluation of suspected traumatic aortic injury.
- Traumatic mediastinal hemorrhage is often venous; however, aortic injury is the primary concern. Direct CT signs of traumatic aortic injury include a dissection flap, pseudoaneurysm, and intramural hematoma.

  Mediastinal hemorrhage that is separated from an intact aorta by a fat plane can be presumed to be venous, and treatment is conservative. In contrast, hemorrhage in contact with the aortic wall is suggestive of aortic injury and necessitates surgical treatment.

THORACIC AORTIC ANEURYSM

Thoracic aortic aneurysm (TAA)

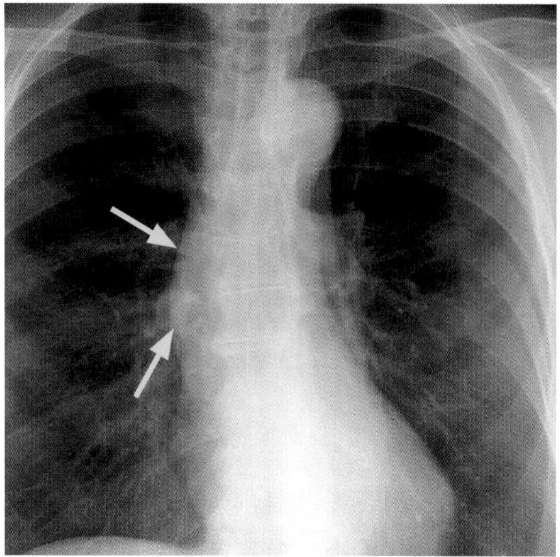

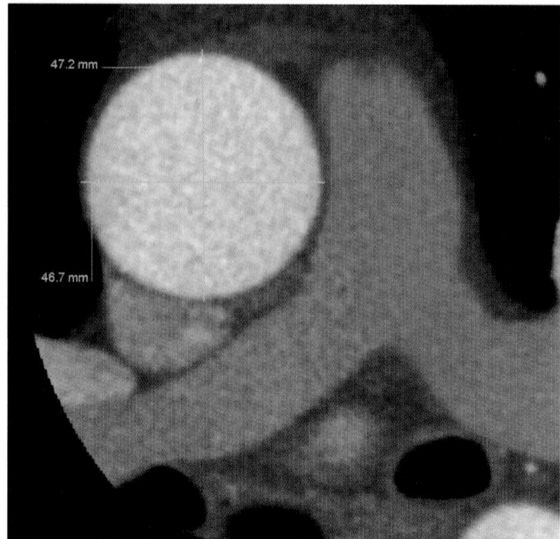

Thoracic aortic aneurysm: Frontal chest radiograph demonstrates ectasia of the right aortic border (arrows). Gated contrast-enhanced CT with a double-oblique short-axis reformation demonstrates an ascending aortic diameter of 4.7 cm, representing an aneurysm.

Case courtesy Michael Steigner, MD, Brigham and Women's Hospital.

- A thoracic aortic aneurysm (TAA) is defined as an ascending aortic diameter >4 cm or a descending thoracic aorta >3 cm in diameter. Aortic size may also be normalized to body surface area and compared to reference values.
- Double-oblique short-axis multiplanar reformatted images perpendicular to the aortic lumen (i.e., true short-axis) should always be used to measure aortic diameter.
- Most thoracic aortic aneurysms are caused by atherosclerosis, with the descending thoracic aorta affected more commonly. Almost one third of patients with atherosclerotic TAA will have an associated abdominal aortic aneurysm.
- Non-atherosclerotic causes of TAA include connective tissue disorders (such as Marfan and Ehlers–Danlos syndromes), bicuspid aortic valve (BAV) associated aortopathy, vasculitis (including Takayasu arteritis, giant cell arteritis, ankylosing spondylitis, and relapsing polychondritis), cystic medial necrosis, and infectious aortitis.
- Annuloaortic ectasia represents dilated sinuses of Valsalva and ascending aorta with effacement of the sinotubular junction, resulting in a tulip bulb-shaped aorta. Annuloaortic ectasia is associated with Marfan and Ehlers–Danlos syndromes.
- Surgical treatment is recommended for an ascending TAA >5.5 cm in diameter and a descending TAA >6 cm in diameter. However, patients with connective tissue disorders and BAV aortopathy (meeting criteria for valve replacement) have a lower surgical threshold of 4.5 cm. Beyond simple size criteria, annual growth rate >1 cm/year (or >5 mm/6 months) is an indication for surgical repair.
- A sign of impending rupture is the *draped aorta* sign, which describes drooping of the posterior aorta against the spine on an axial image.
- Complications of TAA treatment include rupture, dissection, infection, endoleak, and paraplegia (caused by artery of Adamkiewicz occlusion).

Abdominal aortic aneurysm (AAA)

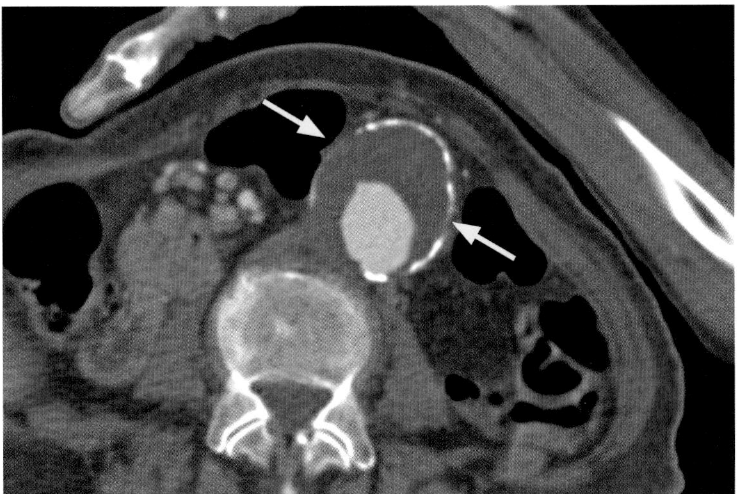

Abdominal aortic aneurysm: Axial CT of the infrarenal aorta demonstrates a large, peripherally calcified abdominal aortic aneurysm (arrows) containing extensive mural thrombus.

Case courtesy Michael Hanley, MD, University of Virginia Health System.

- Abdominal aortic aneurysm (AAA) is relatively prevalent in older men (seen in up to 5.9% of men by age 80) and less common in women. Rupture of abdominal aortic aneurysm is the 13th leading cause of death in older men. Risk factors for development of an abdominal aortic aneurysm include age, male sex, smoking, and family history.
- An abdominal aortic aneurysm is defined as an aortic diameter ≥3 cm. Similar to measurement of thoracic aortic aneurysms, double-oblique reformatted images should be used to obtain a true cross-sectional diameter. Volume measurement can also be used to monitor for endoleak on follow-up.
- The natural history of abdominal aortic aneurysm is progressive enlargement and eventual rupture.

> The annual risk of rupture for an AAA between 5.5 and 5.9 cm is **9.4%.**
>
> The annual risk of rupture for an AAA between 6.0 and 6.5 cm is **10.2%**.
>
> The annual risk of rupture for an AAA between 6.5 and 6.9 cm is **19.2%**.
>
> The annual risk of rupture for an AAA greater than 7 cm is **32.5%**.

- Ultrasound screening of high-risk patients is approved by Medicare in the US for patients older than age 65. If an aneurysm is detected on screening, follow-up is recommended:

> Aneurysm **<4 cm**: Follow-up in 6 months; if no change → **annual surveillance**.
>
> Aneurysm **4–4.5 cm**: Follow-up in 6 months; if no change → **6-month surveillance**.
>
> Aneurysm **5–5.5 cm**: **Consider surgery**.
>
> Aneurysm **>5.5 cm**: **Surgery recommended**.

- In addition to a size >5.5 cm, repair is recommended when the AAA is expanding at a rapid rate (>5 mm/year) or is symptomatic.
- The mortality of elective open AAA repair is >3%, while the mortality for urgent repair is 19%. A ruptured AAA has a mortality of at least 50%.
- Repair of abdominal aortic aneurysm can be performed with a traditional open or endovascular technique. Endovascular repair is preferred for patients with high surgical risks and is associated with reductions in major morbidity and hospital time. Long-term outcomes are equivalent between endovascular and open repair, but endovascular repair often requires repeat interventions.
- Complications of endovascular repair of AAA include rupture, dissection, infection, endoleak, and aorto-enteric fistula.

- An endoleak is persistent flow into an excluded aneurysm sac after endovascular treatment with a stent graft.

Type I endoleak: Inadequate seal of graft

- Type I endoleak is inadequate graft seal. Type IA is a proximal leak and IB is distal.

Type IA endoleak: Inadequate proximal seal allows blood into the excluded aneurysm sac.

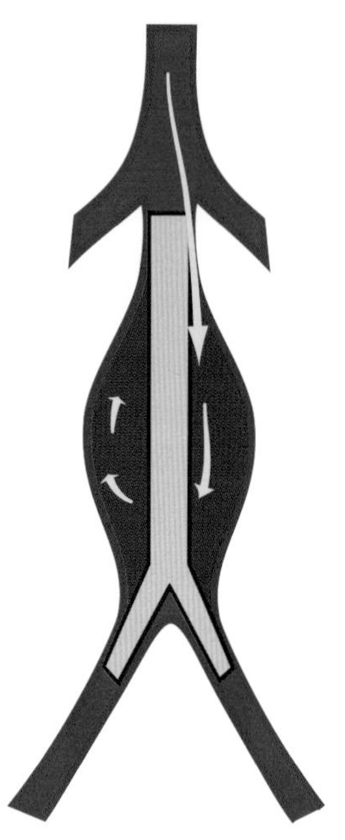

Inadequate proximal seal leads to enhancement in the proximal aneurysm sac (yellow arrow).

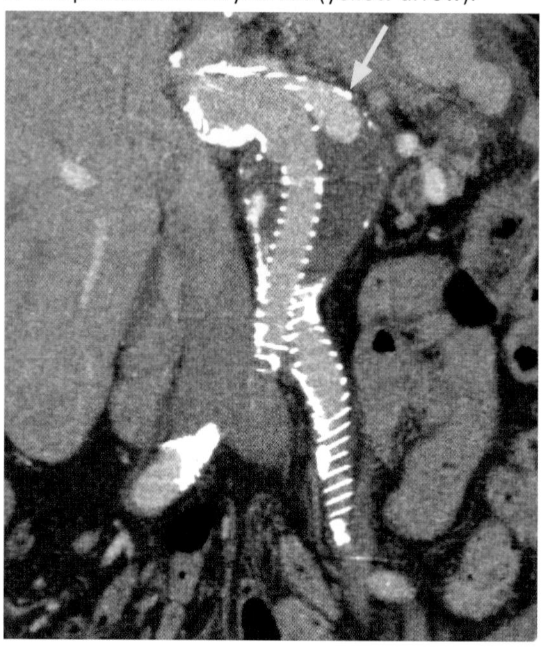

Type II endoleak: Persistent collateral flow to excluded aneurysm

- Type II endoleak is persistent collateral flow to the excluded aneurysm sac, which typically arises from the lumbar arteries or the inferior mesenteric artery (IMA).

Type II endoleak: Communication from either the IMA or a lumbar artery causes blood to flow into the excluded aneurysm sac.

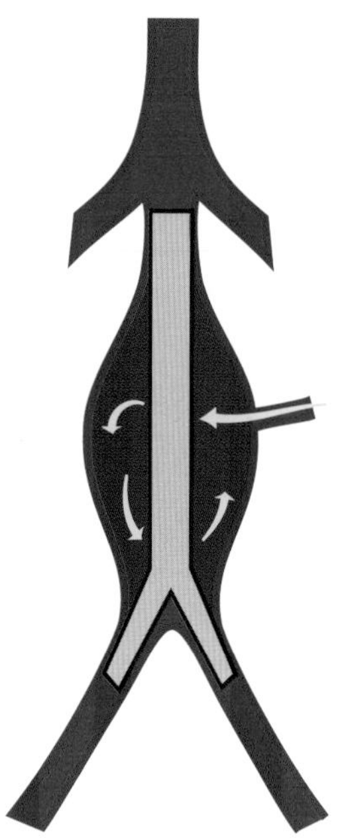

Axial image shows focal enhancement in the excluded aneurysm sac (yellow arrow), with faint communication (red arrow) leading to the IMA.

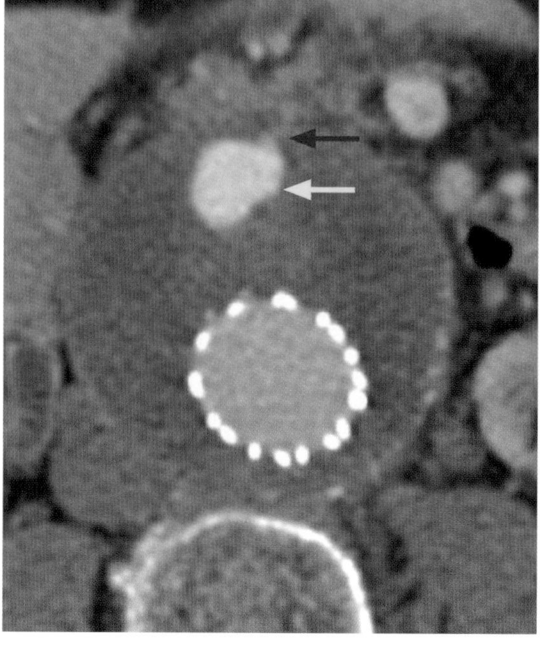

Type III endoleak: Device failure causing leakage

- Type III endoleak represents device failure causing leakage through graft fabric or segments of a modular graft.

Type III endoleak: Blood enters the excluded aneurysm sac via a defect in the graft.

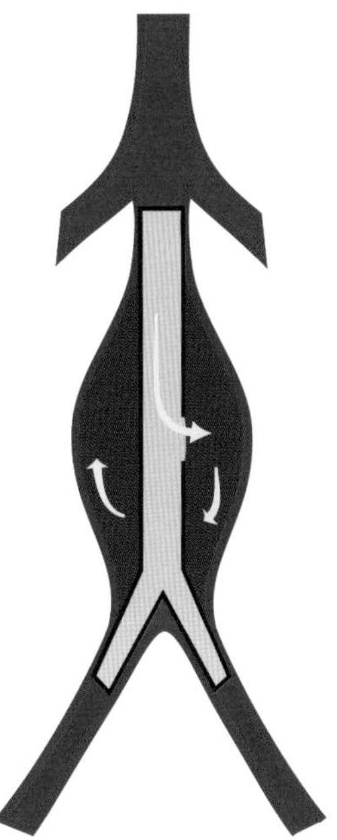

Coronal CT demonstrates contrast extravasating (yellow arrow) through the angulation of a modular aortic graft.

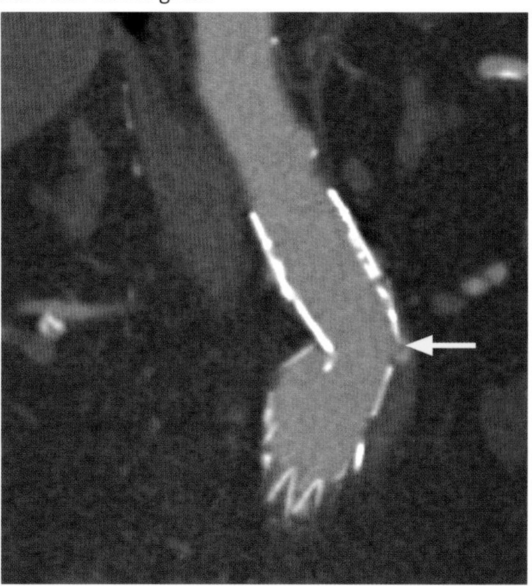

Types IV and V endoleaks

- Both type IV and type V endloeaks are diagnoses of exclusion as no endoleak can be visualized by imaging although the sac continues to increase in size.

- **Type IV endoleak:** Type IV endoleak is caused by a porous graft and is typically transient and seen intra-procedurally. Type IV endoleak usually resolves within one month after withdrawal of anticoagulation. It is rarely seen with modern grafts.

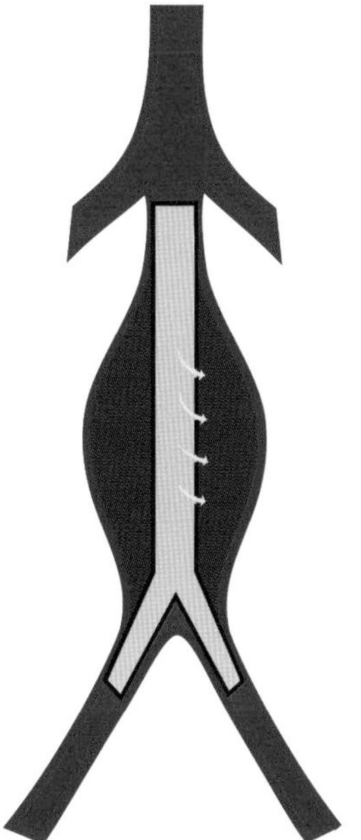

- **Type V endoleak:** Also called endotension, type V endoleak is continued expansion of the aneurysm without any other endoleak present, thought to be due to an endoleak below the resolution of imaging.

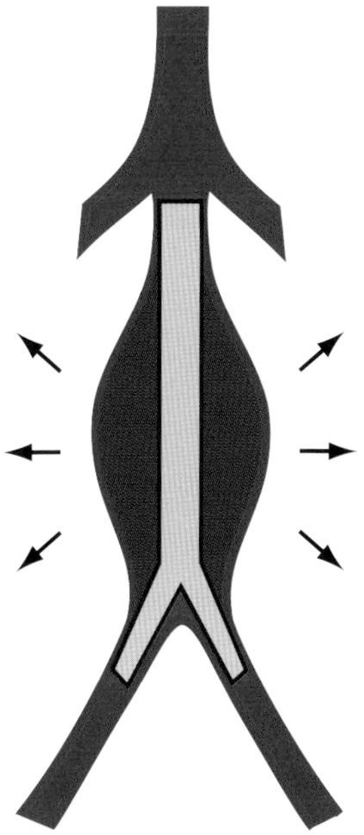

Aortitis

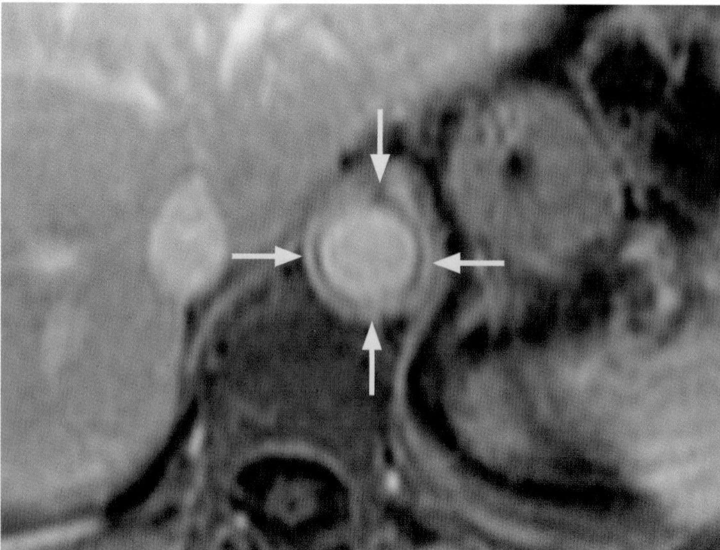

Active aortitis: T1-weighted post-contrast fat saturated MRI demonstrates circumferential mural thickening and enhancement of the aortic wall (arrows).

Case courtesy Michael Steigner, MD, Brigham and Women's Hospital.

- Aortitis is inflammation of the aorta, which may be either infectious or inflammatory.
- A complication of infectious aortitis is the development of a mycotic aneurysm.

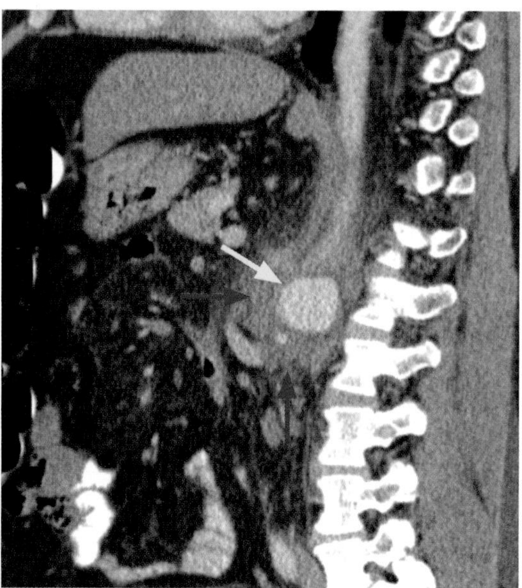

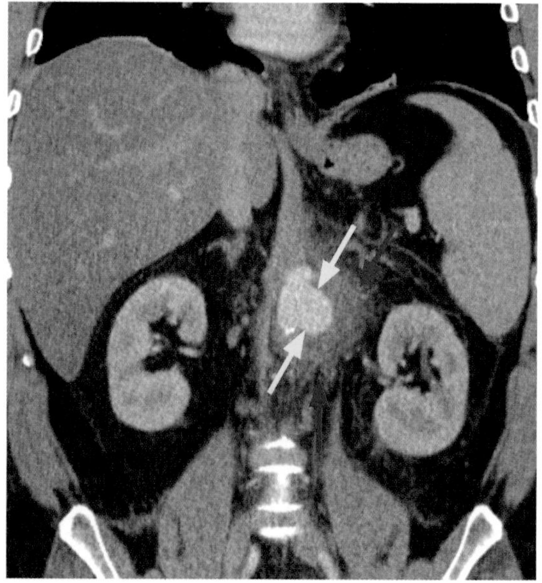

Mycotic aneurysm due to *Staphylococcus aureus*: Sagittal (left image) and coronal (right image) contrast-enhanced CT shows marked periaortic inflammatory change (red arrows) associated with a saccular aortic aneurysm (yellow arrows).

- Inflammatory aortitis can be due to Takayasu arteritis, giant cell arteritis, ankylosing spondylitis, polyarteritis nodosa, rheumatoid arthritis, and immune complex disease. Inflammatory aortitis is treated with corticosteroids.
- The acute phase of aortitis will show circumferential mural thickening and enhancement. There may be an associated aneurysm, dissection, or intramural hematoma. In contrast to intramural hematoma, aortitis tends to cause circumferential thickening rather than the eccentric, crescentic thickening of IMH.

  MRI findings of active aortitis include an aortic wall thickness >2 mm and enhancement of the aortic wall.

- In the chronic phase of the disease, there can be long segmental stenoses and/or aneurysms.

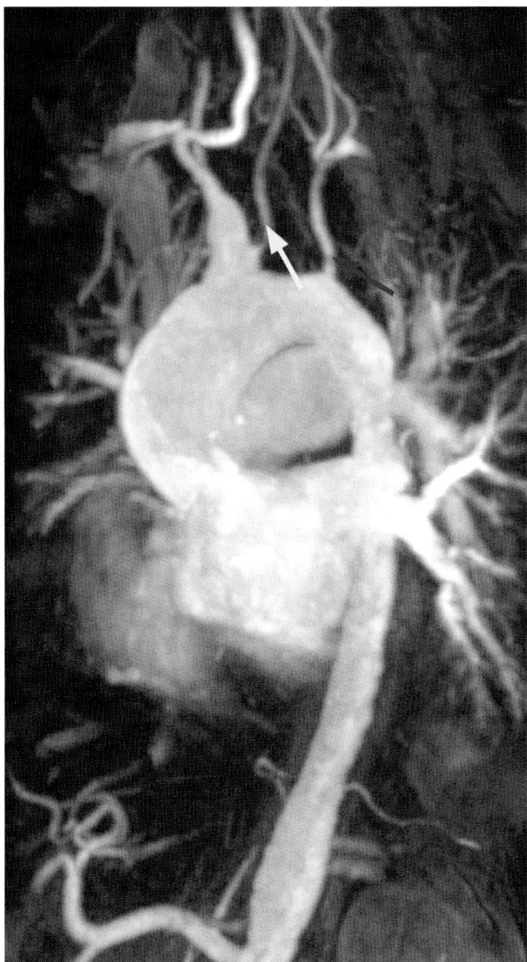

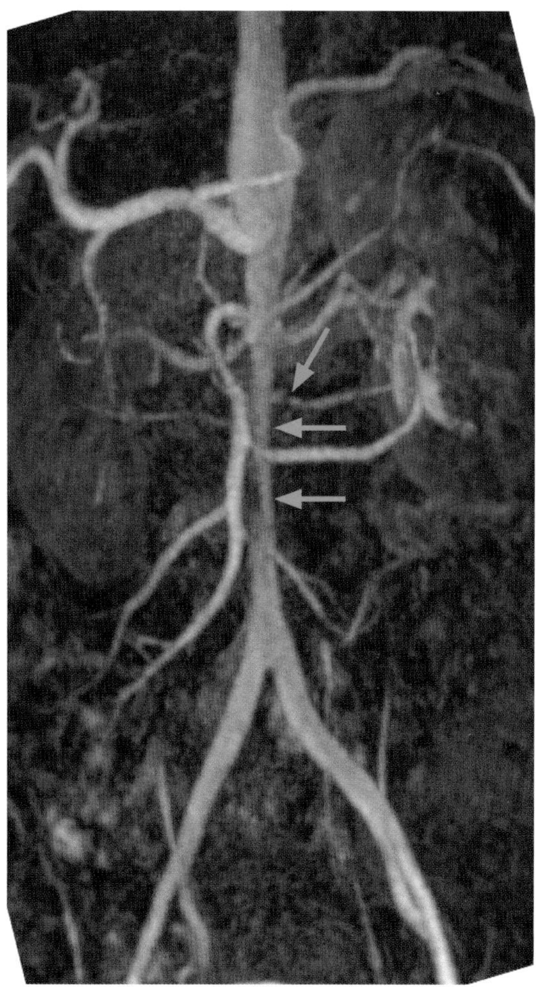

Takayasu arteritis:

Sagittal-oblique maximum intensity projection MR angiogram (left image) of the aortic arch shows narrowing of the left common carotid artery (yellow arrow) and left subclavian artery (red arrow). Note the incidental common origin of the brachiocephalic trunk and the left common carotid artery.

Coronal maximum intensity projection MR angiogram (right image) of the abdominal aorta in the same patient shows a long smooth stenosis of the infra-celiac abdominal aorta (blue arrows), with a focal stenosis of the accessory left renal artery (green arrow).

Case courtesy Michael Hanley, MD, University of Virginia Health System.

- Also known as *pulseless disease,* Takayasu arteritis is an idiopathic, inflammatory, large-vessel vasculitis that involves the thoracic and abdominal aorta, subclavian arteries, carotid arteries, pulmonary arteries, and large mesenteric arteries.
- Takayasu arteritis typically affects young to middle-aged women.
- On imaging, long smooth stenoses are classic. Imaging is often indistinguishable from giant cell arteritis, with the patient's age being the main distinguishing factor. Takayasu arteritis occurs in relatively younger patients and giant cell arteritis is rare in patients under age 50.
- During the acute phase, treatment is with steroids. If symptomatic stenoses occur, endovascular treatment can be performed, but only when the active inflammation has resolved, as measured by normalization of the erythrocyte sedimentation rate.

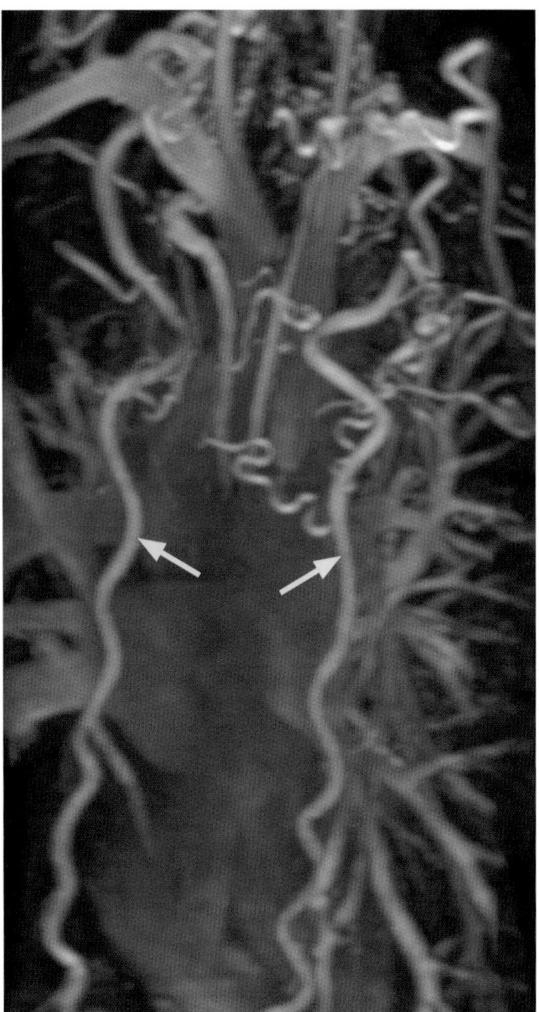

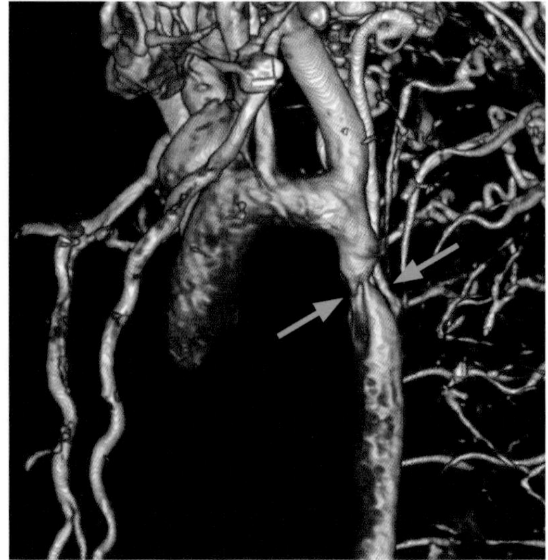

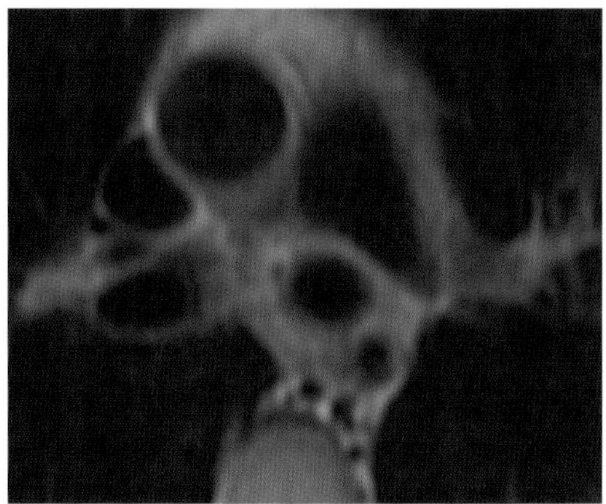

Aortic coarctation: Coronal maximum intensity projection MR angiogram (left image) shows extensive collateral vessels throughout the thorax, with prominent internal thoracic arteries (yellow arrows). 3D volume rendered CT of the aorta (top right image) demonstrates the coarctation (blue arrows) distal to the aortic isthmus. Double inversion recovery fast spin echo MRI (bottom right image) also demonstrates the coarctation.

Case courtesy Michael Steigner, MD, Brigham and Women's Hospital.

- Aortic coarctation is congenital focal narrowing of the proximal descending aorta.
- The adult form of coarctation is usually juxtaductal (at the junction of the ductus arteriosus), leading to upper extremity hypertension. In contrast, an infant presenting with congestive heart failure due to coarctation is usually due to a preductal variant, which functions as a left ventricular obstructive lesion.
- In the setting of coarctation, prominent collaterals develop between the internal thoracic arteries to both the epigastric vessels and intercostal arteries.
- The radiographic findings of coarctation include the *3* sign of the left upper heart border, which represents a double bulge from the focal aortic narrowing and post-stenotic dilation. Rib notching is frequently seen from collateral intercostal vessels.
- Phase contrast MRI can be used to measure the gradient of flow across the coarctation. Calculation of the flow differential between the proximal descending aorta and the aorta at the hiatus aids in determining hemodynamic significance.
- A pseudocoarctation represents focal narrowing of the aorta, similar in morphology to a true coarctation; however, there is no pressure differential and thus no collaterals.

Coronary CT angiography

Evidence for using coronary CT to evaluate for ischemic cardiac disease

- Coronary CT angiography (CCTA) is an excellent test to rule out hemodynamically significant coronary artery disease. Meta-analyses of multiple trials have shown the negative predictive value for CCTA to be in the high 90s.
- The ACRIN-PA and ROMICAT-II clinical trials (both published 2012 NEJM) evaluate the use of CCTA in the emergency room setting for acute chest pain in low to medium risk patients. Both trials conclude that early CCTA improves efficiency, clinical decision making, and leads to a shorter hospitalization, although the ROMICAT-II trial did note increased radiation exposure in the CCTA group and no significant cost difference.
- Coronary CT is very sensitive for hemodynamically significant (>50% lumenal diameter) stenoses; however, a stenosis found on CT may be overcalled, especially if there is calcified plaque, which can cause a blooming artifact.

ECG gating and radiation dose

- ECG gating is used to minimize cardiac motion. The choice of ECG gating has a large effect on patient radiation dose.

  To estimate the radiation dose, the dose–length product (DLP) should be multiplied by a conversion factor of 0.017 to arrive at the dose in millisieverts.
- In a retrospectively gated exam, continuous CT scanning is performed throughout the cardiac cycle and the images are correlated to the ECG cycle afterwards.

  The main advantage of retrospective gating is the ability to create cine reconstructions to evaluate cardiac and valvular function, typically with 10–20 frames per cardiac cycle.

  The main disadvantage of retrospective gating is a significant increase in radiation exposure compared to a prospectively gated study.
- For prospective gating, the ECG is used to time image acquisition at a specific phase of the cardiac cycle, exposing the patient to radiation only during this segment of the cardiac cycle.

  The main advantage of prospective gating is decreased radiation exposure.

  However, since only a fraction of the cardiac cycle is acquired, cine reconstructions are not possible.

Spatial resolution and grading of stenoses

- Coronary arteries have an average luminal diameter of approximately 3 mm.
- CT has an isotropic voxel resolution of 0.35 to 0.5 mm, which allows only 6 to 9 voxels to image the entire coronary artery lumen. This is insufficient resolution to grade a stenosis with accuracy greater than approximately 20% of the diameter.
- In contrast, catheter angiography has a spatial resolution of approximately 0.16 mm, to depict the average lumen of a coronary artery over approximately 18 pixels.
- Due to the limited spatial resolution of CT, a stenosis is classified into categories: <20%; 20–50%; 50–70%, or >70%. A >50% stenosis is considered potentially hemodynamically significant. Conversely, a <50% stenosis is considered not hemodynamically significant.

Temporal resolution and "freezing" of cardiac motion

- A CT scanner requires slightly more than 180 degrees of gantry rotation for image acquisition: For a complete rotation time of 330 ms, the temporal resolution is ~175 ms.
- Dual source CT has two X-ray sources oriented 90 degrees to each other and needs to rotate only 90 degrees to complete a reconstruction, with a temporal resolution of ~75 ms.

Procedure

- A low heart rate (typically below 60 bpm) is desired in order to maximize the R–R interval.

- Beta-blockade is usually necessary to achieve this target heart rate. Oral metoprolol is administered (between 5 and 25 mg, typically administered in 5 mg doses). Oral beta blocker gives better heart rate control and decreased heart rate variability compared to IV.
- Just prior to scanning, sublingual nitroglycerin (0.5–0.8 mg) is administered to dilate the coronary arteries.

Coronary artery anatomy

RCA, right coronary artery
SAN, SA nodal branch
PDA, posterior descending artery
PLA, posterolateral artery
AVN, AV nodal branch

LMCA, left main coronary artery
LAD, left anterior descending
LCx, left circumflex
OM, obtuse marginal
Diag, diagonal

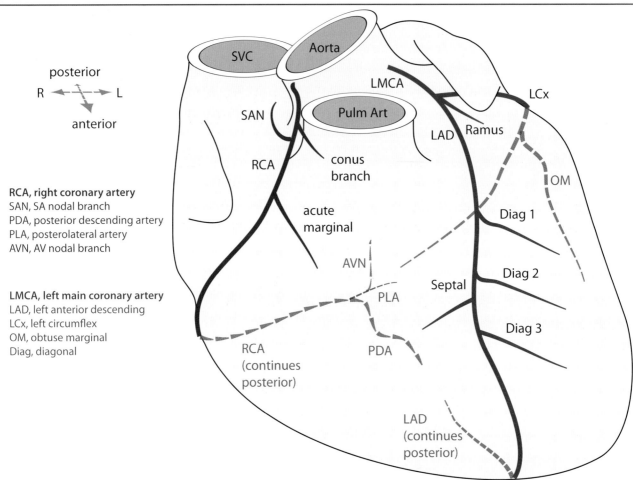

- The diagram above is in anatomic orientation, as if one were looking directly at the patient from the front.

Coronary artery origination

- Most commonly, there are two coronary artery origins off the proximal aorta at the sinuses of Valsalva. The most common anomaly is a high take-off from the sinotubular junction or above.
- There are three coronary sinuses. The right coronary artery arises from the right coronary sinus (located anterior); the left main coronary artery arises from the left coronary sinus (located left-posterior); and no coronary artery arises from the noncoronary sinus (located right-posterior).

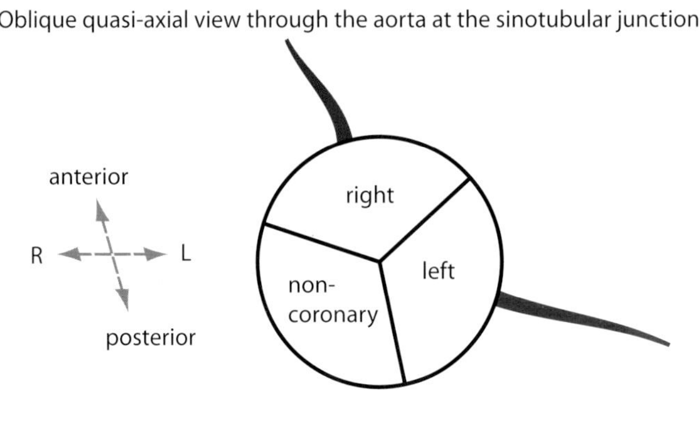

Oblique quasi-axial view through the aorta at the sinotubular junction

Left main coronary artery (LMCA)

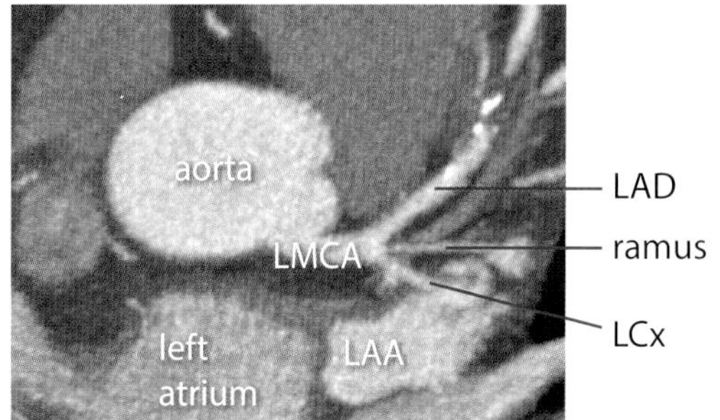

- The left main coronary artery (LMCA) courses between the pulmonary artery and the left atrial appendage (LAA).
- The LMCA bifurcates into left anterior descending (LAD) and left circumflex (LCx) arteries. A ramus branch may be present to form a trifurcation.

Left anterior descending (LAD) coronary artery

- The left anterior descending (LAD) coronary artery courses in the anterior interventricular groove, which is the anatomic groove between the right and left ventricles.
- The LAD gives off the diagonal branches (LA***D*** - ***D***iagonal) and septal branches, which penetrate the interventricular septum to supply blood to the anterior half of the septum.

Left circumflex (LCx) coronary artery

- The left circumflex (LCx) coronary artery courses underneath the left atrial appendage (LAA) in the left atrioventricular groove (between the left ventricle and left atrium).
- The LCx artery gives off the obtuse marginal (OM; circ***OM***flex) branch, which supplies the posterolateral wall of the left ventricle. The angle of the lateral wall of the obtuse marginal artery is obtuse, hence the name.
- The LCx uncommonly (~7%) supplies the posterior descending artery (PDA), which is the criteria for a left-dominant system. In the anatomic diagram on the previous page, the more common right-dominant system is shown, where the right coronary artery supplies the PDA.

Right coronary artery (RCA)

Axial

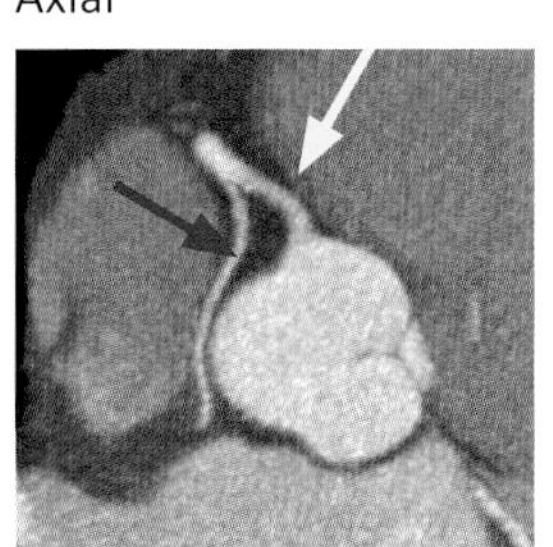

RCA (yellow arrow) arises from the right coronary cusp and gives off the SA nodal branch (red arrow).

Axial

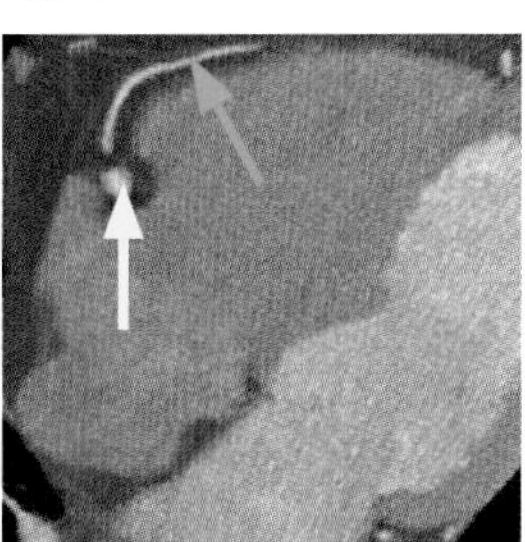

RCA (yellow arrow) gives off acute marginal (blue arrow), which courses along the anterior RV wall.

Axial

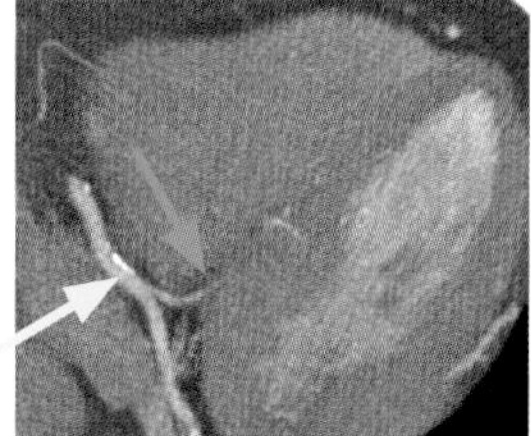

RCA (yellow arrow) gives off PDA (green arrow) in this right-dominant system.

Sagittal

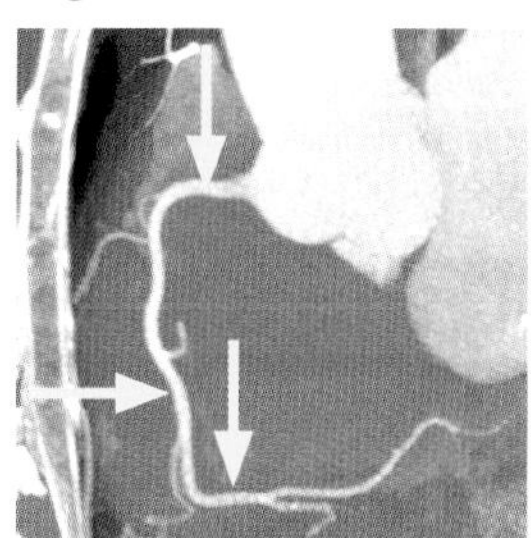

Sagittal thick-slice MIP shows the complete course of RCA (yellow arrows).

- The right coronary artery (RCA) mirrors the LCx in course, sitting within the right atrioventricular groove.
- The first branches of the RCA are the conal branch, anteriorly (supplies the right ventricular outflow tract) and the sinoatrial node branch posteriorly.
- The RCA gives off an acute marginal branch, which courses anterior to the right ventricular (RV) free wall and muscular branches to supply the RV free wall (not drawn).
- The atrioventricular node branch (AVN) branches off at the crux (junction of all four chambers where the atrioventricular and interventricular grooves intersect).
- The posterior descending artery (PDA) arises from the RCA in approximately 85% to supply the posterior half of the ventricular septum.
- The terminal branch of the RCA is most commonly the posterolateral artery (PLA) that supplies the posterior left ventricle.

Determination of dominance

- Whichever side supplies the PDA, PLA, and AV nodal branch (AVN) is considered the dominant coronary artery. Most commonly, in about 85% of cases, the RCA is the dominant artery.
- Left-dominant anatomy is uncommon, occurring in approximately 7% of cases. In left-dominant anatomy, the LCx supplies the PDA, PLA, and AVN.
- Codominant anatomy can also be seen in approximately 7% of cases, typically with the RCA supplying the PDA, while the LCx supplies the PLA.

STRUCTURAL CORONARY ARTERY ANOMALIES

Coronary artery anomalies: Overview

- Anomalies of the coronary arteries are rare. A *malignant* coronary artery anomaly carries an increased risk of sudden death (in up to 40% of patients), often associated with exercise.
- Multidetector CT is the best modality to evaluate anomalous coronary artery anatomy.
- Anomalies of coronary artery **origin** may be always malignant (if arising from the pulmonary artery) or potentially malignant (depending on the course):

Coronary artery arising from the pulmonary artery which is malignant. Either the right or left main coronary artery may arise from the pulmonary artery. Both are very rare.

Anomalous left coronary artery from the pulmonary artery (**ALCAPA**).

Anomalous right coronary artery from the pulmonary artery (**ARCAPA**).

RCA arising from left coronary sinus.

Left main coronary artery (LMCA) arising from right coronary sinus.

Left circumflex (LCx) or left anterior descending (LAD) arising from right coronary sinus.

Any artery arising from the noncoronary sinus.

- Anomalies of coronary artery **course** may be benign or malignant and include:

Interarterial course (between the aorta and pulmonary artery) of an anomalous coronary artery is malignant.

Retroaortic, prepulmonic, and septal coronary artery course are all considered benign.

- An intramural course of a coronary artery is seen when the vessel courses through the wall of the aorta for a short segment. This anomaly is associated with sudden death. There is typically a slit-like configuration of the coronary artery on CCTA. The treatment of intramural coronary artery is bypass, reimplantation, or the unroofing procedure, which opens and enlarges the ostium from inside the aorta.

Benign coronary artery anomaly

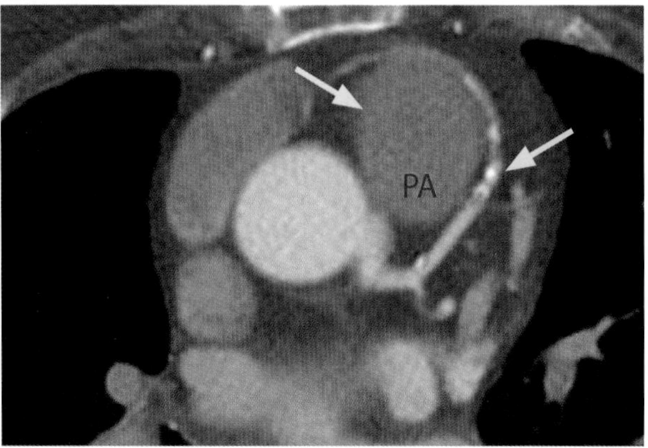

Prepulmonic (benign) course of the left anterior descending (LAD) coronary artery:

Axial image from a gated coronary CT shows an anomalous course of the LAD, which runs anterior (arrows) to the pulmonary artery (PA).

Case courtesy Michael Hanley, MD, University of Virginia Health System.

- An aberrant coronary artery course is considered clinically benign if the coronary artery does not course between the aorta and the pulmonary artery.

Malignant coronary artery anomaly

Malignant: Anomalous origin of LEFT coronary artery arising from the RIGHT coronary sinus, passing between the aorta and the PA.

Malignant: Anomalous origin of RIGHT coronary artery arising from the LEFT coronary sinus, passing between the aorta and the PA.

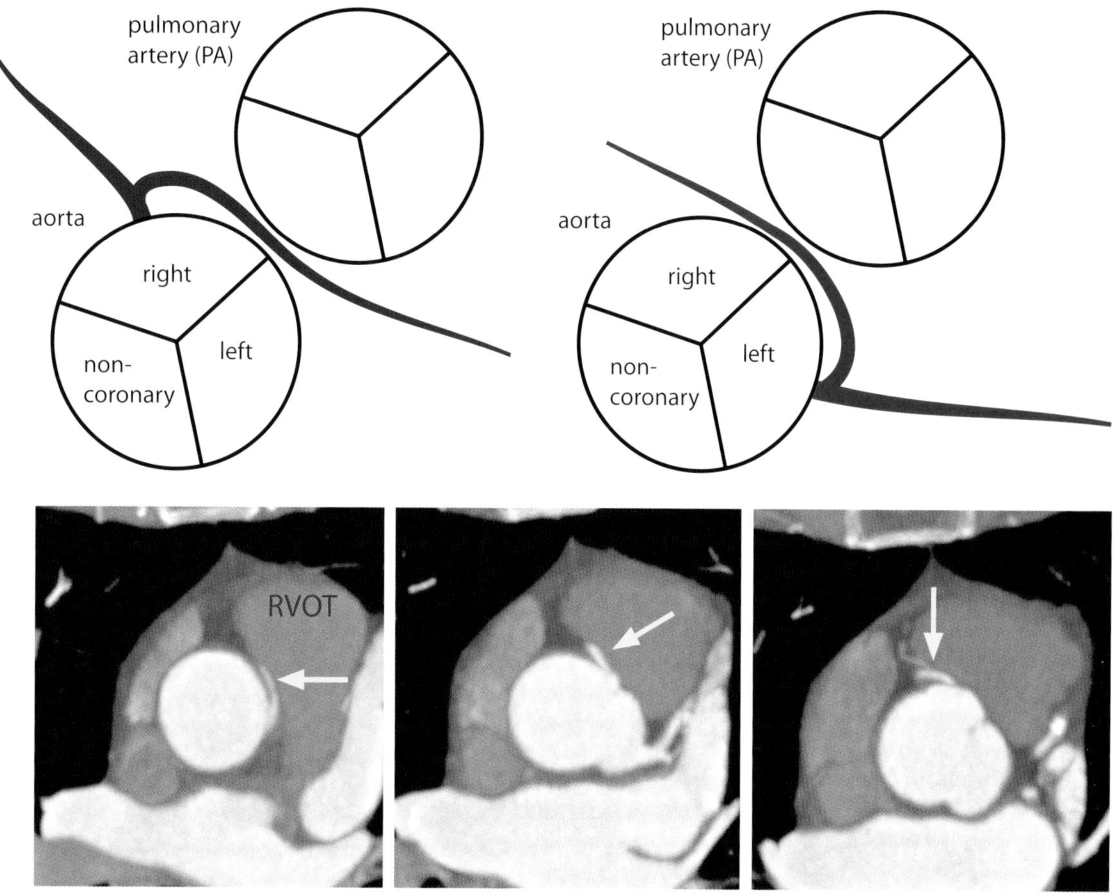

Malignant course of anomalous right coronary artery:

Sequential axial images from a coronary CT show anomalous origin of the right coronary artery (arrow) from the left coronary sinus, which then courses between the aorta and the right ventricular outflow tract (RVOT).

Case courtesy Michael Hanley, MD, University of Virginia Health System.

- Anomalous interarterial (between the pulmonary artery or right ventricular outflow tract and the aorta) course of a coronary artery carries a high risk of sudden death of up to 40%, associated with exercise. It is thought that dilation of the aorta occurs during exercise, which may compress the anomalous vessel resulting in myocardial infarction.
- Either an anomalous left coronary artery or anomalous right coronary artery may take a malignant interarterial course.
- Treatment is surgical bypass grafting.

Anomalous left coronary artery from the pulmonary artery (ALCAPA)/Bland–White–Garland syndrome

- Also called Bland–White–Garland syndrome, anomalous left coronary artery from the pulmonary artery (ALCAPA) is a very rare but serious coronary artery anomaly, where the left coronary artery arises from the pulmonary artery. Most affected patients are infants, with over 90% mortality in the first year of life if untreated.
- Treatment is surgical, with either direct implantation of the anomalous coronary artery (in children) or ligation of the anomalous vessel in conjunction with bypass grafting (in adults).
- Less commonly, the RCA may arise from the pulmonary artery, which is known as anomalous right coronary artery from the pulmonary artery (ARCAPA). Treatment is similar.

Myocardial bridging

- Myocardial bridging describes a band of myocardium overlying a segment of a coronary artery, most commonly seen in the mid LAD.
- Myocardial bridging is usually asymptomatic; however, it may be a cause of angina, myocardial infarction, or even death.
- If bridging is present and thought to be the source of the patient's symptoms, further evaluation is recommended with exercise myocardial perfusion.

Cardiac MRI

Overview of cardiac MRI

- Cardiac MRI provides high-resolution dynamic imaging of the heart using primarily segmented steady-state free precession (SSFP) and/or gradient echo cine sequences.
- SSFP is a "white blood" sequence that provides excellent contrast between myocardium and blood pool. It is well-suited for cardiac MRI due to its high temporal resolution and excellent contrast.
- Cine MRI provides quantitative assessment of cardiac morphology and function. Real-time images can be used for subjective analysis in poor gating situations.
- Tissue characterization is typically performed with double or triple inversion fast spin echo sequences.

Contrast-enhanced perfusion MRI

- First-pass contrast-enhanced perfusion MRI is performed pre and post vasodilator stress to evaluate myocardial perfusion. Normal myocardium enhances, while areas of decreased perfusion will be relatively hypoenhancing.

Delayed contrast-enhanced MRI (DE-MR)

- Delayed contrast-enhanced MRI (DE-MR) is used to image changes in the myocyte to interstitial space ratio. This ratio decreases most commonly after a myocardial infarction where myocytes are replaced with scar tissue.
- In distinction to contrast-enhanced perfusion described above where first-pass enhancement is normal, any delayed enhancement in DE-MR is abnormal and represents an increase in the extracellular volume fraction.
- Although delayed enhancement is most commonly due to prior infarct, abnormal enhancement may also be due to nonischemic etiologies, depending on the pattern of enhancement.
- Normal myocardium is nulled out with an inversion time of approximately 300 milliseconds and therefore appears black, although the inversion time varies with delay time, excretion rates, contrast relaxicity, and volume.

Delayed enhancement: Ischemic cardiomyopathy

- Delayed enhancement post infarction will extend from the subendocardium to the epicardium in a vascular distribution.

Subendocardial delayed enhancement

- Since the endocardium is the most susceptible to ischemia, ischemic-type delayed enhancement will always involve the subendocardial surface and should have a vascular territory. After remodelling, a chronic infarct will demonstrate delayed enhancement.

Transmural delayed enhancement

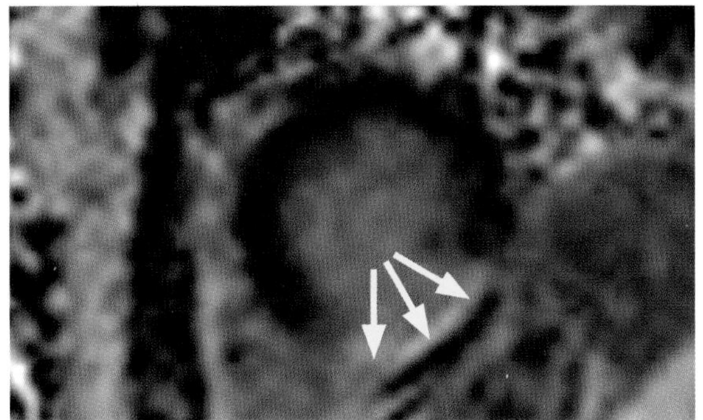

Transmural delayed enhancement due to infarct:

Delayed contrast-enhanced short-axis cardiac MRI shows transmural enhancement (arrows) of the inferior wall of the left ventricle, consistent with transmural infarction in the right coronary artery territory.

Case courtesy Michael Hanley, MD, University of Virginia Health System.

- Ischemic-type delayed enhancement may involve the endocardium only or may be transmural. Transmural enhancement extends across the entire myocardial thickness.
- Transmural delayed enhancement represents nonviable scar from prior transmural infarct.
- Evaluation of the cine images will usually demonstrate hypokinesis in the region of abnormal delayed enhancement.

Delayed enhancement: Nonischemic

- Delayed enhancement not following a vascular territory is not due to ischemia. Several distinct patterns of nonischemic delayed enhancement have been described.

Mid-myocardial delayed enhancement

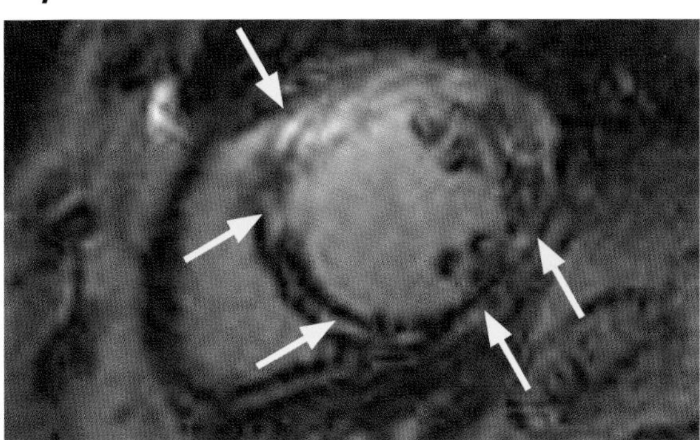

Mid-myocardial delayed enhancement due to Chagas disease:

Delayed contrast-enhanced short-axis cardiac MRI shows patchy mid-myocardial enhancement (arrows) throughout the left ventricle myocardium. This is a nonischemic distribution, but is nonspecific.

Case courtesy Michael Hanley, MD, University of Virginia Health System.

- **Dilated cardiomyopathy (DCM)** is the most common nonischemic cardiomyopathy. Most commonly idiopathic, DCM may also be caused by alcohol abuse, myocarditis, or drug toxicity. MRI imaging of DCM will show mid-myocardial delayed enhancement. Additional MRI findings of DCM include diffuse chamber enlargement and reduced ejection fraction.
- **Sarcoidosis** is a systemic disease of noncaseating granulomas with cardiac manifestations of arrhythmias, left ventricular dysfunction, and restrictive cardiomyopathy. Cardiac findings are usually seen in conjunction with other manifestations of sarcoid, including lung disease and adenopathy. Cardiac MRI of sarcoid typically shows either mid-myocardial or subepicardial delayed enhancement in a nodular or patchy pattern.
- **Chagas disease** is caused by the protozoan *Trypanosoma cruzi,* and can lead to a cardiomyopathy. On cardiac MRI, there is typically epicardial or mid-myocardial delayed enhancement, which can be seen even before the development of symptoms.
- **Hypertrophic cardiomyopathy** is characterized by abnormal left ventricular myocardial thickening without dilation. Pathologic thickening may be diffuse or focal. In severe cases, hypertrophic cardiomyopathy may be a cause of sudden death. On cardiac MRI, there can be mid-myocardial delayed enhancement in the regions of hypertrophied myocardium and at the junctions of the interventricular septum and the right ventricular free wall, due to myofibril disarray. Evaluation of the cine images will show reduced diastolic filling of the left ventricle.

Epicardial/subepicardial delayed enhancement

- **Myocarditis** is inflammation of the myocardium, which may be secondary to multiple causes. Viral infection is the most common cause of myocarditis, followed by autoimmune disorders and drug toxicity. In addition to subepicardial delayed enhancement, cardiac MRI of myocarditis also shows wall motion abnormalities in the affected regions.
- **Chagas** disease may cause epicardial or mid-myocardial delayed enhancement.
- **Sarcoidosis** may cause either mid-myocardial or subepicardial delayed enhancement in a nodular or patchy pattern.

Circumferential subendocardial delayed enhancement

- **Amyloidosis** is a disorder of glycoprotein deposition throughout the extracellular spaces. In the heart, amyloidosis causes biventricular myocardial thickening, which leads to diffuse ventricular subendocardial delayed enhancement.
- **Cardiac transplant** patients may demonstrate circumferential subendocardial delayed enhancement, thought to correlate with the presence of myocardial fibrosis pathologically.

Summary of delayed enhancement MRI

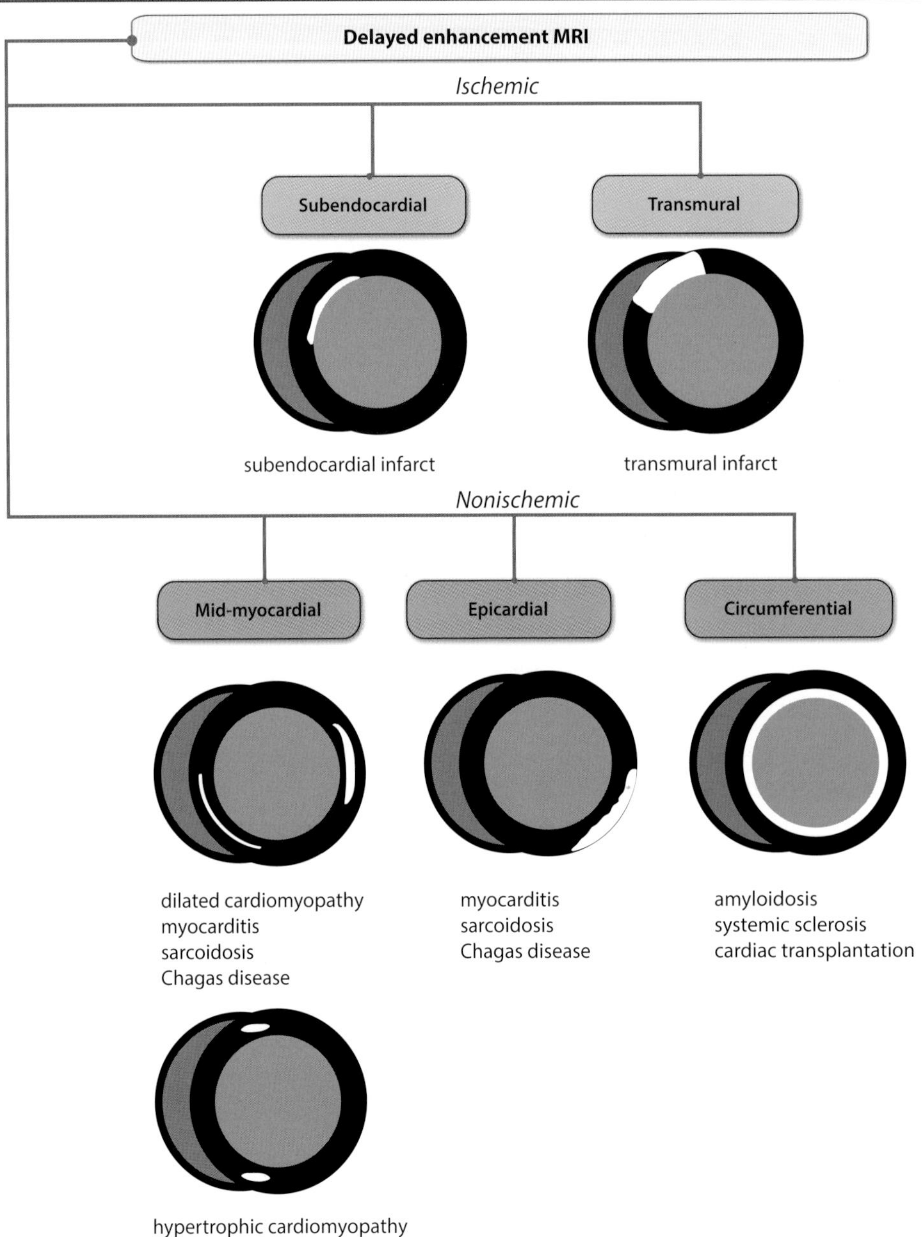

- By applying a systematic approach, the standard chest radiograph can offer valuable information about the presence or severity of heart disease.
- The radiographic evaluation of heart disease begins with an assessment of the size of the cardiac silhouette. Radiographically evident heart disease can be divided into two categories: Those with a **normal**-sized cardiac silhouette and those with an **enlarged** cardiac silhouette.
- A ratio of the cardiac silhouette to the inner diameter of the thorax (the cardiothoracic ratio) of 0.55 or greater (on a PA projection) suggests enlargement of the cardiac silhouette.
- Cardiovascular diseases with an enlarged cardiac silhouette include cardiomyopathy secondary to congestive heart failure, valvular regurgitation (aortic, mitral, or tricuspid regurgitation), high-output or volume overload states, dilated cardiomyopathy, pericardial effusion, and paracardiac mass.
- To distinguish between the various causes of enlarged heart cardiac disease, the key structures to evaluate are the left atrium and the aorta.

> If the **left atrium is enlarged** and the cardiac silhouette is enlarged, that suggests **mitral regurgitation**.
>
> If the **aorta is enlarged** and the cardiac silhouette is enlarged, that suggests **aortic regurgitation**.
>
> If neither the left atrium nor the aorta is enlarged, that suggests one of the other etiologies.

- Cardiovascular diseases with a normal-sized cardiac silhouette include valvular stenosis (aortic or mitral stenosis), pulmonary artery hypertension, hypertrophic cardiomyopathy, restrictive physiology, and acute myocardial infarction.
- Similar to evaluation of diseases with an enlarged cardiac silhouette, the key structures to evaluate in the presence of a normal cardiac silhouette are the left atrium and the aorta.

> If the **left atrium is enlarged** and the cardiac silhouette is normal, that suggests **mitral stenosis**.
>
> If the **aorta is enlarged** and the cardiac silhouette is normal, that suggests **aortic stenosis** or aortic aneurysm.
>
> If neither the left atrium nor the aorta is enlarged, that suggests one of the other etiologies.

- Other structures to always evaluate include the pulmonary vascularity, thoracic wall, chamber enlargement, and the great vessels (pulmonary arteries, ascending aorta, aortic arch, and descending aorta).

Right ventricular enlargement

- The right ventricle is the most anterior cardiac chamber. Right ventricular enlargement causes displacement of the cardiac apex in a leftward direction (in contrast to left ventricular enlargement, which causes displacement in a left-inferior direction).
- Right ventricular enlargement may cause opacification of the retrosternal clear space on the lateral radiograph.

Right atrial enlargement

- The right atrium forms the right heart border. Right atrial enlargement causes lateral bulging or elongation of the right heart border.

Left ventricular enlargement

- The left ventricle forms the left heart border. Left ventricular enlargement typically causes displacement of the cardiac apex in a left-inferior direction.
- Note that hypertrophic cardiomyopathy does *not* cause enlargement of the external contour of the ventricle.

Left atrial enlargement

- The left atrium is the most posterior cardiac chamber. An enlarged left atrium may be caused by mitral regurgitation (with an enlarged cardiac silhouette) or mitral stenosis (with a normal cardiac silhouette).
- An enlarged left atrium can splay the carina, seen on the frontal view. On the lateral radiograph, an enlarged left atrium can elevate the left upper lobe bronchus.

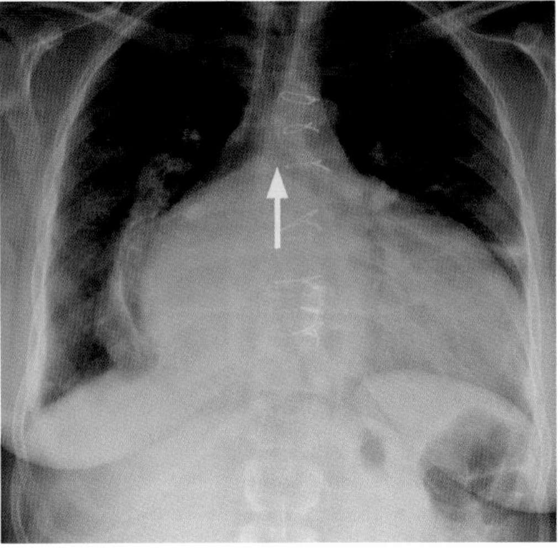
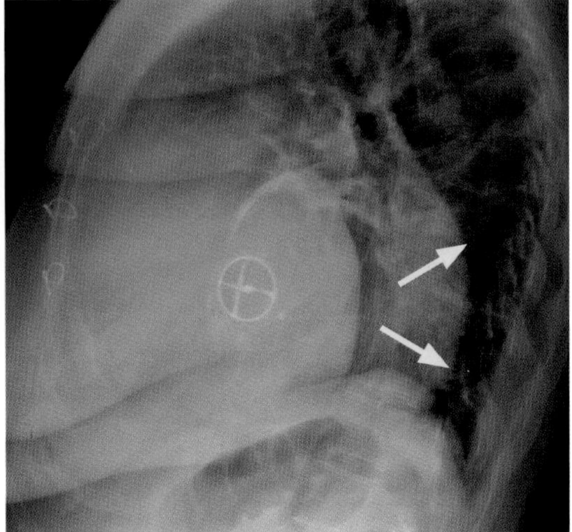

Left atrial enlargement with cardiomegaly (due to mitral regurgitation): Frontal chest radiograph (left image) demonstrates massive cardiomegaly with marked enlargement of the left atrium, as evidenced by splaying of the carina (arrow). Lateral radiograph shows marked posterior displacement of the esophagus (arrows). A prosthetic mitral valve is present.

Case courtesy Ritu Gill, MBBS, Brigham and Women's Hospital.

- An important clue to the presence of left atrial enlargement is the *double density* sign, seen over the right heart. The *double density* represents the right aspect of the enlarged left atrium visualized through the right atrium.

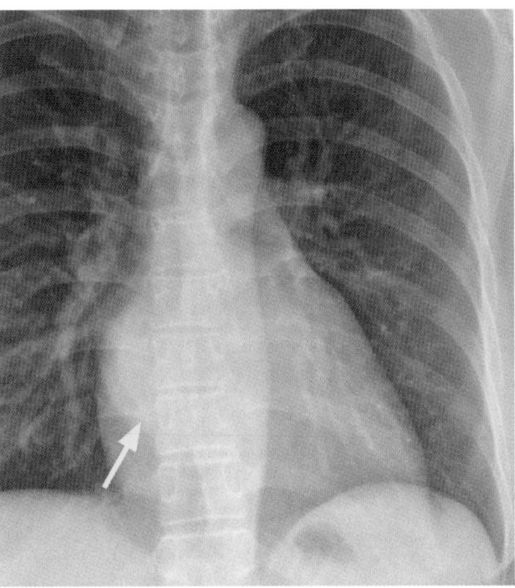
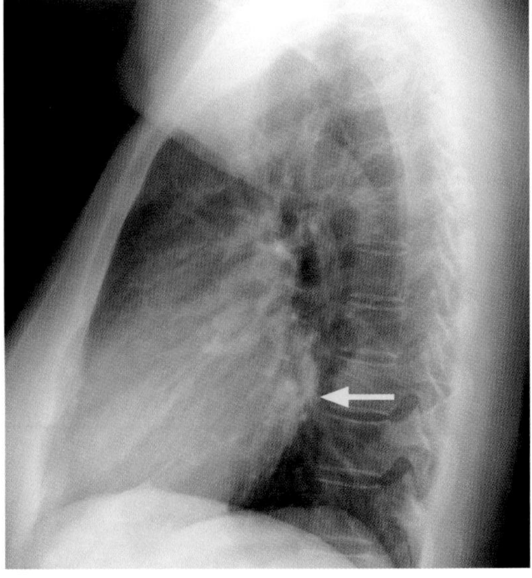

Left atrial enlargement without cardiomegaly (due to mitral stenosis): Frontal chest radiograph (left image) demonstrates the *double density sign* (arrow) with the left atrial border visualized through the right atrium. Lateral radiograph demonstrates posterior protrusion of the left atrium (arrow).

Case courtesy Ritu Gill, MBBS, Brigham and Women's Hospital.

- On a lateral esophogram, an enlarged left atrium can displace the esophagus posteriorly and may be a cause of dysphagia.

IMAGING AND COMPLICATIONS OF MYOCARDIAL INFARCTION

Plain film evaluation of myocardial infarction (MI)

- The majority of initial plain chest radiographs obtained in patients with acute myocardial infarction (MI) are normal; however, the most common abnormality seen is increased pulmonary venous pressure (or overt pulmonary edema).

  The presence of pulmonary edema after MI is a poor prognostic indicator.

  Papillary muscle rupture due to myocardial infarction typically produces acute pulmonary edema. A classic radiographic finding is isolated right upper lobe pulmonary edema due to acute papillary muscle rupture.
- The plain chest radiograph can evaluate for some complications of acute MI such as pericardial effusion, left ventricular aneurysm, and papillary muscle rupture.
- In a patient with acute chest pain, the initial chest radiograph can often suggest an alternative cause for the patient's acute chest pain, such as pneumothorax or pneumonia.

True left ventricular aneurysm

- A true left ventricular aneurysm is a focal outpouching of the ventricular wall, with all layers of the muscular wall affected.
- True aneurysms are associated with occlusion of the left anterior descending coronary artery.
- The most common location of a true left ventricular aneurysm is along the anterolateral or apical wall of the left ventricle. Plain film findings of a true LV aneurysm include an abnormal contour along the midportion of the left cardiac border near the apex.
- A true aneurysm may calcify.
- True ventricular aneurysms are associated with wall motion dyskinesia but they rarely rupture. Management is medical.

False aneurysm (pseudoaneurysm)

- A false cardiac aneurysm (pseudoaneurysm) is a contained ventricular rupture, with only pericardial adhesions preventing a complete rupture. There is no myocardium in the wall of a false aneurysm.
- False aneurysms are associated with occlusion of the circumflex or right coronary arteries.
- The most common location of a false aneurysm is the upper diaphragmatic and posterior wall. Plain film findings suggestive of a false LV aneurysm include a retrocardiac density seen on the frontal view and an abnormal posterior contour on the lateral radiograph.
- False aneurysms may rupture at any time. An increase in size over sequential films is especially worrisome for impending rupture.
- Treatment of a left ventricular pseudoaneurysm is surgical.

Dressler syndrome

- Dressler syndrome is an autoimmune pericarditis, often associated with pericardial and pleural effusions.

VALVULAR DISEASE

Endocarditis

- Endocarditis is infection of the cardiac valves. Risk factors for development of endocarditis include intravenous drug abuse, poor dental hygiene, diabetes, and prosthetic valves.
- Valvular vegetations are usually diagnosed by echocardiography, although CT angiography is routinely able to depict vegetations >1 cm in diameter. CT can also evaluate for the presence of a perivalvular abscess and assess for extracardiac complications of endocarditis, such as septic pulmonary emboli.

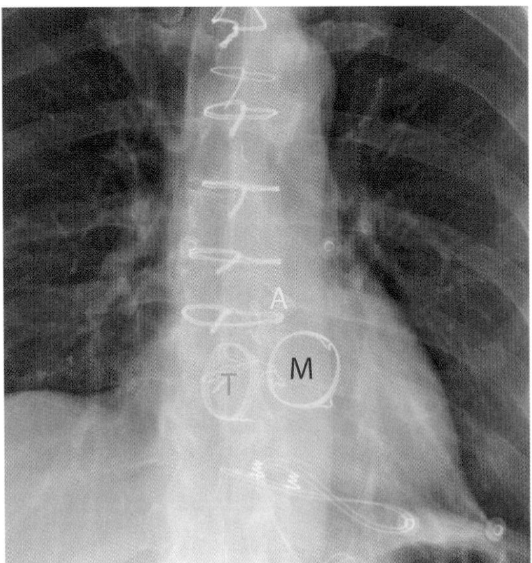

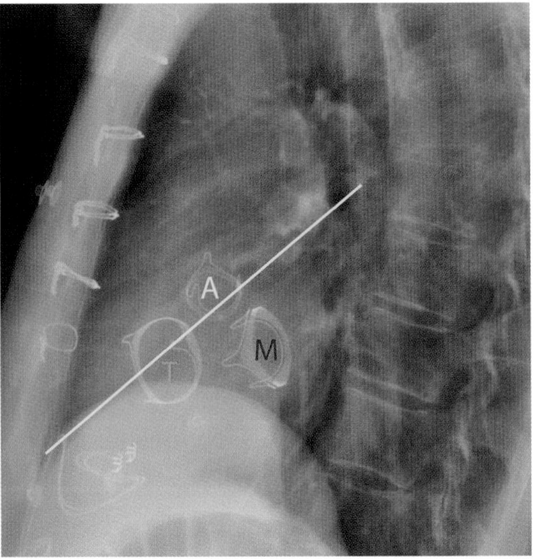

Prosthetic aortic (A), mitral (M), and tricuspid (T) valves. Note that on the lateral radiograph (right image) the aortic valve is located on a plane drawn from the sternal/diaphragmatic junction and the carina (yellow line).

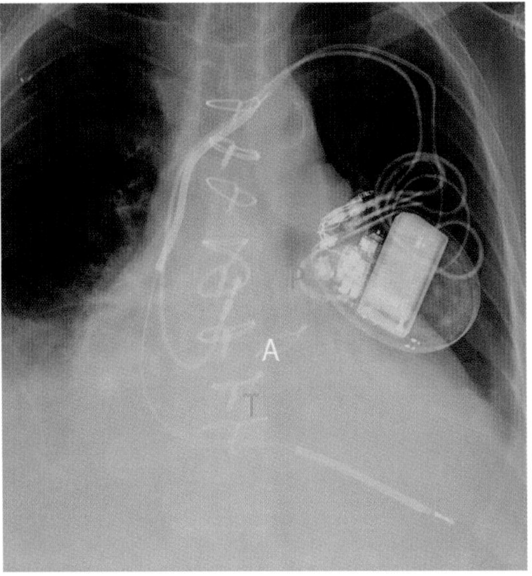

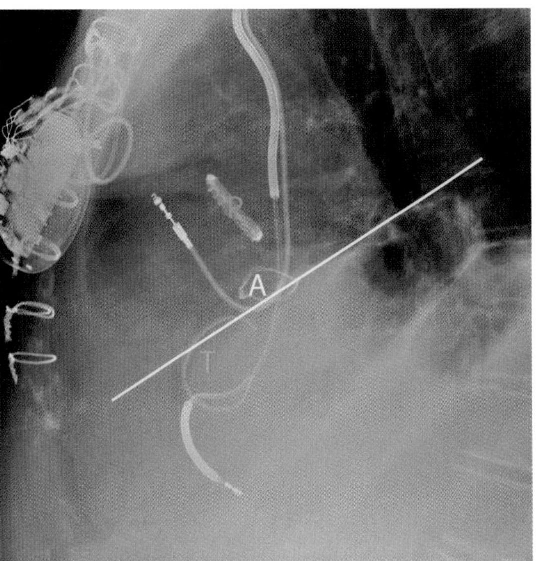

Prosthetic aortic (A), pulmonic (P), and tricuspid (T) valves in a different patient. The tricuspid prosthesis is a ring annuloplasty. The aortic valve is seen on the plane connecting the sternal/ diaphragmatic junction with the carina on the lateral radiograph.

- On the lateral radiograph, the aortic valve is centered on the plane drawn from the sternal/diaphragmatic junction and the carina.
- The tricuspid valve is to the right and anterior to the mitral valve.
- The pulmonic valve is the most superior and most leftward valve.
- Evaluation of prosthetic valves can be challenging in patients with abnormal chamber enlargement or cardiac rotation.
- The atrioventricular valves (mitral and tricuspid) are open in diastole.

Mitral regurgitation

- Acute mitral regurgitation secondary to myocardial infarction can present as acute pulmonary edema with a normal size heart.
- Chronic mitral regurgitation can lead to enlargement of the cardiac silhouette and left atrial enlargement.

  The left atrial appendage (LAA) is often enlarged in patients with rheumatic disease; however, the LAA is typically not enlarged in nonrheumatic mitral regurgitation.

Mitral stenosis

- Mitral stenosis appears as a normal size heart with left atrial enlargement.
- Pulmonary venous pressures are typically elevated.

Mitral annular calcification

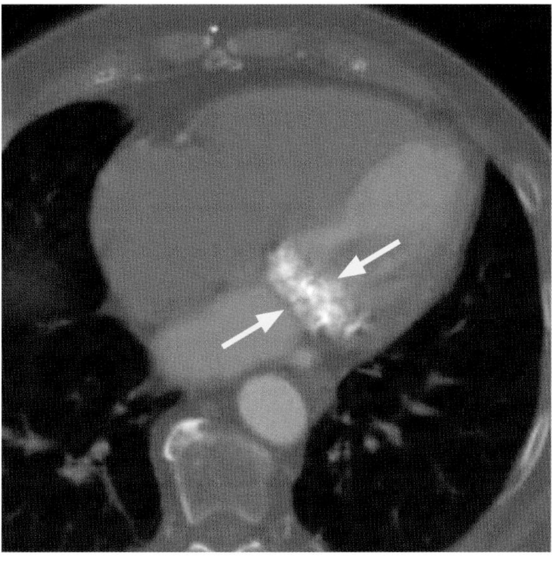

Mitral annular calcification:

Contrast-enhanced axial CT in bone windows demonstrates extensive calcification of the mitral valve annulus (arrows).

Case courtesy Michael Hanley, MD, University of Virginia Health System.

- Mitral annular calcification (MAC) is a degenerative process where calcium is deposited along the fibrous annulus encircling the mitral valve.
- MAC may be associated with increased risk of stroke, adverse cardiovascular events, and atrial fibrillation. MAC is considered a risk marker for cardiovascular disease.
- MAC can be associated with mitral regurgitation, but unlike mitral *valve* calcifications, MAC is not associated with mitral stenosis.

Aortic stenosis

- Aortic stenosis causes left ventricular hypertrophy; however, the heart size does not change.
- The ascending aorta is usually enlarged in long-standing aortic stenosis.
- The pulmonary vascularity is typically normal.

Aortic regurgitation

- Long-standing aortic regurgitation causes left ventricular enlargement, which is apparent on radiographs as cardiomegaly. There is typically enlargement of the ascending aorta.
- Similar to aortic stenosis, the pulmonary vasculature is typically normal.

Right-sided valvular disease

- The right side of the heart is preferentially involved in patients with carcinoid disease, leading to tricuspid and pulmonic valve dysfunction, although the left-sided valves can be involved as well.

Catecholamine induced (takotsubo) cardiomyopathy

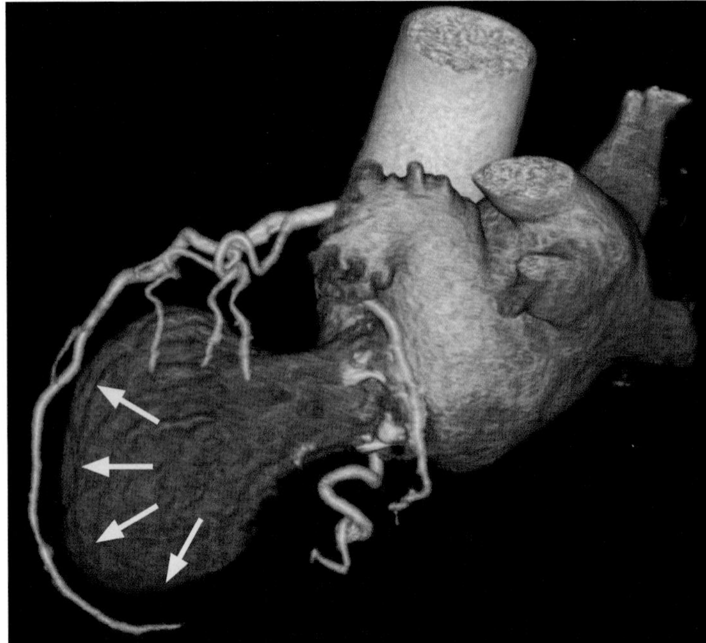

Catecholamine induced cardiomyopathy:

3D volume rendered image from a cardiac CT (with the myocardium removed) demonstrates marked ballooning of the left ventricular apex (arrows). The coronary arteries are normal.

Case courtesy Michael Steigner, MD, Brigham and Women's Hospital.

- Catecholamine induced cardiomyopathy, also known as takotsubo cardiomyopathy and broken heart syndrome, can clinically mimic acute myocardial infarction.
- Typically affecting older women in the setting of acute emotional stress, catecholamine induced cardiomyopathy can present with chest pain, abnormal ECG, and elevation of cardiac enzymes. Cardiac catheterization is normal.

  One theory is that men may suffer catecholamine induced cardiomyopathy as well but typically don't survive. There may be a protective effect of estrogen.
- Catecholamine induced cardiomyopathy is typically self-limited.
- On cardiac MRI or coronary CT, there is a characteristic ballooning of the cardiac apex. The shape of the heart is similar to a Japanese octopus pot, hence the name *takotsubo.* There is no abnormal delayed enhancement on MRI.

Arrhythmogenic cardiomyopathy

- Arrhythmogenic cardiomyopathy (previously called arrhythmogenic right ventricular dysplasia, as it was thought to only affect the right ventricle) represents fibrofatty replacement of ventricular myocytes, causing focal contraction abnormalities and/or aneurysm formation.
- Diagnosis is usually difficult and depends on major and minor criteria from EKG, imaging, and biopsy findings, as determined by task force in 2010. Imaging plays a supportive role in the diagnosis. Imaging findings may contribute 1 major and 1 minor criterion based on the presence of right ventricular enlargement or presence of focal aneurysm. The presence of myocardial fat is no longer in the criteria as fat can be seen in normal individuals with aging.
- Left ventricular involvement can be seen in up to three quarters of patients.
- Patients may suffer lethal arrhythmias and therefore require ICD placement once diagnosis is confirmed.

Myocardial noncompaction

- Myocardial noncompaction is a developmental defect in embryologic formation of the left ventricle, due to failure of part of the left ventricle to form a solid myocardium.
- Patients with noncompaction have an increased risk of adverse cardiac events, including arrhythmias, thrombus formation, stroke, and cardiomyopathy.
- On imaging, the left ventricle appears as heavily trabeculated as the right ventricle with a relatively thin left ventricular wall.

Hypertrophic cardiomyopathy (HCM)

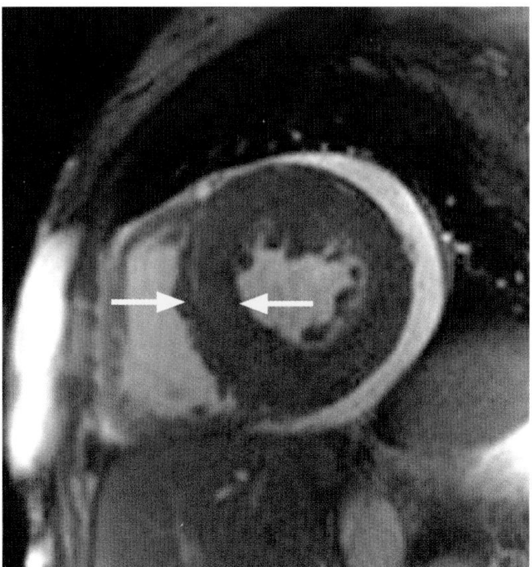

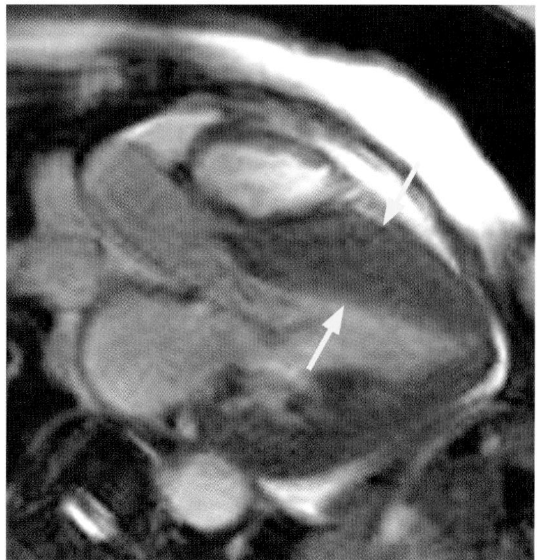

Hypertrophic cardiomyopathy: Short-axis (left image) steady-state free precession MRI shows concentric hypertrophy of the left ventricular myocardium (yellow arrows), without chamber enlargement. A small pericardial effusion is present. Three-chamber view (right image) from the same study better shows the septal predominance of the ventricular hypertrophy (arrows).

Case courtesy Michael Hanley, MD, University of Virginia Health System.

- Hypertrophic cardiomyopathy (HCM) is an autosomal dominant cardiomyopathy, characterized by hypertrophic left ventricular myocardium. HCM is the most common cardiomyopathy.
- The asymmetric septal hypertrophy variant, known as idiopathic hypertrophic subaortic stenosis (IHSS), may cause left ventricular outflow tract obstruction. Criteria for diagnosis include a wall thickness of ≥15 mm and a ratio of ≥1.5 compared to the lateral wall. A wall thickness ≥30 mm is an indication for ICD placement.
- Systolic anterior motion of the anterior leaflet of the mitral valve can cause mitral regurgitation and resultant left atrial enlargement.
- Although diagnosis is usually made by echocardiography, indications for MRI are to confirm the diagnosis of HCM, to measure the left ventricular mass, and to quantify the degree of subvalvular stenosis.

Restrictive cardiomyopathy

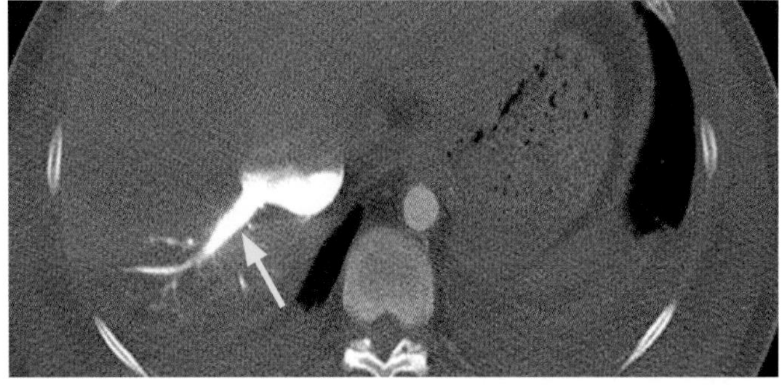

Impaired diastolic filling: Contrast-enhanced CT demonstrates dilation and reflux of contrast into the IVC and hepatic veins (arrow), indicative of impaired right ventricular filling and resultant dilation of the right atrium, IVC, and hepatic veins.

Case courtesy Michael Hanley, MD, University of Virginia Health System.

- Restrictive cardiomyopathy is characterized by small, stiff, thickened ventricles that impair diastolic filling. This results in dilated atria and ultimately a dilated IVC. The etiology of the restrictive cardiomyopathy may be idiopathic or due to sarcoidosis, hemochromatosis, or myocardial deposition diseases (e.g., amyloidosis).
- Note that restrictive cardiomyopathy and constrictive physiology are different entities, although both conditions may feature identical ventricular pressure tracings and both are characterized by impaired diastolic filling.
- Constrictive physiology (subsequently discussed under pericardial disease) is secondary to increased pericardial pressure from thickened (often calcified) pericardium or pericardial effusion, causing impaired diastolic filling.
- The main role of imaging the heart in impaired diastolic filling is to exclude constrictive pericarditis as the etiology of the diastolic dysfunction. Constrictive pericarditis can be treated surgically by removing the pericardium; however, there is no effective treatment for restrictive cardiomyopathy and patients tend to have a poor prognosis.

Dilated cardiomyopathy

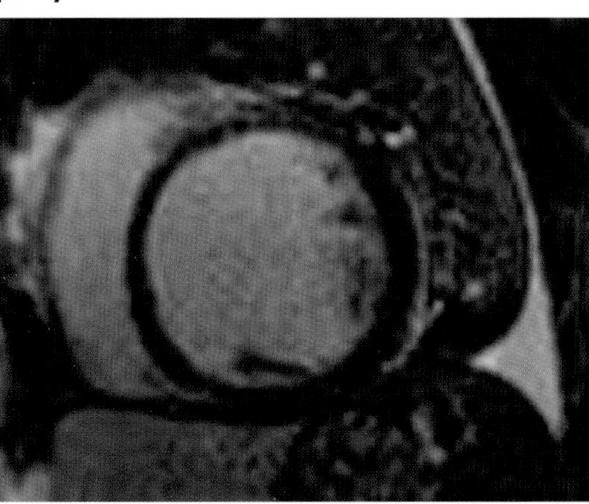

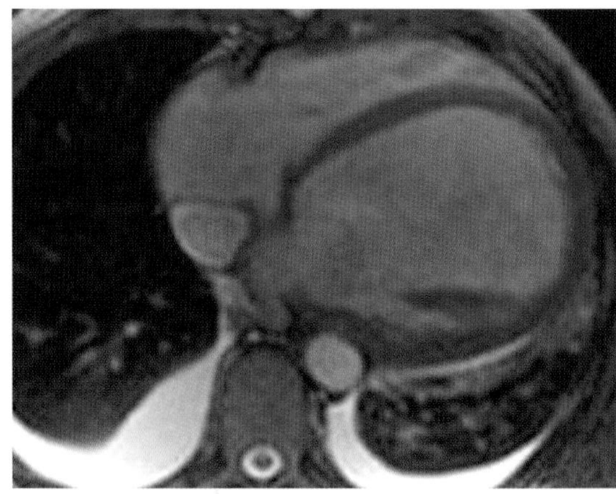

Nonischemic dilated cardiomyopathy: Delayed-enhancement short-axis cardiac MRI (left image) shows no abnormal enhancement, but there is diffuse concentric dilation of the left ventricular and right ventricular cavities, which is also appreciated on the axial image (right image). Bilateral small pleural effusions are present.

Case courtesy Michael Hanley, MD, University of Virginia Health System.

- Dilated cardiomyopathy represents concentric ventricular chamber enlargement with impaired systolic function. Typically, both ventricles are involved.
- Dilated cardiomyopathy can be ischemic or idiopathic in etiology, and evaluation by MRI or CT is useful to determine the etiology. An ischemic cause can be suggested by delayed enhancement in a vascular distribution on MRI or coronary disease seen on CCTA.
- Catheter angiography is recommended to exclude coronary artery disease in a new diagnosis of dilated cardiomyopathy.

- Up to 41% of patients with idiopathic DCM demonstrate abnormal enhancement in a nonischemic distribution in the mid-ventricular wall. The significance of this enhancement in patients with idiopathic DCM is uncertain.

Lipomatous hypertrophy of the interatrial septum

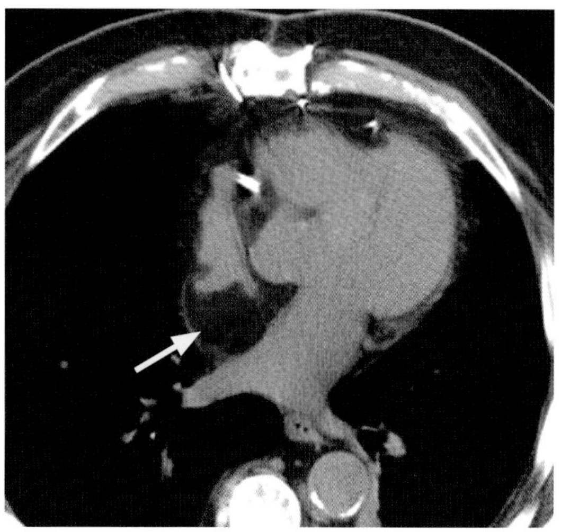

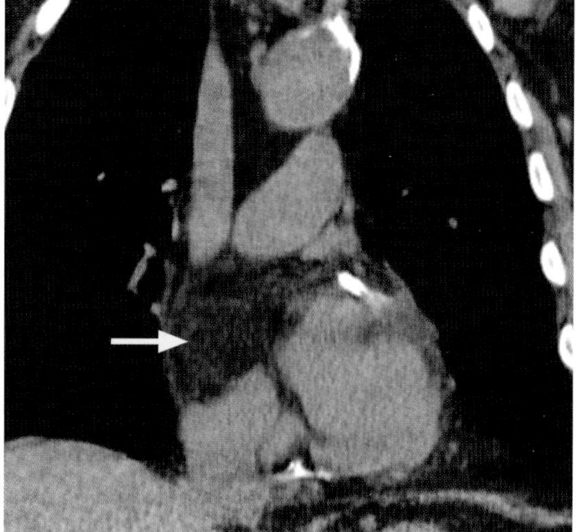

Lipomatous hypertrophy of the interatrial septum: Axial and coronal noncontrast CT demonstrates a focal area of fat attenuation at the interatrial septum, along the right heart border (arrows).

Case courtesy Michael Hanley, MD, University of Virginia Health System.

- Lipomatous hypertrophy of the interatrial septum represents proliferation of fatty deposits within the interatrial septum, typically along the lateral right heart border.
- Lipomatous hypertrophy is an incidental finding that does not require treatment. It is important not to mistake it for a cardiac mass. An exceedingly rare differential consideration of a fatty cardiac mass is liposarcoma.

Pericardial disease

Pericardial anatomy

- The pericardium consists of two layers (the visceral and parietal pericardium), which are separated by approximately 40 mL of pericardial fluid.
- The visceral pericardium is too thin to be visualized on imaging. The pericardial apparatus (combination of the visceral and parietal layers and pericardial fluid) measures <1 mm on cadaveric studies and can be seen on CT and MRI, with a normal thickness <2 mm. A pericardial thickness of ≥4 mm on imaging is considered clearly abnormal.

Pericardial effusion

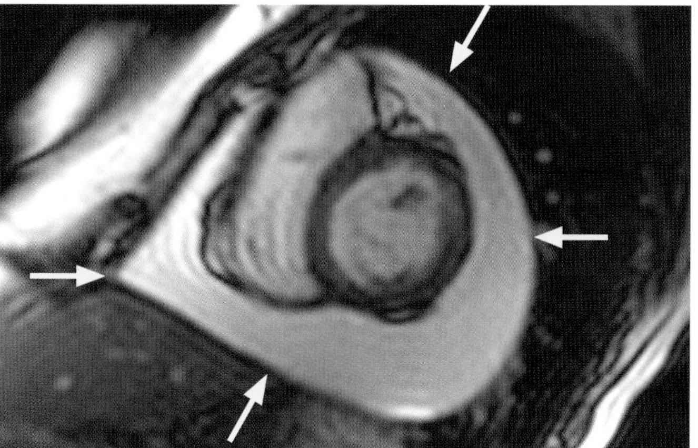

Pericardial effusion:

Short-axis image from a steady state free precession cardiac MRI demonstrates a large pericardial effusion (arrows).

Case courtesy Michael Steigner, MD, Brigham and Women's Hospital.

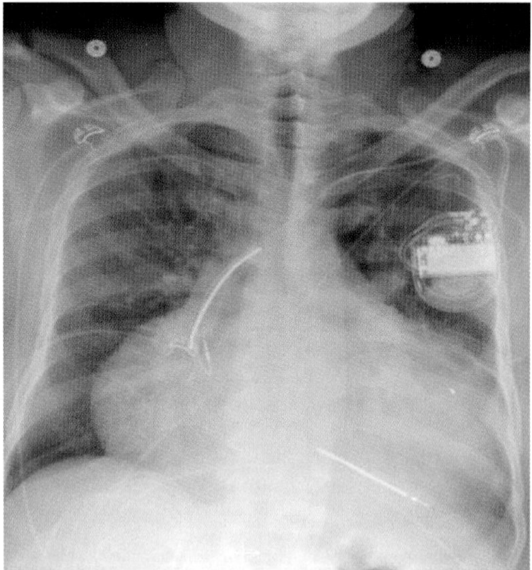

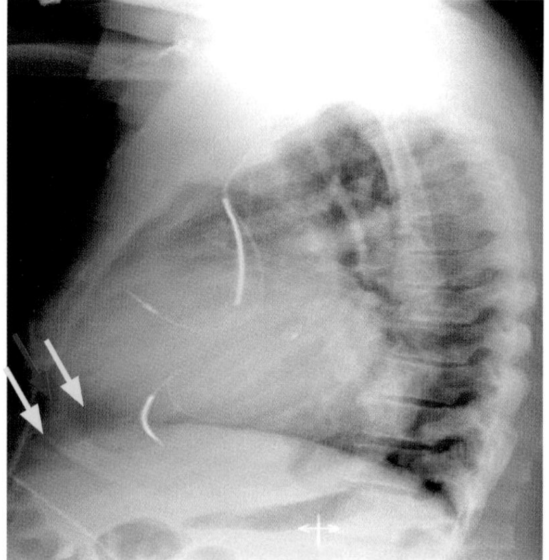

Pericardial effusion and *oreo cookie* sign (in a different patient): Frontal radiograph (left image) demonstrates a markedly enlarged heart, which is nonspecific but can be seen in pericardial effusion. Lateral radiograph demonstrates the *oreo cookie* sign with two parallel lucencies (yellow arrows) indicating the epicardial and pericardial fat stripes surrounding a white "filling" indicating the pericardial effusion (red arrow).

Case courtesy Michael Hanley, MD, University of Virginia Health System.

- The primary clinical concern of a pericardial effusion is cardiac tamponade. As little as 100–200 mL of pericardial fluid can impede diastolic filling if it accumulates quickly.
- The classic plain film finding of pericardial effusion is the *oreo cookie* sign, which represents the parallel lucent epicardial and pericardial fat stripes (the cookies) and the radiopaque pericardial effusion (the white filling).

Pericardial calcification

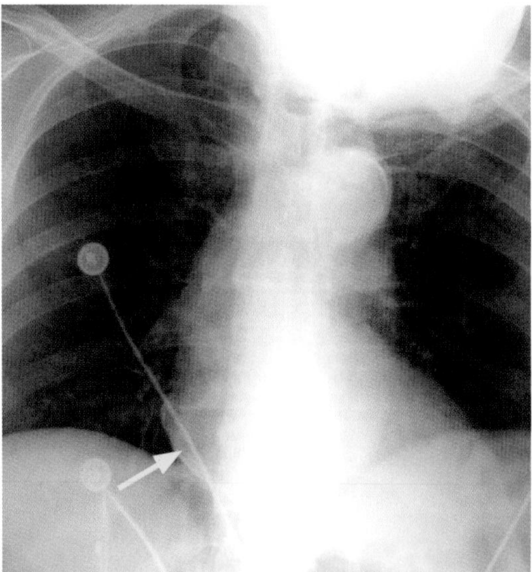

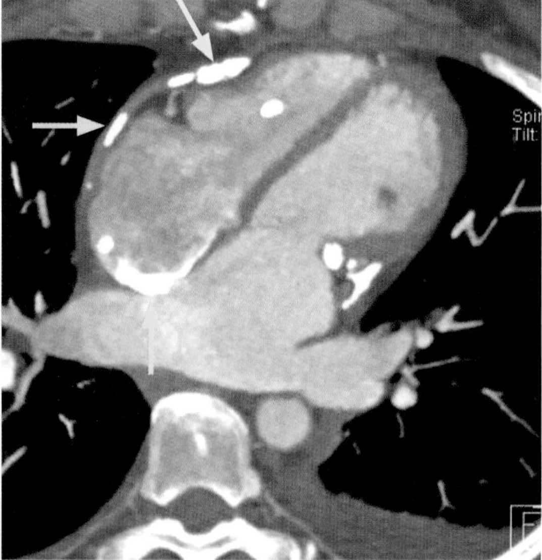

Pericardial calcification: Chest radiograph shows faint peripheral calcification of the right heart border (arrow). Axial contrast-enhanced CT shows multifocal calcification throughout the pericardium (arrows).

Case courtesy Michael Hanley, MD, University of Virginia Health System.

- Pericardial calcification can be a result of prior pericarditis, most commonly viral or uremic in etiology. Pericardial calcification can be associated with constrictive physiology.
- The main differential of pericardial calcification is myocardial calcification due to old infarct.

Congenital absence of the pericardium

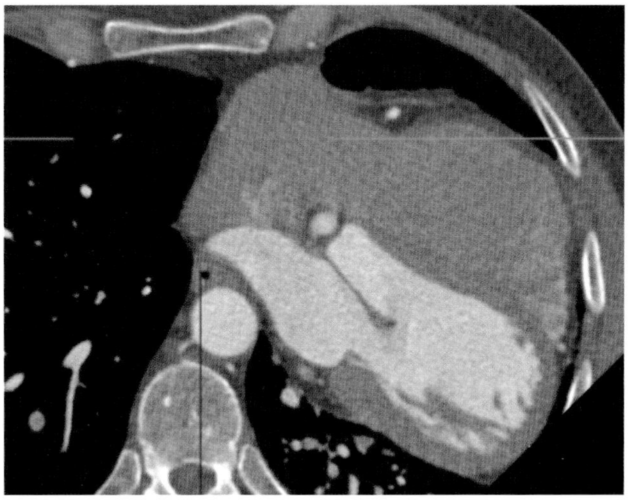

Congenital absence of the left pericardium:

Axial image from a coronary CT shows an abnormal axis of the heart, which is displaced left-posteriorly into the left hemithorax.

Although a pericardial defect is not directly visualized on this image, the characteristic abnormal cardiac axis should lead one to consider congenital absence of the left pericardium.

Case courtesy Michael Steigner, MD, Brigham and Women's Hospital.

- Congenital absence of the pericardial is a spectrum of disorders ranging from a focal pericardial defect to complete absence of the right and left pericardium. Total absence of the pericardium is very rare.
- The most common form of pericardial absence involves the left pericardium in the region of the left atrial appendage and adjacent pulmonary artery.
- Patients with partial absence of the pericardium are at risk for herniation of a portion of the heart through the pericardial defect.
- On imaging, a clue to the presence of a pericardial defect is a lucent notch between the aorta and pulmonary artery (sometimes seen on radiography, but generally better appreciated on CT), which represents interposed lung between these vascular structures.
- Defects of the left pericardium cause leftward displacement of the heart, which may in some cases be the only imaging finding.

References, resources, and further reading

General References:

Miller, S.W., Abbara, S. & Boxt, L.B. Cardiac Imaging: The Requisites (3rd ed.) Mosby. (2009).

Webb, W.R. & Higgins, C.B. Thoracic Imaging – Pulmonary and Cardiovascular Radiology. Lippincott Williams & Wilkins. (2005).

Aorta:

Agarwal, P.P., Chughtai, A., Matzinger, F.R.K. & Kazerooni, E.A. Multidetector CT of thoracic aortic aneurysms. Radiographics, 29(2), 537-52(2009).

Bashir, M.R., Ferral, H., Jacobs, C., McCarthy, W. & Goldin, M. Endoleaks after endovascular abdominal aortic aneurysm repair: management strategies according to CT findings. AJR. American Journal of Roentgenology, 192(4), W178-86(2009).

Chao, C.P., Walker, T.G. & Kalva, S.P. Natural history and CT appearances of aortic intramural hematoma. Radiographics, 29(3), 791-804(2009).

Gotway, M.B. et al. Imaging findings in Takayasu's arteritis. American Journal of Roentgenology, 184(6), 1945(2005).

Hayashi, H. et al. Penetrating Atherosclerotic Ulcer of the Aorta: Imaging Features and Disease Concept. Radiographics, 20(4), 995-1005(2000).

Jeudy, J., Waite, S. & White, C.S. Nontraumatic thoracic emergencies. Radiologic Clinics of North America, 44(2), 273-93, ix(2006).

Layton, K. & Kallmes, D. Bovine Aortic Arch Variant in Humans: Clarification of a Common Misnomer. American Journal of Neuroradiology, 1541-2(2006).

Ledbetter, S., Stuk, J.L. & Kaufman, J.A. Helical (spiral) CT in the evaluation of emergent thoracic aortic syndromes. Radiologic Clinics of North America, 37(3), 515-89(1999).

Rakita, D. et al. Spectrum of CT findings in rupture and impending rupture of abdominal aortic aneurysms. Radiographics, 27(2), 497-507(2007).

Cardiac CT:

Heffernan, E.J., Dodd, J.D. & Malone, D.E. Cardiac multidetector CT: technical and diagnostic evaluation with evidence-based practice techniques. Radiology, 248(2), 366-77(2008).

Hoffmann, U. et al. Coronary CT angiography versus standard evaluation in acute chest pain. The New England Journal of Medicine, 367(4), 299-308(2012).

Kim, S.Y. et al. Coronary Artery Anomalies: Classification and ECG-gated Multi-Detector Row CT Findings with Angiographic Correlation. Radiographics, 26, 317-34(2006).

Litt, H.I. et al. CT angiography for safe discharge of patients with possible acute coronary syndromes. The New England Journal of Medicine, 366(15), 1393-403(2012).

O'Brien, J.P. et al. Anatomy of the heart at multidetector CT: what the radiologist needs to know. Radiographics, 27(6), 1569-82(2007).

Raff, G.L. et al. SCCT guidelines for the interpretation and reporting of coronary computed tomographic angiography. Journal of Cardiovascular Computed Tomography, 3(2), 122-36(2009).

Sparrow, P. et al. CT and MRI Imaging Findings in Patients with Acquired Heart Disease at Risk for Sudden Cardiac Death. Radiographics, 29, 805-23(2009).

Miscellaneous:

Chen, J.J., Manning, M.A., Frazier, A.A., Jeudy, J. & White, C.S. CT Angiography of the Cardiac Valves: Normal, Diseased, and Postoperative Appearances. Radiographics, 29, 1393-412(2009).

Marcus, F.I. et al. Diagnosis of arrhythmogenic right ventricular cardiomyopathy/dysplasia: proposed modification of the task force criteria. Circulation, 121(13), 1533-41(2010).

Cardiac MRI:

Boxt, L.M. Cardiac MRI Imaging: A Guide for the Beginner. Radiographics, 19(4), 1009-25(1999).

Mahrholdt, H., Wagner, A., Judd, R.M., Sechtem, U. & Kim, R.J. Delayed enhancement cardiovascular magnetic resonance assessment of non-ischaemic cardiomyopathies. European Heart Journal, 26(15), 1461-74(2005).

Vogel-Claussen, J. et al. Delayed Enhancement MRI Imaging: Utility in Myocardial Assessment 1. Radiographics, 26(3), 795 (2006).

Pericardium:

Broderick, L.S., Brooks, G.N. & Kuhlman, J. Anatomic Pitfalls of the Heart and Pericardium. Radiographics, 25, 441-53(2005).

10 Interventional radiology

Contents

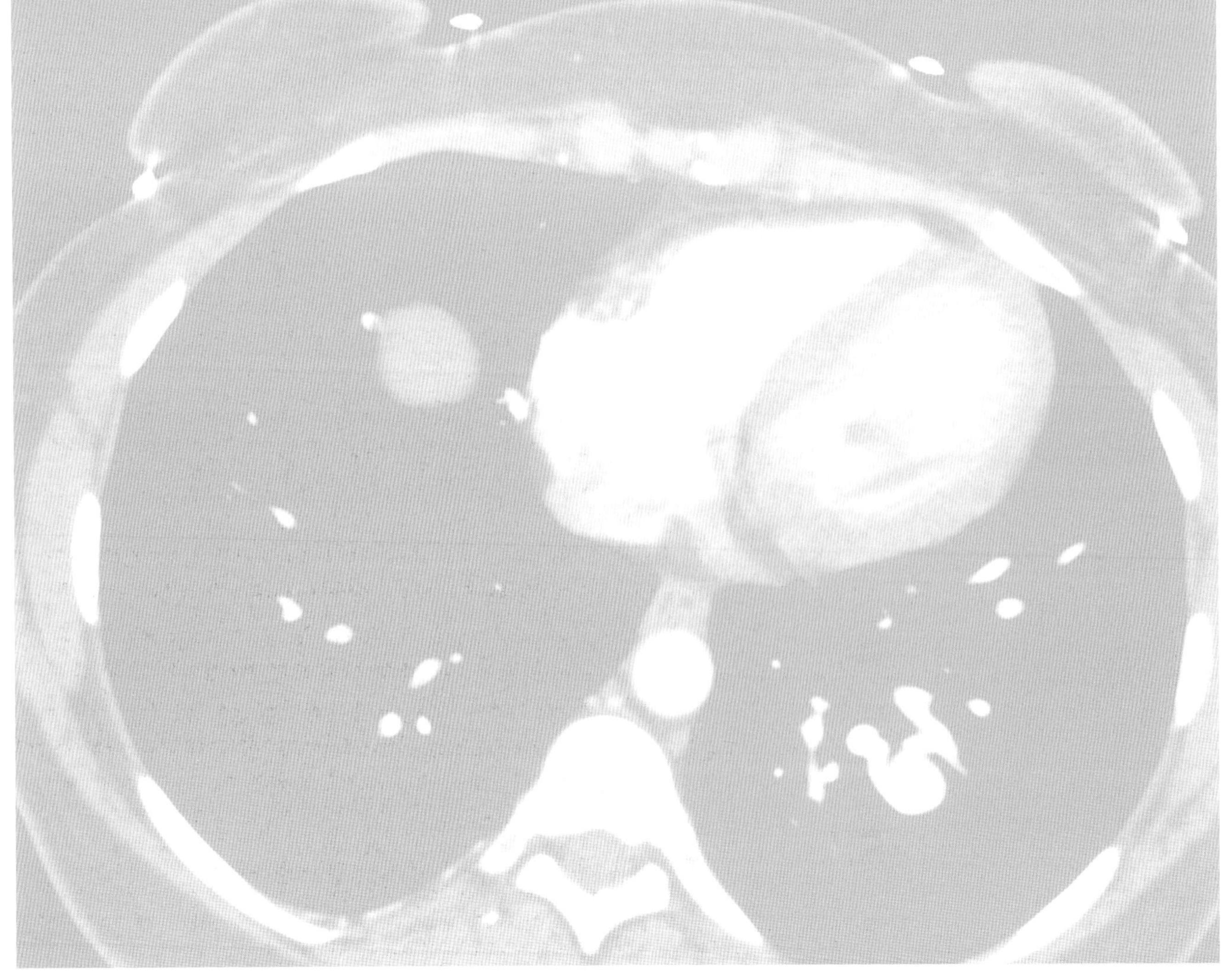

APPROACH TO INTERPRETING AN ANGIOGRAM

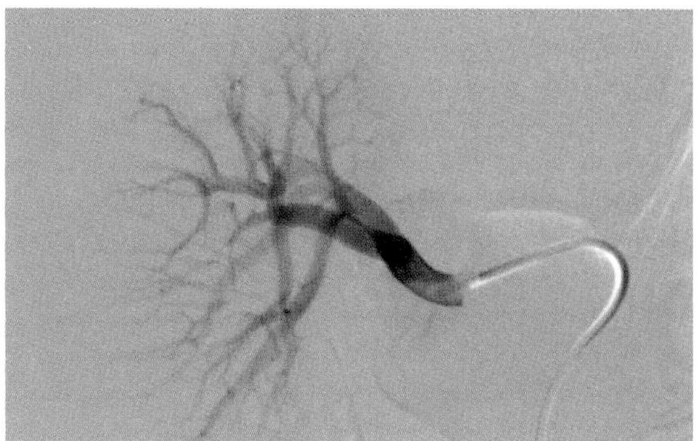

Early arterial phase

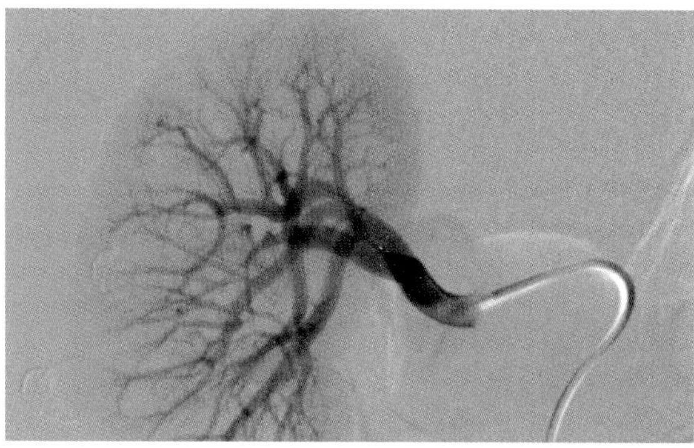

Late arterial phase

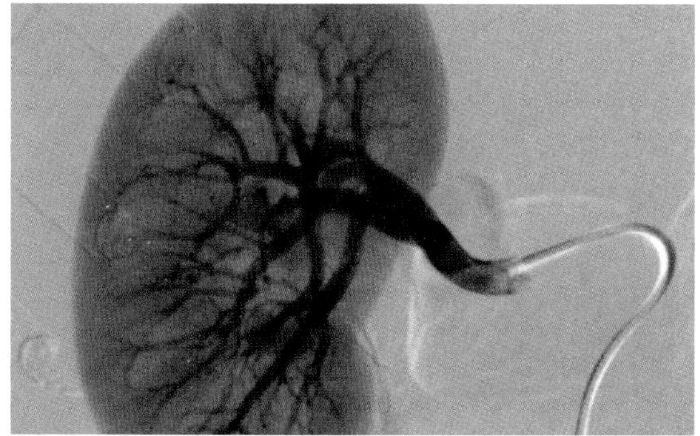

Parenchymal phase

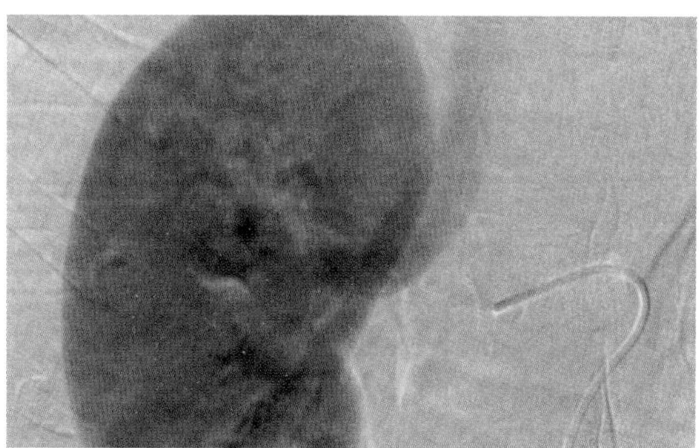

Venous phase (renal vein drains into IVC)

Normal selective digital subtraction angiogram of the right renal artery demonstrates four phases of vascular opacification.

- The mnemonic "what, where, when, VIA (vessels, interventions, anything else)" can be helpful to remember the comprehensive approach to evaluating a vascular case.

What?

- What type of study is it — angiogram, digital subtraction angiogram (DSA), venogram?

Where?

- Where in the body is the catheter and in which vessel?
- Is a flush catheter in a large vessel or is it a selective/superselective angiogram?

When?

- Early arterial phase, late arterial phase, parenchymal phase, or venous phase?
- Is there opacification of any veins during an arterial phase? If so, that suggests a shunt.

Vessels?

- Is there any contrast going where it shouldn't, such as active extravasation or neovascularity?
- Do the vessels have a normal contour? Is there any dissection, irregularity, stenosis, or encasement (external compression)?

Interventions?

- Any previously placed stents, grafts, filters, coils, surgical clips, or drains?

Anything else?

- Any other finding on the film? Bony fracture to suggest trauma?

Femoral arterial access technique

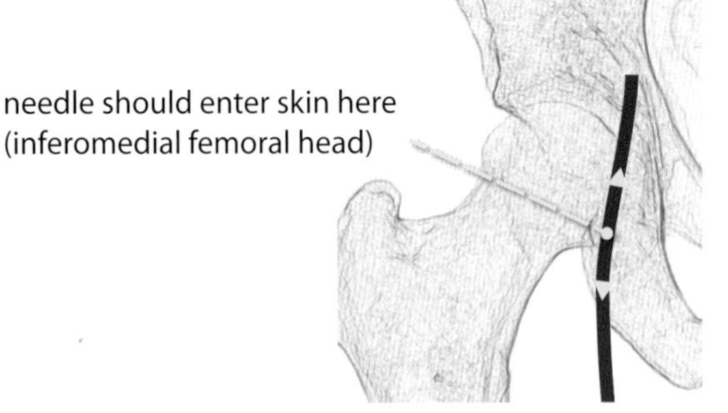

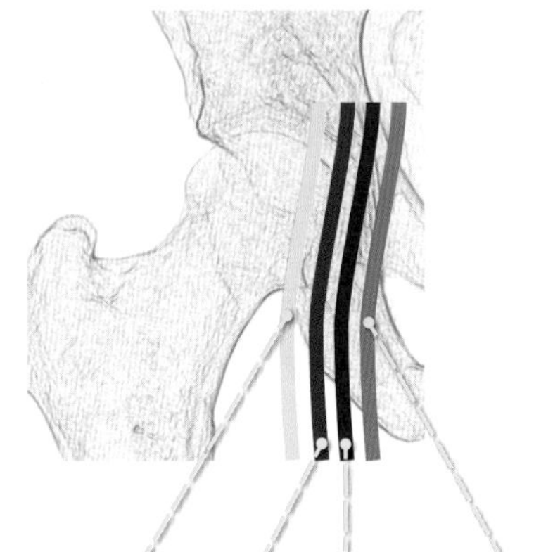

- The common femoral artery begins inferior to the inguinal ligament. From lateral to medial, the mnemonic **NAVL** helps to localize the femoral nerve, artery, vein, and lymphatics.
- The ideal position to access the femoral artery is the inferomedial margin of the femoral head, for two reasons. First, the femoral head provides a hard surface to press against to provide adequate hemostasis. Second, at the level of the femoral head, the femoral artery and nerve are side by side. If arterial puncture is performed too low, the femoral vein may be traversed with possible formation of arteriovenous fistula.

Hematoma

- A hematoma may be superficial or retroperitoneal. A superficial subcutaneous hematoma has a generally benign clinical course, while a retroperitoneal hematoma carries a risk of fatal hemorrhage.
- There is increased risk of retroperitoneal hematoma with a high (more cranial) arterial puncture above the pelvic brim.

Pseudoaneurysm

- Pseudoaneurysm formation occurs in approximately 1% of arterial punctures. On color Doppler, a pseudoaneurysm appears as a swirling *yin-yang* with high-velocity flow at the site of communication with the femoral artery.
- Watchful waiting can be performed for a small pseudoaneurysm <1 cm in size. Ultrasound-guided thrombin injection is the treatment of choice for a pseudoaneurysm >1 cm. Less commonly, ultrasound-guided compression of the neck of the pseudoaneurysm can be performed to thrombose the pseudoaneurysm.

Arteriovenous fistula (AVF)

- An arteriovenous fistula (AVF) is an anomalous connection between an artery and a vein. AVFs are usually asymptomatic but may enlarge and ultimately cause high-output cardiac failure.
- There is increased risk of developing an iatrogenic AVF with a low (inferior/distal) femoral arterial puncture. The femoral vein often passes deep to (instead of medial to) the femoral artery distal to the standard puncture site.
- On Doppler ultrasound, an AVF demonstrates arterial flow within a vein and there is loss of the normal triphasic waveform in the artery. Increased diastolic flow is often seen in the artery proximal to the fistula.

Air embolism

- Air embolism is a rare but potentially life-threatening complication of vascular procedures.
- The most dangerous portion of a venous access procedure is the insertion of the catheter into the peel-away sheath.
- If air embolism is suspected (e.g., if the patient becomes acutely hypoxic as the catheter is inserted into the peel-away sheath), the patient should be immediately placed in the left-lateral decubitus (left side down) position so the air bubble remains antidependent in the right heart. 100% oxygen should be administered. If practical, fluoroscopy can be used to identify the air bubble. Catheter aspiration can be considered if the air bubble is large.

Injection rates

- The terminology for injection rates for angiographic runs is "*cc/sec* for *total cc.*" For instance, "25 for 50" means an injection rate of 25 cc/sec for a total of 50 cc.
- The diameter in mm of a vessel is a rough guide to the injection rate (in cc/sec), and the total volume of contrast injected depends on the intravascular volume of the vascular bed.

Aortogram (aortic arch): 20 for 30.	Mesenteric artery: 5 for 25.
Abdominal aorta: 20 for 20.	Renal artery: 5 for 15.
Inferior vena cavogram: 20 for 30.	Distal artery: 3 for 12.

Percutaneous transluminal angioplasty (PTA)

- Percutaneous transluminal angioplasty (PTA) is the first-line technique for treatment of a stenosis, where a balloon is inflated across the stenosis to create a controlled stretch injury and increase the luminal cross-sectional area.
- When treating a stenosis caused by atherosclerotic plaque, angioplasty widens the luminal diameter due to disruption of the intima and extension of the plaque into the media.
- Most balloons are *non-compliant.* That is, they have a fixed diameter that does not expand no matter the air pressure. If a non-compliant balloon is inflated above its rated maximum pressure, the balloon will burst.
- In general, a balloon should be selected that is 10–20% larger than the vessel diameter.
- Balloons are sized by diameter in millimeters and length in centimeters. For instance, a 10 × 6 balloon is 10 mm in diameter and 6 cm in length.
- Risks of angioplasty include distal emboli, vessel rupture, and dissection. Anticoagulation (typically heparin) should always be used with angioplasty.

Stents

- The two broad categories of stents are balloon-expandable and self-expandable stents.
- In general, balloon-expandable stents have a higher radial force upon deployment but will not rebound if crushed. Thus, balloon-expandable stents are suboptimal for sites prone to external compression, such as around joints or the adductor canal in the leg.
- Self-expandable stents are more flexible and trackable through vessels than balloon-expandable stents. Their use is favored when the route to the lesion is tortuous or when the anatomy is prone to external compression.
- In general, a stent should be selected that is 1–2 cm longer than the stenosis, with a diameter that is 1–2 mm wider than the unstenosed vessel lumen. A rule of thumb is 10% oversizing of an arterial stent and 20% oversizing of a venous stent.
- Most stents are fenestrated and provide only a scaffolding-like support; however, covered stents are employed for treatment of pseudoaneurysm, dissection, and TIPS.

PRINCIPLES OF EMBOLIZATION

Embolic materials

- The two main categories of embolic materials are permanent (coils, particles, glue, and sclerosing agent) and temporary (absorbable gelatin sponge and autologous clot).
- Coils create thrombosis by inducing vascular stasis. The main advantage of coils is the ability for precise and quick placement, without distal embolization. The primary disadvantage is sacrifice of distal access: Once a vessel is coiled, it cannot be re-accessed for retreatment.

  When using coils for embolization of a specific lesion, the general technique is to first coil *distal* to the lesion, then proximal to it. This prevents recurrent bleeding from retrograde collaterals.
- Particles flow distally to occlude the small capillaries. Two types of particles are tris-acyl gelatin microspheres (*Embospheres*, BioSphere Medical) and polyvinyl alcohol.
- Absorbable gelatin sponge (*Gelfoam*, Pfizer) is the most commonly used *temporary* embolic agent, lasting 2–6 weeks. Of important note, because Gelfoam is dissolved foam, post-procedural CT imaging can show numerous gas locules in the embolized organ. This appearance can mimic abscess and careful clinical observation is necessary to prevent unnecessary interventions.
- Sodium tetradecyl sulfate is a sclerosing agent used for vascular malformations and varices.
- Cyanoacrylate is a special glue that rapidly hardens when it comes in contract with blood.

Complications of embolization

- **Post-embolization syndrome** usually occurs within the first day after embolization and clinically presents with pain, cramping, fever, and nausea/vomiting, thought to be due to release of endovascular inflammatory modulators by infarcted tissue. Treatment is NSAIDS, opioids when appropriate, and IV fluids.
- **Non-target embolization** is unintentional embolization of structures other than the target. For instance, during uterine fibroid embolization there is a risk of non-target embolization of the ovaries. During bronchial artery embolization, there is a risk of non-target embolization to the brain causing stroke and to the spinal arteries causing paralysis.

CATHETERS

Catheter sizing

- Catheters are sized in French (Fr), where 1 Fr = 0.33 mm. For instance, a 6 Fr catheter has an external diameter of 2 mm. The luminal diameter will be slightly smaller
- *Sheath versus catheter:* A *sheath* has a defined *luminal* diameter; however, the overall diameter of the catheter will be slightly larger. For instance, a 6 Fr sheath can by definition fit a 6 Fr catheter inside, but will be 7 or 8 Fr in external diameter.

High-flow catheters

- High-flow (also known as flush) catheters have multiple sideholes and may be coiled (most commonly; known as a pigtail/omniflush catheter), curved, or straight.
- High-flow catheters are used for large vessel angiography, such as the aorta and vena cava.

Selective and superselective catheters

- Selective and superselective catheters have a single hole at the end of the catheter. There are numerous shapes of the distal portion, each tailored towards a specific situation or general purpose use.
- *C2* and *SOS* are reverse curved-tip catheters; and *Berenstein* is an angled-tip catheter.

Wires

Wire sizing

- Wires are sized in inches, with a standard wire measuring 0.035" in diameter and a microwire measuring 0.018" in diameter.

Standard floppy tip wires

- Standard wires have a floppy tip or J-tip, which allows the wire to be safely inserted blindly (although once in the vessel the course should be followed on fluoroscopy).
- A *Bentson* wire is a typical floppy tip wire; *Rosen* is a J-tip wire.

Hydrophilic wires

- Hydrophilic wires are used to cross a stenosis or for initial cannulation of an indwelling device, as would be performed for a routine check and change.
- *Roadrunner* (Cook) and *Glidewire* (Terumo) wires are hydrophilic.

Stiff wires

- Stiff wires are used when structural rigidity is required. For instance, a devices that dilates the subcutaneous tissues (such as a sheath, biliary drain, nephrostomy tube, etc.) needs to be inserted over a stiff wire.
- An *Amplatz* (Boston Scientific) wire is a commonly used superstiff wire.

Thoracic angiography

Giant cell arteritis (GCA)

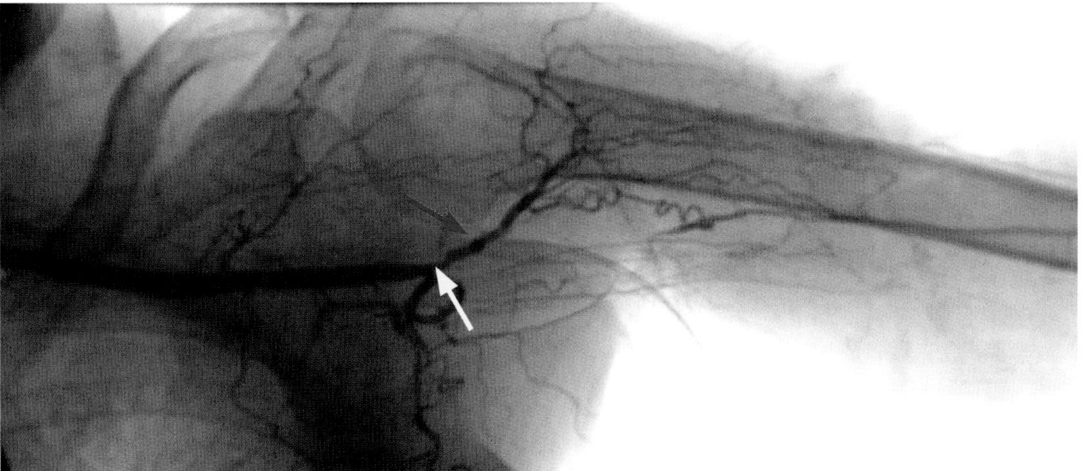

Giant cell arteritis: Selective angiogram of the axillary artery (catheter is not visible) shows mild narrowing of the axillary artery, complete occlusion of the axillary/brachial artery at the origin of the brachial artery (yellow arrow), and an irregular appearance of the posterior circumflex humeral artery (red arrow).

Case courtesy Timothy P. Killoran, MD, Brigham and Women's Hospital.

- Giant cell arteritis (GCA) is a medium and large-vessel vasculitis that has overlapping imaging findings with Takayasu arteritis. GCA tends to affect older patients (typically greater than 50 years of age) compared to Takayasu arteritis.
- The medium-sized upper extremity arteries are most commonly affected in GCA, including the subclavian, axillary, and brachial arteries. The aorta is rarely involved, unlike in Takayasu arteritis. GCA typically produces long smooth stenoses and occlusions.
- Definitive diagnosis is with temporal artery biopsy. Treatment is steroids.

Aorta

- Aortic disease is discussed in the cardiovascular imaging section.

Superior vena cava (SVC)

Congenital anomalies of the superior vena cava (SVC)

- Normally, the embryologic left anterior cardinal vein regresses and the right anterior cardinal vein develops into the SVC.
- **Left-sided SVC** is due to persistence of the embryological left anterior cardinal vein and regression of the right anterior cardinal vein.

  The left SVC usually drains directly into the coronary sinus → right atrium.

  Rarely, the left SVC drains directly into the left atrium causing a right to left shunt.

  Left-sided SVC is weakly associated with congenital heart disease (CHD). Left SVC is an incidental finding in 0.5% of the population but is seen in 4% of patients with CHD.

- A **duplicated SVC** is due to persistence of both the right and left anterior cardinal veins.

  Duplicated SVC also carries an association with congenital heart disease.

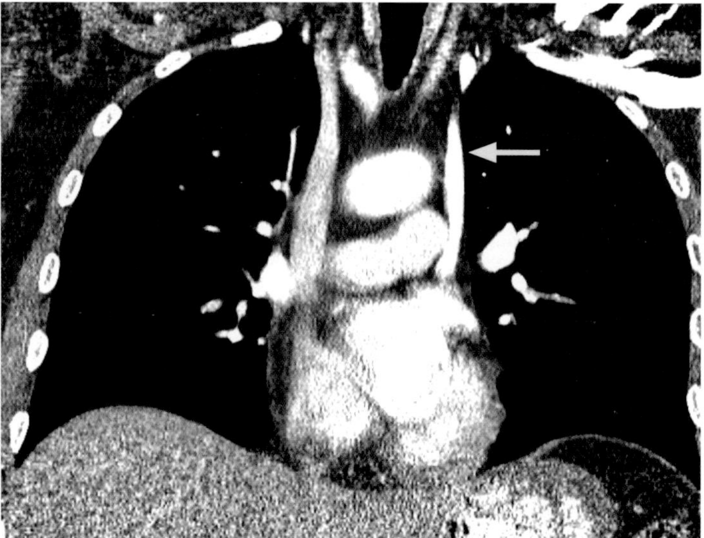

Duplicated SVC:

Coronal CT shows right and left SVCs. The left SVC (arrow) is more opacified with contrast because of the left-sided contrast injection.

SVC obstruction

- Acute obstruction of the SVC causes SVC syndrome, which clinically presents as facial and upper extremity edema and cyanosis. Acute SVC syndrome is a vascular emergency.
- In contrast to acute SVC syndrome, chronic occlusion or stenosis of the SVC may be asymptomatic. If symptoms are present, facial edema that improves with standing is characteristic.
- The most common causes of SVC obstruction are compression by thoracic malignancy, catheter-associated thrombosis, and mediastinal fibrosis after histoplasmosis exposure.
- A classic cross-sectional abdominal imaging finding in SVC obstruction is increased enhancement of hepatic segment IVa due to collateral opacification of the vein of Sappey.

  The vein of Sappey drains the liver in the region of the falciform ligament and communicate with internal thoracic veins, which act as collateral vessels in the setting of SVC occlusion.

- Combined internal jugular and femoral approaches may be necessary for treatment of SVC occlusion. Stenting is often necessary.

Pulmonary artery angiography technique

- Before performing a pulmonary angiogram, it is essential to evaluate an EKG to ensure that a left bundle branch block (LBBB) is not present. If the pulmonary artery catheter were to cause temporary right bundle branch block in the presence of a LBBB, the lack of left-sided conduction may cause complete heart block, which can be fatal. A temporary pacer should be placed prior to pulmonary arteriography in the presence of a LBBB.
- Normal right-sided pressures:

  Right atrium: 0–8 mm Hg.

  Right ventricle: 0–8 mm Hg diastolic; 15–30 mm Hg systolic.

  Pulmonary artery: 3–12 mm Hg diastolic; 15–30 mm Hg systolic.

Pulmonary arteriovenous malformation (AVM)

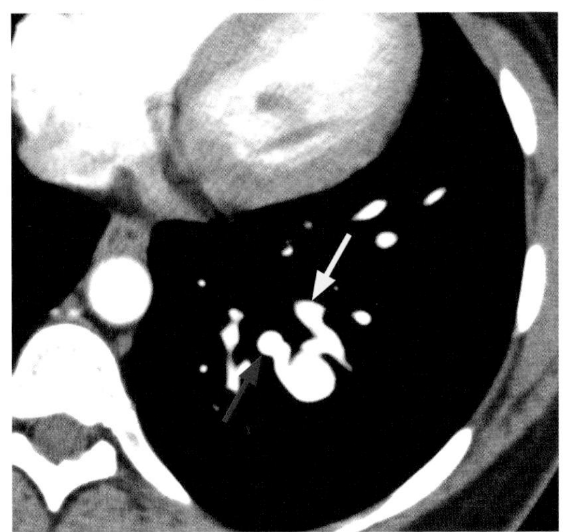

Contrast-enhanced CT demonstrates a pulmonary AVM with the feeding artery (yellow arrow) and draining vein (red arrow). Although not shown on this image, the feeding artery arises from the pulmonary artery and the draining vein drains to the left atrium.

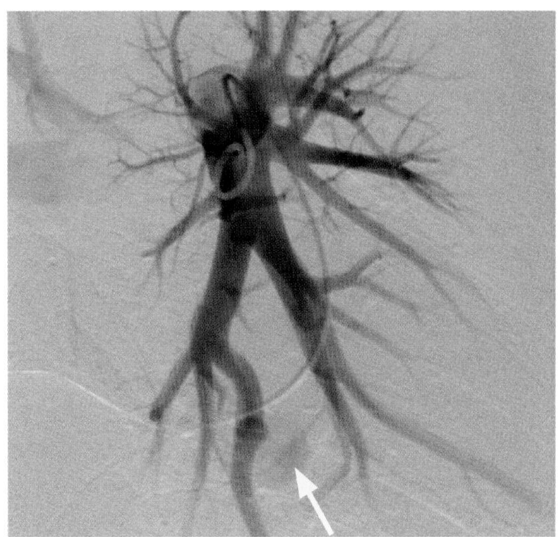

Nonselective DSA early arterial phase angiography of the left pulmonary artery in LAO orientation with a pigtail catheter in the left PA shows a faint contrast blush representing the AVM nidus (arrow). Venous drainage is not yet visible. This was treated with coils.

Case courtesy Alisa Suzuki Han, MD, Brigham and Women's Hospital.

- A pulmonary arteriovenous malformation (AVM) is an abnormal connection between the pulmonary artery and pulmonary veins, causing a right to left shunt.
- Patients with hereditary hemorrhagic telangiectasia (HHT), also known as Osler–Weber–Rendu syndrome, may have multiple pulmonary AVMs. HHT can clinically present with brain abscess, stroke, or recurrent epistaxis (due to nasal mucosa telangiectasia).
- Coils must be used to embolize a pulmonary AVM. Particles are contraindicated as the right to left shunt would cause brain emboli and infarction.
- Most pulmonary AVMs have a single feeding artery and coiling of this inflow artery (via a pulmonary arterial approach) is usually sufficient treatment.

  Note that the treatment of peripheral (e.g., in a limb) AVM generally requires elimination of the entire nidus, which is often fed from multiple arterial branches.
- An asymptomatic lesion with a feeding artery size >3 mm or a symptomatic lesion (i.e., prior infarct or brain abscess) is an indication for treatment.

Bronchial artery embolization for hemoptysis

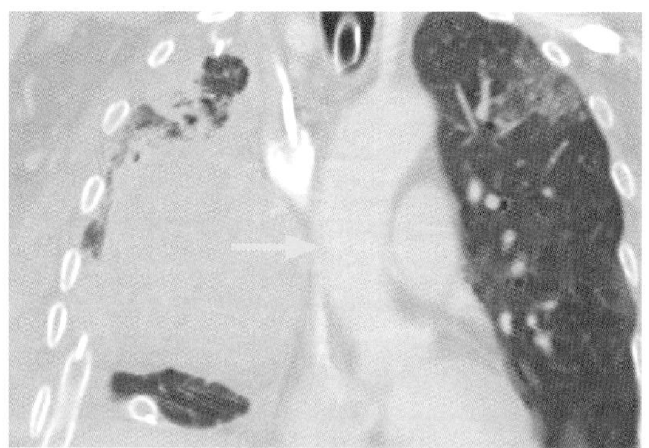

Coronal CT in a patient with hemoptysis shows a dominant right-sided thoracic mass abutting the mediastinum, causing narrowing of the SVC (arrow).

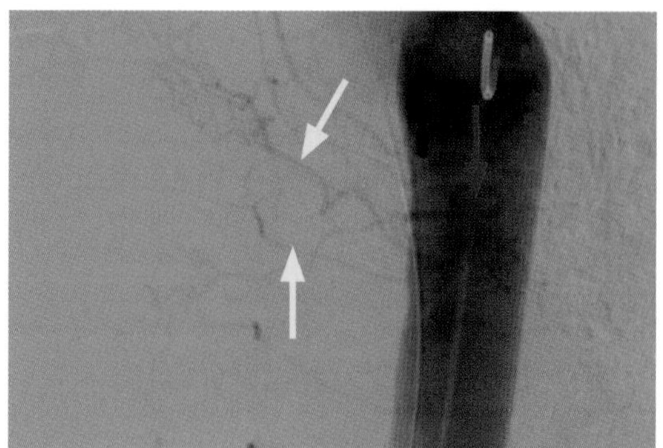

Initial nonselective DSA aortography faintly opacifies the common bronchial trunk (red arrow) and the two right bronchial arteries (yellow arrows).

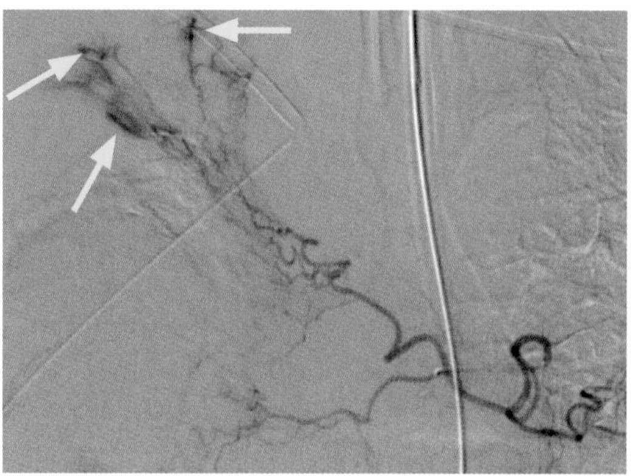

Selective angiography of the common bronchial trunk shows multiple foci of active extravasation in the right upper lobe (arrows).

Massive hemoptysis caused by thoracic malignancy treated with particle embolization of the common bronchial artery trunk (post embolization images not shown): In this case, the right bronchial arteries were not able to be accessed. Due to the emergent nature of the hemoptysis, the common bronchial trunk was embolized to complete stasis with particles. There was complete resolution of the active extravasation. The mass was later shown to be a thymoma.

Case courtesy Alisa Suzuki Han, MD, Brigham and Women's Hospital.

- Massive hemoptysis (hemoptsysis of >300 mL/24 h) has a very high mortality, most commonly due to asphyxiation. The vast majority (90%) of cases of hemoptysis involve the bronchial arteries, with the pulmonary arteries involved in most of the rest of the cases. Occasionally, other systemic arteries may be involved, so if a patient continues to bleed after evaluation of the bronchial and pulmonary arterial circulation, the subclavian, internal mammary, inferior phrenic, and celiac arteries should be evaluated as well.
- Chronic inflammation can lead to hypertrophied bronchial arteries and subsequent hemoptysis. In the USA, cystic fibrosis and thoracic malignancy are the most common causes of hemoptysis. Worldwide, tuberculosis and fungal infection are more common.
- The bronchial arteries arise from the thoracic aorta at T5–T6, although the arterial anatomy is quite variable. There are usually one or two bronchial arteries on each side.
- Embolization is performed with a distal embolic agent, most commonly particles. Initial angiography should carefully evaluate for the rare presence of a left to right shunt prior to particle embolization to prevent inadvertent cerebral embolization. Embolization is usually performed to near-stasis.

  Because rebleeding after treatment is common, coils are rarely used to treat hemoptysis. Because coils prevent repeat access, the use of coils would preclude retreatment.

- A potentially devastating complication is nontarget embolization of the spinal cord via the anterior spinal artery or smaller tributaries arising from bronchial and intercostal arteries. A complete neurological exam should be documented prior to the procedure.

NORMAL ANATOMY

Osseous landmarks

- Celiac artery: Arises from the aorta at the level of the T12 vertebral body.
- Superior mesenteric artery (SMA): Arises at the level of the T12–L1 disk space.
- Renal arteries: Arise at the level of the L1–L2 disk space.
- Inferior mesenteric artery (IMA): Arises to the left of midline at the L2–L3 disk space.

Celiac axis anatomy

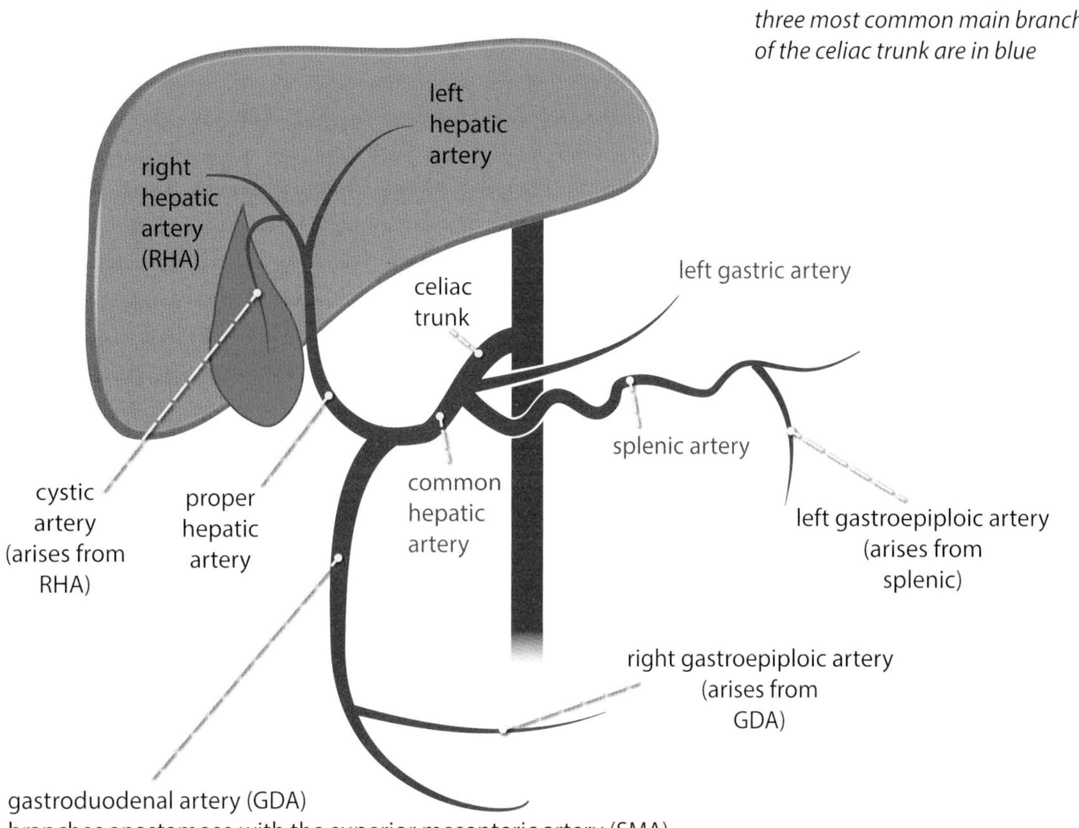

- The anatomy of the celiac axis and abdominal viscera is highly variable.
- Approximately 75% of the time the celiac artery demonstrates normal arterial anatomy with three main branches: The left gastric, the common hepatic, and the splenic artery.
- The left gastric artery may be the source of bleeding in esophageal Mallory–Weiss tear.
- The left gastroepiploic artery arises from the splenic artery and anastomoses with the right gastroepiploic artery along the greater curvature of the stomach. The right gastroepiploic artery arises from the gastroduodenal artery.

normal early-arterial subtraction celiac artery digital selective angiogram

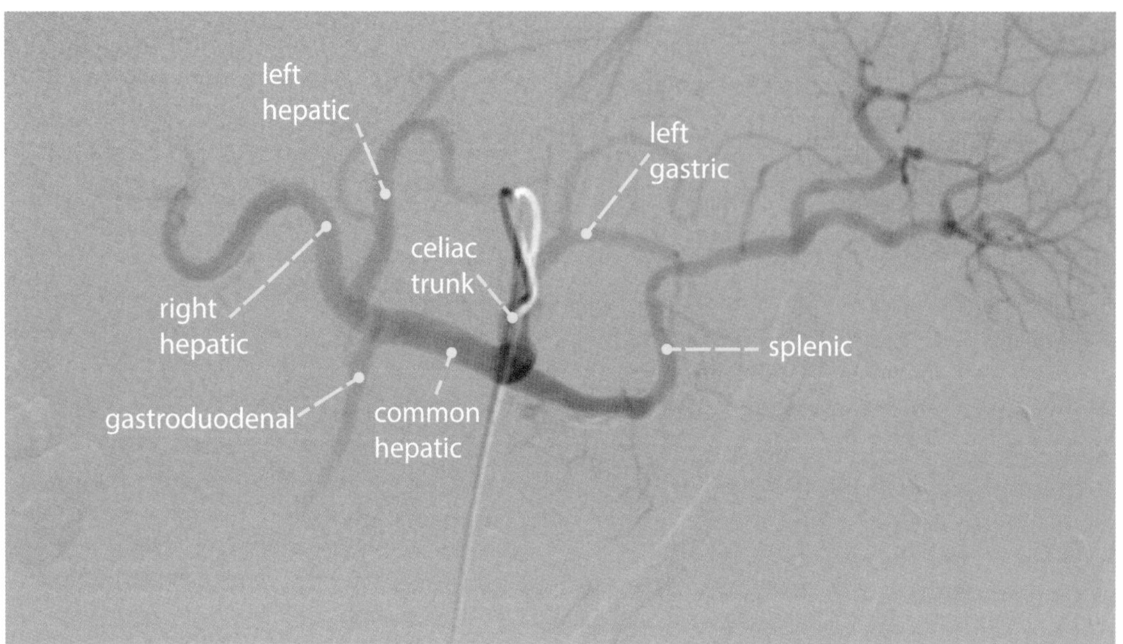

normal late-arterial subtraction celiac artery digital selective angiogram

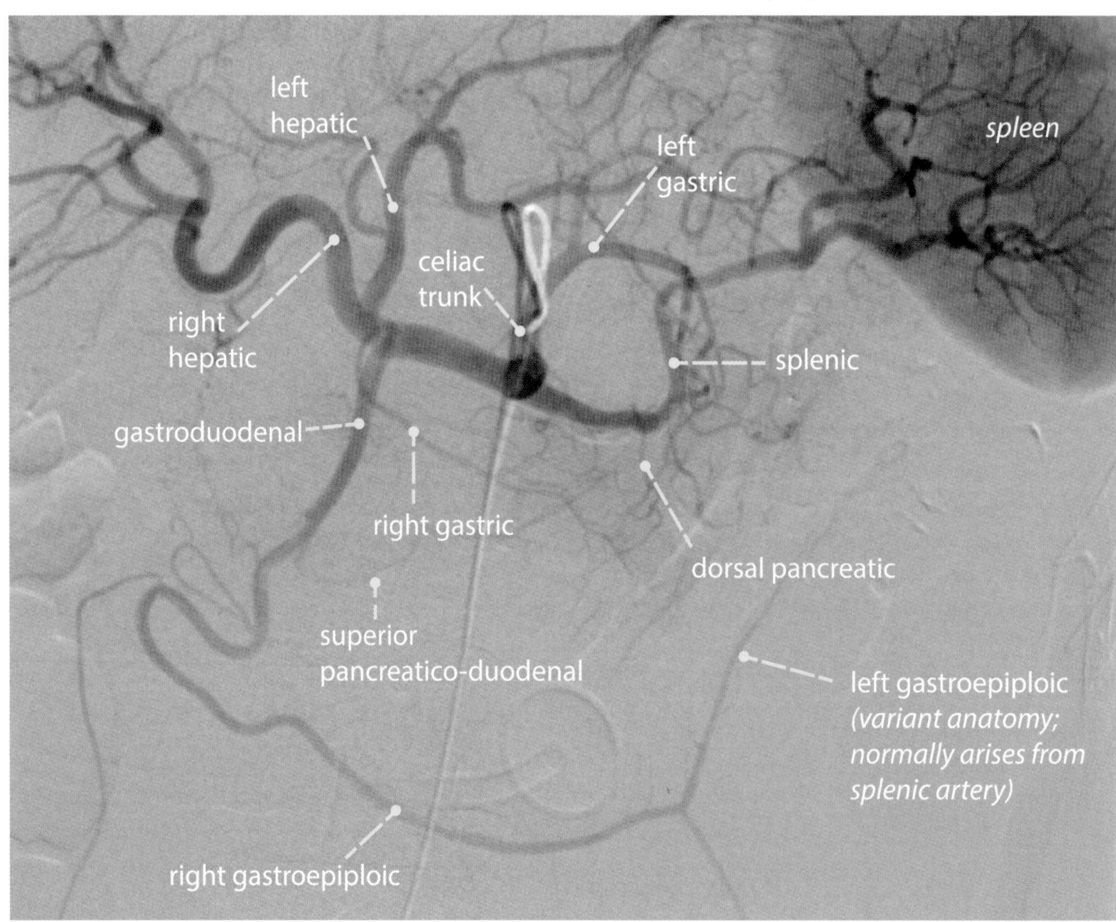

- Most commonly (75%), the proper hepatic artery supplies blood to the liver. The proper hepatic artery is the continuation of the common hepatic artery after the takeoff of the gastroduodenal artery. The proper hepatic artery divides into the right and left hepatic arteries. The cystic artery arises from the right hepatic artery to supply the gallbladder.
- A **replaced right hepatic artery** (RRHA) is present in 10–18% of patients, where the right hepatic artery arises from the SMA. An RRHA may become clinically significant in the setting of SMA disease or during abdominal surgery.

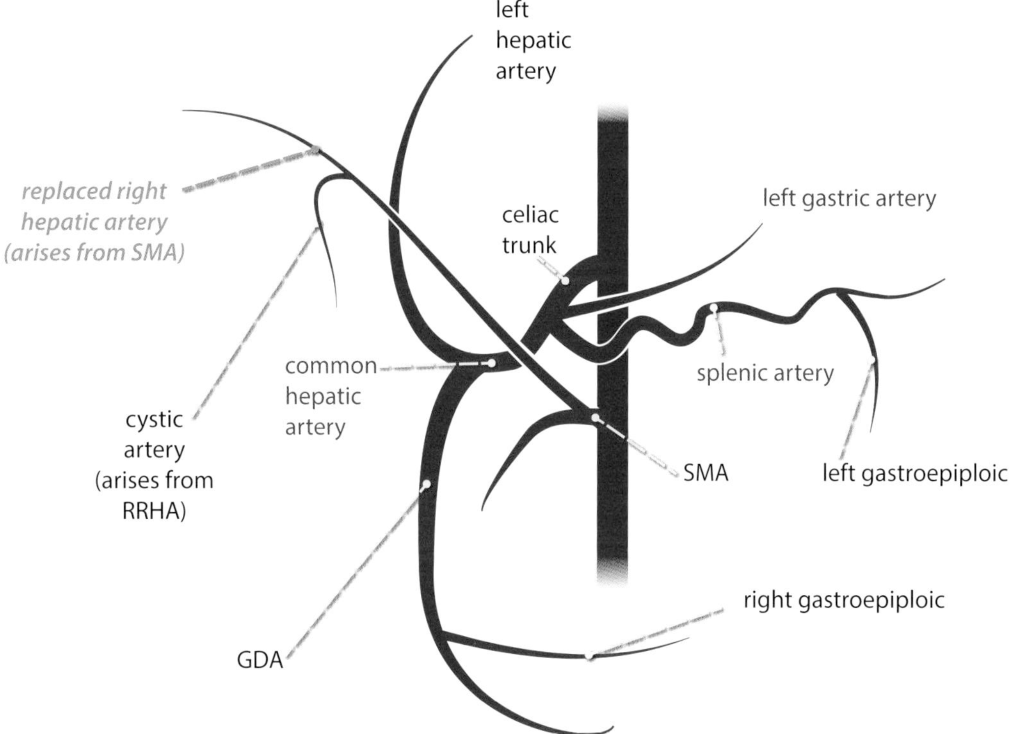

It is essential for the surgeon to be aware of an RRHA prior to laparoscopic cholecystectomy to prevent inadvertent arterial injury.

RRHA is beneficial in case of a living right hepatic donor, as the RRHA is longer and larger than a regular RHA. This allows a better anastomosis to the recipient vasculature. In contrast, there may be increased arterial complications if the hepatic transplant recipient has an RRHA, due to reduced diameter of the common hepatic artery.

In the setting of an RRHA, SMA stenosis may theoretically predispose the right lobe of the liver to ischemia, although this is usually not clinically relevant due to intrahepatic collaterals and portal vein supply.

- An **accessory right hepatic artery** is an artery arising from the SMA that supplies the right hepatic lobe in the presence of a normal right hepatic artery (arising from the proper hepatic artery).

- A **replaced left hepatic artery** (RLHA) is present in 11–12% of patients, where the left hepatic artery arises from the left gastric artery.

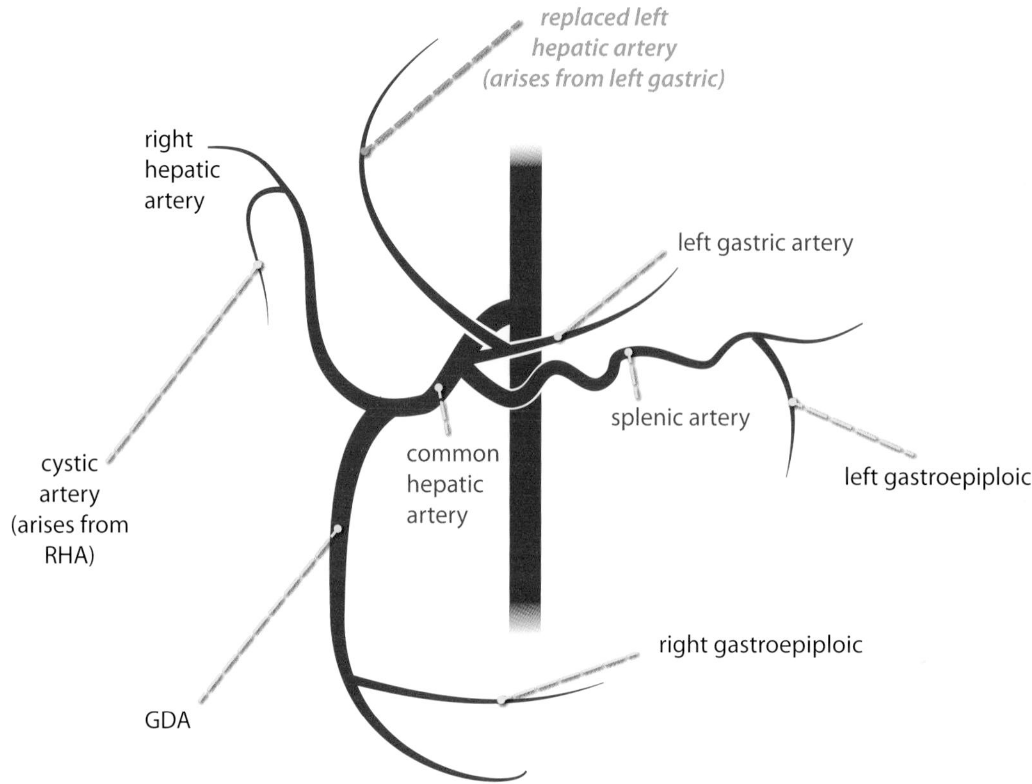

The presence of an RLHA is clinically significant during gastrectomy, as resection of the RLHA may predispose to liver injury.

- An **accessory left hepatic artery** is an artery arising from the left gastric artery that supplies the left hepatic lobe in the presence of a normal left hepatic artery (arising from the proper hepatic artery).

Superior mesenteric artery (SMA)

- The superior mesenteric artery (SMA) arises from the anterior aorta at about the level of T12–L1 to supply the distal duodenum, the entire small bowel, and the proximal large bowel from the cecum to the mid-transverse colon.
- The **inferior pancreaticoduodenal artery** is the first branch of the SMA. The inferior pancreaticoduodenal artery forms collaterals with the celiac artery.
- The **middle colic artery** arises from the SMA and supplies the transverse colon. The middle colic artery anastomoses with the **marginal artery of Drummond**.
- The **right colic artery** courses retroperitoneally, where it supplies the right colon and the hepatic flexure.
- The terminal artery of the SMA is the **ileocolic artery**, which sends arterial branches to the terminal ileum, cecum, and appendix.

Inferior mesenteric artery (IMA)

- The inferior mesenteric artery (IMA) originates at the left anterior aspect of the aorta at L3–L4.
- The IMA gives off the **left colic artery** to supply the descending colon.
- The **sigmoid arteries** are variable in number. They run in the sigmoid mesocolon to supply the sigmoid.
- The IMA terminates as the **superior rectal (hemorrhoidal) artery**, which supplies the upper rectum.

Internal iliac branches

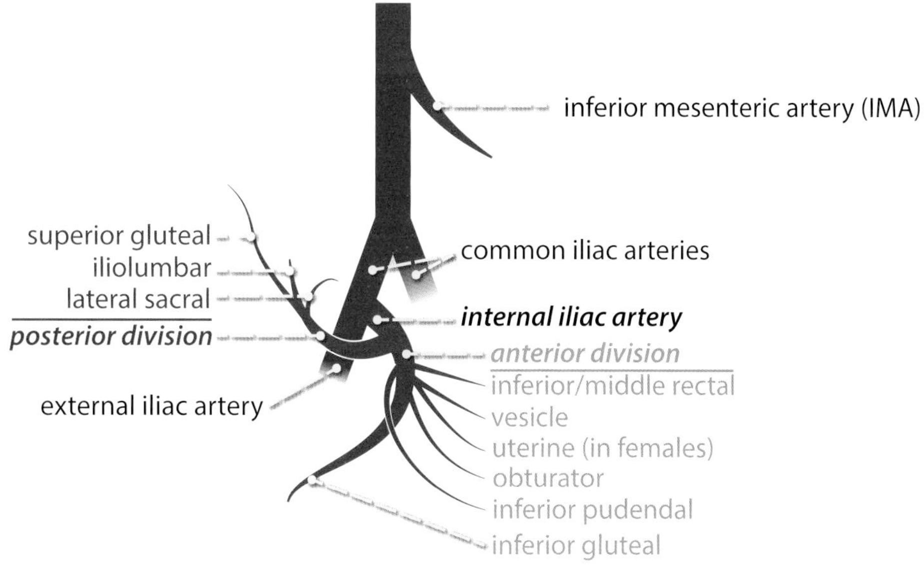

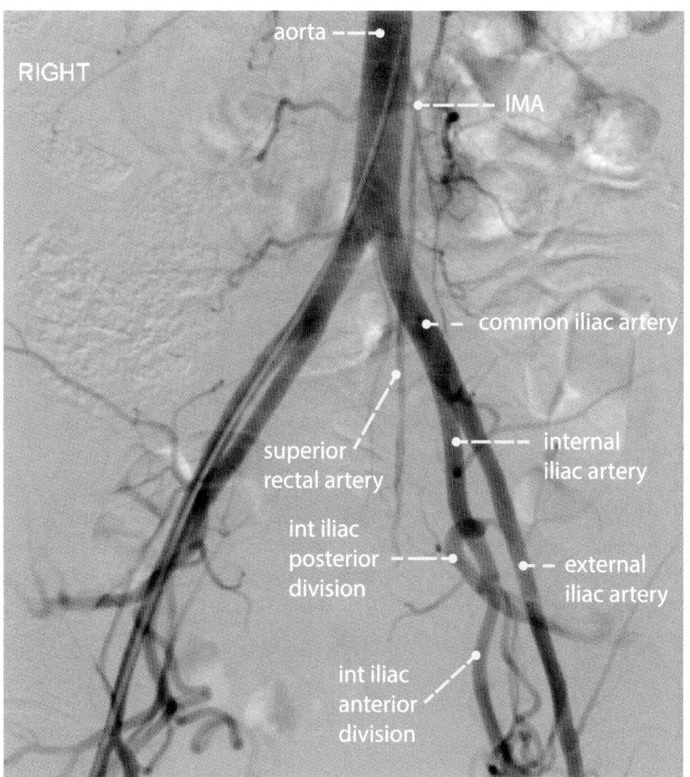

- The anterior division of the internal iliac artery supplies most of the pelvic viscera.

  The branches of the anterior division include the **inferior/middle rectal artery** (anastomoses with the IMA via the pathway of Winslow), the **uterine artery**, the **obturator artery**, and the **inferior gluteal artery**.

- The posterior division of the internal iliac artery supplies the musculature of the pelvic and gluteal regions.

  The branches of the posterior division include the **lateral sacral artery**, the **iliolumbar artery** (anastomoses with external iliac via the deep circumflex iliac artery), and the **superior gluteal artery**.

External iliac branches

- The **inferior epigastric artery** anastomoses with the superior epigastric artery.
- The **deep circumflex iliac artery** anastomoses with the internal iliac via the iliolumbar artery.
- The **femoral artery** continues distally to supply the leg.

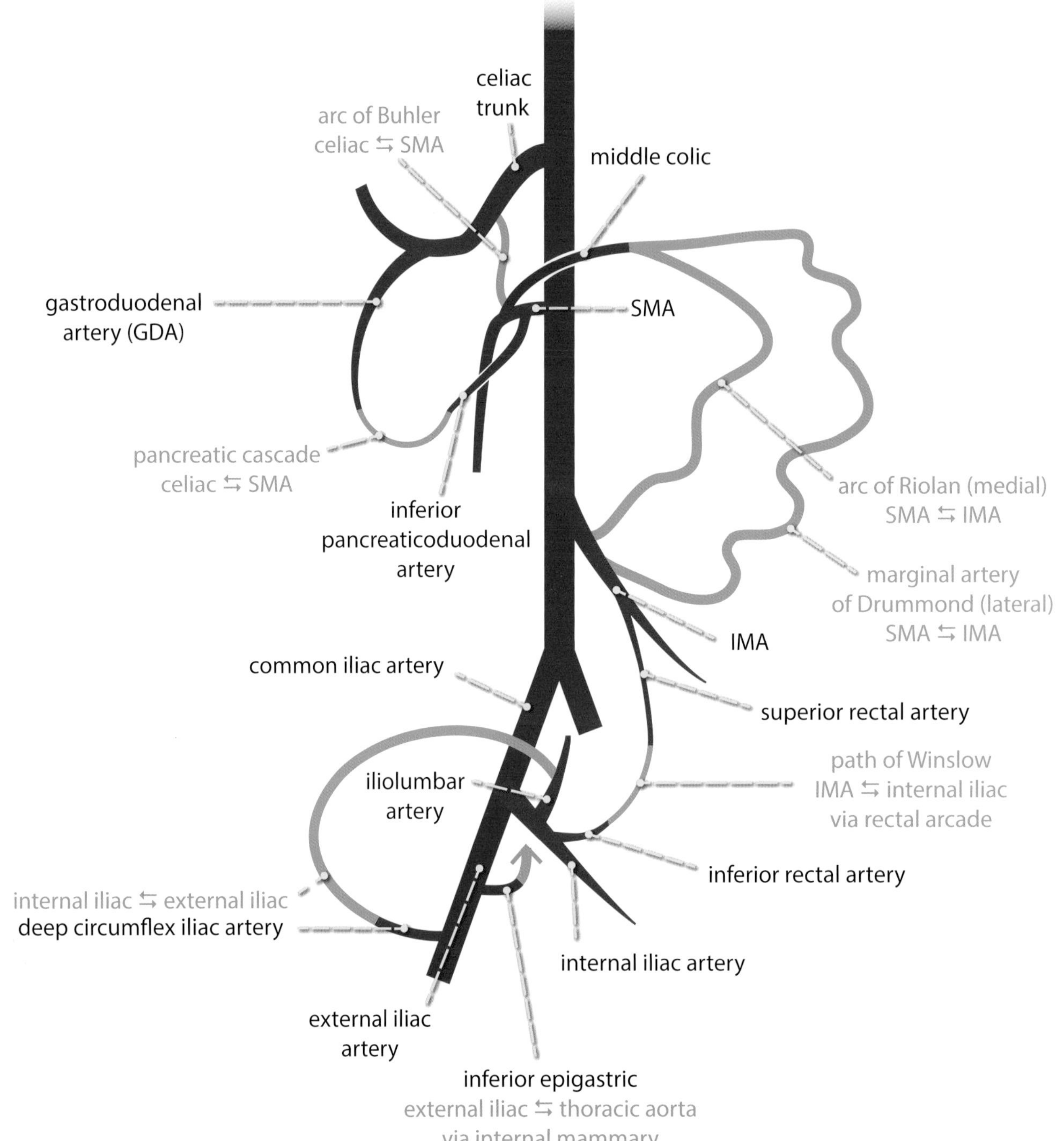

Celiac ⇆ SMA anastomoses

- The **arc of Buhler** is an uncommon short-segment direct connection between the celiac artery and the SMA. It is a persistent embryologic remnant and not an acquired collateral pathway.
- The inferior **pancreaticoduodenal artery** is the first SMA branch. It forms a rich collateral network with the celiac about the pancreatic head, called the pancreatic cascade.
- The **arc of Barkow** (not drawn) connects the SMA to the celiac axis via the right and left epiploic arteries.

SMA ⇆ IMA anastomoses

- The **marginal artery of Drummond** is the major SMA ⇆IMA anastomosis. It lies in the peripheral mesentery of the colon, adjacent to the mesenteric surface of the colon. The marginal artery of Drummond is comprised of branches from the ileocolic, right, middle, and left colic arteries. Normally, the marginal artery of Drummond is small in caliber, but it may become prominent in the setting of IMA or SMA disease.
- The **arc of Riolan** is an inconstant SMA ⇆IMA anastomosis. The arc of Riolan also runs through the colonic mesentery, but more medial compared to the marginal artery of Drummond.
- The Cannon–Böhm point is the point of transitional blood supply to the colon between the SMA (proximal) and IMA (distal), at the splenic flexure. This watershed zone is susceptible to ischemia in case of systemic arterial insufficiency.

Iliac artery anastomoses

- **External iliac ⇆ thoracic aorta**: The inferior epigastric artery arises from the external iliac artery and anastomoses with the thoracic aorta via the internal mammary artery.
- **External iliac ⇆ internal iliac**: The deep circumflex iliac artery arises from the external iliac artery and anastomoses with the posterior division of the internal iliac artery via the iliolumbar artery.
- **Internal iliac ⇆ IMA**: The inferior/middle rectal arteries arise from the internal iliac artery and anastomose with the IMA via the superior rectal artery. This collateral pathway is the path of Winslow (rectal arcade).

Mesenteric vasculopathy and aneurysms

Polyarteritis nodosa (PAN)

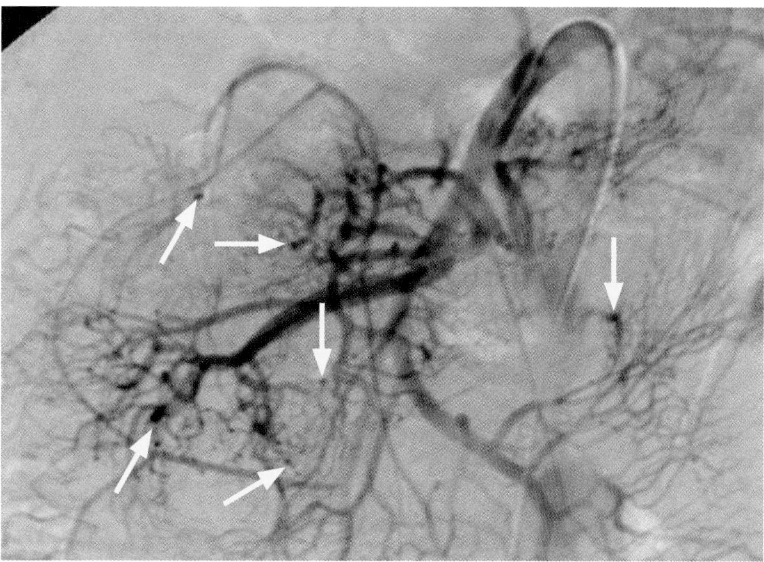

Polyarteritis nodosa:

Selective digital substraction angiogram of the superior mesenteric artery shows numerous tiny peripheral aneurysms (arrows).

Case courtesy Dmitry Rabkin, MD, Brigham and Women's Hospital.

- Polyarteritis nodosa (PAN) is a systemic necrotizing vasculitis of small and medium-sized arteries that causes multiple small visceral aneurysms. P-ANCA is usually elevated.
- The differential diagnosis of multiple renal artery aneurysms includes multiple septic emboli, *speed kidney* (due to chronic methamphetamine abuse), and Ehlers–Danlos.
- PAN typically affects renal, hepatic, and mesenteric end-arterioles.
- PAN is associated with several medical conditions remembered with the mnemonic CLASH (**c**ryoglobulinemia, **l**eukemia, rheumatoid **a**rthritis, **S**jögren syndrome, and **h**epatitis B).
- Treatment of PAN is with steroids, not procedures.

Splenic artery aneurysm

- Splenic artery aneurysm is the most common visceral aneurysm. Multiparous females and patients with portal hypertension are at increased risk of developing splenic artery aneurysms. Splenic artery aneurysms have an increased risk of rupture during pregnancy.
- A splenic artery *pseudo*aneurysm may be the result of trauma or pancreatitis.
- Indications for treatment of a splenic artery aneurysm include presence of symptoms (such as left upper quadrant pain), aneurysm size >2.5 cm, and prior to expected pregnancy.
- Endovascular coil embolization is the preferred approach. Coils are first placed distal to the aneurysm neck (to exclude retrograde collateral flow), then placed proximally.

Hepatic artery aneurysm

- Hepatic artery aneurysm is the second most common visceral aneurysm.
- Embolization of the right hepatic artery distal to the cystic artery (which arises from the right hepatic artery) is preferred, as embolization proximal to the cystic artery increases the risk of ischemic cholecystitis, which may be seen in up to 10% of cases.

Cirrhosis

- The classic angiographic finding of liver cirrhosis is corkscrewing of the hepatic artery branches, caused by liver fibrosis. A hypervascular mass in a cirrhotic liver may represent hepatocellular carcinoma.

MESENTERIC ISCHEMIA

- Mesenteric ischemia is inadequate blood supply to the bowel. It is seen most commonly in the elderly and has multiple causes, including acute arterial embolism, chronic arterial stenosis, venous occlusion, and low-flow states. For the purposes of interventions, the etiologies can be divided into **acute** or **chronic.**

Acute mesenteric ischemia

- Acute mesenteric ischemia typically presents as catastrophic abdominal pain, often with lactic acidosis. Acute mesenteric ischemia is most commonly caused by an SMA embolus.
- An SMA embolism distal to the middle colic artery carries the highest risk of intestinal ischemia, as there are few native distal collaterals. The middle colic artery anastomoses with the IMA via the marginal artery of Drummond and the arc of Riolan.
- In most patients with acute mesenteric ischemia, treatment is surgical revascularization (embolectomy or bypass), direct inspection of bowel, and resection of necrotic bowel.
- In select patients with acute embolic mesenteric ischemia (patients without peritoneal signs or clinical findings suggestive of bowel necrosis), endovascular therapy with thrombolysis or suction embolectomy may be performed.
- **Nonocclusive mesenteric ischemia (NOMI)** is a highly lethal (70–100% mortality) form of acute mesenteric ischemia. NOMI is also known as "intestinal necrosis with a patent arterial tree" and features spasm and narrowing of multiple branches of the mesenteric arteries. Direct arterial infusion of the vasodilator papaverine (60 mg bolus, then 30–60 mg/h) is the primary treatment of NOMI.

Chronic mesenteric ischemia

- Chronic mesenteric ischemia is usually caused by atherosclerosis. The classic clinical presentation is postprandial abdominal pain out of proportion to the physical exam.
- Mesenteric angiography shows ostial narrowing of the mesenteric vessels, often with post-stenotic dilation. The lateral aortagram is the most useful view to evaluate the origins of the celiac and superior mesenteric arteries.

- Because mesenteric collaterals are so extensive, at least two of three mesenteric arteries (celiac, SMA, and IMA) must be diseased to produce symptoms in chronic disease.
- Chronic mesenteric ischemia can be treated endovascularly with angioplasty and stenting.

Gastrointestinal (GI) bleeding

Role of interventional radiology in gastrointestinal (GI) bleeding

- Gastrointestinal (GI) bleeding can be classified as **upper GI** (bleeding source proximal to the ligament of Treitz), **lower GI** (bleeding source distal to the ligament of Treitz), and **variceal**. Variceal bleeding is due to portal hypertension and is treated by reducing portal pressure, discussed subsequently.
- Endoscopy is the best initial procedure for acute upper GI bleeding. Endoscopy can be both diagnostic and therapeutic.
- For lower GI bleeding, a hemodynamically stable patient should first be evaluated by mesenteric CT angiogram or nuclear medicine tagged red blood cell scan to localize the bleed, as these tests are thought to be more sensitive than angiography. A bleeding rate of 0.5 to 1.0 mL/min is generally required to be angiographically positive.

  A tagged red blood cell scan can detect bleeding rate as low as 0.2 to 0.4 mL/min.

  Many institutions now favor mesenteric CT angiography as the first test for evaluation of acute lower GI bleeding because CT is rapid, easy to perform, and readily available. On CTA, acute bleeding is seen as contrast extravasation. CTA may be able to detect bleeding rates as low as 0.35 mL/min.
- A hemodynamically unstable patient with clinical evidence of current GI bleeding may go straight to angiography.
- Due to the copious collaterals between the celiac axis and the SMA, it is often reasonable to perform empirical (in absence of visualized extravasation) embolization of the left gastric artery in upper GI bleeding. However, lower GI collaterals are much less well developed and there is a significant risk of bowel infarct with indiscriminate lower GI embolization.
- Intraarterial infusion of vasopressin (antidiuretic hormone) can often control active lower GI bleeding, but there is a very high rebleeding rate once the infusion is stopped. Vasopressin is most useful in cases of bleeding from antimesenteric vessels, which are more difficult to reach directly by catheter. Major complications of vasopressin are seen in up to 20% including arrhythmia, pulmonary edema, and hypertension.

  Vasopressin is directly infused into the SMA or IMA. The dose of vasopressin is 0.2–0.4 units per minute (100 units mixed in 500 mL saline given at 1 mL/minute), given as a continuous infusion for up to 24 hours.

  Vasopressin can only be used for 24 hours before tachyphylaxis (lack of further response) develops.

Angiodysplasia

- Angiodysplasia is an acquired vascular anomaly that is a common cause of chronic intermittent lower GI bleeding, most typically located in the right colon or cecum. Because angiodysplasia is so prevalent (identified in up to 15% of patients incidentally), the presence of angiodysplasia in a bleeding patient should not stop the hunt for other possible sources.
- Even when angiodysplasia is the cause of bleeding, active extravasation is rarely seen.
- On imaging, angiodysplasia is a tangle of vessels with early filling of an antimesenteric draining vein. The typical *tram-track* appearance is caused by simultaneous opacification of the parallel artery and vein.
- Endovascular treatments, such as vasopressin or embolization, are generally not effective due to the abnormal vessels of angiodysplasia. Treatment is endoscopy with electrocoagulation, laser therapy, or other techniques. Surgery can be performed for recurrent or uncontrollable bleeding, but is usually not necessary.

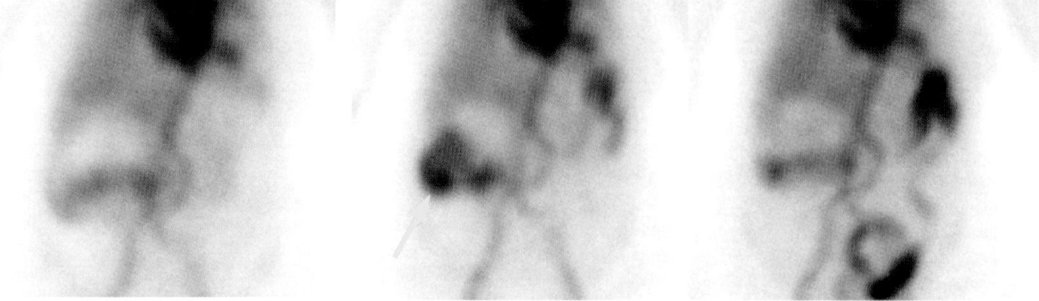

Tagged red blood cell scan at 15, 30, and 45 minutes shows abnormal tracer accumulation at the hepatic flexure (arrow) with rapid transit into the distal colon by 45 minutes.

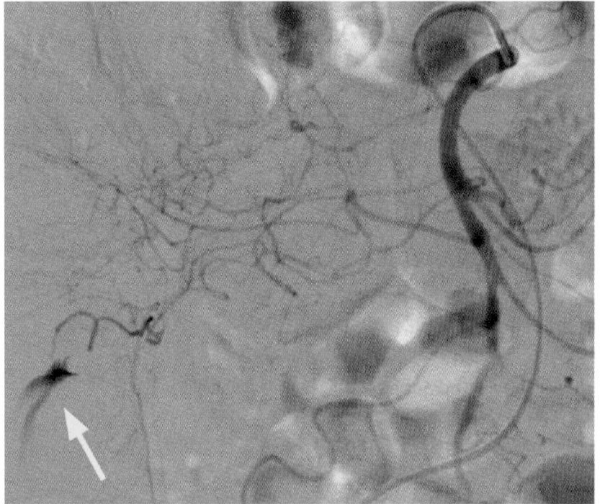

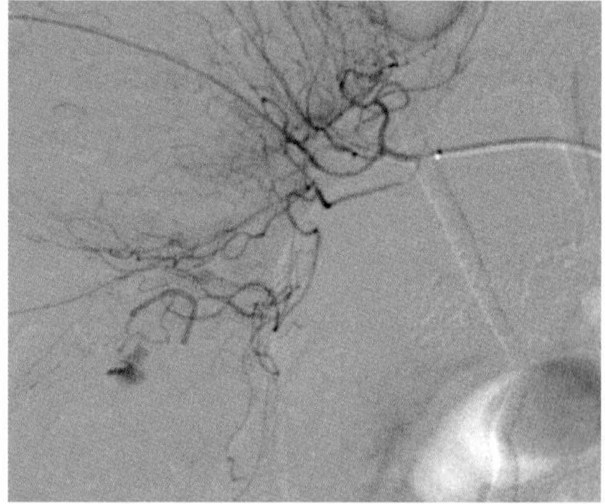

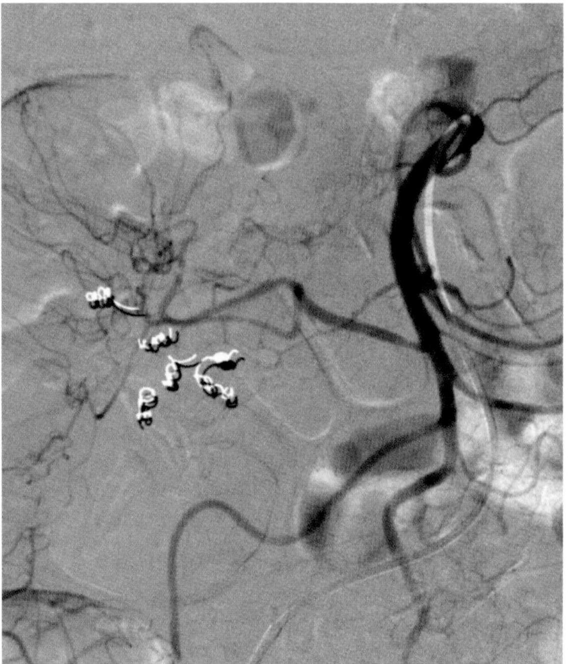

Diverticular bleed: Initial selective DSA angiogram of the SMA (top left image) shows an area of active extravasation (arrow) in a distal right branch of the middle colic artery.

Superselective DSA angiogram of the middle colic artery (top right image) shows that the area of active extravasation is too distal to be reached by catheter. At this point, the surgery team was consulted and it was determined that the patient was not a good operative candidate. The decision was made to embolize as selectively as possible, knowing the possible risk of bowel ischemia.

After placement of several coils in the middle colic branches, follow-up selective SMA angiogram (left image) demonstrates resolution of the active extravasation. There was no post-procedural evidence of bowel ischemia.

Case courtesy Alisa Suzuki Han, MD, Brigham and Women's Hospital.

- Diverticulosis is the most common cause of lower GI bleeding in older adults.
- Most patients respond to conservative management, but angiography can be used for stable or unstable patients who fail medical management.
- If active extravasation is seen, potential therapies include superselective embolization (most commonly with coils) or vasopressin infusion.

Atherosclerotic renal artery stenosis

- Atherosclerosis is most common cause of renal artery stenosis in older adults.
- Atherosclerosis tends to affect the ostia (origin) of the renal arteries.
- Angioplasty and stenting have greater long-term patency compared to angioplasty alone.
- The overall clinical benefit of endovascular revascularization is controversial. In 2009, the ASTRAL trial published in the New England Journal of Medicine compared medical therapy alone to medical therapy and endovascular renal artery revascularization. This study found no benefit of endovascular treatment with respect to blood pressure, renal function, or mortality. The criticisms of the ASTRAL trial are that there was a lack of severe lesions in the patient population and the patients receiving medical treatment did better than in previous studies.

Fibromuscular dysplasia (FMD)

- Fibromuscular dysplasia (FMD) is an idiopathic vascular disease affecting primarily the renal and carotid arteries. FMD is bilateral two thirds of the time.
- FMD is predominantly seen in young or middle-aged women.
- In contrast to the ostial involvement of renal artery atherosclerosis, FMD tends to affect the mid or distal third of the renal arteries.
- The most common form of FMD is the medial fibroplasia subtype (80%), which features the classic *string of pearls* or *string of beads* appearance on angiography.
- A less common form is intimal fibroplasia, which is more common in children and appears as a smooth stenosis, not the string of pearls typical of medial fibroplasia.

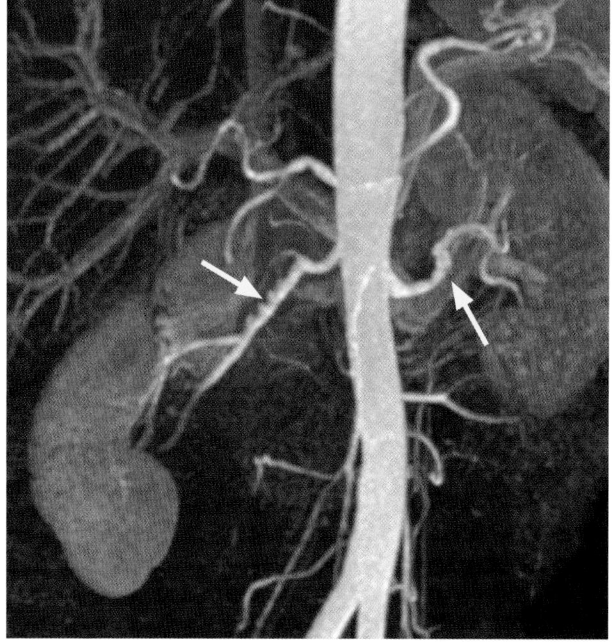

Fibromuscular dysplasia (medial fibroplasia subtype): MIP image from an MR-angiogram of the abdominal aorta shows the classic "beaded" appearance of both renal arteries (arrows) predominantly in the mid portion of the renal arteries, with sparing of the ostia.

- Perimedial and adventitial fibroplasia are less common variants.
- FMD clinically responds well to angioplasty alone, with improved blood pressure control in 97%, including a 42% cure rate and a 90% patency rate at 5 years. The high clinical success rate is thought to be due to mechanical disruption of the fibrous tissue by the angioplasty balloon. Restenosis following angioplasty occurs relatively frequently, in 10–15% of patients.
- Stenting of FMD is not recommended, as stenting can complicate retreatment with angioplasty and lead to in-stent stenosis due to intimal hyperplasia.

Neurofibromatosis

- Neurofibromatosis may cause renal artery stenosis in children.

Renal cell carcinoma (RCC)

- Most renal cell carcinomas (RCC) are hypervascular. The tumors often feature arteriovenous shunting and venous lakes, with a classic angiographic appearance of *bizarre neovascularity*.

Oncocytoma

- Oncocytoma is a benign renal mass that cannot be reliably distinguished from renal cell carcinoma on cross-sectional imaging.
- Angiography classically shows a *spokewheel* appearance with a peritumoral halo. In contrast to RCC, bizarre neoplastic vessels are absent.

Angiomyolipoma (AML)

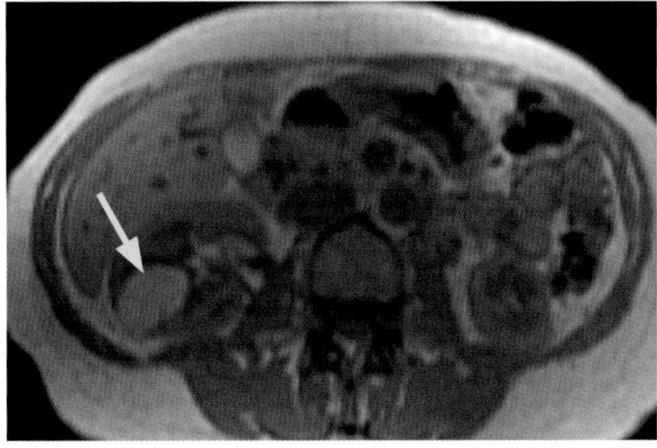

Axial T1-weighted MRI shows a mass in the lower pole of the right kidney, which is isointense to fat (arrow).

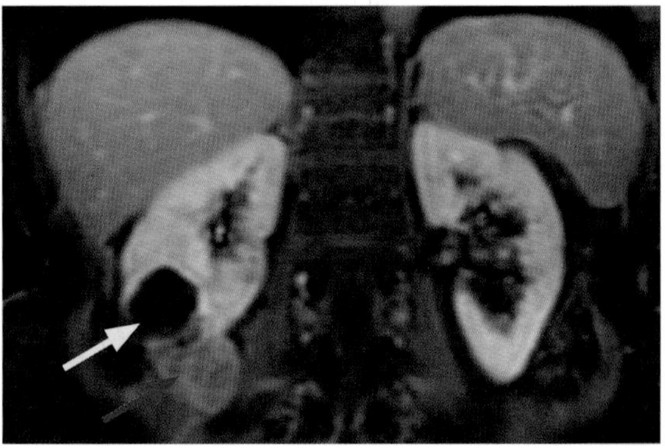

Coronal T1-weighted post-contrast fat-saturated MRI shows saturation of the upper component of the mass (yellow arrow), consistent with macroscopic fat. An inferior enhancing component is present (red arrow).

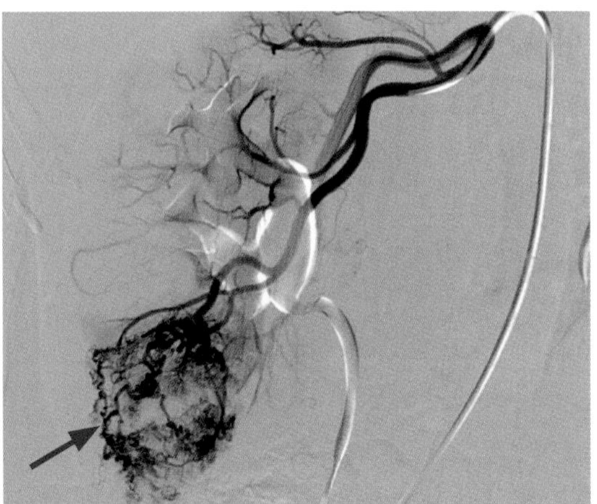

Superselective digital subtraction arteriogram of a right renal artery branch shows intense tumor blush in the lower pole (red arrow). There is no AV shunting.

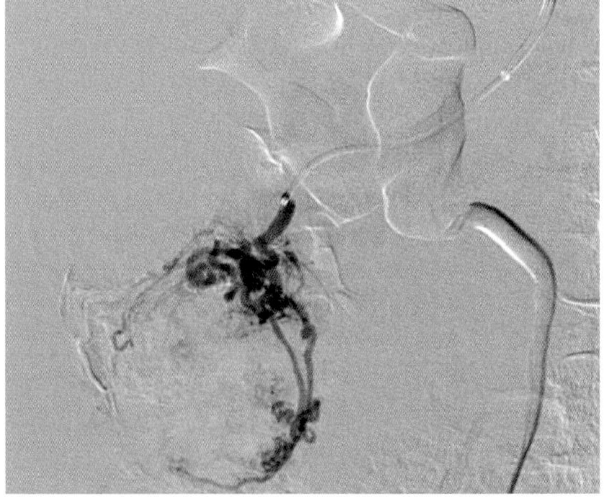

After super-selective embolization with particles, there is markedly reduced flow. Tortuous feeding arteries are still present peripherally.

Angiomyolipoma: *Case courtesy Bela Kis, MD, Brigham and Women's Hospital.*

- Renal angiomyolipoma is a hypervascular hamartoma containing blood vessels (angio), smooth muscle (myo), and fat (lipoma). An AML is diagnosed on cross-sectional imaging as a renal mass containing macroscopic fat.
- Angiography shows tortuous feeding arteries, which have a sunburst appearance on the parenchymal phase. Occasionally, small aneurysms are visible, which predispose to risk of hemorrhage, especially if the AML is >4 cm in diameter. In contrast to a renal arteriovenous fistula, AMLs do not feature arteriovenous shunting – that is, no veins will be opacified during arterial phase imaging.

- It is not always possible to differentiate an AML from RCC on angiography, so cross-sectional imaging is usually indicated if a suspected AML is diagnosed incidentally.

Renal trauma

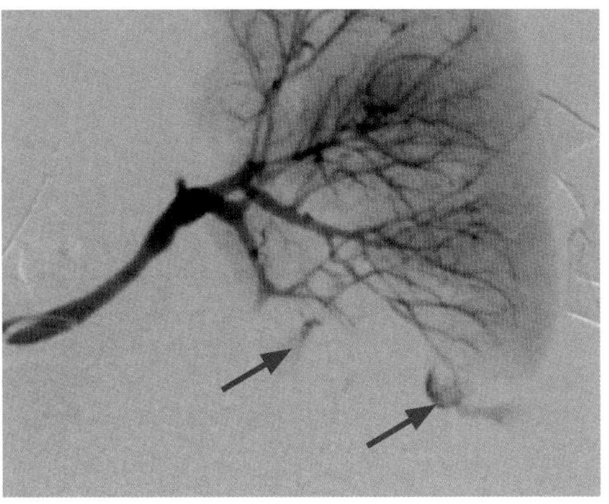
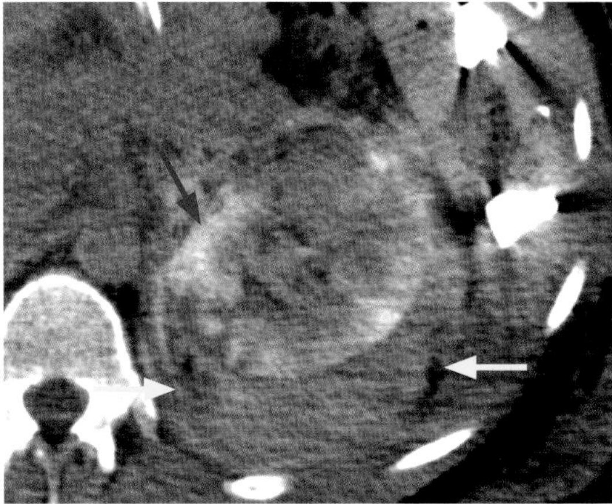

Grade IV renal injury: Selective DSA angiogram of the left kidney (left image) shows lack of vascularization of the lower pole of the kidney and two foci of active contrast extravasation (red arrows). These were treated super selectively with coiling. Post-embolization unenhanced CT (right image) shows residual irregular pooling of contrast in the renal cortex (red arrow) and a large perinephric urinoma (yellow arrows), diagnostic of grade IV injury. There are bullet fragments in the left hemiabdomen.

Case courtesy Alisa Suzuki Han, MD, Brigham and Women's Hospital.

- Renal trauma can be classified as blunt (>80% of injuries), penetrating (such as gunshot or stab wound), or iatrogenic. Hematuria is usually present with renal trauma, regardless of etiology. A horseshoe kidney is especially susceptible to traumatic injury as it is not protected by the inferior ribs and may be compressed against the vertebral column.
- The Organ Injury Scale (OIS) from the American Association for the Surgery of Trauma (AAST) classification is the most widely used classification of renal injury. This scale is further discussed in the genitourinary imaging section.

  Grades I–III include nonexpanding hematomas or parenchymal laceration without collecting system injury. These injuries are usually managed conservatively.

  Grade IV includes a deep parenchymal laceration that extends to the collecting system, causing the CT finding of extravasation of opacified urine on delayed imaging. Injury to the renal artery or vein with contained hemorrhage is also OIS grade IV, and is often treated with endovascular coil embolization as in the case above.

  Grade V (most severe) injury is a shattered kidney with avulsion of the renal hilum. Treatment is usually surgical.

- Other important vascular injuries not included in the OIS classification include traumatic renal artery thrombosis and renal artery pseudoaneurysm.
- Indications for endovascular treatment of renal trauma include active extravasation, dissection, or pseudoaneurysm. Treatment is usually superselective coil embolization.

Renal arteriovenous fistulas and malformations

- Renal arteriovenous fistulas (AVFs) are almost always acquired, secondary to trauma or renal biopsy. Congenital intrarenal arteriovenous malformations are rare.
- The majority of renal AVFs are asymptomatic and often heal spontaneously. When symptomatic, hematuria is the most common complaint. Less commonly, a renal AVF can lead to high-output cardiac failure or spontaneous retroperitoneal hemorrhage.
- Angiography of an AVF shows venous opacification during the arterial phase.
- Treatment is with embolization (coils, glue, or alcohol).

Median arcuate ligament syndrome (MALS)

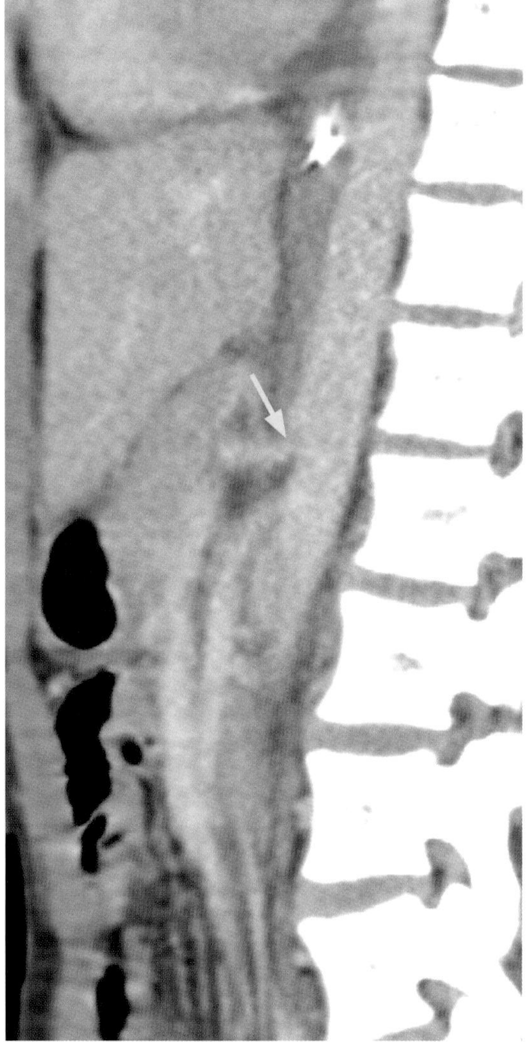

Contrast-enhanced portal-venous phase sagittal CT demonstrates kinking at the origin of the celiac artery (arrow), suggestive of median arcuate ligament syndrome. This was an incidental finding as the CT was performed for trauma.

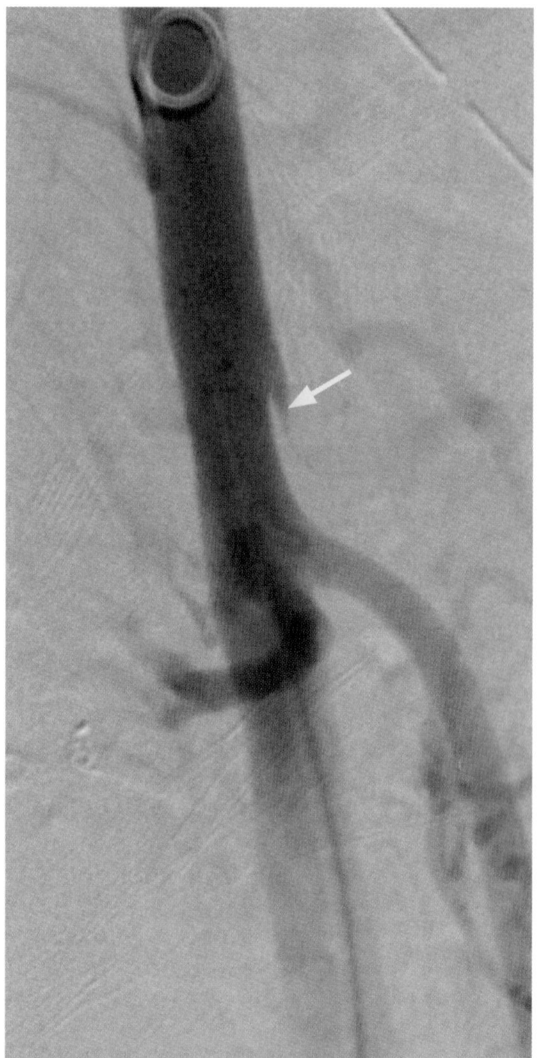

Nonselective lateral DSA aortagram with the pigtail catheter near the diaphragmatic hiatus shows an acute tapering of the celiac artery (arrow). The SMA is well-opacified. Delayed images (not shown) showed retrograde filling of the celiac artery through the SMA.

Median arcuate ligament syndrome found incidentally. The patient was asymptomatic and no treatment was performed. Of note, angiography was performed for embolization of a renal injury (not pictured).

Case courtesy Alisa Suzuki Han, MD, Brigham and Women's Hospital.

- Median arcuate ligament syndrome (MALS) is celiac artery compression by the median arcuate ligament, a part of the diaphragmatic crura. Arterial compression worsens with expiration.
- While most patients are asymptomatic, MALS may clinically present with crampy abdominal pain. MALS tends to occur in young, thin women.
- Angioplasty is not effective and stents are controversial due to high risk of device failure. Definitive treatment is surgical release of the median arcuate ligament to enlarge the diaphragmatic hiatus.

Superior mesenteric artery (SMA) syndrome

- SMA syndrome is compression of the ***duodenum*** between the aorta and the SMA, and is also known as Wilkie syndrome.
- SMA syndrome occurs in thin children, burn victims, and patients who have lost weight.

Nutcracker syndrome

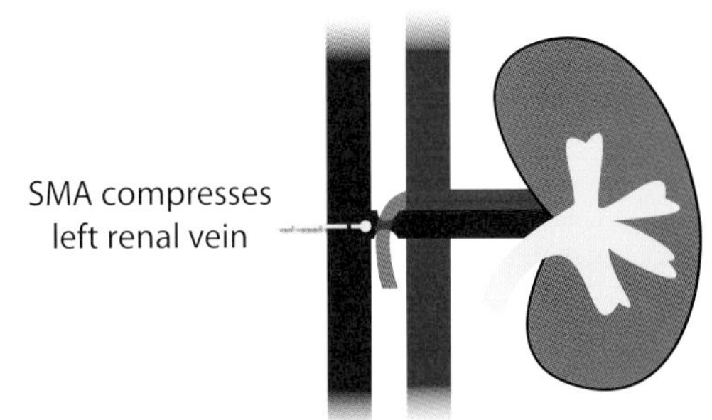

- Nutcracker syndrome is compression of the left renal vein between the aorta and the SMA. This is similar to SMA syndrome, but the renal vein is compressed instead of the duodenum.
- A posterior variant, called *posterior nutcracker*, is the compression of a retroaortic (or circumaortic) renal vein between the aorta and the vertebral body.
- Nutcracker syndrome can present with variable clinical symptoms including pain, hematuria, orthostatic proteinuria, pelvic congestion, and varicocele (in a male).
- Treatment depends on the symptoms. The majority of cases of hematuria resolve within two years of observation. If treatment is desired, angioplasty and stenting of the renal vein can be performed.

May–Thürner

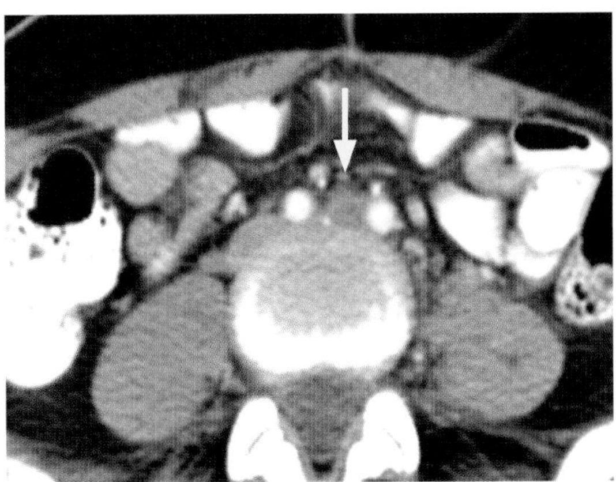

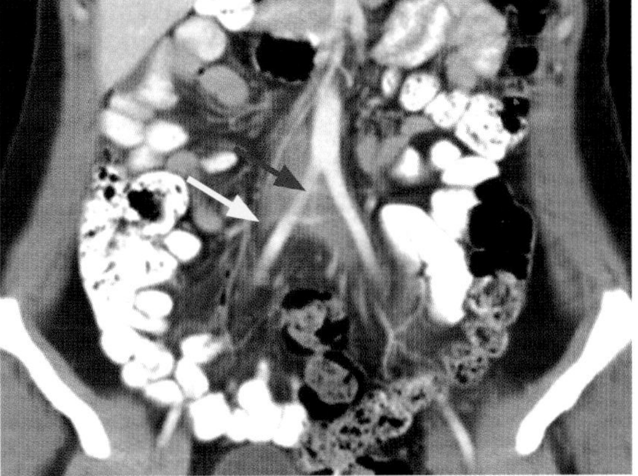

May–Thürner: Axial contrast-enhanced CT (left image) shows a distended and hypoattenuating left common iliac vein (yellow arrow), suggestive of thrombosis. Coronal CT (right image) shows the right common iliac artery (red arrow) crossing the bifurcation of the IVC and right common iliac vein (yellow arrow). The venous thrombosis is not apparent on the coronal view.

Case courtesy Michael Hanley, MD, University of Virginia Health System.

- May–Thürner syndrome is venous thrombosis of the left common iliac vein caused by compression from the crossing right common iliac artery.
- Chronic compression leads to a fibrous adhesion in the vein, predisposing to thrombosis.

LEFT common iliac VEIN compressed by RIGHT common iliac ARTERY

- Treatment is endovascular thrombolysis followed by stenting.

PORTAL HYPERTENSION

Measuring portal pressure

- Direct portal vein (PV) pressure measurement requires traversing the hepatic parenchyma and is thus invasive and impractical. Wedged hepatic vein pressure is routinely measured via an internal jugular vein catheter and is thought to equal PV pressure in most patients.
- The **portosystemic gradient** (also known as the corrected sinusoidal pressure) represents the actual sinusoidal resistance to portal flow and is calculated as:

  (Wedged hepatic vein pressure) – (free hepatic vein pressure)
- Portal hypertension is defined as a portosystemic gradient >5 mm Hg.

Collateral pathways seen in portal hypertension

- *Light blue represents portal veins → dark blue represents systemic veins*
- Esophageal varices: Coronary vein → azygos/hemiazygos veins
- Gastric fundal varices: Splenic vein → azygos veins
- Splenorenal shunt: Splenic or short gastric → left adrenal/inferior phrenic → left renal vein
- Mesenteric varices: SMV or IMV → iliac veins
- Caput medusa: Umbilical vein → epigastric veins
- Hemorrhoids: IMV → inferior hemorrhoidal veins

Transjugular intrahepatic portosystemic shunt (TIPS)

- Transjugular intrahepatic portosystemic shunt (TIPS) lowers elevated portal pressures by the creation of a direct connection between the portal vein and the hepatic vein.
- The most common indication for TIPS is treatment of variceal hemorrhage that cannot be controlled endoscopically. Other indications for TIPS include refractory ascites and Budd–Chiari (hepatic vein thrombosis).
- Assessment of hepatic dysfunction is performed pre-procedure with either the Child–Pugh classification or Model for End-Stage Liver Disease (MELD) score.

  The **Child–Pugh** classification of hepatic dysfunction combines lab values (INR, bilirubin, and albumin) with clinical assessment (ascites and hepatic encephalopathy).

  The **MELD** score of hepatic dysfunction combines INR, bilirubin, and creatinine in a complex logarithmic formula. The higher the MELD score, the higher the post-TIPS mortality.
- Absolute contraindications to TIPS include:

  Right-sided heart failure, which will be worsened by TIPS, as right sided venous return increases.

  Severe active hepatic failure, as the post-TIPS shunting of blood beyond the hepatic sinusoids can cause liver function to worsen further.

  Severe hepatic encephalopathy, which TIPS can worsen.
- Portal vein patency should be established pre-procedure with cross-sectional or US imaging.
- Usually the right hepatic vein is connected with the right portal vein via a covered stent. The right hepatic vein has relatively constant anatomy and tends to be larger than the left.
- After the right hepatic vein is cannulated, wedged balloon CO_2 occlusion venography is performed and the portal vein is retrogradely opacified. CO_2 is the preferred contrast agent as it is 400 times less viscous than iodinated contrast and is therefore easily able to pass through the hepatic sinusoids.
- The most demanding portion of the procedure is establishing access into a portal vein. Once a tract between the hepatic and portal circulation is secured, the tract is sequentially dilated and stented, aiming for a reduction of the portosystemic gradient to <12 mm Hg.
- TIPS patency is followed by Doppler ultrasound, discussed in the ultrasound section.

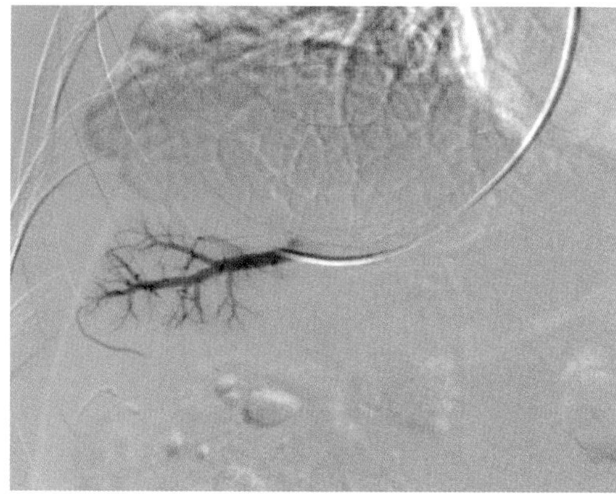

1) Right hepatic venography is performed through an internal jugular access.

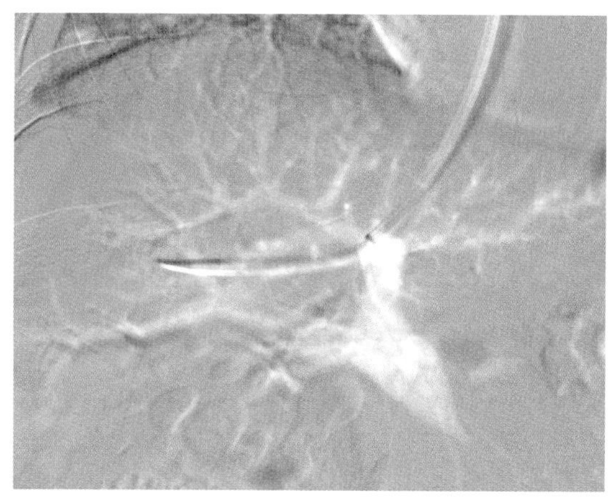

2) The catheter is wedged in a distal hepatic vein and an occlusion balloon inflated. Indirect CO_2 venography of the portal veins is performed.

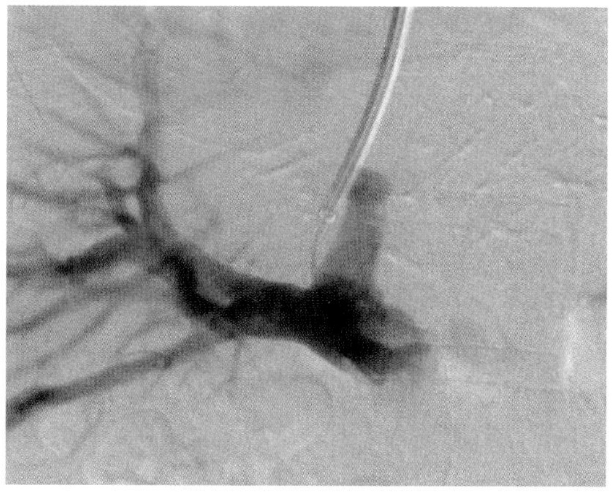

3) Direct cannulation of the portal vein (usually the right portal vein) through the liver parenchyma is the most challenging portion of the procedure. Indirect CO_2 venography is used as a guide.

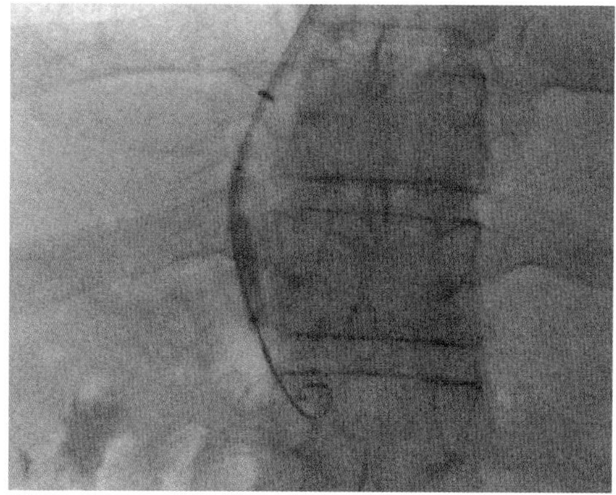

4) After the portal vein is cannulated, the tract is dilated with an 8 mm × 3–4 cm balloon to allow placement of the stent-graft.

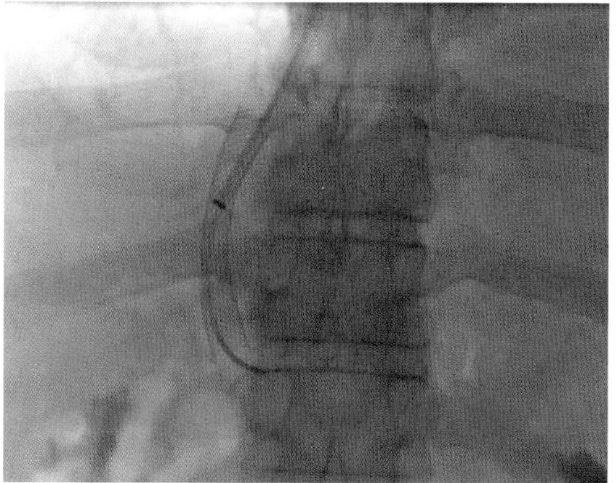

5) Once the tract is dilated, a covered stent-graft is deployed (usually a self-expanding stent). The stent-graft should be dilated until a pressure gradient between the portal vein and inferior vena cava of <12 mm Hg is reached.

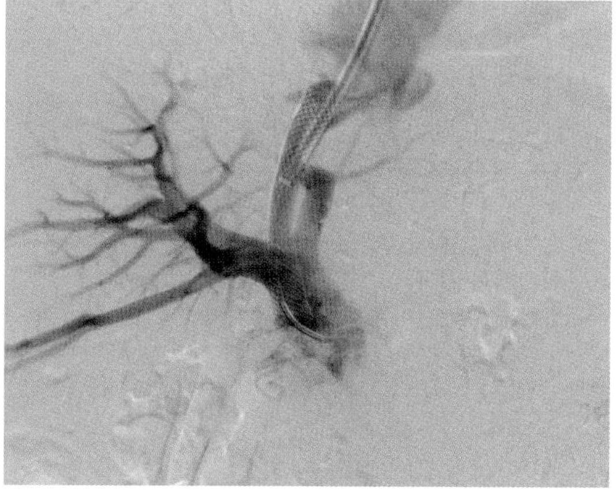

6) Completion portal venogram is performed. At this point, any varices present may be embolized.

Inferior vena cava (IVC) filter placement

- The purpose of an IVC filter is to reduce the risk of pulmonary embolism (PE) originating from a lower extremity deep venous thrombosis (DVT). Indications for filter placement include DVT and contraindication to anticoagulation; recurrent PE while anticoagulated; and high risk of developing DVT/PE in a patient with contraindication to anticoagulation, such as a multi-trauma patient.
- The most common complication of IVC filter placement is access site thrombosis, followed by IVC thrombosis. IVC perforation occurs not uncommonly, but is almost always inconsequential. Filter fracture or embolization is rare.
- The first step of the procedure is an inferior vena cavogram, performed with a high-flow (pigtail) catheter. The cavogram guides the selection of filter type and placement location.
- If a duplicated IVC is present, in order to prevent a clot from circumnavigating the filter, either a single filter is placed above the IVC confluence or a filter is placed in each duplicated IVC. If pre-procedural imaging is not available, a clue to the presence of a duplicated IVC on initial cavography is the absence of iliac vein influx contralateral to the side injected.

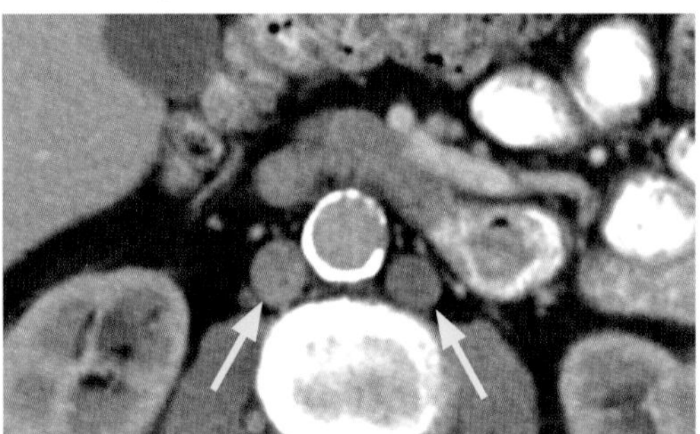

Duplicated IVC: Pre-procedure contrast-enhanced CT (left image) shows duplicated IVCs on either side of the aorta (arrows).

The presence of duplicated IVCs is confirmed by cavography of the left IVC (bottom left image), where the left renal vein (arrow) drains into the left IVC.

Post-procedure radiograph (bottom right image) shows the IVC filter (arrow at filter tip) placed above the confluence of the duplicated IVC.

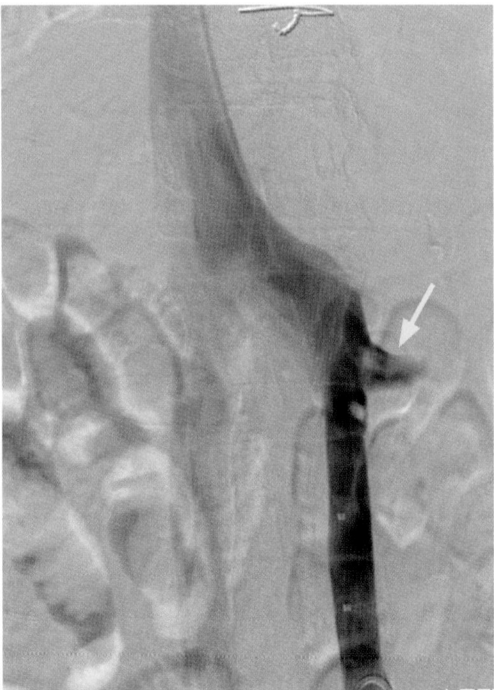

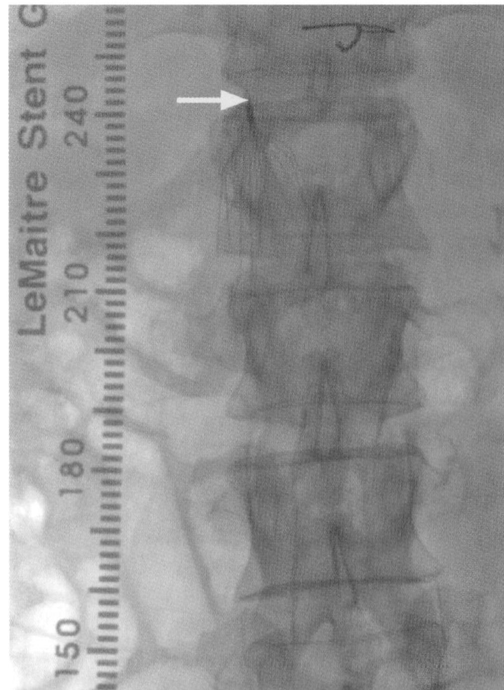

Case courtesy Alisa Suzuki Han, MD, Brigham and Women's Hospital.

- An IVC diameter >28 mm generally requires a special *bird's nest* filter, which can be placed in IVCs ranging from 28–40 mm. If the IVC is >40 mm in diameter, separate IVC filters can be inserted in each common iliac vein.

- The preferred location of the IVC filter is immediately inferior to the lowest renal vein, including any variant renal veins (circumaortic or retroaortic). Placement inferior to the lowest renal vein prevents the anomalous vein from acting as a conduit for clot propagation.

  Circumaortic left renal vein is an anatomic variant seen in 2–10% of the population, where the left renal vein is composed of two separate components. One component passes anterior to the aorta (the normal configuration) and a second retroaortic component passes posterior to the aorta to meet the IVC.

  Retroaortic left renal vein is a slightly less common variant (seen in 2–7% of the population), where a single renal vein passes posterior to the aorta. A retroaortic left renal vein usually joins the IVC more inferiorly than the right renal vein.

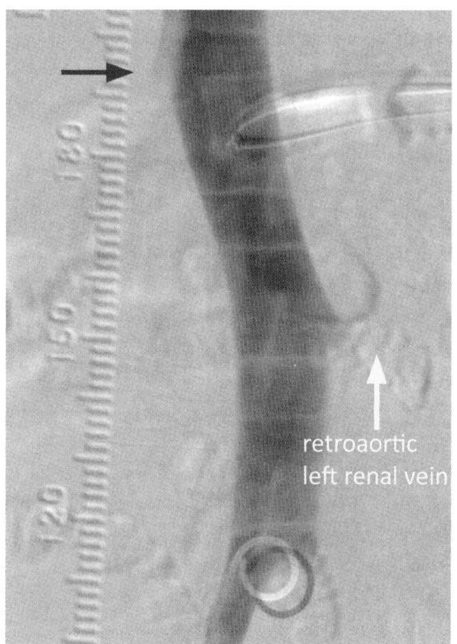

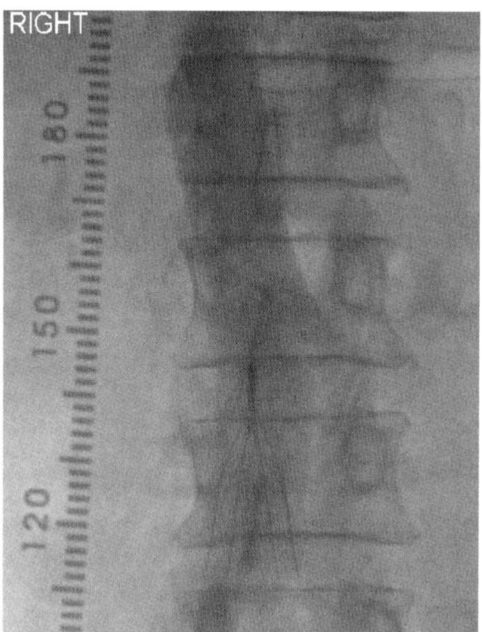

Retroaortic left renal vein: Initial digital subtraction inferior vena cavography (left image) shows the left renal vein (yellow arrow) entering the IVC markedly inferior to the right renal vein (red arrow), indicating that the left renal vein is likely retroaortic. Post-procedure radiograph shows the filter tip placed a few mm inferior to the confluence of the left retroaortic renal vein, as indicated by the ruler (top of the filter at 148; retroaortic left renal vein at 152).

Case courtesy Alisa Suzuki Han, MD, Brigham and Women's Hospital.

  Interruption of the IVC with azygos continuation is a rare anomaly where blood from the lower IVC flows into the azygos and hemiazygos veins, into the thorax, and then into the right atrium. Interruption of the IVC with azygos continuation is associated with polysplenia and congenital heart disease. It is caused by embryologic failure of the right subcardinal vein to join the intrahepatic venous complex.

- The presence of preexisting IVC thrombus may interfere with the positioning of IVC filter, requiring higher than normal placement.

Varicocele

- A varicocele is dilation of the pampiniform venous plexus. Primary varicocele (most common) is due to absent or incompetent valves in the proximal gonadal vein causing venous reflux. Secondary varicocele is due to a mass obstructing venous return. Primary varicoceles are a highly prevalent and treatable cause of infertility.
- The vast majority of varicoceles are left sided as the left gonadal vein drains into the left renal vein, while the right gonadal vein drains directly into the IVC. A solitary right varicocele should prompt the workup for an obstructing retroperitoneal mass.
- Diagnosis by scrotal ultrasound shows a dilated (>2 mm) venous plexus with a *bag of worms* appearance, which worsens on Valsalva maneuver.
- Treatment is coil embolization or surgical ligation of the gonadal vein; these have been shown to be equivalent in outcome.

CHOLANGIOGRAPHY

PERCUTANEOUS TRANSHEPATIC CHOLANGIOGRAPHY (PTC)

Biliary intervention overview and technique

- Percutaneous transhepatic cholangiography (PTC) is the injection of contrast into the biliary tree through a percutaneous approach, traversing the hepatic parenchyma.
- The two most common indications for PTC are relief of biliary obstruction and to provide biliary diversion in the case of ductal injury, which may be post traumatic or post surgical.
  - Less common indications include percutaneous treatment of biliary calculi (endoscopic treatment is much more common) and adjunctive pre-surgical treatment prior to a biliary anastomosis. A biliary anastomosis is technically facilitated by having a pre-placed catheter to sew around.
- Pre-procedure prophylactic antibiotics are administered, as biliary stasis predisposes to bacterial overgrowth. Gram-negative coverage is needed, typically with levofloxacin.
- The right and left biliary trees are accessed using slightly different techniques.
- The **right biliary tree** is accessed via a right midaxillary line two-puncture approach. The needle should be inserted directly over the ribs, as the neurovascular bundle runs underneath each rib.
  - A 22 gauge needle is inserted, parallel to the table and to the inferior border of the liver.
  - Contrast is injected as the needle is withdrawn in an attempt to opacify the biliary tree.
  - Once a bile duct is opacified, the needle is temporarily left in place and a second puncture is made with a 21 gauge needle as low as possible to access the duct.
  - Once the second needle has accessed a duct, a 0.018" wire is advanced, exchanged for a 5 or 6 Fr sheath, and subsequently a hydrophilic wire (such as a Roadrunner or Glidewire) is guided into the small bowel.
  - The hydrophilic wire is exchanged for a stiff wire (e.g., Amplatz) and the biliary drain is placed.
  - Extra sideholes may be manually cut, if necessary, to allow sideholes to extend from the biliary puncture site to the bowel.
  - The role of regular flushing is controversial. Some institutions advocate regular forward flushing, while others do not routinely flush. Regardless, a biliary drain should never be aspirated, as aspiration could draw up bowel contents into the biliary system and risk the development of cholangitis.
  - Three-month preventative maintenance is recommended.
- The **left biliary tree** is accessed by a left subxiphoid approach The left side is accessed in a similar manner to the right; however, ultrasound can often visualize dilated ducts, obviating the need for two punctures.
- If stent placement is required to treat a stricture, a metallic stent is usually only placed in patients with a life expectancy of less than 6 months. Most metallic stents cannot be removed and have a median patency of 6–8 months, although newer covered metal stents can be removed.
- Plastic stents, which are placed endoscopically, do allow regular exchange.
- An alternative to stent placement is an internal/external biliary drain, although this option is less comfortable for the patient due to the external drain.
- Most contraindications to PTC are relative. For instance, although an intrahepatic tumor (primary or metastasis) should not be traversed, a directly accessible bile duct may still be present. Similarly, ascites is a contraindication but therapeutic paracentesis can be first performed.
- Complications of percutaneous biliary drainage include sepsis, hemorrhage, bile leak, hemobilia (due to arterial–biliary fistula), and abscess.

Bile duct injury

- The most common cause of bile duct injury is iatrogenic from a laparoscopic cholecystectomy. A less common cause of bile duct injury is from orthotopic liver transplant.
- Treatment is to provide biliary diversion to a drainage bag to allow the leak to heal.

Sclerosing cholangitis

- Sclerosing cholangitis is a chronic inflammatory and fibrosing process leading to multifocal strictures of the intra- and extrahepatic biliary tree. Sclerosing cholangitis clinically presents with obstructive jaundice, malaise, and abdominal pain. It occurs more commonly in men and is associated with inflammatory bowel disease (ulcerative colitis).
- Sclerosing cholangitis ultimately leads to biliary cirrhosis and increases the risk of developing cholangiocarcinoma.
- Treatment of sclerosing cholangitis is liver transplant, although percutaneous biliary drainage can provide palliative relief for the symptoms of obstructive jaundice.
- Cholangiogram shows multifocal biliary strictures throughout the intra- and extrahepatic biliary tree. The differential diagnosis of multifocal biliary strictures includes:

Sclerosing cholangitis.
Primary biliary cirrhosis.
Multifocal cholangiocarcinoma.
Chronic bacterial cholangitis.
AIDS cholangitis (usually associated with papillary stenosis).

Malignant biliary obstruction

- Unilateral biliary obstruction of either the right or left hepatic ductal system may be due to metastatic disease or primary malignancy of the bile ducts. In the majority of cases, only the affected biliary system requires treatment.
- Hilar obstruction, in contrast, is due most commonly to a hilar cholangiocarcinoma (Klatskin tumor), which most often requires two biliary drains, one each in the right and left ducts. Occasionally an anatomic anomaly, such as anomalous drainage of the right duct directly into the left duct, may allow complete drainage of a hilar obstruction with a single biliary drain. Pre-procedure MRCP may be helpful to delineate biliary anatomy.

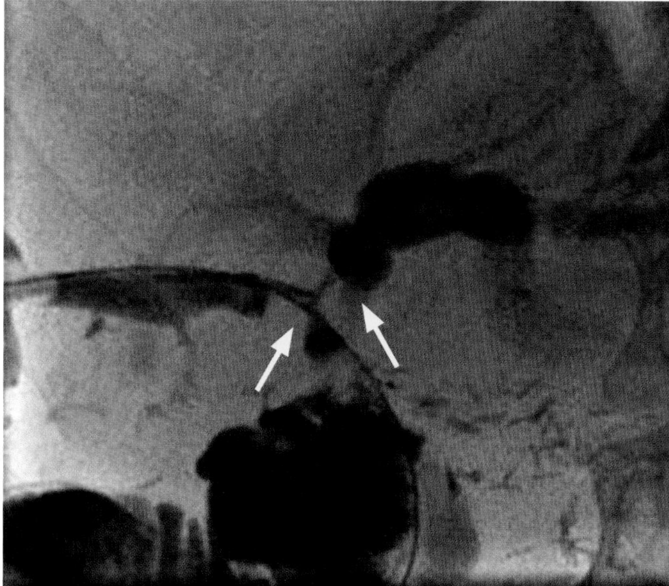

Klatskin tumor: Cholangiogram demonstrates bilateral marked dilation of the right and left hepatic ducts, with shouldering of the ducts at the hilum (arrows). A wire is in place in the right-sided ducts.

Case courtesy Timothy P. Killoran, MD, Brigham and Women's Hospital.

Acute cholecystitis

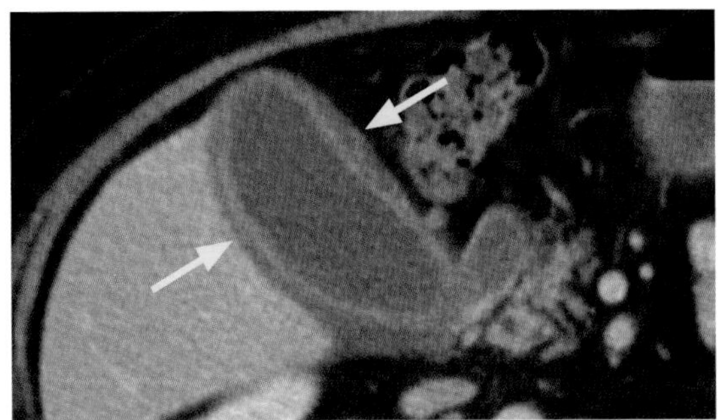

Contrast-enhanced CT shows diffuse gallbladder wall thickening (arrows). There are no radiopaque gallstones.

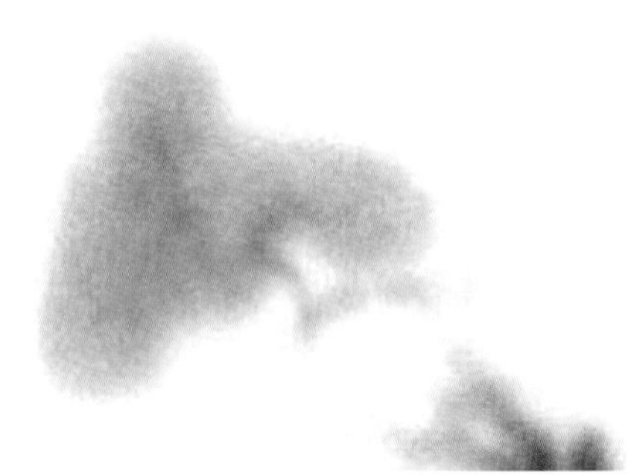

HIDA scan shows no gallbladder uptake, consistent with cystic duct obstruction.

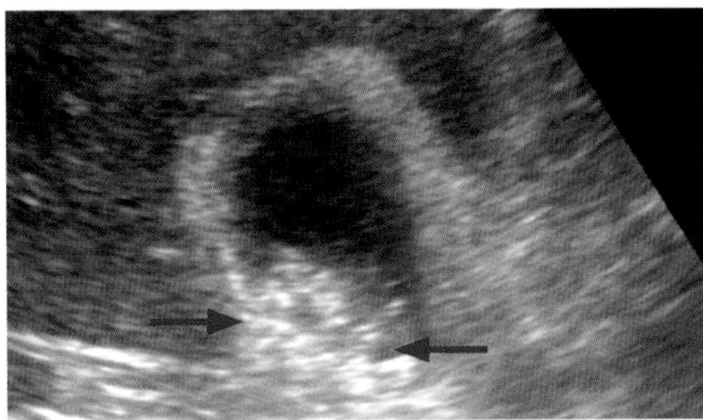

Pre-procedural ultrasound confirms thickened gallbladder wall, with numerous dependent echogenic gallstones (red arrows) not seen on CT.

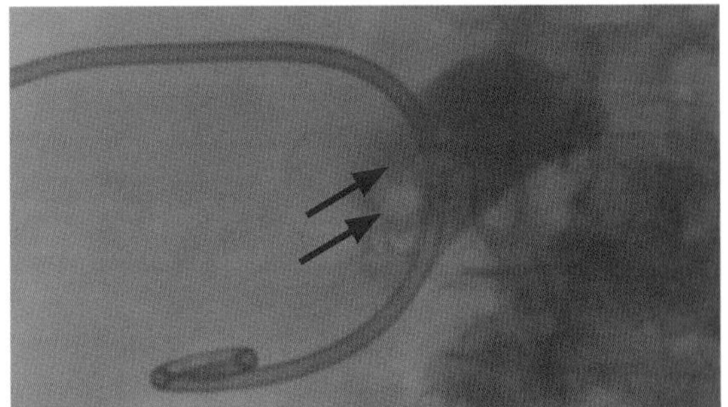

Post-cholecystostomy opacification of the gallbladder shows numerous gallbladder filling defects (red arrows), representing multiple stones.

Acute calculous cholecystitis. *Case courtesy Alisa Suzuki Han, MD, Brigham and Women's Hospital.*

- Percutaneous gallbladder drainage (cholecystostomy) is indicated for the treatment of acute calculous or acalculous cholecystitis in patients who are not surgical candidates.
- Cholecystotomy is a temporizing measure for treatment of calculous cholecystitis prior to cholecystectomy, but it may cure acalculous cholecystitis without surgery.
- Of note, cultures are negative in 40% of acute cholecystitis.
- Similar to percutaneous transhepatic cholangiography, prophylactic antibiotics are given.
- The two percutaneous approaches to the gallbladder are transhepatic and transperitoneal.

  Transhepatic (through the liver): In the transhepatic approach, a needle is inserted in the midaxillary line (either intercostal or subcostal) and directed towards the bare area of the gallbladder fossa through the liver under sonographic guidance. Transhepatic cholecystostomy has decreased risk of peritoneal bile leak, but increases the risk of liver laceration. The transhepatic approach is more commonly performed.

  Transperitoneal (avoiding the liver): In the transperitoneal approach, the needle is directed into the gallbladder from a subcostal approach in the right anterior abdomen, beneath the liver margin. While there is less risk of damaging the liver, a transperitoneal approach carries an increased risk of peritoneal bile leak. Additionally, a transperitoneal approach necessitates penetration of the gallbladder fundus, which is the most mobile portion.

- The drainage tube must remain in place until the following criteria are met:

  Patient is clinically improved. There is a risk of sepsis if the tube is removed prematurely.

  Cystic duct and common bile duct are demonstrated to be patent on repeat cholangiogram.

  At least six weeks have passed since placement (regardless of transhepatic or transperitoneal approach), to allow a fibrous tract to develop extending from the gallbladder to the skin puncture. If the tube is removed prematurely there is a risk of bile peritonitis.

PERCUTANEOUS NEPHROSTOMY (PCN)

PERCUTANEOUS NEPHROSTOMY INDICATIONS AND TECHNIQUE

Percutaneous nephrostomy (PCN) indications

- The most common indication for percutaneous nephrostomy (PCN) is urinary diversion of an obstructed kidney due to stone, malignancy, or stricture. Pyonephrosis (pus in the collecting system) is an emergent indication for percutaneous nephrostomy.
- Less commonly, PCN may be used to place an anterograde ureteral stent if a retrograde ureteral stent is unable to be placed cystoscopically.

Percutaneous nephrostomy technique

- Direct visualization of the collecting system is necessary. In most cases, urinary obstruction will lead to hydronephrosis, allowing ultrasound-directed puncture. If there is no dilation of the collecting system, intravenous contrast can be administered to opacify the nondilated collecting system and allow fluoroscopic guidance.
- The patient is positioned prone and a 22 gauge needle is used for direct posterior access. Bleeding complications can be minimized by entering the kidney in the relatively avascular *zone of Brödel,* which is defined as the plane between the ventral and dorsal renal artery branches. The optimal entry plane is therefore in the posterolateral kidney directed towards a posterior calyx.
- Complications most commonly include bleeding and infection. Although transient hematuria occurs in nearly every patient, serious bleeding complications are rare. Of particular concern in cases of preexisting infection is the risk of sepsis caused by extensive manipulation.

PERCUTANEOUS GASTROSTOMY

PERCUTANEOUS GASTROSTOMY INDICATIONS AND TECHNIQUE

Percutaneous gastrostomy indications

- Esophageal, head and neck, and neurologic disease may necessitate percutaneous gastrostomy. Of note, there is strong evidence that gastrostomy does not improve survival or quality of life in elderly patients with dementia and decreased oral intake.
- A less common indication for gastrostomy is for long-term bowel decompression, for instance due to palliation of malignant bowel obstruction or prolonged ileus.

Percutaneous gastrostomy technique

- Absolute contraindications to percutaneous gastrostomy include lack of appropriate window (such as colonic interposition), extensive gastric varices, and uncorrectable coagulopathy.
- A nasogastric tube is inserted under fluoroscopic guidance, through which the stomach is insufflated with air.
- Under fluoroscopic guidance, three T-fastener gastropexy clips are deployed to pexy the anterior wall of the stomach to the anterior abdominal wall. After each deployed T-fastener, intra-gastric position is confirmed with a small amount of contrast injected into the stomach.
- After the pexy clips are in place and the stomach is firmly fastened against the anterior abdominal wall, the definitive gastrostomy puncture is made and serially dilated. The gastrostomy can be used 24 hours after the patient is evaluated for peritoneal signs.
- The G-tube must remain in place for at least a month to form a mature transperitoneal tract.

NORMAL ANATOMY OF THE LEG VASCULATURE

Arterial anatomy of the leg

- The femoral artery is the continuation of external iliac artery distal to the inguinal ligament.
- The femoral artery branches include:

  Deep femoral artery, the terminal branch to supply the deep muscles of the thigh.

  Superficial circumflex iliac artery.

  Superficial femoral artery (SFA), which continues to supply the leg and foot.
- After passing posteriorly through the adductor hiatus, the SFA becomes the popliteal artery. From medial to lateral, the branches of the popliteal artery are:

  Posterior tibial artery (most medial).

  Peroneal artery (arises from the tibioperoneal trunk, along with the posterior tibial artery).

  Anterior tibial artery (most lateral; the only anterior artery of the lower leg). It is easy to remember that the *anterior tibial* artery is *lateral* because the only muscle bulk of the anterior lower leg is the *lateral* compartment and that muscle is the *anterior tibialis*.

MRA and schematic of the arteries of the lower leg

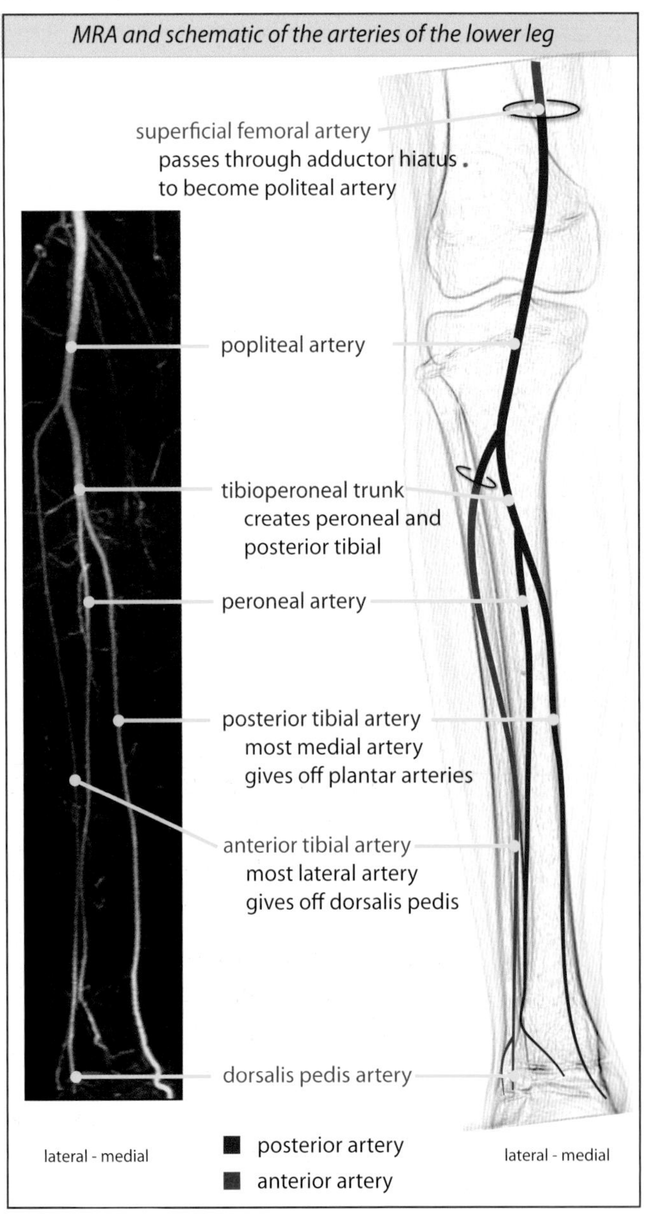

Venous anatomy of the leg

- The venous anatomy of the leg is discussed in the ultrasound section.

Distal aorta, iliac, pelvic, and leg arteries

Atherosclerotic distal aortic occlusive disease (Leriche syndrome)

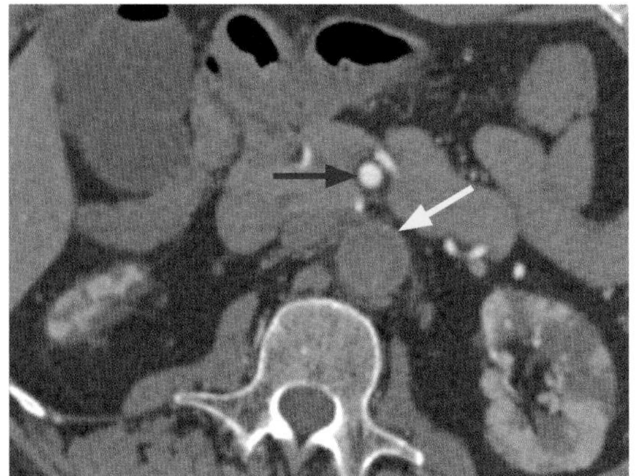

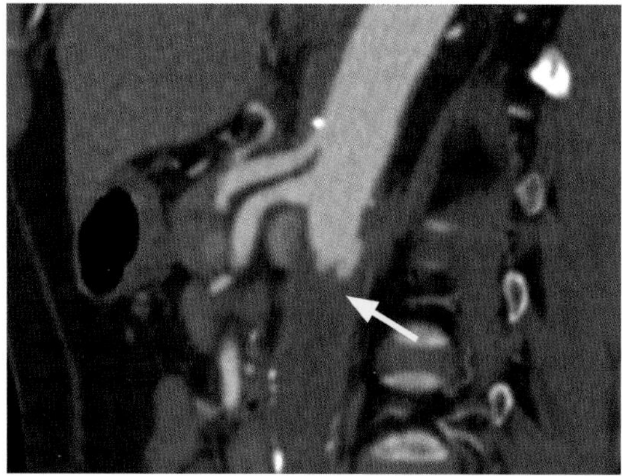

Leriche syndrome: Axial CT angiogram (left image) shows no opacification of the aorta (yellow arrow), while there is good opacification of the superior mesenteric artery (red arrow). There is patchy enhancement of the kidneys. Sagittal oblique MIP shows occlusive thrombus of the aorta (yellow arrow).

Case courtesy Michael Hanley, MD, University of Virginia Health System.

- Leriche syndrome is chronic occlusive atherosclerotic disease of the distal abdominal aorta, producing the classical quartet of impotence, buttock claudication, absent femoral pulses, and cold lower extremities.
- Over time, extensive collaterals develop from the thoraco-abdominal aorta to the external iliac arteries, most commonly the *anterior, middle,* and *posterior* pathways:

> ***Anterior:*** Thoracic aorta → internal thoracic artery → superior epigastric artery → inferior epigastric artery → external iliac artery
>
> ***Middle:*** Abdominal aorta → SMA → IMA → superior rectal artery (terminal branch of IMA) → middle/inferior rectal arteries (via the path of Winslow) → retrograde through the internal iliac artery anterior division → external iliac artery
>
> ***Posterior:*** Abdominal aorta → intercostal and lumbar arteries → superior gluteal and iliolumbar arteries (branches of internal iliac artery posterior division) → deep circumflex iliac artery → external iliac artery

Iliac atherosclerotic disease

- Percutaneous interventions are efficacious and well-tolerated for treatment of appropriate aortoiliac atherosclerotic flow-limiting disease. The 2006 second TransAtlantic Inter-Society Consensus (TASC-II) recommendations for treatment of aortoiliac and infrainguinal occlusive disease classify lesions as Types A through D (most severe).
- Percutaneous transluminal angioplasty (PTA) is the treatment of choice for noncalcified, concentric iliac stenoses <3 cm in length (Type A).
- For lesions between 3 and 10 cm in length (Types B and C), either PTA or surgery could be performed. Although the TASC-II guidelines advocate surgery, many institutions would perform primary proximal iliac stenting for lesions >3 cm in length.
- In contrast, PTA has only a limited role in treating stenoses >10 cm (Type D) and in treating occlusions >5 cm after thrombolysis.
- Subsequent to angioplasty, stenting is indicated if there is >30% residual stenosis or >10 mm Hg systolic pressure gradient at rest.

Iliac artery aneurysm

- An iliac artery aneurysm is defined as an iliac artery diameter >1.5 cm. Repair is recommended once the diameter is >3.0 cm.
- Iliac artery aneurysms are typically seen in older men and are associated with abdominal aortic aneurysms. They are most commonly associated with atherosclerosis. Iliac aneurysms may also be due to connective tissue diseases, such as Marfan syndrome.
- Cross-sectional imaging is recommended if an iliac stenosis is seen first on angiography. An iliac aneurysm with intra-luminal thrombus can simulate an atherosclerotic stenosis on angiography.
- In appropriate candidates, endovascular stent-graft is the preferred treatment for an iliac artery aneurysm.
- Mass effect from the aneurysm may cause neurologic and urologic symptoms, in which case surgical treatment is recommended. Endovascular aneurysm repair cannot rapidly decreased aneurysm size, although endovascularly treated aneurysms do gradually decrease in size.

Persistent sciatic artery

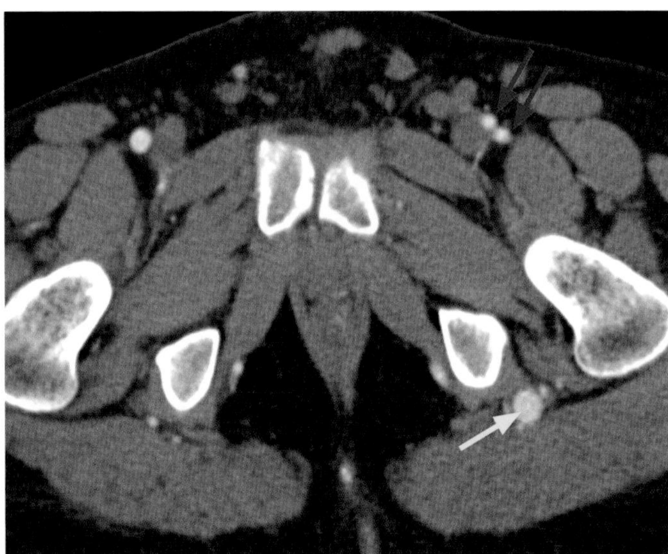
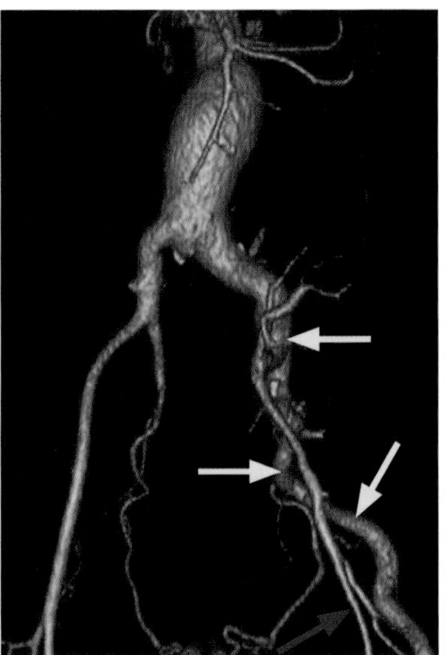

Persistent sciatic artery: Axial CT angiogram (left image) shows an enlarged vessel in the left gluteal region (yellow arrow) between the ischial tuberosity and the gluteus maximus. Two small vessels are present in the left inguinal region (red arrows) instead of a normal common femoral artery.

Three-dimensional volume-rendered reconstruction from the same study (right image) shows an enlarged left internal iliac artery, which continues distally as the persistent sciatic artery (yellow arrows). This patient also has a left femoral artery, although decreased in caliber (red arrow).

Case courtesy Michael Hanley, MD, University of Virginia Health System.

- A persistent sciatic artery is a very rare vascular anomaly where the fetal sciatic artery persists to supply the majority of blood supply to the leg.
- The persistent sciatic artery arises from the internal iliac artery (usually from the inferior gluteal artery) and continues distally to the popliteal artery. A rudimentary femoral artery may be present.
- A persistent sciatic artery may predispose to aneurysm formation.

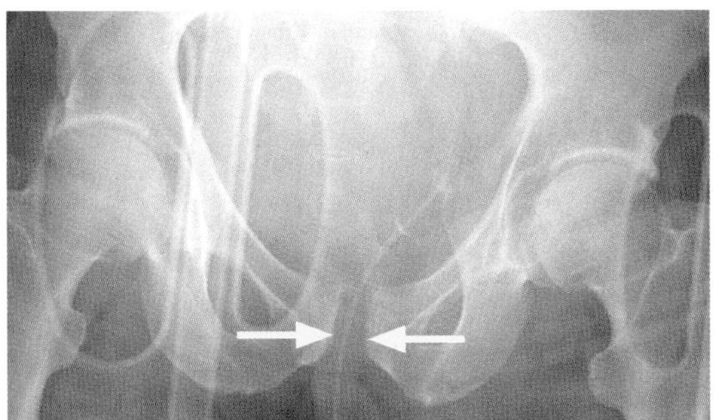

Initial trauma-board pelvic radiograph shows diastasis of the pubic symphysis (arrows).

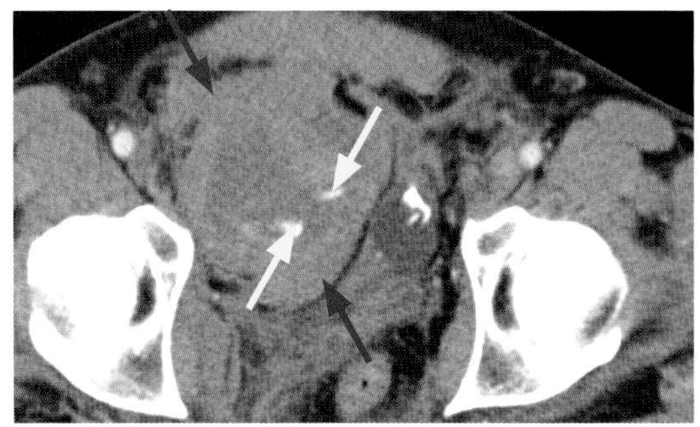

Contrast-enhanced CT shows a large hematoma in the right hemipelvis (red arrows) with foci of active extravasation (yellow arrows).

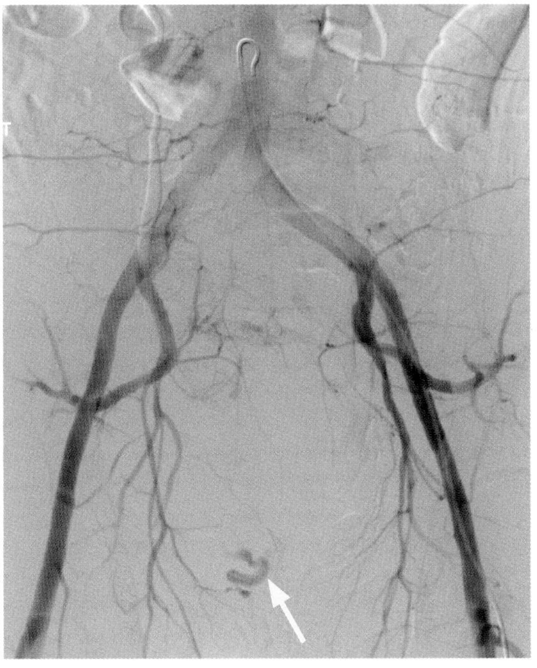

Nonselective arterial-phase DSA angiogram of the internal iliac arteries with the flush catheter in the distal aorta shows a focus of active extravasation (arrow) arising from the right pudendal artery.

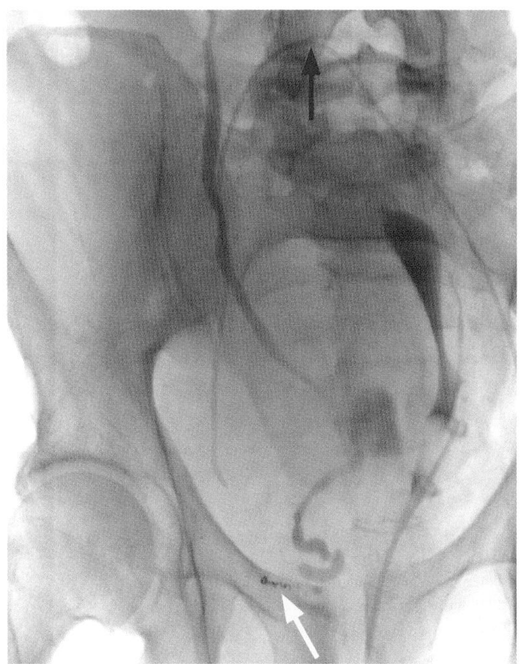

Post-coiling, intra-procedural radiograph shows coils within the right pudendal artery (yellow arrow). Note the catheter (red arrow) in the right internal iliac artery via a left femoral approach.

Case courtesy Alisa Suzuki Han, MD, Brigham and Women's Hospital.

- Pelvic trauma can lead to catastrophic hemorrhage from arterial injury. It is possible to exsanguinate completely within the pelvis: A 3 cm diastasis of the symphysis pubis doubles the potential intra-pelvic volume to approximately 8 liters.
- In the setting of active pelvic bleeding and pelvic fractures, angiography is usually performed *prior* to orthopedic surgery. Active bleeding can be difficult to control surgically.
- The first step in treating a pelvic arterial injury is to perform a nonselective pelvic arteriogram, followed by selective bilateral internal iliac arteriograms of the anterior and posterior divisions.
- Because of the rich collateral supply in the pelvis, rapid nonselective gelfoam embolization of either the entire anterior or posterior division of the internal iliac artery is often acceptable. A potentially time-consuming superselective embolization should be avoided in the setting of life-threatening hemorrhage.

Uterine artery embolization (UAE)

- The two primary indications for uterine artery embolization (UAE) are symptomatic treatment of fibroids and postpartum hemorrhage. Polyvinyl chloride particles are used.
- The goal of fibroid treatment is to produce hemorrhagic infarction of the hypervascular fibroids while still maintaining adequate perfusion to the endometrium and myometrium, thus preserving future fertility.

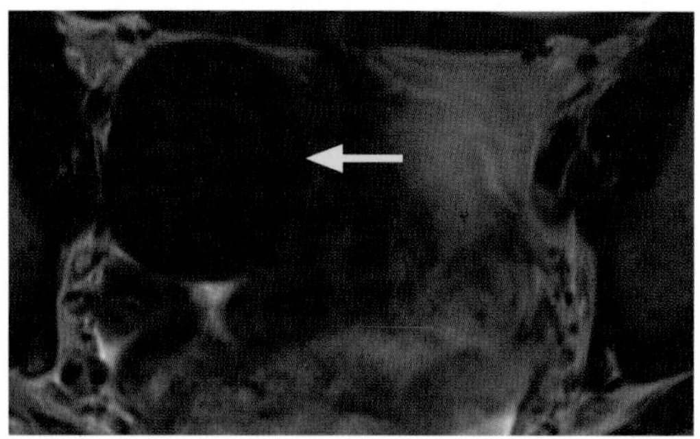

Axial T2-weighted MRI shows a large, hypointense fibroid (arrow).

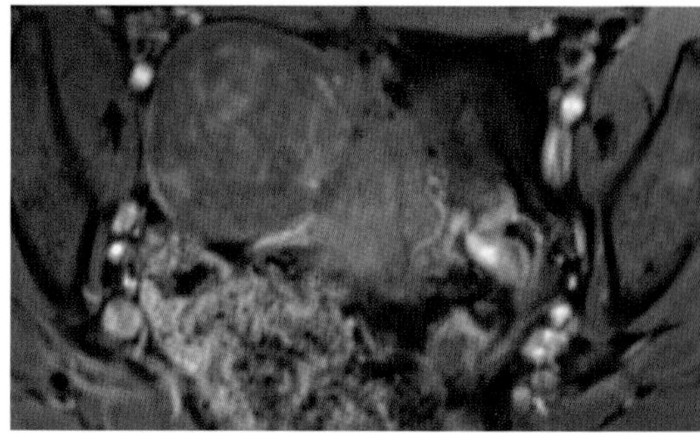

Post-contrast axial T1-weighted MRI shows the avid heterogeneous enhancement of the fibroid.

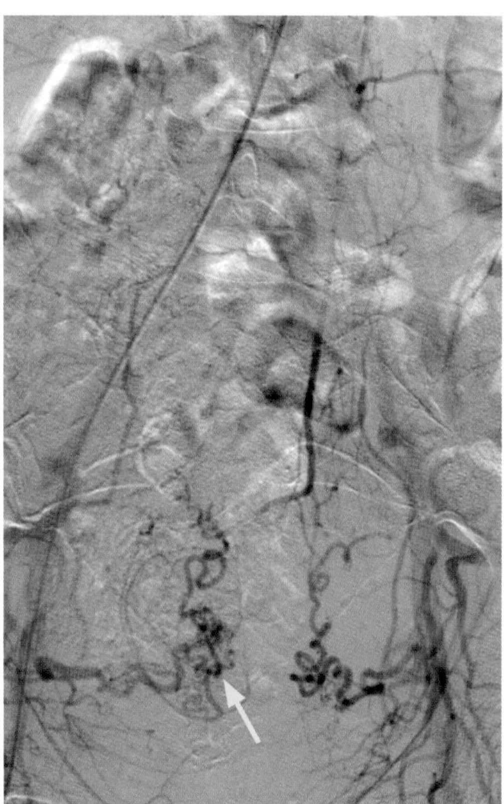

Nonselective late arterial phase digital subtraction angiogram of the internal iliac arteries with the flush catheter in the distal aorta (not visualized) shows the bilateral hypertrophied uterine arteries, more prominent on the right (arrow).

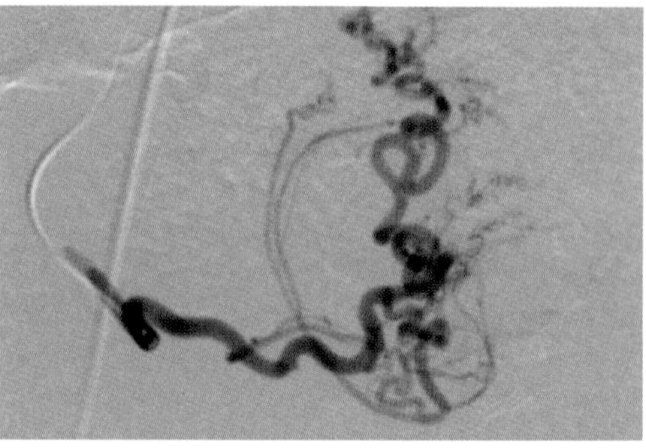

Pre-embolization selective digital subtraction angiogram of the right uterine artery demonstrates the enlarged, tortuous vessels.

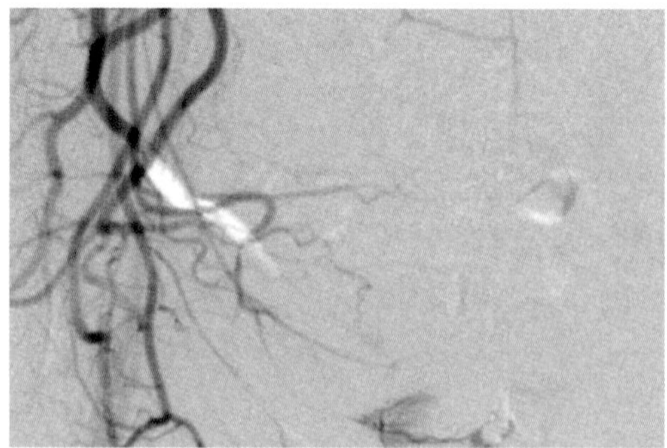

Post-treatment nonselective angiogram of the right internal artery anterior division (catheter not visualized) demonstrates near-stasis of the uterine artery, which is the desired end-point. A small amount of contrast is seen medially in the bladder.

Case courtesy Alisa Suzuki Han, MD, Brigham and Women's Hospital.

- There is approximately a 1.25% serious complication rate for UAE, which is especially important to consider as many of these patients are otherwise healthy reproductive-age women. Serious complications include abscess, endometritis, and ovarian necrosis due to non-target embolization, leading to subsequent premature menopause.

THROMBOEMBOLIC AND ATHEROSCLEROTIC LOWER EXTREMITY DISEASE

Chronic arterial occlusive disease

- Peripheral vascular disease shares risk factors with coronary artery disease, including smoking, diabetes, hypertension, hyperlipidemia, lack of exercise, and family history.
- Clinically, chronic peripheral atherosclerosis presents initially with claudication, which can progress to ischemic rest pain or tissue loss in severe cases.
- Claudication is usually first treated conservatively, with risk factor control, exercise, aspirin, and/or cilostazol (a platelet-aggregation inhibitor with vasodilator action).
- The most common locations for lower extremity atherosclerotic stenoses include the common iliac arteries (discussed previously), superficial femoral artery, popliteal artery, tibioperoneal trunk, and origins of the tibial arteries.
- The Rutherford classification clinically categorizes chronic limb ischemia. Category 0 is asymptomatic, category 1 is mild claudication, categories 2–3 are moderate to severe ischemia, category 4 is ischemic rest pain, and categories 5–6 are minor or major tissue loss, respectively. Revascularization should not be attempted if the limb is not viable.
- An ankle–brachial index (ABI) should be performed in every patient with suspected arterial occlusive disease. The ABI is the ratio of systolic blood pressure (SBP) in the ankles compared to the arms, and is calculated as: ankle SBP/brachial SBP.

  A decreased ABI suggests a hemodynamically significant stenosis between the great vessels and the ankles since the ankle blood pressure is less than the upper extremity blood pressure.

  An ABI <0.9 is abnormal. An ABI between 0.5 and 0.9 usually correlates with intermittent claudication. Rest pain is usually present with an ABI <0.4.
- Pulse-volume recordings characterize the Doppler waveform at multiple levels. The anatomic location of a lesion can be deduced by the change from a normal triphasic waveform to a biphasic (moderate stenosis) or flat waveform (severe stenosis/occlusion).

Femoropopliteal disease

- Similar to aortoiliac disease, the second TransAtlantic Inter-Society (TASC-II) consensus classifies femoropopliteal lesions and gives associated recommendations for intervention.

  Type A: Single stenosis ≤10 cm: ***Endovascular treatment is the treatment of choice.***

  Type B: Multiple lesions (stenosis or occlusion), each <5 cm; single lesion <15 cm: ***Endovascular treatment is preferred, depending on patient's comorbidities and preference.***

  Type C: Multiple stenoses or occlusions >15 cm: ***Surgery is preferred, depending on patient's comorbidities and preference.***

  Type D: Chronic total occlusion: ***Surgery is treatment of choice.***

Acute thromboembolic disease

- Acute limb ischemia is an emergency, with a very different clinical and angiographic presentation compared to chronic atherosclerotic disease. In acute thromboembolic disease, symptom onset is acute, with pain, pallor, poikilothermia (coldness), pulselessness, and paresthesias. *Blue toe syndrome* is acute thromboembolism in the toes.
- The most common embolic source is a left atrial thrombus, with atrial fibrillation a significant risk factor. Echocardiography is indicated in the workup.
- Angiography shows an acute cutoff of the affected vessel, often with a *meniscus* sign. Significant atherosclerotic disease may be absent.
- Treatment options include surgical embolectomy, surgical bypass graft, and endovascular thrombolysis. When attempting to treat endovascularly, a hydrophilic wire is used to cross the lesion. A multi-sidehole infusion catheter is placed across the thrombus and tissue plasminogen activator (tPA) is infused at 0.5 mg/h for 48–72 hours.

- While receiving intra-arterial tPA, the patient must be cared for in the ICU, with regular monitoring of hematocrit and fibrinogen. TPA infusion should be slowed if the fibrinogen decreases to <150 mg/dL and stopped if it reaches <100 mg/dL.

Popliteal aneurysm

- A popliteal artery aneurysm is defined as a popliteal artery measuring 8 mm or more.
- Popliteal aneurysms are almost always due to atherosclerosis and are associated with other atherosclerotic aneurysms. Approximately 20% of patients with a popliteal aneurysm also have an aortic aneurysm, and up to half have bilateral popliteal aneurysms.
- Popliteal aneurysms are usually asymptomatic. When symptomatic, the typical presenting symptom is distal ischemia due to embolism. Popliteal aneurysm rupture is rare.
- Treatment is recommended for all symptomatic popliteal artery aneurysms and asymptomatic aneurysms >2 cm in diameter.
- Treatment is with endovascular stent-graft or surgical bypass.

NON-ATHEROSCLEROTIC LOWER EXTREMITY ARTERIAL DISEASE

Buerger disease

- Buerger disease is a medium and small vessel occlusive vasculitis that affects the lower extremities (most commonly) and the hands (less commonly). It is seen in adult male smokers and should be clinically suspected in a middle-aged male presenting with claudication.
- On angiography, there are segmental stenoses of the medium and small arteries in the leg, with typical *corkscrew* collaterals in the vasa vasorum.
- The larger arteries, including the common femoral artery, superficial femoral artery, and popliteal artery, are typically spared.
- Primary treatment of Buerger disease is smoking cessation.

Popliteal entrapment syndrome

- Popliteal entrapment syndrome is compression of the popliteal artery by a calf muscle or fibrous band, most commonly an aberrant medial head of the gastrocnemius. It is an important cause of exercise-induced claudication in healthy young males. Bilateral involvement is common.
- There are six different types of popliteal entrapment, depending on the deviation of the aberrant muscle and the popliteal artery. However, by far the most common anomalies involve the medial head of the gastrocnemius, with either medial deviation (type I) or no deviation (type II) of the popliteal artery.
- Treatment is surgical release of the offending muscle (usually the medial head of the gastrocnemius). Angiography is only used for diagnosis, not therapy.

Cystic adventitial disease

- Cystic adventitial disease is a rare cause of distal claudication where one or more mucoid cysts in the adventitia surrounding the popliteal artery leads to lumenal compression.
- Clinically, most patients are middle-aged men presenting with claudication.
- MRI is the best diagnostic tool, as the cystic component can be readily identified with typical T2 hyperintensity.
- Treatment is surgical resection of the cyst or surgical bypass. Cyst aspiration can also be performed, but the cyst almost always recurs.

NORMAL VASCULAR ANATOMY OF THE UPPER EXTREMITY

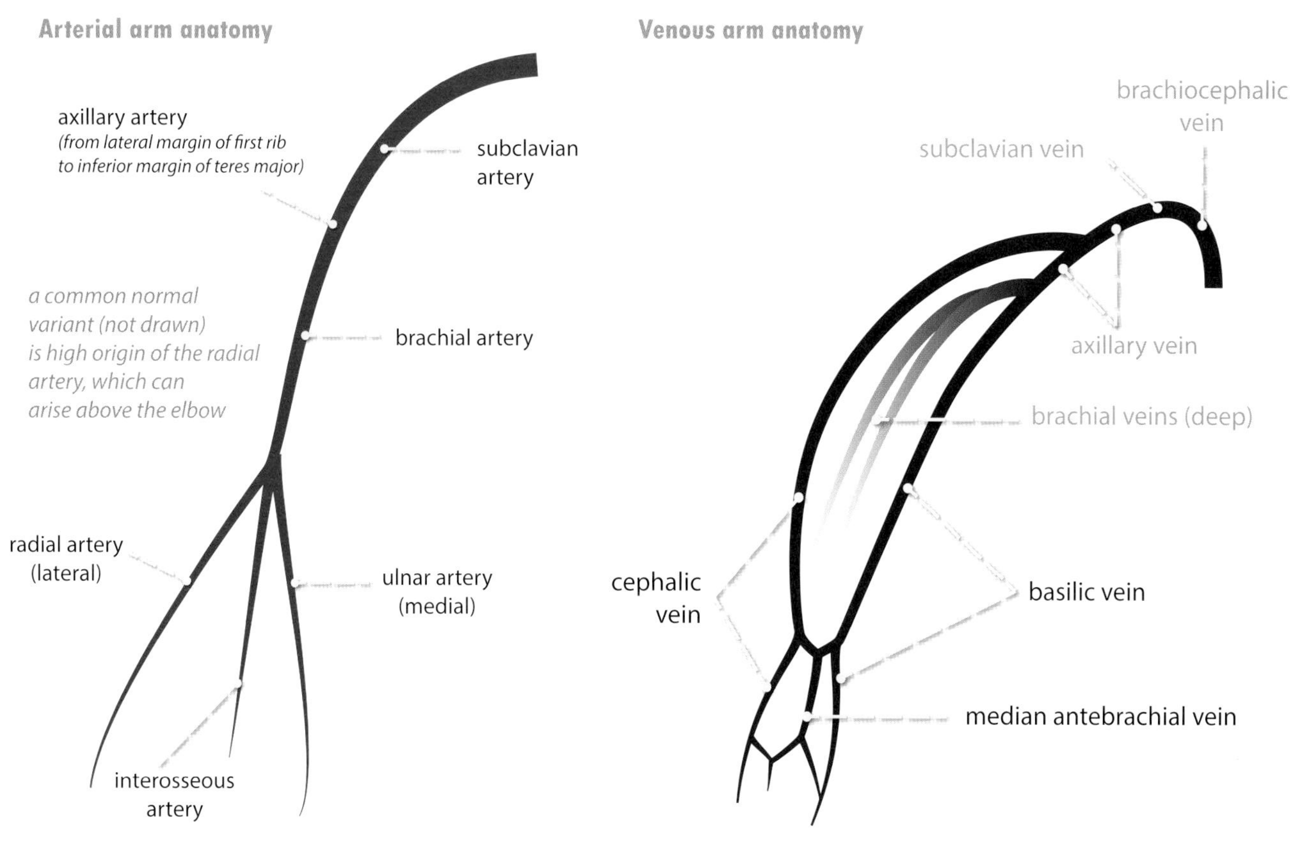

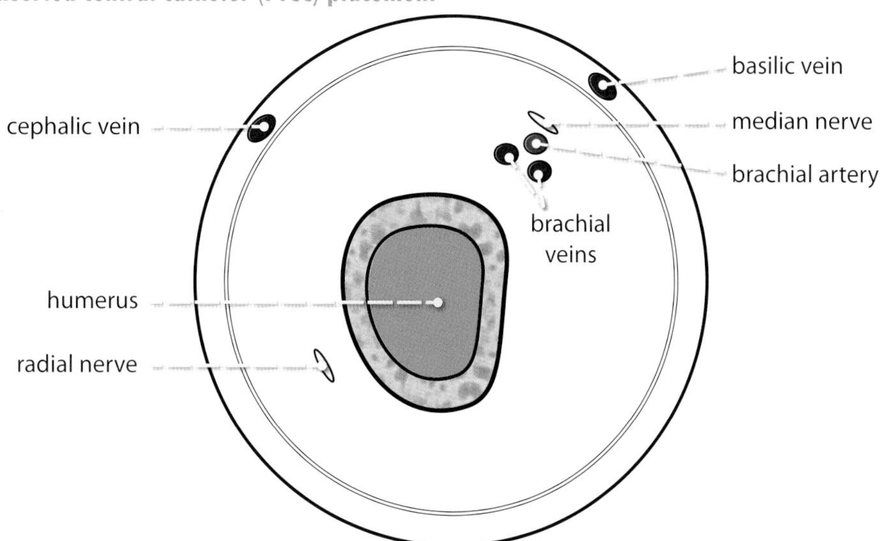

- The basilic vein, located medial and superficial to the brachial veins, is the first choice for peripherally inserted catheter (PICC) placement. The cephalic vein adds an extra curve as it joins the axillary/subclavian vein, but is generally the second choice if the basilic is not available. There is risk of damaging the median nerve with placement in a brachial vein as the median nerve lies superficial to the brachial veins.
- A PICC should not be placed in a patient with chronic renal failure who may need a fistula in the future. Central access using the neck veins should be used instead.

THORACIC OUTLET SYNDROMES (TOS)

Overview of thoracic outlet syndromes

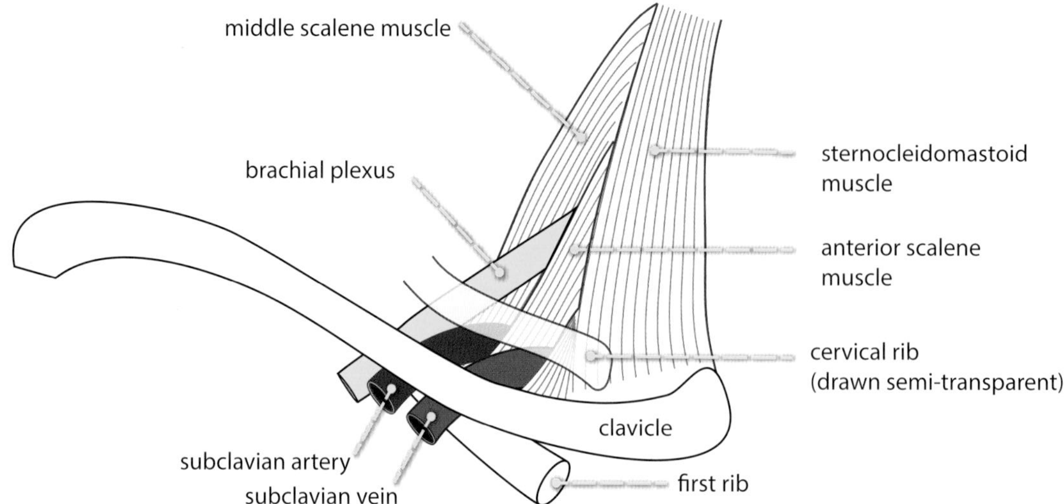

- *Thoracic outlet* syndromes are a controversial spectrum of disorders caused by compression of either the brachial plexus, subclavian artery, or subclavian vein, clinically presenting with upper extremity paresthesias, pain, numbness, and/or coolness.
- The interscalene triangle is the space bounded by the anterior scalene muscle, the middle scalene muscle, and the first rib. The brachial plexus and subclavian artery pass through the interscalene triangle.
- In contrast, the subclavian vein does not pass through the interscalene triangle, but instead runs anterior to the anterior scalene muscle.

Neurogenic thoracic outlet syndrome

- The neurogenic form of thoracic outlet syndrome is the most common manifestation, due to mechanical compression of the brachial plexus.

Subclavian artery compression

- Compression of the subclavian artery clinically presents with hand or finger pain, numbness, paresthesias, or coolness. Raynaud phenomenon is common. Raynaud phenomenon is intermittent distal vasospasm caused by cold temperature or other external stimuli.
- Symptoms worsen with arm abduction.
- **Adson's maneuver** is a test for subclavian artery compression at the thoracic outlet. First, the radial artery is palpated in neutral position. Then, the patient's head is turned to the contralateral side while they inhale. In arterial thoracic outlet syndrome, the radial pulse will be reduced with this maneuver.
- A mechanical compression is almost always present. Over 70% of patients with subclavian artery compression have a cervical rib. Other causes of subclavian artery compression include an accessory scalene muscle (scalenus minimus), enlargement of the anterior scalene muscle, and well-developed musculature.
- Potential complications include arterial mural thrombus, aneurysm, and distal embolization. The hands should always be evaluated for signs of distal emboli.
- The preferred treatment of subclavian artery compression is surgical thoracic outlet decompression (e.g., resection of a cervical rib) and repair of the subclavian artery if an aneurysm is present. Endovascular arterial thrombolysis may be performed adjunctively, weighed against the risk for distal embolization.

Paget-Schroetter syndrome (subclavian vein compression)

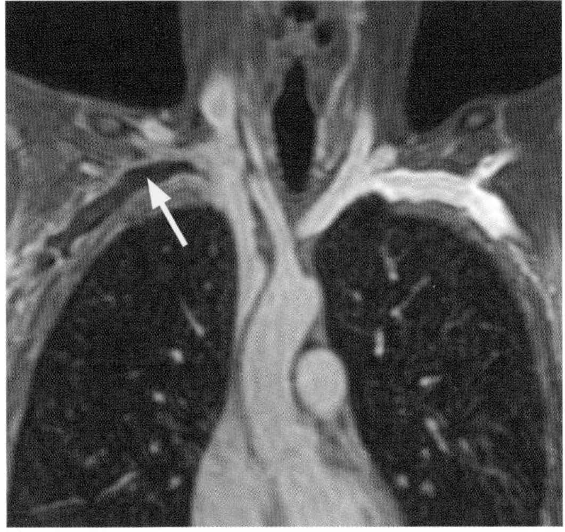

Coronal contrast-enhanced MR venography with arms abducted demonstrates right subclavian vein thrombus (arrow). The MRI did not demonstrate a mechanical cause for the thrombosis.

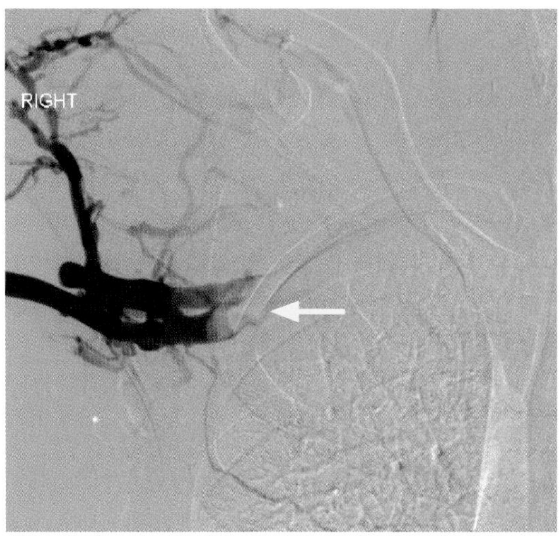

Diagnostic venography confirms complete occlusion of the right subclavian vein (arrow) with complete lack of opacification of the SVC and the formation of numerous collaterals.

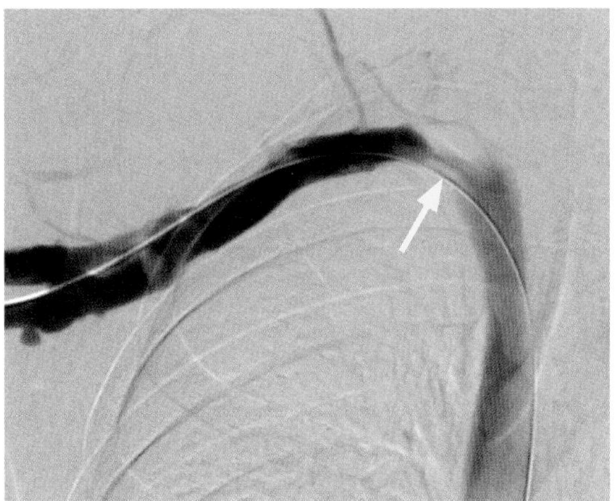

24 hours after continuous thrombolysis infusion, the subclavian vein is patent, with a residual stenosis at the subclavian/brachiocephalic confluence (arrow).

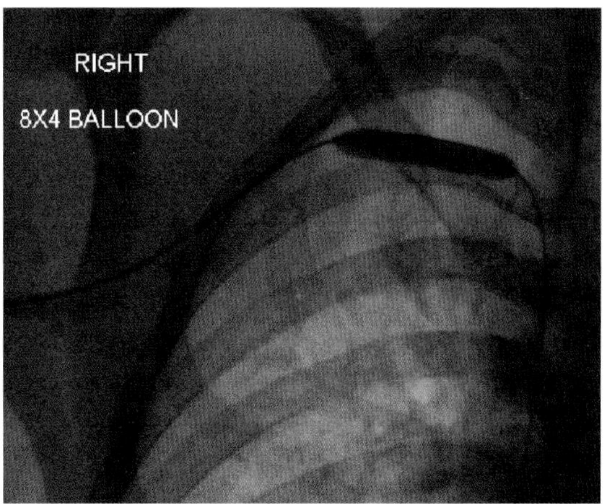

Because the MRI confirmed lack of mechanical obstruction, an 8 mm x 4 cm angioplasty balloon was used at the site of stenosis.

Case courtesy Alisa Suzuki Han, MD, Brigham and Women's Hospital.

- Paget–Schroetter syndrome is compression and thrombosis of the subclavian vein as it enters the thorax and is usually seen in muscular young men. Chronic compression causes intimal hyperplasia, which leads to subclavian vein thrombosis. Paget–Schroetter syndrome clinically presents with upper-extremity swelling or pain worsened with effort.
- During diagnostic venography, it is necessary to evaluate the arm both in neutral position and abducted. Both sides should be evaluated. Frequently, both subclavian veins are compressed, even if only one side is symptomatic.
- Treatment is thrombolysis, then subsequently surgical thoracic outlet decompression.
- If there is residual stenosis following thrombolysis, surgical decompression should generally be performed prior to angioplasty. However, if pre-procedure imaging demonstrated no mechanical cause, then angioplasty can be performed, as in the case above.
- Stents should generally not be used, especially if there is a mechanical obstruction, due to high risk of device failure.

MISCELLANEOUS PROXIMAL UPPER EXTREMITY DISEASE

Subclavian steal syndrome

- Subclavian steal syndrome is a proximal stenosis or occlusion of the subclavian artery, which leads to retrograde flow from the vertebral artery into the subclavian artery distal to the flow-limiting lesion.
- Subclavian steal syndrome clinically presents with vertebrobasilar insufficiency or syncope exacerbated by arm exercise. There may occasionally be direct signs of brachial artery insufficiency, such as extremity coolness or even fingertip necrosis.
- Subclavian steal is best diagnosed with angiography. The early arterial phase shows the proximal subclavian flow-limiting lesion and the later arterial phase shows retrograde flow from the vertebral artery into the subclavian.
- Treatment options include surgical bypass or angioplasty of the flow-limiting lesion.

SURGICAL DIALYSIS ACCESS

Arteriovenous fistula

- A surgical fistula for dialysis access provides good long-term patency (85% at two years), but requires several months to "mature" and about 30% of fistulas fail to mature. A fistula is mature when the veins have enlarged sufficiently to allow the high flow rates for dialysis.
- Once mature, a fistula can remain patent even with relatively low flow rates.
- The two common fistula locations are:

  Radial artery → cephalic vein at the wrist

  Brachial artery → variable veins in the forearm
- Common causes of late fistula failure include venous outflow stenosis and perianastomotic venous stenosis.

Polytetrafluorethylene (PTFE) graft

- A polytetrafluorethylene (PTFE) graft is a short bridge of synthetic graft material placed surgically between an adjacent artery and vein. Grafts have only 50% patency at 2 years, but are able to be used sooner than fistulas. Grafts require higher flow rates to remain patent compared to fistulas.
- Similar to a fistula, the most common cause of graft failure is a venous stenosis, either at the venous anastomosis or outflow vein.

Clinical evaluation of surgical dialysis access

- A pulsatile fistula with lack of thrill suggests venous outflow obstruction.
- High access recirculation at dialysis suggests venous outflow stenosis.
- Weak pulse and poor thrill suggests arterial inflow stenosis.
- A pulseless fistula suggests thrombosed fistula.

Venous stenosis of surgical dialysis access

- Venous outflow stenoses are typically treated with angioplasty, often requiring high-pressure or cutting balloons to dilate the fibrotic lesions.
- The goal of the procedure is to restore a palpable thrill and pulse, or to restore the venous to brachial artery pressure ratio to less than 0.4.

Thrombosis of surgical dialysis access

- Both arteriovenous fistulas and PTFE grafts may become thrombosed. In general, PTFE grafts are simpler to declot compared to fistulas as the thrombus is usually limited to the graft.

- Thrombosis is often secondary to venous stenosis, which must be treated as well.
- Either pharmacologic or mechanical thrombolysis can be performed.

Hand

Hypothenar hammer

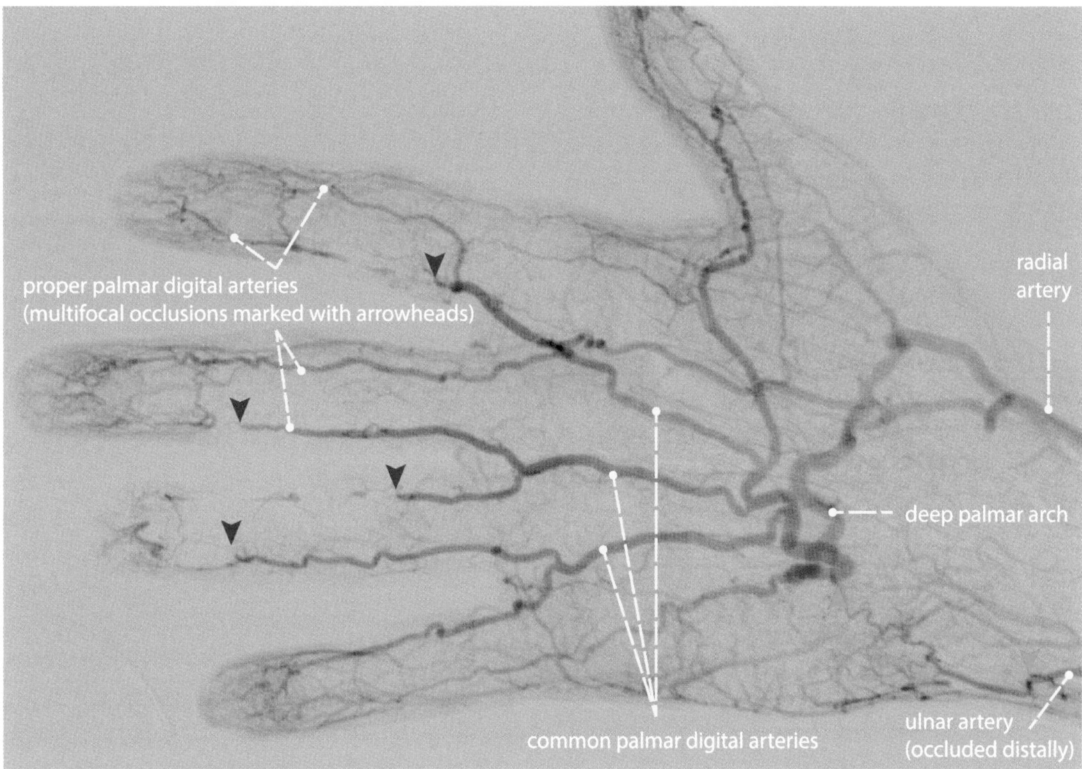

Hypothenar hammer: Digital subtraction angiogram of the hand shows an approximately 2–3 cm occlusion of the ulnar artery (between the blue arrowheads), and multifocal occlusions of the proper palmar digital arteries in the 2nd through 4th digits (red arrowheads).

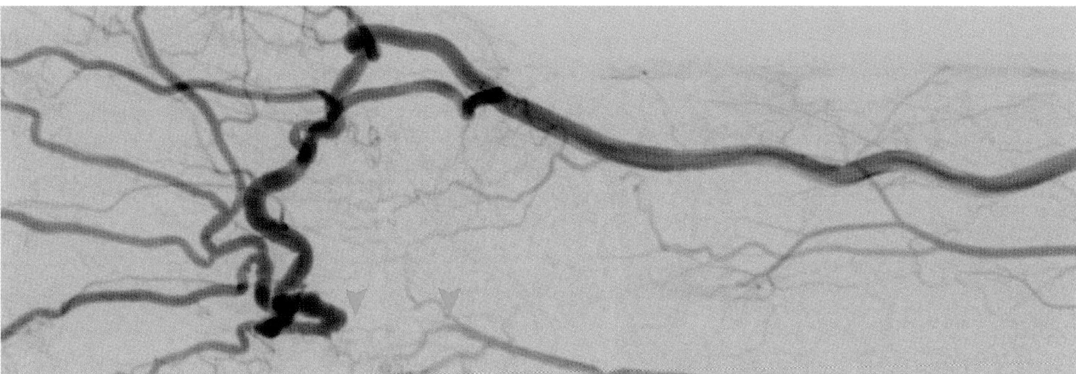

Digital subtraction angiogram of the wrist better shows the segmental occlusion of the ulnar artery (between the blue arrowheads). At surgery, an ulnar artery aneurysm (not visible on angiography) was found and treated.

Case courtesy Alisa Suzuki Han, MD, Brigham and Women's Hospital.

- Hypothenar hammer syndrome represents injury to the ulnar artery as it crosses the hamate bone. Chronic repetitive trauma causes the ulnar artery to be chronically traumatized at the hamate, leading to intimal injury, thrombus, aneurysm, or pseudoaneurysm.
- The classic clinical history of hypothenar hammer syndrome is a jackhammer operator with ischemia of the fourth and fifth digits.

- Imaging shows occlusion of the ulnar artery, often with distal embolic occlusions due to distal thrombi, usually in the 4th and 5th fingers (but 3rd finger also seen in the case above).
- Treatment is surgical, as there is often ulnar artery injury not apparent on angiography.

Buerger disease

- As previously discussed, Buerger disease is a small and medium vessel vasculitis that typically occurs in male smokers. It more commonly involves the legs but may also involve the hands, where it may present with ischemia, ulcerations, and even gangrene.
- Small vessel occlusions and prominent *corkscrew* collaterals are the typical angiographic features.

Raynaud disease

- Raynaud disease is small arterial vasospasm triggered by cold temperature.
- On imaging, there is decreased perfusion of the distal digital arteries, with improvement upon warming or vasodilator administration.
- Reynaud disease is associated with scleroderma and other connective tissue disorders.

Thromboembolic disease

- Thromboembolic disease of the upper extremities is most commonly caused by cardiac emboli (of which atrial fibrillation is a common cause). Less commonly, a subclavian artery aneurysm may be the source of the thrombus.
- If the source of emboli is central (such as the heart), bilateral disease would be expected, while a unilateral lesion would show unilateral emboli.
- The characteristic imaging feature of distal thromboembolic disease is occlusion of distal small arteries of the hand.

General References:

Kaufman, J. & Lee, M. Vascular and Interventional Radiology. The requisites (1st ed.). Mosby. (2004).

Mauro, M., Murphy, K., Thomson, K., Zollikofer, C. Image-Guided Intervention. Elsevier. (2008).

Valge, K. Vascular and Interventional Radiology (2nd ed.). Saunders. (2006).

Thoracic Angiography:

Pelage, J.P. et al. Pulmonary Artery Interventions: An Overview 1. Radiographics, 25(6), 1653–67(2005).

Yoon, W. et al. Bronchial and Nonbronchial Systemic Artery Embolization for Life-threatening Hemoptysis: A Comprehensive Review. Radiographics, 22(6), 1395-409(2002).

Mesenteric Vascular Anatomy:

Einstein, A.J. et al. Images in vascular medicine the Arc of Riolan: diagnosis by magnetic resonance angiography. Vascular medicine (London, England), 10(3), 239(2005).

Lange, J.F. et al. Riolan's arch: confusing, misnomer, and obsolete. A literature survey of the connection(s) between the superior and inferior mesenteric arteries. American Journal of Surgery, 193(6), 742-8(2007).

Moon, J.J., Wijdicks, C.A. & Williams, J.M. Right hepatic artery branching off the superior mesenteric artery and its potential implications. International Journal of Anatomical Variations, 2, 143-5(2009).

Ozbülbül, N.I. CT angiography of the celiac trunk: anatomy, variants and pathologic findings. Diagnostic and Interventional Radiology (Ankara, Turkey), 17(2), 150-7(2011).

Rosenblum, J.D., Boyle, C.M. & Schwartz, L.B. The Mesenteric Circulation: Anatomy and Physiology. Surgical Clinics of North America, 77(2), 289-306(1997).

Walker, T.G. Mesenteric Vasculature and Collateral Pathways. AJR. American Journal of Roentgenology, 1(212), 167-74(2009).

Splenic and Renal Arteries:

Cianci, R. et al. Revascularization versus medical therapy for renal artery stenosis: antihypertensive drugs and renal outcome. New England Journal of Medicine, 361, 1953-62(2009).

Lee, Y.J., Oh, S.N., Rha, S.E. & Byun, J.Y. Renal trauma. Radiologic Clinics of North America, 45(3), 581-92, ix(2007).

Madoff, D.C. et al. Splenic arterial interventions: anatomy, indications, technical considerations, and potential complications. Radiographics, 25 Suppl 1, S191-211(2005).

Non-variceal GI Bleeding:

Geffroy, Y. & Rodallec, M. Multidetector CT angiography in acute gastrointestinal bleeding: why, when, and how. Radiographics, 31, 32–6(2011).

Green, B.T. & Rockey, D.C. Lower gastrointestinal bleeding–management. Gastroenterology Clinics of North America, 34(4), 665-78(2005).

Hastings, G.S. Angiographic localization and transcatheter treatment of gastrointestinal bleeding. Radiographics, Inc, 20(4), 1160-8(2000).

Loffroy, R. et al. Embolization of acute nonvariceal upper gastrointestinal hemorrhage resistant to endoscopic treatment: results and predictors of recurrent bleeding. Cardiovascular and Interventional Radiology, 33(6), 1088-100(2010).

Millward, S.F. ACR Appropriateness Criteria on treatment of acute nonvariceal gastrointestinal tract bleeding. Journal of the American College of Radiology: JACR, 5(4), 550-4(2008).

Arterial, Venous, and Visceral Abdomo-Pelvic Compression Syndromes:

Gander, S., Mulder, D.J., Jones, S. & Ricketts, J.D. Recurrent abdominal pain and weight loss in an adolescent: Celiac artery compression syndrome. Canadian Journal of Gastroenterology, 24(2), 2009-11(2010).

Horton, K.M., Talamini, M.A. & Fishman, E.K. Median Arcuate Ligament Syndrome: Evaluation with CT Angiography 1. Radiographics, 25(5), 1177–82(2005).

Kurklinsky, A.K. & Rooke, T.W. Nutcracker phenomenon and nutcracker syndrome. Mayo Clinic Proceedings. Mayo Clinic, 85(6), 552-9(2010).

Manghat, N.E., Mitchell, G., Hay, C.S. & Wells, I.P. The median arcuate ligament syndrome revisited by CT angiography and the use of ECG gating – a single centre case series and literature review. The British Journal of Radiology, 81(969), 735-42(2008).

Portal Hypertension and TIPS:

Kumar, A., Sharma, P. & Sarin, S.K. Hepatic venous pressure gradient measurement: time to learn! Indian Journal of Gastroenterology, 27(2), 74-80(2008).

Madoff, D., Hicks, M. & Vauthey, J. Transhepatic Portal Vein Embolization: Anatomy, Indications, and Technical Considerations. Radiographics 1, 22, 1063-76(2002).

Owen, A.R., Stanley, A.J., Vijayananthan, A. & Moss, J.G. The transjugular intrahepatic portosystemic shunt (TIPS). Clinical radiology, 64(7), 664-74. (2009).

Percutaneous Nephrostomy:

Dyer, R., Regan, J. & Kavanagh, P. Percutaneous Nephrostomy with Extensions of the Technique: Step by Step. Radiographics, 22, 503-25(2002).

Lower Extremity Angiography:

Hai, Z. et al. CT angiography and MRI in patients with popliteal artery entrapment syndrome. AJR. American Journal of Roentgenology, 191(6), 1760-6(2008).

Dieter, R.S., Dieter, R.A.J. & Dieter, R.A.I. Peripheral Arterial Disease. New York: McGraw Hill. (2009).

Norgren, L. et al. Inter-Society Consensus for the Management of Peripheral Arterial Disease (TASC II). Journal of Vascular Surgery, 45 Suppl S(Tasc li), S5-67(2007).

Sakamoto, I. et al. Endovascular treatment of iliac artery aneurysms. Radiographics, 25, S213-27(2005).

Uterine Artery Embolization:

Kitamura, Y., Ascher, S. & Cooper, C. Imaging Manifestations of Complications Associated with Uterine Artery Embolization 1. Radiographics, 25, 119-33(2005).

Upper Extremity Angiography:

Bittl, J.A. Catheter interventions for hemodialysis fistulas and grafts. JACC. Cardiovascular Interventions, 3(1), 1-11(2010).

Hooper, T.L., Denton, J., McGalliard, M.K., Brismée, J.-M. & Sizer, P.S. Thoracic outlet syndrome: a controversial clinical condition. Part 1: anatomy, and clinical examination/diagnosis. The Journal of Manual & Manipulative Therapy, 18(2), 74-83(2010).

Hooper, T.L., Denton, J., McGalliard, M.K., Brismée, J.-M. & Sizer Jr, P.S. Thoracic outlet syndrome: a controversial clinical condition. Part 2: non-surgical and surgical management. Journal of Manual & Manipulative Therapy, 18(3), 132-8(2010).

Huang, J.H. & Zager, E.L. Thoracic Outlet Syndrome. Neurosurgery, 55(4), 897-903(2004).

11 Pediatric imaging

Contents

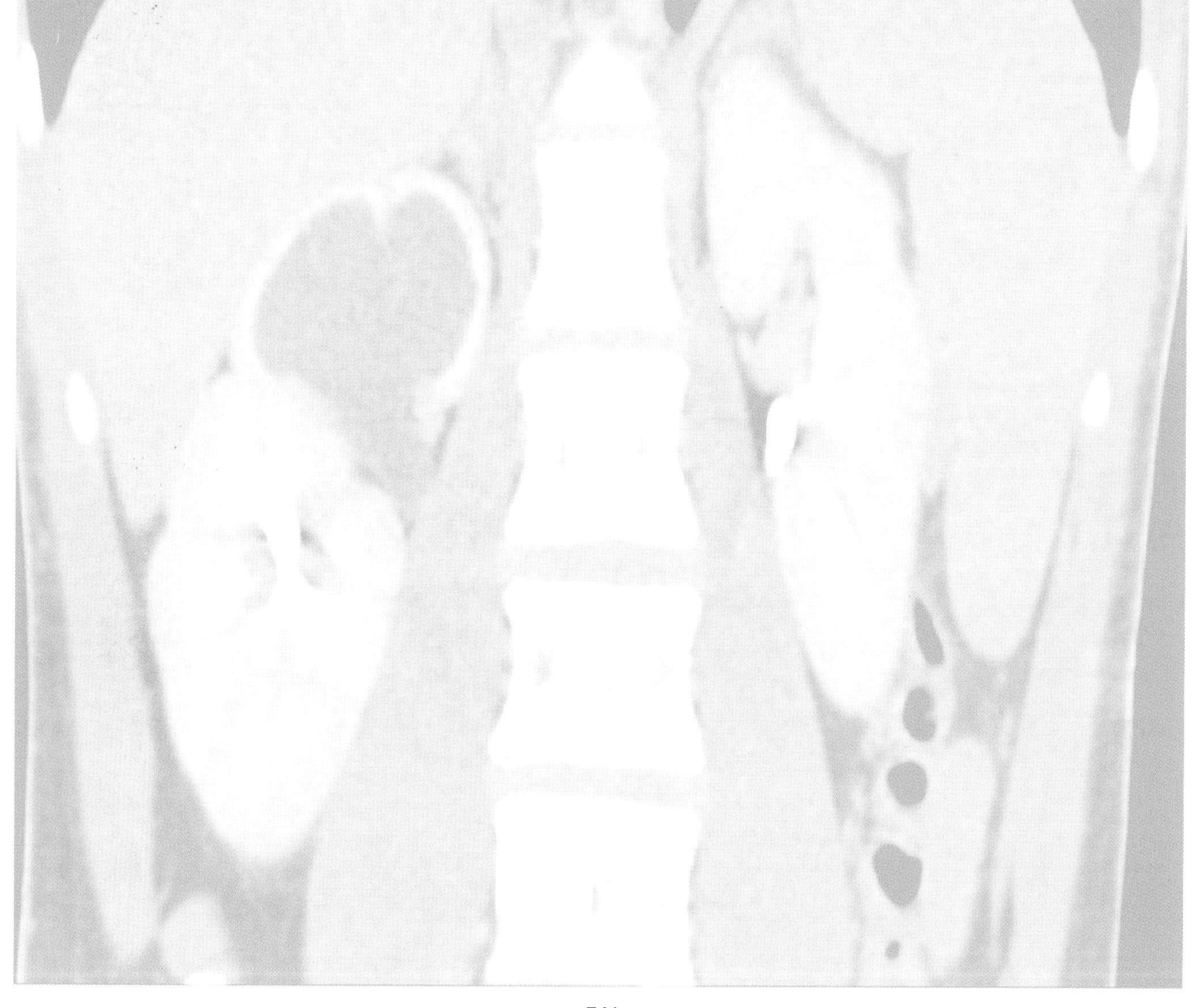

ANATOMY

normal lateral neck radiograph

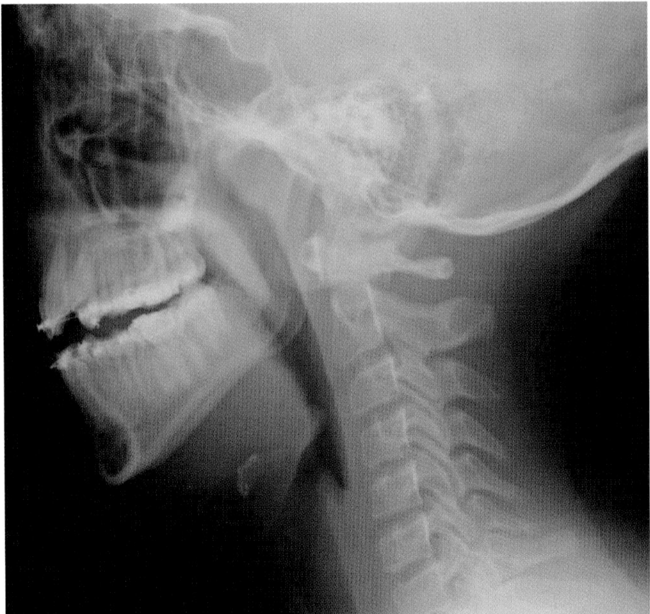

normal lateral neck radiograph with labels

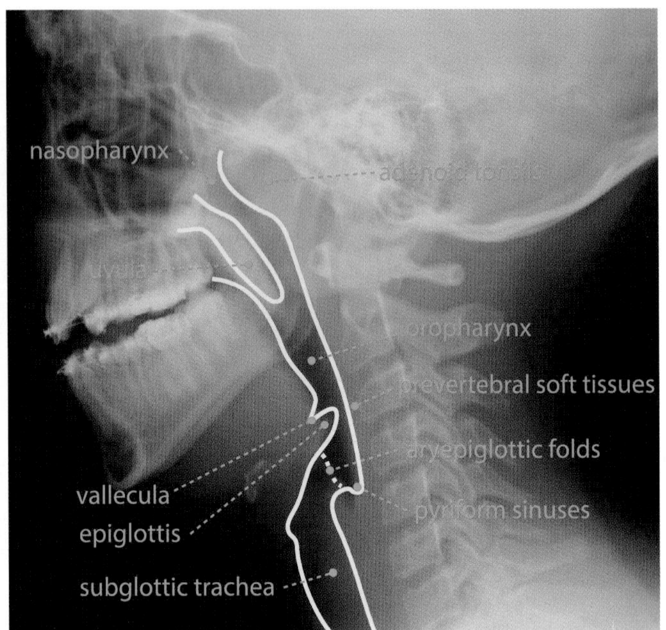

sites of pathology that can be seen on the lateral neck radiograph

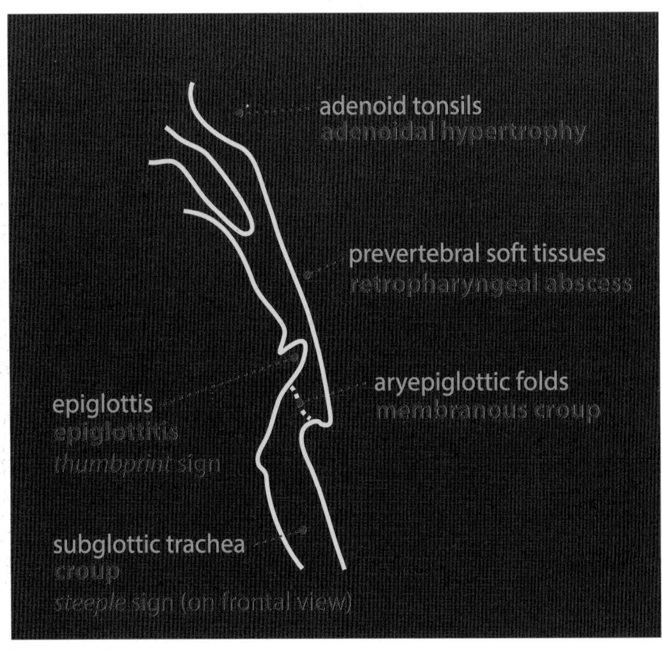

Pediatric upper airway obstruction

- Upper airway obstruction above the level of the trachea can be congenital (choanal atresia), neoplastic (rhabdomyosarcoma), or infectious (peritonsillar abscess).
- Upper airway obstruction can also be classified by anatomic level: Nasal and nasopharyngeal (choanal atresia, rhabdomyosarcoma, adenoidal hypertrophy), or oropharyngeal (peritonsillar abscess, thyroglossal duct cyst).

Choanal atresia

- Choanal atresia is congenital occlusion of the choanae in the posterior nasal cavity.

  Choanal atresia can be osseous, membranous, or mixed. There is almost always some degree of osseous abnormality, with approximately 70% of cases mixed and 30% of cases being a pure bony atresia.

- Choanal atresia is often associated with other congenital malformations, most commonly **CHARGE syndrome**:

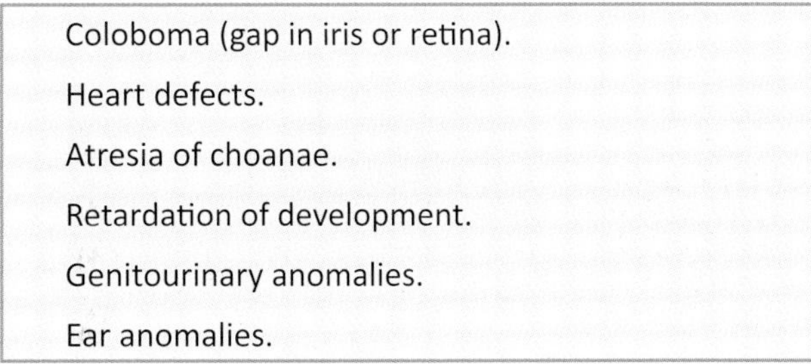

Coloboma (gap in iris or retina).
Heart defects.
Atresia of choanae.
Retardation of development.
Genitourinary anomalies.
Ear anomalies.

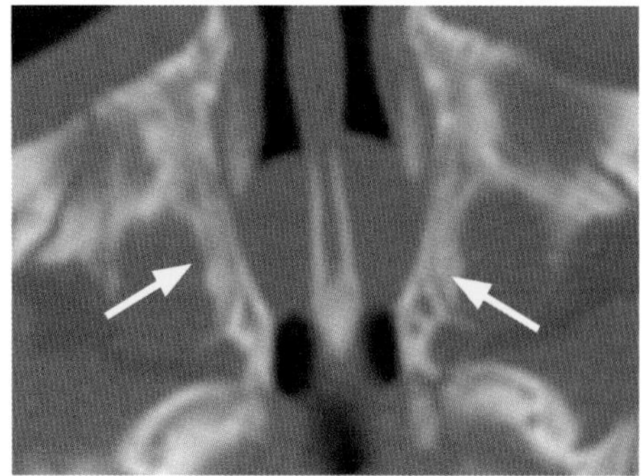

Choanal atresia, mixed membranous and bony: Axial noncontrast CT shows complete obstruction of both choanae by soft tissue, with medial bowing of the thickened lateral nasal walls (arrows) and medialization of the pterygoid plates. This child had CHARGE syndrome.

Case courtesy Sanjay Prabhu, MBBS, Boston Children's Hospital.

Juvenile nasopharyngeal angiofibroma (JNA)

- Juvenile nasopharyngeal angiofibroma is a highly vascular, benign hamartomatous lesion seen in adolescent males. It typically originates at the sphenopalatine foramen and spreads into the nasopharynx and pterygopalatine fossa, causing bony remodeling along the way.

  The primary differential is nasal rhabdomyosarcoma, which causes bony destruction.

  For an image of JNA, please refer to the head and neck chapter in the neuroimaging section.

Nasal rhabdomyosarcoma

- Nasal rhabdomyosarcoma is the most common childhood soft-tissue sarcoma, with the head and neck a common primary site. It presents as a highly aggressive mass.

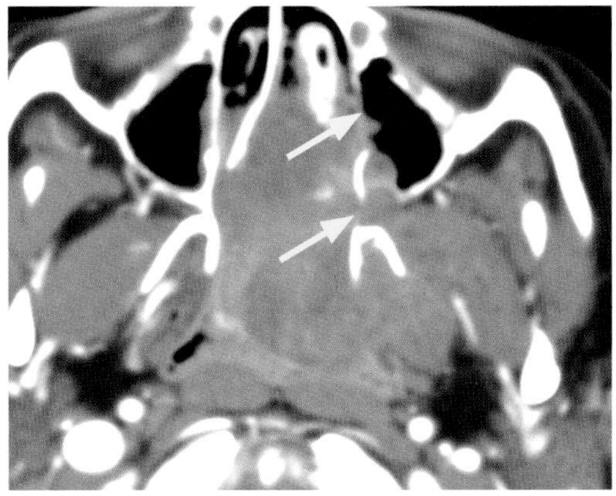

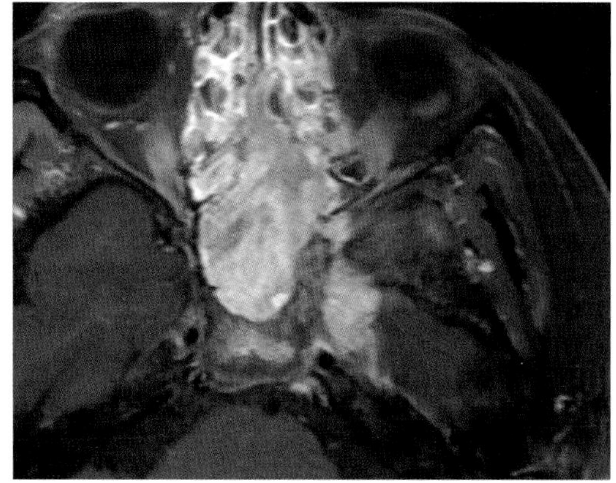

Nasal rhabdomyosarcoma: Axial contrast-enhanced CT (left image) and axial fat-suppressed post-contrast T1-weighted MRI at a higher level (right image) shows a destructive, avidly enhancing mass invading the nasopharynx and causing bony destruction of the left posterior wall of the maxillary sinus and pterygoid plates (yellow arrows). There is invasion into the left medial temporal lobe (red arrow) apparent on MRI.

Epiglottitis

- Epiglottitis is infectious inflammation of the epiglottis. A very rare disease in the era of *Haemophilus influenza* immunization, epiglottitis is a true emergency as the airway can obstruct without warning. Modern cases tend to be seen in immunosusceptible individuals, such as HIV patients or transplant recipients.
- The classic radiographic findings of epiglottitis are thickening of the epiglottis seen on the lateral view (the *thumbprint* sign) in conjunction with thickening of the aryepiglottic folds.

Croup (laryngotracheobronchitis)

- Croup is a viral (usually parainfluenza) infection with characteristic inspiratory stridor and barking cough. It affects infants and toddlers. Croup is a clinical diagnosis. The purpose of radiography is to evaluate for other causes of stridor.
- The *steeple* sign is seen on the frontal view and represents loss of the normal shouldering of the subglottic trachea. There may be "ballooning" of the hypopharynx on the lateral view.

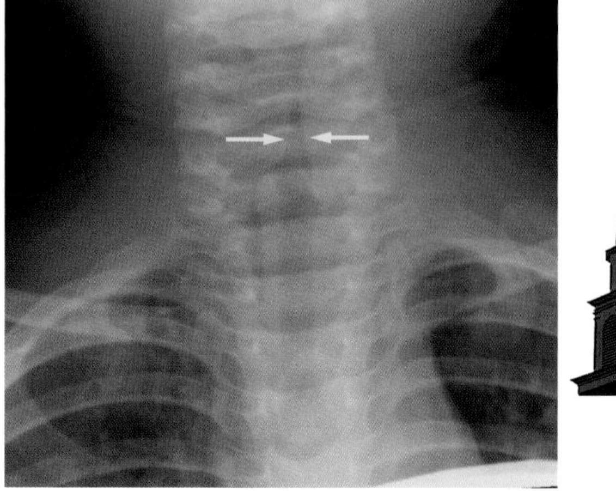
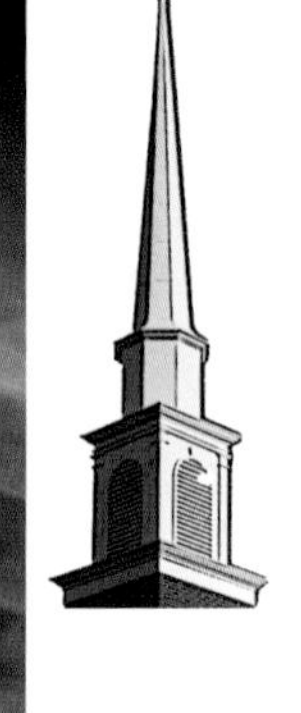

Steeple sign in croup: Frontal radiograph shows symmetric narrowing of the subglottic trachea and loss of the normal shouldering, simulating a steeple.

Aspirated foreign body

- Radiography can't directly visualize a radiolucent foreign body, although secondary signs of air trapping can suggest the diagnosis.
- Decubitus radiographs can be performed to look for non-physiologic persistent expansion of the dependent lung, signifying an obstruction on the persistently expanded side.

Retropharyngeal abscess

- Retropharyngeal abscess is purulent infection of the retropharyngeal space and is one of the more common causes of nontraumatic prevertebral soft tissue swelling in children.
- Retropharyngeal *pseudothickening* can be seen if a radiograph is obtained in neck flexion.
- A retropharyngeal abscess rarely presents with air in the retropharyngeal tissues unless a foreign body has perforated the esophagus.
- CT is usually necessary to determine the nature of radiographic retropharyngeal swelling. In addition to retropharyngeal abscess, the differential of nontraumatic prevertebral swelling includes retropharyngeal cellulitis, lymphoma, and foregut duplication cyst.

  Retropharyngeal cellulitis appears similar to pharyngeal abscess on radiography, but no drainable fluid collection is seen on CT.

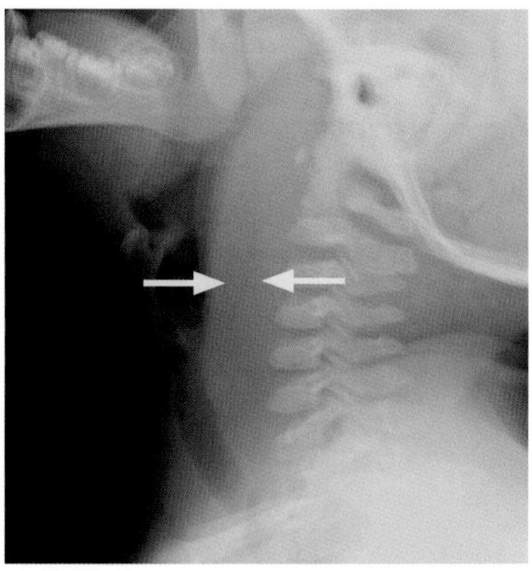

Retropharyngeal abscess: Lateral neck radiograph shows marked thickening of the prevertebral tissues (arrows). Although nonspecific, this patient had a retropharyngeal abscess.

Exudative (bacterial) tracheitis

- Exudative tracheitis may clinically present similarly to epiglottitis with fever, stridor, and respiratory distress, and is also potentially life-threatening.
- In contrast to croup, exudative tracheitis tends to affect older children and is bacterial in etiology (most commonly *S. aureus*).
- On imaging, intraluminal membranes may be visible in the subglottic and cervical trachea.

Subglottic hemangioma

- A subglottic hemangioma is a benign vascular neoplasm that produces stridor in infancy. It is the most common pediatric subglottic tracheal mass.
- Subglottic hemangioma is often associated with cutaneous hemangiomata.
- The classic radiographic finding is **asymmetric** narrowing of the subglottic trachea on the frontal view, although a hemangioma may also cause symmetric narrowing.

Laryngeal papillomatosis

- Laryngeal papillomatosis is a cause of multiple laryngeal nodules due to HPV infection, resulting in thick and nodular vocal cords. Papillomatosis increases the risk of laryngeal squamous cell carcinoma (analogous to cervical cancer risk from HPV).
- Papillomas may rarely seed the lungs, causing multiple cavitary nodules.

Tracheal stenosis

- Iatrogenic tracheal stenosis (e.g., due to prolonged intubation) may be a cause of stridor.
- Congenital tracheal stenosis is usually associated with vascular anomalies, discussed in the following section.

Tracheobronchomalacia

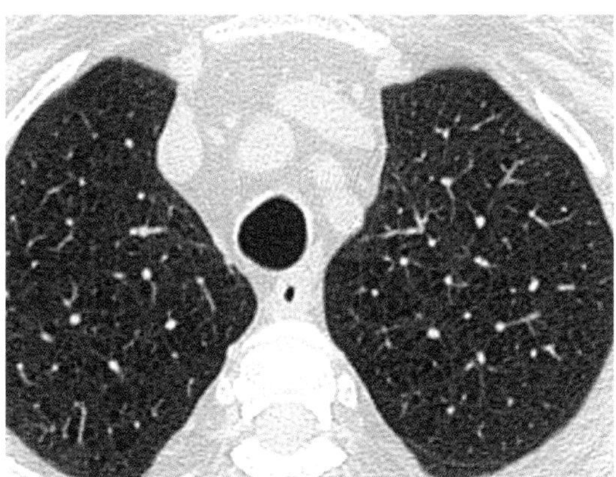

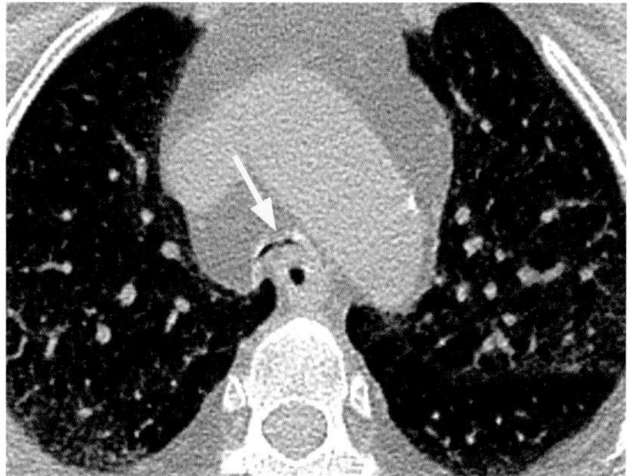

Tracheomalacia: Inspiratory CT (left image) demonstrates the normal, slightly ovoid shape of the trachea. Expiratory CT (right image) in the same patient shows excessive tracheal collapse (arrow). This example is from an adult with mild emphysema.

Case courtesy Michael Hanley, MD, University of Virginia Health System.

- Tracheobronchomalacia causes excessive expiratory airway collapse from weakness of the tracheobronchial cartilage. Tracheobronchomalacia may be either congenital or acquired secondary to intubation, infection, or chronic inflammation.
- A standard inspiratory CT may be normal. Either expiratory CT or dynamic airway fluoroscopy is necessary to diagnose tracheobronchomalacia.
- Greater than 50% reduction in cross-sectional area of the airway lumen is suggestive of tracheomalacia, although normal patients may achieve this threshold with a forceful expiration.

VASCULAR RINGS AND SLING

- Rings and slings are important vascular causes of stridor in infancy and childhood. The typical initial evaluation is with barium esophagram, followed by CT or MRI if abnormal.
- Complete encircling of the trachea and esophagus by the aortic arch or great vessels is a vascular *ring*.
- A vascular *sling* refers to an anomalous course of the left pulmonary artery, which arises aberrantly from the right pulmonary artery and traps the trachea in a “sling” on three sides.
- An important clue to a potential vascular cause of stridor is a **right sided aortic arch** visualized on the frontal radiograph.

  The pulmonary artery sling is the only vascular anomaly that causes stridor in a patient with a normal (left) aortic arch.
- The three most important vascular causes of stridor are double aortic arch, right arch with aberrant left subclavian artery, and pulmonary sling. Each of these will show abnormality on the lateral radiograph or esophagram.

  The double aortic arch and right arch with aberrant left subclavian artery look the same on radiography/esophagram, each producing a posterior impression on the esophagus.

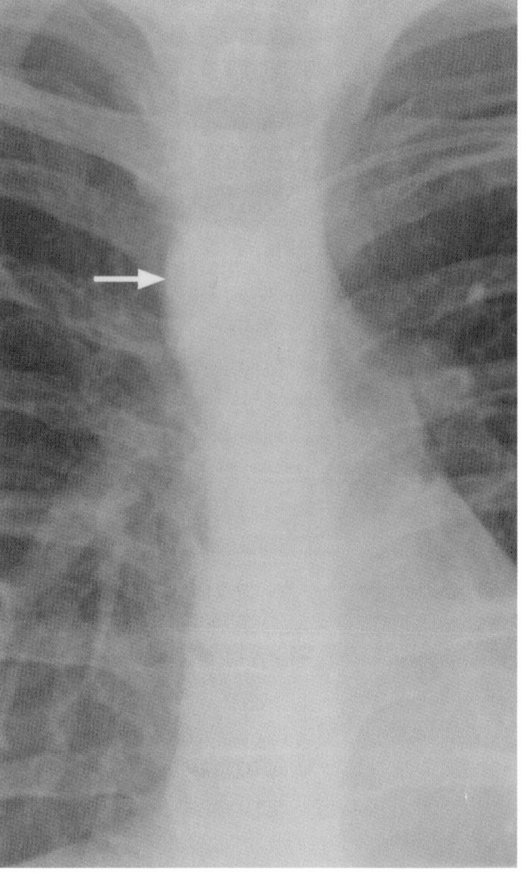

Frontal chest radiograph shows a right-sided aortic arch (arrow), which could be a clue to a vascular cause of stridor.

Normal anatomy

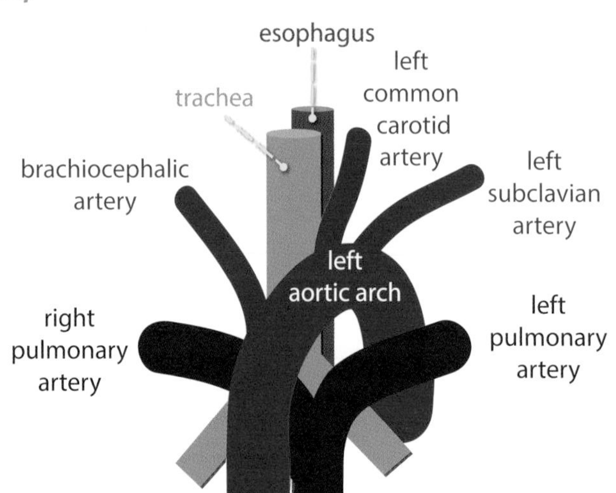

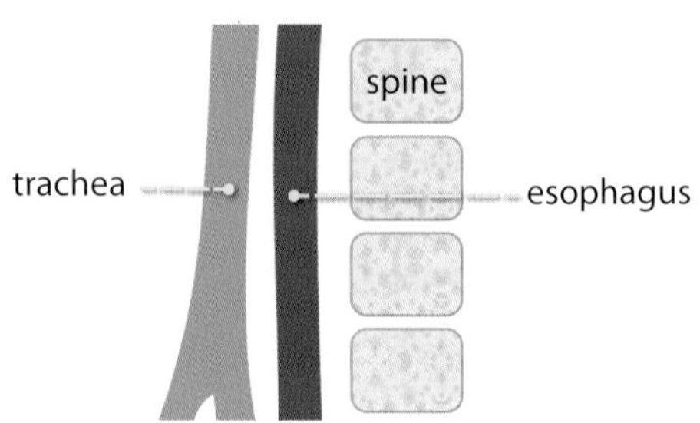

A normal lateral view (either esophagram or radiograph, diagrammed above) shows a smooth contour of the esophagus and trachea, without any abnormal impressions.

Double aortic arch

- Double aortic arch is the most common vascular ring. The arches encircle both the trachea and esophagus, and may cause stridor.
- The right arch is usually superior and larger in caliber than the left.
- For presurgical planning, the goal of the radiologist is to determine which arch is dominant, typically with MR; the surgeon will then ligate the non-dominant arch to alleviate the stridor.

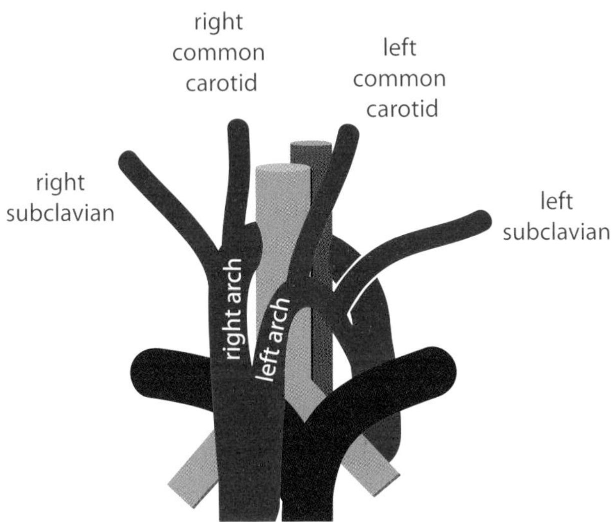

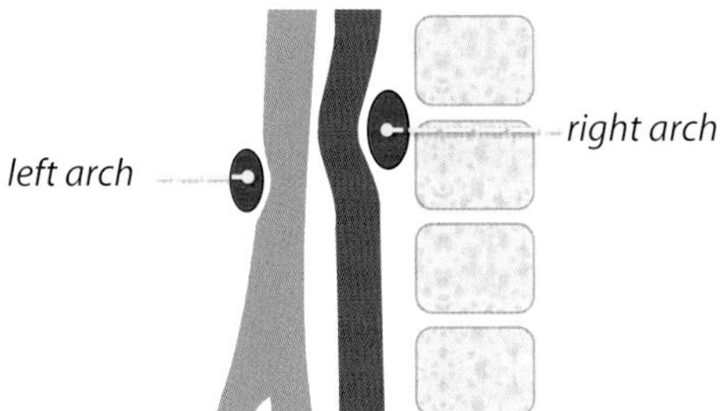

On the lateral schematic (above), there is a posterior indentation of the esophagus (caused by the right arch) and an anterior indentation of the trachea (caused by the left arch).

The anatomic schematic to the left shows complete encircling of both the trachea and the esophagus by the double arches. There may be bilateral impressions on both the trachea and esophagus from the arches.

Right arch with aberrant left subclavian artery

- The second most common vascular ring is a right aortic arch with an aberrant left subclavian artery. The right arch indents the anterior trachea while the aberrant left subclavian artery wraps posteriorly around the esophagus. The ring is completed by the ligamentum arteriosum.

  In contrast, the more common anatomical variant of a **left** arch with an aberrant **right** subclavian artery (discussed on the next page) is a (usually) asymptomatic normal variant that is not a vascular ring.

- On the frontal view, a right arch with aberrant left subclavian artery produces a leftward impression/deviation of the trachea by the right aortic arch.

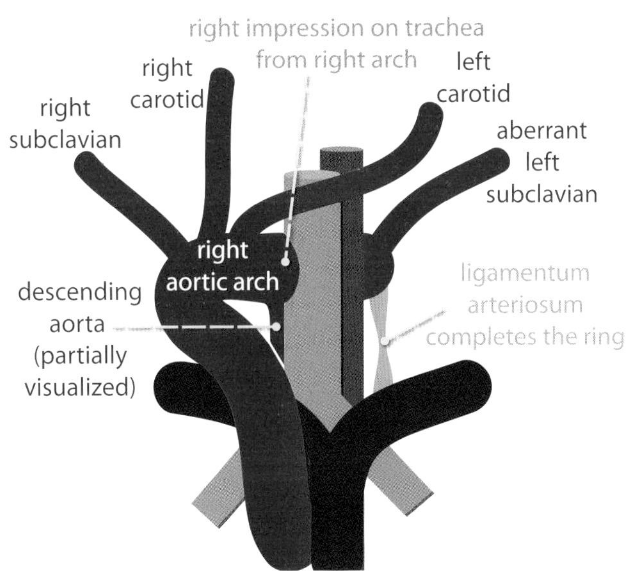

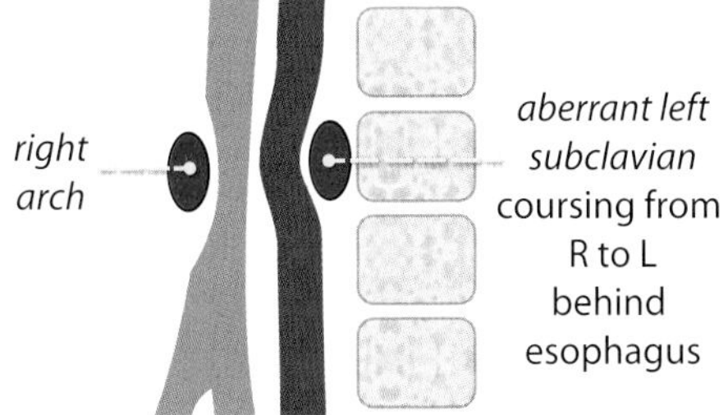

The lateral esophagram shows anterior not reliably dentation of the trachea (by the impression of the right arch) and posterior impression on the esophagus (by the aberrant left subclavian artery).

Radiographic and fluoroscopic findings are not reliably indistinguishable from the double aortic arch described above. CT or MRI is necessary for definitive diagnosis.

Pulmonary sling: Anomalous origin of the left pulmonary artery from the right pulmonary artery

- An anomalous *left* pulmonary artery, arising from the right pulmonary artery, forms a sling by coursing in between the trachea and esophagus. Usually only the trachea is trapped in the sling, but occasionally the bronchus intermedius may also be compressed.
- Pulmonary artery sling is the only vascular cause of stridor in a patient with a left arch. The aortic branching pattern is normal.
- Pulmonary artery sling is associated with tracheal anomalies including tracheomalacia and bronchus suis (RUL bronchus originating from trachea).

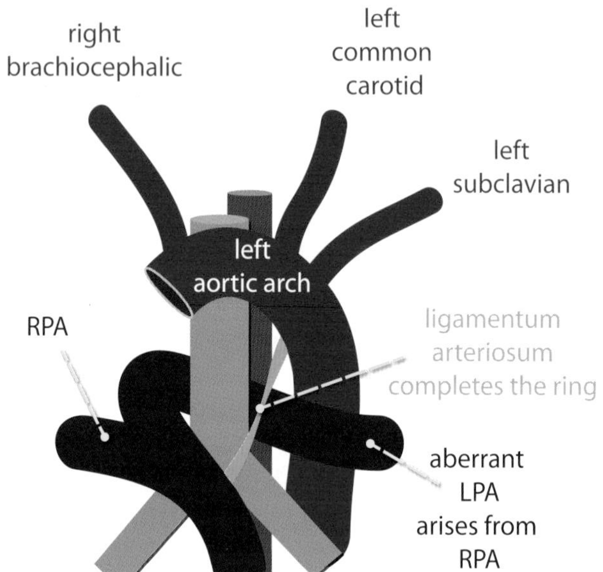

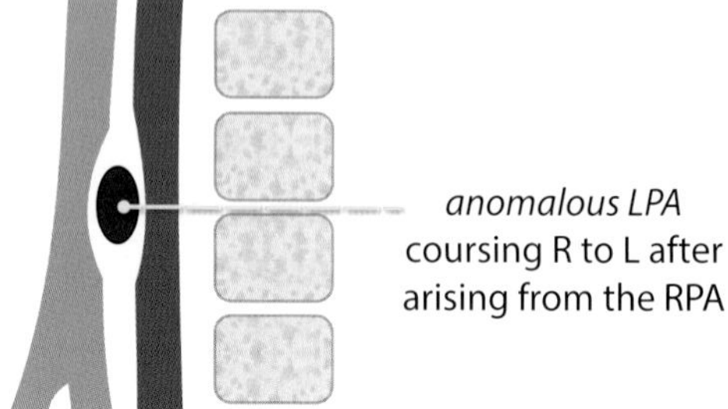

The key radiographic finding of pulmonary artery sling, seen on a lateral esophagram, is posterior indentation of the trachea and anterior indentation of the esophagus. The anomalous left pulmonary artery (LPA) runs in between the trachea and the esophagus.

(RPA = right pulmonary artery; LPA = left pulmonary artery)

Left aortic arch with aberrant right subclavian artery

- A left aortic arch with an aberrant right subclavian artery is not a ring or a sling, and is not a cause of stridor. It almost never causes symptoms, but in the rare case that it does, dysphagia may result, which is called *dysphagia lusoria*.

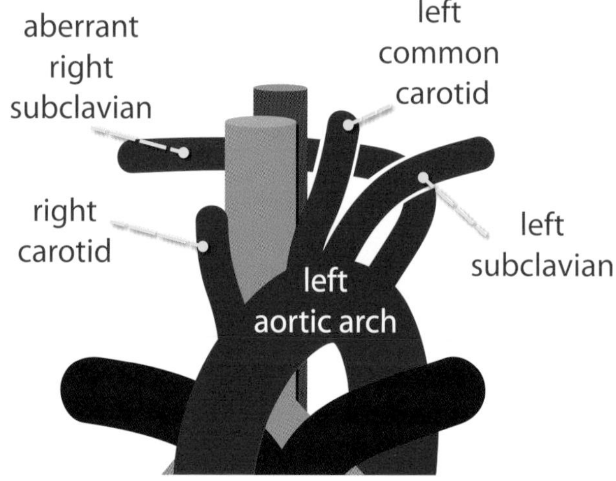

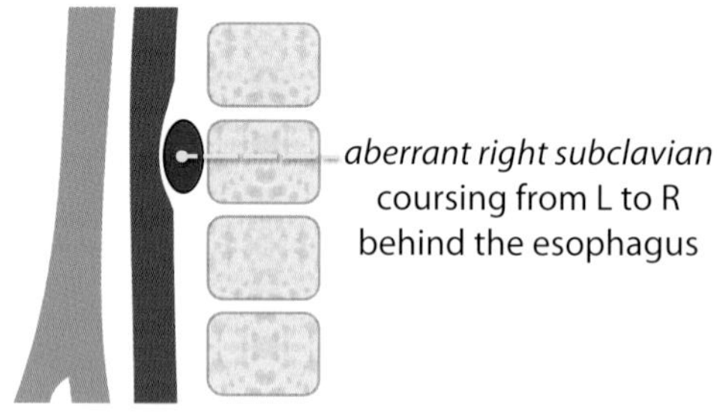

The lateral esophagram (above) shows a small posterior indentation on the esophagus.

Schematic diagram (left) demonstrates the aberrant right subclavian coursing posterior to the esophagus.

Innominate artery syndrome

- In infants, the large thymus can occasionally cause the normal innominate artery to press against the anterior trachea, potentially producing innominate artery syndrome.
- Innominate artery syndrome is not a vascular ring, and it is controversial whether this entity is a clinically relevant form of breathing difficulty.

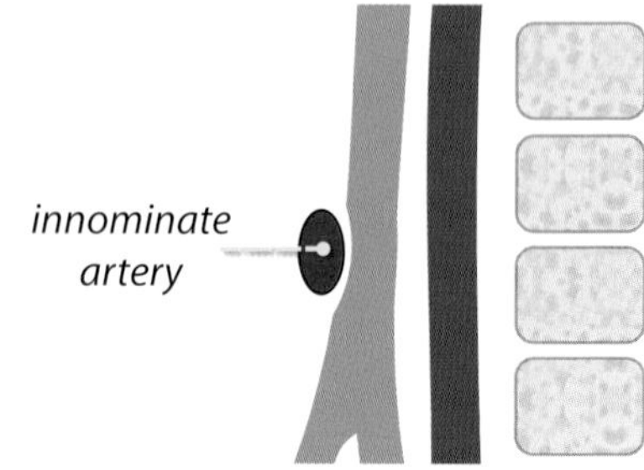

Summary of vascular impressions with a posterior esophageal impression

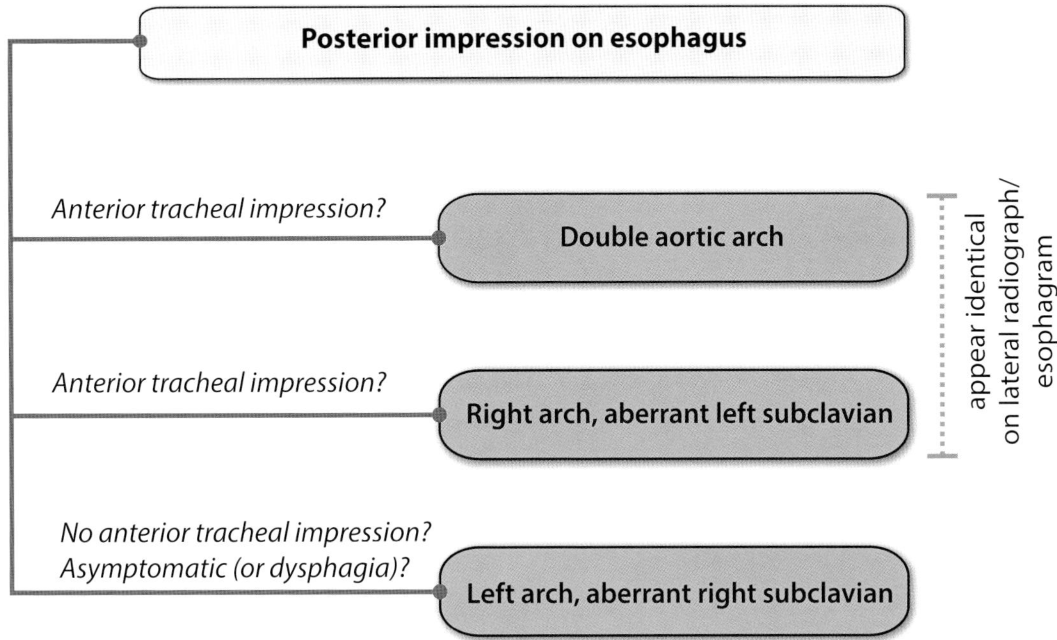

- Double aortic arch or right arch with aberrant left subclavian artery:

  These two rings may appear identical on the lateral esophagram or radiograph. In addition to a posterior esophageal impression, both will also feature an anterior impression on the trachea.

  Both entities may cause stridor.

- Left aortic arch with aberrant right subclavian artery:

  This entity is rarely symptomatic. It would cause dysphagia if it produced any symptoms at all.

  Esophageal impression is often *smaller* compared to the other two above entities.

Summary of vascular impressions with an anterior esophageal impression

- Pulmonary artery sling:

  Pulmonary artery sling is the only vascular ring or sling to produce an *anterior* impression on the esophagus. Since the aberrant pulmonary artery runs between the trachea and esophagus, it also produces a *posterior* tracheal impression.

  Pulmonary artery sling is also the only congenital vascular cause of stridor with a left aortic arch.

MEDICAL RESPIRATORY DISTRESS IN THE NEWBORN

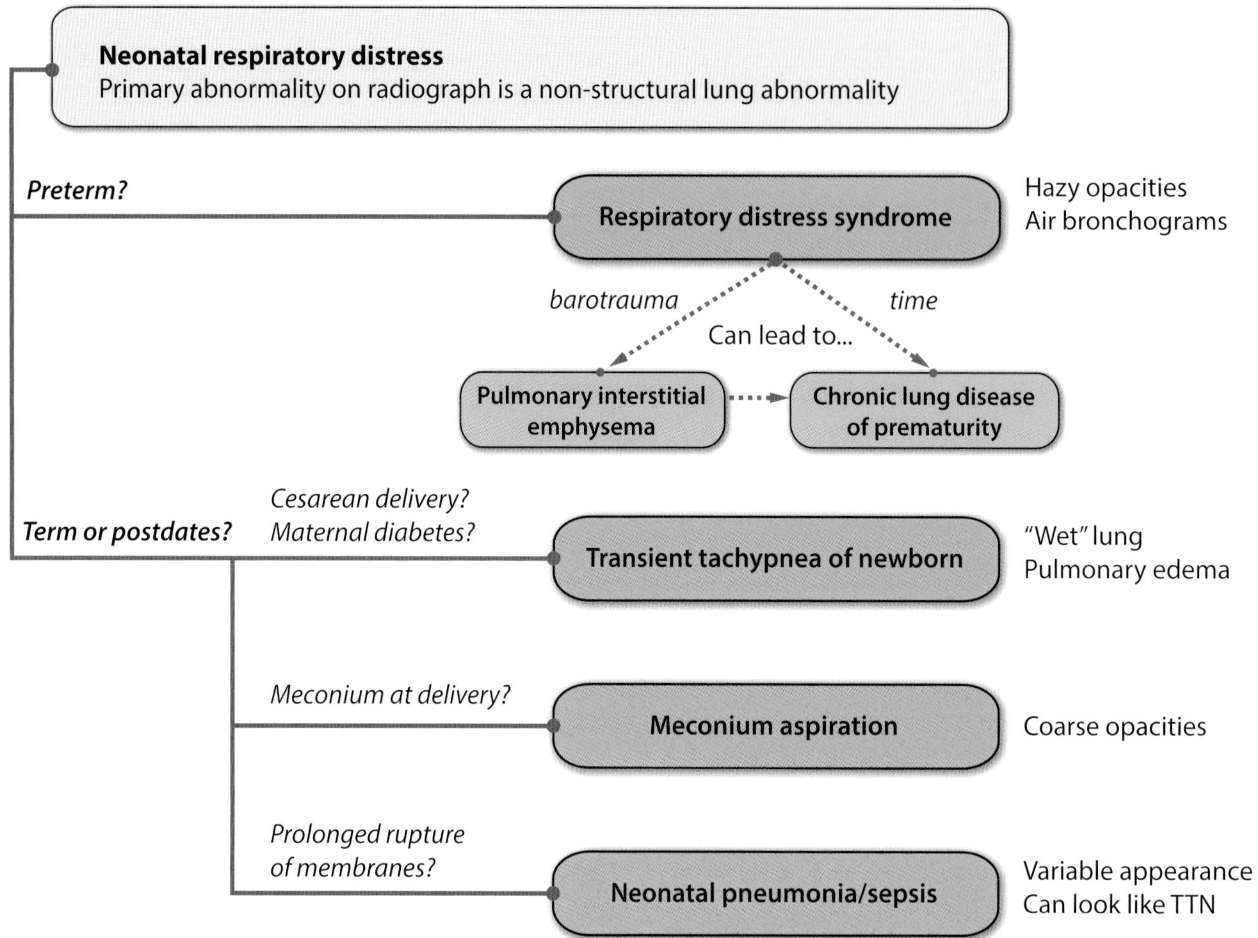

- Multiple processes can cause respiratory distress in a neonate, including pulmonary disease, congenital heart disease, thoracic mass, airway disorders, skeletal abnormalities, vascular anomalies, etc.
- Despite this broad range, there are four classic differentials for a newborn with "medical respiratory distress" — that is, a baby that appears to be anatomically normal by radiograph (i.e., without cardiomegaly or thoracic mass), but has a diffuse pulmonary abnormality.

Transient tachypnea of the newborn (TTN)

- Transient tachypnea of the newborn (TTN) is the most common cause of neonatal respiratory distress. It is caused by lack of clearance of fetal lung fluid.
- Normally, prostaglandins dilate pulmonary lymphatics to absorb excess fluid. When pulmonary fluid persists, TTN may result. The etiology of the excess fluid may relate to prostaglandin imbalance, potentially worsened by maternal asthma or diabetes, male sex, or Cesarean delivery (lack of vaginal "squeeze").
- Chest radiograph shows pulmonary edema, often with fluid tracking in the minor fissure.
- TTN can be clinically and radiographically difficult to differentiate from neonatal pneumonia. Therefore, antibiotics are often given initially, although there is no specific treatment necessary for TTN. TTN resolves spontaneously after a few hours or days.

Respiratory distress syndrome (RDS)/Hyaline membrane disease

- Respiratory distress syndrome (RDS), also called hyaline membrane disease, is the most common cause of respiratory distress in pre-term infants.
- RDS is caused by insufficient surfactant (due to immature type II pneumocytes) and resultant decreased lung compliance.
- Greater than 95% of cases are seen in pre-term infants born before 34 weeks. Less commonly, term babies born to diabetic mothers have increased prevalence of RDS.
- Imaging is characterized by hazy pulmonary opacities, often with air-bronchograms. A key imaging feature that may be seen is **decreased lung volumes** if the baby is not intubated.

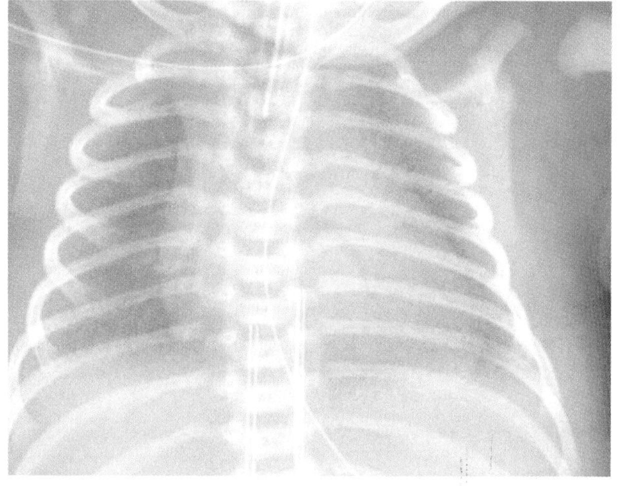

Respiratory distress syndrome: Frontal radiograph in a premature infant shows hazy, granular pulmonary opacities and low lung volumes. The baby is intubated, with partially visualized nasogastric tube, umbilical venous, and umbilical arterial catheters.

Case courtesy Michael Hanley, MD, University of Virginia Health System.

- **Pulmonary interstitial emphysema** (PIE) is a condition often associated with RDS, where barotrauma causes air to dissect through the immature alveoli into the interstitial space and spread along the lymphatic pathways.

  The radiographic appearance of PIE is hyperinflated lungs with many small cysts representing dissecting air bubbles. PIE may lead to pneumomediastinum or pneumothorax.

  Special ventilator settings unique to pediatrics, such as high-frequency oscillating ventilation, reduce the severity of PIE.

Bronchopulmonary dysplasia (BPD)/chronic lung disease of prematurity

- Respiratory distress syndrome (with or without PIE) lasts for a few days to a week. Beyond that, persistent lung disease is called bronchopulmonary dysplasia, also called chronic lung disease of prematurity.
- Bronchopulmonary dysplasia (BPD) is clinically defined as abnormal chest radiograph and persistent need for oxygen at 36 post-conceptual weeks or at 28 days of life, although one may suspect BPD prior to 28 days of life.
- Unlike RDS, BPD features mild hyperinflation and coarse opacities.
- BPD is the most common cause of chronic respiratory failure in pediatrics.

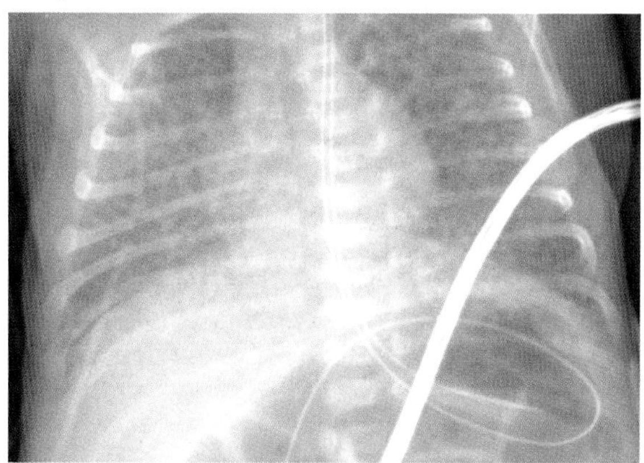

Bronchopulmonary dysplasia: Chest radiograph in a 28-day-old infant with a history of prior respiratory distress syndrome shows coarse interstitial opacities and normal to slightly increased lung volumes. An endotracheal tube and two nasogastric tubes are partially visualized.

Case courtesy Michael Hanley, MD, University of Virginia Health System.

Meconium aspiration syndrome

- Peripartum aspiration of meconium is typically seen in full-term and post-term neonates. Meconium is a highly irritating mixture of desquamated cells, bile pigments, and pancreatic enzymes that can cause significant respiratory distress.
- Imaging is characterized by ropy, coarse interstitial opacities. The lungs lose compliance and become especially susceptible to barotrauma and pneumothoraces.
- Outcome is variable, with much worse prognosis in the presence of a pneumothorax.

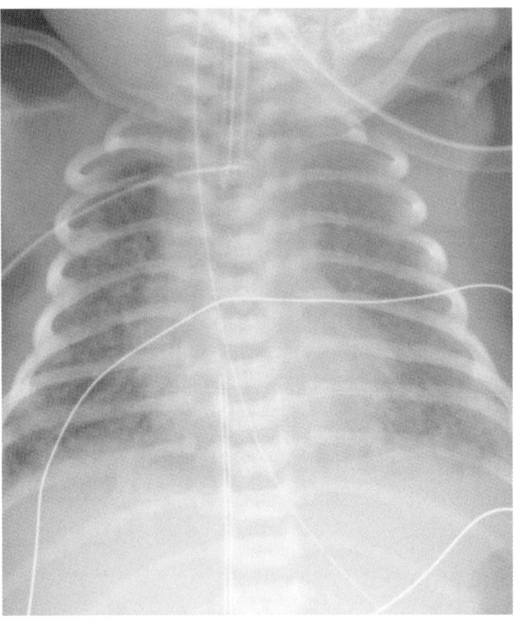

Meconium aspiration: Chest radiograph shows coarse interstitial opacities. Endotracheal tube, nasogastric tube, and umbilical venous catheter are partially seen. Although initially intubated, this baby was extubated and did well.

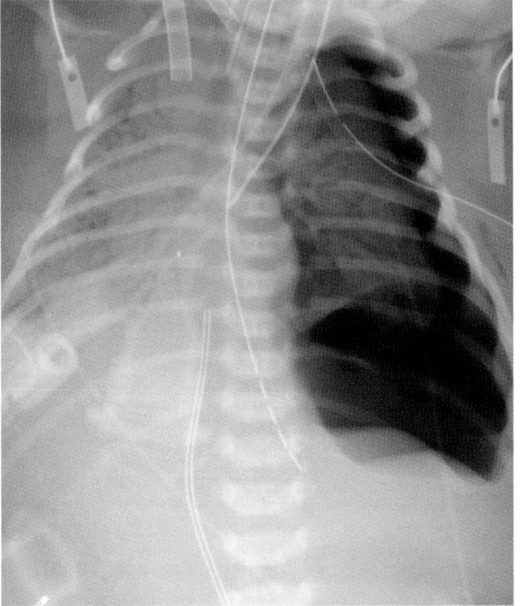

Severe meconium aspiration in a different patient: There is a large left pneumothorax and dense opacifications in the right hemithorax. This baby is receiving extracorporeal membrane oxygenation (ECMO). This infant did not survive.

Neonatal pneumonia

- Unlike the previously described entities, which present with immediate respiratory distress, neonatal pneumonia takes hours to days to develop. The most common pathogens are group B streptococcus, *S. aureus*, and *E. coli*, which are acquired at birth from the vaginal flora.
- In neonatal pneumonia, the infection is not confined to the lung and is thought to represent neonatal sepsis.
- Typical signs of adult pneumonia, such as fever or elevated white count, are not reliable in neonates. Therefore it can be difficult to distinguish between neonatal pneumonia and TTN. A history of prolonged rupture of membranes or known maternal infection may suggest neonatal pneumonia.
- Neonatal pneumonia may lead to post-infectious pneumatocele, especially if the organism is *S. aureus*.

Congenital diaphragmatic hernia (CDH)

- Congenital diaphragmatic hernia (CDH) represents herniation of abdominal contents into the thorax, most commonly through a left posterior defect in the diaphragm (Bochdalek).
- The primary complication is pulmonary hypoplasia on the affected side.
- Right-sided lesions with liver herniations are rare and have a poor prognosis.
- The key imaging finding is a mass in the thorax displacing the mediastinum. At birth, the herniated bowel may be fluid-filled and appear solid. However, shortly after birth, air fills the bowel to create the typical appearance shown to the right.
- CDH is associated with bowel malrotation (95%), neural tube defects, and congenital heart disease.

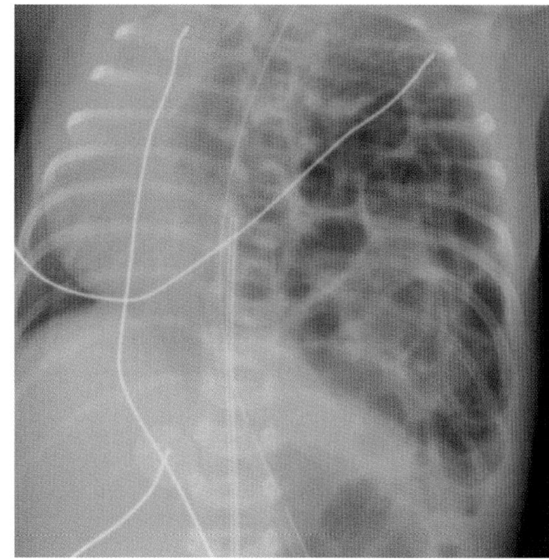

Congenital diaphragmatic hernia: Chest radiograph in a neonate shows multiple loops of air-filled bowel herniated into the left thorax, producing rightwards displacement of the heart.

Overview of bronchopulmonary foregut malformations

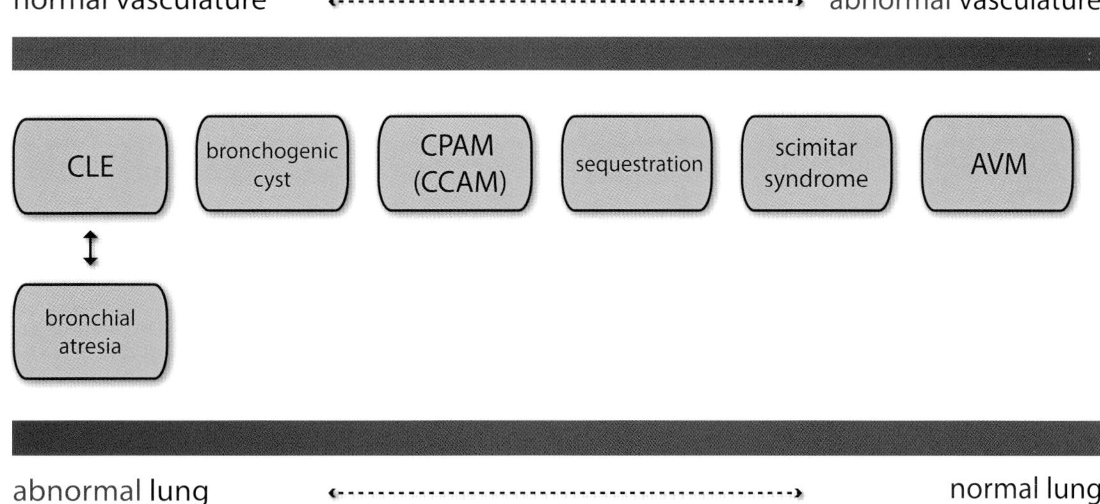

- Bronchopulmonary foregut malformations describe a range of congenital abnormalities of the embryonic foregut, which represent an inverse spectrum of normal to abnormal vasculature with normal to abnormal pulmonary parenchyma.

Congenital lobar emphysema (CLE), a lesion of abnormal lung development without an associated vascular anomaly. **Bronchial atresia** is typically diagnosed later in life, and has been postulated by some authors to represent previously undiagnosed congenital lobar emphysema.

Bronchogenic cyst.

Congenital pulmonary airway malformation (CPAM), previously called congenital cystic adenomatoid malformation.

Scimitar syndrome, a form of partial anomalous pulmonary venous return.

Pulmonary arteriovenous malformation (AVM), an anomalous connection between the pulmonary artery and pulmonary veins, is a purely vascular malformation without any abnormal lung development.

Congenital lobar emphysema (CLE)

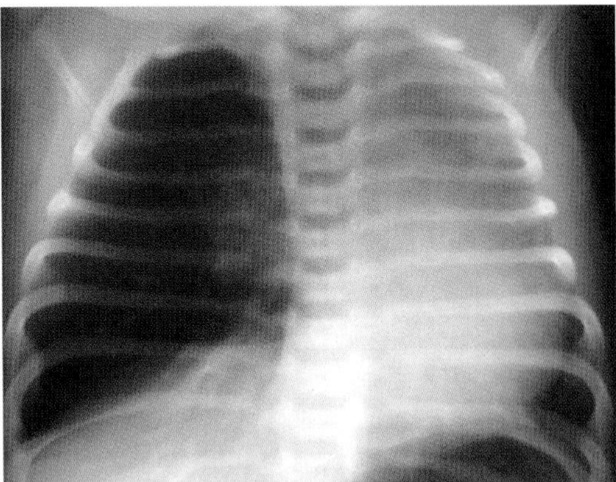

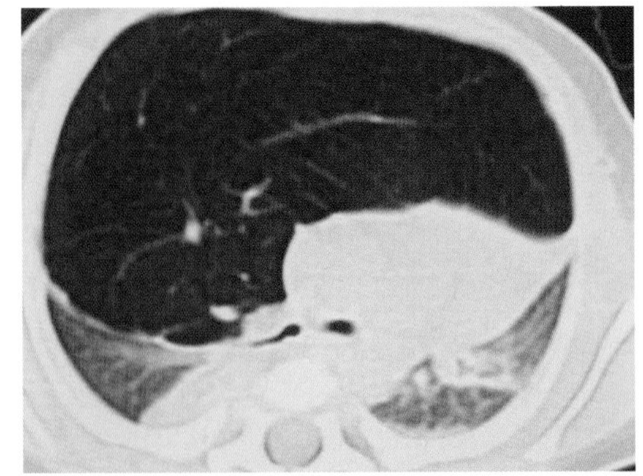

Congenital lobar emphysema: Chest radiograph (left image) shows a hyperlucent right lung with scant vascular markings and mediastinal shift to the left. Axial CT shows a massively hyperexpanded right middle lobe, which has herniated across the midline and exerts mass effect on the heart and bilateral lower lobes.

Case courtesy Michael Callahan, MD, Boston Children's Hospital.

- Congenital lobar emphysema (CLE) is a syndrome of lobar air trapping. CLE has no affiliation with pulmonary interstitial emphysema (PIE), despite similar names.
- The most common cause of CLE is bronchomalacia, which results in airway collapse on expiration, leading to hyperinflation. CT can be performed to evaluate for a cause of bronchial obstruction, which is only found in about half of the cases of CLE.
- CLE usually involves the upper and middle lobes.
- In the perinatal period, CLE is initially fluid-filled, but becomes radiolucent as the fluid clears. Eventually, lobar hyperexpansion can exert mass effect on surrounding structures. The involved lobe may herniate across the midline. It is essential not to mistake CLE for a tension pneumothorax, as a chest tube will increase respiratory distress.

Bronchial atresia

- Bronchial atresia is interruption of a bronchial branch with associated distal mucus impaction and hyperinflation.
- The left upper lobe is the most commonly affected.
- Bronchial atresia is usually incidentally diagnosed in adults and may be etiologically related to CLE.
- The bronchi distal to the atretic segment become filled with mucus that cannot be cleared, ultimately forming a tubular mucocele. The distal airways are ventilated through collateral pathways and demonstrate air trapping, resulting in local hyperinflation.
- Imaging shows a geographic region of hyperlucent lung with air trapping. A mucous plug may be visible just distal to the obstructed bronchial segment.

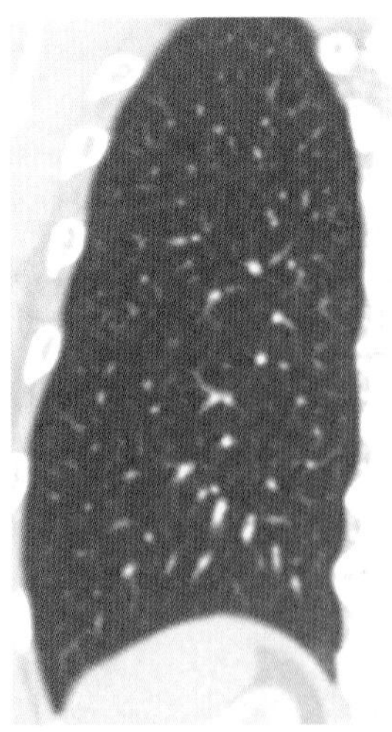

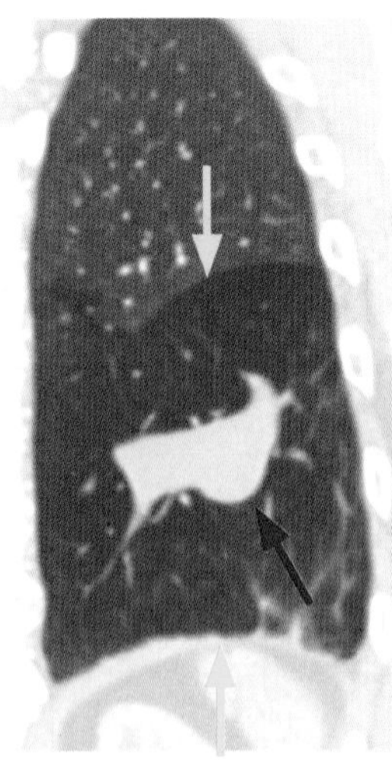

Bronchial atresia: Coronal CT shows hyperlucency of the left lower lobe (yellow arrows). There is a globular, well-defined opacity (red arrow) in the left lower lobe representing a mucocele of the atretic left lower lobe bronchus. This case is slightly atypical in that the left *lower* lobe is affected.

Case courtesy Ritu R. Gill, MD, MPH, Brigham and Women's Hospital.

Congenital pulmonary airway malformation (CPAM)/Congenital cystic adenomatoid malformation (CCAM)

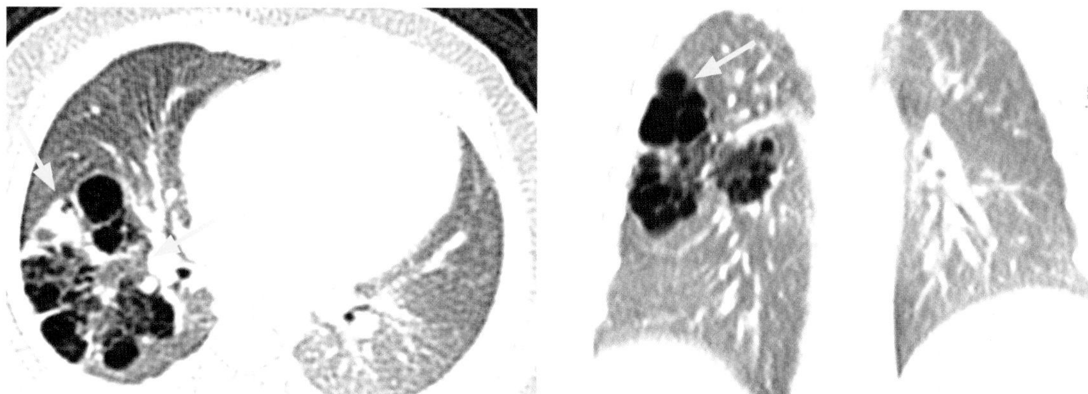

CPAM: Axial (left image) and coronal CT images show a large, multicystic mass in the right upper lung (arrows) with both large and small cysts, representing a mixed type I and type II CPAM.

- Congenital pulmonary airway malformation (CPAM) is a hamartomatous proliferation of terminal bronchioles that communicate with the bronchial tree. Congenital cystic adenomatoid malformation (CCAM) is an older term for the same entity.
- The arterial supply of CPAM arises from the pulmonary circulation. In contrast, sequestration (discussed below) derives its blood supply from the systemic circulation.
- The original classification (Stocker, revised in 2002) is important to be aware of, but the prognosis of CPAM depends more on the size of the lesion rather than its classification.

Type I: One or more large cysts >2 cm. Most common form.

Type II: Multiple small cysts. Can be associated with renal agenesis.

Type III: Innumerable tiny cysts too small to see, which appear solid.

Type IV: Single large cyst, may be indistinguishable from a cystic pleuropulmonary blastoma, which is a rare malignancy that is the most common primary childhood lung tumor.

- CPAM may exert mass effect and is prone to infection. Surgery is usually recommended.

Sequestration

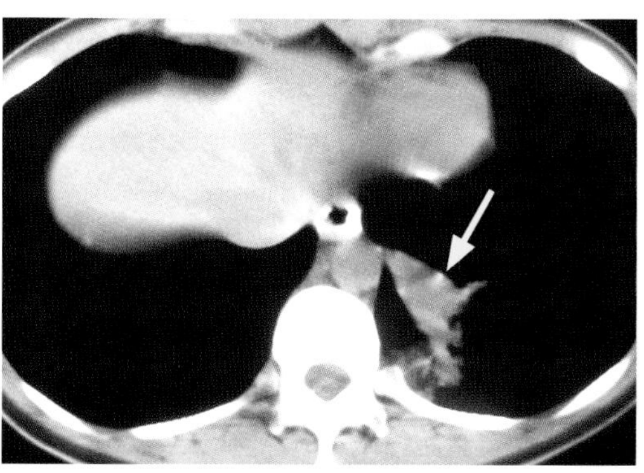

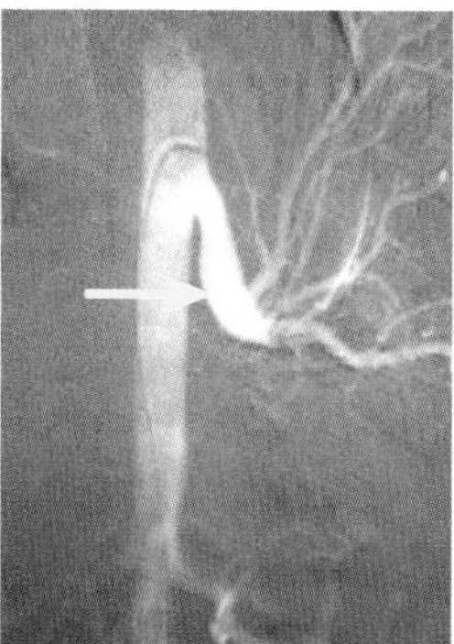

Sequestration: Axial CT shows a left lower lobe soft tissue mass abutting the aorta (arrow).

Thoracic aortogram demonstrates a large feeding artery arising directly off the aorta (arrow).

Case courtesy Michael Callahan, MD, Boston Children's Hospital.

- Sequestration is aberrant lung tissue with **systemic blood supply**, usually arising from the aorta. The key imaging finding is a systemic arterial vessel, which can be seen by Doppler ultrasound prenatally, or by CTA or MRA postnatally. The most common location is the left lower lobe. In contrast to CPAM, sequestration is usually solid.
- Two types of sequestration, intralobar and extralobar, are usually distinguished by CT or MR:

Extralobar: External to the pleura, with primarily systemic venous drainage. May occasionally be below the diaphragm near the adrenal gland, where it may mimic an adrenal mass.

Intralobar: Inside pleura, usually with pulmonary venous drainage.

Scimitar syndrome

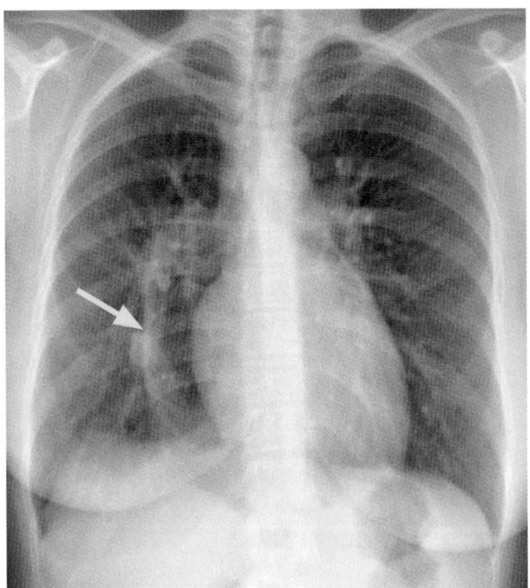

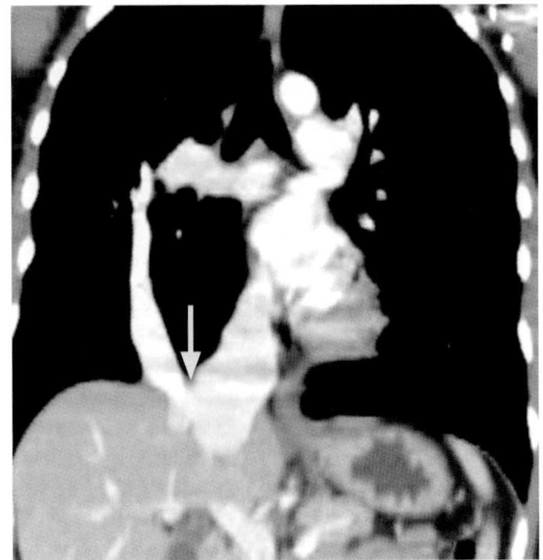

Scimitar syndrome: Frontal chest radiograph (left image) shows a curvilinear opacity extending from the right hilum towards the diaphragm, representing the *scimitar* sign (arrow). Coronal contrast-enhanced CT (right image) shows the anomalous scimitar vein draining into the inferior vena cava, consistent with partial anomalous pulmonary venous return.

Case courtesy Michael Hanley, MD, University of Virginia Health System.

- Scimitar syndrome represents partial anomalous pulmonary venous return (PAPVR) from right lower lobe pulmonary veins into either the right atrium or IVC.

  In contrast to PAPVR, in *total* anomalous pulmonary venous return (TAPVR), all four pulmonary veins return blood to the right atrium, and an obligate right-to-left shunt is necessary for survival.

- The anomalous vein appears like a "scimitar" on the frontal radiograph, representing the *scimitar* sign.
- Scimitar syndrome can be associated with hypoplasia and hyperlucency of the right lung (although this finding is not demonstrated in the case above).

SMALL AIRWAYS DISEASE

Bronchiolitis

- Bronchiolitis is an infection of the lower respiratory tract, most commonly caused by respiratory syncytial virus (RSV). It is the leading cause of infant hospitalization in the US.
- Inflammation of bronchiolar epithelium leads to peribronchial infiltration by inflammatory cells. The resultant necrotic debris may lead to small airway obstruction, which is the hallmark of bronchiolitis.
- Clinically, bronchiolitis presents as increased work of breathing and wheezing in a child less than two years of age, usually with a viral upper respiratory prodrome. Bronchiolitis is primarily a clinical diagnosis.
- Radiographic findings include hyperexpanded lungs (best seen as flattening of the diaphragms) and increased peribronchial markings. These findings are subjective, with high variability among even experienced pediatric radiologists.

Bronchiolitis obliterans syndrome (BOS) = constrictive bronchiolitis

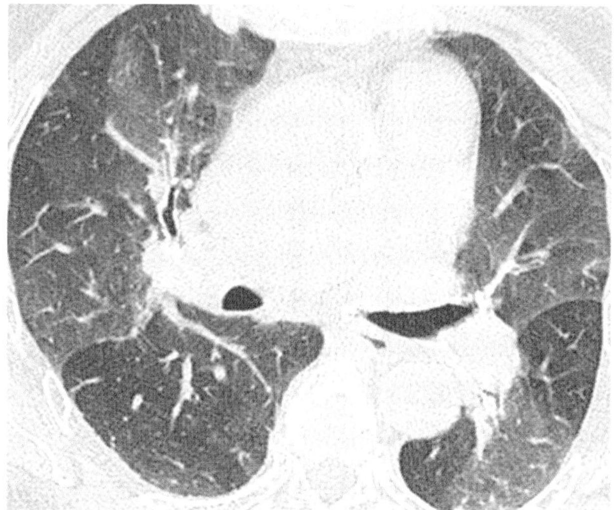

Bronchiolitis obliterans: Axial CT shows mosaic perfusion with geographic regions of ground glass attenuation.

This is an example in an adult; however, the findings are similar in children.

Case courtesy Ritu R. Gill, MD, MPH, Brigham and Women's Hospital.

- Bronchiolitis obliterans syndrome (BOS) is the final common pathway of small airway obstruction by inflammatory and fibrous tissue, which may be due to multiple etiologies. BOS may be post-transplant in origin, postinfectious (typically following viral or atypical bacterial pneumonia), or related to toxin or drug exposures.
- BOS is one of the most clinically important complications of pediatric allogeneic lung and bone marrow transplantation.
- Chest radiographs are usually normal or may show mild hyperinflation.
- CT demonstrates findings of small airways obstruction, including:

  Air trapping on expiratory views.

  Mosaic perfusion.

  Bronchiectasis and bronchial wall thickening.

- One complication seen in up to one third of young patients with post-infectious BOS is **Swyer–James–MacLeod** syndrome. Swyer–James–MacLeod syndrome is an acquired abnormality of pulmonary development secondary to BOS, which leads to a unilateral hyperlucent lung with volume loss.

  In particular, adenovirus infection is implicated in the etiology of Swyer–James–MacLeod.

  The key radiographic feature of Swyer–James–MacLeod is a unilateral, small, hyperlucent lung on the affected side.

  Note that Swyer–James–MacLeod is *not* a sequela of viral *bronchiolitis* (of which RSV is the most common cause), but is only seen after *bronchiolitis obliterans*, classically triggered by adenovirus infection.

Cryptogenic organizing pneumonia (COP) = bronchiolitis obliterans organizing pneumonia (BOOP)

- Cryptogenic organizing pneumonia (COP) is a disorder of the distal airways characterized by filling of the bronchioles and alveoli with granulation tissue polyps. Bronchiolitis obliterans organizing pneumonia (BOOP) is an older term for the same entity and many authors recommend against using the term BOOP because of its potential confusion with bronchiolitis obliterans. BOOP is a completely different disease from bronchiolitis obliterans.
- The underlying histologic changes of COP are referred to as organizing pneumonia (OP). COP is the clinical syndrome of OP of unknown cause. OP may be secondary to infection, drug reaction, or inhalation. OP may also be a complication of stem cell transplant, but much less commonly than BOS.
- Radiographic features of COP/OP include multifocal migratory consolidations, ground glass opacities, and nodules. The *atoll* or *reverse halo* sign is thought to be relatively specific for OP and features a central lucency surrounded by ground glass.

Bronchiectasis

- Bronchiectasis is bronchial dilation, most commonly due to inflammation.
- Bronchiectasis can have a variety of causes in the pediatric population:

> Cystic fibrosis.
>
> Allergic bronchopulmonary aspergillosis.
>
> Post-infectious.
>
> Tracheobronchomegaly (Mounier–Kuhn).
>
> Aspiration.
>
> Intralobar sequestration, possibly due to recurrent infections.

- The *signet-ring* sign describes enlargement of the bronchiole, which appears larger than the adjacent pulmonary artery branch.

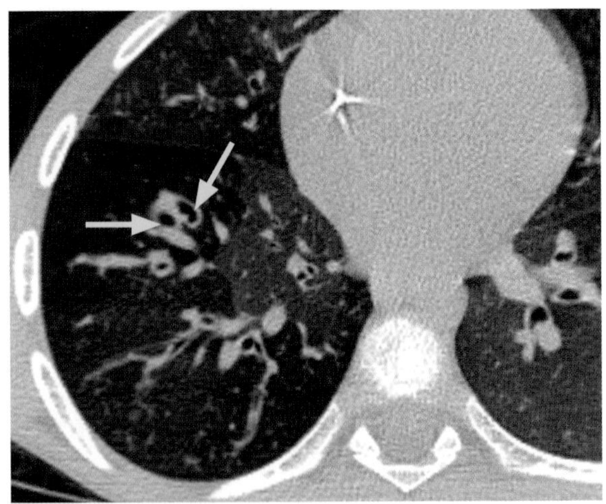

Bronchiectasis in cystic fibrosis: Axial CT demonstrates relative enlargement of numerous subsegmental bronchi with associated bronchial wall thickening (arrows).

Case courtesy Michael Hanley, MD, University of Virginia Health System.

UNILATERAL HYPERLUCENT LUNG

- A unilateral hyperlucent lung is a common finding in pediatric chest radiology. The two most important acute diagnoses are endobronchial foreign body and pneumothorax.

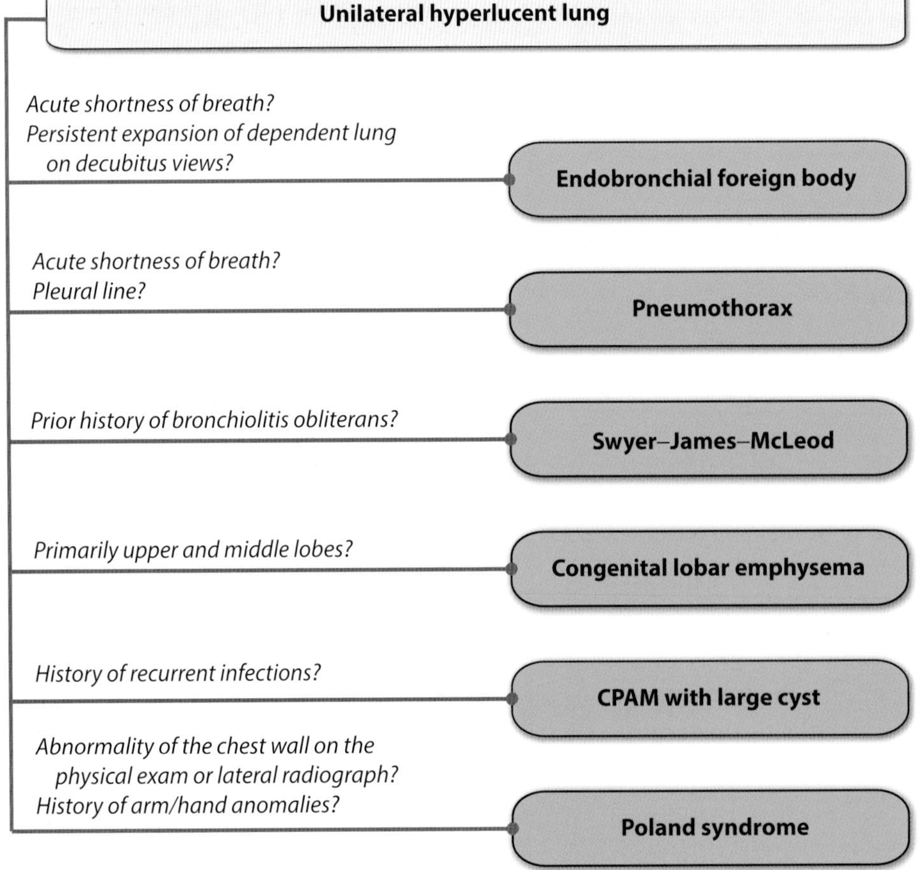
Unilateral hyperlucent lung
Acute shortness of breath? Persistent expansion of dependent lung on decubitus views?
Endobronchial foreign body
Acute shortness of breath? Pleural line?
Pneumothorax
Prior history of bronchiolitis obliterans?
Swyer–James–McLeod
Primarily upper and middle lobes?
Congenital lobar emphysema
History of recurrent infections?
CPAM with large cyst
Abnormality of the chest wall on the physical exam or lateral radiograph? History of arm/hand anomalies?
Poland syndrome

Poland syndrome

- Poland syndrome is an autosomal recessive syndrome of unilateral congenital absence (complete or partial) of the pectoralis major muscle. Associated anomalies of the ipsilateral arm and hand, including short metacarpals and syndactyly (joined fingers), may be present.

Pediatric mediastinal masses

- An approach to mediastinal masses, including the relevant anatomy and division of the three main compartments (anterior, middle, and posterior), is discussed in the thoracic imaging section.
- This brief differential highlights the common mediastinal masses in children.

Anterior mediastinum

- Normal thymus is sometimes mistaken as an anterior mediastinal mass. A special case is thymic rebound, which is physiologic regrowth of the thymus after chemotherapy, and should also not be mistaken for an anterior mediastinal mass.
- Lymphoma.
- Germ cell tumor.
- Thymoma (very rare in children).

Middle mediastinum

- Foregut duplication cyst.
- Neurenteric cysts, which are often associated with vertebral anomalies.
- Lymphadenopathy.

Posterior mediastinum

- Neurogenic tumors, including neuroblastoma, ganglioneuroblastoma, and ganglioneuroma.

Miscellaneous

Pneumomediastinum

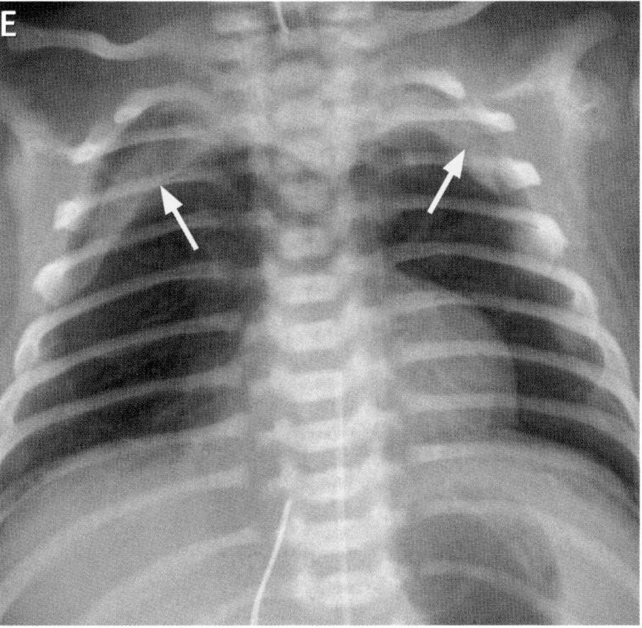

Spinnaker sail sign of pneumomediastinum:

Frontal chest radiograph in an intubated neonate demonstrates elevation of both thymic lobes (arrows).

Case courtesy Michael Hanley, MD, University of Virginia Health System.

- The *spinnaker sail* sign is seen in pneumomediastinum and represents the thymus lifted off the mediastinum by the ectopic air.
- The *spinnaker sail* sign should not be confused with the *sail* sign, which is the rightward extension of the normal thymus.

APPROACH TO THE PLAIN FILM OF CONGENITAL HEART DISEASE

Plain film evaluation of congenital heart disease: Of historical interest only?

- Most congenital heart disease is diagnosed in utero during routine fetal ultrasound.
- If a newborn has unexpected shortness of breath with clinical concern for a cardiac cause, a cardiac echo is typically the imaging study of choice. Advanced imaging, such as CTA or MRI, may also be helpful in certain clinical situations.
- Even though the specific diagnosis of congenital heart disease may not be determined from the plain radiograph, there is value in describing the plain radiographic findings (e.g., increased pulmonary vascularity, cardiomegaly, etc.).

Plain film evaluation of congenital heart disease: One piece of clinical history and two things to look at

- The critical piece of the clinical history is whether the patient is cyanotic or acyanotic.
- After that's been established, the first imaging feature to evaluate is the pulmonary vascularity, which can be characterized as increased venous flow, increased arterial flow, or decreased arterial flow. Increased vascularity can be determined by examining the peripheral third of the lungs. Normally, there is very little blood flow peripherally; increased peripheral vasculature suggests either increased pulmonary arterial or pulmonary venous flow.

1) **Increased** pulmonary **venous** flow (pulmonary edema) is seen when the left ventricular outflow tract can't keep up with venous return.

Can be caused by left heart insufficiency, an obstructive lesion of the left heart, or congestive heart failure.

Peripheral 1/3 of the lungs shows *indistinct* vessels and septal markings.

2) **Increased** pulmonary **arterial** flow, also called "shunt vascularity" tends to present in childhood rather than infancy. Increased arterial flow is caused by a left → right shunt, as the right side of the heart (which pumps blood to the lungs via the pulmonary arteries) is pumping too much blood.

The peripheral 1/3 of the lungs shows *distinct*, large-caliber vessels.

3) **Decreased** pulmonary **arterial** flow is due to right ventricular outflow tract insufficiency.

Any lesion causing decreased pulmonary arterial flow is ALWAYS cyanotic because not enough blood is being oxygenated in the lungs.

Peripheral 1/3 of the lungs shows decreased vasculature.

- The second imaging feature to evaluate is the heart size. The heart can be normal in size, slightly enlarged, or massively enlarged. It is never smaller than normal (even in hypoplastic left heart syndrome).
- Additional findings, such as specific contour to the aorta and cardiac chambers, orientation of the aortic arch, and side of stomach bubble can help refine the diagnosis.

Plain film evaluation of congenital heart disease: Can it be anything else?

- It is important to remember that an apparently enlarged heart and abnormal pulmonary vasculature can be due to other diseases in addition to congenital heart disease, including:

Intracardiac tumor, such as a rhabdomyoma.

CHF due to a peripheral shunt (e.g., vein of Galen malformation or hepatic hemangioendothelioma).

Mediastinal mass.

Congenital diaphragmatic hernia with unaerated bowel.

Bronchiolitis may also mimic pulmonary edema, particularly in children with congenital heart disease.

Overview of radiographic differential diagnosis for congenital heart disease

Acyanotic congenital heart disease

- Neonatal **increased pulmonary venous flow** (pulmonary edema) may be caused by:

> **Hypoplastic left heart,** similar in physiology to CHF (left ventricle cannot keep up with venous return).
>
> **Aortic coarctation**, which is a left ventricular outflow tract lesion.
>
> **Congestive heart failure (CHF)**, which may be due to a primary cardiac anomaly or an extra-cardiac arteriovenous shunt, such as a vein of Galen malformation or hepatic hemangioendothelioma.
>
> **Neonatal sepsis**, typically seen in the setting of neonatal pneumonia.

- Increased **pulmonary arterial flow** (shunt vascularity) tends to present in childhood rather than the neonatal period. Increased pulmonary arterial flow can be caused by:

> **Atrial septal defect (ASD).**
>
> **Ventricular septal defect (VSD).**
>
> **Patent ductus arteriosus (PDA).**
>
> **Endocardial cushion defect (ECD)**, also known as an AV canal defect, has a strong association with Down syndrome.

Cyanotic congenital heart disease

- **Decreased pulmonary vascularity with cardiomegaly**:

> **Ebstein anomaly**.

- **Decreased pulmonary vascularity without cardiomegaly**:

> **Tetralogy of Fallot.**

- **Usually increased pulmonary vascularity without cardiomegaly** (but variable): "T" lesions (excluding Tetralogy of Fallot):

> **Transposition of the great arteries.**
>
> **Truncus arteriosus.**
>
> **Tricuspid atresia.**
>
> **Total anomalous pulmonary venous return (TAPVR)**.
>
> **Single** ("Tingle" to keep the T-theme consistent) **ventricle**, and variants including double outlet left ventricle and double outlet right ventricle.

Normal anatomy

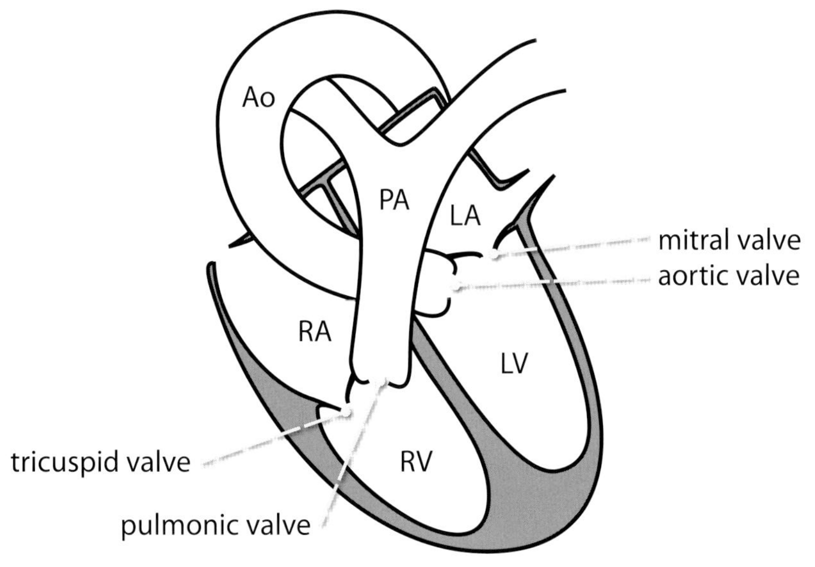

Ao = aorta
PA = pulmonary artery
RA = right atrium
LA = left atrium
RV = right ventricle
LV = left ventricle

Acyanotic: pulmonary edema (increased pulmonary venous flow)

Hypoplastic left heart (HLH)

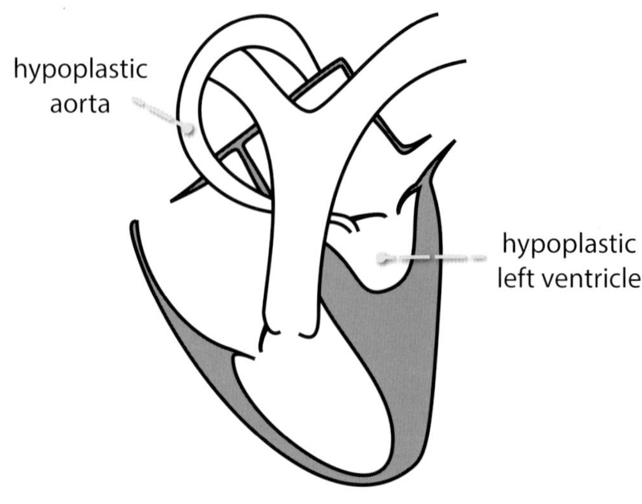

- Hypoplastic left heart (HLH) syndrome represents a spectrum of congenital heart anomalies characterized by underdevelopment of any part of the left heart including left atrium, mitral valve, left ventricle, aortic valve, or aorta.
- Survival is dependent on a patent ductus arteriosus with resultant right to left shunting to supply the systemic circulation.
- Immediately after birth, the ductus arteriosus remains patent and pulmonary arterial resistance remains high, so blood continues to flow to the systemic circulation. After a few days, however, the ductus begins to close and pulmonary arterial resistance falls, leading to cardiogenic shock without operative management.
- The neonatal chest radiograph in HLH is usually normal, but HLH is classified as a "pulmonary edema" lesion. With a patent ductus and high pulmonary vascular resistance, the pulmonary blood flow is in the normal range, but as pulmonary resistance decreases, pulmonary blood flow increases. As the ductus closes, blood clearance from the lungs is delayed and pulmonary edema may result.
- Note that despite the left heart hypoplasia, the heart does not appear small on imaging.
- The surgical treatment of hypoplastic left heart is the **Norwood** procedure, performed in three sequential stages. A staged repair is necessary since the high pulmonary vascular resistance in the neonatal period precludes immediate definitive repair.

> **Stage 1**: The first stage of the Norwood procedure has three main components. First, the right ventricle is redirected to supply the systemic circulation, by reconstructing the aorta using the main pulmonary artery (**Damus–Kaye–Stansel procedure**). Second, the atrial septum is excised and the PDA is ligated, to redirect pulmonary venous return to the right heart via the atrial septal defect. Third, pulmonary arterial circulation is provided via a modified **Blalock–Taussig shunt** (BTS), which **connects the right subclavian artery to the right pulmonary artery** via a prosthetic graft. This stage is performed within the first few days of life.
>
> **Stage 2**: The BTS is replaced with a **bidirectional Glenn** (BDG) shunt, where the **SVC is connected to the right pulmonary artery**. This procedure is performed once pulmonary arterial resistance has fallen to normal levels, approximately 3–6 months after stage 1. The goal of stage 2 is to begin to separate systemic and pulmonary circulations.
>
> **Stage 3**: A **modified Fontan** is performed once the patient cannot supply adequate oxygenated blood to the systemic circulation. In this procedure, a tunneled conduit **connects the IVC to the pulmonary artery**. The SVC continues to empty into the right pulmonary artery via the BDG constructed in stage 2.

Extracardiac shunt causing CHF

- The two most common lesions to cause neonatal CHF are vein of Galen malformation and hepatic hemangioendothelioma.

Aortic coarctation

- Aortic coarctation may cause CHF in infants due to left ventricular obstruction, leading to cardiomegaly and increased pulmonary venous flow.

- It is rare for shunt lesions to present in the neonatal period because pulmonary vascular resistance is high and left to right shunting is limited. In long-standing shunting, progressive volume overload causes the typical "shunt" vascularity (very prominent distinct pulmonary arteries without the haziness of pulmonary edema) and cardiomegaly.

Atrial septal defect (ASD)

- Although atrial septal defect (ASD) is a common intracardiac left-to-right shunt, it is rarely diagnosed in infants or young children. ASD usually presents in later childhood or early adulthood, twice as commonly in females. Although most are an isolated abnormality, ASD may rarely be associated with syndromes, such as Holt–Oram (ASD and upper extremity bone deformities, including absence or hypoplasia of the thumb).
- Ostium secundum ASD is the most common type of ASD (accounting for 75% of cases), caused by incomplete covering of the ostium secundum by the septum secundum.
- Ostium primum ASD is the second most common type of ASD (15% of cases), caused by incomplete fusion of the septum primum to the endocardial cushion.
- Sinus venosus ASD occurs either near the superior vena cava or inferior vena cava. Although only accounting for 10% of ASDs, sinus venosus ASD is important to remember because of its association with anomalous pulmonary venous drainage.
- **An ASD causes right heart volume overload.** The left atrium is usually normal because blood is decompressed from the left atrium to the right atrium during both systole and diastole. However, if mitral regurgitation is present, secondary left atrial enlargement may result.
- Initially, the right atrium enlarges, followed by right ventricular enlargement (which may be visible on the lateral radiograph as filling of the retrosternal clear space). In late-stage disease the pulmonary artery also becomes enlarged.
- Shunt vascularity is usually present on radiography by the time the lesion is symptomatic.
- Treatment is ASD closure, typically with an Amplatzer or similar device.

Ventricular septal defect (VSD)

- Ventricular septal defect (VSD) is typically diagnosed earlier than ASD, with many children presenting after the first month of life as pulmonary vascular resistance falls. A VSD may occur in the membranous (70%) or muscular interventricular septum.
- **VSD primarily causes dilation of the left heart.** Left-to-right shunting occurs in systole, causing volume overload of the left heart and resulting in left atrial and left ventricular dilation.

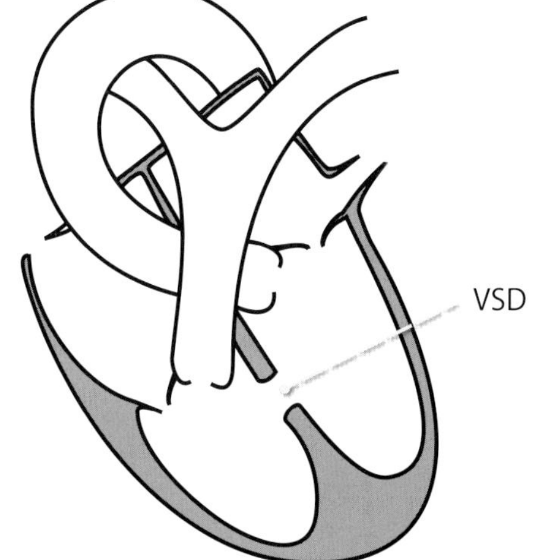

- Imaging findings are variable, depending on the size of the VSD. The classic imaging findings of shunt vascularity and cardiomegaly typically take a few years to develop, although there may be mild cardiomegaly and increased pulmonary vascular flow shortly after birth. The left atrium is often enlarged, which may splay the main stem bronchi at the carina.
- If unrepaired, Eisenmenger syndrome may develop, which represents pulmonary hypertension and reversal of the shunt direction. Eisenmenger syndrome is rare as most patients undergo surgery before pulmonary flow reversal occurs.

Patent ductus arteriosus (PDA)

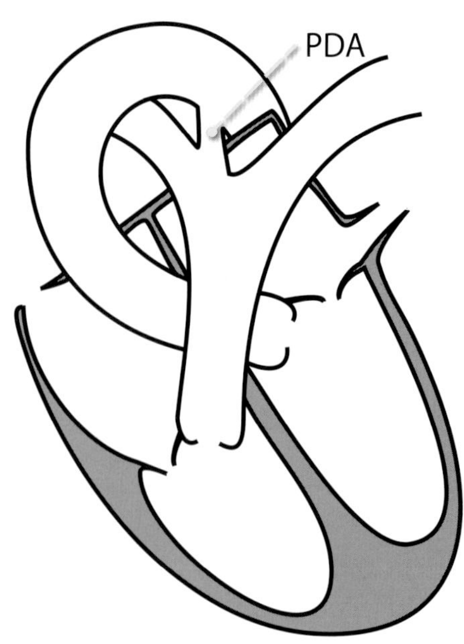

- The ductus arteriosus is a normal vascular structure of the fetal circulation, connecting the proximal left pulmonary artery to the descending aorta. The ductus normally closes within the first days of life. A patent ductus arteriosus (PDA) results in a persistent left-to-right shunt. PDA is much more common in premature infants, thought to be due to the presence of fetal prostaglandins, which inhibit closure of the ductus.
- A small PDA is usually asymptomatic. A large PDA may produce a characteristic *machine-like murmur* and cause CHF in infancy.
- The classic clinical presentation of PDA is a premature infant who develops radiographic evidence of CHF at 7–10 days of life, as pulmonary vascular resistance begins to fall.
- Treatment of PDA is medical (indomethacin) or surgical (clip placement). Eisenmenger syndrome may develop if untreated.

Endocardial cushion defect (ECD), also called AV canal defect

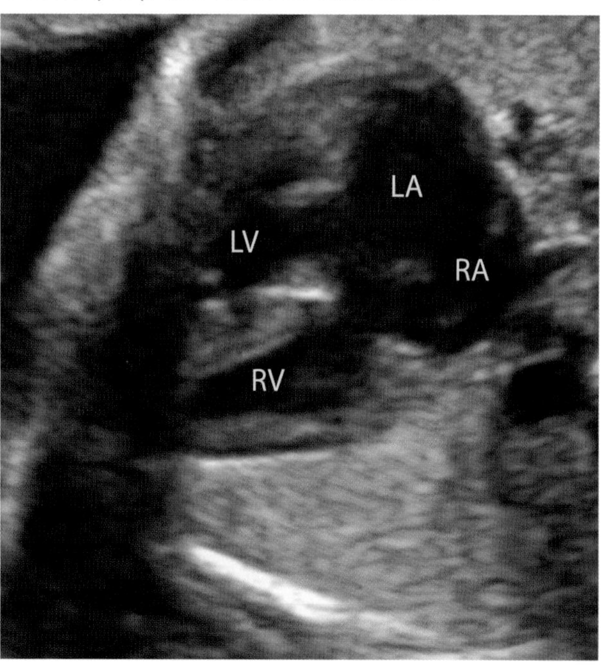

Endocardial cushion defect:

Four-chamber view of the heart from a prenatal ultrasound at 32 weeks gestation demonstrates complete absence of the interatrial septum and a large defect in the upper part of the interventricular septum.

Case courtesy Beryl Benacerraf, MD, Diagnostic Ultrasound Associates, Boston.

- Endocardial cushion defects, also known as AV canal defects, encompass a spectrum of abnormalities including ostium primum ASD, VSD, and mitral or tricuspid anomalies. Endocardial cushion defects are strongly associated with trisomy 21.
- The primitive endocardial cushion is responsible for the formation of several structures in fetal development, including:

  Posterior and membranous ventricular septum.

  Anterior leaflet of the mitral valve.

  Septal leaflet of tricuspid valve.

  Responsible for closure of the ostium primum.

Ebstein anomaly

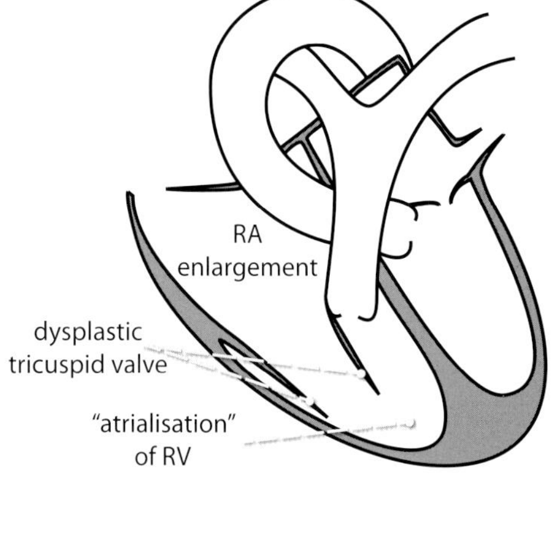

- Ebstein anomaly is a severe malformation of the tricuspid valve characterized by apical displacement of the septal and posteroinferior leaflets, resulting in obstruction of the pulmonic valve and right ventricular outflow tract obstruction. These changes lead to morphologic "atrialization" of the RV.
- An ASD is always present.
- Imaging typically shows a huge heart, with massive right atrial enlargement and decreased pulmonary vascularity. The classic description for Ebstein anomaly is a *box-shaped* heart.

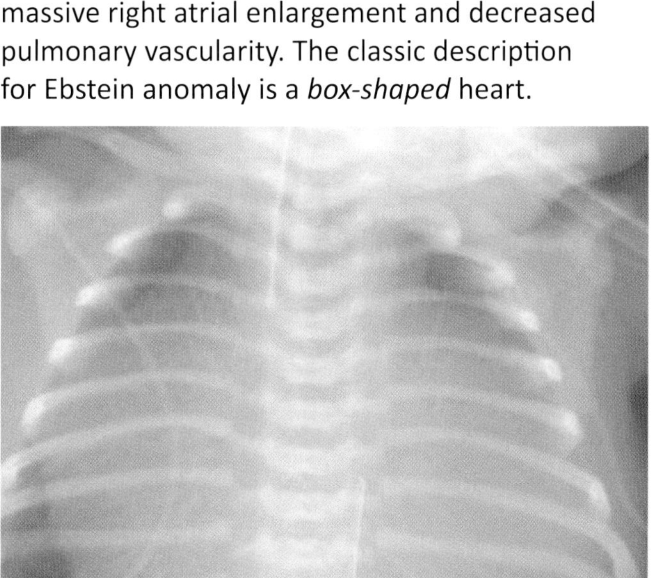

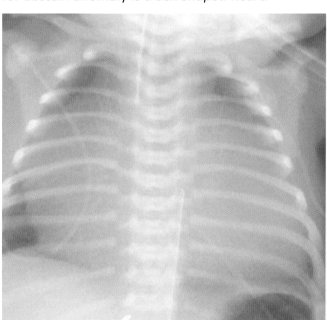

Ebstein anomaly: Frontal chest radiograph in a neonate shows massive cardiomegaly. Although the enlarged heart obscures most of the lungs, there are hardly any vascular markings in the visualized periphery.

An endotracheal tube and umbilical artery catheter are in place.

Pulmonary atresia with intact ventricular septum would appear identical.

Pulmonary atresia with intact ventricular septum

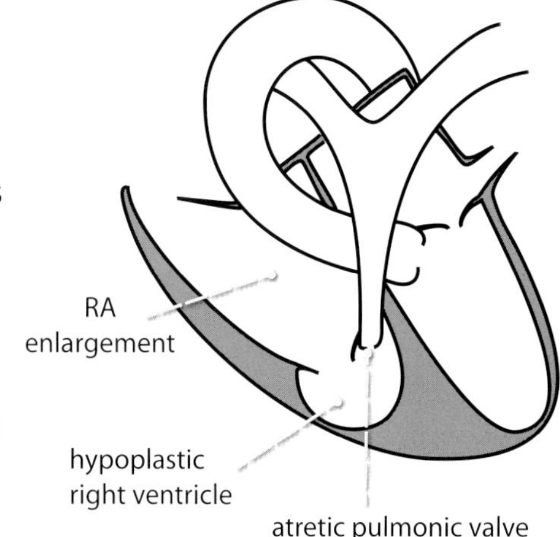

- Pulmonary atresia with intact ventricular septum appears identical to Ebstein anomaly on radiography, with massive right atrial enlargement and decreased pulmonary blood flow. Because the lack of VSD markedly reduces blood flow to the lungs, pulmonary blood flow depends on a left to right shunt, such as a patent ductus.
- Pulmonary atresia with intact ventricular septum is completely different from pulmonary atresia *with* a VSD, which is in the spectrum of tetralogy of Fallot and most commonly has a normal-sized heart.

Cyanotic: Decreased pulmonary vascularity without cardiomegaly

Tetralogy of Fallot (ToF)

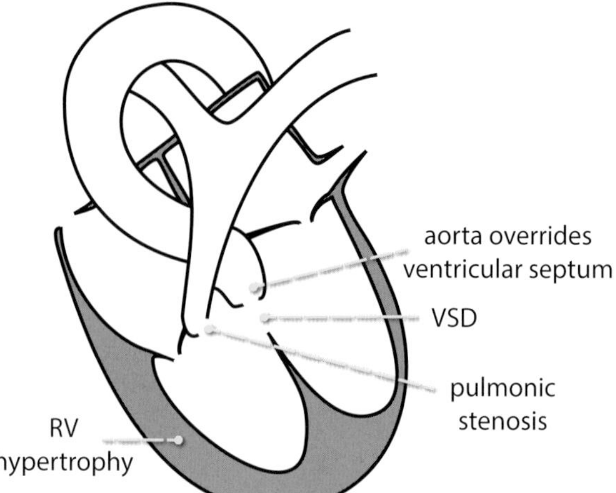

- The four components of ToF are:

  1. Right ventricular outflow tract obstruction.
  2. Right ventricular hypertrophy.
  3. VSD.
  4. Aorta is "over-riding" the VSD.

  A variation of ToF is the pentalogy of Fallot, which also has an ASD.
- The degree of cyanosis depends on degree of right ventricular outflow tract obstruction.
- Tetralogy of Fallot (ToF) is the most common cyanotic heart disease of children and adults.

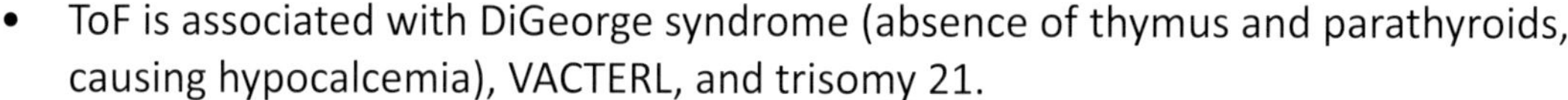

- ToF is associated with DiGeorge syndrome (absence of thymus and parathyroids, causing hypocalcemia), VACTERL, and trisomy 21.
- Classic radiographic findings of ToF are a *boot-shaped heart* (cardiac apex uplifted by RV hypertrophy, although the heart is normal in size) and decreased pulmonary vascularity.
- 25% of cases of ToF have a right-sided aortic arch.
- Surgical repair involves closure of VSD and opening of the right ventricular outflow tract obstruction, which is usually performed in infancy.
- Pulmonary atresia with a VSD is a severe form of ToF.

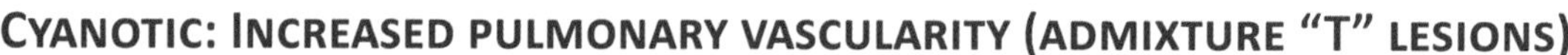

Cyanotic: Increased pulmonary vascularity (admixture "T" lesions)

Transposition of the great arteries (TGA)

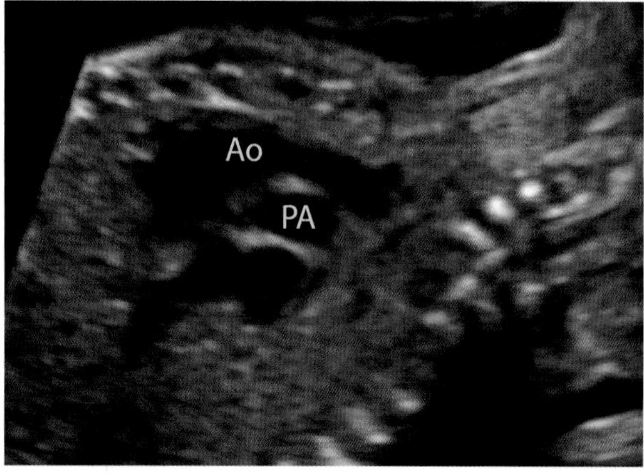

Transposition of the great arteries:

Antenatal ultrasound at an oblique plane through the great vessels demonstrates the aorta (Ao) is anterior to the pulmonary artery (PA), as the aorta arises from the right ventricle (the most anterior cardiac chamber).

Case courtesy Beryl Benacerraf, MD, Diagnostic Ultrasound Associates, Boston.

- In transposition of the great arteries (TGA), the right ventricle pumps blood to the aorta and the left ventricle pumps blood to the pulmonary arteries. TGA is the most common cause of cyanotic heart disease in newborns.

  Since the atria and ventricles are properly paired but the ventricles pump to the wrong great vessels, this configuration is termed atrioventricular concordance and ventriculoarterial discordance.
- The "strict" form of TGA is incompatible with life: There must be a site for admixture, either ASD, VSD, PDA, or a combination of left-to-right shunts.

- Prenatal ultrasound diagnosis of TGA requires evaluation of the short- or long-axis of the great vessels. TGA is usually inapparent on a four-chamber view. Sonographic diagnosis shows the aorta anterior to the heart and the great vessels exiting the heart in parallel (rather than crossing in the normal fashion).
- The classic radiographic findings of TGA are an "egg-on-a-string" appearance to the heart with a narrow mediastinal waist (caused by the configuration of the great vessels and thymic involution secondary to stress), lack of main pulmonary artery bulge, and parallel course of the aorta and PA. Although described in the literature, the "egg-on-a-string" appearance is uncommonly seen. A more typical radiographic appearance of TGA is a slightly narrow mediastinum and increased pulmonary vasculature; however, the radiographic picture can be varied depending on the nature of the coexisting shunt. A right aortic arch is seen in 5%.
- Surgical treatment is the arterial switch (Jatene) procedure, which swaps the aorta and pulmonary artery, and relocates the coronary arteries to the neo-aorta.

Tricuspid atresia

- Tricuspid atresia is absence of the tricuspid valve, which may have a variable appearance depending on the size of the associated VSD.

  Small VSD: Normal size heart, with decreased pulmonary vasculature.

  Large VSD: Enlarged heart with increased pulmonary flow.

Truncus arteriosus

- In truncus arteriosus, a single great artery arises from the base of the heart to supply the systemic, pulmonary, and coronary circulations. The single great artery usually over-rides a VSD.
- Truncus arteriosus is the most common type of congenital heart disease to have a right arch (21–36% of cases).
- The classic radiograph appearance is cardiomegaly, narrow mediastinum, and pulmonary edema.

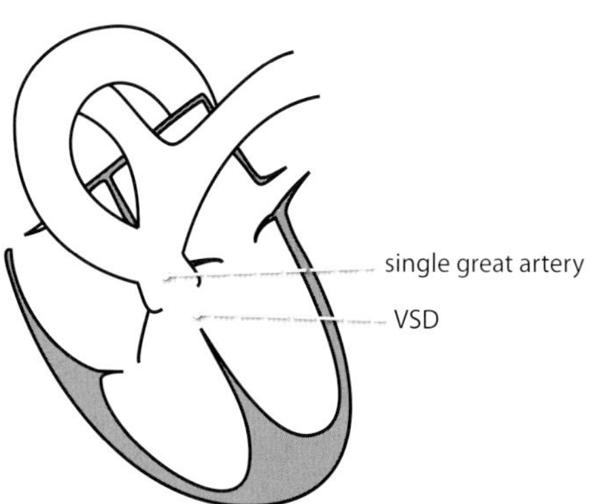

Total anomalous pulmonary venous return (TAPVR)

- In total anomalous pulmonary venous return (TAPVR), all pulmonary veins connect anomalously to the systemic venous circulation instead of draining into the left atrium.
- There is an obligate interatrial right-to-left communication enabling blood to reach the left heart, typically an ASD.
- Classification of TAPVR is based on the position of the venous drainage relative to the heart:

  Supracardiac (50%): Anomalous venous return is at or above the level of the SVC. The common confluence of the pulmonary veins drains into the left inominate vein via a **vertical** vein. Chest radiograph shows the characteristic *snowman* sign, with the dilated vertical vein making up the left border of the snowman. The snowman sign is seen in older patients without pulmonary venous obstruction.

  Cardiac (20%): Anomalous drainage is into the coronary sinus or right atrium.

  Infracardiac (20%): The anomalous drainage passes through the diaphragm via the esophageal hiatus and then drains into the hepatic IVC, hepatic vein, or portal venous system.

  Mixed (20%): Anomalous venous drainage is a combination of the above types.

- Clinical and radiographic findings depend on the degree of pulmonary venous obstruction and admixture. A typical radiographic appearance of obstructed TAPVR appearance is a normal-sized heart and pulmonary edema in an infant.

Single ("tingle") ventricle

- There are multiple variations of the single ventricle anomaly, which are all characterized by arteriovenous admixture at the level of a shared monoventricle.
- Double outlet right ventricle (DORV) can be considered a form of single ventricle.

SUMMARY OF CONGENITAL HEART DISEASE

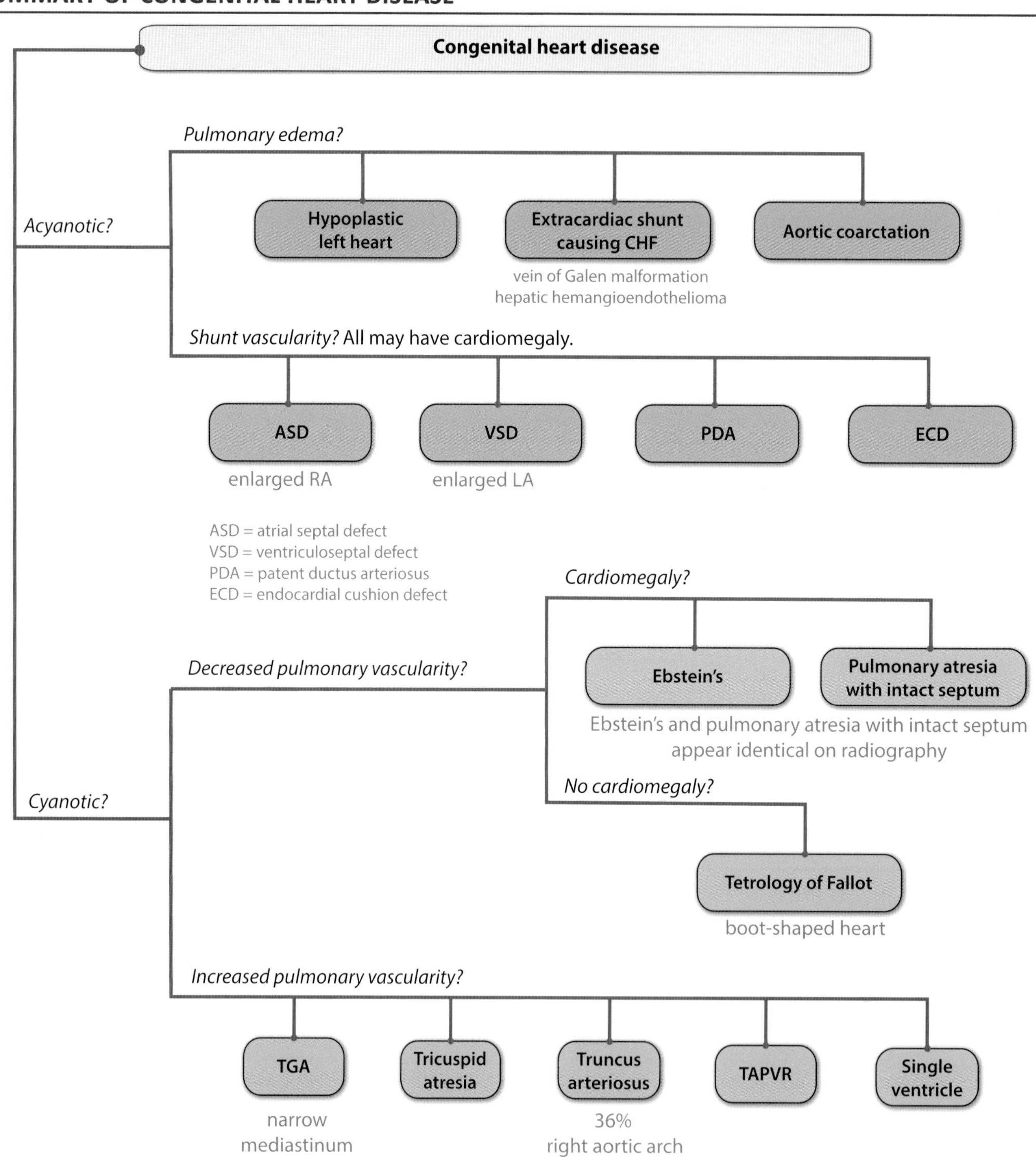

MISCELLANEOUS

Aortic coarctation

- Aortic coarctation is congenital focal narrowing of the aorta in the region of the ductus arteriosus. It may be preductal (proximal to the ductus, illustrated on the right), periductal, or postductal.
- The preductal form may cause congestive heart failure (CHF) in infants due to left ventricular obstruction. In contrast, the juxtaductal or postductal variants present later in life in the teenage or early adult years as upper extremity hypertension.
- Aortic coarctation is associated with bicuspid aortic valve, which may become stenotic and cause post-stenotic aortic dilation proximal to the site of coarctation.

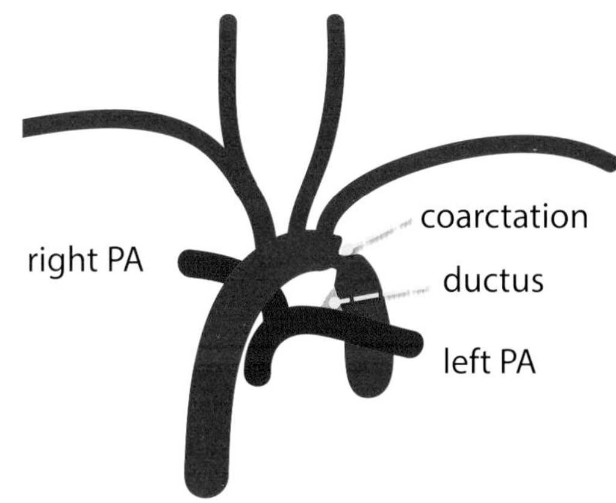

Diagram demonstrates infantile-type preductal aortic coarctation, with the coarctation located proximal to the ductus.

- Aortic coarctation is associated with Turner syndrome (XO).
- In infants, aortic coarctation may produce acyanotic CHF. In adults, the classic radiographic finding is the *3* sign representing the contour of the coarcted aorta in the left upper mediastinum. Although rib notching is described as a classic finding, this is rarely seen.

CARDIAC MASSES

Rhabdomyoma

- Rhabdomyoma is the most common cardiac tumor, and primarily affects babies under 1 year old with tuberous sclerosis. Rhabdomyoma is the earliest sign of tuberous sclerosis that can be diagnosed in utero.
- Rhabdomyoma has a varied clinical presentation, including arrhythmia and obstruction.
- The most common radiographic appearance of rhabdomyoma is cardiomegaly. Pulmonary vasculature is variable.

Teratoma

- Cardiac or pericardial teratoma is the second most common cardiac tumor detected in utero. A common location is attached to the root of pulmonary artery and aorta.
- Teratoma may cause pleural effusion when arising from the pericardium. Pericardial teratoma is one of the primary causes of massive perinatal pericardial effusion, with potential for tamponade.

Fibroma

- Fibroma is a rare, benign cardiac tumor of infancy and early childhood, arising from fibroblasts and myofibroblasts.
- Fibroma has a similar clinical presentation to rhabdomyoma, with rhythm disturbances and outflow obstruction. The interventricular septum is the most common site of origin, where a fibroma is especially likely to cause arrhythmia due to disruption of the conduction system.
- Cardiomegaly is the most common imaging finding.

Hemangioma

- Similar to teratoma, neonatal cardiac hemangioma is also associated with massive pericardial effusion.

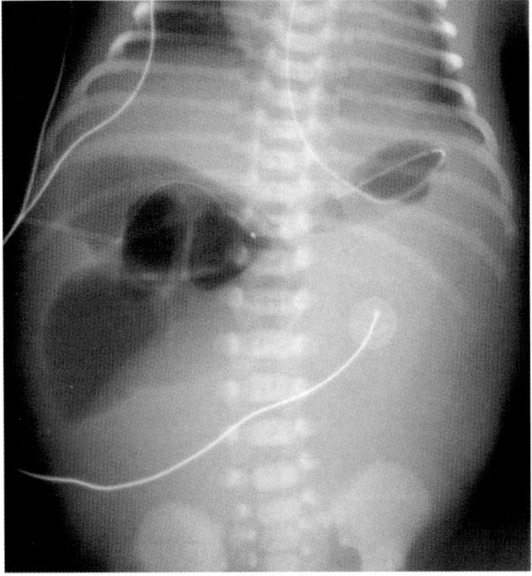

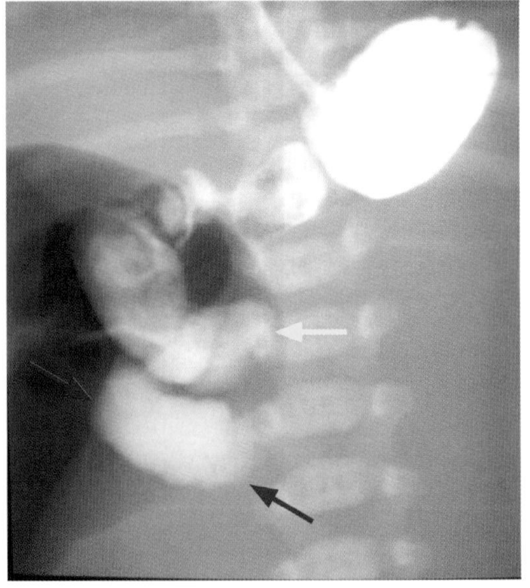

Malrotation with midgut volvulus: Abdominal radiograph (left image) shows a high bowel obstruction, with dilated proximal bowel and absence of distal bowel gas. Upper GI (right image) of the same patient demonstrates a duodenal–jejunal junction to the right of midline (yellow arrow) and a corkscrew appearance of the distal duodenum and proximal jejunum (red arrow).

Case courtesy Michael Callahan, MD and Carlo Buonomo, MD, Boston Children's Hospital.

- Malrotation is the failure of normal rotation of the bowel during embryogenesis, which predisposes to volvulus due to abnormal mesenteric fixation.
- Volvulus is a true surgical emergency, with a high mortality rate due to bowel ischemia if the diagnosis is delayed. Most infants with volvulus present with **neonatal bilious emesis**.

  Although bilious emesis may be due to several entities including non-obstructive gastroenteritis, malrotation with volvulus must be ruled out emergently with an upper GI.

- It is possible to have malrotation without volvulus, and symptoms without volvulus can be vague or nonspecific, including feeding intolerance, cyclic vomiting, and malabsorption. Therefore, it is essential to consider malrotation in a child with abdominal symptoms.

  75% of infants with malrotation present within the first month of life and 90% become symptomatic within one year.

- In order to diagnose malrotation (with or without volvulus), it is important to understand the anatomy of the normal upper gastrointestinal tract. In normal embryologic development, the bowel rotates 270 degrees counterclockwise around the superior mesenteric artery, causing the characteristic retroperitoneal course of the duodenum.

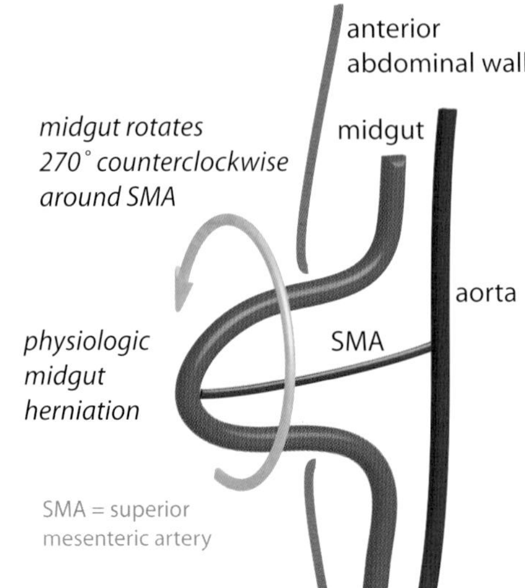

Normal rotation of the midgut about the superior mesenteric artery (SMA) during organogenesis.

Normal bowel rotation occurs between the 5th and 11th weeks of gestation.

- The most important anatomy to demonstrate on every upper GI is the C-sweep of the duodenum and position of the duodeno-jejunal junction (DJJ). The normal DJJ is evaluated on the frontal view and should be to the **left of the left-sided pedicle at the level of the duodenal bulb (L1).**

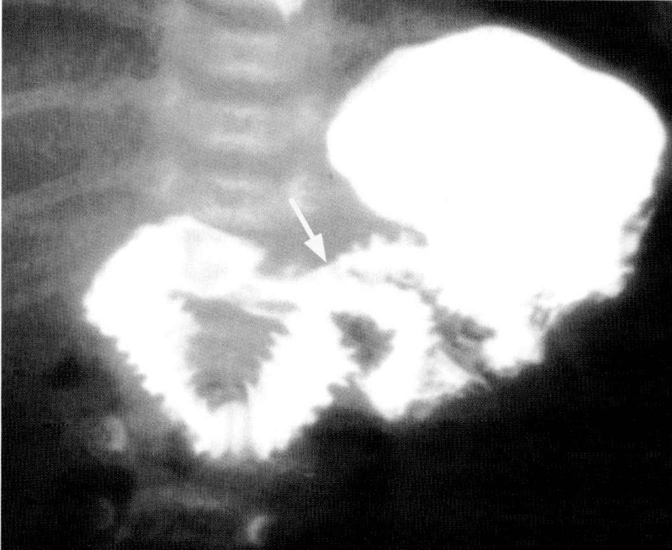

Normal upper GI: Spot image shows the duodeno-jejunal junction (arrow) to the left of midline, beyond the left pedicle of the vertebral body.

Case courtesy Michael Callahan, MD, Boston Children's Hospital.

On the lateral view, the normal duodenum first courses posteriorly into the retroperitoneum, inferiorly while retroperitoneal, anteriorly across the spine (remaining in the retroperitoneum), and then superiorly to meet the jejunum at the DJJ in the peritoneal space.

- On abdominal radiography, midgut volvulus most commonly appears as multiple dilated loops of bowel. Less commonly, midgut volvulus may produce a *double bubble* sign from duodenal obstruction. However, plain films can also be entirely normal in the setting of malrotation and vomiting.
- The classic upper GI finding of midgut volvulus is the *corkscrew* appearance of twisted bowel.
- In the absence of midgut volvulus, the diagnosis of malrotation can be challenging. The DJJ is a mobile structure and can be manipulated during the upper GI exam. Even experienced pediatric radiologists may occasionally disagree. Some clues to the presence of malrotation include:

  DJJ inferior to the duodenal bulb.

  DJJ to the right of the left pedicle.

  Cecum either more midline than typical or frankly in the left lower quadrant.

  On CT or US: Inversion of normal relationship of SMA and SMV (normally SMV to the right of the SMA). Color Doppler ultrasound or CT studies of the twisted mesenteric vessels demonstrate the *whirlpool* sign.

- The treatment of malrotation with volvulus is the Ladd procedure:

  Volvulus reduction, resection of necrotic bowel, and lysis of mesenteric adhesions ("Ladd" bands).

  The small and large bowel are separated, with the small bowel positioned primarily on the patient's right and the large bowel on the patient's left.

  Appendectomy may be performed.

Intussusception

- Intussusception is caused by two telescoping bowel loops prolapsing into each other. The most common location is ileocolic where the ileum prolapses into the colon.
- Intussusception is common and classically presents with colicky abdominal pain, "currant jelly stool," and a palpable right lower quadrant abdominal mass.
- Most children between 3 months and 3.5 years old have idiopathic intussusceptions caused by lymphoid tissue from a preceding viral illness. In contrast, both newborns and children older than 3.5 years often have a pathologic lead point, which may be an intestinal polyp, Meckel diverticulum (infants), or lymphoma (children).
- A transient, asymptomatic, incidental, short-segment intussusception in older children or adults seen on CT performed for another reason is likely clinically insignificant.
- Radiographs are nonspecific, but may show a soft tissue mass in the right lower quadrant.
- Ultrasound is the primary modality for diagnosis, which shows a characteristic *target* or *pseudokidney* sign with alternating layers of bowel wall and mesenteric fat.
- The differential diagnosis of bloody stool and thick-walled bowel on ultrasound includes intussusception, colitis, and much less commonly intramural hematoma (e.g., due to trauma or Henoch–Schönlein purpura).

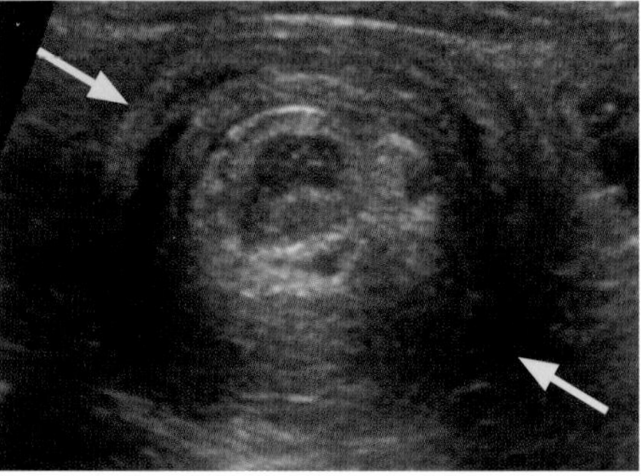

Ilio-colic intussusception: Right lower quadrant ultrasound shows the *target* sign (arrows) with alternating layers of bowel wall and interposed mesenteric fat.

Case courtesy Michael Hanley, MD, University of Virginia Health System.

- The first line treatment is reduction with an air or contrast enema. The choice of air or contrast varies by institution, but air enemas are generally considered safer.

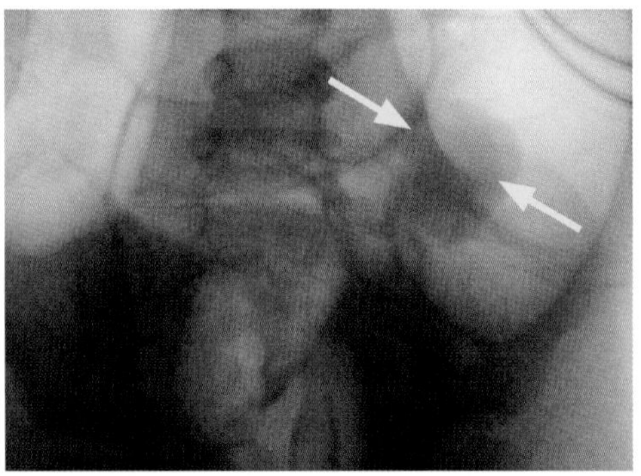

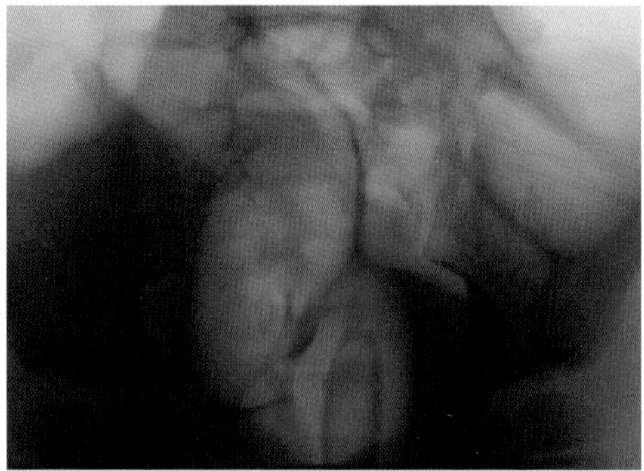

Intussusception reduction (same patient as the ultrasound above): Initial prone spot radiograph (left image) from an air enema shows a mass in the right lower quadrant (arrows), which spontaneously reduces after continued insufflation of air (right image).

A surgeon should be present. IV antibiotics are sometimes, but not universally, administered.

A large-bore needle (16 gauge angiocatheter) must be available to decompress a potential tension pneumoperitoneum, which may cause fatal compression of the IVC if untreated.

A large enema tip should be used to prevent leakage, which may need to be taped to the skin.

Air should be insufflated up to 120 mm Hg (between cries; reading during cries will be artificially high).

A successful reduction will show rush of air into the small bowel.

The "rule of 3's" applies to hydrostatic reduction: Up to 3 attempts can be performed, up to 3 minutes each. If unsuccessful, the patient must go to surgery.

- Contraindications to pneumatic reduction include free air, peritoneal signs, and septic shock.

Esophageal atresia and tracheoesophageal fistula (TEF)

- Esophageal atresia is a blind-ending esophagus caused by faulty embryologic separation of the primitive trachea from the esophagus. In embryologic development, the trachea and esophagus initially form as one structure.
- Esophageal atresia is almost always associated with tracheoesophageal fistula (TEF).
- 50% of patients with TEF have associated anomalies, most commonly the **VACTERL** association:

> **V**ertebral segmentation anomalies.
>
> **A**nal atresia.
>
> **C**ardiac anomalies.
>
> **T**racheo**E**sophageal fistula.
>
> **R**enal anomalies.
>
> **L**imb (radial ray) anomalies.

- A classic radiographic finding of the most common A type (82%) TEF (with proximal esophageal atresia and a distal tracheoesophageal fistula) shows an NG tube terminating in the mid-esophagus with air-filled bowel from a distal TEF.
- The much less common B type (8%) may present with a gasless abdomen, due to esophageal atresia without fistula.
- The H type (6%) features a continuous esophagus without esophageal atresia, but with an upper esophageal TEF. This type may present later in childhood with recurrent aspiration.
- Esophageal atresia should be considered in utero if there is polyhydramnios and lack of visualization of the stomach.

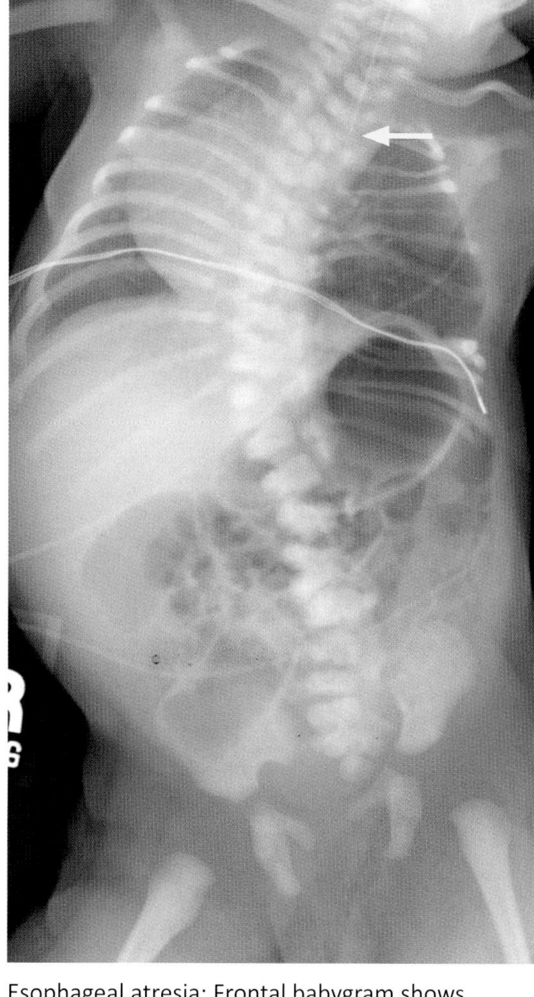

Esophageal atresia: Frontal babygram shows high position of the esophageal catheter (arrow) with distal bowel gas, consistent with tracheoesophageal fistula.

This neonate has VACTERL, with multiple vertebral segmentation anomalies and dextrocardia visible on this radiograph. Not visible on this image are this baby's anal atresia, unilateral renal agenesis, and a missing thumb.

- TEF is often associated with tracheal anomalies including tracheomalacia and bronchus suis (right upper lobe bronchus arising directly from trachea).

Gastric atresia

- Gastric atresia represents congenital obstruction of the distal stomach.
- Gastric atresia causes non-bilious vomiting. In contrast to hypertrophic pyloric stenosis, the vomiting does not get progressively worse.
- A diagnostic imaging finding is the *single* bubble, with a large bubble of air (or contrast) in the proximal stomach.
- A less severe variant is a nonobstructive antral web.

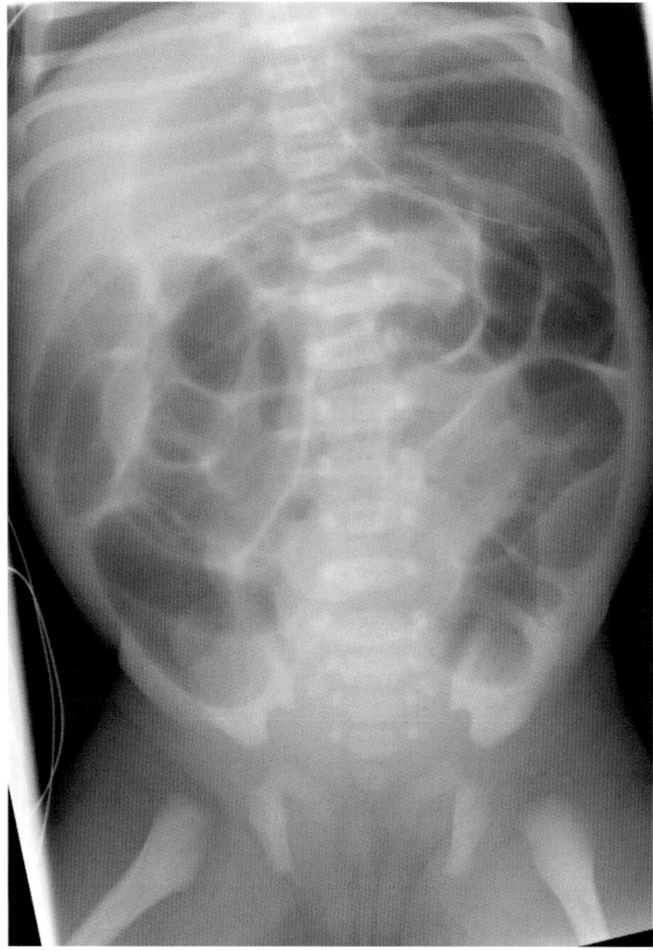

Neonatal distal bowel obstruction: Abdominal radiograph shows numerous dilated loops of bowel throughout the entire abdomen. A nasogastric tube is in the stomach.

- Neonatal bowel obstruction, occurring within the first 24–48 hours of life, is a completely different entity from childhood or adult obstruction, with different workup and different etiologies. Unlike in adults, CT plays no role in the workup of neonatal bowel obstruction.
- In the neonate, small bowel cannot be distinguished from large bowel based on location or size of the bowel loops.
- When loops of distended bowel are seen and obstruction is suspected, it is possible to divide the differential into *proximal/high* obstruction (proximal to the distal jejunum) or *distal/low* obstruction (distal to the distal jejunum) based solely on the number of dilated loops seen.
- All cases of proximal obstruction are surgical.
- The goal of imaging is to differentiate surgical from non-surgical causes of distal obstruction.
- If the initial radiograph does not provide a definite diagnosis, the imaging test of choice for a **proximal** obstruction is typically an **upper GI**. Midgut volvulus must be ruled out.

  A patient with characteristic clinical and imaging findings of duodenal atresia can be diagnosed on radiograph alone. For instance, a baby with known Down syndrome and a double bubble on radiograph is considered diagnostic of duodenal atresia.

- Subsequent to the initial radiograph, the imaging test of choice for a **distal obstruction** is a **contrast enema**, which can be both diagnostic and therapeutic.

  A neonatal contrast enema is performed with a relatively low-osmolar, water-soluble contrast material, such as a 17% solution of iothalamate meglumine (400 mOsm/kg water; *Cysto-Conray II*, Covidien).

- All causes of congenital proximal bowel obstruction are surgical. The primary purpose of an upper GI is to distinguish between midgut volvulus (requiring emergent surgery) and the atresias, which require a non-emergent repair.

Malrotation and midgut volvulus

- Discussed in GI emergencies.

Duodenal atresia, stenosis, and web

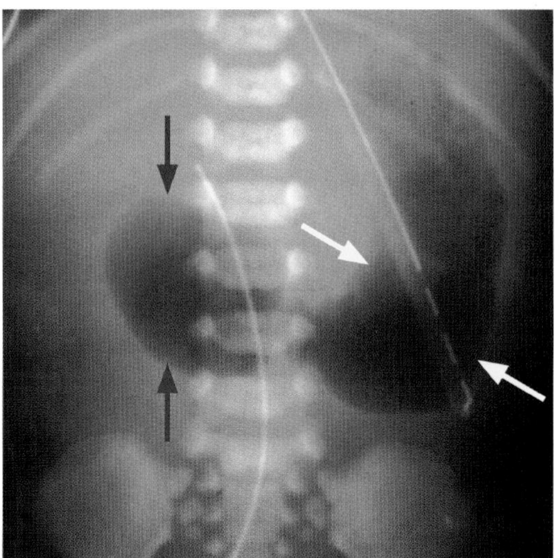

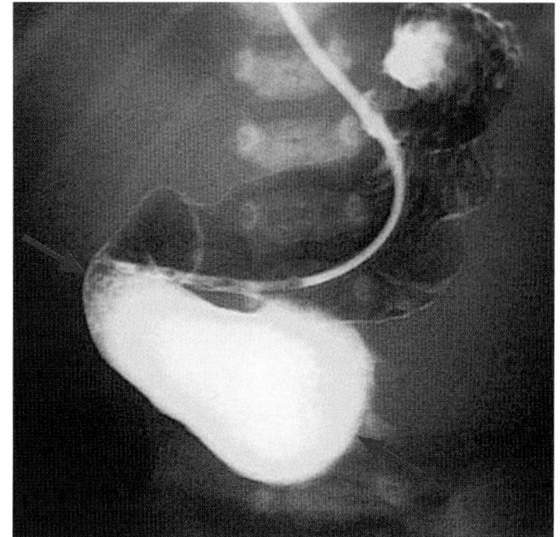

Duodenal atresia: Abdominal radiograph (left image) shows the classic *double bubble* sign, with a distended stomach (yellow arrows) and a distended duodenal bulb (red arrow). Upper-GI study (right image) shows a markedly distended duodenum (red arrows) and no contrast passage into the jejunum.

Case courtesy Michael Callahan, MD and Carlo Buonomo, MD, Boston Children's Hospital.

- During embryogenesis, the duodenum forms as a solid tube. Lack of recanalization causes the spectrum of diseases ranging from duodenal atresia (most severe; complete lack of recanalization) to duodenal stenosis (least severe; partial recanalization).
- A less severe variant, the duodenal web, allows liquids to pass, but causes the *windsock deformity* after the child begins to eat solid foods, which get stuck in the web.
- Even a complete atresia does not preclude distal bowel gas. In the presence of a rare congenital bifid common bile duct, bowel gas can travel through the ampulla of Vater and enter the distal bowel.
- Duodenal anomalies are associated with additional abnormalities in 50% of cases, most commonly Down syndrome; 30% of babies with duodenal atresia have Down syndrome. Other associated anomalies include:

  VACTERL.

  Shunt vascularity cardiac lesions (ASD, VSD, PDA, and endocardial cushion defect).

  Malrotation.

  Annular pancreas, which is seen in 20% of babies with duodenal atresia.

- The classic radiographic appearance of duodenal atresia is the *double bubble* sign caused by dilation of both the stomach and the proximal duodenum, without distal bowel gas. A patient with a *double bubble* and no distal bowel gas can be presumed to have duodenal atresia.
- If distal bowel gas is present with a *double bubble* sign, the differential diagnosis includes midgut volvulus, annular pancreas (pancreas wraps around the duodenum), and the less severe variants of duodenal atresia including duodenal stenosis and web.

Jejunal atresia and stenosis.

- Unlike duodenal atresia, jejunal atresia is most commonly caused by an in-utero vascular insult. Jejunal atresia is more common than stenosis.
- The *triple bubble* has been described to represent proximal jejunal atresia, which may present on radiography as dilated stomach, duodenum, and proximal jejunum.

Congenital low/distal bowel obstruction

- A contrast enema is performed to differentiate surgical causes (distal atresias and Hirschsprung disease) from medical causes (meconium ileus and functional immaturity) of low/distal bowel obstruction.
- When performing a contrast enema, isotonic or mildly hypertonic water-soluble contrast is used, such as a 17% solution of cysto-Conray II (400 mOsm). High osmolar contrast may cause fluid shifts and resultant destabilization of the patient.

Differential diagnosis of microcolon

- Microcolon is a colon of abnormally small caliber (typically <1 cm), secondary to disuse. A relatively distal obstruction is necessary to develop a microcolon, as the succus entericus secreted by the proximal bowel prevents microcolon. The two most common causes of microcolon are meconium ileus and ileal atresia.

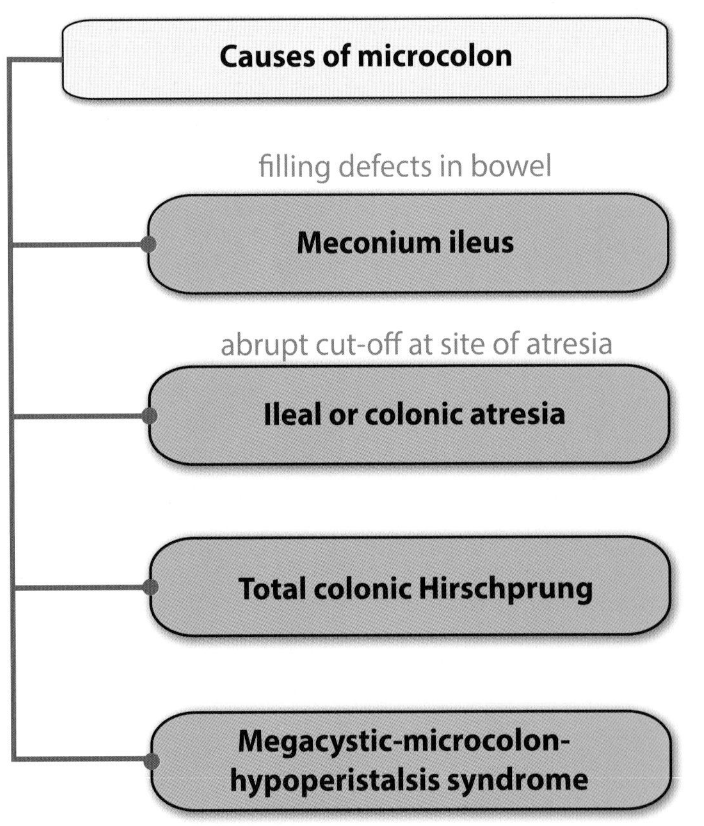

Peritoneal/scrotal calcifications may be seen in association with meconium ileus. In contrast to meconium ileus, small left colon syndrome (also confusingly called meconium plug syndrome; subsequently discussed) does NOT cause a microcolon.

Jejunal atresia does NOT cause microcolon as there is enough succus entericus produced to nourish the colon.

Total colonic Hirschsprung is rare. The much more common segmental involvement does not cause microcolon.

Meconium ileus

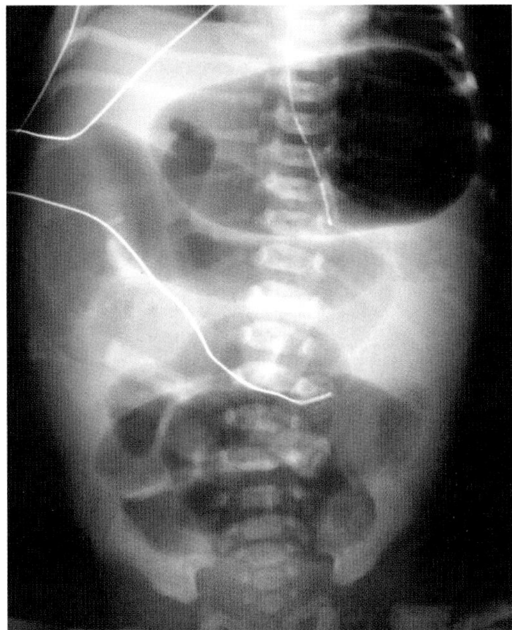

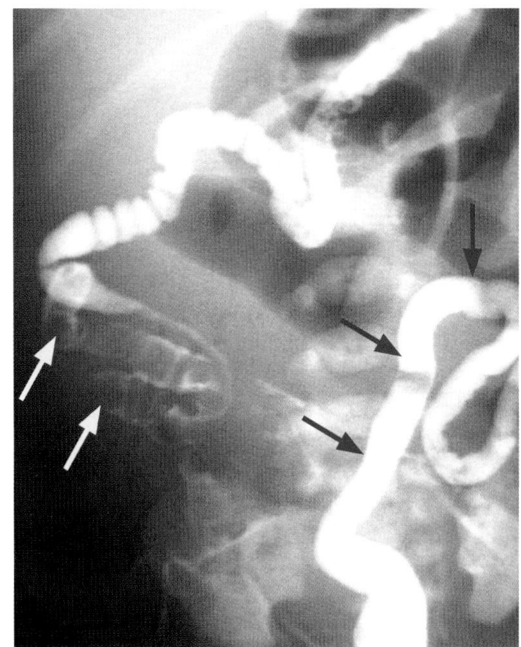

Meconium ileus: Neonatal abdominal radiograph (left image) shows a low/distal small bowel obstruction, with a dilated stomach and numerous dilated loops of bowel extending to the pelvis. Contrast enema (right image) shows a very small caliber colon (*microcolon;* red arrows), with numerous rounded filling defects in the distal ileum (yellow arrows), representing inspissated meconium.

Case courtesy Michael Callahan, MD and Carlo Buonomo, MD, Boston Children's Hospital.

- Meconium ileus causes bowel obstruction from inspissated meconium in the distal ileum and colon. Meconium ileus may be complicated by perforation and resultant meconium peritonitis, which can cause abdominal and scrotal calcifications.
- Meconium ileus is the earliest manifestation of cystic fibrosis: Almost 100% of babies with meconium ileus have cystic fibrosis, while ~10% of babies with cystic fibrosis have meconium ileus.
- The classic radiographic appearance of meconium ileus is a distal obstruction (multiple loops of dilated bowel), with *soap-bubble* lucencies in the right lower quadrant.
- Contrast enema shows a microcolon (meconium ileus has the smallest of all microcolons) with a distended ileum containing multiple rounded filling defects representing inspissated meconium.
- Meconium ileus is both diagnosed and treated with therapeutic water-soluble gastrografin enema, which functions to loosen the inspissated meconium. It often takes multiple attempts to fully clean out the meconium, and carefully increasing the contrast osmolality may be helpful. Uncommonly, resistant cases may need to be treated surgically.

Ileal atresia/colonic atresia

- Atresia of the ileum or colon features a microcolon distal to the atretic segment.
- Colonic atresia is rare.
- Unlike meconium ileus, ileal and colonic atresia demonstrate an abrupt cutoff at the site of atresia, and there are no filling defects within the bowel.

Small left colon/functional immaturity of the colon (FIC)/meconium plug syndrome

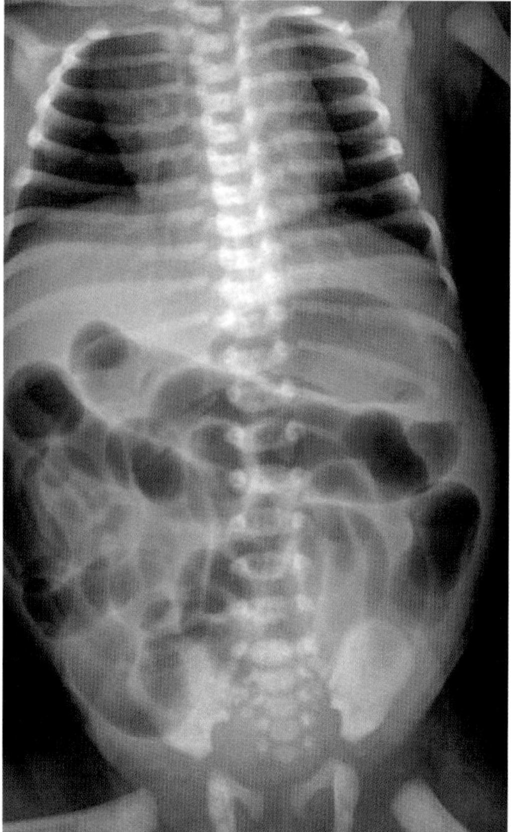

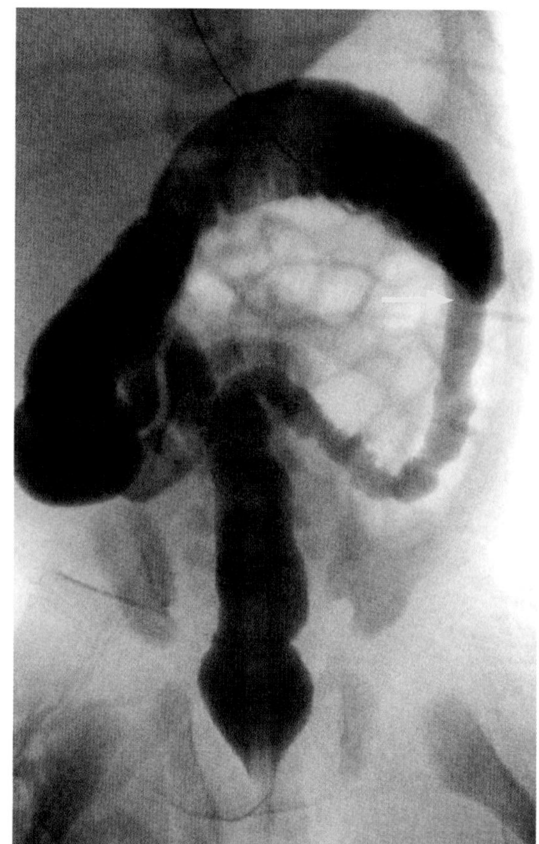

Small left colon: Babygram (left image) shows numerous loops of dilated bowel, suggestive of a distal obstructive pattern. Contrast enema (right image) shows a moderately reduced caliber of the left colon, with an abrupt transition (arrow) at the splenic flexure. The rectum is normal in caliber.

Case courtesy Michael Hanley, MD, University of Virginia Health System.

- Small left colon, also known as functional immaturity of the colon or meconium plug syndrome, is the most common diagnosis in neonates who fail to pass meconium. Small left colon is caused by temporary functional immaturity of the colonic ganglion cells, which causes the distal colon to have abnormal motility right after birth.
- Small left colon is seen more commonly in pre-term neonates, neonates born to mothers who received magnesium for (pre)eclampsia, and infants born to diabetic mothers. Infants with small left colon are almost always otherwise normal.
- In contrast to meconium ileus, small left colon is *not* a cause of microcolon. Small left colon is *not* associated with cystic fibrosis/meconium ileus despite the confusing name of "meconium plug syndrome."
- The imaging appearance on an abdominal radiograph is of a distal obstructive pattern.
- Contrast enema shows a small left colon, typically with a discrete transition in caliber at the splenic flexure. There may be filling defects within the small left colon representing meconium plugs.
- Similar to meconium ileus, water-soluble enema is diagnostic and therapeutic, and small left colon resolves with conservative therapy.
- The primary differential consideration is Hirschsprung disease with a transition at the splenic flexure. In contrast to small left colon, Hirschsprung disease would not feature a distensible rectum and would not resolve after an enema treatment.

Hirschsprung disease

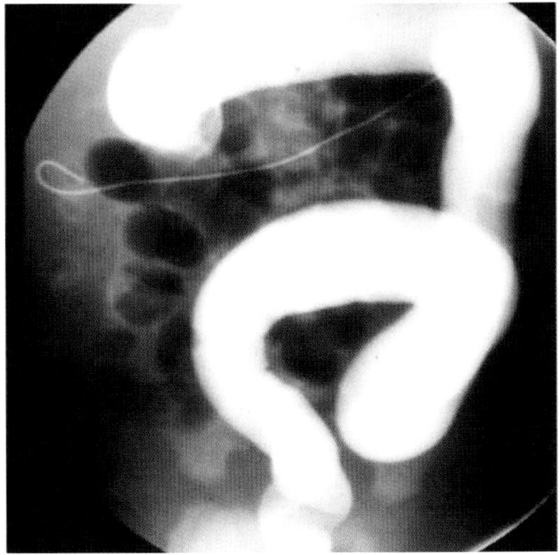

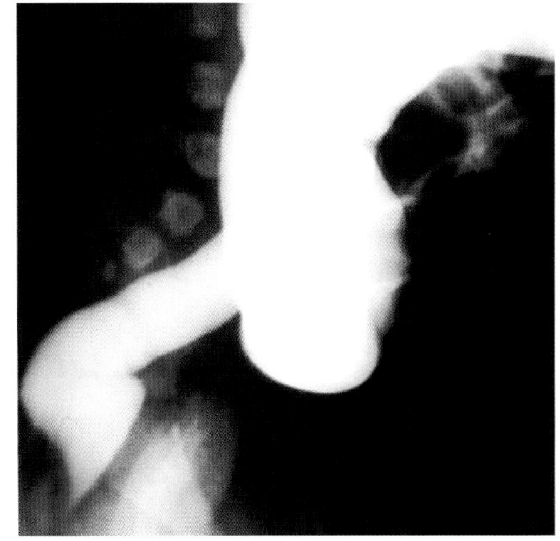

Hirschsprung disease: Frontal (left image) and lateral (right image) spot radiographs from a contrast enema show a narrowed rectum, which has a smaller diameter than the sigmoid colon.

Case courtesy Michael Callahan, MD and Carlo Buonomo, MD, Boston Children's Hospital.

- Hirschsprung disease is aganglionosis of the distal bowel, resulting in lack of relaxivity of the involved bowel. Hirschsprung disease is caused by arrest of the normal craniocaudal (proximal-to-distal) migration of vagal neural crest cells to the distal bowel wall. The anus is therefore always affected and the involved bowel is continuous distal to proximal. Hirschsprung disease ranges in severity from isolated internal anal sphincter involvement (ultrashort segment) to involvement of the entire colon (very rare, approximately 1–3% of cases, and typically genetic).
- Up to one third of cases of Hirschsprung develop a form of enterocolitis similar to necrotizing enterocolitis, with toxic megacolon being the fulminant form. It is therefore important to consider Hirschsprung in a neonate with bowel obstruction and colitis.
- There are multiple congenital anomalies associated with Hirschsprung disease. Five percent have trisomy 21, but there is much less of an association with Down syndrome compared to duodenal atresia.
- Radiography of Hirschsprung disease shows a distal bowel obstruction pattern.
- Contrast enema typically shows a *cone-shaped* transition zone at the junction of the spastic, narrowed distal colon and the dilated proximal colon, which is best seen on the lateral view.

  The rectum normally has a larger diameter than the sigmoid. When Hirschsprung involves the rectum, the rectum will be in spasm and the sigmoid will be dilated, caused an abnormal rectum:sigmoid ratio less than 1 (i.e., rectum is smaller than the sigmoid).

  The initial contrast enema may be normal in neonates with ultrashort segment involvement.
- In contrast to functional immaturity of the colon, Hirschsprung disease tends to cause a tapered, rather than an abrupt, transition zone.
- Definitive diagnosis is with suction biopsy of the bowel wall. Treatment is surgical.

Megacystis microcolon intestinal hypoperistalsis syndrome

- Megacystis microcolon intestinal hypoperistalsis syndrome is a rare congenital loss of bladder and bowel smooth muscle function causing absent intestinal peristalsis, microcolon, and distended non-obstructed urinary bladder. It is usually fatal.

Malrotation

- Although uncommon, the Ladd bands of malrotation may cause a distal obstruction.

- The etiologies and imaging of childhood bowel obstruction overlap with those of adults. Adult bowel obstruction is most commonly caused by adhesions and hernia, both of which may also cause obstruction in a child.
- The most common causes of childhood bowel obstruction can be remembered with the mnemonic **AAIIMM** (appendicitis, adhesions, internal/inguinal hernia, intussusception, Meckel's, and malrotation). Most causes of childhood obstruction are treated surgically.

Appendicitis

- Appendicitis is one of the more common causes of ileus or partial bowel obstruction in children.

Inguinal hernia

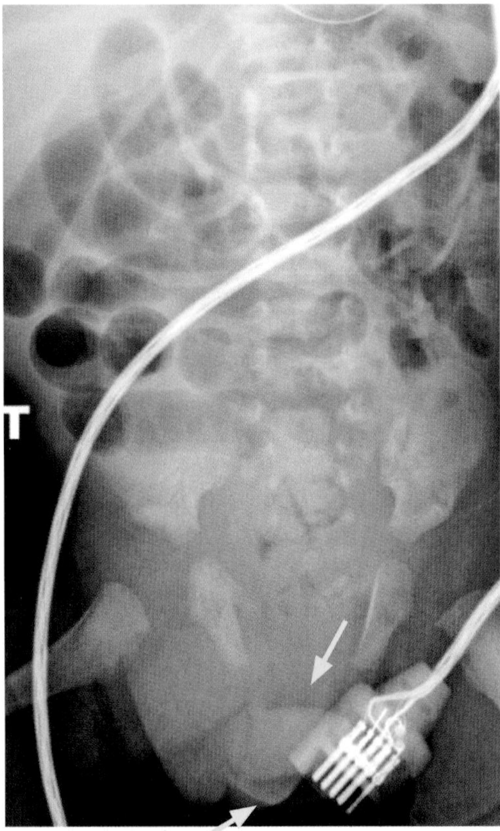
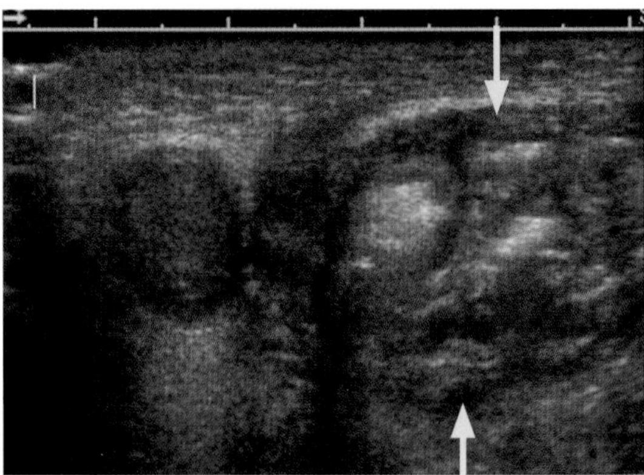
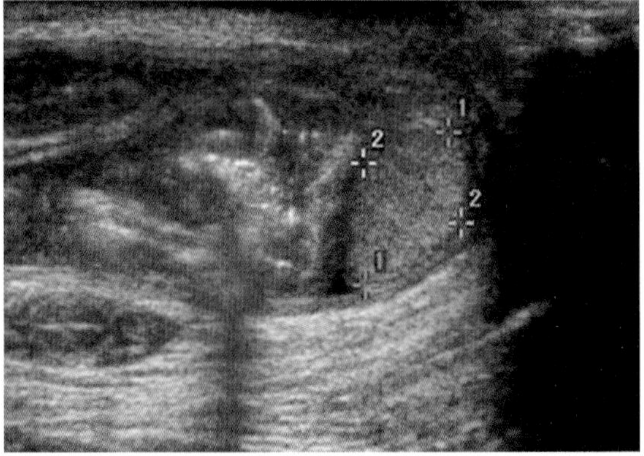

Inguinal hernia: Frontal radiograph (left image) shows numerous dilated loops of bowel, with the suggestion of increased opacification in the region of the left hemiscrotum (arrows). Transverse ultrasound of the scrotum (top right image) shows numerous loops of bowel in the left hemiscrotum (arrows). A sagittal ultrasound of the left testis (bottom right image) shows that the testis is normal (calipers) but is displaced by the intra-scrotal bowel loops.

Case courtesy Michael Callahan, MD, Boston Children's Hospital.

- Indirect inguinal hernia is due to a patent processus vaginalis, which maintains a peritoneal communication to the scrotum via the inguinal ring.
- Imaging of an inguinal hernia causing obstruction shows bowel in the inguinal canal or scrotum. There is risk of bowel incarceration in an irreducible hernia.

Crohn disease

- Crohn disease may be a cause of bowel obstruction. Up to 30% of newly diagnosed Crohn disease presents in the pediatric population.

Imperforate anus

- Imperforate anus is a clinical diagnosis, but radiology plays a role to evaluate the level of the obstruction, which is classified as high or low in relation to the puborectalis sling.

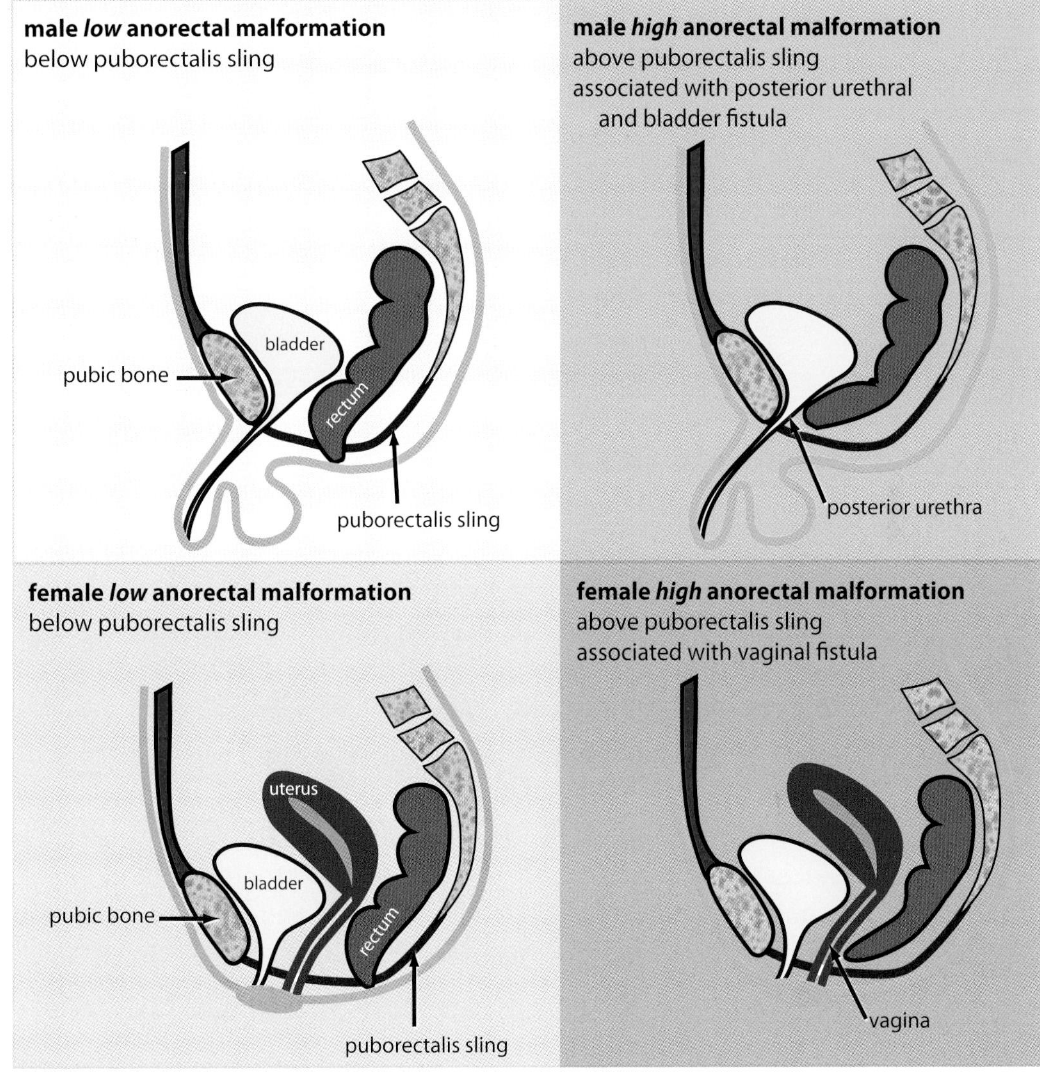

- A high lesion (above the puborectalis sling) is associated with genitourinary–rectal fistula, lumbosacral anomalies or VACTERL association, and requires a more complex treatment.

  Males may have a fistula between the rectum and posterior urethra or bladder.

  Females may have a rectovaginal fistula.

  In either sex, treatment is initial colostomy followed by definitive repair.

- A low lesion (below the puborectalis sling) is associated with perineal fistula and is treated with single-stage perineal anoplasty.
- The determination of high or low lesion is usually made clinically, based on passage of meconium, and is dependent on sex.

  In males, if meconium is passed in the urine → high lesion.

  In females, if meconium is passed in the vagina and a fistula is not visualized → high lesion. Low lesions may cause distal vaginal fistulas, which can be visualized by physical exam.

- Previously, prone radiographs were used to determine if a lesion was high or low; however, infracoccygeal ultrasound is thought to be a more accurate method to determine the level of the imperforate anus.

Neonatal cholestatic jaundice

Approach to pathologic neonatal jaundice

- In contrast to the unconjugated hyperbilirubinemia of the benign and self-limited physiologic jaundice of the newborn, conjugated hyperbilirubinemia is never normal and is due to hepatic or biliary dysfunction.
- There are innumerable causes of conjugated hyperbilirubinemia, including biliary atresia, Alagille syndrome, bile acid synthetic defects, metabolic disease, alpha-1-antitrypsin deficiency, and infectious etiologies.
- The goal of imaging is to differentiate between biliary atresia (approximately 25% of neonatal conjugated hyperbilirubinemia) and "neonatal hepatitis," which is a wastebasket diagnoses for all other causes combined. Tc-99m-HIDA hepatobiliary scintigraphy is the test of choice to distinguish between these two entities.

  Patients may be premedicated with 5 days of phenobarbital to stimulate hepatocyte activity prior to hepatobiliary scintigraphy, although this varies by institution.

  The HIDA agent is actively transported into the hepatocyte and excreted (not conjugated) into the bile.
- Biliary atresia requires prompt repair to prevent irreversible liver damage. The treatment of neonatal hepatitis is nonsurgical.

Biliary atresia

- Biliary atresia is characterized by an obliterative cholangiopathy that affects the intra- and extra-hepatic bile ducts, leading to obstructive (conjugated) jaundice. Biliary atresia leads to progressive cirrhosis and death in early childhood if untreated.
- Hepatobiliary scintigraphy shows normal hepatic tracer uptake and clearance but **no excretion into the small bowel.** Ultrasound is not able to distinguish between biliary atresia and neonatal hepatitis. The absence of a gallbladder on ultrasound is suggestive of biliary atresia, but a gallbladder is seen in 20% of cases.
- Treatment of biliary atresia is the Kasai portoenterostomy, a palliative procedure. The entire extrahepatic biliary tree is excised and a jejunal Roux loop is anastomosed to the cut surface of the liver capsule. 80% of children with a successful surgery survive 10 years, at which point a liver transplant is necessary.

Neonatal hepatitis

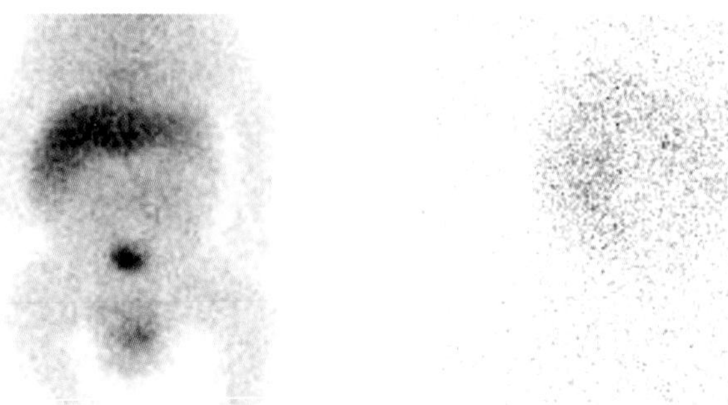
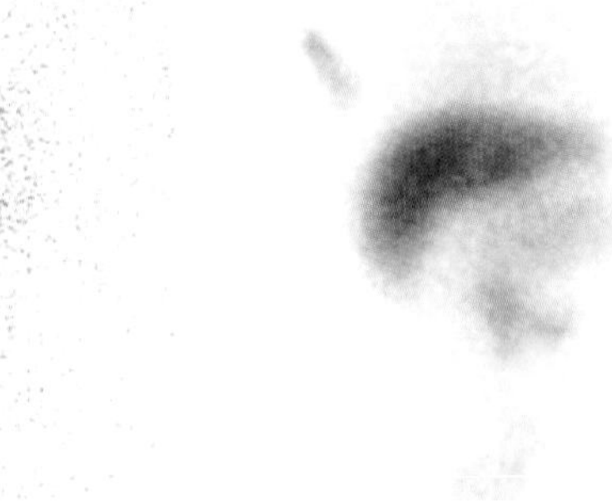

Neonatal hepatitis: 60-minute delay HIDA (left image) shows uptake in the liver but with a large amount of blood pool activity. There is uptake in the bladder and the diaper, but no bowel uptake. Delayed 24-hour image (middle image) also does not show bowel uptake, but there is abnormal persistent hepatic uptake, which is suggestive of hepatitis. A follow-up exam was performed a few weeks later (right image), which showed normal hepatic uptake and small bowel excretion, confirming resolution of neonatal hepatitis.

Case courtesy Michael Hanley, MD, University of Virginia Health System.

- Hepatobiliary scintigraphy shows poor hepatic excretion, delayed hepatic clearance (beyond 12 hours), and variable bowel excretion.
- Biliary atresia can be effectively ruled out if there is any excretion into the GI tract.

Pediatric hepatobiliary neoplasia and masses

- Primary pediatric liver tumors may be classified pathologically as epithelial (hepatocyte-derived) or mesenchymal, with benign and malignant tumors in each category. Liver metastases may be seen in the setting of neuroblastoma, Wilms tumor, sarcoma, and Burkitt lymphoma.
- It is usually possible to narrow the differential based on imaging appearance (cystic or solid), age of the patient, and tumor markers (AFP and endothelial growth factor).
- Benign epithelial lesions also seen in adults, including focal nodular hyperplasia and adenoma, are discussed in the gastrointestinal imaging section.

Cystic Liver/biliary masses

Mesenchymal hamartoma

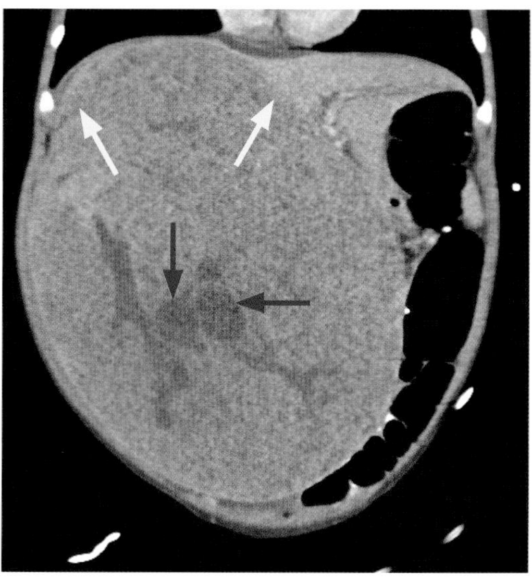

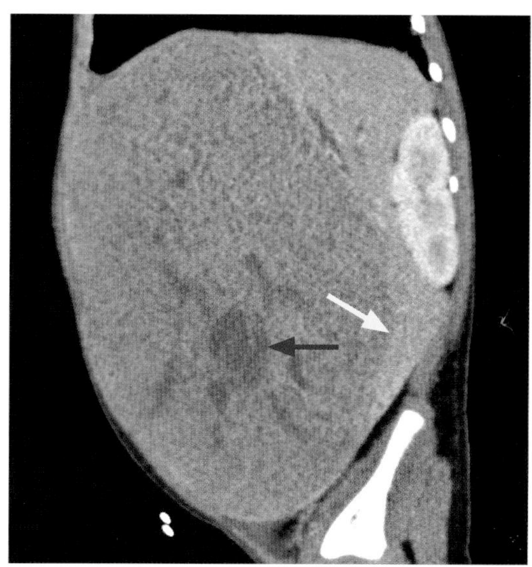

Mesenchymal hamartoma: Coronal (left image) and sagittal contrast-enhanced CT shows a massive, heterogeneous mass arising from the right lobe of the liver. The displaced liver parenchyma forms a *claw* sign around the mass (yellow arrows). There are cystic spaces (red arrows) and portal venous fragments within the mass; however, the mass appears predominantly solid, which may be secondary to numerous tiny cysts below the resolution of CT.

Case courtesy Michael Hanley, MD, University of Virginia Health System.

- Mesenchymal hamartoma is a benign, multicystic, hamartomatous lesion, which contains malformed bile ducts, portal vein fragments, and often extramedullary hematopoiesis. It is considered a developmental anomaly rather than a neoplasm.
- Most children present in the neonatal period with an enlarging abdominal mass, with 80% diagnosed by 2 years of age.
- In contrast to hepatoblastoma, tumor markers are not elevated.
- Imaging of mesenchymal hamartoma typically shows a large, multicystic, abdominal mass. The cysts can be of various sizes, can contain debris, and can be divided by septae of variable thickness. Hemorrhage and calcification are rare. Occasionally, the cysts may be so small that the mass appears solid. When large, the mass may displace vasculature.
- Surgical resection is almost always curative.

Choledochal cyst/Caroli disease

- Choledochal cysts (including Caroli disease) represent saccular or fusiform dilation of bile ducts, which may be segmental or diffuse. The Todani classification of choledochal cysts is discussed further in the gastrointestinal imaging section.

Gallbladder hydrops

- Gallbladder hydrops is a pathologically distended gallbladder, usually associated with infection or a systemic inflammatory process such as Kawasaki disease.

Solid liver/biliary masses

Terminology of "hemangioma" in pediatric radiology

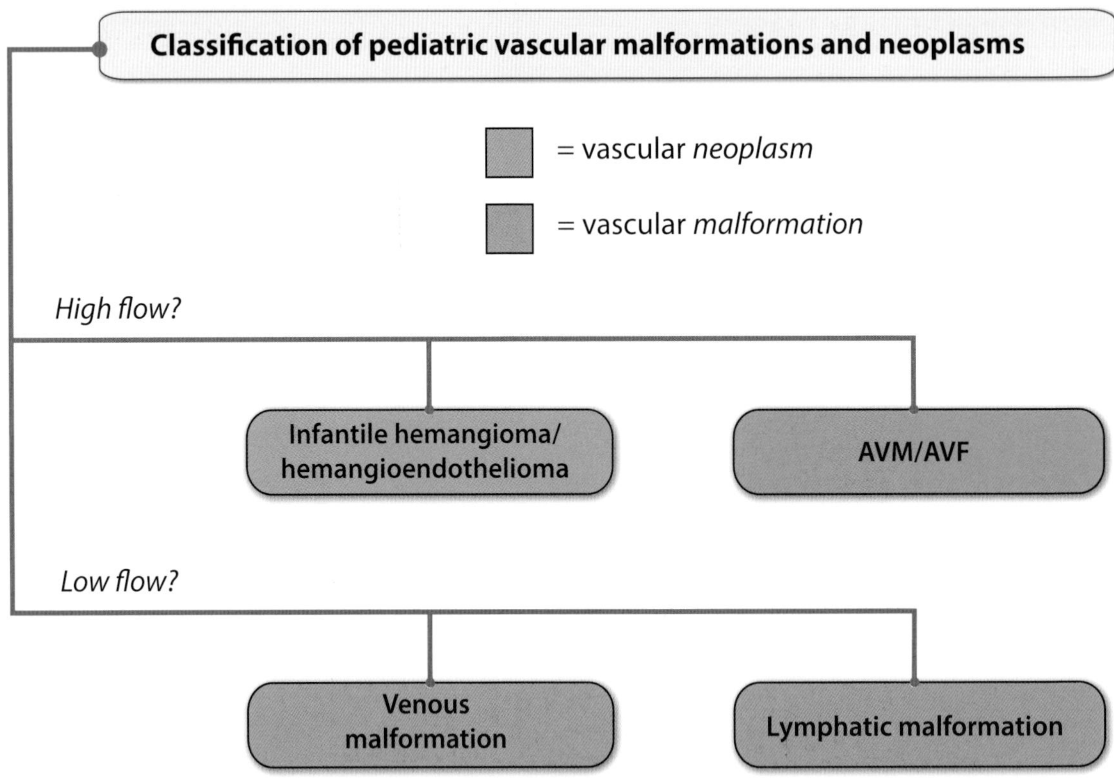

- Pediatric vascular anomalies can be divided into vascular neoplasms and vascular malformations, where neoplasms feature new cell growth and malformations feature disorganized vasculature without cell growth.
- Pediatric vascular anomalies can also be classified physiologically as high-flow or low-flow lesions. High-flow vascular malformations include arteriovenous malformations (AVM) and arteriovenous fistulas (AVF), while low-flow vascular malformations include venous malformations and lymphatic malformations.
- The term "hemangioma" is a common source of confusion. In particular, the term "hepatic hemangioma" is often used to describe multiple unrelated vascular lesions including infantile hemangioma, potentially malignant hemangioendotheliomas, and benign venous malformations.
- The common adult hepatic "hemangioma" is actually a venous malformation in the classification above. Similarly, the soft tissue "hemangiomas" of Maffucci syndrome are also venous malformations.
- Infantile hemangioma and hemangioendothelioma, discussed on the next page, are high-flow vascular neoplasms. Hemangioendotheliomas have the potential to metastasize.

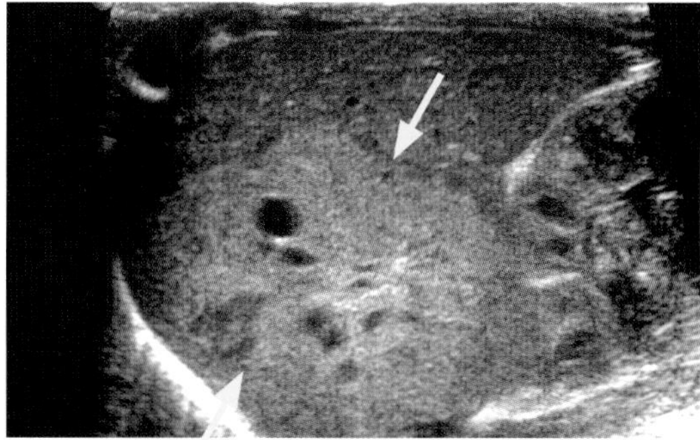

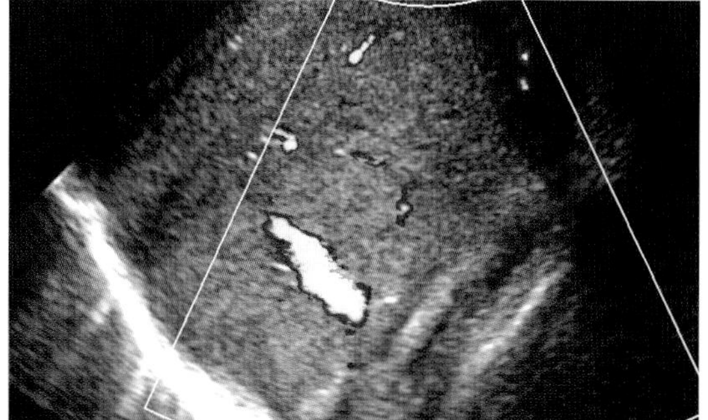

Grayscale (left image) and power Doppler (right image) ultrasound images of the liver show a highly vascular mass in the right hepatic lobe (arrows), containing numerous dilated vascular spaces.

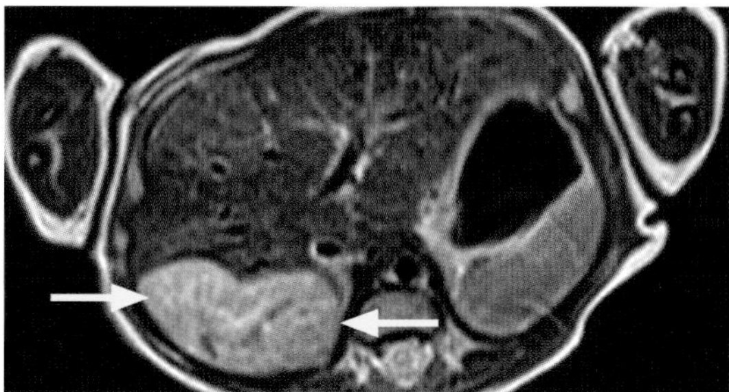

T2-weighted MRI shows a T2 hyperintense, predominantly solid mass (arrows) in the right liver.

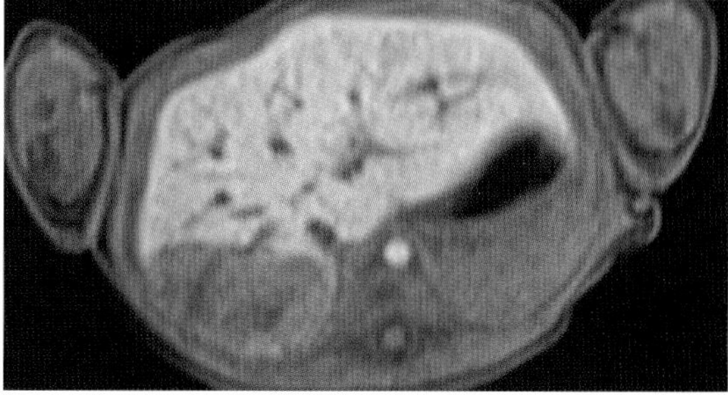

T1-weighted fat-saturated MRI shows the mass to be predominantly T1 hypointense relative to liver.

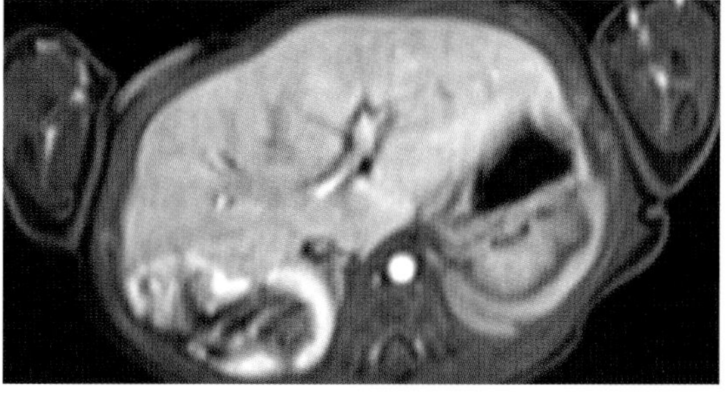

Post-contrast early-phase T1-weighted fat-saturated MRI shows intense enhancement of the tumor periphery.

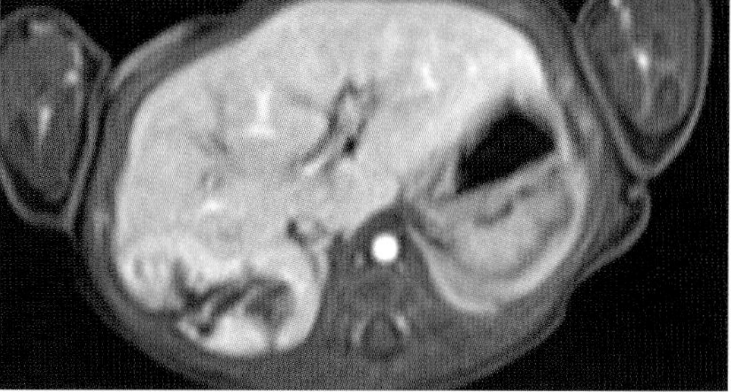

Post-contrast later-phase T1-weighted fat-saturated MRI shows lack of contrast opacification of the central tumor, consistent with tumor necrosis.

Infantile hemangioma. *Case courtesy Michael Hanley, MD, University of Virginia Health System.*

- Infantile hemangioma and hemangioendothelioma are related vascular neoplasms that are the most common vascular hepatic tumors and which may cause congestive heart failure in up to 25%. Tumor markers are not elevated.

  Infantile hemangioma is benign. While hemangioendothelioma is usually benign, it has the potential to metastasize. This text will use the term "infantile hemangioma" to include both of these entities.

  Infantile hemangioma is associated with Kasabach–Merrit syndrome, which is a syndrome of vascular neoplasm, hemolytic anemia, and consumptive coagulopathy.

- Infantile hemangioma may be focal, multifocal, or diffuse. Lesions are highly vascular, T2 hyperintense, and tend to enhance peripherally with delayed fill-in. There may be calcification, central necrosis, and hemorrhage.

  Angiography (which can be performed prior to embolization) classically shows an enlarged celiac artery, with a decreased caliber of the aorta distal to the celiac axis.

- Similar to cutaneous infantile hemangiomas, most hepatic infantile hemangiomas will spontaneously involute in the first year of life, especially if GLUT-1 positive. The beta-blocker propranolol may accelerate involution. Surgery may be necessary for lesions causing CHF.

Hepatoblastoma

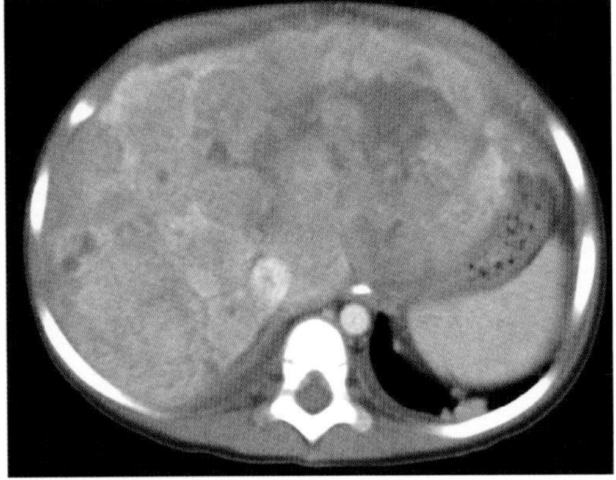

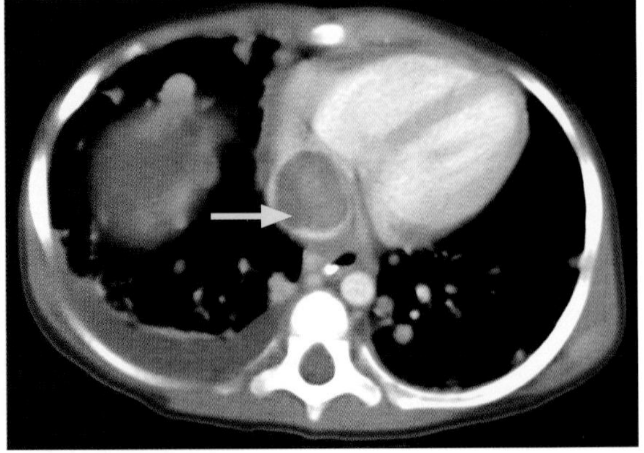

Hepatoblastoma: Contrast-enhanced axial CT shows a heterogeneous mass with mixed areas of enhancement and necrosis completely replacing the liver parenchyma. There is a hypoattenuating lesion expanding the IVC (arrow), representing tumor thrombus.

- Hepatoblastoma is a malignant embryonal neoplasm that is the most common liver tumor of early childhood and the third most common childhood abdominal malignancy overall (third to neuroblastoma and Wilms tumor).

  Hepatoblastoma occurs in children slightly older than those affected by infantile hemangioma and mesenchymal hamartoma. Less than 10% of cases occur during the neonatal period.

- Hepatoblastoma is associated with several genetic anomalies and syndromes, including:

  Beckwith–Wiedemann (Q6 month screening ultrasound screening is performed).

  Familial adenomatous polyposis syndrome.

  Fetal alcohol syndrome.

- Alpha fetoprotein (AFP) is elevated.
- A classic radiographic finding of hepatoblastoma is right upper quadrant calcification.
- Cross-sectional imaging shows a heterogeneous, predominantly solid, enhancing liver mass, which demonstrates a propensity for portal vein and hepatic vein invasion.

Hepatocellular carcinoma (HCC)

- Similar to adults, hepatocellular carcinoma (HCC) is usually seen in the background of cirrhosis.
- Pediatric causes of cirrhosis include alpha-1-antitrypsin deficiency, glycogen storage disease, tyrosinemia, biliary atresia, and chronic viral hepatitis.
- AFP (alpha fetoprotein) is elevated, similar to hepatoblastoma.
- Imaging is similar to adult HCC, appearing as a heterogeneous hepatic mass with early arterial enhancement and rapid washout. Similar to hepatoblastoma, HCC also commonly demonstrates venous invasion.

Undifferentiated embryonal sarcoma (malignant mesenchymoma)

- Undifferentiated embryonal sarcoma is a highly aggressive mesenchymal neoplasm occurring in school-age children 6–10 years old.
- Unlike hepatoblastoma and HCC, AFP is negative.

Metastatic disease

- Wilms tumor and neuroblastoma are common pediatric tumors with a propensity to metastasize to the liver.

Meckel diverticulum

- Meckel diverticulum is an omphalomesenteric duct remnant. In young children, the most common manifestation of a Meckel diverticulum is gastrointestinal bleeding (if the Meckel contains ectopic gastric mucosa). Less commonly, a Meckel may cause intussusception by acting as a lead point.
- In adults, small bowel obstruction is the most common complication of a Meckel diverticulum, followed by Meckel diverticulitis.

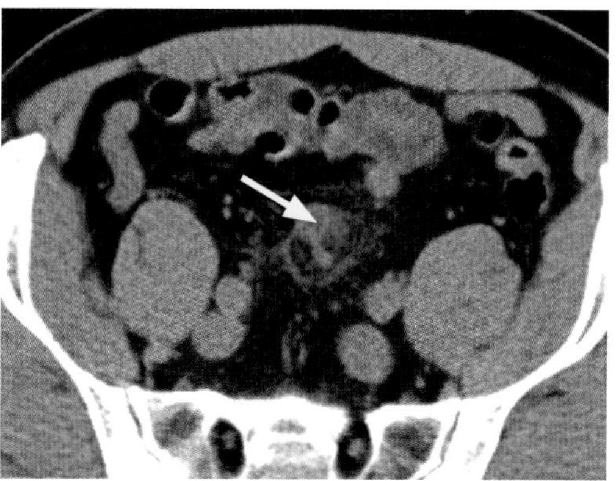

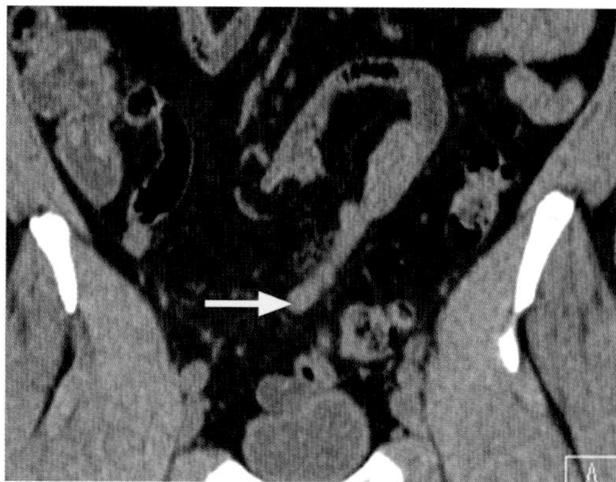

Meckel diverticulitis in an adult: Axial (left image) and coronal noncontrast CT shows a blind-ending, tubular structure (arrows) arising from the mid to distal ileum, with associated mild inflammatory change.

Case courtesy Michael Hanley, MD, University of Virginia Health System.

- The omphalomesenteric duct connects the fetal intestine to the yolk sac via the umbilicus. Incomplete regression of the duct leads to a spectrum of anomalies, ranging from an umbilico-ileal fistula (fecal drainage from the umbilicus) to a Meckel diverticulum. Meckel diverticulum is by far the most common anomaly (approximately 95%) caused by remnant of the omphalomesenteric duct. A Meckel diverticulum is located at the antimesenteric aspect of the distal ileum.

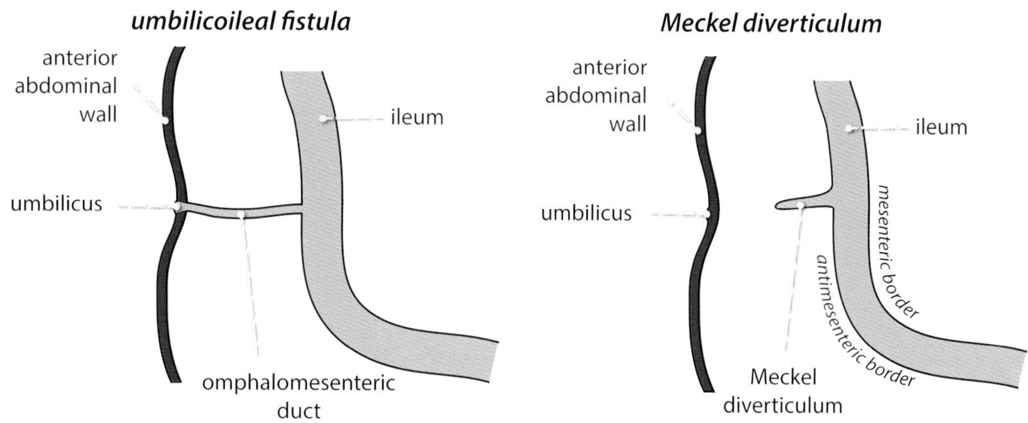

- Although there are often exceptions, the "rule of 2s" states that Meckel diverticula are present in 2% of the population, located 2 feet from the ileocecal valve, and become symptomatic before age 2.
- A Meckel diverticulum causing rectal bleeding can be diagnosed with a Tc-99m-pertechnetate scan. The scan is only positive if the Meckel contains ectopic gastric mucosa; however, these are the Meckels that are most likely to bleed.

  Approximately 50% of Meckels contain ectopic gastric (less commonly pancreatic) mucosa.

  On pertechnetate scan, uptake kinetics of the ectopic mucosa is equal to gastric mucosa.

Spectrum of meconium

- **Meconium aspiration** causes respiratory distress in term neonates.
- **Meconium Ileus** is the earliest manifestation of cystic fibrosis and only occurs in patients with cystic fibrosis. It causes a microcolon.
- **Meconium plug syndrome** (small left colon) is a self-limited cause of distal neonatal bowel obstruction. Unlike meconium ileus, meconium plug syndrome is not associated with cystic fibrosis, and is not a cause of microcolon.
- **Meconium ileus-equivalent syndrome** can be the presenting symptom of previously undiagnosed cystic fibrosis, typically in an adolescent or young adult. Meconium ileus-equivalent syndrome clinically presents with recurrent abdominal pain and chronic constipation.
- **Meconium peritonitis** is caused by in-utero small bowel perforation and meconium spillage, resulting in peritonitis, secondary calcification, and meconium pseudocyst formation.

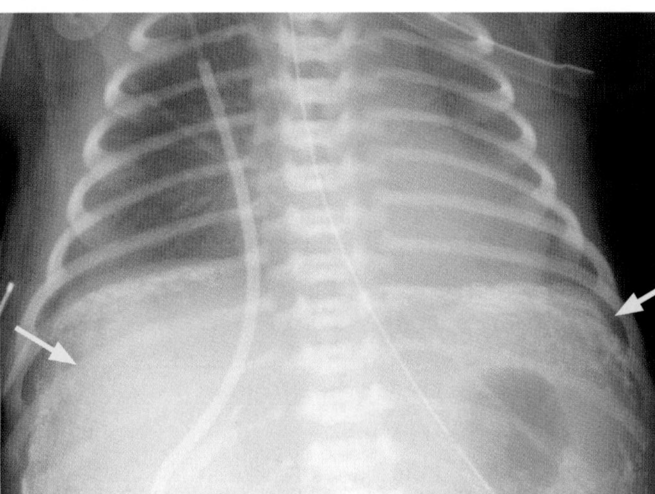

Meconium peritonitis: Frontal radiograph shows diffuse coarse calcifications abutting the peritoneal surface (arrows) in the right and left upper quadrants.

Case courtesy Michael Callahan, MD, Boston Children's Hospital.

Abdominal calcification

- Abdominal calcification seen on radiography can be an important clue to the presence of underlying pathology, including:

Meconium peritonitis.
Several pediatric neoplasms may contain calcifications, including neuroblastoma, teratoma, and hepatoblastoma.
Adrenal hemorrhage may cause calcification of the adrenal glands.
Right upper quadrant calcifications can be seen with gallstones, hepatoblastoma, and hepatic TORCH infections (e.g., CMV and toxoplasmosis).

HYDRONEPHROSIS AND HYDROURETER

Vesicoureteral reflux (VUR)

- Vesicoureteral reflux (VUR) is abnormal retrograde reflux of urine from the bladder into the ureter, which predisposes to acute pyelonephritis, renal scarring, and irreversible loss of renal function. VUR can be primary (due to an abnormally short intravesicular portion of the distal ureter) or secondary (due to distal obstruction, such as from posterior urethral valves or neurogenic bladder).
- The typical imaging evaluation of a child with a febrile UTI is controversial and may involve renal ultrasound and voiding cystourethrogram (VCUG). Renal ultrasound is not sensitive for the detection of reflux, although some institutions perform ultrasound as a screening modality. Recent studies suggest that approximately 5% of children with a UTI and a normal ultrasound have VUR.
- Siblings of patients diagnosed with reflux are typically screened with ultrasound: Up to 45% may have reflux, the majority being asymptomatic.
- The goal of any treatment of VUR is to prevent pyelonephritis and the resultant renal scarring, which can lead to irreversible loss of renal function. The treatment can be either medical (prophylactic antibiotics) or surgical, depending on the grade.

  Grades I–III are initially treated medically (prophylactic antibiotics).

  Higher grade reflux often is treated surgically.
- Approximately 90% of grade I and II reflux will spontaneously regress after a few years.
- Grading of reflux is based on voiding cystourethrogram (VCUG):

I: Reflux into ureter only, with normal ureteral and calyceal morphology.

II: Reflux into non-dilated renal calyces, with normal ureteral and calyceal morphology.

III: Reflux into renal collecting system, with blunting of the calyces (loss of normal "spiky" appearance of calyces).

IV: Reflux into moderately dilated ureter.

V: Reflux into severely dilated and tortuous ureter.

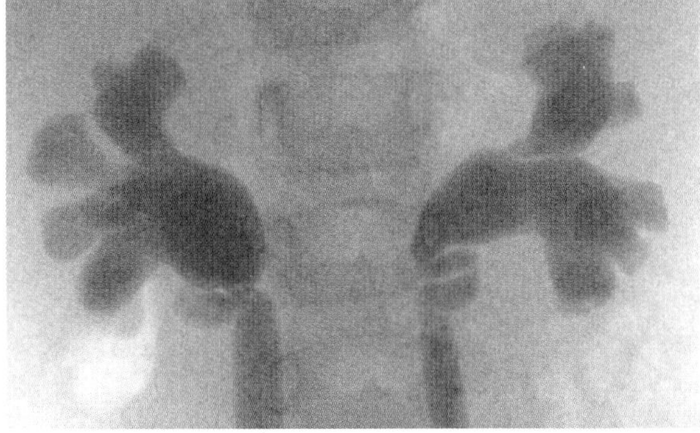

Bilateral grade IV reflux: Fluoroscopic stored image from a VCUG shows moderate calyceal and ureteral dilation.

- VCUG is often preferred as the initial study for evaluation of reflux because it provides anatomic details about the upper tract and also allows evaluation of the urethra.

  In boys, partial posterior urethral valves may be a cause of UTI.
- Two nuclear studies are often used for the evaluation and follow-up of reflux:

  Radionuclide cystogram (RNC) involves the instillation of approximately 1 mCi of Tc-99m-pertechnetate into the bladder through a catheter. RNC is the most sensitive test to evaluate for reflux. RNC is often used for follow-up of reflux once the anatomy is established by VCUG. RNC grading is 3-stage:

  RNC grade 1: Ureteral reflux only (VCUG I).

  RNC grade 2: Reflux reaches renal calyces (VCUG II–III).

  RNC grade 3: Ureteral dilation (VCUG IV–V).

  Tc-99m-DMSA renal scintigraphy (DMSA scan) is the gold standard for detection of renal cortical scarring.

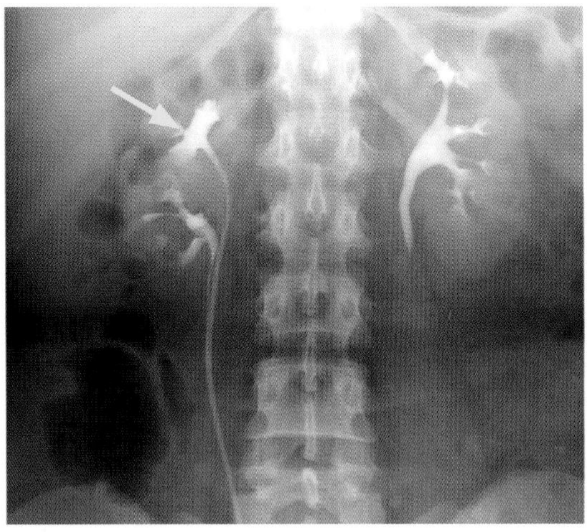

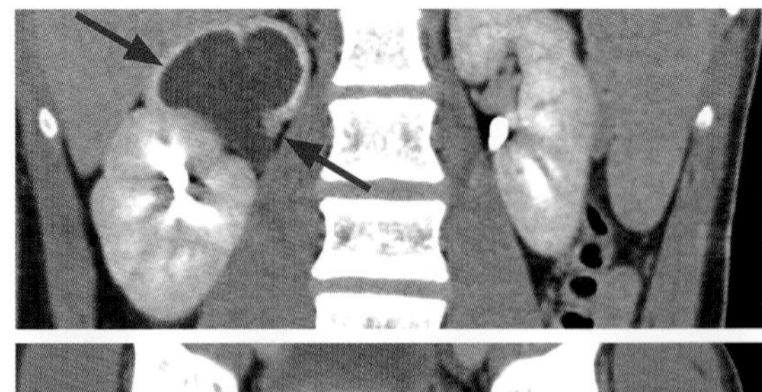

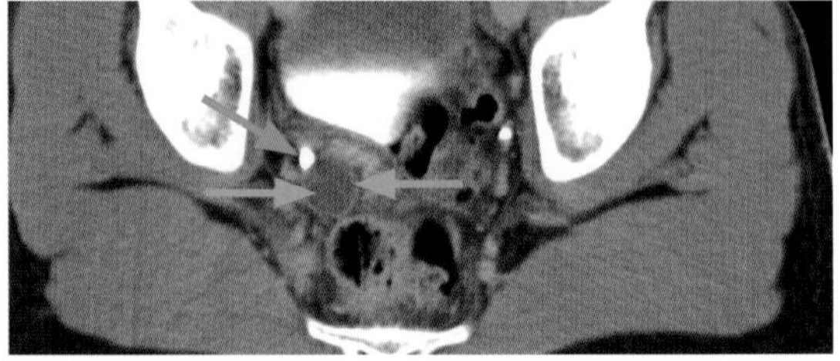

Two patients with duplicated collecting systems: Intravenous pyelogram (left image) shows a duplicated right collecting system, with mild blunting of the upper pole calyces (yellow arrow).

In a different patient, coronal (top right image) and axial (bottom right) contrast-enhanced pyelographic phase CT shows severe hydronephrosis of the obstructed right upper pole (red arrow). The dilated unopacified upper pole ureter (blue arrow) courses medially to the opacified normal-caliber lower pole ureter (green arrow).

Cases courtesy Michael Hanley, MD, University of Virginia Health System.

- A duplex collecting system contains two separate pelvicalyceal systems and two ureters. A duplex system may be of no clinical significance if the ureters fuse. However, if the ureters insert separately into the bladder, there is an increased risk of obstruction (in the upper pole moiety) and reflux (in the lower pole moiety), as described by the Weigert–Meyer rule.
- **The *Weigert–Meyer* rule:** In a duplicated system, the upper pole ureter inserts ectopically (inferomedially) into the bladder and is prone to obstruction, often due to a ureterocele. The lower pole ureter inserts orthotopically (normally) but is prone to reflux.

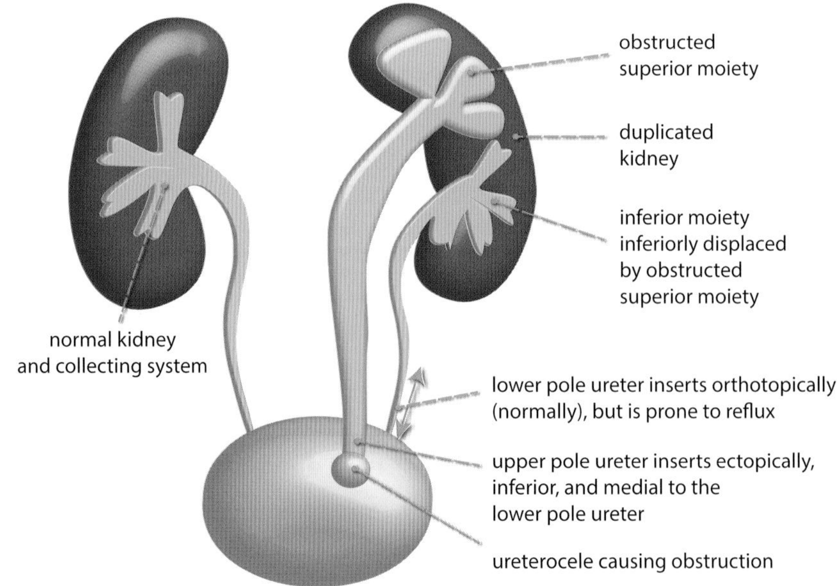

- Although hydronephrosis in an obstructed upper pole system would be apparent on ultrasound, a completely obstructed system may not be seen on VCUG at all since contrast cannot flow retrograde into the obstructed ureter. The *drooping lily* sign is seen on VCUG where the "invisible" obstructed upper moiety compresses the refluxed contrast in the lower moiety collecting system.

  The differential diagnosis of a *drooping lily* is renal ptosis, which would be expected to show a normal number of calyces. In contrast, the obstructed upper pole of the *drooping lily* has fewer calyces.

Ureteropelvic junction (UPJ) obstruction

- Ureteropelvic junction (UPJ) obstruction is the most common cause of unilateral hydronephrosis in children. UPJ obstruction may be caused by an aberrant renal artery compressing the ureter, aperistaltic segment of the ureter, or can be idiopathic.

Posterior urethral valves (bladder outlet obstruction)

- Posterior urethral valves are the most common cause of congenital bladder outlet obstruction, caused by an obstructing web in the posterior (prostatic) urethra.
- Ultrasound shows dilation of the posterior (prostatic) urethra, a dilated and trabeculated bladder, and hydronephrosis. The appearance of the dilated posterior urethra and dilated bladder produces the characteristic *keyhole* appearance on ultrasound.
- The main differential consideration is prune belly syndrome, which would show dilation of the entire ureter rather than only the prostatic portion.

Prune belly syndrome

- Prune belly syndrome is a congenital muscular disorder that affects the abdominal wall musculature and the smooth muscles of the entire urinary collecting system.
- Prune belly may be associated with cryptorchidism.
- The muscular defect leads to dilation of the entire collecting system, including the bladder and both ureters. In contrast to posterior urethral valves, the entire urethra is dilated.

Ureterocele (UVJ obstruction)

- A ureterocele is focal dilation of the distal ureter within the bladder wall, where the ureter infolds between the mucosal and muscular layers of the bladder wall.
- An *ectopic ureterocele* is almost always associated with ectopic insertion of the upper pole ureter in a duplicated system. A *simple ureterocele* is seen with an orthotopically (normally) inserting ureter.
- The typical ultrasound appearance of an ectopic ureterocele is a cystic lesion within the bladder wall, usually associated with hydroureter and hydronephrosis of an obstructed upper pole moiety in a duplex system. Ectopic ureteroceles are almost always located inferior and medial to the lower pole ureteral insertion site.
- VCUG typically shows the ureterocele as a rounded filling defect.

Summary of levels of obstruction

- This schematic diagram of the genitourinary system demonstrates the anatomic locations for various causes of hydronephrosis or hydroureter:

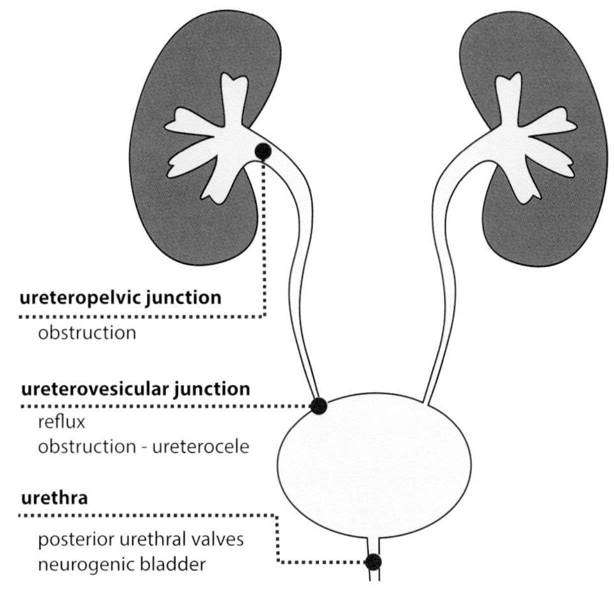

CYSTIC RENAL LESIONS

Hydronephrosis

- Hydronephrosis is the most common cystic abdominal mass in a neonate.

Multicystic dysplastic kidney (MCDK)

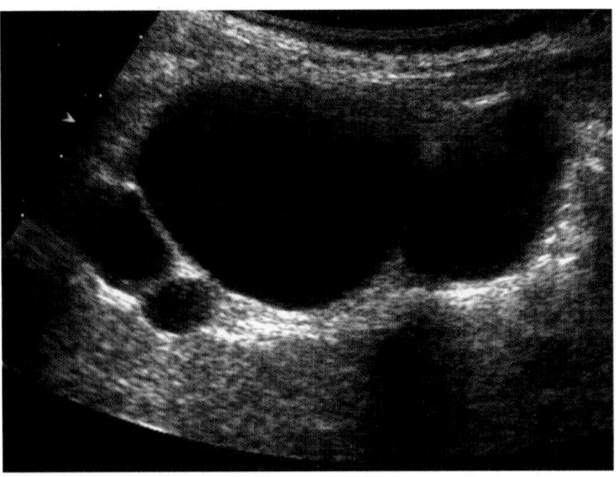
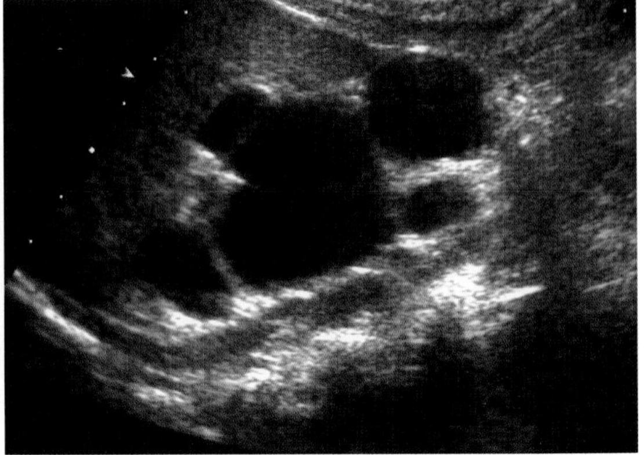

Multicystic dysplastic kidney: Two longitudinal ultrasound images of the kidney show multiple separate cystic structures that do not connect. The main differential consideration is hydronephrosis, in which case the cystic spaces would demonstrate continuity.

- Multicystic dysplastic kidney (MCDK) is the most common *neonatal* cystic renal mass, characterized by a progressive renal dysplasia thought to be a result of fetal urinary obstruction.
- MCDK is typically unilateral, but bilateral abnormalities may be present in 20–30%.
- The natural progression of MCDK is gradual involution. It is thought that many adults with a solitary kidney may have had a previously undiagnosed, involuted MCDK.
- The risk of Wilms tumor in MCDK is controversial. Although an association between MCDK and Wilms tumor has been reported, there is no strong evidence to support a link.
- Imaging of MCDK shows a multicystic "mass" replacing the renal parenchyma. The cystic elements do not communicate with each other, which is in contrast to hydronephrosis.

Simple renal cyst

- An isolated simple renal cyst is rare in children. When seen, renal cysts are more likely to be syndromic, in association with tuberous sclerosis or von Hippel–Lindau.

Tuberous sclerosis: In addition to renal cysts, patients may have:

Renal angiomyolipomas.

Cardiac rhabdomyoma.

CNS cortical hamartomas, subependymal nodules, and subependymal giant cell astrocytoma.

von Hippel–Lindau (VHL): In addition to renal cysts, patients have:

Renal cell carcinoma (RCC): Up to 30% of VHL patients die from RCC.

Adrenal pheochromocytoma.

Pancreatic cysts, islet cell tumors, and serous cystadenomas.

Brain and spinal cord hemangioblastomas.

Multilocular cystic nephroma

- Multilocular cystic nephroma is a benign, multiseptated cystic neoplasm. It has a bimodal age distribution, seen in young boys age 3 months to 2 years and middle-aged women.
- Multilocular cystic nephroma is a multiseptated cystic renal mass with enhancing septa. Its appearance may mimic cystic Wilms tumor. A characteristic imaging finding is its propensity to herniate into the renal pelvis, causing hydronephrosis.

Autosomal dominant polycystic kidney disease (ADPKD)

- Autosomal dominant polycystic kidney disease (ADPKD) usually manifests in adulthood, although 50% develop some cysts within the first decade of life.
- ADPKD is associated with hepatic cysts and less commonly pancreatic cysts.

Autosomal recessive polycystic kidney disease (ARPKD)

- Autosomal recessive polycystic kidney disease (ARPKD) features tiny cysts that develop in infancy due to generalized dilation of the collecting tubules. The cysts are typically too small to be resolvable by imaging, producing a characteristic appearance on ultrasound of bilaterally enlarged, echogenic kidneys.
- Earlier presentations have worse prognosis, with fetal diagnosis often causing severe oligohydramnios and pulmonary hypoplasia. ARPKD is associated with hepatic fibrosis, especially when ARPKD manifests later in childhood.

Malignant solid renal masses

Wilms tumor

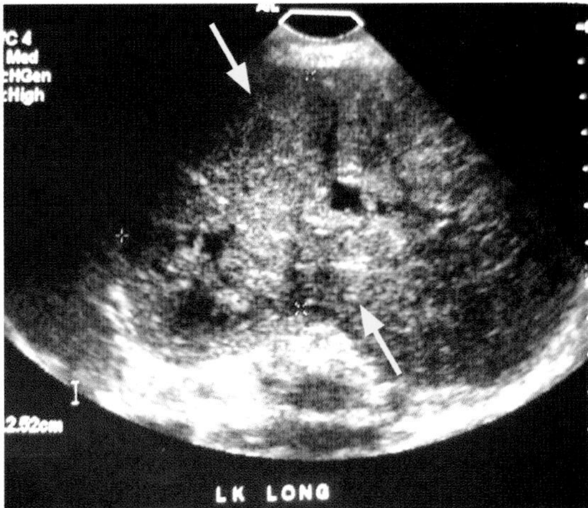

Sagittal ultrasound of the left kidney shows near-complete replacement of the renal parenchyma by a large, heterogeneous mass (arrows).

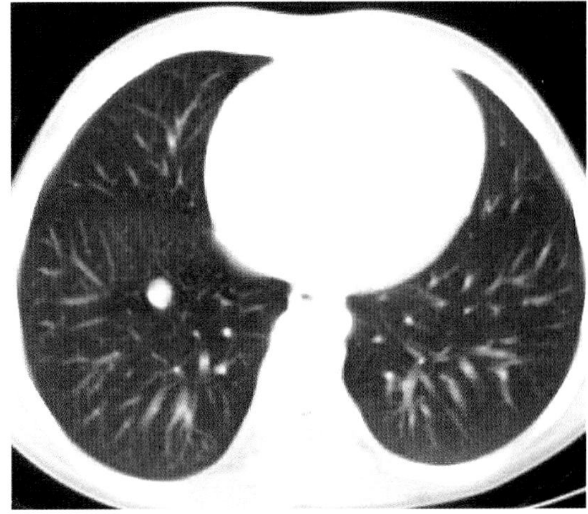

Axial chest CT shows a right lower lobe nodule, suspicious for metastasis.

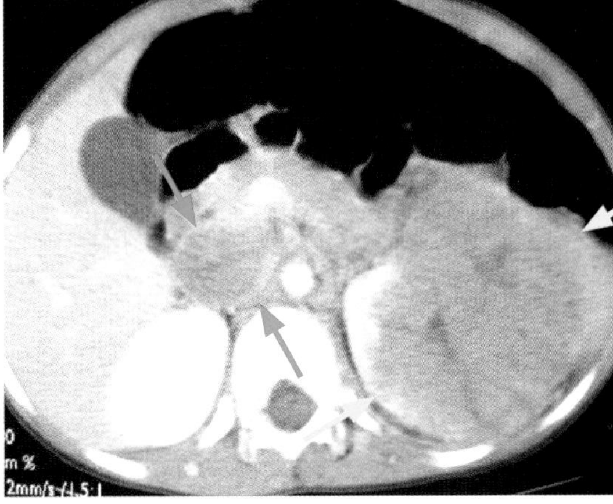

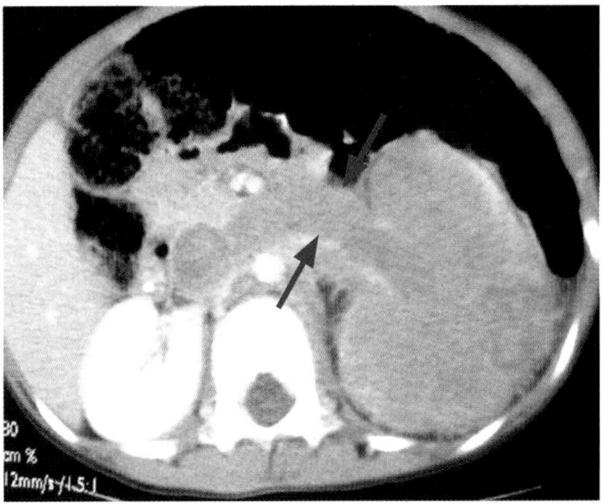

Contrast-enhanced axial CT images through the kidneys show near complete replacement of the left kidney by a dominant mass (yellow arrows) containing central foci of necrosis. There is extension into and expansion of the left renal vein (red arrows) and inferior vena cava (blue arrows). Given the presence of lung metastasis, this represents Stage IV Wilms tumor.

Case courtesy Michael Callahan, MD, Boston Children's Hospital.

- Wilms tumor is the most common childhood renal neoplasm. It typically affects children between 3 and 5 years of age. Wilms arises from persistent metanephric blastema.
- Patients with increased risk for Wilms tumor are screened with regular ultrasound until school age, and include patients with:

> **Beckwith–Wiedemann syndrome** (hemihypertrophy, macroglossia, omphalocele, neonatal hypoglycemia (due to insulin overproduction by pancreatic β-cells), and increased risk of childhood malignancies, including Wilms tumor and hepatoblastoma).
>
> **WAGR syndrome** (Wilms tumor, aniridia, genitourinary anomalies, and mental retardation).
>
> **Horseshoe kidney**: Approximately 2x incidence of Wilms tumor.
>
> **Trisomy 18.**

- The classic imaging appearance of Wilms is a heterogeneous, solid renal mass. The *claw* sign indicates renal parenchyma origin. Tumor venous extension is seen in 5–10%. Calcifications may be present. A cystic variant may mimic benign multilocular cystic nephroma.
- Liver or lung metastases are each seen in approximately 10%, and bone metastases (typically lytic) are seen in approximately 5% of cases
- Staging of Wilms tumor uses the National Wilms Tumor Study (NWTS) system, which is a combination of radiologic and post-surgical findings:

> **Stage I**: Completely resected mass confined to the kidney.
> Two-year survival: 95%
>
> **Stage II**: Completely resected mass with spread to nearby structures (e.g., renal capsule or blood vessels).
> Two-year survival: 90%
>
> **Stage III**: Incompletely resected mass with spread to nearby structures.
> Two-year survival: 85%
>
> **Stage IV**: Hematogenous metastases (e.g., to lung, liver, bone, or brain) or lymphatic metastasis outside of the abdomen or pelvis.
> Two-year survival: 55%
>
> **Stage V** (unique to Wilms): Bilateral Wilms at the time of diagnosis (approximately 5–10%).
> Two-year survival: Variable.

Renal cell carcinoma (RCC)

- Although far more common in adults, renal cell cancer (RCC) does occur in older children and adolescents. Overall, <1% of all RCCs occur in children, typically in the setting of von Hippel–Lindau syndrome.
- Renal medullary carcinoma is an especially aggressive variant of renal cell carcinoma affecting patients with sickle cell trait.

Rhabdoid tumor

- Rhabdoid tumor is a rare, aggressive malignancy that may occur in the brain or kidney.
- Imaging shows an ill-defined, aggressive renal mass. Renal and CNS lesions may be concurrent.

Clear cell sarcoma

- Clear cell sarcoma is an uncommon renal cancer with propensity to metastasize to bone.

Renal metastases

- The most common primary malignancies to metastasize to the kidneys in children are neuroblastoma, leukemia, and lymphoma.
- Leukemia is characteristically infiltrative, diffuse, and bilateral.
- Lymphoma has multiple imaging presentations, including multiple masses or diffuse infiltration.

Mesoblastic nephroma

- Mesoblastic nephroma is a benign tumor that appears identical to Wilms by imaging, but occurs in younger children typically ≤1 year old.
- Although benign, mesoblastic nephroma is always removed surgically since it cannot be differentiated from Wilms.
- Like Wilms tumor, mesoblastic nephroma arises from persistent metanephric blastema.
- Mesoblastic nephroma should not be confused with multilocular cystic nephroma, which is a cystic renal mass with a bimodal age distribution, and is not related to the metanephric blastema.

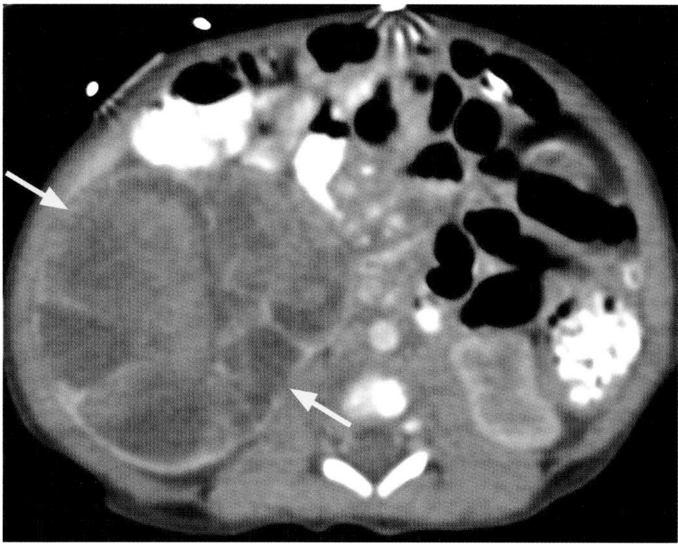

Mesoblastic nephroma: Axial contrast-enhanced CT in a neonate shows a large mass replacing the right renal parenchyma (arrows), containing numerous foci of necrosis.

Case courtesy Michael Callahan, MD, Boston Children's Hospital.

Nephroblastomatosis

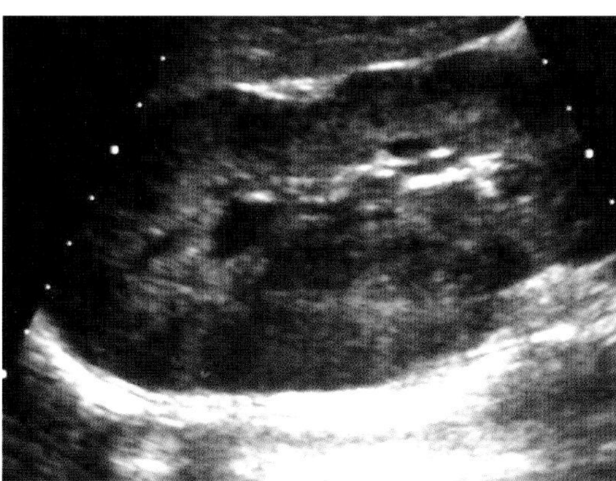

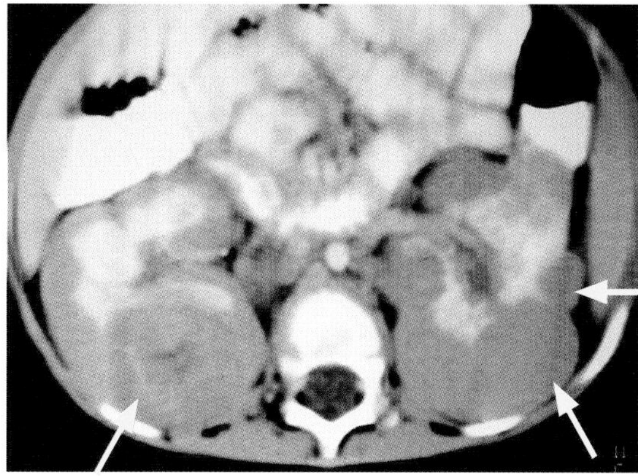

Nephroblastomatosis: Sagittal ultrasound (left image) of the right kidney shows marked lobular enlargement of the kidney and reduced echogenicity of the renal cortex. Axial contrast-enhanced CT shows bilateral nephromegaly and numerous lobulated, relatively low attenuation rounded nodules and masses (arrows).

Case courtesy Michael Callahan, MD, Boston Children's Hospital.

- Nephroblastomatosis is the persistence of metanephric blastema. The term nephrogenic rest is used when metanephric blastema persists beyond 36 weeks gestation.
- On imaging, nephroblastomatosis may appear as a discrete, homogeneous, nonenhancing renal mass. Nephroblastomatosis is commonly multifocal, confluent, and bilateral.
- Nephroblastomatosis is a precursor to Wilms tumor, so frequent screening is performed. Worrisome findings on screening include rapid growth, inhomogeneity, and enhancement.

Angiomyolipoma (AML)

- Angiomyolipoma (AML) is a benign renal tumor with elements of blood vessels (angio), muscle (myo), and fat (lipoma). Multiple AMLs are associated with tuberous sclerosis.
- Most AMLs feature macroscopic fat, which is visible on CT or MRI. An AML larger than 4 cm has a risk of hemorrhage.

Confusing names

Metanephric blastema

- Metanephric blastema is one of the two embryologic tissues that forms the genitourinary system. Metanephric blastema develops into the renal parenchyma, while the ureteric bud forms the collecting system.
- If metanephric blastema persists after embryogenesis, it can lead to:

> **Mesoblastic nephroma**, a benign tumor that arises from persistent metanephric blastema. Its appearance mimics Wilms but it occurs in neonates.
>
> **Nephroblastomatosis**, which is benign persistent metanephric blastema manifesting as single, multiple, or confluent homogeneous renal masses. Nephroblastomatosis has an increased risk of Wilms tumor.
>
> **Wilms tumor**, an aggressive renal malignancy that is the most common childhood renal neoplasm. It typically occurs in children between the ages of 3 and 5 years old.

Multilocular cystic nephroma

- Multilocular cystic nephroma does not arise from mesonephric blastema and is not related to mesoblastic nephroma.
- Multilocular cystic nephroma is a cystic renal mass with a bimodal age distribution, seen in young boys and middle-aged women.

Differential diagnosis of multiple renal masses

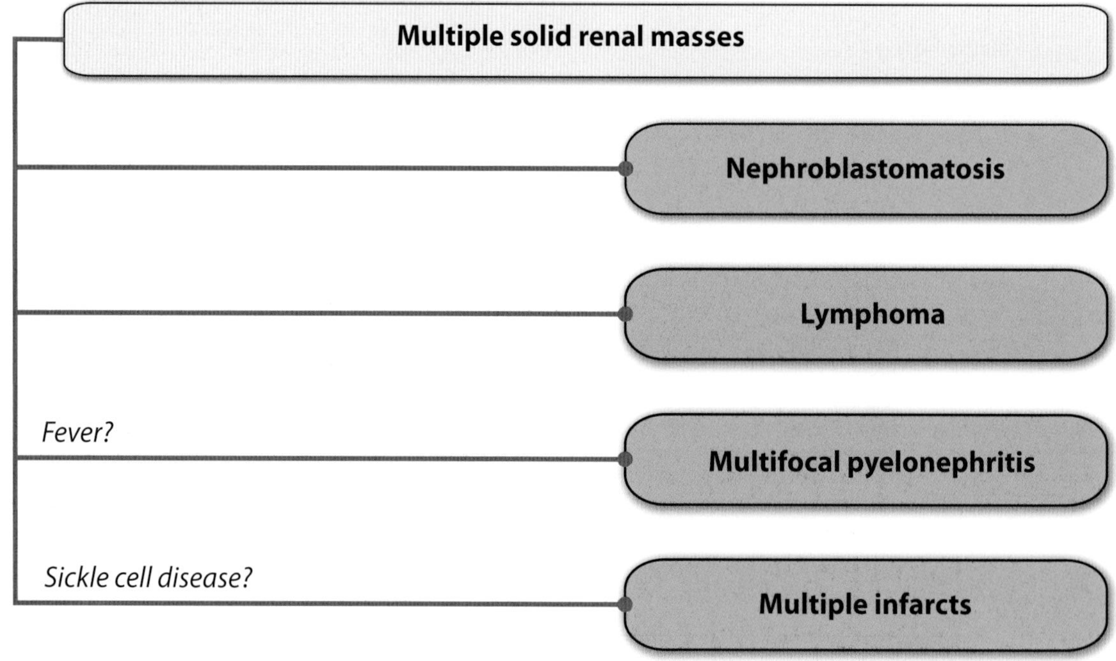

Neuroblastoma

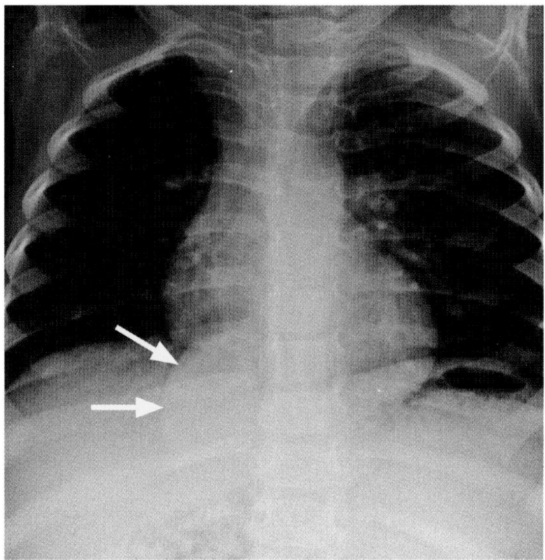

Chest radiograph shows a subtle abnormal right paradiaphragmatic contour (arrows), which does not silhouette with the heart, suggestive of a posterior mediastinal mass.

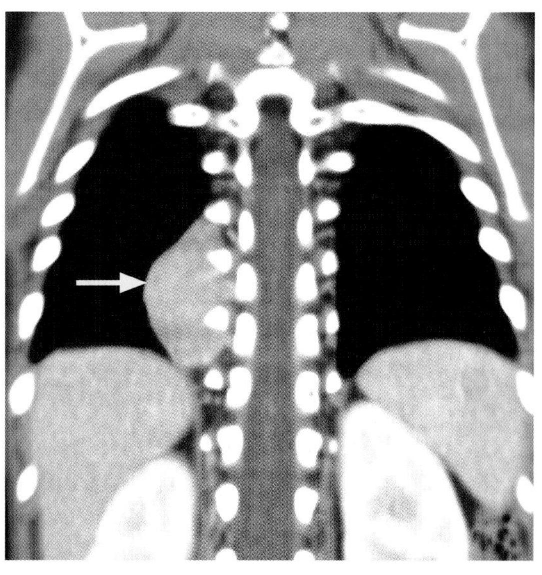

Coronal contrast-enhanced CT shows a diffusely enhancing right paraspinal mass (arrow), without calcification or expansion into the spinal canal.

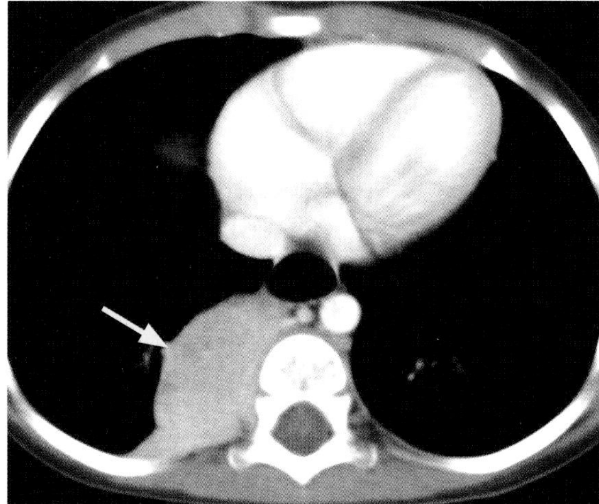

Axial contrast-enhanced CT (from the same study as the coronal image above) confirms the paraspinal location of the enhancing mass (arrow).

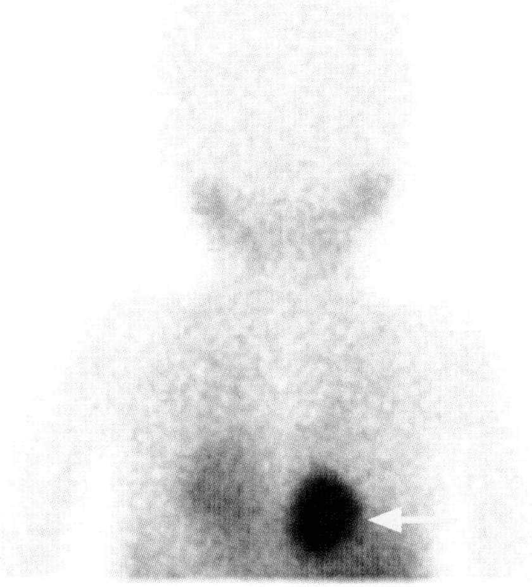

Posterior planar imaging from a I-123 MIBG scan shows avid tracer uptake in the right paraspinal region (arrow).

- Neuroblastoma is a primitive neural crest cell malignancy that arises from the sympathetic chain, most commonly from the adrenal gland. The mean age at diagnosis is 2 years.
- A typical CT appearance of an adrenal neuroblastoma is a suprarenal mass, with calcifications seen in ~50%. Neuroblastoma tends to encase vessels, while Wilms tumor is known to displace vessels.
- On MRI, neuroblastoma often invades into neural foramina and the spinal canal. Diffusion is often restricted, reflecting hypercellularity.
- Neuroblastoma is positive on I-123 MIBG scintigraphy.
- Metastases may be found in 75% of patients and commonly involve the bone marrow (typically permeative and lytic). A classic presentation of metastatic neuroblastoma is an intracranial, subdural mass originating from the marrow.

- For purposes of neuroblastoma staging, "midline" is defined as the contralateral edge of the vertebral body (i.e., for a left neuroblastoma, "midline" is the right lateral edge of the vertebral body).

> **Stage I**: Tumor limited to organ of origin (e.g., adrenal).
> Two-year survival: 75%
>
> **Stage II**: Local spread (nodes may be positive), but no disease crossing midline.
> Two-year survival: 75%
>
> **Stage III**: Local spread, crosses midline.
> Two-year survival: 25%
>
> **Stage IV**: Distant metastases.
> Two-year survival: 25%
>
> **Stage 4S**: Stage I or II with metastases confined to skin, liver, and bone marrow, and age <1 year (better prognosis than Stage 3 or 4). Stage 4S may also apply to children up to 18 months.
> Two-year survival: 75%

Ganglioneuroma and ganglioneuroblastoma

- Ganglioneuroma is a benign neurogenic tumor that appears similar to neuroblastoma on imaging. Ganglioneuroblastoma is intermediate in biological behavior between benign ganglioneuroma and malignant neuroblastoma.
- In contrast to neuroblastoma, ganglioneuroma affects slightly older children (most common age of a ganglioneuroma patient is 6 years old) and only 50% of ganglioneuromas are positive on I-123 MIBG scintigraphy. MRI classically shows restricted diffusion of a neuroblastoma, but not in ganglioneuroma.

Adrenal hemorrhage (in neonates)

- Adrenal hemorrhage is typically diagnosed by ultrasound as a hypoechoic, avascular, suprarenal mass. Hemorrhage may appear similar to neuroblastoma on initial ultrasound, but a follow-up scan would demonstrate involution. Old hemorrhage may calcify.

Adrenal cortical carcinoma

- Adrenal cortical carcinoma is an extremely rare disease, with a prevalence of approximately 1–2 cases per million per year. When occurring in children, it may be associated with Beckwith–Wiedemann and Li–Fraumeni syndromes.
- Adrenal cortical carcinoma has a bimodal age distribution, seen in children younger than 5 years old and adults in their 4th and 5th decades.

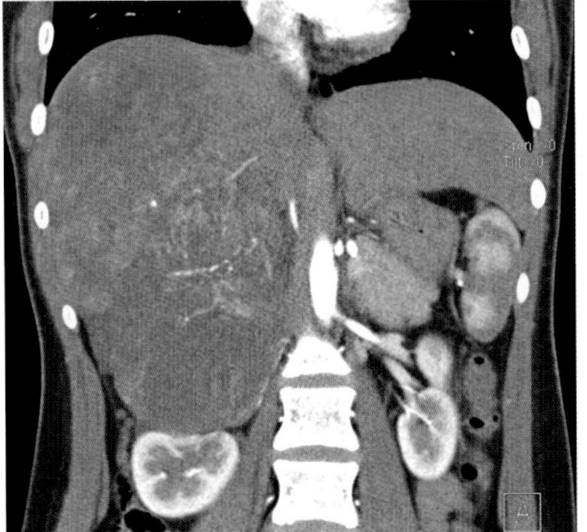
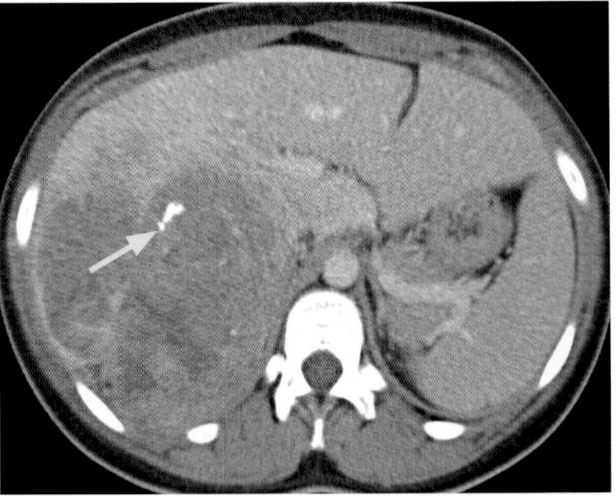

Adrenocortical carcinoma: Coronal and axial contrast-enhanced CT shows a heterogeneously enhancing suprarenal mass invading into the liver parenchyma with a focus of coarse calcification (arrow).

Cystic pelvic masses

- The differential diagnosis for cystic pediatric pelvic masses depends on the sex of the child. A pediatric cystic pelvic mass is most likely due to a congenital genitourinary anomaly.

Either sex

- **A urachal anomaly** results from incomplete obliteration of the embryologic allantois. The urachus is the remnant of the allantois, which connects the urinary bladder to the umbilical cord. There is a risk of adenocarcinoma if a urachal anomaly is not resected.

  Patent urachus (most common): Connection between bladder and umbilicus (vesico-cutaneous fistula).

  Urachal cyst: Noncommunicating cyst between the bladder and umbilicus.

  Urachal sinus: Blind-ending sinus at umbilicus.

  Vesicourachal diverticulum: Blind-ending bladder diverticulum.

- A **rectal duplication** cyst is a rare type of gastrointestinal duplication cyst, usually occurring in the retrorectal space. They are typically resected due to malignant potential.

Girls only

- A **dilated fluid or blood-filled vagina and/or uterus** may be in response to hormonal stimulation and outflow obstruction, either in the neonatal period (fluid-filled) or at puberty (blood-filled).

  Hydrometrocolpos: Vagina and uterus dilated with fluid. **Hydrocolpos**: Vagina dilated with fluid.

  Hematometrocolpos: Dilated vagina and uterus filled with blood; occurs at menarche with vaginal outflow tract obstruction (e.g., congenital imperforate hymen).

- **Ovarian dermoid cyst**, otherwise known as a mature cystic teratoma.

Boys only

- A **Müllerian duct cyst** is caused by incomplete regression of the Müllerian ducts. In a normal male, the Müllerian ducts regress. A persistent Müllerian duct remnant can cause a Müllerian duct cyst.

  In a normal **female**, Müllerian ducts (paramesonephric ducts) develop into the fallopian tubes, uterus, cervix, and upper vagina.

- The **prostatic utricle** is a normal midline structure that is the terminal remnant of the Müllerian duct. It arises from the posterior urethra near the verumontanum (ridge of the posterior urethra near the seminal vesicle insertion). When associated with hypospadia (urethra opens along the ventral penile shaft), a prostatic utricle can become very large.

Solid pelvic masses

- Solid pelvic masses are less likely to represent genitourinary anomalies, and are more concerning for neoplasm.

Rhabdomyosarcoma

- Rhabdomyosarcoma is the most common sarcoma of childhood, occurring equally commonly in the pelvis and head and neck (together making up almost 80% of cases).
- Imaging features a characteristic lobulated, *bunch of grapes* appearance.

Sacrococcygeal teratoma

- Sacrococcygeal teratoma is usually apparent on prenatal imaging. When detected after birth the characteristic clinical appearance is a skin-covered mass extending from the midline buttocks.
- Sacrococcygeal teratoma has a heterogeneous imaging appearance with cystic, solid, and fatty components.

PHYSIOLOGY OF THE PHYSIS

- The physis, commonly known as the growth plate, consists of four histological zones of cartilage arranged in layers.
- The zone closest to the metaphysis is the *zone of provisional calcification*, composed of chondrocytes that undergo apoptosis after preparing the matrix for calcification. New bone subsequently forms along the scaffolding formed by these chondrocytes, leading to longitudinal growth.

FRACTURES IN CHILDREN

Salter Harris classification

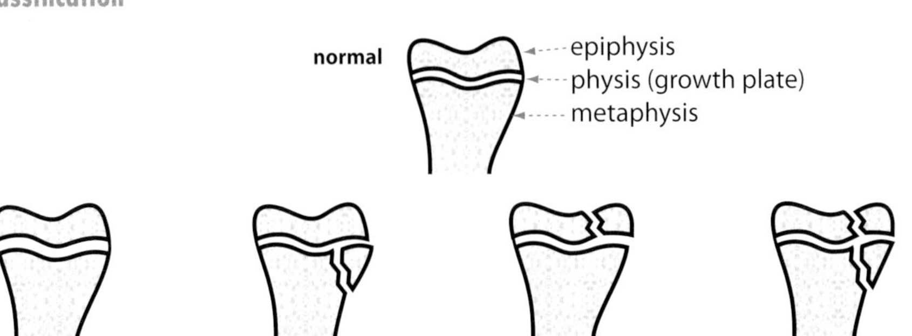

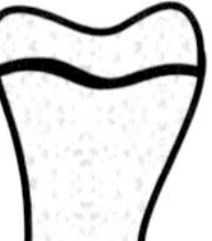

Type I
physeal injury only
may be radiographically occult, or may show subtle physeal widening

Type II
fracture through metaphysis

Type III
fracture through epiphysis

Type IV
fracture through metaphysis and epiphysis

Type V
physis completely crushed

- The unfused physis is the weakest part of the developing skeleton. An injury that can cause a ligament sprain in an adult may result in physeal fracture in a child.
- The Salter Harris (SH) system classifies physeal fractures based on involvement of physis and adjacent epiphysis and metaphysis. In general, the higher the classification, the greater the chance of growth disturbance.
- Type I: Injury limited to the physis.

  SH I injuries are often radiographically occult if the epiphysis is not displaced. The physis may be asymmetrically widened. In the absence of physeal widening, the diagnosis of a SH I injury can be suggested based on soft-tissue swelling around the physis.

  Examples: **Slipped capital femoral epiphysis** and **gymnast's wrist** (physeal widening caused by chronic stress on the wrist, which may mimic rickets).
- Type II: Fracture extends to metaphysis.

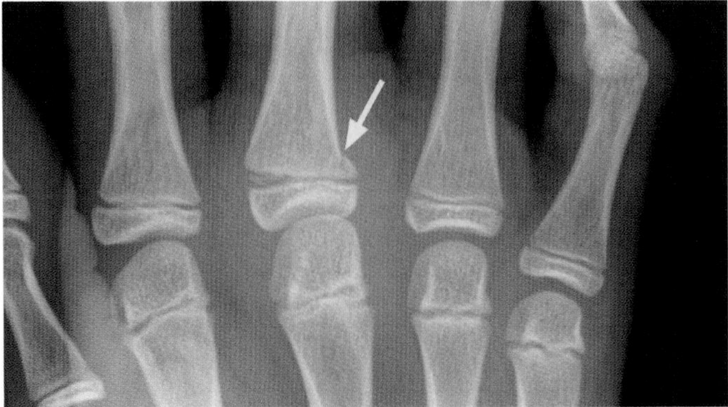

Salter Harris II fracture:

Radiograph of the hand shows a nondisplaced fracture of the ulnar aspect of the base of the third proximal phalanx (arrow), which extends to the physis.

Case courtesy Michael Hanley, MD, University of Virginia Health System.

- Type III: Fracture extends to epiphysis.

  Example: **Juvenile tillaux fracture**, a distal tibial epiphyseal fracture.

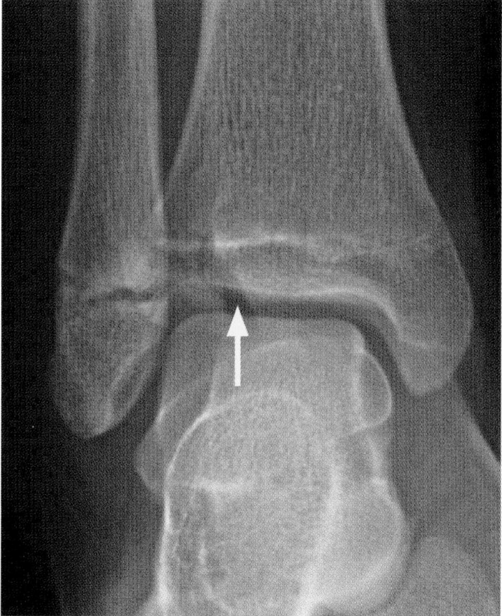

Frontal ankle radiograph shows a fracture through the lateral distal tibial epiphysis (arrow), with lateral displacement of the epiphyseal fragment.

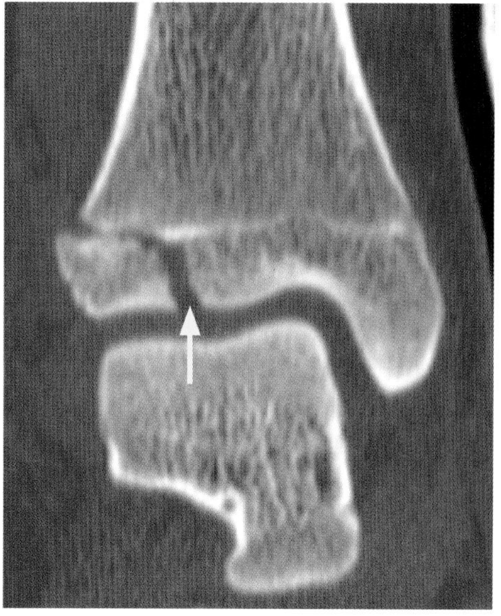

Coronal CT confirms the longitudinal fracture through the lateral distal tibial epiphysis, with lateral displacement of the epiphyseal fragment.

- Type IV: Fracture goes through metaphysis, physis, and epiphysis.

  Example: **Triplane fracture**, comprised of 3 fractures of the distal tibia: Oblique fracture through the metaphysis, vertical fracture through the epiphysis, and horizontal fracture through the physis.

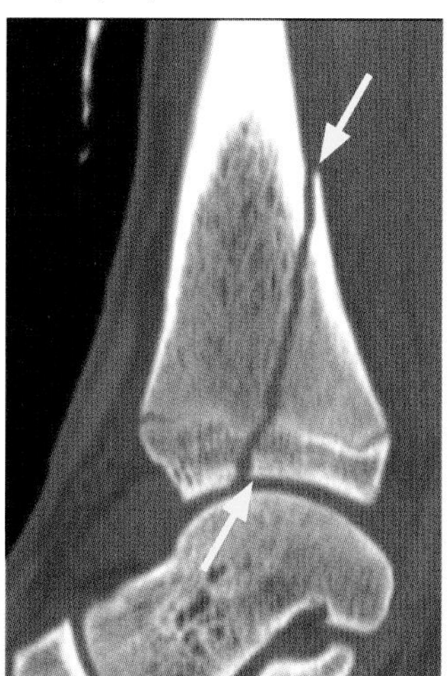

Sagittal ankle CT shows an oblique Salter IV fracture through the distal tibial metaphysis, physis, and epiphysis (arrows).

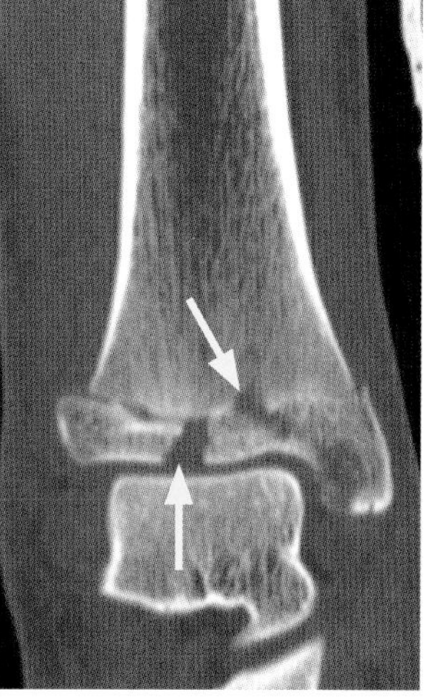

Coronal ankle CT shows a complex injury to the epiphysis including a vertical component and lateral displacement of the epiphyseal fragment.

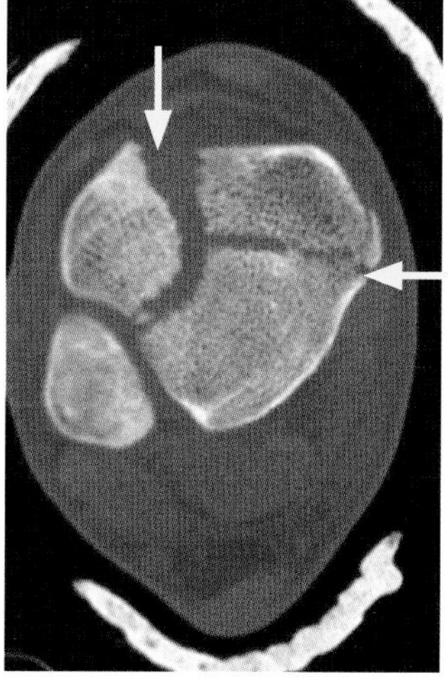

Axial CT through the level of the physis shows two perpendicular horizontal epiphyseal fractures.

- Type V: Physis is crushed.
- Mnemonic: **SALTR**

  Slip

  Above

  Lower

  Through

  Ruined or Rammed

- Alternative mnemonic: **SMETC**

  Slip

  Metaphysis

  Epiphysis

  Through

  Crushed

- Six separate ossification centers, each appearing at different stages of development, make evaluation of the pediatric elbow challenging. However, the cartilaginous ossification centers always ossify in the same order, which can be remembered with the mnemonic **CRITOE**:

> **C**apitellum (typically ossifies between 6 months and 1 year of age).
>
> **R**adial head.
>
> **I**nternal (medial) epicondyle.
>
> **T**rochlea.
>
> **O**lecranon.
>
> **E**xternal (lateral) epicondyle (typically ossifies between 10 and 14 years of age).

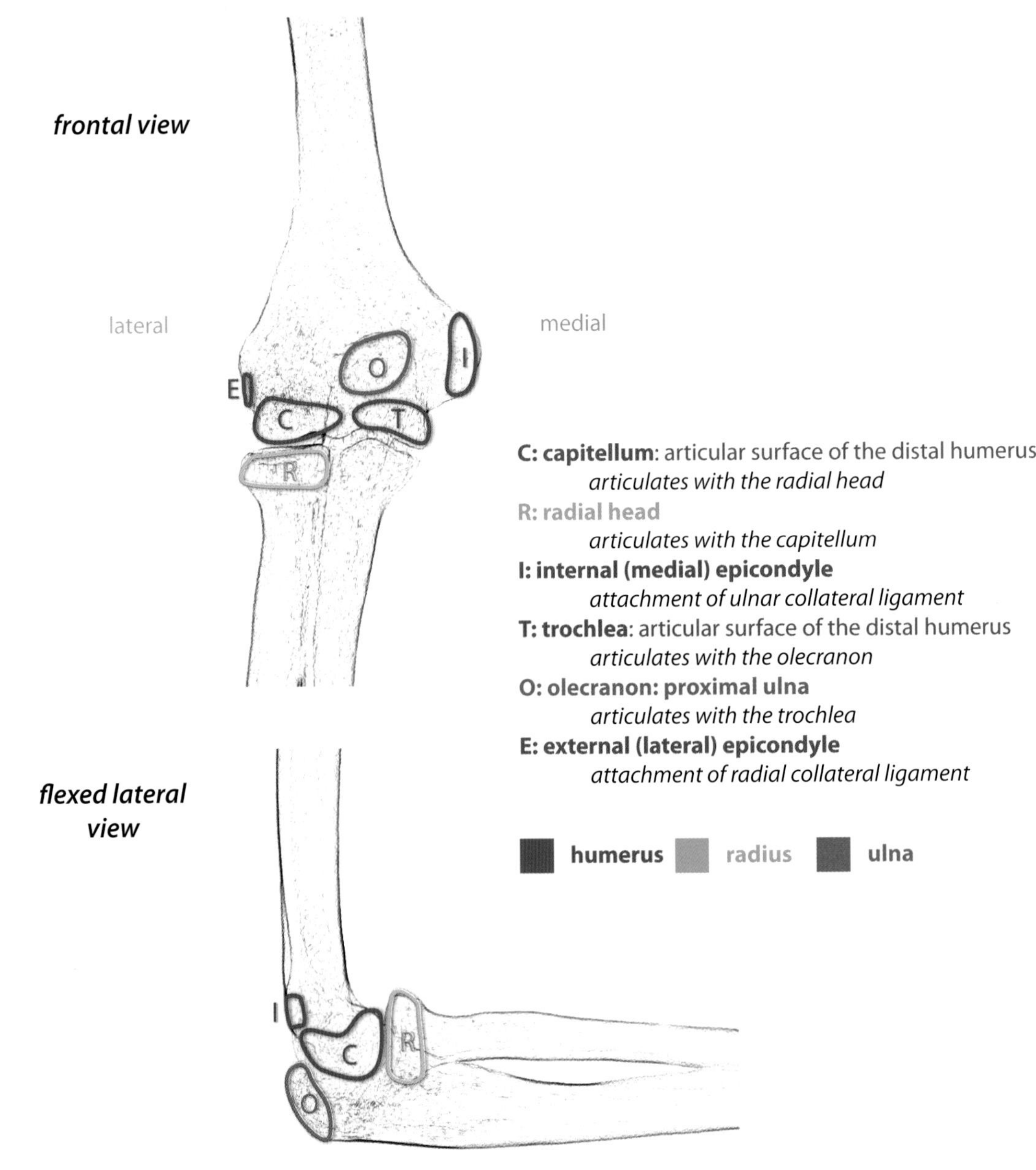

- An elbow effusion, as evidenced by displacement of the anterior and/or posterior fat pads (posterior more sensitive), is pathognomonic of a fracture, even if no fracture is visible.

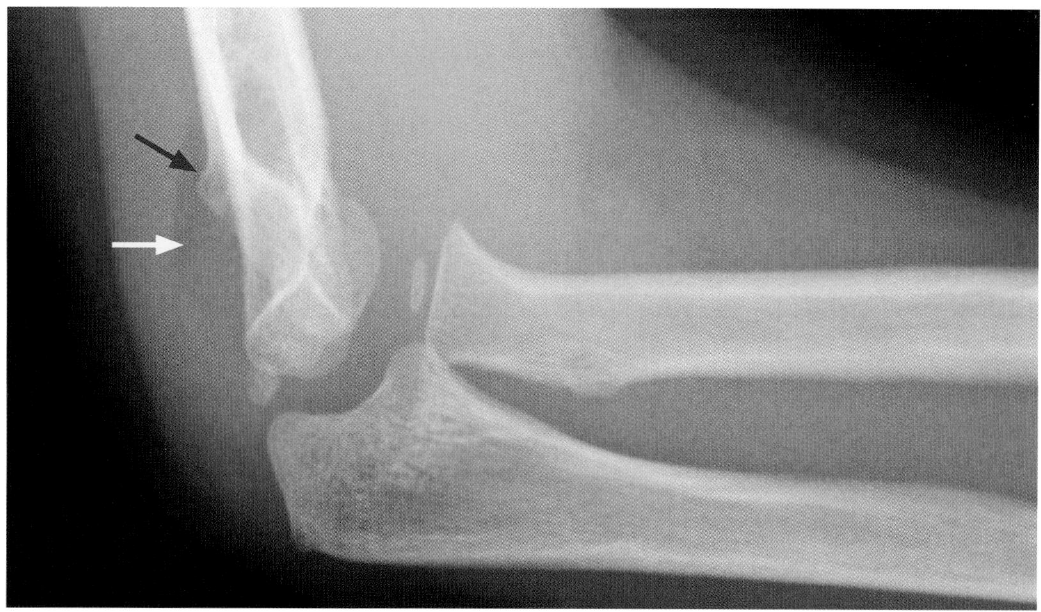

Lateral radiograph of the elbow shows a posterior *fat pad* sign indicative of an elbow effusion (yellow arrow). Bony protuberance along the posterior humerus (red arrow) represents a supracondylar fracture.

- The elbow alignment is evaluated with the anterior humeral and radiocapitellar lines.

> **Anterior humeral line:** Drawn along the anterior humeral cortex, the anterior humeral line should pass through the middle of the ossified capitellum on the lateral view. If abnormal, suggests supracondylar fracture.
>
> **Radiocapitellar line:** Drawn through the radial shaft, the radiocapitellar line should pass through the capitellum on all views. If abnormal, suggests elbow dislocation.

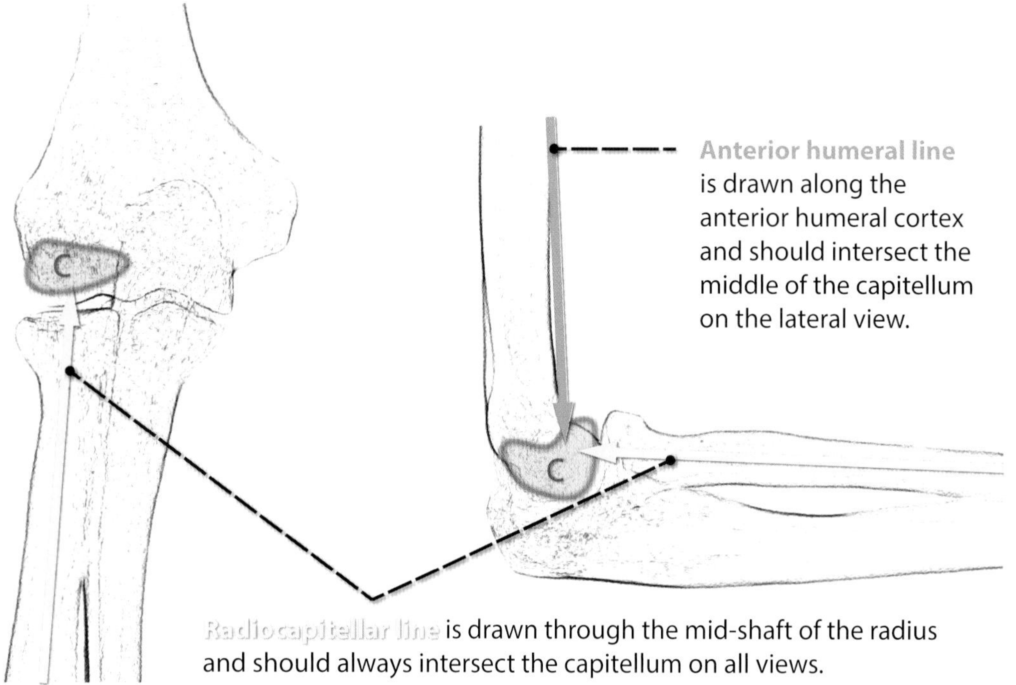

C
C
Anterior humeral line
is drawn along the
anterior humeral cortex
and should intersect the
middle of the capitellum
on the lateral view.
Radiocapitellar line is drawn through the mid-shaft of the radius
and should always intersect the capitellum on all views.

- Supracondylar fracture is the most common pediatric elbow fracture.

  Lateral condyle fracture is the second most common fracture.

  In contrast, the most common adult elbow fracture is of the radial head.

Toddler's fracture

- Toddler's fracture is a nondisplaced spiral fracture through the tibial metadiaphysis, caused by a rotational force to the leg.
- Toddler's fracture may be clinically difficult to diagnose.
- Radiograph shows a hairline spiral lucency through the distal tibia.
- Nondisplaced fractures of the cuboid and calcaneus may appear similar, with a faint sclerotic band sometimes the only sign of a fracture.

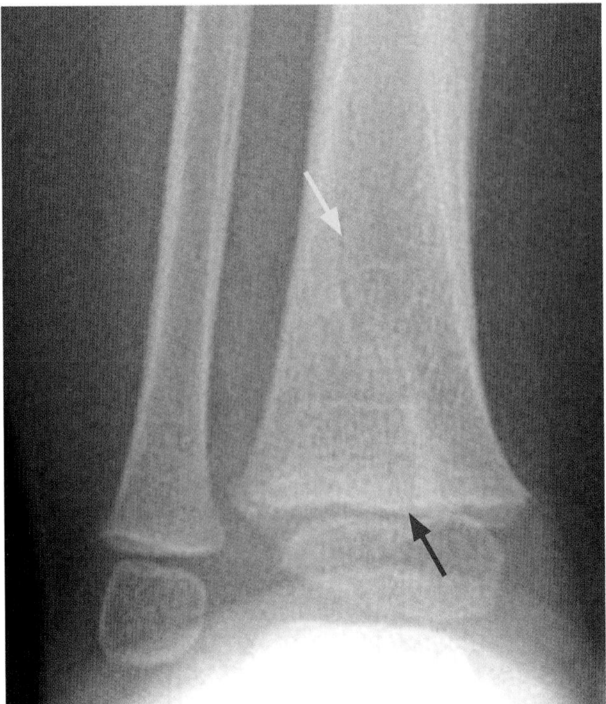

Toddler's fracture: Frontal radiograph of the lower leg shows a spiral lucent line through the distal tibia (yellow arrow), with a sclerotic component extending to the epiphysis (red arrow).

Radial buckle fracture

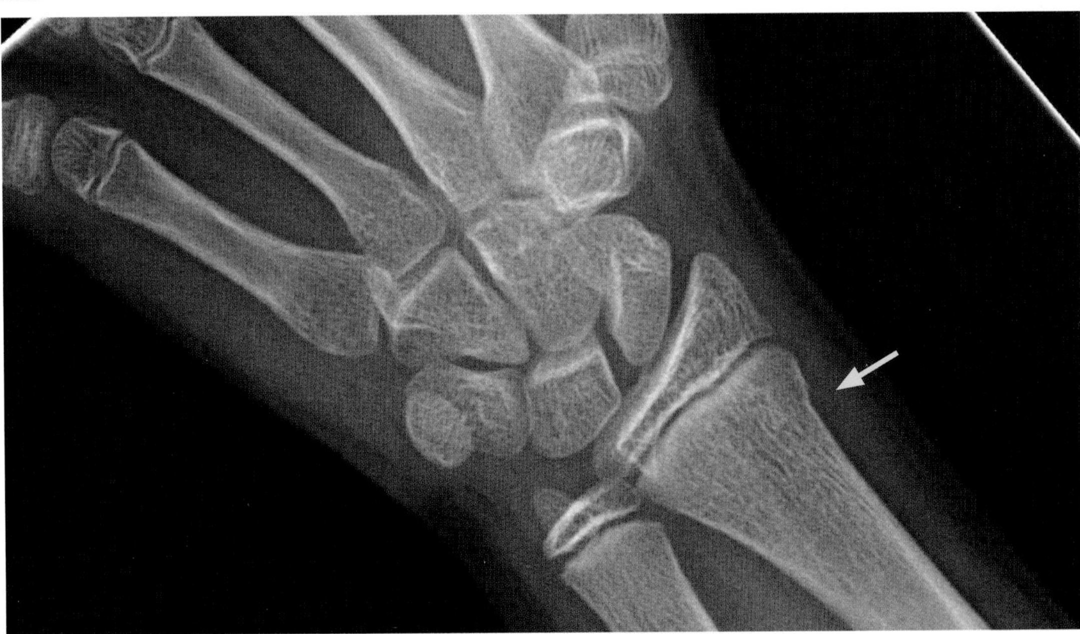

Distal radial buckle fracture: Frontal wrist radiograph demonstrates subtle irregularity and angulation of the distal radial cortex (arrow), representing an angled buckle fracture.

- Buckle fractures are unique to the pediatric skeleton, representing a buckling of cortex rather than a true break.
- Buckle fractures can be subtle on imaging and sometimes are only detected by careful inspection of the cortex. Normally, the cortex should be so smooth that a virtual marble can roll down the cortex without bouncing off. Any focal cortical irregularity in a child should raise concern for a buckle fracture.

Pelvic apophyseal avulsion injuries

- An apophysis is a growth plate that does not contribute to longitudinal growth. There are five pelvic apophyses and two proximal femoral apophyses, which arise in puberty and fuse by the third decade. The apophyses are the weakest link of the myotendinous unit. Pelvic apophyses close relatively late in skeletal development and are therefore susceptible to avulsion. Apophyseal avulsion fractures occur most commonly in athletic adolescents, who have strong muscles and open apophyses.
- Acute injuries appear as an avulsed bone fragment. Subacute avulsions are more complex appearing, as the donor site may undergo mixed lytic and sclerotic change in an attempted reparative response.
- Avulsion injuries may be subtle as they are Salter Harris I equivalent fractures. There is often minimal or no displacement of the otherwise normal-appearing apophyseal ossification.

Attachment of muscles to pelvic apophyses	*Attachment of muscles to femoral apophyses*
• Iliac crest apophysis: Abdominal muscles. • Anterior superior iliac spine (ASIS): Sartorius. • Anterior inferior iliac spine (AIIS): Rectus femoris. • Ischial tuberosity apophysis: Hamstrings. • Pubic ramus: Hip adductors and gracilis.	• Greater trochanter: Gluteus medius and minimus. • Lesser trochanter: Iliopsoas.

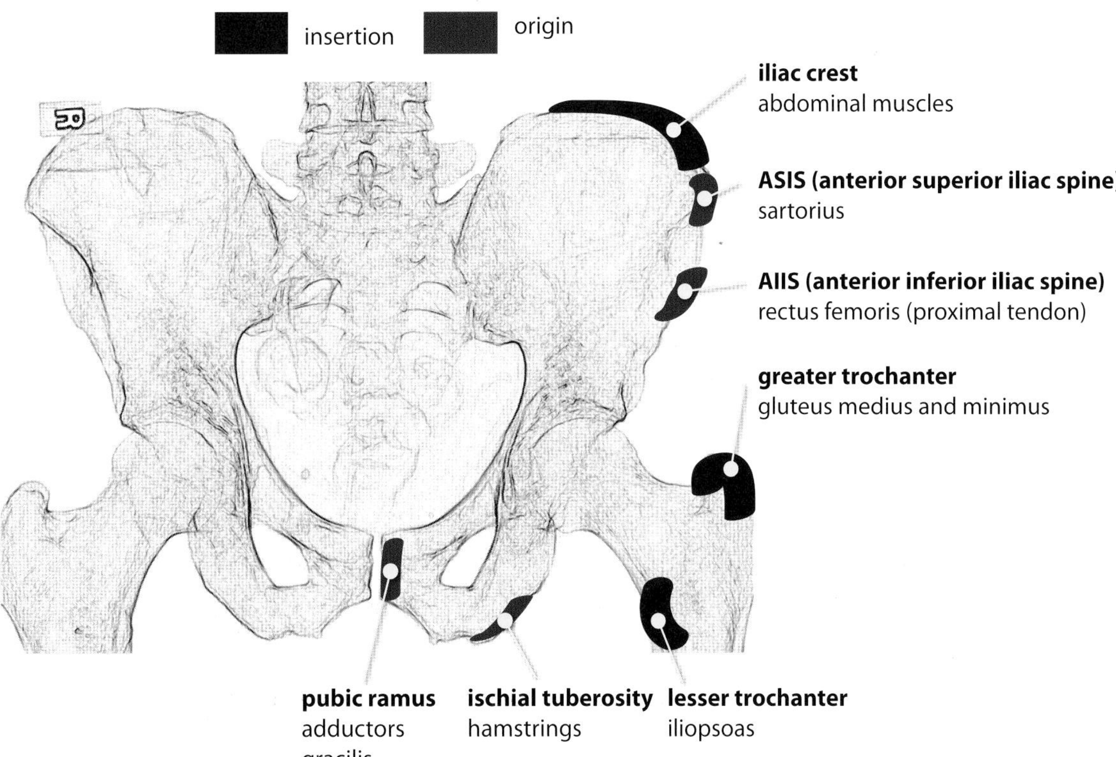

- Although a lesser trochanter avulsion may occur in an athletic adolescent due to avulsion of the iliopsoas insertion, in an adult a lesser trochanteric fracture is suspicious for a pathologic fracture.

CHILD ABUSE

Overview of imaging for child abuse

- If there is clinical or radiographic concern for child abuse, a complete skeletal survey using high-resolution bone technique (for children under 2 years of age) should be performed, including frontal views of all long bones, rib views with obliques, skull, pelvis, hands/feet, and entire spine. The images are reviewed by the radiologist while the child is still in the department.
- Bone scintigraphy is more sensitive for posterior rib fractures, but has higher radiation dose than radiography, is insensitive for skull fractures, and cannot evaluate fracture morphology for age.
- The age of fractures is estimated by the presence of callus formation. In general, a fracture is less than two weeks old if there is no callus, and at least one week old if there is callus.

  These estimates are rough guidelines. A younger child will form callus and heal more quickly.

Highly specific fractures (but not the most common fractures)

- These fractures are highly specific for child abuse, but are not always seen. If any of these fractures are seen, immediate concern must be raised for child abuse.

Highly specific fractures for child abuse

- **Classic metaphyseal lesion** (also called metaphyseal corner fracture or bucket handle fracture) is highly specific for abuse, and is a circumferential fracture through the peripheral spongiosa bone of the distal metaphysis, most commonly around the knee or ankle. A classic metaphyseal lesion is thought to be due to violent shaking.

  The classic metaphyseal lesion typically heals quickly (within 10 days) without callus formation, so prompt radiography is essential for diagnosis.
- **Posterior rib fracture** is also highly specific for abuse, but may be very difficult to diagnose when acute. A repeat chest radiograph with bone technique can be performed in the acute setting, or follow-up radiograph after one week to view interval callus formation.

  Unlike in adults, rib fractures are *not* typically seen after CPR in children. In the rare case of rib fractures from CPR, fractures tend to be anterior and lateral, not posterior.
- **Scapula fracture**.
- **Sternum fracture**.
- **Spinous process fracture**.

Suspicious fractures (but not highly specific)

- These fractures should raise suspicion for child abuse, but are not highly specific.
- **More than one fracture**.
- **Fracture out of proportion** to the history.
- **Digital fracture in infants**.
- **Long bone fracture in non-ambulatory child**.
- **Complex skull fracture**.

Nonspecific (but frequently seen)

- These fractures are commonly seen, both in the setting of child abuse and accidental trauma, but are not specific for child abuse when seen in isolation.
- **Linear skull fracture**.
- **Long bone fracture in ambulatory child**.

Skeletal dysplasias

Overview of skeletal dysplasias

- Bone dysplasias are characterized by impairment of normal growth of bone yielding an abnormal skeleton. The impairment can involve growth slowing down, speeding up, or can cause the bones to grow in an unusual manner.
- Several terms used to describe abnormal limb growth include:

  Rhizomelia: Proximal limb shortening (e.g., humerus is too short).

  Mesomelia: Middle limb shortening (e.g., radius is too short).

  Acromelia: Distal limb shortening (e.g., hand or wrist is too short).

  Micromelia: Entire limb is shortened.

  Amelia: Limb is absent.

Achondroplasia

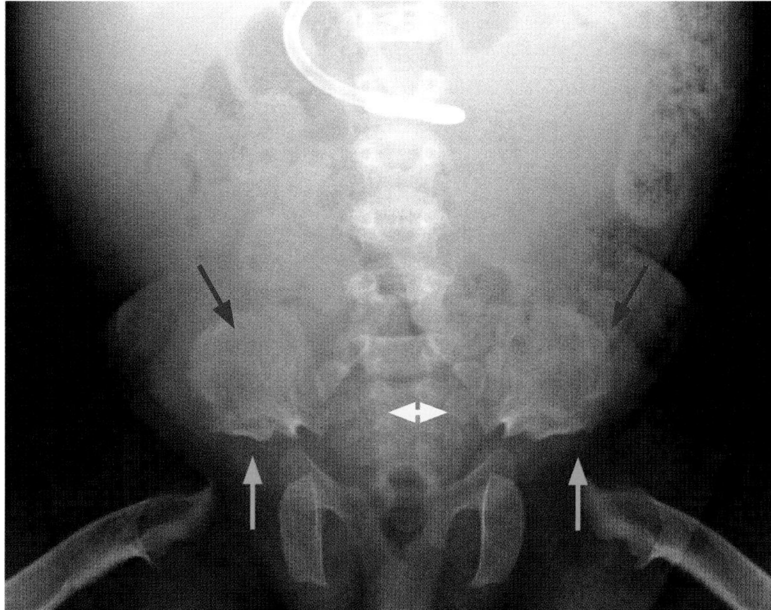

Achondroplasia: Abdominal radiograph shows narrowing interpedicular distances in the lower lumbar vertebra (yellow double arrows), *tombstone* iliac wings (red arrows), and flat acetabula (blue arrows).

This child also has a nasogastric tube.

- Achondroplasia is the most common cause of dwarfism. Affected individuals have normal intelligence.
- Key radiographic findings include abnormal morphology of the lumbosacral spine and pelvis:

> Narrowing of interpedicular distances in the lower spine causes spinal stenosis that is compensated for by a characteristic lumbar lordosis as the child learns to walk.
>
> Posterior scalloping of vertebral bodies.
>
> Characteristic *tombstone* iliac wings.
>
> Flat acetabula, with short femoral necks.

- Other findings include frontal bossing of the skull.

Thanatophoric dysplasia (lethal)

- Thanatophoric is most common **lethal** skeletal dysplasia. It is inherited in an autosomal dominant manner.
- Key radiographic findings are focused on the vertebral bodies and femur:

> Flattening of vertebral bodies (platyspondyly), causing H-shaped vertebral bodies with diffuse narrowing of interpedicular distance.
>
> Curved *telephone receiver* femurs.

Osteogenesis imperfecta (OI)

- Osteogenesis imperfecta (OI) represents a varied spectrum of disorders due to abnormal type I collagen. OI type II is lethal.
- Key radiographic findings include multiple fractures in the ribs (causing characteristic *accordion ribs*), vertebral bodies, and long bones. Additional findings include:
  - Bowed long bones.
  - Osteopenia.
  - Wormian bones in skull, which are secondary to non-coalesced ossification centers in the skull.
- The differential diagnosis for multiple fractures includes OI, rickets and child abuse. Of these three, OI is the only entity to cause antenatal fractures.
  - With rickets one would not expect antenatal injury. Fractures and osteopenia may be present.
  - With child abuse one would not expect osteopenia or antenatal injury. Fractures may be present.

Asphyxiating thoracic dystrophy (Jeune syndrome)

- Asphyxiating thoracic dystrophy is an autosomal recessive disorder of a congenitally small thorax causing respiratory distress.
- In addition to the small thorax and associated pulmonary dysplasia, bony findings include:
  - Short ribs that are bulbous anteriorly.
  - High-riding *handlebar* clavicle.
  - *Trident* acetabulum.

Cleidocranial dysostosis

- Cleidocranial dysostosis is a skeletal dysplasia characterized primarily by abnormalities in the clavicles. Affected patients are of normal intelligence but tend to be short.
- The key radiographic finding is complete or partial absence of the clavicles.
- Cleidocranial dysostosis is strongly associated with wormian bones in the skull.

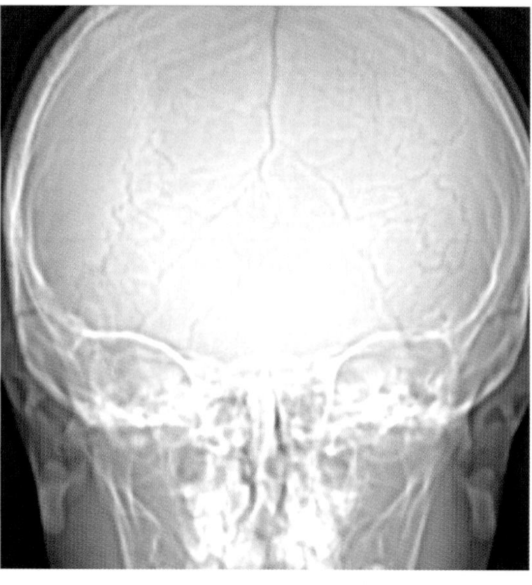
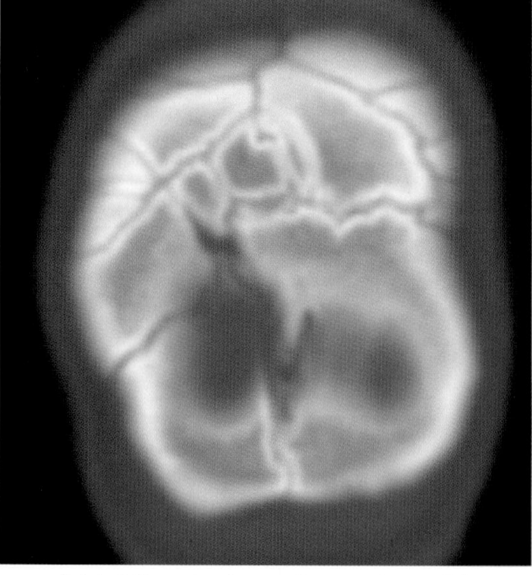

CT scout (left image), and coronal CT (right image) show multiple Wormian bones in a patient with cleidocranial dysostosis.

Case courtesy Sanjay Prabhu, MBBS, Boston Children's Hospital.

  - Wormian bones are nonspecific, and are also seen in hypothyroidism, osteogenesis imperfecta, healing rickets, and Down syndrome.
- Additional radiographic findings of cleidocranial dysostosis include:
  - Delayed ossification of the skull (neonatal).
  - Widened pubic symphysis (typically not seen until later in life).

Stippled epiphyses

- Several skeletal dysplasias and metabolic bone diseases can cause stippling of the epiphyses, including:

  Chondrodysplasia punctata, a short-limbed dwarfism (usually rhizomelic).

  Multiple epiphyseal dysplasia (Fairbank disease), a mildly short-limbed, autosomal dominant skeletal dysplasia that usually manifests in late childhood or adolescence.

  Hypothyroidism.

  Complications of **maternal warfarin use** in a newborn.

Enchondromatoses

- The enchondromatoses are characterized by multiple intra-osseous benign cartilaginous tumors in an asymmetric distribution. These syndromes are associated with an increased risk of malignant transformation to chondrosarcoma (Maffucci > Ollier).
- **Ollier disease** is an enchondromatosis without associated abnormalities.
- **Maffucci syndrome** is an enchondromatosis with venous malformations, which cause phleboliths that are evident on radiography.

Multiple hereditary exostoses (osteochondromatosis)

- Multiple hereditary exostoses is an autosomal dominant disorder of multiple benign osteochondromas (also called exostoses) growing from the metaphyses of long bones.
- Complications include pain, deformity, and malignant transformation into low-grade chondrosarcoma (between 5 and 25% of cases).
- In contrast to enchondromatosis, skeletal involvement is usually symmetric bilaterally.

MUCOPOLYSACCHARIDOSES

Overview of mucopolysaccharidoses

- Mucopolysaccharidoses are a group of lysosomal storage disorders including Hurlers, Morquio, and Hunters. These disorders share common radiographic findings and are typically distinguished clinically and biochemically.
- Key radiographic findings include anterior vertebral body beaking, thickened ribs, and undertubulated bones. Other findings include:

  Madelung deformity of the wrists (wedge-shaped proximal carpal row, with radius shifted towards ulna).

  Thickened calvarium with a *J-shaped* sella.

Hurlers

- Hurlers features anterior beaking of the vertebral bodies, primarily **inferiorly.**

Morquio

- Morquio also features anterior beaking of **middle** portion of the vertebral body (mnemonic: **M**orquio/**m**iddle).
- Morquio is associated with spinal stenosis and atlantoaxial instability.

- A limp (abnormal gait pattern caused by pain) should be carefully evaluated and may be secondary to trauma, septic arthritis, chronic fracture, avascular necrosis, or lymphoma.

Septic hip arthritis

- Infection of the synovium and joint space is an orthopedic emergency as joint destruction and growth arrest may occur without prompt washout and antibiotics.
- Any hip effusion must be urgently aspirated to evaluate for septic arthritis.
- The primary differential consideration for septic arthritis is aseptic toxic synovitis, which is a self-limited noninfectious diagnosis of exclusion. Less common causes of hip effusion and limp include hemarthrosis in trauma or hemophilia (history is usually evident).
- Septic arthritis is usually secondary to hematogenously seeded metaphyseal osteomyelitis that breaks through the periosteum to infect the joint capsule. *S. aureus* is the most common cause.
- Plain film findings are not sensitive or reliable for evaluation of effusion, but include:

Displacement or distortion of gluteal or psoas fat planes. The gluteus medius and minimus insert on the greater trochanter. The psoas inserts on the lesser trochanter.

Widening of the *teardrop* distance (space between the lateral margin of the pelvic *teardrop* and the medial margin of the femoral head). The *teardrop* is the antero-inferior acetabulum.

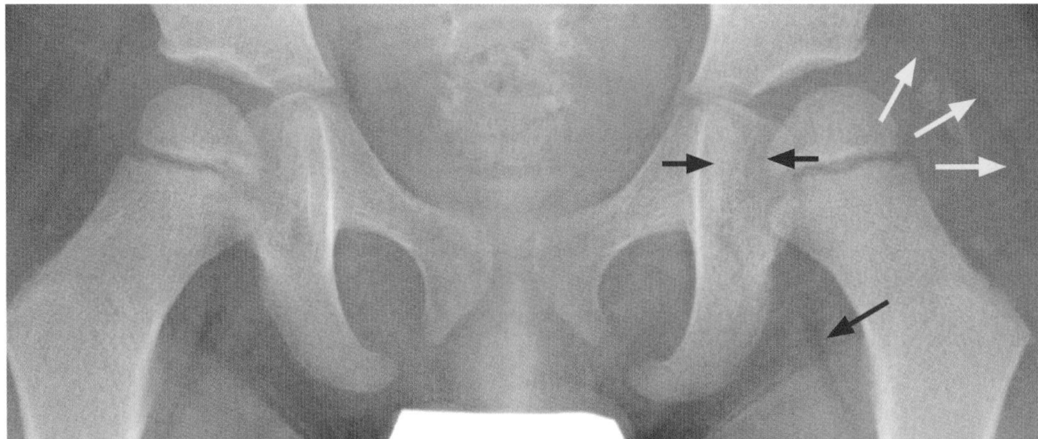

Hip effusion: AP radiograph shows lateral displacement of the left gluteal fat plane (yellow arrows) and subtle medial bowing of the psoas fat plane (red arrow). The teardrop distance (blue arrows) is not widened, emphasizing the relative insensitivity of these radiographic findings to detect effusion.

- Ultrasound is the imaging modality of choice. Both sides should be compared for symmetry.

The presence of internal echoes within an effusion does not have clinical significance.

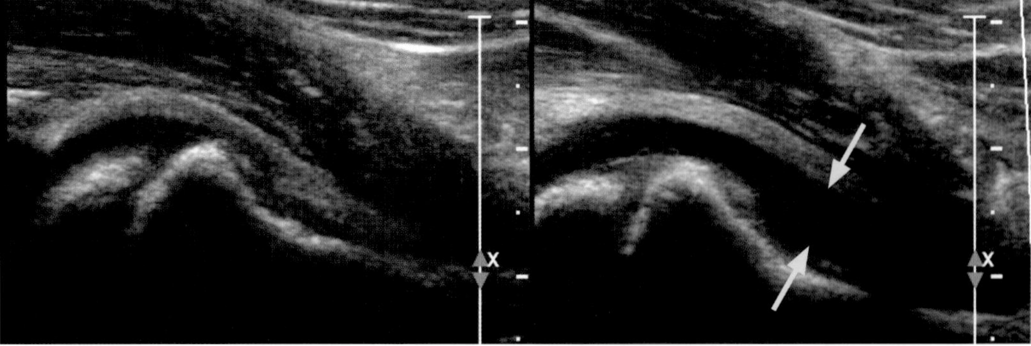

Bilateral hip ultrasound in the same patient shows increased anechoic fluid in the left hip joint (right panel; arrows) relative to the normal right hip. This child ended up having aseptic toxic synovitis, but the radiographic and ultrasound findings are identical to septic arthritis.

Slipped capital femoral epiphysis (SCFE)

- Slipped capital femoral epiphysis (SCFE) is a Salter I fracture of the proximal femoral epiphysis (displacement of the epiphysis from the metaphysis) seen in obese preadolescents (most affected children are between 10 and 16 years old). SCFE typically affects children slightly older than those with Legg–Calvé–Perthes disease, which is discussed on the following page.
- Initial findings on an AP view can be subtle, including asymmetric widening of the proximal femoral growth plate and lack of intersection of Klein's line with the femoral head.

  Klein's line is a line drawn along lateral margin of the femoral neck, which should normally intersect the femoral head, as in the normal right hip below. A radiographic clue to SCFE is lack of intersection of Klein's line with the femoral head.

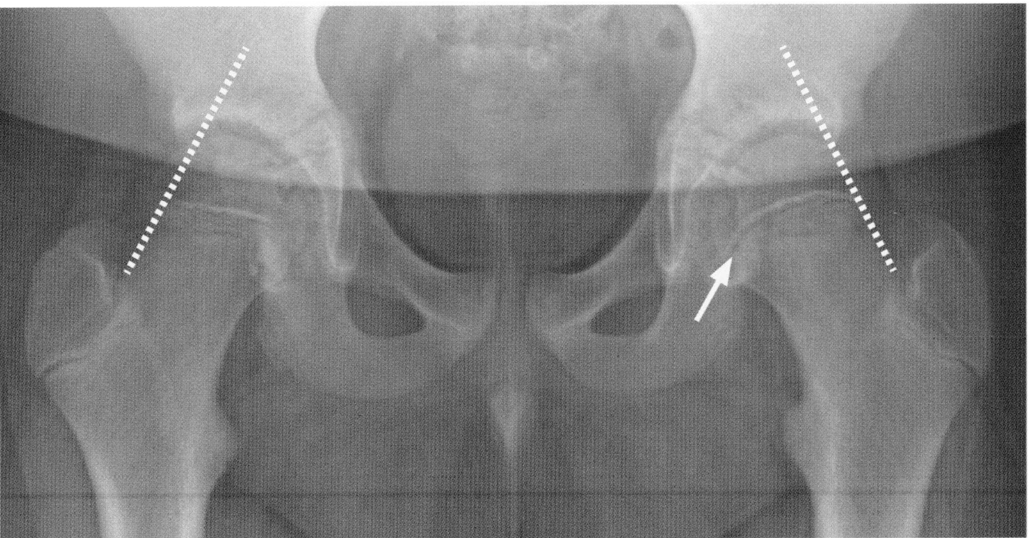

Early left SCFE: There is minimal widening of the left physis (arrow) without physeal displacement. There is minimal asymmetry in the alignment of the Klein's lines (dashed yellow lines). These findings are very subtle.

- Although Klein's line is drawn on the AP view, the physeal widening and displacement is best evaluated on the frog-leg lateral projection.

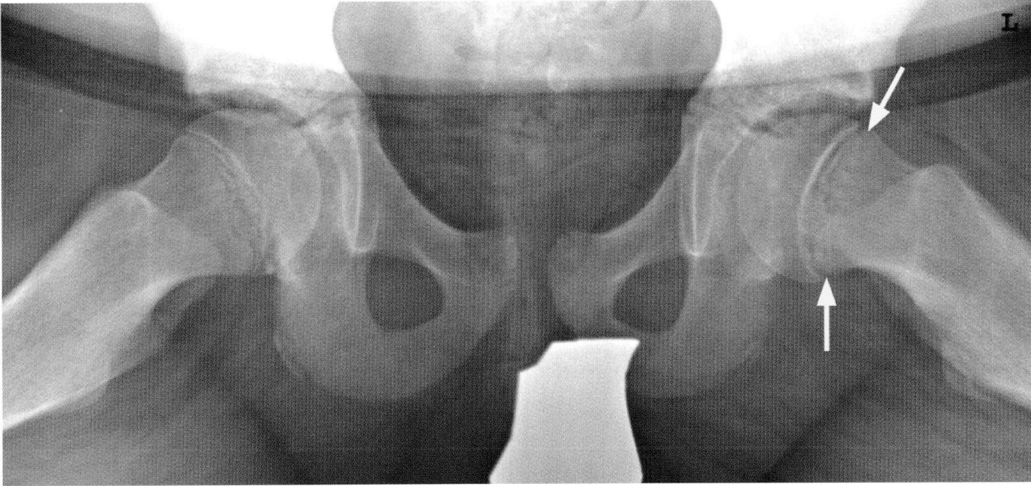

Frog-leg lateral radiograph in the same patient shows very slight medial slippage of the left femoral head and more apparent physeal widening (arrows), suggesting early SCFE.

- The contralateral hip should always be carefully evaluated. SCFE may be bilateral, but is usually asymmetric.

Legg–Calvé–Perthes (LCP)

- Legg–Calvé–Perthes (LCP) disease is avascular necrosis of the capital femoral epiphysis ossification center. LCP is of unknown etiology and typically occurs in children between the ages of 4 and 8 years.
- LCP is usually unilateral. A systemic cause should be sought when bilateral, such as sickle cell disease or steroids.
- Imaging findings are dependent on stage and chronicity.
- **Early LCP** can be subtle, and often multiple modalities are used for initial diagnosis. Early LCP may show subtle sclerosis of the femoral head on radiography. There is typically decreased uptake on bone scan.

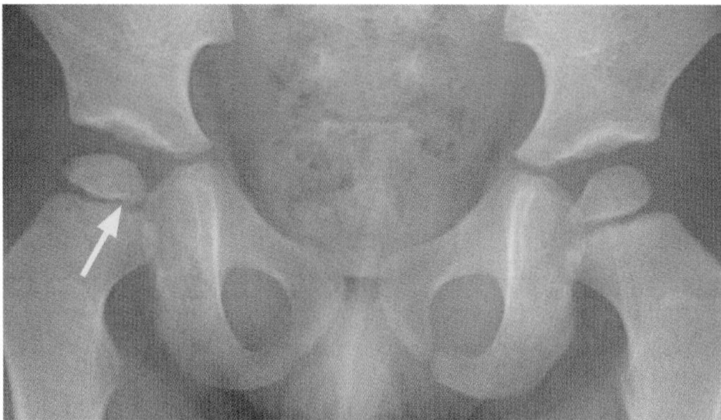

Early Legg–Calvé–Perthes. Frontal radiograph of the pelvis shows subtle irregularity and sclerosis of the inferior aspect of the right femoral epiphysis ossification center (arrow).

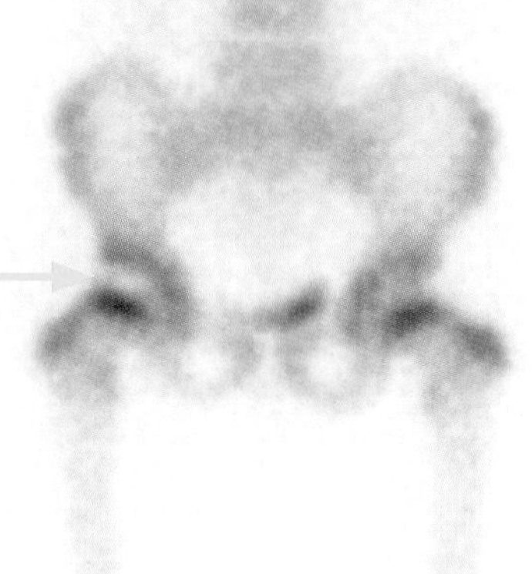

Anterior planar Tc-99m MDP bone scan in the same patient with early LCP shows a photopenic defect (arrow) in right femoral epiphysis.

- **Late LCP** shows secondary signs of osteonecrosis. The femoral head becomes flattened and distorted, with secondary changes of osteoarthritis. Bone scan of late LCP typically shows increased uptake due to attempted repair.

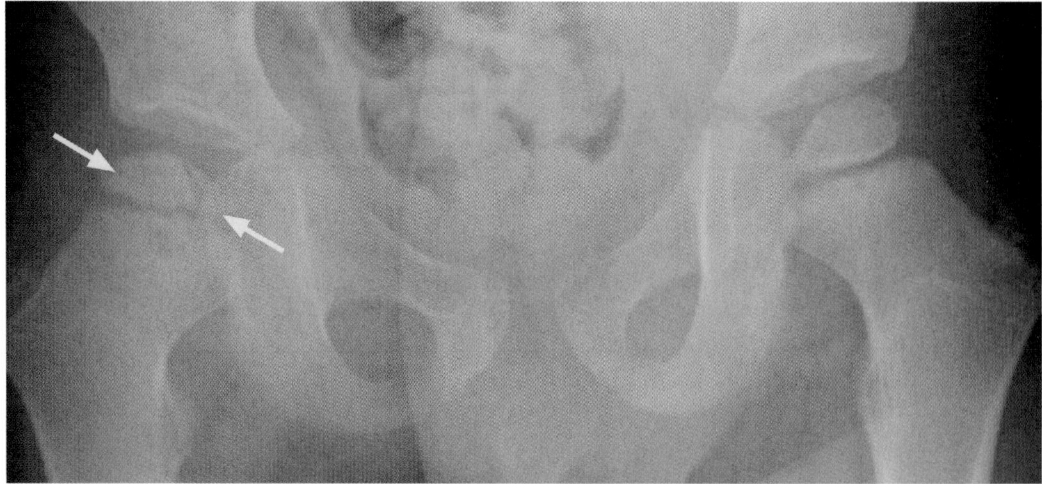

Later stage of LCP in the same patient. This follow-up slightly obliqued frontal radiograph shows increased sclerosis and irregularity of the right femoral head, with new fragmentation (arrows).

Osteosarcoma

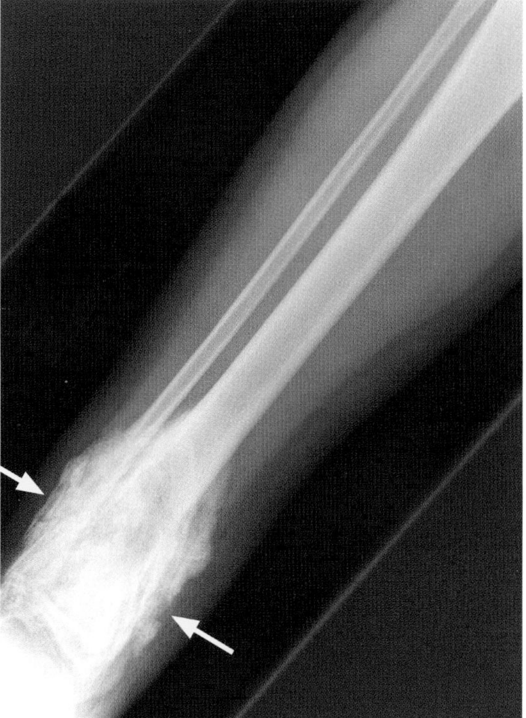

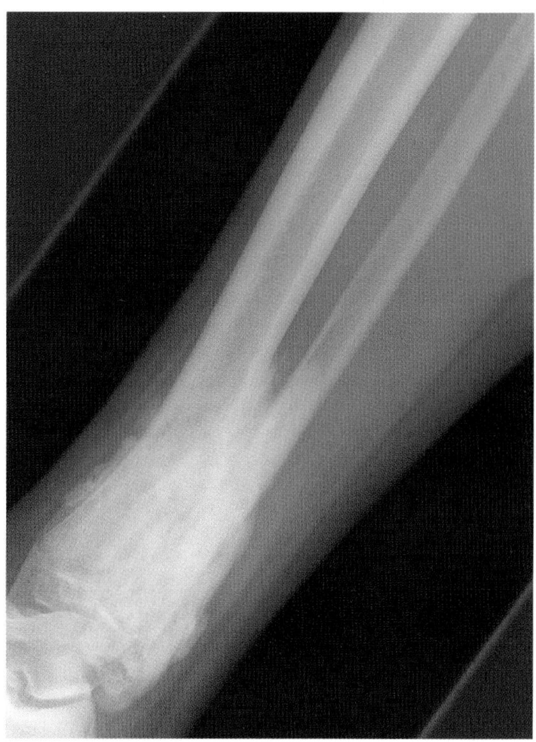

Conventional osteosarcoma: Frontal (left image) and oblique (right image) radiographs of the tibia and fibula show a sclerotic lesion of the distal tibia (arrows) associated with cloud-like ossification extending into the soft tissue. This appearance is of a highly aggressive mass.

Case courtesy Michael Hanley, MD, University of Virginia Health System.

- Osteosarcoma is the most common primary pediatric bone tumor. There are over 10 types of osteosarcoma, with the most common subtype the conventional (intramedullary) type, representing 75% of all osteosarcomas. Conventional osteosarcoma is seen most commonly about the knee in the distal femur or proximal tibia.
- The characteristic radiographic appearance of conventional osteosarcoma is a destructive lesion often invading the cortex, with extensive osteoid matrix.
- Osteosarcoma is further discussed in the musculoskeletal imaging section.

Ewing sarcoma

- Ewing sarcoma is the second most common primary pediatric bone tumor. It is an aggressive, small round blue cell tumor of neuroectodermal differentiation.
- Ewing sarcoma most commonly arises from the femoral diaphysis, followed by the flat bones of the pelvis. Ewing may also develop in the tibia, humerus, and ribs.
- The lung is the most common site of metastasis.
- The characteristic radiographic appearance is a permeative lesion in the medullary cavity with wide zone of transition and associated aggressive **lamellated (onion-skinning)** or spiculated periosteal reaction.
- Ewing often causes a soft-tissue mass, which can be difficult to see by radiography due to lack of ossification.

Osseous Langerhans cell histiocytosis (LCH)

- Langerhans cell histiocytosis (LCH) is abnormal proliferation of Langerhans cells with a variety of clinical manifestations, ranging from an isolated lytic bony lesion to fulminant systemic disease.

  Langerhans cells are dendritic cells (histiocytes) that normally live in the epidermis and lymph nodes, where they act as antigen-presenting cells.

  Histopathologically, **Birbeck** bodies are seen on electron microscopy within the histiocytes.

- Clinical subtypes of LCH have varied presentations.

  Eosinophilic granuloma (osseous LCH) features skeletal involvement only. It may be mono- or polyostotic. Despite the name, the involvement of eosinophils is variable.

  Hand–Schüller–Christian (multifocal, unisystem) is a clinical triad of pituitary hypophysitis (causing diabetes insipidus), exophthalmos, and lytic bone lesions (typically affecting the skull).

  Letterer–Siwe (multifocal, multisystem) is a fulminant disease with multisystem involvement, primarily seen in young infants and toddlers under age 2. Prognosis is poor.

  Pulmonary LCH (PLCH) is a disease of adult smokers, discussed in the thoracic imaging section. Osseous LCH is occasionally seen in conjunction with PLCH.

  In clinical practice, the most important factor is thought to be determination of unifocal or multifocal disease rather than the classification above.

- The eosinophilic granuloma variant of LCH is relatively common and may present clinically with pain, tenderness, and fever, often mimicking osteomyelitis. Children between ages 5 and 15 are typically affected.

- The appearance of the affected bone depends on the bone involved:

  Skull: *Beveled edge* lytic lesion.

  Flat bones (e.g., pelvis): *Hole within a hole* lytic lesion.

  Long bone (diaphysis most common, but may occur anywhere including rarely the epiphysis): Permeative destruction, with later lytic lesion and faint rim of sclerosis.

  Spine: Complete vertebral body collapse (vertebra plana), pictured to the right.

  Maxilla: *Floating* teeth.

- Along with infection, eosinophilic granuloma should be considered in the differential diagnosis in any patient under 30 with a lytic lesion anywhere.

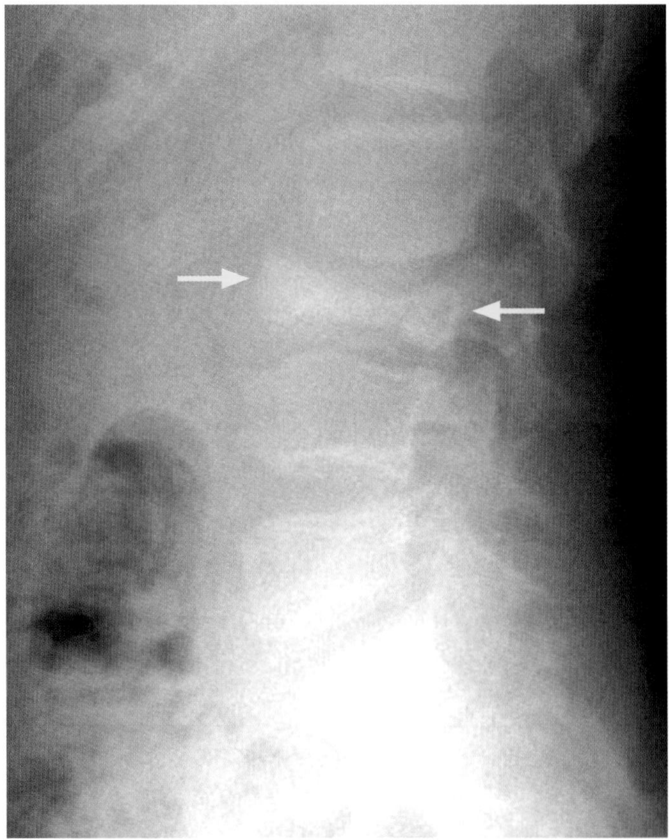

Eosinophilic granuloma (osseous LCH) causing vertebra plana (complete collapse) of L2 (arrows).

Osteomyelitis

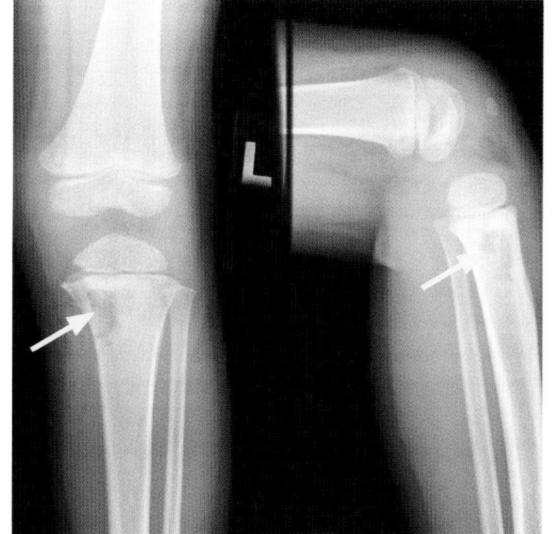

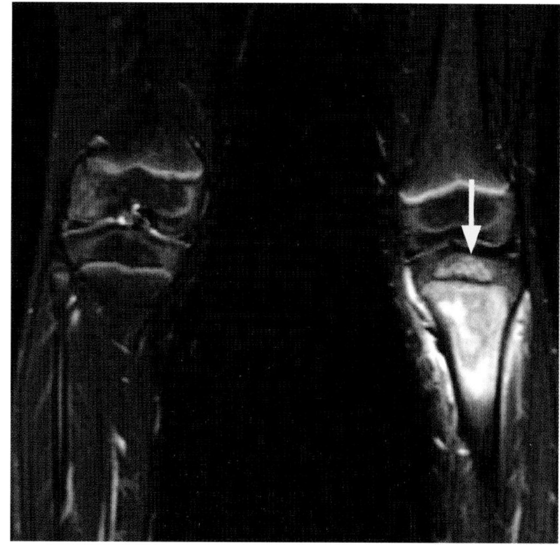

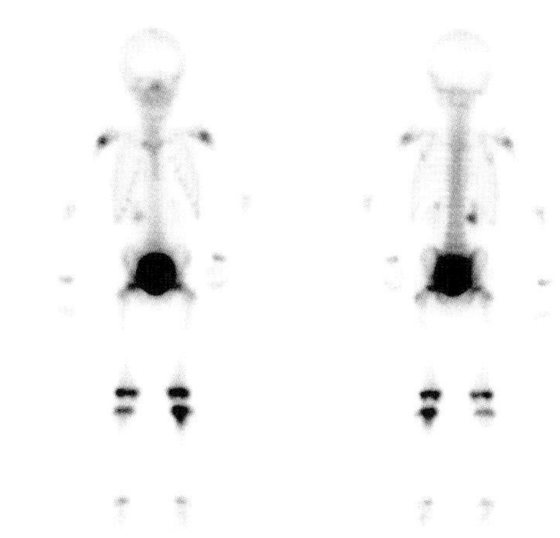

Osteomyelitis: Frontal and lateral radiographs of the knee (top left panel) show an irregular lucency (arrows) of the medial proximal tibial metaphysis.

Coronal fluid-sensitive T2-weighted MRI of both knees shows extensive marrow edema of the proximal left tibial metaphysis extending across the physis into the epiphysis (arrow) and into the soft tissues. The right knee appears normal.

Anterior and posterior Tc-99m MDP bone scan (bottom left panel) shows increased proximal left tibial uptake (arrow). The bone scan was positive on all three phases (angiographic and blood pool phases not shown).

Case courtesy Michael Hanley, MD, University of Virginia Health System.

- The initial findings of osteomyelitis are often subtle on radiography and may require a combination of plain radiographs, MRI, and scintigraphy for accurate early diagnosis.
- Osteomyelitis in children is most commonly hematogenous, with the metaphyseal marrow the most common site of initial seeding.

  In infants, the epiphysis receives blood supply from transphyseal vessels arising from metaphysis, so infection can cross the physis. In older children, capillaries do not cross the physis, so transphyseal extension of a metaphyseal infection is uncommon.
- The most common organism implicated in hematogenous osteomyelitis is *S. aureus*, with *Salmonella* seen in sickle cell patients.
- The imaging findings on radiography, MRI, and scintigraphy follow the anatomic progression of infection. The initial hematogenous infection is intramedullary and then subsequently spreads through the cortex and uplifts the periosteum. The pediatric periosteum is only loosely adherent to bone, and the purulent infection is able to dramatically uplift the periosteum, causing a prominent periosteal reaction.
- It usually takes 10–15 days for findings to become evident on radiography. The initial finding may be focal osteopenia due to hyperemia. Subsequently, a lucent, often aggressive-appearing medullary lesion can erode through the cortex and cause periosteal reaction. MRI and scintigraphy are much more sensitive for the detection of early osteomyelitis. Osteomyelitis is further discussed in the musculoskeletal imaging section.

Spinal osteomyelitis/discitis

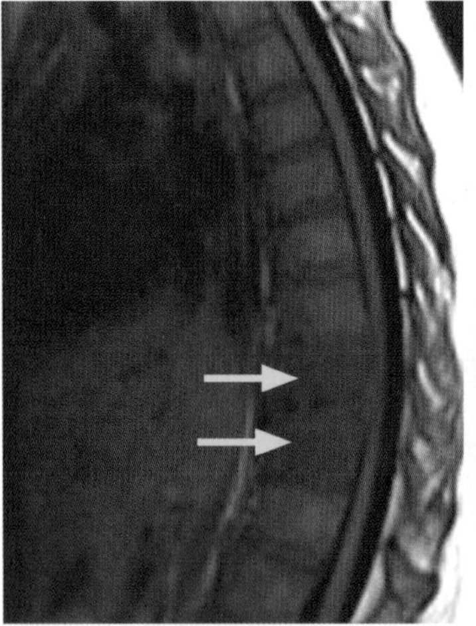

Sagittal T1-weighted MRI shows hypointense marrow signal of two adjacent vertebral bodies in the lower thoracic spine (yellow arrows).

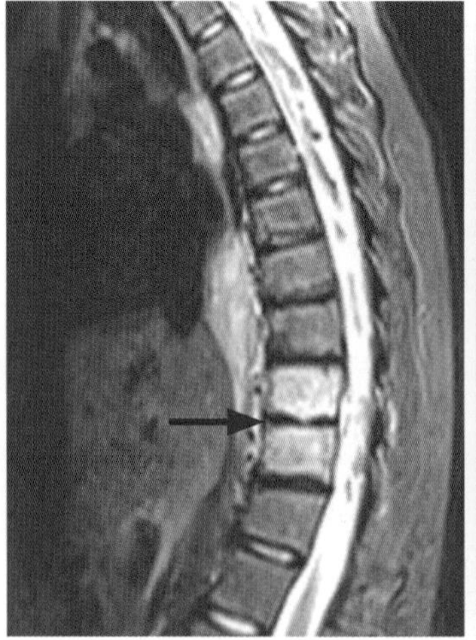

Sagittal T2-weighted fat-suppressed MRI shows hyperintense marrow edema in the affected vertebral bodies with subtle focal narrowing of the disk space (red arrow).

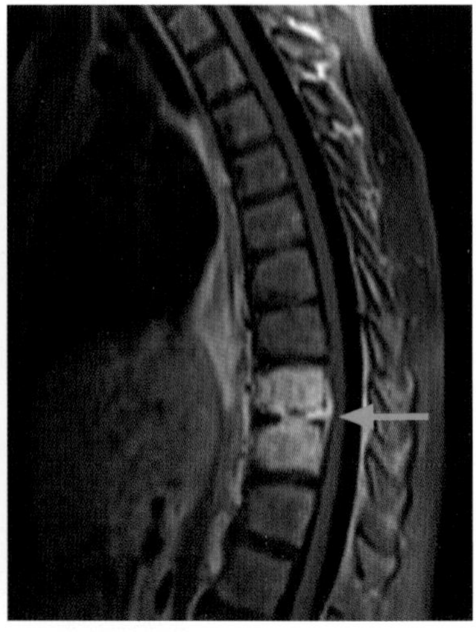

Sagittal T1-weighted post-contrast MRI with fat suppression shows avid enhancement of the affected vertebral bodies and mild epidural enhancement (blue arrow) traversing the disk space.

Discitis with epidural extension: *Case courtesy Michael Hanley, MD, University of Virginia Health System.*

- Isolated discitis is unique to children, due to the presence of blood vessels directly feeding the intervertebral disk. In adults, infection can spread through the disk, but in children infection begins in the disk.
- A typical clinical history of discitis is a young child up to 4 years old with preceding upper respiratory tract infection and back pain or refusal to sit. Discitis most commonly occurs in the lumbar spine in young children.
- Less commonly, discitis may occur in pre-teen children in the thoracic spine.
- The initial radiographic findings are disk space narrowing and vertebral end plate irregularity. These findings may be subtle. Plain films may also be normal. Because persistent back pain is never normal in children, further evaluation with MRI is recommended if clinical suspicion for discitis is high.
- MRI shows narrowing of the disk space, with bone marrow edema of two adjacent vertebral bodies. The affected vertebral bodies may enhance, and enhancement and edema may extend into the soft tissues and epidural space.

Chronic recurrent multifocal osteomyelitis (CRMO)

- Chronic recurrent multifocal osteomyelitis (CRMO) is a nonpyogenic, inflammatory disorder that can mimic osteomyelitis. It tends to occur in lower extremity long bones.
- CRMO is typically a self-limited diagnosis. Biopsy may need to be performed to exclude pyogenic infection.
- The key imaging finding is migratory lytic and sclerotic lesions in time and space. CRMO may be indistinguishable from pyogenic osteomyelitis on radiographs and MRI. Unlike infectious osteomyelitis, CRMO does not feature soft tissue abscess, bony sequestra, or fistula.
- CRMO is associated with SAPHO syndrome, characterized by:

Synovitis	Hyperostosis
Acne	Osteitis
Pustulosis	

Leukemia

- Leukemia is the most common pediatric malignancy, with bony changes seen in >50% of patients.
- Imaging findings can be varied. One of the most distinctive radiographic features of leukemia is the *metaphyseal lucent band*.
- The etiology of the lucent bands is controversial, thought to be possibly due to malnutrition or vitamin deficiency in young children. The differential diagnosis of metaphyseal lucent bands includes:

> Leukemia, lymphoma.
>
> Severe illness.
>
> TORCH infections.
>
> Scurvy.

- Other osseous findings of leukemia include generalized osteopenia or permeative lytic lesions.

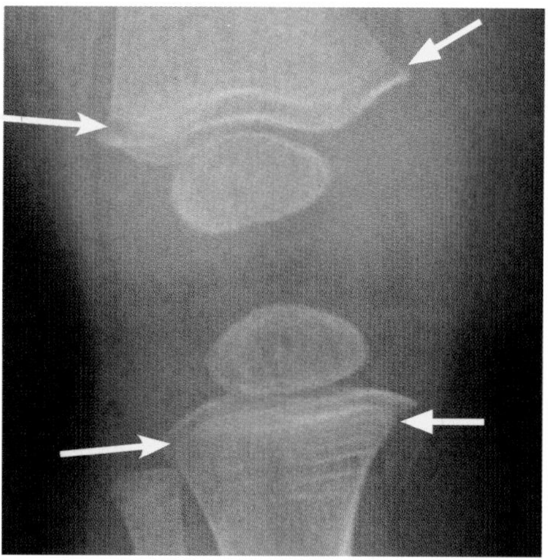

Frontal knee radiograph shows lucent metaphyseal bands in the distal femur and proximal tibia in a child with leukemia.

Case courtesy Michael Callahan, MD, Boston Children's Hospital.

Metabolic bone disease

Rickets

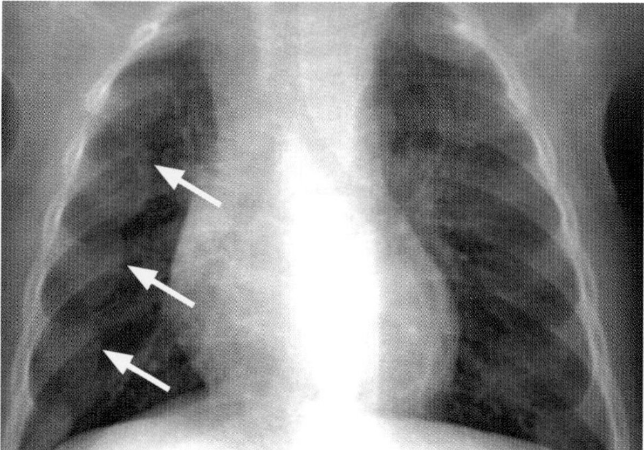

Chest radiograph in a child with rickets shows widening of the rib epiphyseal cartilage, creating the classic *rachitic rosary* appearance (yellow arrows).

Case courtesy Michael Callahan, MD, Boston Children's Hospital.

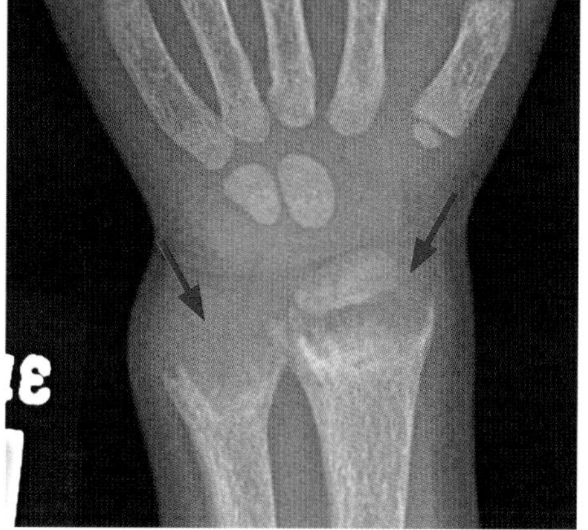

Frontal radiograph in the wrist of a different patient shows metaphyseal fraying and cupping (red arrows).

Case courtesy Michael Hanley, MD, University of Virginia Health System.

- Rickets is a metabolic bone disorder caused by inadequate vitamin D or abnormal vitamin D metabolism. It is characterized by abnormal calcification at the zone of provisional calcification, leading to abnormal physeal development.
- Radiographs show expansion, fraying, and cupping of the long bone metaphyses, often associated with adjacent metaphyseal periosteal new bone.
- Other findings of rickets include bowing of the legs, osteopenia, and fractures. The classic *rachitic rosary* represents anterior cupping of the ribs with widening of the rib epiphyseal cartilage. The skull may become demineralized.
- **Oncogenic rickets** is a variant of rickets seen with hemangiopericytoma or nonossifying fibroma due to tumor metabolites that cause deranged vitamin D metabolism.

Torch infections

Syphilis

- Syphilis is caused by the spirochete *Treponema pallidum.* Syphilis can be transmitted in utero through the placenta to cause congenital syphilitic osteomyelitis.
- The *Wimberger* sign is destructive erosion of the medial aspect of the proximal tibial metaphysis. The *Wimberger* sign is not to be confused with the *Wimberger ring* sign of scurvy, which is increased density of the ossification centers.
- Syphilis is one of many causes of symmetric periosteal reaction in a child.

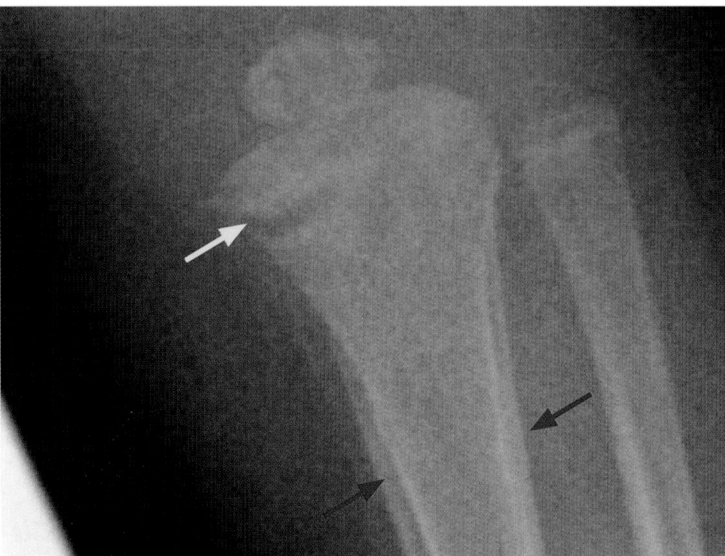

Wimberger sign in congenital syphilis:

Magnified frontal leg radiograph shows a deep erosion of the medial aspect of the proximal tibia (yellow arrow), representing the *Wimberger* sign. There is also periosteal reaction along the partially visualized tibial diaphysis (red arrows).

Childhood arthritis

Juvenile idopathic arthritis (JIA)/juvenile rheumatoid arthritis (JRA)/juvenile chronic arthritis (JCA)

- Juvenile idiopathic arthritis (JIA), also known as juvenile rheumatoid arthritis (JRA) and juvenile chronic arthritis (JCA), is the most common chronic arthropathy of childhood. It is a systemic idiopathic disease defined as being present for more than 6 weeks in a patient younger than 16 years old. JIA is usually rheumatoid-factor negative.
- The most common subtype of JIA is pauciarticular disease, typically affecting young girls. Regardless of subtype, the knee is the most commonly affected joint, but any joint can be affected.
- The imaging appearance reflects the underlying pathophysiology of synovitis, as the earliest radiographic changes are joint effusion, soft tissue swelling, and osteopenia. Later changes include periostitis and erosions.
- Chronic disease leads to eventual joint ankylosis, which is in contrast to adult rheumatoid arthritis, where ankylosis is rare. The most common sites of ankylosis are in the wrist, at the carpometacarpal joints, and the cervical spine.

  Cervical spine ankylosis in a child may appear similar to Klippel–Feil syndrome. In contrast to Klippel–Feil, JIA does not feature segmentation anomalies.
- Accelerated skeletal maturation and accelerated bone growth are caused by synovitis and hyperemia, which lead to premature fusion of the physes and/or abnormal bone growth.
- Still disease is an acute systemic subtype of JIA affecting children under the age of five. Still disease presents with fever, anemia, leukocytosis, hepatosplenomegaly, and polyarthritis. Boys and girls are affected equally in Still disease.

Developmental dysplasia of the hip (DDH)

- Developmental dysplasia of the hip (DDH) is abnormal development of the femoral head–acetabular relationship. An abnormally shallow acetabular angle results in uncovering of the femoral head by the acetabulum. There is an increased incidence of DDH in breech births, so all breech births are typically screened by ultrasound.
- Ultrasound is performed a few weeks after birth. Imaging is delayed because of the effects of perinatal maternal hormones on neonatal ligamentous laxity.
- The alpha angle is the angle formed by the bony ilium and acetabular roof, obtained from the coronal hip ultrasound. A normal alpha angle is greater than 60 degrees. The bony portion of the acetabular roof should cover at least 50% of the cartilagineous femoral head.
- An alpha angle less than 60 degrees or less than 50% coverage of the femoral head by acetabulum is abnormal, suggesting DDH.

hip dysplasia: same coronal image with different annotations
alpha angle <60 degrees
femoral head less than 50% covered by bony acetabulum

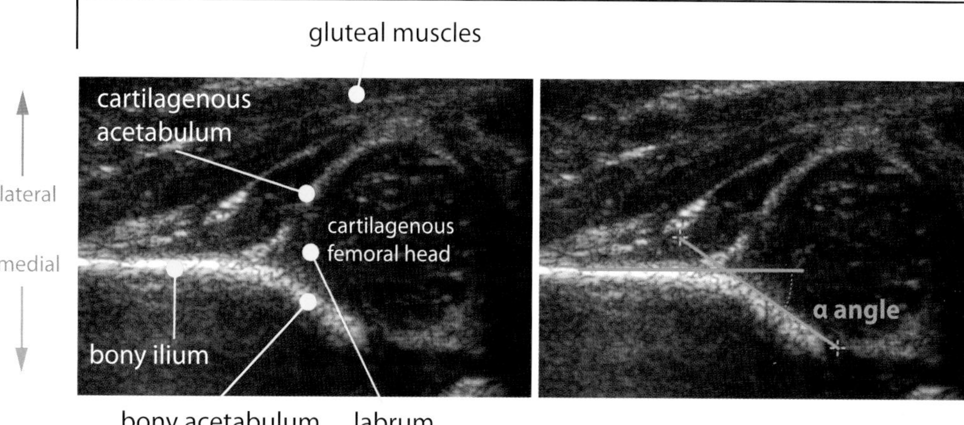

- After femoral head ossification (typically after 6 months of age) radiographs are performed.
- On pelvic radiography, the ossified femoral head should normally sit in the inner lower quadrant formed by the intersection of the Hilgenreiner and Perkins lines.

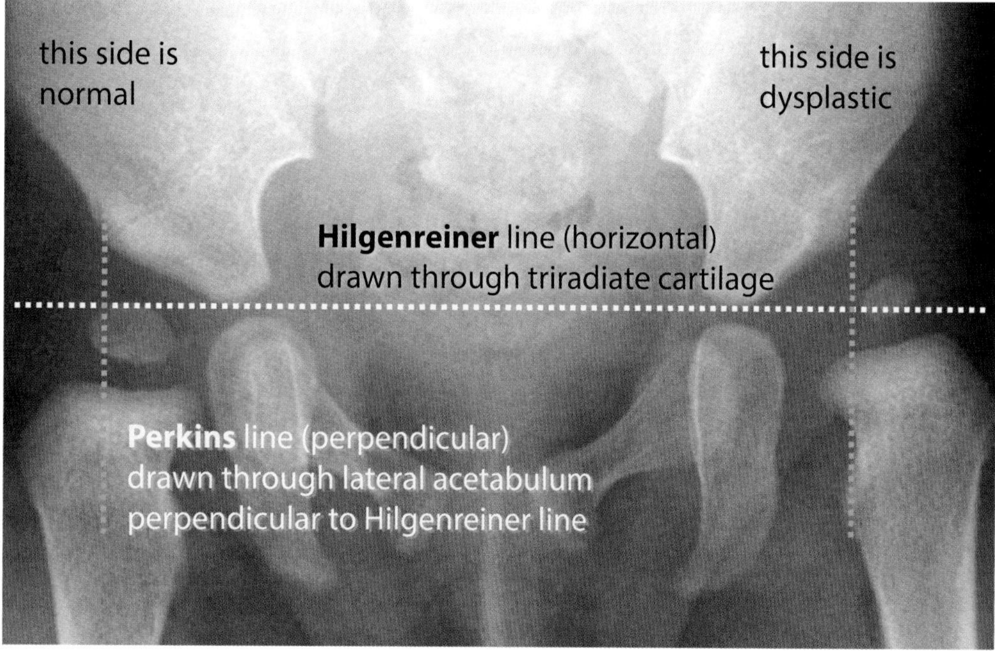

Osteochondroses

- The osteochondroses are a heterogeneous group of disorders that were at one point thought to be initiated by avascular necrosis. The current understanding is that most of these disorders are secondary to trauma. While many are associated with avascular necrosis, AVN is not thought to be the initiating factor. Most are more common in males.

Blount disease

- Blount disease is an osteochondrosis of the proximal tibial metaphysis, causing tibia varus (bowing) and internal rotation, which eventually leads to progressive deformity, gait deviations, and leg-length discrepancy.
- The infantile form of Blount disease is thought to be due to early walking and obesity, and is typically bilateral.
- The adolescent form is seen in children over 6 years old and is usually unilateral.

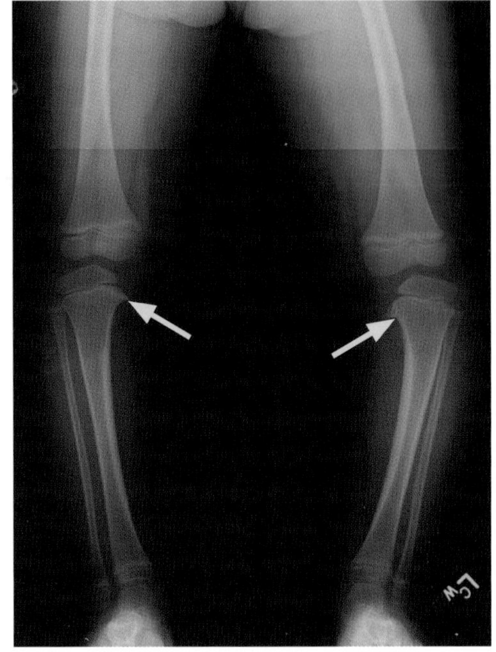

Infantile Blount disease:

Bilateral Blount disease with sloping of the medial portions of the proximal tibial metaphyses (arrows), causing tibia varus.

Madelung deformity

- Madelung deformity is medial sloping of the distal radius caused by dysplasia of the medial distal radial physis and resultant growth disturbance.

Panner disease

- Panner disease is osteochondrosis of the capitellum.

Little league elbow

- Little league elbow is osteochondrosis of the medial epicondyle.

Scheuermann kyphosis

- Scheuermann kyphosis is a syndrome of avascular necrosis of multiple thoracic vertebral bodies leading to multiple compression fractures.

Legg–Calvé–Perthes disease

- Legg–Calvé–Perthes disease is osteochondrosis of the capital femoral epiphysis.

Kienbock disease

- Kienbock disease is osteochondrosis of the carpal lunate.

Osgood–Schlatter disease

- Osgood–Schlatter disease is osteochondrosis of the tibial tuberosity.

Freiberg infraction

- Freiberg infraction is osteochondrosis of the second metatarsal head.

Kohler disease

- Kohler disease is a self-limited osteochondrosis of the navicular bone.

Sever disease

- Sever disease is calcaneal apophysitis (rather than an osteochondrosis) and is a cause of heel pain. Sclerosis of the calcaneal apophysis is nonspecific and can be seen in asymptomatic children, although greater fragmentation of the apophysis may be associated with pain.

Torticollis

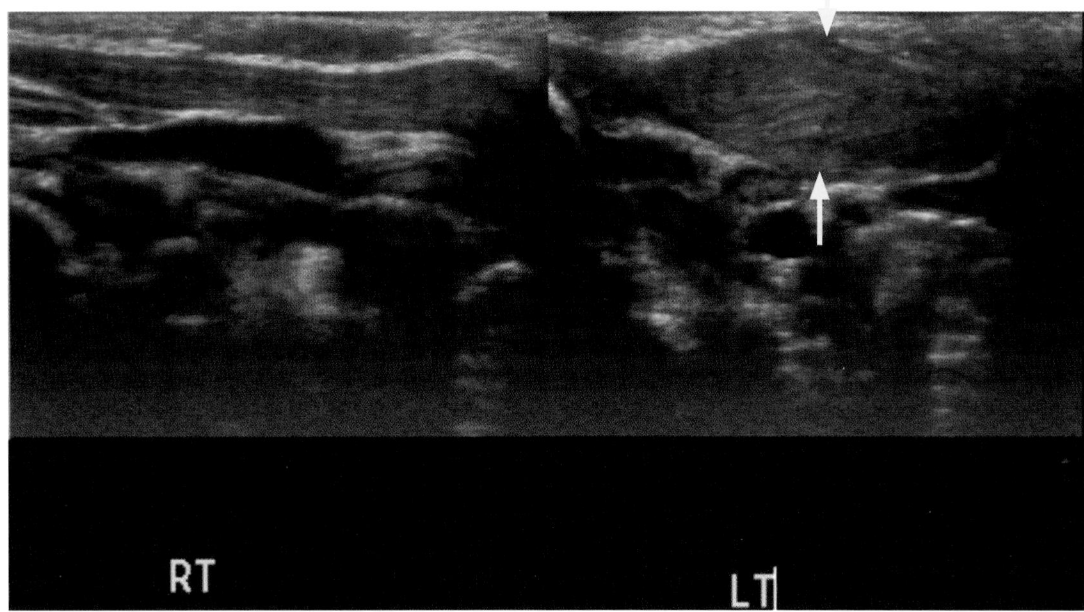

Torticollis: Bilateral neck ultrasound shows fusiform enlargement of the left sternocleidomastoid muscle (arrows). The right side is normal.

- Torticollis is caused by fibromatosis coli (idiopathic sternocleidomastoid enlargement) resulting in an inability to fully straighten the neck. It usually resolves with physical therapy.

Tarsal coalition

- Tarsal coalition is abnormal joining of two normally separate bones in the tarsus. The three types of coalition are fibrous, cartilaginous, and osseous.
- The two most common coalitions (together making up 90% of all tarsal coalitions) are talocalcaneal and calcaneonavicular.
- Tarsal coalition clinically presents as foot pain in the child as the coalition begins to ossify.
- Tarsal coalition is discussed in the musculoskeletal imaging section.

Carpal coalition

- Carpal coalition is abnormal joining of carpal bones.
- Carpal coalition is usually asymptomatic but may be a cause of wrist pain.
- Like tarsal coalition, the coalition may be fibrous, cartilaginous, or osseous.
- Lunotriquetral coalition is the most common carpal coalition.
- Capitohamate is second most common carpal coalition.

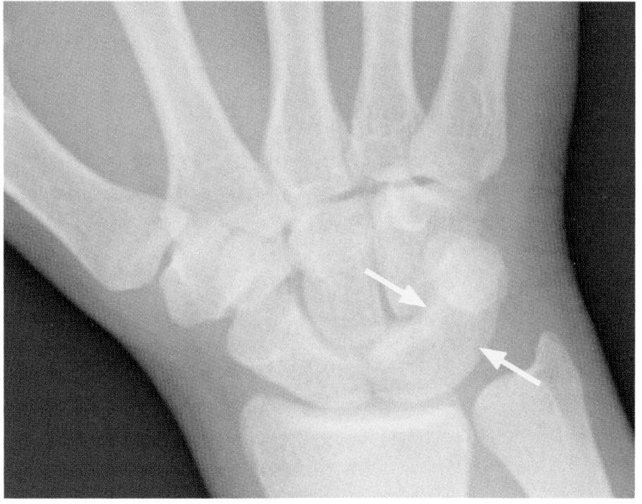

Frontal radiograph of the wrist demonstrates osseous lunotriquetral coalition (arrows).

Case courtesy Michael Callahan, MD, Boston Children's Hospital.

- The periosteum is a thin membrane covering the entire surface of the bone excluding those areas covered by cartilage. It contributes to bone production and remodeling. Irritation of the periosteum, which can be due to trauma, infection, inflammation, neoplasm, or metabolic disturbance, can cause *periosteal reaction*.
- The terms "periosteal reaction," "periostitis," and "periosteal new bone formation" are commonly used as synonyms. Periosteal reaction is simply a nonspecific response to injury resulting in periosteal new bone production.
- Periosteal reaction may also be associated with tumors or infection, typically producing an aggressive appearance in these disorders. The morphology of aggressive periosteal reaction is discussed in the musculoskeletal imaging section.

Physiologic periosteal reaction of the newborn

- Physiologic periosteal reaction occurs in infants 1–4 months old, thought to be due to rapid bone growth and loosely adherent periosteum.
- The periosteal reaction is smooth and thin, and usually only involves the lateral *or* medial aspect of the long bones.

Prostaglandin therapy

- Neonates on prostaglandin therapy for congenital heart disease (to maintain ductal patency) may have periosteal reaction. Prostaglandins are thought to decrease osteoclast bone resorption.

Infectious

- Subperiosteal spread of pyogenic infection elevates the periosteum and irritates it, usually causing an aggressive periosteal reaction.
- Congenital syphilis causes periosteal reaction.

Neoplastic (typically these are aggressive periosteal reactions)

- Multiple malignancies, including leukemia, neuroblastoma, Ewing sarcoma, and osteosarcoma can produce an aggressive periosteal reaction.

Trauma

- Healing fractures (both accidental trauma and child abuse) may cause periosteal reaction.

Metabolic

- Rickets, scurvy (which is also characterized by epiphyseal sclerosis – the *Wimberger rim* sign), and hypervitaminosis A may all cause periosteal reaction.

Syndromic

- Multiple syndromes may cause periostitis. Caffey disease (infantile cortical hyperostosis) is a rare inflammatory disease causing periostitis of the mandible, scapula, and clavicle.

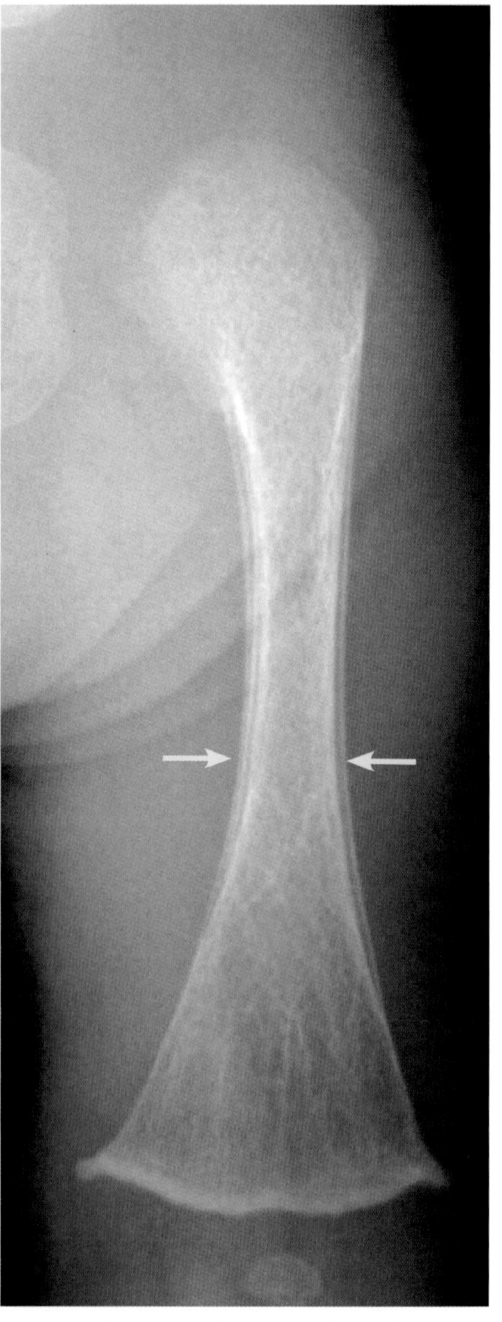

Symmetric periosteal reaction along the femoral diaphysis (arrows). This child was on prostaglandin therapy for congenital heart disease.

NORMAL DEVELOPMENT

Pattern of myelination

- A full-term newborn will have myelination seen in several structures at birth, including: Posterior limb of internal capsule, middle cerebellar peduncle, ventrolateral thalami, dorsal brainstem, and the perirolandic regions.
- Myelination is most apparent on T1-weighted images. On T1-weighted images myelin is bright; on T2-weighted images myelin is dark.
- Myelination generally assumes a mature pattern by age 2 years, although the frontal lobes continue to myelinate through adolescence.

Overview of cortical development

- Primitive brain forms around the primordial ventricular system, which is lined by pluripotent stem cells called germinal matrix cells.
- Development of normal cortex is dependent on both germinal matrix cell ***migration*** and subsequent ***organization*** into the normal six-layered lamination of the cortex.

CONGENITAL MALFORMATIONS

Polymicrogyria

- Polymicrogyria is a malformation of cortical development characterized by a derangement of the normal six-layered organization of the cortex, which leads to abnormally shallow and abnormally numerous sulcation.
- Polymicrogyria is thought to be caused by disturbance either late in neuronal migration or early in cortical lamellar organization.
- Polymicrogyria may be caused by in-utero infection (especially CMV), in-utero ischemia, or genetic causes. Clinical manifestations include developmental delay, quadriparesis, or intractable seizures.
- On MR imaging, sulci appear thick, bumpy, small, and irregular. The junction of the polymicrogyric cortex and the white matter is irregular and less well defined than normal.
- Bilateral perisylvian polymicrogyria is the most common distribution.

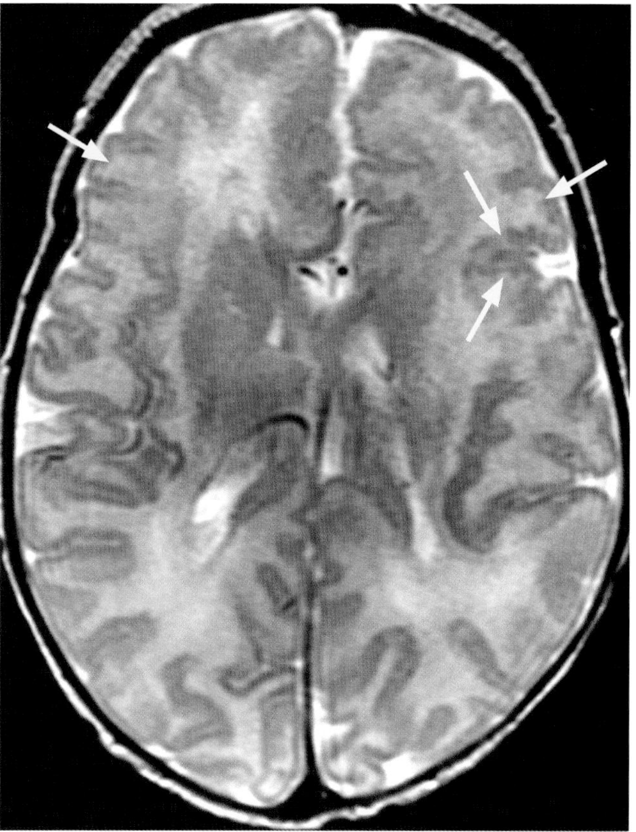

T2-weighted MRI demonstrates bilateral perisylvian and bifrontal polymicrogyria (arrows point to the perisylvian polymicrogyria). The affected regions have an irregular junction of the abnormal cortex and the white matter.

Case courtesy Sanjay Prabhu, MBBS, Boston Children's Hospital.

Lissencephaly

- Lissencephaly is characterized by absent or decreased cortical convolutions causing a smooth, thickened cortical surface. Instead of the normal six-layered cortex, the cortex is arranged into four primitive layers. Lissencephaly is thought to be due to an arrested band of neurons, which have not completed outward migration to the superficial cortex.
- Lissencephaly may be caused by CMV, in which case calcifications are often present.
- Clinically, patients with lissencephaly almost universally have seizures.
- Lissencephaly can be subdivided into type I (classical) and type II (cobblestone). The two forms are genetically and embryologically distinct. Cobblestone lissencephaly is associated with cerebellar and ocular malformations and muscular dystrophy (Walker–Warburg syndrome).
- Type I (classical) lissencephaly is characterized by a smooth cortex and a configuration of the cerebral hemispheres that has been likened to an *hour-glass* or a *figure-of-eight*.

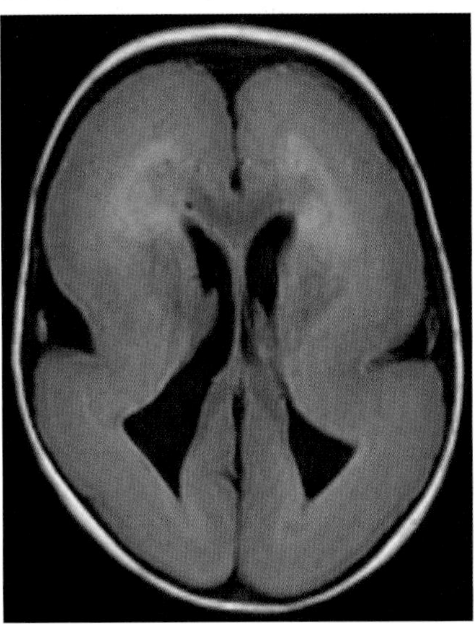
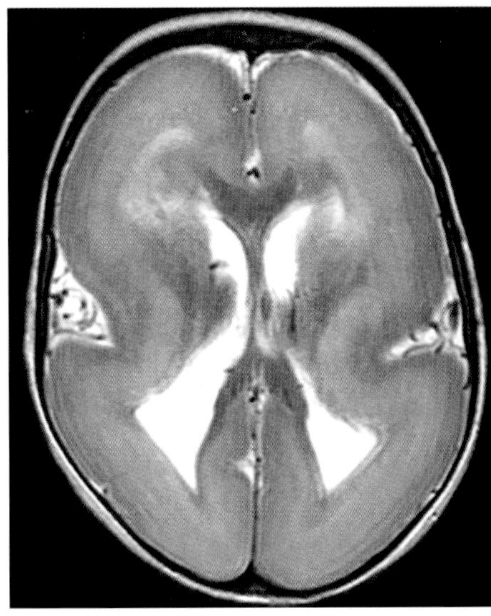

T1-weighted (left image) and T2-weighted (right image) MR images demonstrate **classical** (type I) lissencephaly with a completely smooth cortex and an *hour-glass* or *figure-of-eight* configuration to the cerebral hemispheres.

Case courtesy Sanjay Prabhu, MBBS, Boston Children's Hospital.

- Type II (cobblestone) lissencephaly is characterized by a finely undulating cortex.

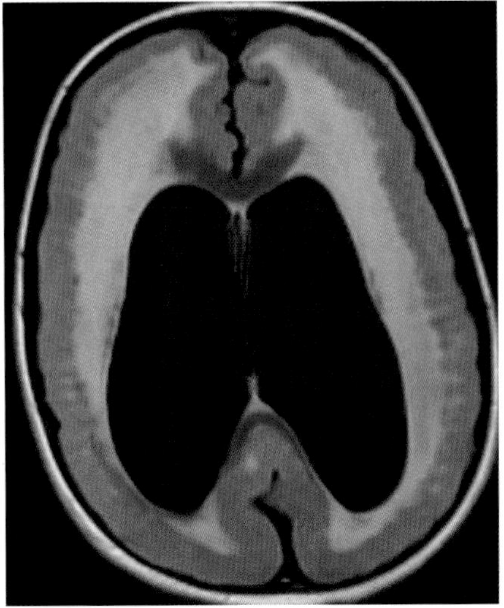
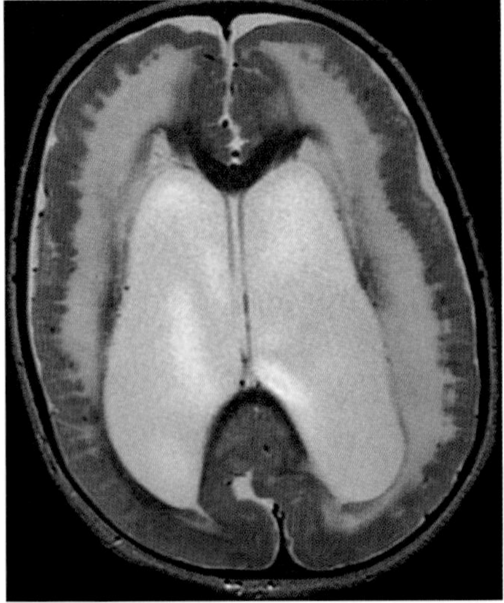

T1-weighted (left image) and T2-weighted (right image) MR images demonstrate **cobblestone** (type II) lissencephaly with a gently lobulated external cortex and a finely undulating or serrated interface at the gray–white junction.

Gray matter heterotopia

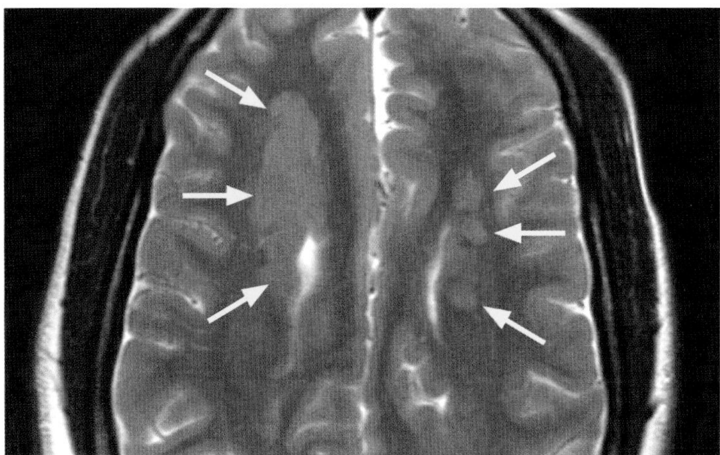

T2-weighted MRI shows extensive bilateral periventricular nodular heterotopia (arrows), most prominent on the right.

Case courtesy Sanjay Prabhu, MBBS, Boston Children's Hospital.

- Gray matter heterotopia is a range of disorders characterized by clusters of normal neurons in abnormal locations.
- Gray matter heterotopia may be a cause of seizures.
- Three main subtypes include periventricular nodular heterotopia, subcortical heterotopia, and marginal glioneural heterotopia.

Agenesis/hypogenesis of corpus callosum

- Agenesis of the corpus callosum is a relatively common congenital abnormality. The most common clinical manifestations of agenesis of the corpus callosum are refractile seizures and/or developmental delay.
- Complete agenesis of the corpus callosum causes secondary abnormalities in ventricular morphology. Colpocephaly (dilation of the occipital horns of the lateral ventricles) may result from decreased white matter volume posteriorly. The lateral ventricles are often parallel in orientation and widely spaced. Medial impressions on the lateral ventricles are caused by *Probst bundles*, which are axons that normally constitute the corpus callosum but instead pursue an aberrant course parallel to the interhemispheric fissure. The third ventricle may be enlarged and high-riding.
- The corpus callosum develops from genu (anterior) to splenium (posterior). Various degrees of corpus callosal hypogenesis may occur, the most common being absence of the splenium.
- Congenital corpus callosal anomalies are often associated with other midline abnormalities including a midline lipoma or interhemispheric cyst.

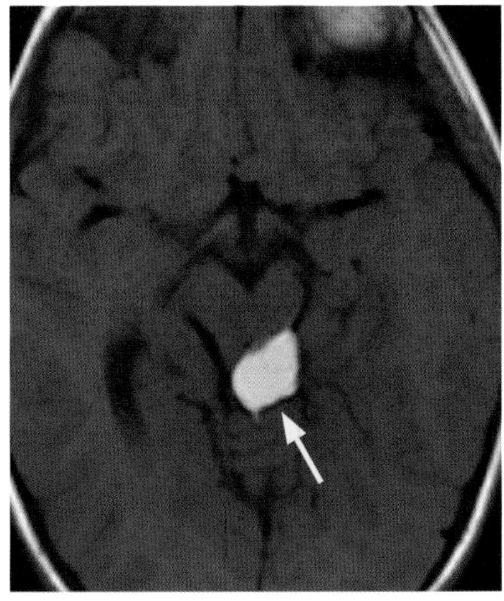

Quadrigeminal plate lipoma: Axial T1-weighted MRI shows a hyperintense lipoma at the left quadrigeminal plate (arrow).

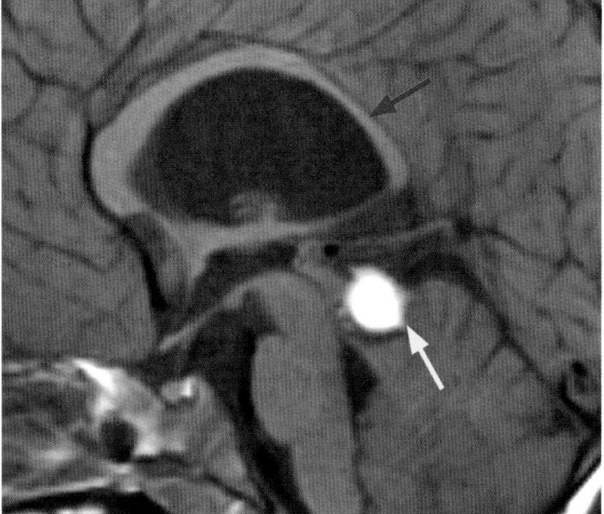

Sagittal T1-weighted MRI shows marked thinning of the posterior body (red arrow) and splenium of the corpus callosum. The third ventricle is enlarged and high-riding. The lipoma (yellow arrow) is reidentified.

Case courtesy Sanjay Prabhu, MBBS, Boston Children's Hospital.

Schizencephaly

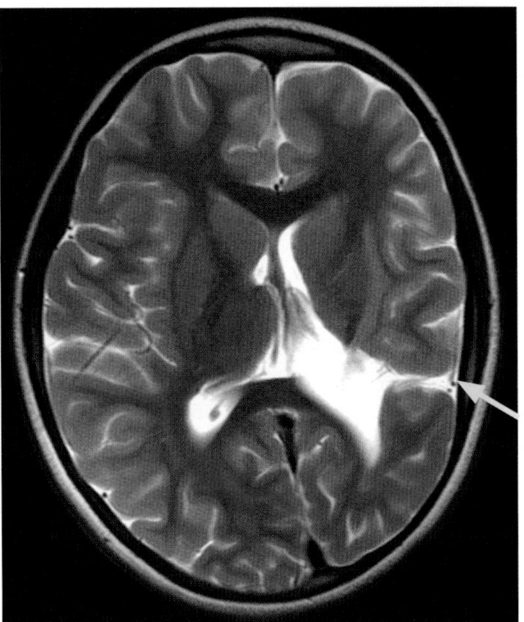

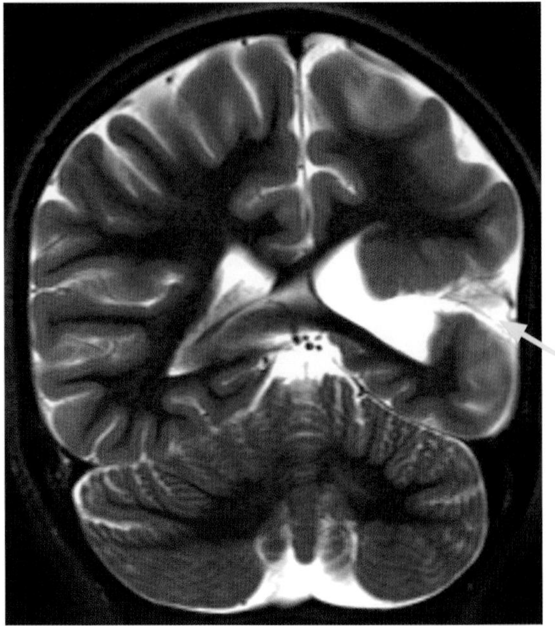

Open-lip schizencephaly: Axial (left image) and coronal T2-weighted images demonstrate a cleft in the left temporoparietal cortex (arrows) extending from the cortical surface to the left lateral ventricle. The cleft is lined by dysplastic-appearing gray matter.

Case courtesy Sanjay Prabhu, MBBS, Boston Children's Hospital.

- Schizencephaly is a malformation characterized by a full-thickness cleft of the cerebral hemisphere lined by dysplastic gray matter (usually from polymicrogyria), forming an abnormal communication between the ventricles and the extra-axial subarachnoid space.
- Schizencephaly is associated with cortical malformations (gray matter heterotopia), with up to 30% of patients with schizencephaly also having cortical malformations.
- Schizencephaly has been morphologically classified into open-lip (walls of the cleft are entirely divided by CSF) and closed-lip (walls of the cleft are apposed or incompletely divided).
- Schizencephaly is associated with septo-optic dysplasia, which is characterized by agenesis of the septum pellucidum and optic nerve hypoplasia.
- The characteristic imaging finding of schizencephaly is a CSF-filled cortical cleft lined by gray matter. Frontal involvement is most common.
- There are several other entities that can cause an interruption or cleft in the cortex, but only a schizencephalic cleft is lined by gray matter. Other cortical clefts include:

Porencephaly, where there is replacement of cortex by a cystic structure.

Encephalomalacia.

Surgical resection cavity.

Holoprosencephaly

- Holoprosencephaly is a complex congenital malformation where the forebrain does not divide into two hemispheres.
- Holoprosencephaly is associated with midline maxillofacial anomalies including a single central incisor. It is commonly said that "the brain predicts the face." Holoprosencephaly is associated with an azygos configuration of anterior cerebral artery (single ACA).
- The three subtypes (from most severe to least severe) are alobar, semilobar, and lobar.

Alobar holoprosencephaly is the most severe form, characterized by complete lack of separation of the cerebral hemispheres. A single large monoventricle almost always communicates with a large dorsal cyst.

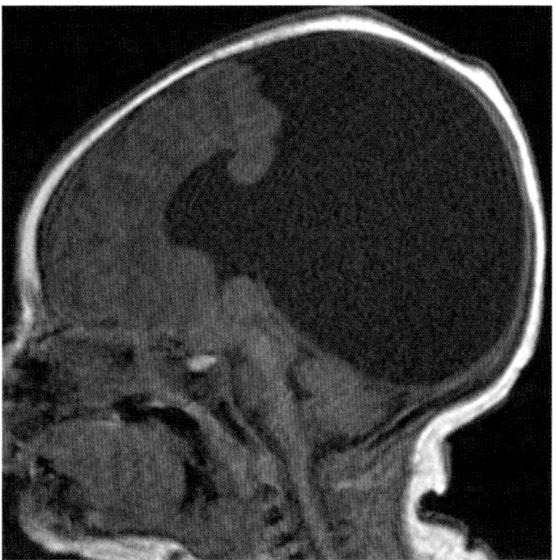

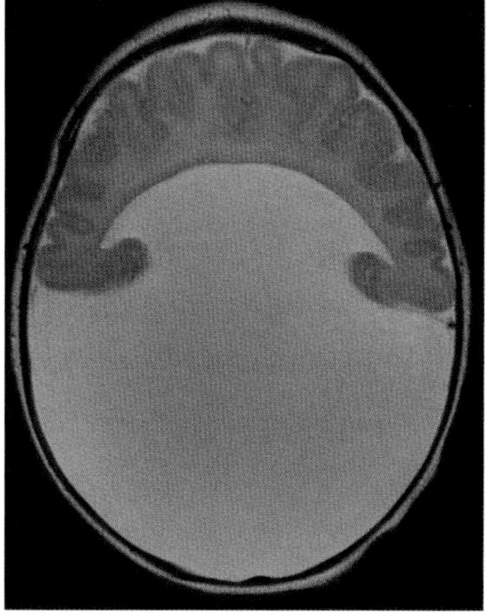

Sagittal T1-weighted (left image) and axial T2-weighted MR images demonstrate severe alobar holoprosencephaly. There is continual frontal lobe cortex across the midline. A midline monoventricle communicates with a dominant dorsal cyst.

Case courtesy Sanjay Prabhu, MBBS, Boston Children's Hospital.

Semilobar holoprosencephaly features at least some degree of separation of the posterior cerebral hemispheres. Similar to alobar holoprosencephaly, the anterior hemispheres also fail to separate.

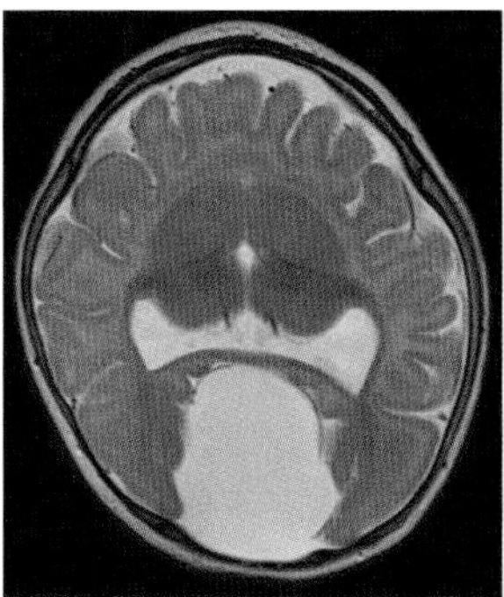

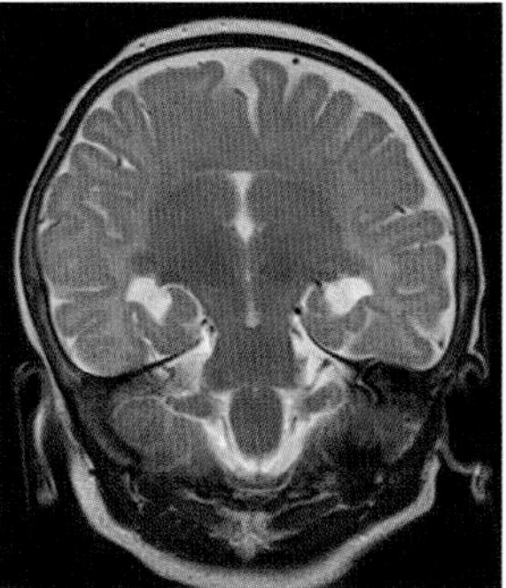

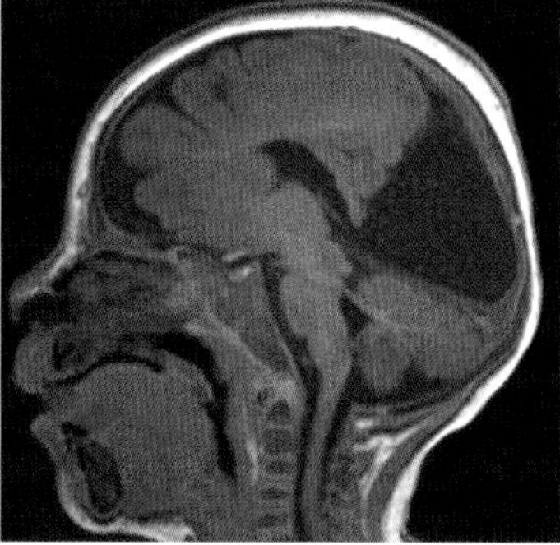

Axial and coronal T2-weighted MRI (left and middle images) and sagittal T1-weighted MRI (right image) shows semilobar holoprosencephaly. There is partial separation of the posterior cerebral cortex, with complete fusion of the frontal lobes. There is a large midline posterior interhemispheric cyst.

Case courtesy Sanjay Prabhu, MBBS, Boston Children's Hospital.

Lobar holoprosencephaly is the mildest form, where only the most rostral aspects of the frontal neocortex are not separated. The corpus callosum is absent in the affected region anteriorly, but the posterior corpus callosum (splenium and posterior body) is present.

Chiari I malformation

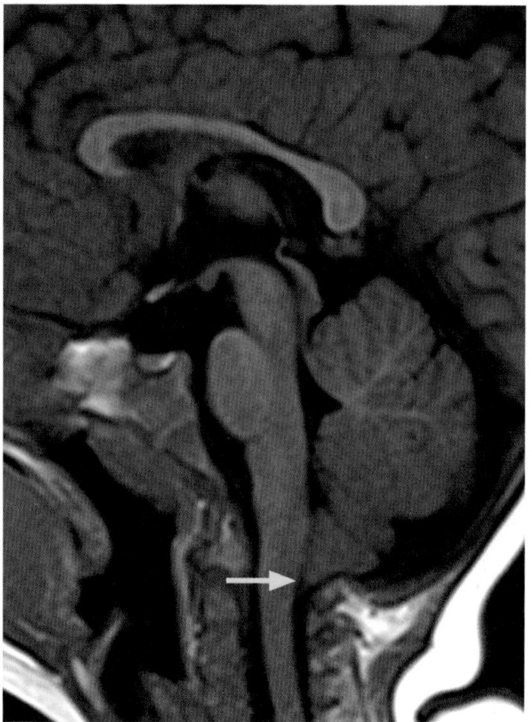

Borderline tonsillar ectopia: Sagittal T1-weighted MRI shows cerebellar tonsils extending inferiorly below the foramen magnum (yellow arrow). There is no hydrocephalus or cervical spine syringomyelia.

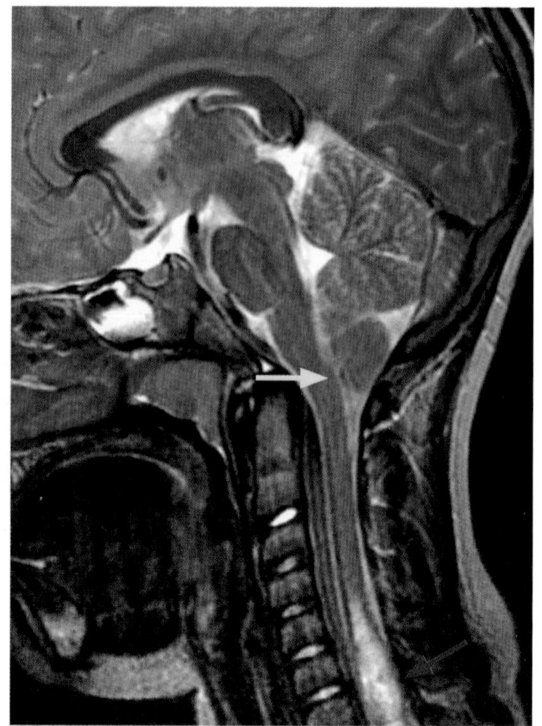

Chiari I in a different patient: Sagittal T2-weighted MRI shows inferior extension of the cerebellar tonsils (yellow arrows). The presence of syringomyelia (red arrow) allows more confident diagnosis of Chiari I.

- Chiari I is inferior displacement of the cerebellar tonsils beyond the foramen magnum.
- The clinical manifestation of Chiari I is variable and ranges from occasional exertional headaches in an otherwise normal individual to severe myelopathy and brainstem compromise. In babies, Chiari I may be associated with sleep apnea and feeding problems.
- The most common complications of Chiari I are cervical syringomyelia and less commonly hydrocephalus.

  Syringomyelia, also called *syringohydromyelia* or *syrinx*, is fluid within the spinal cord. Syringomyelia most commonly represents dilation of the central canal of the spinal cord, which normally extends from the obex of the fourth ventricle to the filum terminale. The syringomyelia associated with Chiari I is fusiform dilation of the central canal that does not typically communicate with the fourth ventricle. Other forms of syringomyelia (typically associated with hydrocephalus) may communicate with the fourth ventricle via the central canal.

- Both clinical diagnosis and diagnostic imaging criteria for Chiari I are controversial. Inferior protrusion of the cerebellar tonsils is a relatively common finding in asymptomatic individuals. Additionally, the clinical symptoms of Chiari I are nonspecific and include headache and malaise, which may not always be attributable to the inferior protrusion of the tonsils.
- The classic criterion for diagnosis is herniation of either cerebellar tonsil by 5 mm, or herniation of both tonsils by 3 mm; however, associated findings allowing a more confident diagnosis include pointing of the cerebellar tonsils, crowding of the posterior fossa, and a complication such as cervical spine syringomyelia or hydrocephalus.
- If the only finding is isolated inferior displacement of the tonsils, the term "borderline tonsillar ectopia" is generally preferred.

Chiari II

- Chiari II is a completely different disease from Chiari I; however, a common feature among all Chiari malformations is inferior displacement of the hindbrain.
- The primary abnormality in Chiari II is herniation of the vermis, cerebellar tonsils, and medulla into the foramen magnum, with resultant *beaking* of the tectum.
- A myelomeningocele is universally present, typically lumbar.
- The fourth ventricle becomes elongated and inferiorly displaced. Approximately 80–90% of children with Chiari II have hydrocephalus necessitating shunt placement, due to fourth ventricular obstruction.
- Associated supratentorial anomalies include corpus callosal dysgenesis, heterotopias, and sulcation abnormalities.

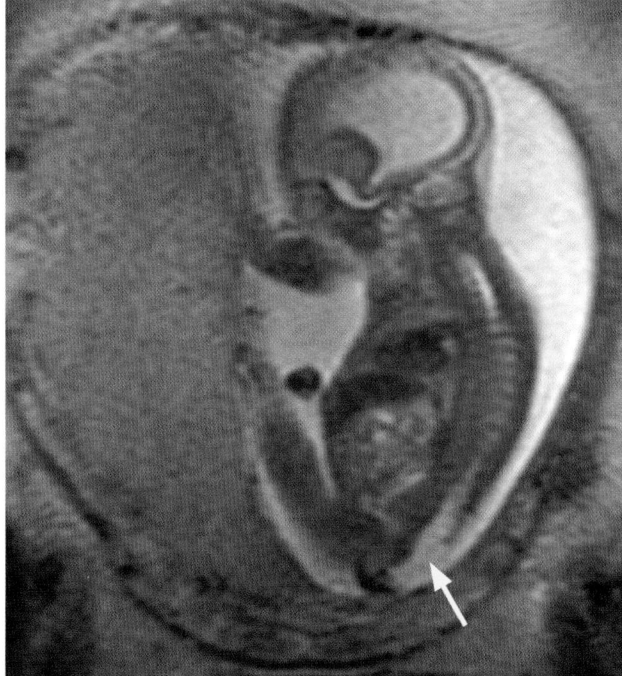

Parasagittal T2-weighted fetal MRI shows a lumbar myelomeningocele (arrow) and marked hydrocephalus.

Case courtesy Sanjay Prabhu, MBBS, Boston Children's Hospital.

Dandy Walker

- The Dandy Walker complex features an enlarged posterior fossa, usually associated with a large posterior fossa cyst. Dandy Walker variants are a continuum of disorders of varying severities.
- An in-utero insult to the developing fourth ventricle is thought to result in fourth ventricular outflow obstruction, cyst-like dilation of the fourth ventricle (which communicates with a retrocerebellar cyst), and resultant inferior vermain hypoplasia.
- Most patients have hydrocephalus.
- Upwards displacement of the tentorium by the enlarged fourth ventricle and posterior fossa cyst causes **torcular–lambdoid inversion.** The torcular herophili is the confluence of the transverse and the straight sinuses, which is pushed superiorly, above the lambdoid suture.

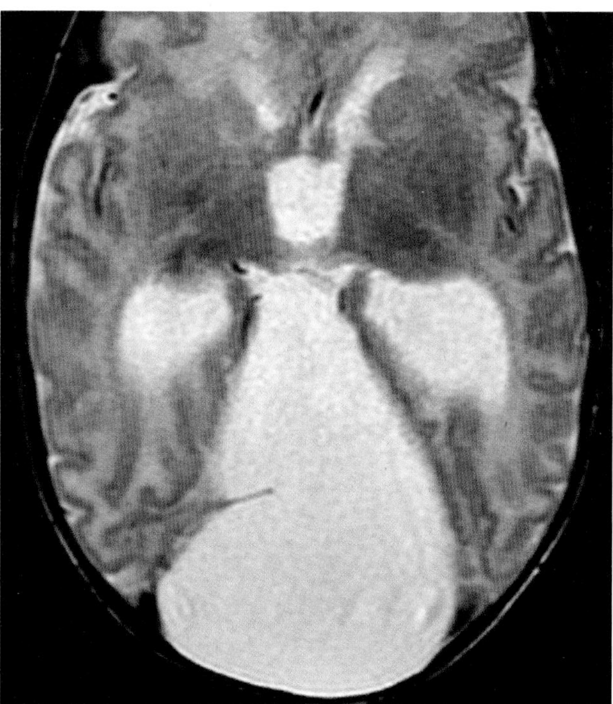

T2-weighted axial MRI shows an enlarged fourth ventricle communicating with a large retrocerebellar cyst, which displaces the tentorium upwards. There is hydrocephalus, with dilation of the temporal horns and third ventricle.

Case courtesy Sanjay Prabhu, MBBS, Boston Children's Hospital.

Neurofibromatosis 1 (NF1)/von Recklinghausen disease

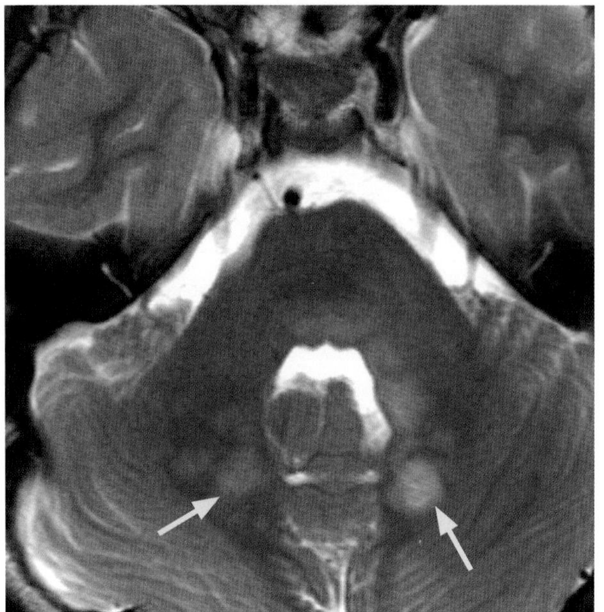

Axial T2-weighted MRI through the cerebellum demonstrates T2 hyperintense "unidentified bright objects" of neurofibromatosis representing myelin vacuolization (yellow arrows).

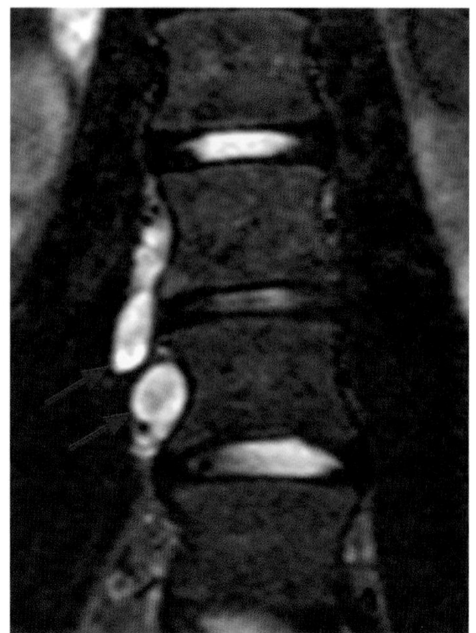

Coronal T2-weighted MRI of the lumbar spine shows the characteristic *target* appearance of plexiform neurofibromas (red arrows), which are T2 hyperintense with central hypointensity.

Case courtesy Sanjay Prabhu, MBBS, Boston Children's Hospital.

- Neurofibromatosis type 1 (NF1), also known as von Recklinghausen disease, is a multisystemic neurocutaneous disorder with prominent skin manifestation (e.g., café au lait spots), peripheral nerve sheath tumors (e.g., plexiform neurofibroma), CNS malignancies (e.g., optic nerve glioma), and bony abnormalities (e.g., sphenoid wing dysplasia).
- NF1 is autosomal dominant in 50% of cases and occurs sporadically in 50%, caused by a defect in chromosome 17.
- In children, "bright spots" or "unidentified bright objects" are almost universally seen on T2-weighted images, thought to be caused by myelin vacuolization. These bright spots are seen most commonly in children ages 4–12 and become less prominent in adults.
- Neurofibromas are WHO grade I nerve sheath tumors. The cutaneous and subcutaneous nerves are more commonly involved than the more proximal peripheral nerves. A *plexiform* subtype is more aggressive and consists of a network of fusiform-shaped masses, with malignant degeneration reported in approximately 5%.

  Like schwannomas, neurofibromas are likely of Schwann cell origin.

  The *target* sign can be seen with either neurofibromas or schwannomas, and reflects central T2 hypointensity thought to be due to a fibrocollagenous core. The *target* sign is suggestive of benignity.

  In contrast to schwannomas, neurofibromas are not encapsulated and involve the entire cross-sectional area of the nerve. If a neurofibroma is resected, the parent nerve must therefore be sacrificed.

- NF1 is associated with multiple brain neoplasms:

  Optic nerve glioma (50% of these tumors are associated with NF1).

  Juvenile pilocytic astrocytoma.

  Brainstem glioma.

- Bone manifestations of NF1 include:

Sphenoid wing dysplasia, which may produce pulsatile enophthalmos or exophthalmos.
Posterior vertebral body scalloping.
Rib notching (*twisted ribbon ribs*) due to erosion from neurofibromas of the intercostal nerves.
Focal gigantism.
Cervical kyphoscoliosis, with a characteristic acute angle.
Neural foraminal enlargement, either due to bony dysplasia or a neurofibroma.
Tibial bowing.

- Eye manifestations of NF1 include hamartomas of the iris, known as Lisch nodules.
- NF1 is also associated with multiple extra-cranial neoplasms:

Wilms tumor.	Angiomyolipoma (renal).
Rhabdomyosarcoma.	Leiomyosarcoma.

Neurofibromatosis 2 (NF2)

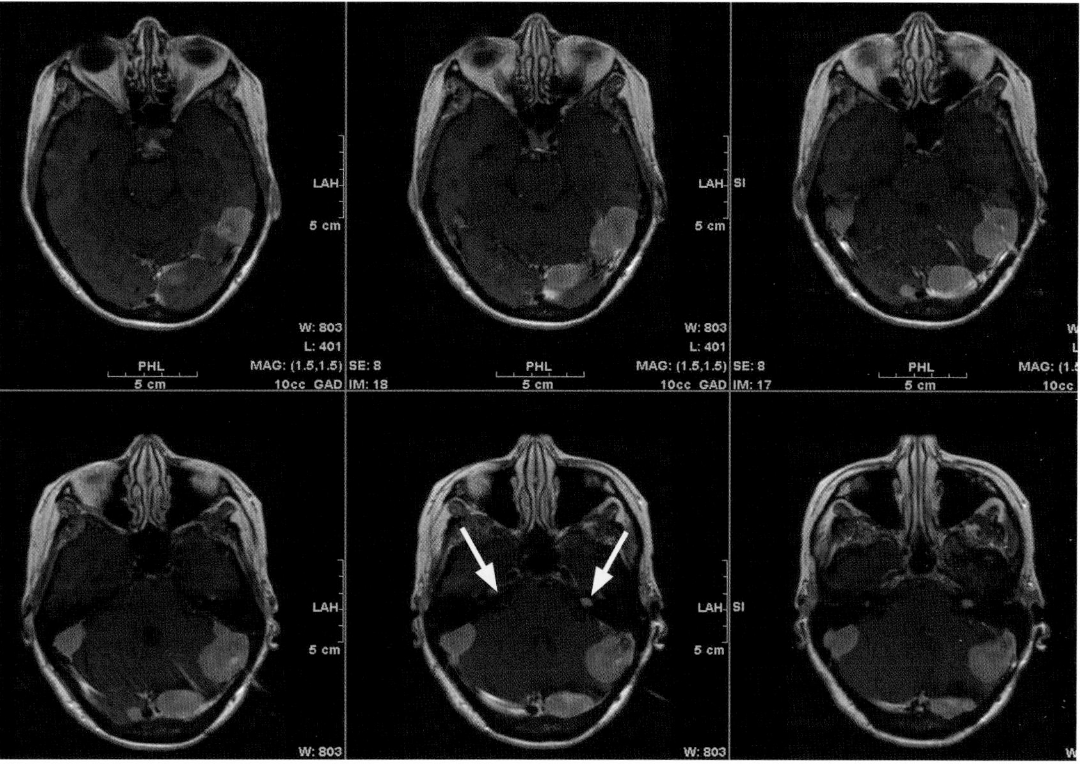

Meningiomatosis and bilateral vestibular schwannomas in neurofibromatosis type 2: Multiple axial post-contrast T1-weighted images show numerous enhancing extra-axial, dural-based masses bilaterally, representing meningiomas. There are bilateral enhancing cranial nerve VIII schwannomas (arrows).

- Neurofibromatosis type 2 (NF2) is an autosomal dominant neurocutaneous disorder completely unrelated to NF1. Despite the name, neurofibromas are not a component of NF2. NF2 is caused by a defect on chromosome 22 and is approximately ten times less common than NF1.
- NF2 is characterized by the **MISME** mnemonic: Multiple Inherited Schwannomas, Meningiomas, and Ependymomas.
- The typical clinical presentation of NF2 is hearing loss caused by bilateral vestibular schwannomas. The presence of bilateral vestibular schwannomas is diagnostic of NF2.

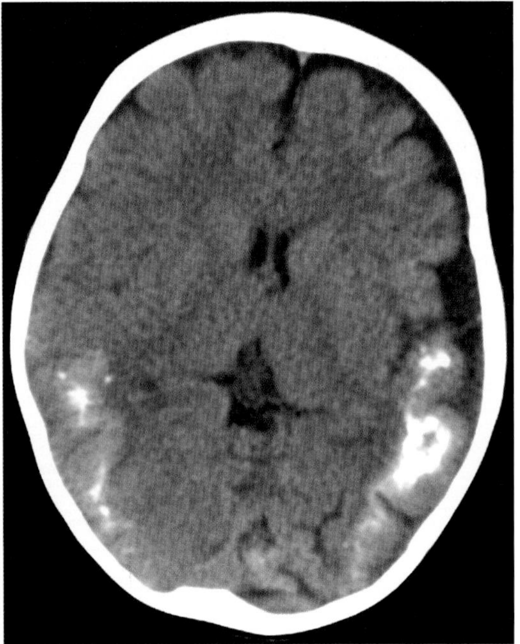

Sturge Weber: Noncontrast CT shows subcortical calcification and cerebral atrophy in a 32-month-old child.

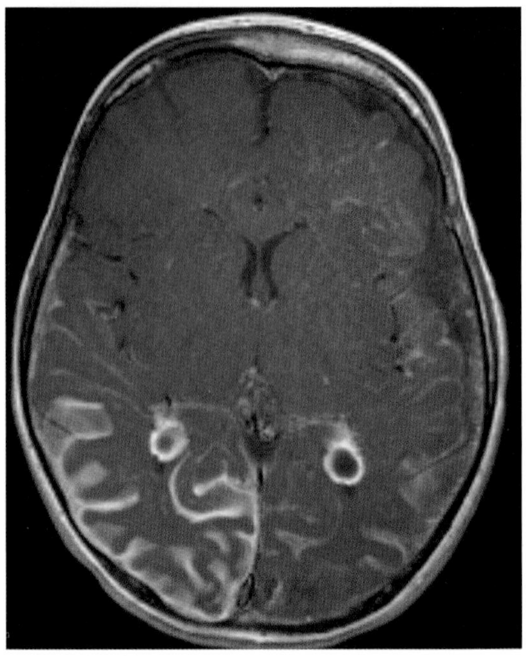

Axial post-contrast T1-weighted MRI of the same patient shows diffuse leptomeningeal enhancement, most prominent in the right occipital lobe, and bilateral choroid plexus engorgement.

Case courtesy Sanjay Prabhu, MBBS, Boston Children's Hospital.

- Sturge Weber is a neurocutaneous disorder characterized by facial port-wine stain (capillary malformation), ocular abnormalities, and failure of normal cortical venous development.

  The port-wine stain typically involves the forehead and upper eyelid, corresponding to the region innervated by the ophthalmic branch of the trigeminal nerve (V^1).

- Sturge Weber is a **vascular** disorder, thought to be caused by failure of regression of the primitive embryologic cephalic venous plexus. This developmental anomaly results in the formation of leptomeningeal venous angiomatosis, which is a vascular malformation characterized by dilated capillaries and venules.
- The underlying vascular anomaly ultimately leads to chronic ischemia, cortical atrophy, and cortical calcification.
- Clinically, patients may have some degree of developmental delay and seizures; however, up to 50% of patients may have normal intelligence. Seizures and developmental delay tend to occur together.
- Characteristic imaging findings are cortical atrophy and subcortical parenchymal calcifications, which are best seen on CT. Contrast-enhanced MRI demonstrates pial enhancement in regions affected by the leptomeningeal venous angiomatosis. The choroid plexi are typically enlarged from compensatory hypertrophy thought to be related to increased flow.

Tuberous sclerosis

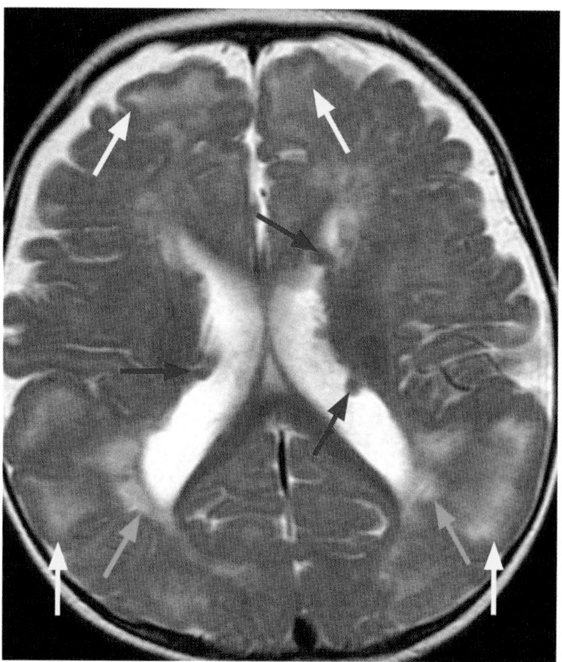

Axial T2-weighted MRI shows numerous bilateral T2 hyperintense cortical tubers (yellow arrows), subcortical tubers (blue arrows), and subependymal nodules (red arrows).

Case courtesy Sanjay Prabhu, MBBS, Boston Children's Hospital.

- Tuberous sclerosis is a hamartomatous disorder affecting several organ systems, with multiple skin manifestations.
- The classical clinical triad of adenoma sebaceum (nodular rash originating in the nasolabial folds), seizures, and mental retardation is not always present.
- Clinically, most patients have epilepsy, neurocognitive dysfunction, and pervasive developmental disorders.
- Neuroimaging features multiple T2 hyperintense white matter cortical or subcortical tubers (hamartomas) and subependymal nodules.
- 15% of patients develop subependymal giant cell astrocytoma (SEGA), which may appear on imaging as a newly enhancing or enlarging subependymal nodule.
- Extracranial manifestations include:

> Renal: Multiple angiomyolipomas.
> Cardiac: Rhabdomyoma.
> Lung: Lymphangioleiomyomatosis.

Midbrain malformations

Joubert and related syndrome

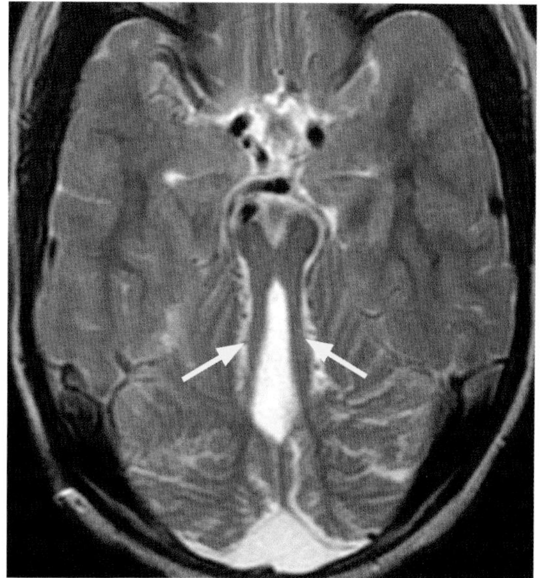

Axial T2-weighted MRI shows a characteristic "molar tooth" configuration of the midbrain (arrows) in a patient with Joubert syndrome. This patient also had a small posterior fossa cyst.

- A "molar tooth" configuration of the midbrain can be seen in several diseases, including Joubert syndrome and related disorders (JSRD).
- JSRD clinically present as a hypotonic child with developmental delay and ataxia. These disorders are often associated with ocular anomalies.
- The primary abnormality of Joubert syndrome is thought to be aplasia or hypoplasia of the cerebellar vermis. Dysplastic cerebellar tissue is often present.
- Unlike Dandy Walker complex, hydrocephalus and a large posterior fossa cyst are uncommon.

Brain tumors

- Brain tumors are discussed in the neuroimaging section.

References, resources, and further reading

General References:

Blickman, J.G., Parker, B.R., & Barnes, P.D. Pediatric Radiology - The Requisites (3rd ed.). Mosby. (2009).

Daldrup-Link, H.E. & Gooding, C.A. Essentials of Pediatric Radiology. Cambridge University Press. (2010).

Donnelly, L. Fundamentals of Pediatric Radiology. Saunders. (2008).

http://pediatricradiology.clevelandclinic.org

Pediatric Airway:

Goodman, T.R. & McHugh, K. The role of radiology in the evaluation of stridor. Archives of Disease in Childhood 81, 456-9(1999).

John, D. Stridor Airway Infants and Upper Obstruction. RadioGraphics, 12, 625-43(1992).

Kussman, B.D., Geva, T. & McGowan, F.X. Cardiovascular causes of airway compression. Paediatric Anaesthesia 14, 60-74(2004).

Pediatric Chest:

Barnes, N.A. & Pilling, D.W. Bronchopulmonary foregut malformations: embryology, radiology and quandary. European Radiology 13, 2659-73(2003).

Gibson, A.T., Steiner, G.M. & Children, S. Review: Imaging the Neonatal Chest. Hernia 172-86(1997).

Hermansen, C.L. & Lorah, K.N. Respiratory distress in the newborn. American Family Physician 76, 987-94(2007).

Kurland, G. & Michelson, P. Bronchiolitis obliterans in children. Pediatric Pulmonology 39, 193-208(2005).

Lobo, L. The neonatal chest. European Journal of Radiology 60, 152-8(2006).

Moonnumakal, S.P. & Fan, L.L. Bronchiolitis obliterans in children. Current Opinion in Pediatrics 20, 272-8(2008).

Visscher, D.W. & Myers, J.L. Bronchiolitis: the pathologist's perspective. Proceedings of the American Thoracic Society 3, 41-7(2006).

Williams, H.J. & Johnson, K.J. Imaging of congenital cystic lung lesions. Pediatric Respiratory Review 3, 120-7(2002).

Zorc, J.J. & Hall, C.B. Bronchiolitis: recent evidence on diagnosis and management. Pediatrics 125, 342-9(2010).

Pediatric Cardiac:

Fayad, L.M. & Boxt, L.M. Chest film diagnosis of congenital heart disease. Seminars in Roentgenology 34, 228-48(1999).

Gaca, A.M. et al. Repair of congenital heart disease: a primer – part 1. Radiology 247, 617-31(2008).

Gaca, A.M. et al. Repair of congenital heart disease: a primer – Part 2. Radiology 248, 44-60(2008).

Strife, J.L. & Sze, R.W. Radiographic evaluation of the neonate with congenital heart disease. Radiologic Clinics of North America 37, 1093-107, vi(1999).

Tonkin, I.L. Imaging of pediatric congenital heart disease. Journal of Thoracic Imaging 15, 274-9(2000).

Wolfson, B. Radiologic interpretation of congenital heart disease. Clinics in Perinatology 28, 1-16(2010).

Pediatric Gastrointestinal:

Applegate, K.E. Evidence-based diagnosis of malrotation and volvulus. Pediatric Radiology 39, 161-3(2009).

Etensel, B. et al. Atresia of the colon. Journal of Pediatric Surgery 40, 1258-68(2005).

Gosche, J.R. et al. Midgut Abnormalities. Surgical Clinics of North America 86, 285-99(2006).

Haddad, M.C. et al. The gamut of abdominal and pelvic cystic masses in children. European Radiology 11, 148-66(2001).

Hartley, J.L., Davenport, M. & Kelly, D.A. Biliary atresia. The Lancet 374, 1704-13(2009).

Isaacs, H. Fetal and neonatal hepatic tumors. Journal of Pediatric Surgery 42, 1797-803(2007).

Lampl, B. et al. Malrotation and midgut volvulus: a historical review and current controversies in diagnosis and management. Pediatric Radiology 359-66(2009).

Panteli, C. New insights into the pathogenesis of infantile pyloric stenosis. Pediatric Surgery International 1043-52(2009).

Vonschweinitz, D. Neonatal liver tumours. Seminars in Neonatology 8, 403-10(2003).

Wootton-Gorges, S.L. et al. Giant cystic abdominal masses in children. Pediatric Radiology 35, 1277-88(2005).

Yousefzadeh, D.K. The position of the duodenojejunal junction: the wrong horse to bet on in diagnosing or excluding malrotation. Pediatric Radiology 39, 172-7(2009).

Pediatric Genitourinary:

Fernbach, S.K., Feinstein, K.A. & Schmidt, M.B. Cystourethrography: A Pictorial Guide 1. RadioGraphics 20, 155-68(2000).

Huang, E. Wilms' tumor and horseshoe kidneys: a case report and review of the literature. Journal of Pediatric Surgery 39, 207-12(2004).

Lee, E.Y. CT imaging of mass-like renal lesions in children. Pediatric Radiology 37, 896-907(2007).

Lopatina, O.A., Berry, T.T. & Spottswood, S.E. Giant prostatic utricle (utriculus masculinis): diagnostic imaging and surgical implications. Pediatric Radiology 34, 156-9(2004).

McLean, T.W. & Buckley, K.S. Pediatric genitourinary tumors. Current Opinion in Oncology 22, 268-73(2010).

Sethi, A. et al. Best Cases from the AFIP: Wilms Tumor in the Setting of Bilateral Nephro blastomatosis. Radiographics 30, 1421-25(2010).

Uetani, N. & Bouchard, M. Plumbing in the embryo: developmental defects of the urinary tracts. Clinical Genetics 75, 307-17(2009).

Pediatric Musculoskeletal:

Bohndorf, K. Infection of the appendicular skeleton. European Radiology 53-63(2004).

Carson, S. et al. Pediatric Upper Extremity Injuries. Pediatric Clinics of North America 53, 41– 67(2006).

Cassart, M. Suspected fetal skeletal malformations or bone diseases: how to explore. Pediatric Radiology 1046-51(2010).

Del Fattore, A., Capannolo, M. & Rucci, N. Bone and bone marrow: the same organ. Archives of Biochemistry and Biophysics 503, 28-34(2010).

Khanna, G., Sato, T.S.P. & Ferguson, P. Imaging of chronic recurrent multifocal osteomyelitis. Radiographics 29, 1159-77(2009).

Legeai-Mallet, L. Hereditary multiple exostoses and enchondromatosis. Best Practice & Research Clinical Rheumatology 22, 45-54(2008).

Maheshwari, A.V. & Cheng, E.Y. Ewing sarcoma family of tumors. Journal of the American Academy of Orthopedic Surgeons 18, 94-107(2010).

Oestreich, A.E. Systematic evaluation of bone dysplasias by the paediatric radiologist. Pediatric Radiology 40, 975-7(2010).

Perry, D.C. & Bruce, C. Evaluating the child who presents with an acute limp. Children 341, 444-9(2010).

Schmit, P., Hugo, V. & Glorion, C. Osteomyelitis in infants and children. European Radiology 44-54(2004).

Silve, C. & Jüppner, H. Ollier disease. Orphanet Journal of Rare Diseases 6, 1-6(2006).

Pediatric Neuroimaging:

Barkovich, A.J. Current concepts of polymicrogyria. Neuroradiology 52, 479-87(2010).

Baselga, E. Sturge-Weber syndrome. Seminars in Cutaneous Medicine and Surgery 23, 87-98(2004).

Colombo, N. et al. Imaging of malformations of cortical development. Epileptic disorders: international epilepsy journal with videotape 11, 194-205(2009).

Comi, A. Pathophysiology of Sturge-Weber Syndrome. Journal of Child Neurology 18, 509-16(2003).

Fernández, A.A. et al. Malformations of the craniocervical junction (Chiari type I and syringomyelia: classification, diagnosis and treatment). BMC Musculoskeletal Disorders 10, S(2009).

Guerrini, R. & Parrini, E. Neuronal migration disorders. Neurobiology of Disease 38, 154-66(2010).

Hahn, J.S. & Barnes, P.D. Neuroimaging advances in holoprosencephaly: Refining the spectrum of the midline malformation. American Journal of Medical Genetics. Part C, Seminars in medical genetics 154C, 120-32(2010).

Stevenson, K.L. Chiari Type II malformation: past, present, and future. Neurosurgical Focus 16, E5(2004).

Tubbs, R.S. et al. The pediatric Chiari I malformation: a review. Child's Nervous System 23, 1239-50(2007).

12 Physics of imaging

Contents

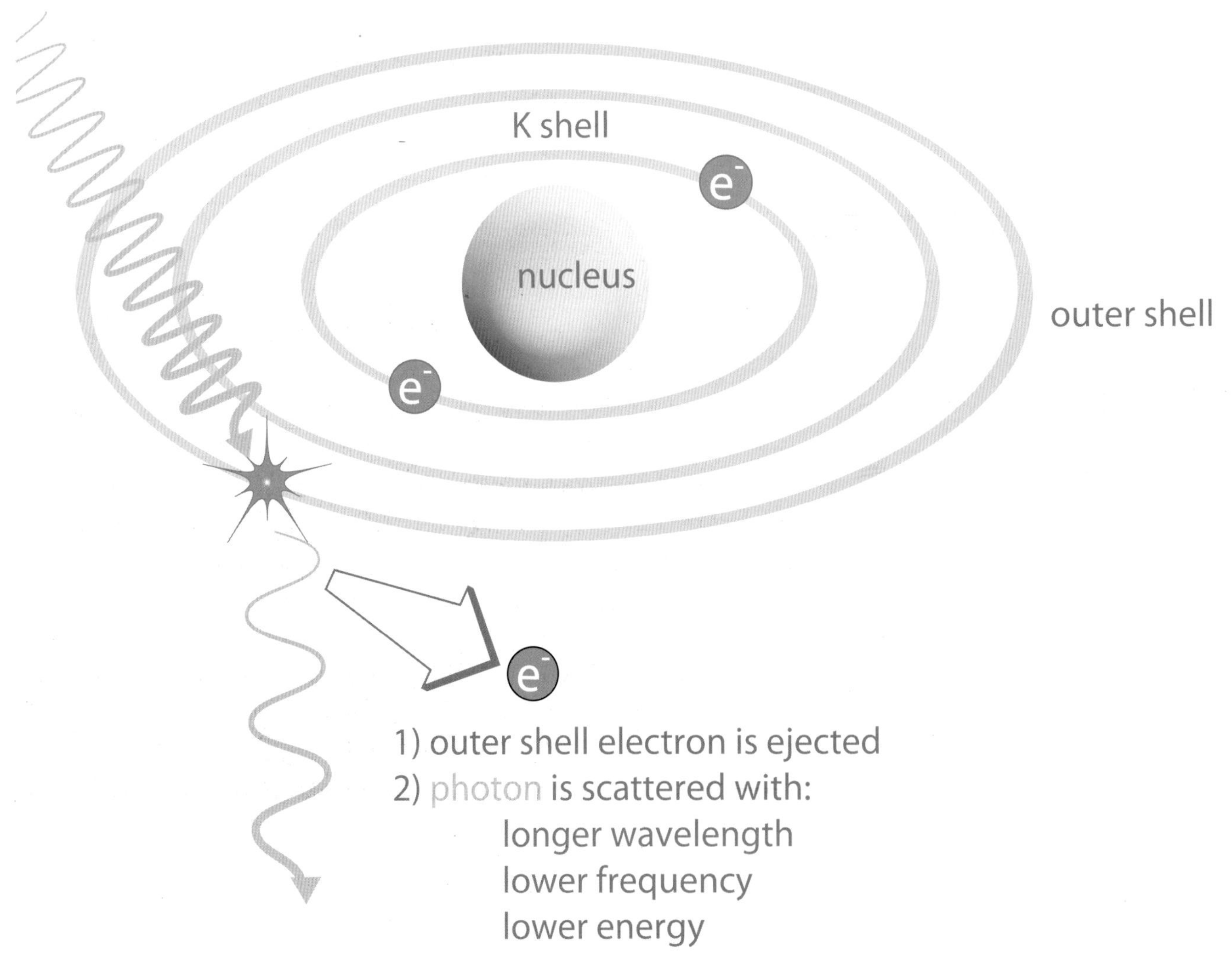

Treatment of Contrast Media Reaction

non-allergic-type acute contrast reactions

mild to moderate non-allergic-type

Hypotension and bradycardia (vasovagal)

1. ECG, pulse oximetry, blood pressure
2. Oxygen via facemask
3. Elevate legs or Trendelenburg
4. Administer IV fluids
5. If poorly responsive, atropine 0.6–1 mg IV
   May repeat up to 0.04 mg/kg (2.8 mg for 70 kg)
6. Call for assistance (at any point)

moderate to severe non-allergic-type

Bronchospasm

1. ECG, pulse oximetry, blood pressure
2. Oxygen via facemask
3. Beta-agonist inhalers
4. If poorly responsive:
   Epinephrine IM 1:1,000, 0.1–0.3 ml (0.1–0.3 mg)
   or
   Epinephrine IV 1:10,000, 1–3 ml (0.1–0.3 mg)
   May repeat up to 1 mg
5. Call for assistance (at any point)

moderate to severe non-allergic-type

Pulmonary edema

1. ECG, pulse oximetry, blood pressure
2. Oxygen via facemask
3. Elevate torso
4. Furosemide 20–40 mg IV
5. Call for assistance (at any point)

moderate to severe non-allergic-type

Seizures

1. ECG, pulse oximetry, blood pressure
2. Oxygen via facemask
3. Consider diazepam 5 mg IV
   or
   midazolam 0.5–1 mg IV
4. Continue to monitor vitals and pulse oximetry
5. Call for assistance (at any point)

allergic-type acute contrast reactions

mild to moderate allergic-type

Urticaria (hives)

1. Discontinue injection if not completed
2. If mild, no treatment
3. If moderate, diphenhydramine PO/IV 25–50 mg
4. If severe:
   Epinephrine IM 1:1,000, 0.1–0.3 ml (0.1–0.3 mg)
5. Call for assistance (at any point)

moderate to severe allergic-type

Facial or laryngeal edema

1. ECG, pulse oximetry, blood pressure
2. Oxygen via facemask
3. Epinephrine IM 1:1,000, 0.1–0.3 ml (0.1–0.3 mg)
   or
   Epinephrine IV 1:10,000, 1–3 ml (0.1–0.3 mg)
   May repeat up to 1 mg
4. Call for assistance (at any point)

severe allergic-type

Hypotension and tachycardia (anaphylaxis)

1. ECG, pulse oximetry, blood pressure
2. Oxygen via facemask
3. Elevate legs or place Trendelenburg
4. IV fluids rapid bolus
5. If poorly responsive:
   Epinephrine IV 1:10,000, 1 ml (0.1 mg)
   May repeat up to 1 mg
6. Call for assistance (at any point)

Iodinated contrast

Iodinated contrast media reaction

Contrast media reaction overview

- Acute reactions to intravenous contrast can be divided into allergic-type and non-allergic-type mechanisms. Both allergic-type and non-allergic-type reactions can range in severity from mild and self-limited to severe and life-threatening.
- Patients with asthma are at increased risk of an allergic reaction to contrast medium.
- A seafood or shellfish allergy is not associated with allergic reaction to contrast.
- Mild nausea, sensation of warmth, and flushing are considered physiologic and are not adverse reactions to contrast.

Mild contrast reactions

- A mild contrast reaction is self-limited and does not require medical management.
- A vasovagal reaction to intravenous contrast is rare and is characterized by bradycardia and hypotension. Mild vasovagal reactions are usually self-limited and are not allergic in etiology.
- Urticarial reactions are mild allergic-type reactions, and include hives and mild angioedema. The symptoms of mild angioedema include scratchy throat, slight tongue or facial swelling, and sneezing, and generally do not require medical management.

Moderate contrast reactions

- Moderate contrast reactions are not immediately life-threatening but may require medical management.
- Moderate allergic-type reactions include severe urticaria, bronchospasm, moderate tongue/facial swelling, and transient hypotension with tachycardia.
- Moderate non-allergic-type reactions include significant vasovagal reaction, pulmonary edema, bronchospasm, and limited seizure.

Severe contrast reactions

- Severe reactions to intravenous iodinated contrast may be immediately life-threatening.
- Allergic-type severe reactions include anaphylaxis and angioedema. Symptoms may be varied and include altered mental status, respiratory distress, diffuse erythema, severe hypotension, or cardiac arrest.
- Non-allergic-type severe reactions include severe pulmonary edema, severe bronchospasm, and severe seizure.

Premedication to prevent contrast reaction

- In a patient with a known contrast allergy, a repeat contrast reaction is most likely to be similar to the prior reaction. However, the repeat reaction may be either more or less severe. Therefore, if IV contrast is necessary for a patient who has had a previous reaction, a premedication regimen is recommended, although contrast reactions may occur despite premedication. Intravenous contrast is generally contraindicated in patients who have had a prior severe allergic-type reaction.
- **Elective premedication**: Prednisone 50 mg PO at 13 hours, 7 hours, and 1 hour before the exam, plus diphenhydramine 50 mg (IV or PO) 1 hour before.
- Emergent premedication: Hydrocortisone 200 mg IV Q4h, 1–2 times prior to administration of IV contrast. Diphenhydramine is given 1 hour prior. Note that IV steroids have *not* been shown to be effective when given sooner than 4 hours before the contrast administration.

CONTRAST-INDUCED NEPHROPATHY (CIN)

Risk of contrast-induced nephropathy (CIN)

- Contrast-induced nephropathy (CIN) is a decrease in renal function of unknown etiology following the intravascular (venous or arterial) administration of iodinated contrast.
- The most important risk factor for development of CIN is preexisting renal insufficiency.
- For patients with eGFR <30 ml/min/1.73m^2, the risk of CIN is between 7.8 and 12.1%.
- For patients with eGFR >30 and <45, the risk of CIN is between 2.9 and 9.8%.
- For patients with eGFR >45 and <60, the risk of CIN is between 0 and 2.5%.
- The development of CIN in patients with normal renal function (eGFR >60 ml/min/1.73m^2) is exceptionally rare.
- Note that gadolinium-based contrast media are not known to cause contrast-induced nephropathy.
- Patients with multiple myeloma are at increased risk of irreversible renal failure after receiving high-osmolality contrast media from tubular protein precipitation. There are no data on the risk of the low or iso-osmolar contrast agents in current use.

Prevention of contrast nephropathy

- The main preventative strategies against CIN are to use the minimal dose of contrast possible and to adequately hydrate the patient. The use of sodium bicarbonate and N-acetylcysteine has been previously advocated but the effectiveness of these agents has not been proven.
- Patients with an eGFR >30 and <60 typically receive approximately 2/3 the standard contrast dose. Administration of intravenous contrast to a patient with an eGFR <30 would require a careful assessment of risks and benefits on a case by case basis.
- The standard dose of intravenous iodinated contrast can generally be given to patients on dialysis. Careful attention should be paid to the volume status in these patients as theoretically the osmotic load increases intravascular volume.

IODINATED CT CONTRAST: GENERAL CONSIDERATIONS

Iodinated contrast and pheochromocytoma

- It is safe to administer nonionic contrast media to patients with pheochromocytoma. Prior studies showed an increased in serum catecholamines after high-osmolality contrast agents, which are no longer in current use.

Iodinated contrast and thyroid uptake

- Thyroid gland uptake of I-131 is reduced to about 50% one week after iodinated contrast injection. Therefore, if radioactive I-131 therapy is planned, iodinated contrast should be avoided for a few weeks prior to I-131 therapy.

Metformin and intravenous contrast

- Metformin is an oral anti-hyperglycemic agent that decreases hepatic glucose production and increases peripheral glucose uptake. Although exceptionally rare, there is an increased risk of metformin-associated lactic acidosis in patients receiving intravenous iodinated contrast, thought to be due to CIN and the resultant accumulation of metformin.
- There is no need to discontinue metformin in patients with normal renal function. In patients with multiple comorbidities, metformin should be discontinued at time of contrast administration and withheld for 48 hours.
- Note that it is not necessary to discontinue metformin prior to gadolinium-based contrast.

Iodinated contrast and pregnancy

- Iodinated contrast crosses the placenta and enters the fetal circulation. No mutagenic or teratogenic effects have been observed; however, no controlled studies in pregnant patients have been performed.
- It is acceptable to administer iodinated contrast to a pregnant patient if medically necessary. It is recommended that a pregnant patient sign an informed consent form prior to undergoing an examination involving ionizing radiation and iodinated contrast.

Iodinated contrast and breast feeding

- The plasma half-life of iodinated contrast is approximately 2 hours. Less than 1% of the administered maternal dose of iodinated contrast is excreted in the breast milk within 24 hours of maternal administration, and 1% of that dose may be absorbed by the infant's gastrointestinal tract. The total infant absorbed dose is therefore approximately 0.01% of the administered maternal dose.
- Breast feeding mothers do not need to halt breast feeding. If the mother is concerned, abstaining from breast feeding for 24 hours (while pumping and discarding milk) would result in effectively zero fetal dose.

Contrast extravasation

- Extravasation is the leakage of contrast into the soft tissues at the injection site. Although the risk of extravasation is not related to the injection flow rate, the use of automatic injectors can lead to a large extravasated volume of contrast media.
- Iodinated contrast is toxic to the soft tissues and skin, although serious adverse events are relatively rare following extravasation. The most common serious injury due to contrast extravasation is compartment syndrome. Less commonly, skin ulceration and tissue necrosis can occur.
- All patients with extravasation should be evaluated by the radiologist. Elevation of the extremity to decrease capillary hydrostatic pressure has been recommended, but is without supporting data. There is no evidence favoring warm or cold compresses, and both are used commonly.
- Surgical consultation should be obtained for progressive swelling and pain, altered tissue perfusion (decreased capillary refill), change in sensation, or skin ulceration or blistering.

Gadolinium-based contrast

Immediate adverse reactions to gadolinium-based contrast

- Both mild and severe adverse reactions to gadolinium-based contrast are much more rare compared to iodinated contrast. Most adverse reactions to gadolinium-based contrast are mild such as nausea, vomiting, headache, or pain at the injection site.
- Allergic-type reactions to gadolinium are rare, seen in 0.004% to 0.7%
- Serious anaphylactic reactions are exceeding rare (<0.01%).

Contrast extravasation

- Gadolinium-based contrast agents are much less toxic to the skin and soft tissues compared to iodinated contrast.
- Evaluation and treatment of extravasation is similar for both types of contrast.

NEPHROGENIC SYSTEMIC FIBROSIS (NSF)

- Nephrogenic systemic fibrosis (NSF) is a highly morbid disease characterized by diffuse fibrosis of the skin and subcutaneous tissues, which may also involve the visceral organs.
- NSF is strongly associated with gadolinium exposure in patients with reduced renal function. The exact mechanism for development of NSF is unknown, but may involve dissociation of toxic free gadolinium in patients with reduced renal clearance. The free gadolinium may bind phosphate and precipitate in tissues, inducing a fibrotic reaction.
- Patients with end-stage renal disease (eGFR <30 ml/min/1.73m^2) have between 1% and 7% chance of developing NSF even after a single exposure to a gadolinium-containing contrast agent. There has been only one established case of NSF developing in a patient with an eGFR >30.
- In general, gadolinium-based contrast should not be given to patients on renal dialysis or with eGFR <30. Although it is exceedingly rare for NSF to develop in a patient with eGFR between 30 and 59, eGFR may fluctuate daily in these patients. For this reason, caution should be employed for patients on the lower end of this spectrum.
- Different brands and formulations of gadolinium-based contrast are associated with varying rates of NSF.

GADOLINIUM-BASED CONTRAST IN PREGNANCY AND BREAST-FEEDING

Gadolinium-based contrast and pregnancy

- Gadolinium-based contrast should not be administered during pregnancy. Gadolinium-based contrast crosses the placenta. Although never demonstrated to cause harm, gadolinium chelates may accumulate in the amniotic fluid and remain there indefinitely, with risk of dissociation of toxic free gadolinium ion.

Gadolinium-based contrast and breast feeding

- The plasma half-life of gadolinium-based contrast is 2 hours. Less than 0.04% of the administered maternal dose is excreted in the breast milk within 24 hours of maternal administration, and 1% of that dose may be absorbed by the infant's gastrointestinal tract. The total infant absorbed dose of gadolinium is therefore approximately 0.0004% of the administered maternal dose.
- It is likely safe for the mother to continue breast feeding. There is no information to suggest that oral ingestion of such a tiny amount of gadolinium-containing contrast may be harmful to the fetus.

Contrast media reference:

ACR Committee on Drugs and Contrast Media (2012). ACR Manual on Contrast Media Version 8. Retrieved from http://www.acr.org/Quality-Safety/Resources/Contrast-Manual, accessed September 2012.

MEASURING RADIATION

Exposure, air kerma, absorbed dose, equivalent dose, and effective dose

- **Exposure** is the charge of electrons liberated per unit mass of air. Exposure is measured in Coulombs/kg.
- **Air kerma** (kinetic energy released per mass) describes the incident X-ray beam intensity as the kinetic energy transferred from uncharged particles (photons) to charged particles (electrons). Air kerma is measured in Gray (J/kg).
- Air Kerma (Gy) can be converted to **absorbed dose** (also quantified in Gy) by the R factor, which depends on kV and the atomic number (Z) of the absorbing tissue.

  Bone (Z = 12) absorbs much more energy than soft tissue (Z ~ 7.6).

  At 10 mGy air kerma, bone absorbs 40 Gy, tissue absorbs 11 Gy.
- The **equivalent dose** (expressed in Sievert; Sv) is the absorbed dose in Gy multiplied by a radiation weighting factor (W_R).

  W_R depends on the linear energy transfer (LET) of the type of radiation. For diagnostic radiology using X-rays, $W_R = 1$. An alpha particle has a high LET.
- The **effective dose** (also expressed in Sv) is an estimation of radiation exposure that takes into account the equivalent dose to all organs exposed and each organ's radiosensitivity.
  Effective dose = the sum of the absorbed dose (Gy) * W_R * W_T for all organs exposed.

  W_T is the tissue weighting factor, which varies from 0.12 for radiosensitive organs (e.g., bone marrow, colon, lung, breast), to 0.01 for less sensitive organs (e.g., bone, brain, and skin).

Radiation units

- SI (Système International) units including Gray and Sievert are almost universally used rather than the older non-SI units. One notable exception is the Curie, which is still commonly used in nuclear medicine (typical dosing ranges are in millicuries).

SI (Système International) units	Non-SI units
• Gray (Gy) quantifies both absorbed dose and air kerma (exposure) as energy absorbed per unit mass. • 1 Gy = 1 J/kg • 1 Gy = 100 Rad	• 1 Rad (radiation absorbed dose) = 10 mGy
• Sievert (Sv) is used to quantify equivalent dose and effective dose. • 1 Sv = 100 Rem	• 1 Rem = 10 mSv
• A Becquerel (Bq) is only used in nuclear medicine for radioactive materials. • 1 Bq = 1 disintegration per second	• 1 Curie = 37 billion Becquerels = $3.7e^{10}$ disintegrations per second

X-ray generator

- X-ray photons are generated when high-energy electrons hit a target at the anode side of the circuit. For general radiography and CT, the target is made of tungsten (atomic symbol W).
  - 99% of the electrons' kinetic energy is converted to heat, and 1% is converted to X-rays.
- 90% of X-rays are produced from bremsstrahlung (nuclear field interaction).
  - The maximum keV (energy) of the X-ray spectrum is the kV of the generator. The average keV ~ 1/3 max.
- 10% of X-rays are produced from characteristic radiation. A characteristic X-ray is produced when a high energy electron knocks a K-shell electron out of orbit.

energetic electron needs to have
keV > K-shell binding energy
high-energy ***electron*** comes in
high-energy ***photon*** comes out
outer shell
K shell
nucleus
2) outer shell electron fills vacancy
3) characteristic X-ray produced
E = E(K-shell) – E(transition shell)
1) K-shell electron ejected
characteristic x-rays are produced with energies just below K-shell binding energy.
No characteristic X-rays are generated when kV < K-edge

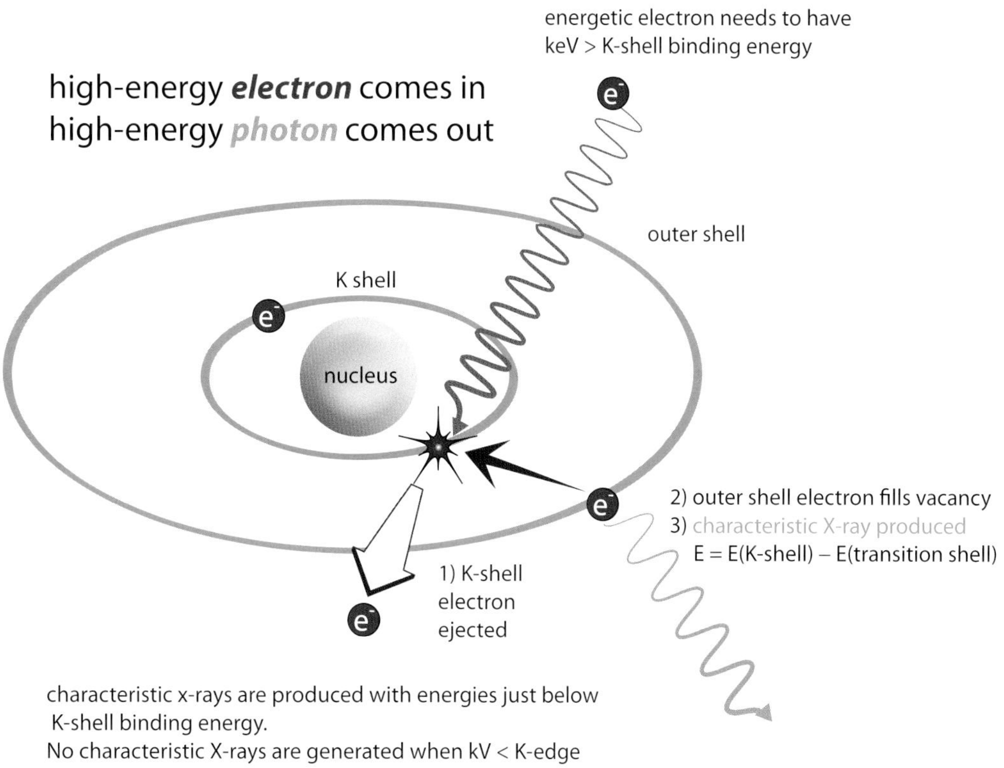

- Tungsten: Atomic weight = 74; K-edge = 70 keV; characteristic X-rays <70 keV.

Effect of kV on tube output

- X-ray production is proportional to $(kV)^2$.
- In practice, changing kV is complicated as a change in kV causes a change in characteristic X-ray, shifts spectrum to the right, and adds photons.
- ↑ kV by 15% → ↑ photons by 100%.
- In general, increasing kV will decrease dose and decrease contrast when automatic exposure control is used.

Heel effect

- The heel effect is due to attenuation at the anode, causing fewer X-rays at the anode side.
- The main contributor to the heel effect is the anode angle (typical anode angle ~15 degrees).
  - ↓ anode angle → ↑ heel effect

X-ray interactions with matter

All of these interactions deal with incoming photons.

- **Coherent scatter**: No exchange of energy, no change in frequency, and no contribution to patient dose. Contributes less than 5% of X-ray interactions.

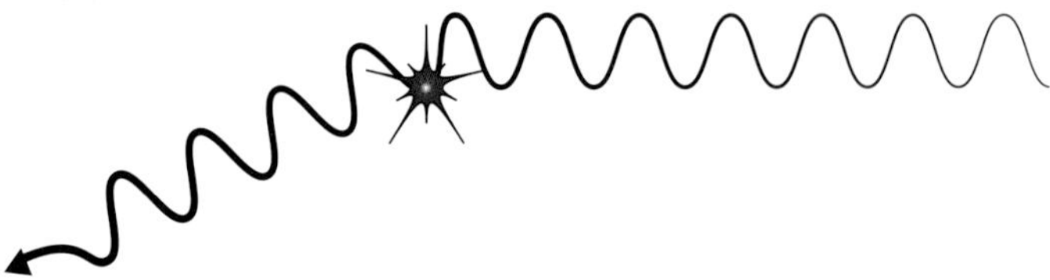

E = energy of incoming photon (keV)

- **Compton scatter**: Proportional to (electron density)/E. Scattered photons go in all directions.

Compton scatter dominates at >25 keV in soft tissue and >40 keV in bone.

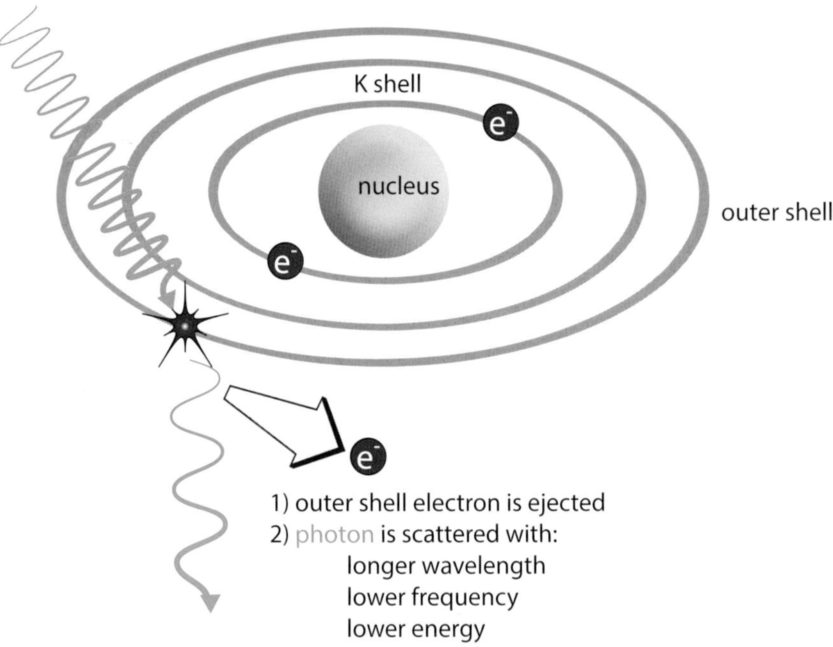
K shell
nucleus
outer shell
1) outer shell electron is ejected
2) photon is scattered with:
longer wavelength
lower frequency
lower energy

Z = electron number

- **Photoelectric effect**: Proportional to Z^3/E^3.

Photoelectric effect dominates at <25 keV in soft tissue and <40 keV in bone.

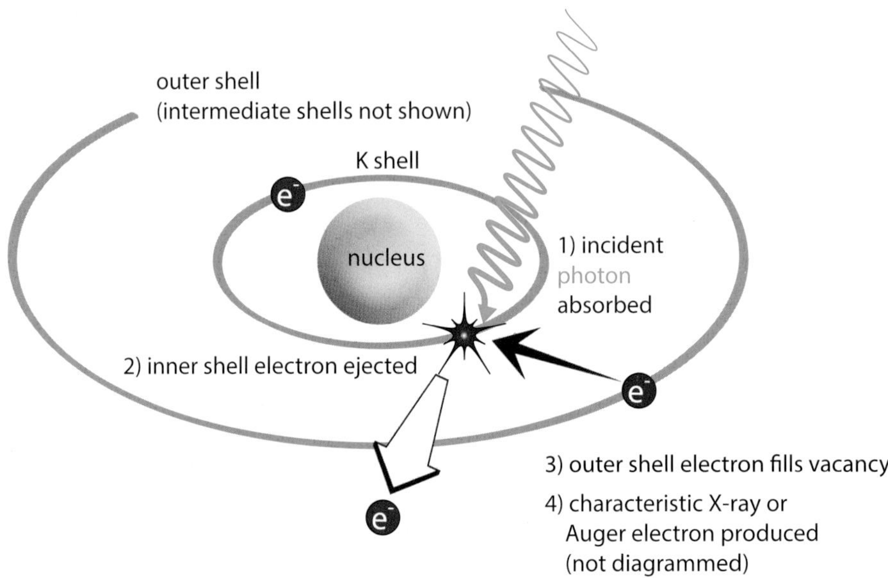
outer shell
(intermediate shells not shown)
K shell
nucleus
1) incident photon absorbed
2) inner shell electron ejected
3) outer shell electron fills vacancy
4) characteristic X-ray or Auger electron produced (not diagrammed)

Energy from the ejected inner shell electron is absorbed locally (energetic electrons don't travel very far); however, a 30 keV electron can cause significant damage via 1,000 ionizations (approximately 30 eV/ionization).

Linear attenuation coefficient

μ (cm^{-1})

- $N = N_0 * e^{-\mu t}$
  fraction transmitted = $e^{-\mu t}$

  N_0 = initial number of photons

  N = transmitted number of photons after thickness **t**

- If μ is "small" (<0.1/cm), then μ is the proportion of photons that interact with matter.

  This is only true for weakly attenuating material.

- If μ is "large" (>0.1/cm), then the formula above is used.

  Example: If μ = 0.5/cm, then $e^{-\mu t}$ = 61% transmitted.

Mass attenuation coefficient

- Mass attenuation coefficient = (μ/ρ), where ρ = density
- Because density is accounted for in the formula above, the mass attenuation coefficient is independent of density.

Scatter and grids

- In radiography, the typical scatter:primary ratio is 5-10:1
- Scatter ↓ contrast
- Grid ratio = height/width

  Typical grid ratios in radiography are between 8 and 12 (the height of the grid is 8–12 times the width between grid elements).

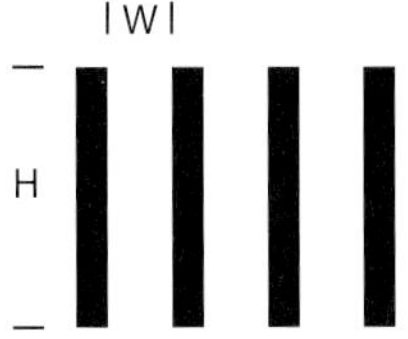

- About 70% of primary radiation passes through the grid.
- Bucky factor is the relative ↑ dose due to grid = incident/transmitted radiation

  The Bucky factor should not be confused with the grid ratio!

  Typical Bucky factor is 5–10 (e.g., ↑ mAs from 40 → 200).

- ↑ kV will ↑ scatter (Compton effects dominate at higher kV).
- Grids not used for extremity radiography (bone is ↑ Z and not very thick).

Beam quality and half value layer (HVL)

- A "high quality" beam has low-energy photons filtered out.
- The half-value layer (HVL) is a measurement of the beam quality and is the thickness of material that attenuates 50% of the incident energy.
- HVL is dependent on photon energy. HVL ↑ with ↑ photon energy.
- Aluminum (Al) is the standard material for measuring HVL.
- Typical HVL for mammography is 0.3 mm Al.
- Typical HVL for radiography is 3 mm Al.

  State regulations require beam quality: HVL >2.5 mm Al at 80 kVp.

- Typical HVL for CT is 8–9 mm Al.

Film optical density (OD) and characteristic curves

- Film optical density (OD) = $\log_{10}(I_0/I_t)$ = $\log_{10}$(incident/transmitted light intensity)

  OD of 1 → 10% photons transmitted through film

  OD of 2 → 1% transmitted

  OD of 3 → 0.1% transmitted
- Film "looks good" if the average OD is ~ 1.5. This occurs after approximately 5 μGy photons hit the film/screen.
- A characteristic curve logarithmically plots the relationship between radiation exposure (air kerma) and film optical density.

  The *toe* is the low-exposure region and the *shoulder* is the high exposure region. *Fog* is the baseline low-level darkening of film that occurs in the absence of radiation exposure.
- Latitude is the range of air kerma with satisfactory film density. A high-latitude film is ideal for imaging body parts with a wide variation of X-ray transmission (e.g., a chest radiograph). A high-contrast (low-latitude) film is ideal for accentuating image contrast in tissues with low subject contrast (e.g., mammography).

- Gamma is steepest part of curve; gradient is average steepness:

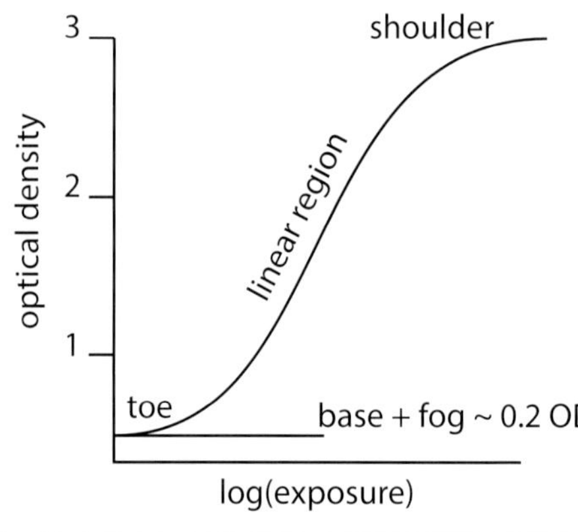

- Effect of latitude on characteristic curve:

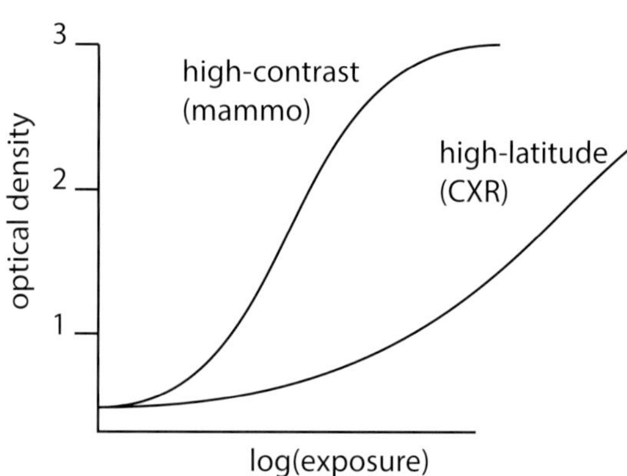

Digital detectors

All except Xe are Solid State detectors.

- **Ionization chamber**: High-pressure Xe (K-edge 35 keV): Used for measuring radiation, not for imaging.
- **Photostimulable phosphor**: Barium fluorohalide (BaFBr); used in computed radiography.

  Read out with red laser light (emits blue light).

  Dynamic range is 10,000:1 (vs. 40:1 for screen-film).

  Can be used with air kerma <0.1 μGy to 1,000 μGy.

CsI and Selenium used without cassette.

- **Scintillator:** Cesium Iodide (CsI); note that CsI also used as input phosphor in an image intensifier.

  Indirect: Absorbed X-rays first converted to light, which is then stored as charge.

  Advantage: K-edge 30-ish, good at absorbing X-rays.

  Disadvantage: Light spreads out → blur
- **Photoconductor**: (Selenium)

  Direct: Absorbed X-rays directly converted to charge.

  Advantage: No light spreading, very sharp.

  Disadvantage: K-edge 13, poor X-ray absorber at standard radiography keV.

  Used in digital mammography.

Contact mammography technique summary	• kV is reduced to ↑ contrast • Focal spot is smaller	• 25 kV; 100 mA (HVL 0.3 mm Al) • 0.3 mm focal spot standard 100 mA tube current • 0.1 mm magnification focal spot 25 mA tube current
	• ↑ ↑ photons deposited on detector, resulting in lower noise	• 200 µGy (vs. 5 µGy for standard radiography)
	• ↑ exposure • ↑ mAs	• 1 s vs. 50 ms for abdominal X-ray • 100 mAs vs. ~20 mAs (abdominal radiograph)
	• Grid ratio smaller	• 5:1 (PE > Compton, less scatter) Bucky factor ~2
	• Film gradient ↑ • Higher luminance viewboxes • Single-emulsion films used • Heel effect taken advantage of	• 3 vs. 2 • 3,000 cd/m^2 is ACR requirement • Cathode side directed to chest wall
Compared to traditional radiography, mammography image quality improved by several factors	• Contrast increased by: ↓ kV, breast compression, ↑ gamma film • Resolution improved by: Single thin screen, small focal spot, compression • Noise (mottle) reduced by: ↑ photons at image receptor (200 µGy vs. 5 µGy for screen-film)	
Mammography X-ray generator and filters	• Molybdenum (Mo) target (K-edge 20 keV) generates characteristic X-rays at 17 and 19 keV. • Mo filter ↓ ↓ low-energy X-rays (which do not contribute to imaging but add to radiation exposure) and ↓ high frequency X-rays (which ↓ contrast). Mo filter lets characteristic X-rays through. • Average energy generated ~ 17 keV (typical rule that average energy ~1/3 to 1/2 max doesn't apply since characteristic X-rays are so much more important). • Rhodium (Rh) filter shifts spectrum to the right, used for thicker/denser breasts. • Rh target/Rh filter used in conjunction for even thicker breasts.	
Breast compression	• Advantages of breast compression: ↑ X-ray penetration ↑ density uniformity ↓ scatter ↓ dose ↓ tissue overlap ↓ focal spot blur	• Disadvantages of compression: May be uncomfortable

Digital mammography

- Pixel size ~80 µm; smallest visible microcalcifications ~ 150 µm
- Resolution ~ 3,000 × 4,000 pixels = 24 MB at 2 byte/pixel
- 5 megapixel monitors needed for viewing

Magnification Mammography

- Magnification = SID/SOD

  SID = source–image distance

  SOD = source–receptor distance

- SID typically 65 cm, SOD typically 35 cm

  In the example below, SID = 65 cm, SOD = 35 cm, and magnification = 65/35 = 1.85

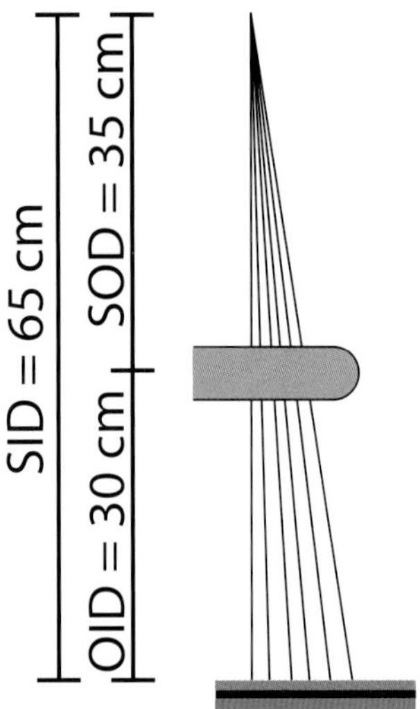

OID = Object–image distance

- If ↑ SID (X-ray tube moved away) then exposure time will be too long.
- If ↓ SID (X-ray tube moved closer) then there will be too much focal spot blur.
- No grid needed (air gap introduced).
- 0.1 mm focal spot used.
- Magnification mammography technique summary:

  25 mA current

  3 second exposure

  70 mAs. Because a grid is not employed, a lower total mAs is needed (compared to 100 mAs with contact mammography using a grid.

MQSA

- The interpreting physician needs to have read 960 mammograms in the prior 24 months.
- A quality control program must be in place.
- Phantom must be tested weekly with an average glandular dose <3 mGy.

Average glandular dose (AGD)

- Federal requirement that AGD <3 mGy per view per breast.

  Note that the fluoroscopic dose limit of 100 or 200 mGy/minute is the only other federal dose regulation.

- A typical AGD is ~ 1.8–1.5 mGy per view per breast (digital slightly lower dose).

Fluoroscopy physics

Electronic magnification

- If field of view (FOV) is ↓ by a factor of two (e.g., from 10 cm to 5 cm), the reduced field of view is projected onto the entire output phosphor of the image intensifier, which will be 4 times dimmer. Therefore, skin exposure will be increased by a factor of 4 by the automatic exposure control.
- Similarly, reducing the exposed area from 10 cm to 7 cm would increase patient entrance air kerma by a factor of two.

Fluoro technique

- Continuous fluoro runs at current of 1 to 5 mA (typically 3 mA), resulting in a very low air kerma/frame of approximately ~0.01 μGy. Compared to a standard chest X-ray exposure of 5 μGy, each fluoro frame has 500 times fewer incident photons.
- There is a federal regulatory limit of 100 mGy/min entrance air kerma.

  High-dose fluoro with audible/visual alarms allows 200 mGy/min for large patients.

Effects of fluoroscopy techniques on dose

- Increasing source to skin distance decreases dose due to inverse-square law.
- Increasing filtration reduces dose by removing low-energy X-rays that would be absorbed.
- Removing grid reduces dose (used in peds), at the risk of increasing scatter.
- Dose spreading (moving the beam around) reduces the maximum skin dose.

  Skin dose rate is about 10–30 mGy/min for continuous fluoroscopy.

  Maximum exposure rate 100 mGy/min or 200 mGy/min in high-level mode.

  At maximum permissible rate in high-level mode, 2 Gy can be delivered in 10 min!

  Large patients are more susceptible to skin injury.
- Magnification *increases* dose, as discussed above.

CT physics

Overview of CT

- Computed tomography (CT) produces images by rotating a fan beam around the patient and determining the linear attenuation coefficients of each individual pixel using a reconstruction algorithm.

Hounsfield units (HU)

- A Hounsfield unit is a measure of relative CT attenuation.

$$HU = 1{,}000 \left(\frac{\mu_x - \mu_{water}}{\mu_{water}} \right)$$

  μ_x = attenuation coefficient of the material being measuring

  μ_{water} = attenuation coefficient of water
- 10 HU = 1% difference in contrast.
- Gray matter and white matter differ in contrast by only 0.5%.
- A material with twice the attenuation of water attenuates 1,000 HU.

RADIATION DOSIMETRY

CT dosimetry

- The computed tomography dose index (CTDI) is the average phantom dose for a single axial slice (one complete rotation without table motion), including scatter, measured in Gy.

  CTDI is measured with 16 cm and 32 cm phantoms. 16 cm will always have higher dose.

- $CTDI_w$ (weighted) = 2/3 $CTDI_p$ + 1/3 $CTDI_c$

  $CTDI_p$ = peripheral

  $CTDI_c$ = central

- $CTDI_{vol} = CTDI_w/\text{pitch}$

  The pitch is related to the table speed. A pitch <1 will overscan and result in increased radiation exposure; conversely, a pitch >1 will skip areas but will decrease exposure.

  $CTDI_{vol}$ is the same for all scans, independent of scan length.

  $CTDI_{vol}$ should be less than reference values:

  - Adult head: 75 mGy (16 cm phantom)
  - Adult abdomen: 25 mGy (32 cm phantom)
  - Pediatric abdomen: 20 mGy (16 cm phantom)

Dose length product (DLP) and effective doses

- The dose length product (DLP) is the best way to estimate radiation risk from CT.
- DLP = $CTDI_{vol}$ * scan length = mGy*cm
- One can obtain an effective dose in mSv from the DLP by using body-part specific conversion factors:

Head	0.0023 mSv/mGy cm
Neck	0.0054
Chest	0.019
Abd	0.017
Pelvis	0.017
Legs	0.0008

- Example conversion: If DLP is 900 mGy*cm for an abdominal CT, the radiation exposure equals (900 mGy*cm) * (0.017 mSv/mGy cm) = 15.4 mSv.

Typical effective doses (mSv) of common diagnostic exams

- Radiography:
  - PA and lateral chest radiograph: 0.1 mSv
  - Cervical spine radiograph: 0.2 mSv
  - Lumbar spine radiograph: 1.5 mSv
  - Abdomen radiograph: 0.7 mSv
  - Pelvic radiograph: 0.6 mSv
  - Mammography: 0.4 mSv
  - Knee radiograph: 0.005 mSv
- Fluoroscopy:
  - Upper GI series: 6 mSv
  - Barium enema: 8 mSv
- Interventional radiology:
  - Cerebral angiography: 1–10 mSv
  - Peripheral angiography: 5 mSv
  - Cardiac cath (diagnostic): 7 mSv
  - TIPS: 100 mSv
- CT:
  - Head CT: 2 mSv
  - Neck CT: 3 mSv
  - Chest CT: 7 mSv
  - Abdomen CT: 8 mSv
  - Pelvis: 6 mSv

IMAGE QUALITY

Contrast

- The most important factor for optimizing contrast is to increase the number of photons that reach the film (film density).
- ↓ scatter → ↑ contrast
- Collimation ↓ scatter and ↓ dose

  Collimation is the rare example of something that ↑ image quality and ↓ dose
- ↑ kV → ↓ contrast with automatic exposure control
- In screen film, contrast is related to screen latitude/gradient.

Resolution and blur

- Only three factors influence blur (resolution), none of which affects image contrast:

  1) Focal spot blur.

  2) Motion blur, which is related to exposure time.

  3) Receptor blur, which is related to intensifying screen thickness. Faster screens ↑ blur.

STATISTICS

Sensitivity, specificity, positive predictive value, and negative predictive value

- Sensitivity = TP/(TP + FN)
- Specificity = TN/(TN + FP)
- Positive predictive value (PPV) = TP/(TP + FP)
- Negative predictive value (NPV) = TN/(TN + FN)

- TP = true positive
- TN = true negative
- FP = false positive
- FN = false negative

ROC curve

- A receiver operator characteristic (ROC) curve compares the diagnostic performance of a test at various thresholds of decision confidence.

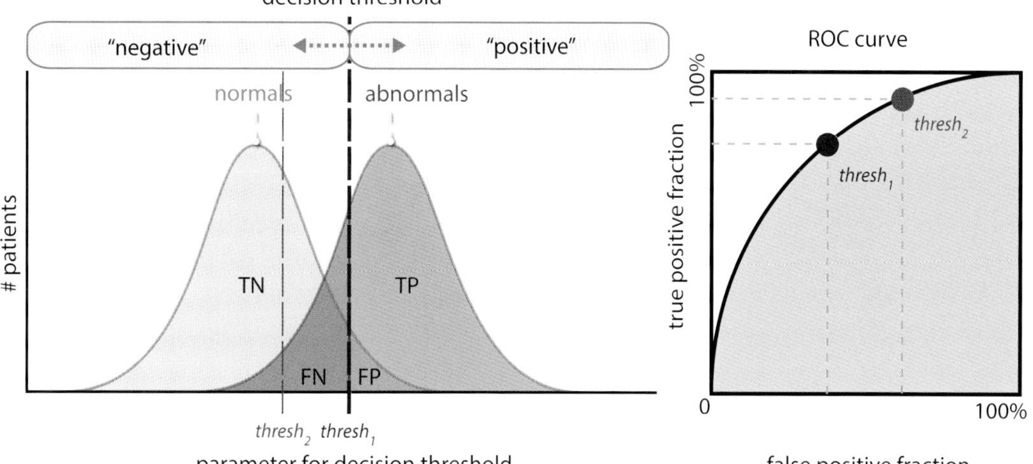

- A patient population includes normals and abnormals. The threshold to determine whether a test parameter is "negative" or "positive" can be set to optimize the ratio of true positives to false positives.
- In threshold 1 (*thresh*$_1$; blue dashed line above), the decision threshold is chosen to balance true positives with false positives. This threshold is visualized on the ROC curve as the blue dot.
- Threshold 2 (*thresh*$_2$; brown dashed line above) is lowered. When plotted on the ROC curve, *thresh*$_2$ moves to the right, which increases the true positive fraction (increases sensitivity) and also increases the false positive fraction.

RADIATION BIOLOGY

DNA damage

- Free radicals mediate the majority of biological damage due to radiation.

Syndromes

- Xeroderma pigmentosa: ↑ sensitivity to UV light
- Ataxia telangiectasia: ↑ sensitivity to X-rays

Deterministic effects

- Deterministic effects occur once the radiation exposure crosses a certain threshold and would not be expected to occur below that exposure.
- A **decrease in peripheral lymphocyte** count can occur after as little as ≥0.5 Gy exposure.
- **Cataracts** may occur after an eye dose of 2 Gy. The posterior pole is preferentially affected. For a given dose, high-LET radiation (neutrons and alpha particles) are much more effective at inducing cataracts compared to X-rays.
- **Radiation-induced erythema** can occur in 1–2 days, but may take up to 10–14 days to develop.

  2 Gy: Transient early erythema

  6 Gy: Robust erythema
- **Epilation** occurs after about 3 weeks.

  3 Gy: Temporary epilation

  7 Gy: Permanent epilation
- **Desquamation** may begin 4 weeks after exposure.

  15 Gy: Moist desquamation
- **Vascular damage** is expected for skin doses >20 Gy.
- **Ulceration** and **depigmentation** are late effects due to dermal damage.
- **Sterility** can be caused in males or females.

  Males: Temporary sterility after >0.15 Gy.

  Females: Permanent sterility and early menopause after >3.5 Gy.

Hereditary effects

- The **doubling dose** is the dose required to double the spontaneous mutation rate when applied to a population. The doubling dose is approximately 1 Gy given to each member of the population.
- The risk of hereditary effects (for an individual) is thought to be approximately 0.2% per Sv. For instance, the risk of a hereditary effect from a gonad dose of 100 mSv = 0.2% * 0.1 Sv = 0.02%.

Death by radiation (whole-body radiation)

Terminology: LD 50/X = lethal dose that kills 50% of the population in X days. For instance, an LD 50/60 will kill 50% of the population in 60 days.

- 3–4 Gy: LD 50/60 due to failure of hematopoietic system.
- 10 Gy: LD 50/5 due to denuding of the GI tract lining (small bowel most sensitive).
- 100 Gy: LD 50/2 due to cerebrovascular syndrome.

Stochastic effects	• Stochastic effects are random and carcinogenic. Stochastic effects arise after a latent period of several years. As the dose to an individual increases, there is an increased risk of developing cancer. Complicating the determination of a stochastic risk is the fact that cancer is a very common disease, there is a low level of background radiation present, and most people who receive medical radiation exposures do not have any ill effects. • The risk of a stochastic effect depends on the dose, dose rate, and type of tissue exposed. • The linear no threshold model is believed to provide the most accurate risk assessment for development of solid tumors, with a latency up to 25 years. The linear no threshold model assumes that there is no threshold required for a stochastic effect, and the risk of cancer increases linearly with increasing exposure. • The linear-quadratic function of dose is thought to best characterize the risk of developing leukemia, with a latency of 5–7 years.
Radiation-induced cancer	• Acute radiation exposure carries a risk of developing cancer of approximately 8%/Gy, based on Japanese nuclear bomb survivors. For instance, a 24% increase in cancer risk would require 4 Gy acutely (8 *4 = 24%). • The risk of leukemia is approximately 1%/Sv for an acute dose. • Chronic exposure (e.g., radiation worker) carries a risk of cancer of 4%/Gy.
Relative radiosensitivities	• The thyroid gland is the most radiosensitive tissue in the human body.
Occupational/ iatrogenic exposures and effects	• Ankylosing spondylitis (treated with X-rays) → leukemia • Fluoroscopy for tuberculosis → breast cancer • Marshall island inhabitants (nuclear weapon testing) → thyroid tumors • Miners (especially uranium) → lung cancer, due to breathing radon • Dial painters → bone sarcomas and nasopharyngeal carcinoma (lick radium on brushes)
Radiation effects on the fetus These effects are for significant exposure (e.g., 2 Gy)	• Weeks 0–2 (pre-implantation): "all-or-nothing": abortion likely after significant exposure • Weeks 2–6: congenital abnormalities ↑ Risk of neonatal death (death at or about the time of birth) • Weeks 8–15: Risk of mental retardation 40%/Sv ↑ Risk of childhood cancer ↑ Risk of reduced head diameter • Weeks 15–25: Risk of mental retardation 10%/Sv ↑ Risk of childhood cancer
Fetal dose (Pregnant radiation workers)	• Dose limit: 0.5 mSv/month allowed (~5 mSv/pregnancy). • Lead apron attenuates externally measured dose by a factor of 20 (fetal dose would be further reduced by factor of 2 due to mother's overlying tissues).

Dose to general public allowed by medical radiation	• 1 mSv/year, which is actually lower than the maximum dose of 5 mSv allowed to the fetus of a radiation worker.
Dose limits by body part	• Eyes: 150 mSv/year • Everything else: 500 mSv/year
Occupational exposure (not pregnant)	• Max permissible effective dose = 50 mSv/year
Background radiation	• Background radiation varies by location, but averages about 3 mSv/year excluding medical radiation. 1 Gy (Sv) is required to double the mutation rate, so 3 mSv = 0.003 Sv = 0.3% increased risk of mutation above the baseline rate. • Radon exposure represents approximately 55% of background radiation. Radon is an alpha emitter with a half-life of 3 days. Its parent radionuclide is radium, with a half life of 1,600 years. Effective dose = Absorbed dose * W_R * W_T W_R = 20 (↑ LET), and W_T = 0.1 (only lung tissue irradiated) Radon exposure is thought to cause ~20,000 deaths/year.

Magnetic resonance imaging (MRI) physics

MRI and pregnancy	• Although no controlled studies have been performed, MRI can be performed at any stage of pregnancy. Gadolinium is contraindicated throughout pregnancy.
MRI quenching	• Quenching causes loss of superconductivity of the MRI scanner magnet coils, which releases helium. Helium displaces O_2 → must evacuate emergently.
Fringe field	• The fringe field surrounds the controlled access area and cannot exceed 5 Gauss.
FDA regulates the following MRI parameters	• Static magnetic field strength >4T. • Time-varying magnetic fields sufficient to produce severe discomfort or painful stimulation. • Radiofrequency power deposition to produce core temperature increase of 1 degree C. • Acoustic noise levels >140 dB.
SAR Specific absorption ratio	• The specific absorption ration (SAR) characterizes the radiofrequency (RF) power absorbed per unit mass. • SAR is proportional to number of images acquired per unit time and depends on patient dimensions, RF waveform, tip angle, and coil type.
MRI noise	• The acoustic noise produced by the MRI scanner is caused by vibrating gradient coils, due to rapidly applied gradient magnetic fields.

Focal heating and thermal injuries

- Conductive loops can cause local heating. Examples of conductive loops include crossed arms, ECG leads, and unconnected surface coil leads in contact with patient's skin.
- Metallic objects can absorb radiofrequency energy and become hot.
- Time-varying magnetic fields can result in peripheral nerve stimulation, muscle movement, and discomfort.

Signal to noise ratio (SNR)

- Signal to noise ratio (SNR) is proportional to: $I * voxel_{x,y,z} * \frac{\sqrt{NEX}}{\sqrt{BW}} * B$

I = intrinsic signal intensity of voxel, dependent on tissue composition and pulse sequence

$voxel_{x,y,z}$ = voxel volume, affected by image matrix and slice thickness

A smaller voxel volume will proportionally decrease signal to noise

NEX = number of excitations; linearly related to time of acquisition

BW = receiver bandwidth (range of frequencies collected by the MRI system; wide BW enables faster data acquisition and reduces chemical shift artifacts but also adds noise → reduces SNR)

B = intrinsic function of magnetic field strength

T1 and T2

- Inherent tissue T1 and T2 characteristics depend on the **longitudinal relaxation (T1)** and **transverse relaxation (T2)** times of the protons in that tissue.
- Tissue signal abnormality is produced by alterations (prolongation or shortening) of the transverse or longitudinal relaxation of the tissue, which may be affected by various pathologic processes.
- MR image weighting (e.g., T1- or T2-weighted images) depends on the repetition time (TR) and echo time (TE) used to obtain images.
- **T1 image contrast is dependent on TR**, which is the interval between sequential radiofrequency pulses. The imaging appearance of specific tissues on T1-weighted images depends on how much longitudinal relaxation occurs between each TR. Images obtained with a short TR and a short TE are T1-weighted.

  Short T1 relaxation times → higher signal on T1-weighted images.

  Fat and subacute blood have short T1 relaxation times and therefore appear hyperintense on T1-weighted images.
- **T2 image contrast is dependent on TE**, which is the interval between the application of the radiofrequency pulse and the collection of the signal. The imaging appearance of tissues on T2-weighted images depends on how much transverse relaxation (loss of proton phase coherence) occurs during each TE. Images obtained with a long TR and a long TE are T2-weighted.

  Slow loss of phase coherence → prolonged T2 relaxation times → hyperintense on T2-weighted images.

  Water has a long T2 relaxation time and therefore is hyperintense on T2-weighted images.

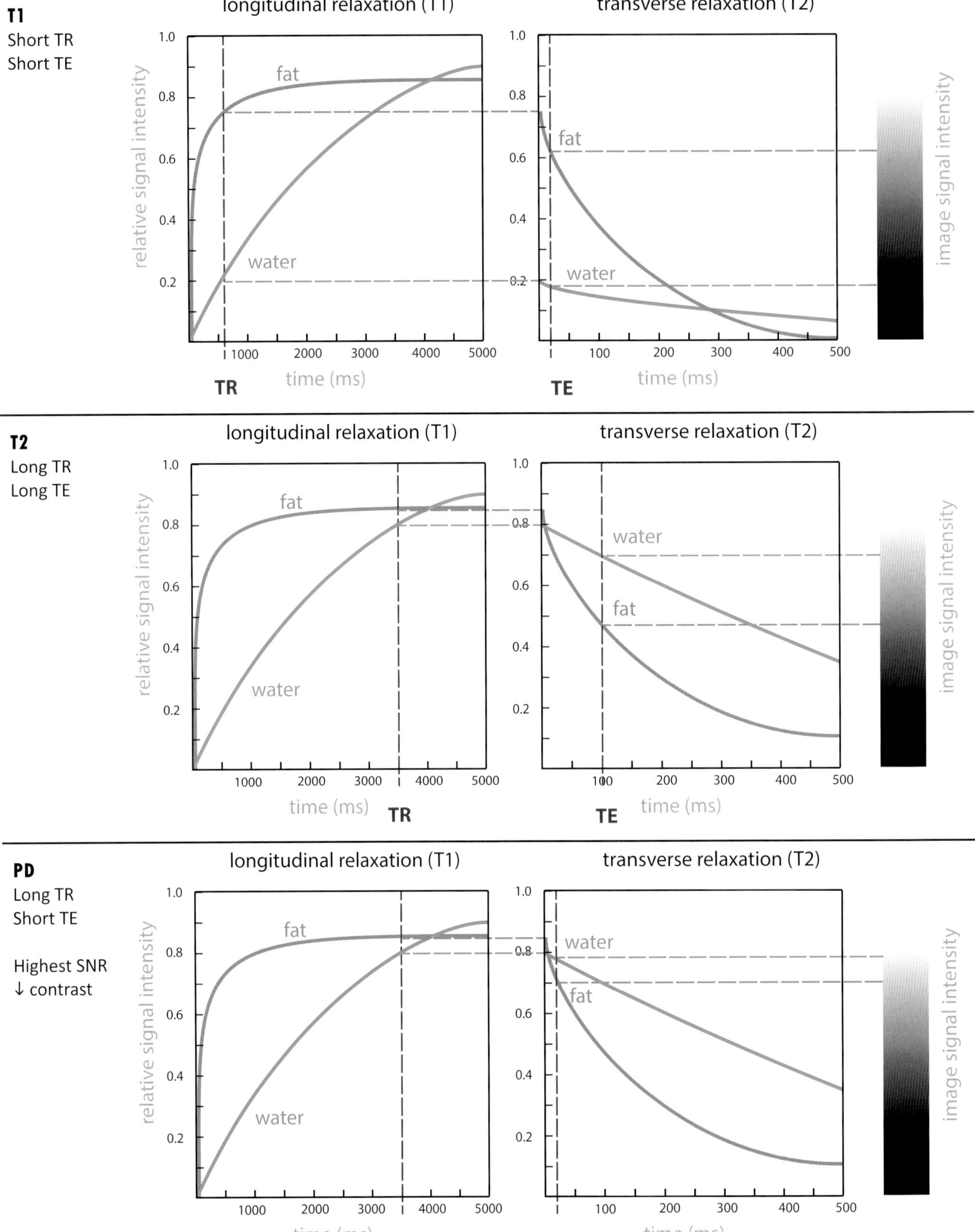
T1
Short TR
Short TE
longitudinal relaxation (T1)
transverse relaxation (T2)
fat
water
relative signal intensity
image signal intensity
time (ms)
TR
TE
T2
Long TR
Long TE
PD
Long TR
Short TE
Highest SNR
↓ contrast

Ultrasound physics

Decibel (dB)	• The decibel is a measure of relative intensity between two sound intensities. • $dB = 10 \log(I/I_{ref})$ • For example, –3 dB is 50% of sound intensity: 10log(0.5) = –3
Thermal index and mechanical index	• The thermal index (TI) is the maximum temperature rise in tissue caused by ultrasound energy absorption. • If TI >1.0, risk benefit analysis should be performed. • The mechanical index (MI) describes the likelihood of cavitation based on peak rarefactional pressure and frequency. • If MI >0.5, risk benefit analysis should be performed.
Factors that affect acoustic output index	• Frame rate • Transmit power • Frequency
Factors that don't affect acoustic output index	• Time-gain compensation • Grayscale mapping *These are both processing techniques*
Cavitation	• Cavitation is the formation of bodies of gas and/or vapor by ultrasound energy. Cavitation is more likely to occur at high pressures and low frequencies. • Stable cavitation is regular pulsation of persistent microbubbles. • Transient cavitation is a more violent form of microbubble dynamics characterized by large size changes in bubbles before collapse.
Safe ultrasound energy	• No biologic effects have been observed with spatial peak temporal average intensities below 1 W/cm^2.
Tissue attenuation	• Tissue attenuation is approximately 0.5 dB per cm per MHz. • For instance, a 4 MHz wave travelling 10 cm is attenuated 20 dB.
Refraction	• Refraction is due to different velocities of sound in different tissues, resulting in apparent bending of the ultrasound wave. • Described by Snell's law.
Wavelength and transducer design	• The transducer thickness = $\lambda/2$, where λ is wavelength. • For a long wavelength (low frequency), the transducer must be made thicker.
Sound waves	• $v = f\lambda$ v = velocity f = frequency λ = wavelength

Axial resolution	• Axial resolution quantifies the ability to separate objects lying along the axis of the beam and is determined by spatial pulse length. Short pulses are achieved by damping of the transducer. The spatial pulse length (SPL) is approximately 2λ. $\text{axial resolution} = \frac{\text{spatial pulse length}}{2}$ For example, at 2 MHz, the SPL is ~ 2 mm and the axial resolution is ~1 mm. at 4 MHz, the SPL is ~1 mm and the axial resolution ~0.5 mm at 8 Mhz, the axial resolution is ~0.25 mm • Axial resolution does not vary with depth.
Lateral resolution	• The lateral resolution is the ability to resolve two adjacent objects. • Lateral resolution improves with beam focusing and ↑ number lines per frame. • Lateral resolution is approximately 4x worse than axial resolution. • Lateral resolution becomes worse with increasing depth.
Elevational resolution	• Elevational resolution is the resolution in the plane perpendicular to the plane of imaging. Elevational resolution is equivalent to slice thickness on cross-sectional imaging. • Elevational resolution is approximately equivalent to lateral resolution and also varies with depth.
Near field and far field	• The near field determines the maximum depth that can be imaged. It is not related to image quality at increasing depths. $\text{near field} = \frac{r^2}{\lambda}$ r = radius of transducer: If r doubles, near field ↑ by 4 λ = wavelength: If λ doubles (↑ freq), near field ↓ by 2 • The near field (where imaging is possible) is called the **Fresnel zone**. • The far field (where the ultrasound beam diverges and imaging is impossible) is called the **Frauenhofer zone**.
Pulse repetition frequency (PRF)	• Pulse repetition frequency (PRF) is the number of times the transducer outputs a pulse of sound waves per second. An increase in PRF causes an inversely proportional decrease in echo listening time. A high PRF therefore limits the maximum depth of tissue that can be imaged. • PRF = **Frame rate** x **lines per frame** • A typical PRF is ~4 kHz → 0.25 ms (250 μsec) between pulses, which allows imaging of approximately 19.3 cm depth.

Definitions

$${}^{A}_{Z}X_{N}$$

A = atomic mass = N + Z

Z = # protons = atomic number

N = # neutrons

X = element

- Isobar: Same atomic mass (e.g., ^{131}I and ^{131}Xe)
- Isoto**P**es: Same number of **P**rotons
- Isoto**N**es: Same number of **N**eutrons

Decay and stability

- The graph below demonstrates that as atomic number (Z) increases, stable elements tend to have slightly increased neutrons relative to protons.
- Isotopes with excess neutrons decay by beta-minus decay, while isotopes with excess protons decay by beta-plus decay.

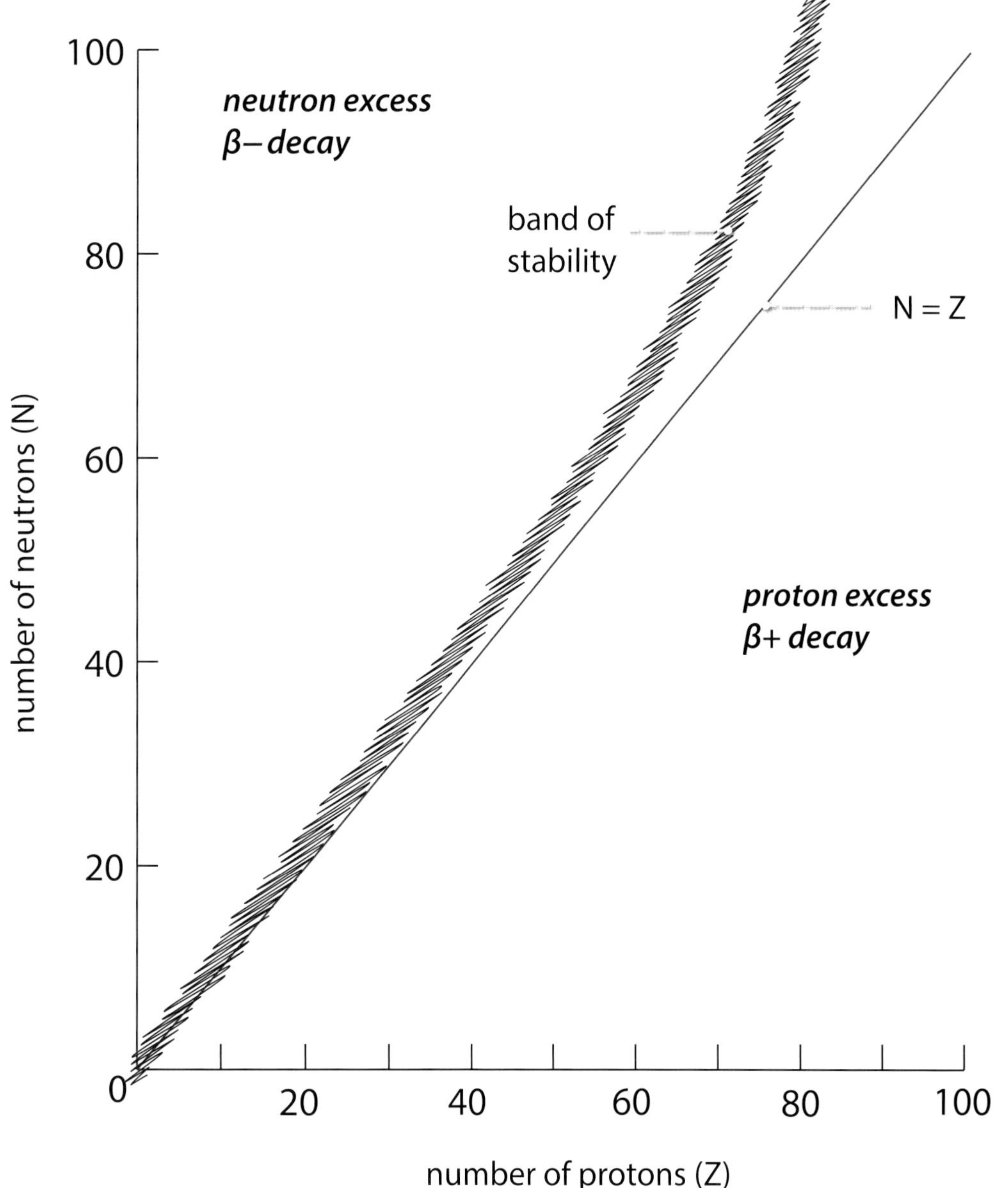

Alpha decay

- An α particle is 2 protons and 2 neutrons = Helium nucleus
- Alpha decay causes loss of an α particle: Atomic mass ↓ by 4; Z ↓ by 2 and N ↓ 2

$$^{A-4}_{Z-2}X_{N-2}$$

Beta minus decay

- β– decay occurs with neutron excess: Neutron converted to proton.

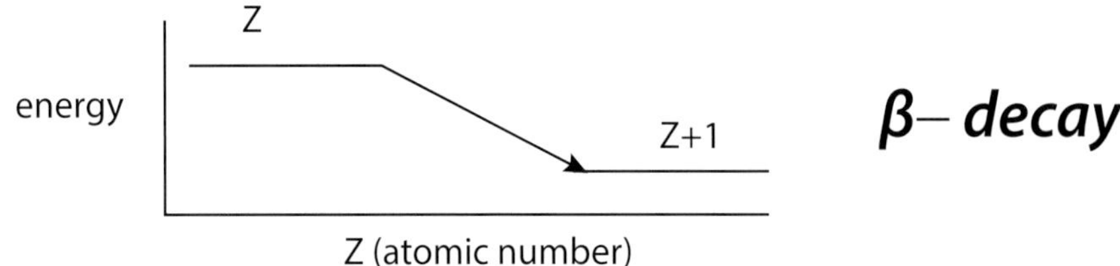

- Elements produced in nuclear reactors are neutron rich.

$$^{A}_{Z+1}X_{N-1}$$

Beta plus decay

- β+ decay occurs with proton excess: Proton converted to neutron.

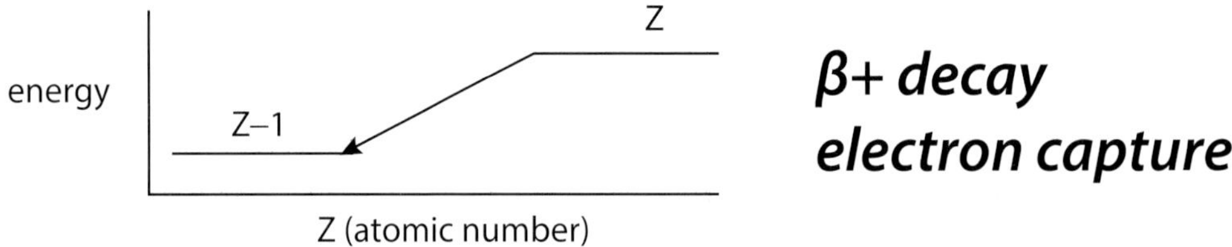

- Elements produced in a cyclotron are proton-rich. β+ decay competes with electron capture (both cause Z ↓ 1 and N ↑ 1). Atomic mass is unchanged.

$$^{A}_{Z-1}X_{N+1}$$

Electron capture

- Electron capture is similar to, and competes with, β+ decay. A proton is converted to a neutron by capturing an e^-, which usually comes from the K-shell. The resultant vacancy is filled by an outer shell e^- and a characteristic X-ray or Auger e^- is released.
- The net change is identical to β+ decay: Z ↓ 1 and N ↑ 1, unchanged mass.
- The following isotopes decay by electron capture (mnemonic: Cowboy says ***"GIIT** over here"* when trying to ***capture*** his horse):

  Gallium-67

  Indium-111

  Iodine-123

  Thallium-201

Activity	• The activity of a radionuclide is the number of decays per unit time. • The activity at time (t) = $N_t = N_0(e^{-\lambda t})$ N_0 = initial activity Decay constant $\lambda = 0.693/T½$, where T½ = half life t = time elapsed
Cumulative activity	• The cumulative activity is the total number of nuclear decays that occur over time. It represents the area under the decay curve plotted over time. • The cumulative activity = $1.44 \times f \times A_0 \times T_E$ f = fractional uptake (assumed to be 1 if not explicitly stated otherwise) A_0 = initial activity T_E = effective half-life
Effective half-life	• The effective half-life is the half-life of a radionuclide within an organ, taking into account the intrinsic physical half-life of the radionuclide and the biological clearance. • The effective half-life = T_E = $\frac{1}{T_E} = \frac{1}{T_B} + \frac{1}{T_{1/2}}$ T_B = biologic half-life $T_{1/2}$ = physical half-life
System resolution	• System resolution is the resolution of the imaging system accounting for the intrinsic resolution of the scintillation camera (without a collimator) and resolution of the collimator. • System resolution = $R = \sqrt{R_i^2 + R_c^2}$ R_i = intrinsic resolution R_c = collimator resolution
Quality control: Dose calibrator	• Constancy: Tested every day ("constantly") with ^{137}Cs (30 year half-life) • Linearity: Tested quarterly with ^{99m}Tc decay • <u>**A**</u>ccuracy: Tested <u>**a**</u>nnually with a calibrated source • These are tests of the *dose calibrator,* not the imaging system!
Quality control: Imaging system	• Uniformity: Tested daily with Co-57

References, resources, and further reading

Reference Textbooks:

Bushberg, J.T., Seibert, J.A., Leidholdt, E.M. & Boone, J.M. The Essential Physics of Medical Imaging (2nd ed.) Lippincott Williams & Wilkins. (2001).

Huda, W. Review of Radiologic Physics (3rd ed.). Lippincott Williams & Wilkins. (2009).

Articles:

Bitar, R. et al. MR pulse sequences: what every radiologist wants to know but is afraid to ask. Radiographics, 26(2), 513-37(2006).

Cody, D.D. AAPM/RSNA physics tutorial for residents: topics in CT. Image processing in CT. Radiographics, 22(5), 1255-68(2002).

Cody, D.D. & Mahesh, M. AAPM/RSNA physics tutorial for residents: Technologic advances in multidetector CT with a focus on cardiac imaging. Radiographics, 27(6), 1829-37(2007).

Hedrick, W.R. & Mahesh, M. Radiation Biology for Diagnostic and Interventional Radiologists (5th ed.). Radiological Society of North America. (2007).

Jacobs, M.A., Ibrahim, T.S. & Ouwerkerk, R. AAPM/RSNA physics tutorials for residents: MR imaging: brief overview and emerging applications. Radiographics, 27(4), 1213-29(2007).

Mahesh, M. The AAPM/RSNA Physics Tutorial for Residents Fluoroscopy: Patient Radiation. Radiographics, 21, 1033-1045(2001).

Mahesh, M. AAPM/RSNA physics tutorial for residents: digital mammography: an overview. Radiographics, 24(6), 1747-60(2004).

McNitt-Gray, M.F. AAPM/RSNA Physics Tutorial for Residents: Topics in CT. Radiation dose in CT. Radiographics, 22(6), 1541-53(2002).

Mettler, F.A., Huda, W., Yoshizumi, T.T. & Mahesh, M. Effective doses in radiology and diagnostic nuclear medicine: a catalog. Radiology, 248(1), 254-63(2008).

Nickoloff, E.L., Lu, Z.F., Dutta, A.K. & So, J.C. Radiation dose descriptors: BERT, COD, DAP, and other strange creatures. Radiographics, 28(5), 1439-50(2008).

Pooley, R.A. AAPM/RSNA physics tutorial for residents: fundamental physics of MR imaging. Radiographics, 25(4), 1087-99(2005).

Schueler, B.A, Vrieze, T.J., Bjarnason, H. & Stanson, A.W. An investigation of operator exposure in interventional radiology. Radiographics, 26, 1533-41 (2006)., discussion 1541.

Zhuo, J. & Gullapalli, R.P. AAPM/RSNA physics tutorial for residents: MR artifacts, safety, and quality control. Radiographics, 26(1), 275-97(2006).

INDEX